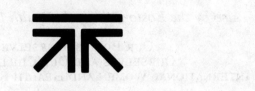

Also by the Boston Women's Health Book Collective

OUR BODIES, OURSELVES
OURSELVES AND OUR CHILDREN
INTERNATIONAL WOMEN AND HEALTH RESOURCE GUIDE

THE NEW OUR BODIES, OURSELVES

A BOOK BY AND FOR WOMEN

The Boston Women's
Health Book Collective

A TOUCHSTONE BOOK

PUBLISHED BY SIMON & SCHUSTER, INC.
New York

Copyright © 1984 by The Boston Women's Health Book Collective
All rights reserved
including the right of reproduction
in whole or in part in any form
Published by Simon and Schuster
A Division of Simon & Schuster, Inc.
Simon & Schuster Building
Rockefeller Center
1230 Avenue of the Americas
New York, New York 10020
SIMON AND SCHUSTER and TOUCHSTONE and colophons are registered trademarks of Simon & Schuster, Inc.
Designed by C. Linda Dingler
Manufactured in the United States of America

3   5   7   9   10   8   6   4

Library of Congress Cataloging in Publication Data

Main entry under title:

The New our bodies, ourselves.

Rev. ed. of: Our bodies, ourselves. 2nd ed.,
completely rev. and expanded. c1976.
Bibliography: p.
Includes index.
1. Women—Health and hygiene. 2. Women—Diseases.
3. Women–Psychology. I. Boston Women's Health Book
Collective. II. Our bodies, ourselves.
RA778.N67   1984   613'.04244   84-5545

ISBN 0-671-46087-0
0-671-46088-9 (pbk)

SPECIAL ACKNOWLEDGMENTS

Editors and Midwives: Jane Pincus and Wendy Sanford worked with each writer to help give the book shape, clarity and unity. In the editing process, they shortened and wrote and/or rewrote parts of every chapter.

Project Coordinators: Nancy Hawley and Wendy Sanford kept in their minds all the people, tasks and stages of this project in the three years from the initial negotiations to the final production of the book.

Resource Coordinators: Pamela Morgan and Judy Norsigian fielded every possible question, sending us to the appropriate resources in order to make the new book as informative and accurate as possible.

Special thanks to:
Ann Godoff, our editor, whose persistence, patience and tactful advocacy pulled us through the last stages of this labor;

Ruth Hubbard, who, red pencil in hand, clarified the language of nearly every chapter in the book;

Jo Polk-Matthews, who relayed many of the chapters to thoughtful outside readers and made sure we got the comments and criticisms we needed;

Gina Prenowitz, who cast her careful eye on the language and politics of important sections of the book;

Nancy Schlick, whose copy editing was respectful, attentive and wonderfully intelligent;

Catherine Shaw, who was an eager, enthusiastic and patient reader of the sprawling first manuscript;

Irv Zola, who had the pleasure of reading and carefully criticizing all our most problematic chapters, and whose advice never failed to be right on the mark;

Our families, lovers and housemates, who lived with us, fed us, complained and loved us anyway and soundly rejoiced when the project was complete.

Sue Ade	Benjamin Doress	Agnes Norsigian	Stephen Salk
Davida Andelman	Hannah Doress	Kyra Zola Norsigian	Toni Sandmaier
Polly Attwood	Caitlin Fisher	Roy Norsigian	Matthew Sanford
Alan Berger	Dan Fisher	Julia Perez	Cheryl Schaffer
Laurel Berger	Philip Hart	Ben Pincus	Jeremy Schwartz
Noah Berger	Gina Hawley	Ed Pincus	Dan Sipe
Belle Brett	Josh Hawley	Sami Pincus	John Swenson
Abraham Brown	Vilma Hunt	Minrose Quinn	Sarah Swenson
Ethel Brown	Kathryn Jewell	Judah Rome	David Wegman
Robert S. Cohen	Patrice Keegan	Micah Rome	Jesse Wegman
Trudy Cox	Cheryl Kennedy	Nathan Rome	Marya Wegman
Aaron Diskin	Philip Kraft	Alan Rosen	Alexi Wolf
Leah Diskin	Nancy Lessin	Megan Crowe-Rothstein	Lea Wolf
Martin Diskin	Jeffrey McIntyre	Natalie Rothstein	Tom Wolf
Bruce Ditzion	Noah McIntyre	Peter Rothstein	Allen Worters
Robbie Ditzion	Halford Meras	Daniel Salk	Amanda Zola
Sammy Ditzion	Nellie Meras	Nikki Salk	Warren Zola

GENERAL ACKNOWLEDGMENTS

Many thanks to the following people for their help:

Bonnie Acker
Lois Alix
Carol Altobelli
Majeeda Amadadeen
Vicky Anderson
Beth Andrews
George Annas
Naomi Armon
Hilde Armour
Harriet Arnoldi
Connie Arsenault
Arthritis and Health
  Resource Center
Gisela Ashley
Diane Austras
Diane Balser
Kim Bancroft
David Banta
Faith Nobuko Barcus
Phoebe Barnes
Kathleen Barry
Pauline Bart
Margaret Belbin
Ruth Bell
Riva Berkovitz
Davi Birnbaum
Alice Bonis
Bea Bookchin
Shafia Bossman
Ursula Bowring-Trenn
Pam Boyle
Almont Bracy
Etta Breit
Jan Brin
Linda Brion-Meisels
Steven Brion-Meisels
Kathy Brownback
Agnes Butcher
Norma Canner
Barbara Carmen
Casa Myrna Vasquez
Robin Casarjian
Mary Rae Cate
Susie Chancey
Wendy Chavkin
Donna Cherniac
Cindy Chin
Aram Chobanian
Ann Chronis
Peggy Clark
Marie Clarke

Savitri Clarke
Yarrow Anne Cleaves
Connie Clement
Cindy Cohen
Deborah Catherine Cohen
Nancy Cohen
Robert S. Cohen
Tom Conry
Liz Coolidge
Betty Corpt
Maria Corsaro
Mary Costanza
Terry Courtney
Belita Cowan
Frannye Crocker
Emily Culpepper
John Cutler
Lynne Dahlberg
William Darrow
Martha Davis-Perry
Caro Dellenbaugh
Catherine DeLorey
Debby DeVaughn
Andrew Dibner
Annette Dickinson
Loretta Dixson
Rose Dobosz
Jan Dodds
Karen Dorman
Barbara Dow
Hugh Drummond
Kim Ducharme
Buffy Dunker
Wendy Dunning
Jane Dwinell
Sally Edwards
Susan Eisenberg
Helen Eisenstein
Carol Englander
Carol Epple
Wendy Roberts Epstein
Kitty Ernst
Tish Fabens
Martha Farrar
Lee Farris
Carolyn Fawcett
Richard Feinberg
Geri Ferber
Fertility Consciousness
  Group
Cynthia Fertman

Ron Fichtner
JoAnne Fischer
Alice Fisher
Maureen Flammer
Mary Flinders
Becky Fowler
Cary Fowler
Dorothy Frauenhofer
Nancy Friedman
Stella Friml
Rose Frisch
Dana Gallagher
Paula Garbarino
Jean Gardella
Linda Gardner
Linda Gaynor
Carole Geddis-Dlugasch
Tobin Gerhardt
Lois Gibbs
Paige Gidney
Cheryl Giles
Betty Gittes
Evelyn Gladu of Omega,
  Somerville, Mass.
Leonard Glantz
Pat Gold
Meg Goldman
Sharon Golub
Mary Moore Goodlett
Jennifer Gordon
Jocelyn Gordon
Ruth Gore and the
  Goldennaires, Freedom
  House, Roxbury, Mass.
Benina Gould
Gray Panthers
Meryl Green
Tova Green
Miriam Greenspan
Betsy Grob
Ione Gunnerson
Joan Gussow
Cynthia Hales
Diana Long Hall
Eleanor Hamilton
Jalna Hanmer
Sandie Harris
Michelle Harrison
Pat Haseltine
Robert Hatcher
Lester Hazell

Muriel Heiberger
Ingeborg Helling
Susan Helmrich
Judy Herman
Curdina Hill
Ruth Hill, Black Women's
  Oral History Project,
  Radcliffe Institute
Hella Hoffman
Kate Hoffman
Beryl-Elise Hoffstein
Joanne Holt
Barbara Homan
Barbara Horgan
Mary Howell
Jeanne Hubbuch
Maile Hulihan
Rick Ingrasci
Jeanne Jackson
Sandy Jaffe
Mary Jane Jarrett
Pat Jerabek
Gail Johnson
Leila Joseph
Myla Kabat-Zinn
Alexandra Kaplan
Peg Kapron
Amy Kasanjian
Linda Katzman
Augusta Kaufman
David Kaufman
Jay Kaufman
Peggy Hershenson
  Kaufman
Lorrie Kendler
Jamie Keshet
Edith Kessler
Nina Kimche
Joanne Klys
Jenny Knaus
Joan Knight
Thurmond Knight
Pat Kraepelian-Bartels
Helen Kramer
Mark Kramer
Karen Kruskal
Ruth Kundsin
Ann LaCasse
Eben LaCasse
Kirsten LaCasse
Marianne LaLuz

GENERAL ACKNOWLEDGMENTS

Hildegarde Lambrom
Nan Lassin
Nancy Lastoff
Tesair Lauve
Stephen Lester
Maggie Lettvin
Debbie LeVan
Jane Levin
Mitch Levine
Myrna Lewis
Heidi Lewitt
Rinchen Lhamo
Frederick Li
Ricky Lieberman
Bonnie Liebman
Dottie Limont
Lee Lindbert
Liz Linderman
Jessica Lipnak
Judy Lipshutz
Mary Logan
Dylan Loman
Carin Layne Lomon
Susan Love
Barbara Low
Ruth Lubic
Brinton Lykes
Peggy Lynch
Ana Machado de Oliveira
P'nina Macher
Howie Machtinger
Catherine MacKinnon
Una MacLean
Brian MacMahon
Elizabeth MacMahon
Carol Mamber
Elizabeth Markson
Lisa Marlin
Irene Marotta
Caroline Marvin
Raquel Matas
Lourdes Mattei
Elizabeth Matz
Charlotte Mayerson
Art Mazer
Katie Mazer
William M. Mazer
Renee Mazon
Maggie McCarthy-Herzig
Bill McCormack
Patty McLean
Martha P. Megee
Jeanne Melvin
Mary Beth Menaker
Barbara Menning
Irma Meridy
Donald Miller
Jean Baker Miller
Miriam Miller
William Minniciello
Denise Minter
Nora Mitchell
Ramona Monteverde
Montreal Health Press

Helen Boulware Moore
Susanne Morgan
Beth Morrison
Marilyn Morrissey
Charlotte Muller
J. B. Mulligan
Sister Angela Murdaugh
Maryann Napoli
Ruth Nelson
Network of Women in
  Trade and Technical Jobs
Holly Newman
Marjorie Newman
Louise Newton
Nancy Nichols
Steve Nickerson
Nine-to-Five Health and
  Safety Committee
Barbara Norfleet
Abigail November
Older Women's League
Oral History Project of the
  Cambridge Arts Council
Pat O'Reilly
Julie Snow Osherson
Patricia Papernow
Jane Patterson
Donald Pedicini
Jackie Petrillo
Robbie Pfeufer
Connie Phillips
Beatrice Pitcher
Jackie Pitullo
Sara Poli
Jane Porcino
Ruth Porham
Clare Potter
Terri Powell
Abraham Press
Helane Press
Janet Press
Rosellen Primrose
Kathleen Quinlan
Pat Rackowski
Jill Rakusen
Carolyn Ramsey
Eloise Rathbone-McCuan
Elsie Reethof
Mira Reicher
Margaret Reid
C. J. Reilly
Erica Reitmayer
Susan Rennie
Ulrike Rettig
Susan Reverby
Naomi Ribner
Marcie Richardson
Claudia Richter
Pat Ricker
Virginia Robison
Lisa Rofel
Eva Rooks
Lynn Rosenberg
Anita Rossien

Alice Rothchild
Donna Roux
Alice Ryerson
Alma Sabatini
Pat Sacry
Jackie Samson
Linda Sanford
Frank Santora
Miriam Schocken
Cyprienne Schroeppel
Allyson Schwartz
Janet Schwartz
Helen Scott
Mary Scully
Barbara Seaman
Eli Shapiro
Rene Shaw
Susan Shaw
Beth Shearer
Helen Sheingold
Karen Sheingold
Sayre Sheldon
Laurie Shields
Andrea Siani
Sergio Siani
Ben Siegel
Jane Siegel
Diane Siegelman
Sandra Signor
Marge Silver
Phyllis Silverman
Yehudit Silverman
Jane Simmons-Nashinoff
Barbara Sindriglis
Joan Sing
Peggy Sloane
Seymour Small
Annette Smith
Barbara Smith
Lee Smith
Mary Smith
Leni Sollinger
Tish Sommers
Ethel Sondik
Heidi Spoerle
Selma Squires
Karen Stamm
Cecilia Stanley
Karen Starr
Judith Stein
Susan Steiner
Sheila Stillman
John Stoekle
Carol A. Stollar
Sheera Strick
Suzanne Stuart

Jana Suchankova
Edith Bjornson Sunley
Carol Sussman
Judy Sutphen
Kate Swan
Chris Sweeney
Cheryl Tabb
Linda Tate
Claire Taylor
Rosemary Taylor
Marsha Tennis
Bernice Thomas
Winnie Thomas
Helen Thornton
Peggy Thurston
Jean Tock
Sally Tom
Barbara Tomaskovic-Devey
Donald Tomaskovic-Devey
Melinda Tuhus
Trude Turnquist
Kathy Ullman
Stephanie Urdang
Carol Doyle Van
  Valkenburgh
Martha H. Verbrugge
Gretchen Von Mering
Margo Wallach
Lila Wallis
Susan Wanger
Gail Washor-Liebhaver
Barbara Waxman
Joan Caplan Weizer
Phoebe Wells
Laura Wexler
Sally Whelan
Beatrice Whiting
Lillian Whitney
Paul Wiesner
Valerie Wilk
Diane Willow Williams
Ann Withorn
Glorianne Wittes
Simon Wittes
Will Wittington
Fran Wiltsie
Alice Wolfson
Jean Wolhandler
Women of the Boston-Area
  Socialist-Feminist Group
WOOSH (Women
  Organizing for
  Occupational Safety and
  Health)
Lisa Yost
Geraldine Zetzel

Coordinator of photographs: Nancy Hawley
Coordinator of graphics: Esther Rome

CONTENTS

PREFACE/INTRODUCTION*

By Jane Pincus and Joan Ditzion

EARLIER PREFACES:
I by Vilunya Diskin and Wendy Sanford
II by Wendy Sanford

In 1969, there was practically no women's health information easily available, and every fact we learned was a revelation. Our first publication of *Our Bodies, Ourselves* helped spark many women to explore the health issues most important to them. Since then, women throughout this country and the world have generated such a wealth of information and resources—research papers, books, health groups and centers, newsletters and journals—that this time around we turned to *them* for help in rewriting the book.

Rewriting has been a challenging, remarkable experience. Every writer (and consultant) ended up working on the book much longer than she ever expected to, with immense goodwill and patience, for very little pay. A typical chapter went through at least three drafts, each commented on and criticized by most Collective members and a wide range of outside readers. Several chapters were themselves written by small groups. Sometimes one person's insight would cause a whole chapter to be rethought. The end result of all this work is an almost totally new *Our Bodies, Ourselves*.

This rewrite reflects our Collective's long-time commitment to keeping the book up to date. Health and medical information changes quickly; new health problems come to the fore; legal and political realities shift, changing people's access to information and care. Equally important, our own political awareness keeps changing: the more we learn, the less we believe that the medical system as it is structured today can or will alter to meet our needs. So in this book, less med-

ically oriented than previous editions, we emphasize what we as women can do for ourselves and for one another, and we often discuss nonmedical perspectives and remedies as well as medical ones. The thousands of women who contact us in person, in letters and by phone have opened up whole new subjects and issues for revisions: "I looked in your book for a discussion of *in vitro* fertilization and couldn't find it." "You've got to include the experiences of differently-abled [disabled] women next time." "This is what happened to me when I got PID [pelvic inflammatory disease]; tell other women about it so they will be forewarned and know how to get the right kind of treatment." "Could you please say more about lesbians and medical care?" Such comments in the past have led to the book becoming denser and longer each time. This edition is no exception. It was difficult to decide what to cut, especially when every chapter turned out to be twice as long as we had room for. To include and condense so much information has meant oversimplifying some subjects and shortchanging others. (Many authors have written long, annotated bibliographies, available from our office upon request.)

We expanded some of the original sections, such as "Women in Motion" and "Violence Against Women," into chapters in their own right. Some entirely new chapters are "Health and Healing: Alternatives to Medical Care"; "Alcohol, Mood-Altering Drugs and Smoking"; "Environmental and Occupational Health"; "New Reproductive Technologies." After noting that in previous editions our discussions of the life cycle always ended with menopause, older women vehemently told us that indeed there *is* life after menopause. Together with them we wrote an all-new chapter on growing older. The chapter on international issues grew out of our correspondence and conversations with

---

*The following chapters were included in prior editions but are not in this current edition: "Our Changing Sense of Selves," by Joan Ditzion; "Considering Parenthood," by Joan Ditzion.

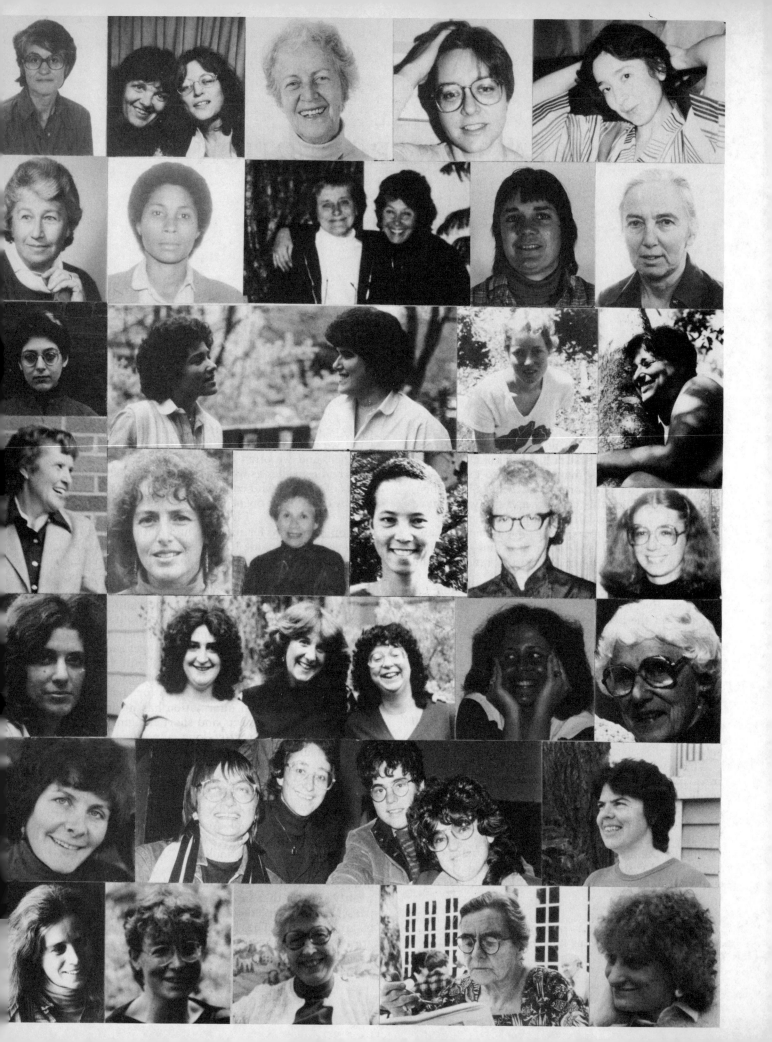

women whom some of us met in Asia, Latin America and Europe, and who visit our office to tell us about the health situations of women in their own countries as they collect information to bring back home. While this continues to be a book written primarily by white women, it includes experiences and information gathered by women of color.

Not all of us in the Collective agree with the content and style of every chapter and section. For instance, we had a long debate about psychotherapy—are women more helped than hurt by it? After many difficult discussions and rewrites we reached a compromise that we could live with. Though we labored over several pages about pornography intended for the "Violence Against Women" chapter, we ended up leaving it out because we couldn't agree about the topic ourselves, and could not do the controversies justice in such limited space. As of this writing, some of us still don't agree with the decision to leave this discussion out of the book.

Our Collective consists of the same core group who worked on the 1973 edition of *Our Bodies, Ourselves* (minus one). One of us now lives in California, another in Vermont. We have been meeting once a week for twelve years and have become a kind of family to one another. We have written together in twos and threes, looked after each other's children, had family picnics and celebrations, played music together and met for meals, given workshops with each other around New England and throughout the country and spent hours in long conversations. Four new babies were born in the past two years, making twenty-one children in all. We have seen one another through four divorces and three marriages, one case of hot flashes and some long, dramatic affairs with men and women. Three children have gone off to college and nine are in the midst of adolescence. We have comforted each other the best we could through four parents' deaths and the illnesses of several others. Most of us have other work in addition to working for the Collective. Now that revisions are over, we plan to do more public speaking nationwide about many of the issues in this book. Most important, we will be raising funds to keep our health information center going and vital. It is located in a large, bright room in the basement of a church in Watertown, Massachusetts, filled wall to wall with all forms of women's health information. Community groups often meet there; women are welcome to come and use our files. The center is staffed by a few Collective members and several terrific women who have worked closely with us over the past years.

It is clear that the same forces which created the need for *Our Bodies, Ourselves* twelve years ago exist today as strongly as ever. The medical system is a vast business, now tied more closely than ever to other businesses in this profit-oriented economy. Rich and poor receive very different types of health and medical care. Preventive health care is not only a low national

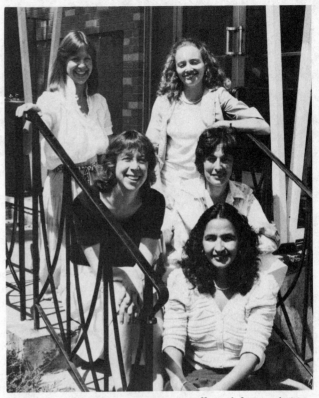

Women's Health Information Center staff: top left, Pamela Morgan; right, Sally Whelan; middle left, Robbie Pfeufer; right, Judy Norsigian; bottom, Maria de Lourdes Mattei   *Nancy Hawley*

priority, but reimbursement policies actually discourage prevention. Industries continue to pollute the environment. Misogynist archconservative mentality, money and policy drive women out of the workforce, deprive women of needed prenatal, abortion and birth control services and cut down access to health information. Drug companies continue to make huge profits by selling products often harmful to women, "dumping" into other countries those drugs judged to be too old or unsafe here. So now, more than ever before, we hold to our original goals:

- to fit as much information on women's health between the covers of this book as we can;
- to let women's different voices and experiences speak out in its pages;
- to reach as many women as possible with the tools which will enable them to take greater charge of their own health care and their lives, deal with the existing medical system and fight whenever possible for improvements and changes;
- to support those women and men working for change both within and outside the existing system of health and medical care;
- to work to create a more just society in which good health is a right, not a luxury, a society which does not perpetuate unequal relationships between the sexes.

Some of the many women who wrote chapters and sections of this book   *Phyllis Ewen*

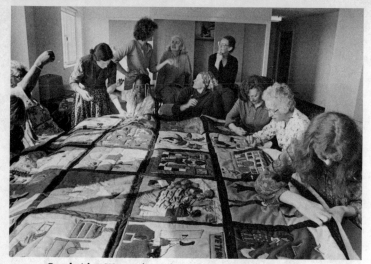

Cambridge Women's Quilting Project   *Bonnie Burt*

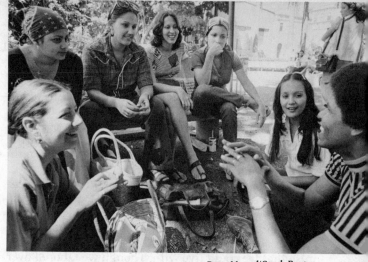

Peter Menzel/Stock Boston

Above all, we want to encourage women to get together—to meet, talk and listen to each other. Most of us in the Collective grew up in the decades after World War Two, when girls' lives centered around finding a man and women's lives around husband and children. Before we began working on this book fourteen years ago, most of us had moved away from our home communities. In 1968–1969, we became active in the early women's movement because of the political ferment of those years, and as a way out of the isolation we were experiencing. As we talked in small groups about our lives, we reclaimed an important part of our heritage, for women in traditional families and small communities have always exchanged experiences and wisdom with one another. In learning to support each other in our daily lives, we were not only continuing a tradition but doing something different too. With only a few exceptions, our own grandmothers and great-grandmothers had not dared speak openly about their feelings and experiences—about sexual feelings, for example, or abortions, which so many of them had had. Religious and cultural taboos had kept too many of them locked in ignorance and silence. Most of them had not felt entitled to protest and resist the circumstances of their lives or had found no context in which to do so. But we began to distinguish between the habits, roles and traditions which nurtured us and gave us strength and those which limited and repressed us. We realized that sexism restricted our options and opportunities. We encouraged each other to change unsatisfactory or painful life situations. We saw the tremendous political strength we gained by identifying common problems and standing in unity with one another. In becoming aware of our own and other women's passions and potentialities, we discovered that we belonged to a family of women, a family larger than we had ever dreamed of.

We are increasingly proud of our dependence upon one another in a culture which so prizes independence. Yet our efforts (along with so many others') to form a community of women are still evolving and, despite their strengths, are quite fragile. A competitive society like ours makes it difficult to work collectively, to be open, to trust one another. It is more difficult to be a feminist these days than it was in the optimistic climate of the early seventies. And when the many women with backgrounds and experiences different from our own speak up and tell the truth about their lives, they make it clear just how diverse this huge community is. Sometimes the great differences between us—race, class, ethnicity, sexual preference, values and strategies—turn us against one another. Keeping in mind our common ground as women must be one of our main tasks. Acknowledging the past and present hurts, the inner fears of difference and the external realities which separate us can enable us to learn to hear each and every woman's voice clearly, to nurture each and every woman's life.

> Remember the dignity
> of your womanhood.
> Do not appeal,
> do not beg,
> do not grovel.
> Take courage,
> join hands,
> stand beside us,
> Fight with us...
>
> CHRISTABEL PANKHURST
> English suffragette, 1858–1928

From

Norma	Nancy	Vilunya	Wendy
Pam	Paula	Esther	Joan
Judy	Ruth	Jane	

465 Mt. Auburn Street
Watertown, MA 02172

xiv

Our Faces Belong to Our Bodies

Our faces belong to our bodies.
Our faces belong to our lives.

Our faces are blunted.
Our bodies are stunted.
We cover our anger with smiles.

Our faces belong to our bodies.
Our faces belong to our lives.

Our anger is changing our faces, our bodies.
Our anger is changing our lives.

Women who scrub have strong faces
Women who type have strong faces
Women with children have strong faces
Women who love have strong faces

Women who laugh have strong faces
Women who fight have strong faces
Women who cry have strong faces
Women who die have strong faces.

Our love is changing our faces, our bodies.
Our love is changing our lives.

Our sisters are changing our faces, our bodies.
Our sisters are changing our lives.

Our anger is changing our faces, our bodies.
Our anger is changing our lives.

Our power is changing our faces, our bodies.
Our power is changing our lives.

Our struggle is changing our faces, our bodies.
Our struggle is changing our lives.

While the information contained in *Our Bodies, Ourselves* will hopefully empower you and give you useful tools and ideas, this book is not intended to replace professional health and medical care.

The Boston Women's Health Book Collective is a nonprofit organization devoted to education about women and health. Our many projects and services include a Women's Health Information Center, open to the public; extensive distribution of free materials to women and organizations in the U.S. and other countries; the publication and distribution of a Spanish-language edition of *Our Bodies, Ourselves (Nuestros Cuerpos, Nuestras Vidas)*; and the operation of a women's health learning center at a nearby women's prison. Royalties income from the sale of *Our Bodies, Ourselves* is not sufficient to support our work. Therefore, the Collective continually needs additional funding from contributions and grants. Tax-deductible donations (made payable to "BWHBC") are welcome. Send to 465 Mt. Auburn Street, Watertown, MA 02172. Thank you.

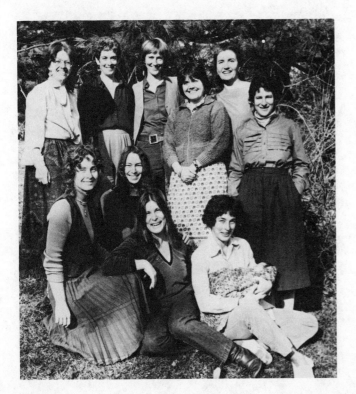

Boston Women's Health Book Collective   *Elizabeth Cole*

PREFACE

I

A GOOD STORY

The history of this book, *Our Bodies, Ourselves*, is lengthy and satisfying.

It began in a small discussion group on "women and their bodies" which was part of a women's conference held in Boston in the spring of 1969, one of the first gatherings of women meeting specifically to talk with other women. For many of us it was the very first time we had joined together with other women to talk and think about our lives and what we could do about them. Before the conference was over, some of us decided to keep on meeting as a group to continue the discussion, and so we did.

In the beginning we called ourselves "the doctors group." We had all experienced similar feelings of frustration and anger toward specific doctors and the medical maze in general, and initially we wanted to do something about those doctors who were condescending, paternalistic, judgmental and non-informative. As we talked and shared our experienced with one another, we realized just how much we had to learn about our bodies. So we decided on a summer project—to research those topics which we felt were particularly pertinent to learning about our bodies, to discuss in the group what we had learned, then to write papers individually or in groups of two or three, and finally to present the results in the fall as a course for women on women and their bodies.

As we developed the course we realized more and more that we really *were* capable of collecting, understanding, and evaluating medical information. Together we evaluated our reading of books and journals, our talks with doctors and friends who were medical students. We found we could discuss, question and argue with each other in a new spirit of cooperation rather than competition. We were equally struck by how important it was for us to be able to open up with one another and share our feelings about our bodies. The process of talking was as crucial as the facts themselves. Over time the facts and feelings melted together in ways that touched us very deeply, and that

is reflected in the changing titles of the course and then the book—from *Women and Their Bodies* to *Women and Our Bodies* to, finally, *Our Bodies, Ourselves*.

When we gave the course we met in any available free space we could get—in day schools, in nursery schools, in churches, in our homes. We wanted the course to stimulate the same kind of talking and sharing that we who had prepared the course had experienced. We had something to say, but we had a lot to learn as well; we did not want a traditional teacher-student relationship. At the end of ten to twelve sessions—which roughly covered the material in the current book—we found that many women felt both eager and competent to get together in small groups and share what they had learned with other women. We saw it as a never-ending process always involving more and more women.

After the first teaching of the course, we decided to revise our initial papers and mimeograph them so that other women could have copies as the course expanded. Eventually we got them printed and bound together in an inexpensive edition published by the New England Free Press. It was fascinating and very exciting for us to see what a constant demand there was for our book. It came out in several editions, a larger number being printed each time, and the time from one printing to the next becoming shorter. The growing volume of requests began to strain the staff of the New England Free Press.* Since our book was clearly speaking to many people, we wanted to reach beyond the audience who lived in the area or who were acquainted with the New England Free Press. For wider distribution it made sense to publish our book commercially.

You may want to know who we are. Our ages range

---

*New England Free Press is no longer in existence.

from twenty-five to forty-one, most of us are from middle-class backgrounds and have had at least some college education, and some of us have professional degrees. Some of us are married, some of us are separated, and some of us are single. Some of us have children of our own, some of us like spending time with children, and others of us are not sure we want to be with children. In short, we are both a very ordinary and a very special group, as women are everywhere. We can describe only what life has been for us, though many of our experiences have been shared by other women. We realize that poor and nonwhite women have had greater difficulty in getting accurate information and adequate health care, and have most often been mistreated in the ways we describe in the book. Learning about our womanhood from the inside out has allowed us to cross over some of the socially created barriers of race, color, income and class, and to feel a sense of identity with all women in the experience of being female.

We are eleven individuals and we are a group. (The group has been ongoing for three years, and some of us have been together since the beginning. Others came in at later points. Our current collective has been together for one year.) We know each other well—our weaknesses as well as our strengths. We have learned through good times and bad how to work together (and how not to, as well). We recognize our similarities and differences and are learning to respect each person for her uniqueness. We love each other.

Many, many other women have worked with us on the book. A group of gay women got together specifically to do the chapter on lesbianism. Other chapters were done still differently. For instance, the mother of one woman in the group volunteered to work on menopause with some of us who have not gone through that experience ourselves. Other women contributed thoughts, feelings and comments as they passed through town or passed through our kitchens or workrooms. There are still other voices from letters, phone conversations, and a variety of discussions that are included in the chapters as excerpts of personal experiences. Many women have spoken for themselves in this book, though we in the collective do not agree with all that has been written. Some of us are even uncomfortable with part of the material. We have included it anyway, because we give more weight to accepting that we differ than to our uneasiness. We have been asked why this is exclusively a book about women, why we have restricted our course to women. Our answer is that we are women and, as women, do not consider ourselves experts on men (as men through the centuries have presumed to be experts on us). We are not implying that we think most twentieth-century men are much less alienated from their bodies than women are. But we know it is up to men to explore that for themselves, to come together and share their sense of themselves as we have done. We would like

to read a book about men and their bodies.

We are offering a book that can be used in many different ways—individually, in a group, for a course. Our book contains real material about our bodies and ourselves that isn't available elsewhere, and we have tried to present it in a new way—an honest, humane and powerful way of thinking about ourselves and our lives. We want to share the knowledge and power that come with this way of thinking, and we want to share the feelings we have for each other—supportive and loving feelings that show we can indeed help one another grow.

From the very beginning of working together, first on the course that led to this book and then on the book itself, we have felt exhilarated and energized by our new knowledge. Finding out about our bodies and our bodies' needs, starting to take control over that area of our lives, has released for us an energy that has overflowed into our work, our friendships, our relationships with men and women, and for some of us, our marriages and our parenthood. In trying to figure out why this has had such a life-changing effect on us, we have come up with several important ways in which this kind of body education has been liberating for us and may be a starting point for the liberation of many other women.

First, we learned what we learned equally from professional sources—textbooks, medical journals, doctors, nurses—and from our own experiences. The facts were important, and we did careful research to get the information we had not had in the past. As we brought the facts to one another we learned a good deal, but in sharing our personal experiences relating to those facts we learned still more. Once we had learned what the "experts" had to tell us, we found we still had a lot to teach and to learn from one another. For instance, many of us had "learned" about the menstrual cycle in science or biology classes—we had perhaps even memorized the names of the menstrual hormones and what they did. But most of us did not remember much of what we had learned. This time when we read in a text that the onset of menstruation is a normal and universal occurrence in young girls from ages ten to eighteen, we started to talk about our first menstrual periods. We found that, for many of us, beginning to menstruate had not felt normal at all, but scary, embarrassing, mysterious. We realized that what we had been told about menstruation and what we had not been told—even the tone of voice it had been told in—had all had an effect on our feelings about being female. Similarly, the information from enlightened texts describing masturbation as a normal, common sexual activity did not really become our own until we began to pull up from inside ourselves and share what we had never before expressed —the confusion and shame we had been made to feel, and often still felt, about touching our bodies in a sexual way.

Learning about our bodies in this way is an exciting kind of learning, where information and feelings are allowed to interact. It makes the difference between rote memorization and relevant learning, between fragmented pieces of a puzzle and the integrated picture, between abstractions and real knowledge. We discovered that people don't learn very much when they are just passive recipients of information. We found that each individual's response to information was valid and useful, and that by sharing our responses we could develop a base on which to be critical of what the experts tell us. Whatever we need to learn now, in whatever area of our lives, we know more how to go about it.

A second important result of this kind of learning is that we are better prepared to evaluate the institutions that are supposed to meet our health needs —the hospitals, clinics, doctors, medical schools, nursing schools, public health departments, Medicaid bureaucracies and so on. For some of us it was the first time we had looked critically, and with strength, at the existing institutions serving us. The experience of learning just how little control we had over our lives and bodies, the coming together out of isolation to learn from each other in order to define what we needed, and the experience of supporting one another in demanding the changes that grew out of our developing critique—all were crucial and formative political experiences for us. We have felt our potential power as a force for political and social change.

The learning we have done while working on *Our Bodies, Ourselves* has been a good basis for growth in other areas of life for still another reason. For women throughout the centuries, ignorance about our bodies has had one major consequence—pregnancy. Until very recently pregnancies were all but inevitable, biology *was* our destiny—that is, because our bodies are designed to get pregnant and give birth and lactate, that is what all or most of us did. The courageous and dedicated work of people like Margaret Sanger started in the early twentieth century to spread and make available birth control methods that women could use, thereby freeing us from the traditional lifetime of pregnancies. But the societal expectation that a woman above all else will have babies does not die easily. When we first started talking to each other about this, we found that that old expectation had nudged most of us into a fairly rigid role of wife-and-motherhood from the moment we were born female. Even in 1969, when we first started the work that led to this book, we found that many of us were still getting pregnant when we didn't want to. It was not until we researched carefully and learned more about birth-control methods and abortion, about laws governing birth control and abortion, and not until we put all this information together with what it meant to us to be female, that we began to feel we could truly set out to control whether and when we would have babies.

This knowledge has freed us to a certain extent from the contant, energy-draining anxiety about becoming pregnant. It has made our pregnancies better because they no longer happen to us, but we actively choose them and enthusiastically participate in them. It has made our parenthood better because it is our choice rather than our destiny. This knowledge has freed us from playing the role of mother if it is not a role that fits us. It has given us a sense of a larger life space to work in, an invigorating and challenging sense of time and room to discover the energies and talents that are in us, to do the work we want to do. And one of the things we most want to do is to help make this freedom of choice, this life span, available to every woman. This is why people in the women's movement have been so active in fighting against the inhumane legal restrictions, the imperfections of available contraceptives, the poor sex education, the highly priced and poorly administered health care that keep too many women from having this crucial control over their bodies.

There is a fourth reason why knowledge about our bodies has generated so much new energy. For us, body education is core education. Our bodies are the physical bases from which we move out into the world; ignorance, uncertainty—even, at worst, shame—about our physical selves create in us an alienation from ourselves that keeps us from being the whole people that we could be. Picture a woman trying to do work and to enter into equal and satisfying relationships with other people—when she feels physically weak because she has never tried to be strong; when she drains her energy trying to change her face, her figure, her hair, her smells, to match some ideal norm set by magazines, movies and TV; when she feels confused and ashamed of the menstrual blood that every month appears from some dark place in her body; when her internal body processes are a mystery to her and surface only to cause her trouble (an unplanned pregnancy, or cervical cancer); when she does not understand or enjoy sex and concentrates her sexual drives into aimless romantic fantasies, perverting and misusing a potential energy because she had been brought up to deny it. Learning to understand, accept, and be responsible for our physical selves, we are freed of some of these preoccupations and can start to use our untapped energies. Our image of ourselves is on a firmer base, we can be better friends and better lovers, better *people*, more self-confident, more autonomous, stronger and more whole.

March, 1973.

PREFACE

II

Some Notes on the Second Edition

When we started to revise *Our Bodies, Ourselves*, we thought it would be a simple two-month job of updating some facts. Now, several months and much hard and exciting work later, we surface for air and rush to get the "new Book" out by February! The revised edition turned out to be 100 pages longer and more than two-thirds revised, because:

1. We ourselves have grown and changed with two more years of living, as we have worked, loved, played, read, heard from others and shared among ourselves.
2. Readers of the first edition have energetically urged us both by letter and in person, to include more of certain kinds of needed information—for instance, on menopause, breast cancer, self-help.
3. Much has changed in the health field, including improvements (like the increased availability of first-trimester abortion and the emergence of various woman-generated health-care alternatives), and setbacks (such as increasing medical intervention in normal childbirth).

These three kinds of change have affected nearly every chapter in the book. Some parts have been almost totally rewritten: Sexuality, Common Medical and Health Problems (Chapter 23), Venereal Disease, Rape, Abortion, Considering Parenthood, Preparation for Childbirth, Some Problems in Childbearing, Menopause and Women and Health Care.

The new book costs two dollars more to cover rising costs of paper and printing. We hope that clinics and other health-care delivery and education groups with IRS tax-exempt status will take advantage of the clinic discount mentioned on the copyright page. (If your group has trouble qualifying for a clinic discount you can write to us.) We have used the royalties from book sales to support health-education work done both by our group and in conjunction with other women's health groups.

We have been together now for more than five years as a work-and-personal-sharing group. Since the book's publication we have experienced some conflict between our work load as authors of a widely selling book and our desire to be a close personal support group for one another. We have been exploring ways of getting our work done more effectively. And we have been learning more about how to ask for help from each other and how to give it. As our interconnectedness grows, we feel increasing love and appreciation for each other.

We feel proud and glad that the book has reached so many people. It has been published in Japan and Italy, and is soon to come out in France, Holland, Sweden, Denmark, Greece and Great Britain. A number of Spanish-speaking women have been working on a Spanish translation for the United States (and possibly other countries) which we hope to have published in 1976. The book has also been put into seven volumes of braille (Braille No. 2328, Library of Congress No. 301).

The work of redefining health education and health care for women is being carried on, expanded and improved by a dramatically increasing number of groups and individuals in the women's health movement. Many women, both as consumers and as health workers, are making a radical challenge to the health-care system as we have known it. The hardest work is ahead: as the challenge has become more effective, most of the medical world has intensified its resistance to change. We urge you to work for change, in any way that feels right for you.

The experience of finding so much of the 1973 edition outdated less than two years later has made us aware that by the time this edition comes out even some of the "revised" material will not be totally up-to-date. Throughout the book we have tried to list resources for the most current information, and we hope you will find them useful tools as you move to take control of your body, your health, your physical, emotional and spiritual well-being—your life.

I
TAKING CARE
OF OURSELVES

INTRODUCTION

By Wendy Sanford

With special thanks to Nancy P. Hawley and Jane Pincus

The following chapters offer some of the basic information we as women need to take care of our health—at home and in the workplace. Though medical care sometimes helps us when we are sick, it does not keep us healthy. To a great extent what makes us healthy or unhealthy is how we are able to live our daily lives—what we eat, how we exercise, how much rest we get, how much stress we live with, how much we use alcohol, cigarettes or drugs, how safe or hazardous our workplaces are, whether we experience the threat or reality of sexual violence. Some of these things are under our control as individuals. Many, however, are not; we can influence them only by working with others to bring changes: pressuring an employer to remove hazards, forming a co-op for cheaper high-quality food, protesting the pollution from a nearby chemical plant, starting a "safelight" network for women alone on the streets at night. Many of these daily health factors are dependent on how much money we have: in an unjust society some people can afford to take better care of their health than others. It is a major aim of the feminist movement to make the crucial tools for health and survival available to everyone.

All through this book we emphasize wherever possible *what women can do*—for ourselves, for each other—in staying healthy, healing ourselves and working for change. Women have a long and proud history as healers. (See p. 589.) Our friends and women's groups are sources of comfort, insight, courage and healing. We *do* need professional help with health problems, even when medical approaches are not always the best, with their excessive emphasis on drugs, surgery and crisis intervention. So we have included a number of nonmedical alternatives in Chapter 5. We have also included a brief discussion of psychotherapy, because so many women use it as a tool for taking care of themselves in a society that presents many barriers to true emotional health.

HEALTHISM

Healthism, simply put, is an overemphasis on keeping healthy. Social critic Robert Crawford believes that many persons today (particularly, he notes, the more affluent) are *too* focused on staying healthy.* He suggests that people have become preoccupied with controlling the more manageable health factors like smoking or diet because they feel powerless to change major factors like financial uncertainty or potential nuclear disaster. When we are overly focused on healthiness or a "healthy lifestyle" as goals to strive for (or as the measure of a "healthy" society), we deflect attention from the more important goals of social justice and peace.

Crawford also points out that even though prevention is crucial, and dangerously glossed over by conventional medicine, it, too, can be overemphasized. In expanding the concept of prevention ever further, we risk defining more and more aspects of life in terms of health and illness—that is, according to a medical model. We may end up seeing exercise, eating, meditation, fresh air, dance, for example—all pleasures in their own right—simply as measures of our potential health or nonhealth. In this way, ironically, we further medicalize our lives.

Keeping healthy can also become a moral issue. Individuals are made to feel guilty for getting sick. People shake their heads disapprovingly over those who "don't take care of themselves." In many cases this amounts to blaming the victim; it shows a failure to recognize the social and economic influences on health habits and illness. With personal habits, too, a certain judgmentalness creeps in: "She *should* have more control over her smoking" or "She *should* get more exercise, stop eating so much sugar." Even when these are matters of personal choice, a moralistic healthism is inappropriate. And it doesn't help people change, even when they may want to.

*See Robert J. Crawford, "Healthism and the Medicalization of Everyday Life," *International Journal of Health Services*, Vol. 10, No. 3 (1980).

STRESS

Common to most of the chapters in this unit is a new understanding of stress as a major health factor. Humans, like all animals, have innate stress-alarm systems originally designed to help us fight or run away when faced with danger. In earlier, simpler times this fight-or-flight response was appropriate. In today's world, however, the dangers are no longer so obvious or so simple. We experience multiple, prolonged, often ambiguous stresses (see below) for which immediate action is often impossible. We squelch the fight-or-flight response over and over again in the course of a single day. It is an increasingly accepted theory that years of failing to discharge the body's stress response can damage the body's immune (disease-fighting) system and result in many different kinds of ill health. Possible long-term consequences of living with too much stress are ulcers, high blood pressure, higher risk of coronary heart disease, rheumatoid arthritis and cancer.

We can minimize the effects of stress in various ways such as exercise, better food, meditation, foot rubs, long hot baths, time to ourselves. It helps to complain when we need to, ask our friends for encouragement, laugh. But it is important, too, to try to identify the *causes* of negative or excessive stress in our lives, and to change as many as we can.* This isn't always easy or possible, especially by ourselves. The following chapters seek to distinguish carefully between what we can do as individuals and the social factors which we must change by working together.

Some Causes of Stress
- financial insecurity
- job loss
- death of somebody we love and/or need
- ending or beginning of a relationship
- job changes; a new job
- having a baby
- moving
- being discriminated against because of race, class, age, looks, sexual preference or physical disability
- an illness for which we can find no appropriate care
- a diet low in fresh foods and high in sugar, white flour, caffeine, additives and salt
- environmental pollution
- the threat of nuclear war

Stresses Specific to Women

- A majority of women now combine outside jobs with full responsibility for home and children. In addition, we may feel—from others, from ourselves—the pressure to be "perfect" at each of these.
- Most jobs pay women little and don't allow us to use our abilities.
- Many women are single parents; many are poor.
- Some of us are at home all day with small children.
- We face sexual harassment and abuse on the street, in workplaces, at home.

Symptoms of Excessive Stress

- headaches
- neck, back and shoulder pains
- nervous twitches, "tics"
- insomnia
- skin rashes
- greater susceptibility to colds, influenza or other illnesses
- worsening of existing conditions or illnesses
- depression, anxiety, irritability, nervousness, despair
- jaw pains and toothaches (from grinding teeth)
- cankers, cold sores
- stomachaches, diarrhea, loss of or increase in appetite
- increased frequency of herpes episodes

---

*Many businesses have introduced "stress reduction" programs for employees. These programs, however, emphasize only what *individuals* can do, and rarely address the *sources* of stress in the workplace, because to do so would mean expensive changes like reducing the workload or eliminating safety hazards.

1

BODY IMAGE

By Wendy Sanford

With special thanks to the women of Boston Self-Help, including Frances Deloatch, Mary Fitzgerald, Jean Gillespie, Oce, Rosemarie Ouilette, Marsha Saxton and Janna Zwerner; and to Joan Lastovica, Judith Stein, Nancy Hawley, Esther Rome, Jane Pincus and Jill Wolhandler

Imagine yourself naked in front of a mirror. Turn around slowly. Do you like what you see? Stroke your body's contours. Do you like what you feel? Try saying something appreciative to each part of yourself. It may be difficult at first. Almost every woman judges some part of her body—sometimes all of it—as "not right," tries to hide it from view, feels ashamed of it even with friends or lovers.

We often feel negative about our physical selves. Our hair is too straight or too curly, nose too small or too large, breasts too big or too small, stomach or thighs too fat, frame too bony. We don't like our body hair or odors. Our genitals—well, we just try to ignore them; after all, they really "belong" to lovers or doctors, not to us. We often compare ourselves to others; we're never okay the way we are. We feel ugly, inadequate. If others say we are beautiful, we don't/can't believe it, or we worry about losing our beauty. We spend precious time and money trying to change our looks. We may also subject ourselves to health hazards: cosmetics and vaginal deodorants which contain dangerous chemicals, low-calorie diets which deprive us of needed nutrients, hair dyes with cancer-causing ingredients, clothes and shoes which severely hamper our freedom of movement, and questionable surgery like the intestinal bypass operation or face-lift. Looks are too often a matter of survival: many employers require that we look a particular way in order to get or keep our jobs. It's hard not to judge ourselves—and each other—on the "acceptability" of our bodies.

Talking with other women about body image helps us see that we can come to think differently about our bodies and come to accept ourselves more fully. It's a process which we can begin at any point in our lives and continue as long as we live.

One freeing step is to take a critical look at the pressures on us to look a certain way. Growing up, we learn to think of our bodies mainly in terms of *how we look*. Early on we get the message: you've got to look good in order to be acceptable, to please men.

My husband gave me a full-length mirror for my thirtieth birthday, to remind me I'd better keep an eye on my looks.

Every society throughout history has had standards of beauty, but at no time before has there been such an intense media blitz telling us what we *should* look like. Magazine covers, films, TV shows, billboards surround us with images which fail to reflect the tremendous diversity among us. Never before have there been hundreds of profitable businesses set up to convince us we don't look good enough. Whole industries depend on selling us products through slick ads depicting "beautiful" women, playing on our insecurities and fears of imperfection.

We naturally want to look and feel good, to wear colors and materials that are beautiful to us, to feel attractive and appreciated. The trouble is that the media defines "looking good" so narrowly that few of us ever feel we have made it. Picture for yourself the "ideal" woman in the dominant culture of America today. She is almost without exception thin, shapely, white, able-bodied, smooth-skinned, young and glamorous. She may change from decade to decade (big breasts are out this year, little breasts are in), yet we always have to measure up to some image.* Media images do have less impact if friends and family like us as we are.

If we are passably close to the current media image of beauty we may not be aware of the intense pressures working on us. But if we are more obviously "different"—fat, old, women of color or physically disabled, for instance—we encounter the pressures more openly

---

*Those of us who are feminists and/or lesbians may not worry so much about pleasing men. Yet we may replace one ideal with another, substituting muscular for shapely, for instance, or Amazon for covergirl, so that there is still an image we feel we have to live up to. Those of us who are nonwhite or non-Anglo Saxon often feel torn between the dominant culture's standards and those of our own community.

and every day. Women who don't "fit" the image experience painfully the negative judgments, fears and hatreds which in subtle or unsubtle ways make it hard for nearly every woman in our society to love and accept herself as she is.

PHYSICAL DISABILITY AND THE PRESSURE TO BE PHYSICALLY "PERFECT"

Authors' Note: Several women from Boston Self-Help (a self-help organization for people with physical disabilities) were generous with their time in talking with us, suggesting books and articles and reading over what we'd written here. Many of us in the Collective had never known women with physical disabilities; our meetings with the Boston Self-Help group began to change both how we see disabled women and how we see ourselves. We have chosen to use the pronouns "we" and "us" in this section because both groups discovered at those meetings that many of the issues we face as women are similar, because the women in the group said that to use the third-person "they" would be too distancing, and because it is important to them that able-bodied women be conscious that they are only "temporarily" able-bodied. By remembering that this state could change at any time through accident or illness, we are more likely to see disabled women as sisters rather than turn away from them in indifference or fear.

This woman is postpolio and has no use of her arms and hands. She takes care of her daughter using her teeth and toes and love. *Jean Gillespie*

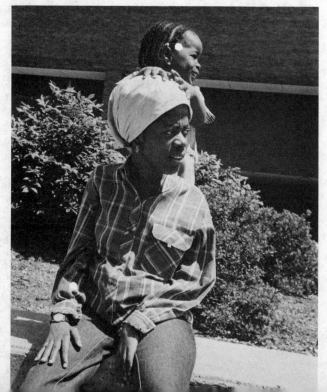

Several million women in this country walk with a limp, move in a wheelchair or with crutches, have impaired sight, speech or hearing, have lost a limb to fire or accident or disease, need special assistance with simple bodily functions or wear the scars of some damaging event. Many of these millions of women are silent and invisible—many of us choose to hide in order to avoid the pain of being stared at and objectified, and the public, in fear, does not acknowledge and accept us.

With a body that doesn't "measure up," we learn pretty quickly what our culture really wants from women.

Having a disability made me very aware at an early age of the messages I was receiving from the larger society about how I was supposed to look and how you're supposed to be. Also, as the doctors poked and studied me endlessly, I learned more quickly than some nondisabled women that I'm seen as an object.

My family's thing was that girls dated in order to find a prospective mate. Since I had cerebral palsy, they assumed I was never going to marry. So why should I date? And I've only just begun to wear a dress this year, because I was always encouraged to wear pants. There was no reason for me to dress like a woman because I wasn't one. That wasn't part of my identity.

The more we vary from the norm, the less families, friends, physicians expect or allow us to be sexual. (See "Sex and Physical Disabilities," p. 182.) If we can't have children, we are pitied for not being "real" women. If we aren't "pleasing" to look at, we are expected to compensate, and we come to expect it of ourselves: we learn to smile a lot and be sweet, or clown around, so people won't feel so uncomfortable around us. Or, believing in our own unworthiness, we fall into the background.

Other "female" stereotypes surface quickly—we are weak, less intelligent, need protection. If we can't control our movements or bodily functions people think we are mentally incompetent. ("My family thinks of epilepsy as a mental illness." "People see my body and don't expect me to be smart.") Like many women, only more so, we are treated like children far into our adult lives. ("People will pinch me on the cheek and use words that you would use to a first- or second-grader." "The doctors still talk to my parents or to the person with me instead of directly to me, as though I'm a child, and I'm sick of it.") As women with physical disabilities, it is difficult but important to assert our adulthood, our power, our individuality and intelligence. This process is crucial for *all* women.

Severe job discrimination penalizes us for having "unacceptable" bodies and creates strong economic incentive for "fitting in" and minimizing differences. This pressure to keep a low profile if we are disabled makes us feel isolated and less free to get the help we need and deserve both physically and emotionally. It also means we have a hard time becoming economically independent. As one woman said, "We are not disabled; it is society which disables us by being so unsupportive."

Sooner or later, if we're lucky, we realize how angry we are at always having had to hide our true feelings and the realities of our lives.

After I got my braces removed at age twelve, I did everything I could to hide my skinny, scarred legs, including wearing knee socks or long pants in the hottest weather. Slowly my anger grew at the restrictions I was accepting. Partly with the help of other disabled women, I came to see my underlying feeling that if people saw my legs they'd not only reject me for being ugly, but they'd somehow see the years in the hospital or how dependent and scared I'd been. I began to reevaluate these experiences as simply things that had happened, not who I am. I wear shorts when I want to now, and I like my legs the way they are.

If coming to love and accept our bodies is a difficult process for every woman in this society, it is especially hard with a disability.

Finally I like my body, and because of my disability that statement has added significance. There is something "WRONG" with my body, so how can I possibly feel good about it or enjoy life in it? Simple answers are: I have no choice and I want to. The more complex answer is that there is nothing wrong with my body. It falls within the wide range of human experience and is therefore both natural and normal. I've been in this body all my life. I was born with it and I'll die with it. It's part of who I am, and I'd be someone else without this body just the way it is.

Dialogue between disabled and nondisabled women reveals that we have much in common. A woman with a brittle bone condition wrote:

...I can't quite pinpoint when I began to listen to the experiences of able-bodied women and relate them to my own. It may have been when someone said that she couldn't go out of the house because her skin was so spotty, or when a beautiful black woman told me how all her life she had wanted to be white and blotchy like her friend at school, or it could have been when a friend of mine who had always been my envy for being followed around by drooling men said that she was so lonely because people only reacted to her stunning body and never to the person inside it. It may have been when my family began to talk about one of its female members who had put on weight and had, in their eyes, become not only unattractive but somehow outrageously undutiful in her role as an ornament. It may have been none of this that made the turning point for me, but instead it could have been the way some of the women put their arms around me and called me their beautiful sister

that made me begin to see that we are not so different after all. We are all made to feel that our role is firstly to be beautiful in a highly stereotyped way, secondly to be interesting and amusing company to men and thirdly, good servants. My experience of finding that I was not necessarily any of those things is the experience of most women sooner or later. I have been lucky enough to discover that I am still a whole and worthwhile person and feel that all those dark years linked me profoundly to other women.[1]

BODY IMAGE AND WEIGHT*

In most cultures and historical periods women have been proud to be large—being fat was a sign of fertility, of prosperity, of the ability to survive. Yet fear of fat and bigness reigns in most sectors of American culture today. Media images of women insist that "Thin is beautiful." The medical world blames a whole range of problems on "overweight." Fat women encounter daily hostility and discrimination.

No wonder so many of us worry about our weight no matter what we weigh, spend precious hours counting calories, feel guilty when we "splurge."

I don't like myself heavy. I want to feel thin, streamlined and spare, and not like a toad. I have taken antifat thinking into myself so deeply that I hate myself when I am even ten pounds "overweight," whatever that means.

Low-calorie dieting has become a national obsession. Fat activists suggest that making women afraid to be fat is a form of social control. Fear of fat keeps women preoccupied, robs us of our pride and energy, keeps us from *taking up space.* Says activist Vivian Mayer, "Mass starvation of women is the modern

*For more on this topic, especially on health issues and low-calorie dieting, see Chapter 2, "Food."

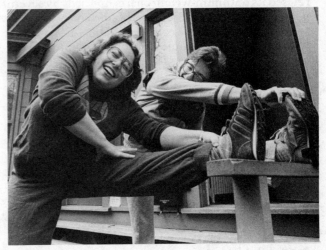

Bonnie Burt

Being Fat in an AntiFat Society*

Being fat in the United States means that we walk down the street to comments like "fat bitch" or "pig." We are expected to laugh at fat jokes. People laugh at us when we try to be physically active or if we show an interest in sex. Friends and family try to get us to diet instead of helping us love ourselves. At public events the seats are too small and uncomfortable. We search for days to find clothes that fit and have a harder time than thin women finding a job or getting into college. Like many other minorities, we never see *our* image on TV or in the movies except as comic or pathetic characters. We often hear that our fatness is the cause of everything that goes wrong in our lives. We are judged as weak-willed or morally lax because we "indulge" ourselves. We live for long stretches in a state of starvation (called "being on a diet") because our appearance touches people's fear of their own appetites.

If we are fat, health practitioners often attribute our health problems to "obesity," postpone treatment until we lose weight, accuse us of cheating if we don't, make us so ashamed of our size that we don't go for help and make all kinds of assumptions about our emotional and psychological state ("She must have emotional problems to be so fat"). In fact, much of our ill health as fat women results from the *stress* of living with fat-hatred—social ridicule and hostility, isola-tion, financial pressures resulting from job discrimination, lack of exercise due to harassment and, perhaps most important, the hazards of repeated dieting.

Fat women have formed various support groups in the past decade. Here are suggestions from women in a local chapter of Fat Liberation:*

No matter what anyone says to you (or what you fear they are saying about you), you have the *right* to go anywhere and do anything you like: to eat whatever you want in restaurants, to go dancing, to enjoy life. If someone or some place makes you feel uncomfortable (by rude remarks, aisles too narrow or chairs too small) it is up to *them* to change, not you.

You have the right to respond angrily to the nasty things people say to you or about you. Practice a few good withering glances or comebacks.

Take up all of the space your body occupies—no more hunching or slumping to try to look smaller. Stand up tall and relax. Practice being big. Or pretend you're a lion afraid of nothing and very, very strong. Move around your house remembering to breathe deeply, keeping your shoulders and back straight. Be loose and big in your movements. Work to create the feeling that you are entitled to go wherever you want and the world should make room for your wonderful presence. Whatever the size of your stomach (thighs, rear end), stop sucking in your stomach muscles. Insist on the right to be comfortable all the way out to your skin. Try to buy clothes that fit easily. Pleated pants or ones with elastic in the waist are less likely to bind your stomach in. Tight clothes don't make us look thinner—but they do make it harder to get out and move around.

American culture's equivalent of foot-binding, lip-stretching and other forms of female mutilation."[2]

Recent research indicates that the "ideal" body weight for each woman is at least ten pounds higher than that stated by medical charts, and that no one at this point *knows* a given woman's "ideal" weight.† The Metropolitan Life Insurance Company recently revised its optimum-weight charts upwards by several pounds. Many health problems blamed on overweight turn out to have a more complex relationship to weight than doctors once assumed. Studies suggest that dieting is usually not successful in the long run, and that repeated low-calorie dieting is in fact a major cause of ill health.

These developments offer women a chance to become more relaxed about weight:

- by experimenting with what weight feels *comfortable* to us rather than trying primarily to be thin;
- by being more accepting of weight variations through the life cycle;

- by developing a clearer understanding of which health problems are truly associated with weight—some (e.g., diabetes and overly high blood pressure) may be, but not others; we must learn to distinguish what facts exist among the many, often damaging fictions;
- by exercising and eating nutritious food to feel healthy, and letting our body weight set itself accordingly;
- if we do diet, by choosing a program which emphasizes exercise and helps us change eating patterns but doesn't starve us.

WORKING TOGETHER FOR CHANGE

In moving toward a more positive self-image, we are stronger if we can talk with other women. We need each other's help to change the deeply entrenched attitudes which make us dislike our bodies. Here are some things groups of women can do together:

---

*See, in particular, William Bennett and Joel Gurin's book *The Dieter's Dilemma*, listed in Resources for Chapter 2, "Food."
†Thanks especially to Judith Stein and Rea Rea Sears of Boston Area Fat Liberation.

*Unpublished manuscript by Judith Stein and others.

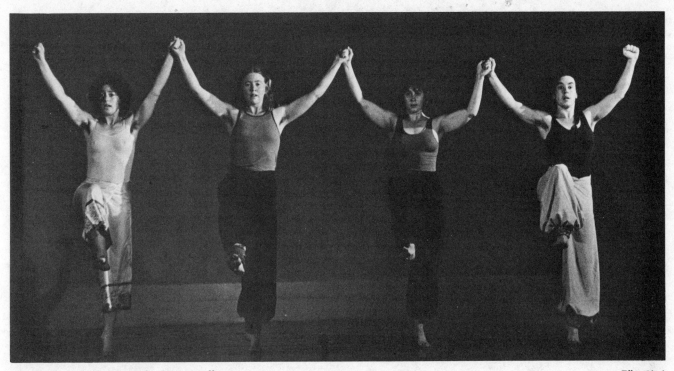

Members of Wallflower Order Dance Collective

Ellen Shub

- Look at ads and criticize how they demean women and limit our ideas of beauty. Find ways to make your protest known to the companies advertised* and to let the media know you want to see more varied and realistic images of women.
- Learn more about how our bodies work, through self-help sessions† and/or discussion.
- Plan together how to challenge men who judge, choose and discard women on the basis of appearance.
- Form or join a working-women's organization; work on ways to pressure employers to accept a wider range of looks and dress.
- Work together on tackling the fears and stereotypes which make us all discriminate against people who are "different." (This is a long process. One step is being painfully honest about our own prejudices; another is learning not to blame ourselves for them; another is getting to know women who are different—in race, age, physical ability.)

If we can begin to eliminate the hatred and ridicule levied against women who don't fit the "norm," we can lessen the stress of "not fitting in" and, with it, a lot of stress-related illness. We also open the possibility of building a social-change movement of many different kinds of women. Working together to change

*See "Today and Tomorrow" in Chapter 8, "Violence Against Women," for an example. See also mailings from a group called Women Against Violence in Pornography and Media, P.O. Box 14635, San Francisco, CA 94114.

†Chapter 24, "The Politics of Women and Medical Care."

the attitudes and conditions which restrict us, we feel proud and more able to take control of our lives.

A better self-image doesn't pay the rent or cook supper or prevent nuclear war. Feeling better about ourselves doesn't change the world by itself, but it can give us more energy to do what we want and can to work for change.

NOTES

1. Jo Campling, ed. "Micheline," *Images of Ourselves: Women with Disabilities Talking*. London: Routledge and Kegan Paul, 1981, pp. 26–27.

2. Vivian Mayer Aldebaran. "Uptight and Hungry: The Contradiction in Psychology of Fat." *The Radical Therapist: Journal of Radical Therapy*, p. 6.

RESOURCES

General

Cambridge Documentary Films. *Killing Us Softly*. Film (16 mm, 30 minutes) based on a lecture/slide show by Jean Killbourne. Available from CDF, P.O. Box 385, Cambridge, MA 02139. Purchase: $550/450 (sliding scale). Rental 1 day: $46 plus postage. Powerful and provocative presentation of the advertising industry's objectification of women's bodies. An excellent film for colleges, schools, church groups, women's centers. Highly recommended.

Campling, Jo, ed. *Images of Ourselves: Women with Disabilities Talking*. London: Routledge and Kegan Paul, 1981. In this excellent book, twenty or more women with varied disabilities write informatively and movingly about their lives.

Chernin, Kim. *The Obsession: Reflections on the Tyranny of Slenderness*. New York: Harper and Row, 1981. Perceptive analysis of our culture's obsession with weight, how it affects every woman's life, and the eating disorders which result.

Corbette, K., A. Cupolo and V. Lewis. *No More Stares: A Role Model Book for Disabled Teenage Girls*. Disability Rights Education Defense Fund, 2032 San Pablo Ave., Berkeley, CA 94702, 1982.

Duffy, Yvonne. *All Things Are Possible*. See "Sexuality and Physical Disabilities" in Resources, Chapter 11, "Sexuality," for details.

Fat Liberator Publications, P.O. Box 5227, Coralville, IA 52241.

Orbach, Susie. *Fat Is a Feminist Issue*. New York: Berkeley Publishing Corp., 1978. This book has some helpful material about accepting your own body weight. It suffers, however, from the underlying assumptions that fat people eat compulsively, that it's better to be thin than fat and that if you're healthy you must be thin.

Schoenfielder, Lisa, and Barb Wieser, eds. *Shadow on a Tightrope: Writings by Women About Fat Oppression*. Aunt Lute Book Co., P.O. Box 2723, Iowa City, IA 52244. Anthology of all the best articles about fat liberation.

2

FOOD

By Esther Rome

With special thanks to Marsha Butman and Vivian Mayer

This chapter in previous editions was called "Nutrition and the Food We Eat" and was written by Judy Norsigian.

Food touches practically every aspect of our lives and affects how we feel physically and emotionally. By eating well we take care of ourselves on the most basic level. Eating has enormous emotional importance for women because we are still usually the ones who have the responsibility for budgeting, planning and cooking for others in our households. Food often takes on magical powers of nurturance.

I like baked chicken, mashed potatoes, jellied cranberry sauce, salad, milk—they make me feel cared for. When I cook it for myself I become both my mother and me as a child.

Because we don't control food production, food can be a source of problems as well as joy. It's hard to get practical, reliable information about what is best to eat, and often hard to find what we need. Even when we know how to make good choices we may not have enough money to eat well.

I know I should buy fresh fruits and vegetables, but I can't afford them since I lost my job. We eat canned goods since they are cheaper and don't spoil.

About 80 percent of the poor in this country are women and children. Budget cutbacks increase the dependency of women and children on food subsidy programs like food stamps, school breakfast and lunch programs, meals for the elderly, etc. These programs, even when most heavily funded, have never been adequate.*

Many of us want to share the responsibility for choosing, buying and preparing food in our households. This may mean changing our eating and cooking patterns, encouraging a husband or partner to learn to shop and cook, getting teenage children to cook once a week and sharing meals with friends.

*The Women, Infant and Children supplement program (WIC) at its height covered only 39 percent of the people eligible for it. (One study estimated that for every dollar spent on this program, three dollars was later saved in reduced medical costs.) Food stamps cover about half the cost of an adequate meal for healthy people and make no provision if special diets are needed.

When my husband and I first decided to take turns cooking it was very hard for me to let him take the responsibility. I would suggest recipes and look over his shoulder while he cooked, giving him helpful hints. Since he was unsure of himself, that only encouraged him to ask me how to do something every few minutes. When I realized that I might as well have been cooking myself, I decided to make sure I stayed in a different room and answered most questions with "Why don't you experiment?" Now he's just as good a cook as I am. We have the added benefit of more variety since he makes different kinds of things than I do.

EATING WELL

Our Changing Diet*

With the abundance and variety of food in this country, you might be surprised that many nutritionists think we eat more poorly now than at the turn of the

*For an analysis of the development of "food science," see Naomi Aaronson, "Fuel for the Human Machine: The Industrialization of Eating in America" (Dissertation, Brandeis University, Waltham, MA 02154, 1978). Also excerpted in Kaplan. (See Resources.)

James R. Holland/Stock Boston

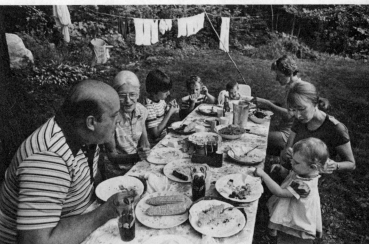

century. Even today 40 to 50 percent of middle-class Americans, who have enough money to buy whatever food they want, suffer from deficiencies of one or more nutrients. [1] We eat too much fat, salt and sugar. We used to eat more whole foods, such as whole-wheat rather than white flour. Food generally was minimally processed; that is, changed little from its original state. This change usually involved the kind of cooking or preserving that could be done in a home kitchen. Now we have technology to refine and process food; that is, to change it radically in ways we never could before, by splitting it into its components and sometimes transforming, rearranging and adding to these parts. We also used to eat more complex carbohydrates, food with a lot of starch and/or natural sugars and fiber. Now we eat fewer carbohydrates (starches and sugars) and more is refined, like cane sugar.

Diet and Illness

Because of the dietary changes mentioned above we may be making ourselves more susceptible to various diseases; current research suggests many links. Many of us have found this research compelling enough to change what we eat. Others of us who have had health problems have found that changing what we eat improves our health.

Disease	Possible Causes from Eating Patterns
Italics means there is a lot of research supporting these connections.	
Exercise and hereditary predisposition are other important factors for many of these problems.	
Some cancers	Too many *fats*; lack of *fiber*
Benign breast conditions	Caffeine-containing compounds
High blood pressure	Too much *salt*, alcohol, saturated fats; too little calcium, potassium
Heart disease	Too many *saturated fats*, *cholesterol* and sugar; lack of fiber
Cavities	Too much *sugar*
Diabetes and hypoglycemia	Too much sugar; lack of fiber
Osteoporosis	Lack of *calcium* and Vitamin D
Gallstones	Lack of fiber

Government Regulations for Good Eating

Nutrient Guidelines

We still do not know what an optimum diet is but the government is making some attempt to determine this. The U.S. Recommended *Daily* Allowances (U.S. RDAs) set by the U.S. Department of Agriculture (USDA) that you see on food packages under "Nutritional Information per Serving" are based on the Recommended *Dietary* Allowances determined by a board of respected scientists, the Food and Nutrition Board of the National Academy of Sciences. The U.S. RDAs are not fixed; the numbers of nutrients and amounts recommended change from time to time with new information. The U.S. RDAs can be valuable for comparing the nutritional value of foods. However, those foods which are enriched or fortified look deceptively nutritious since the manufacturer is required to report only those vitamins and minerals which have a U.S. RDA.

Many people take the U.S. RDAs too literally, thinking that if they follow them, they are protected. The U.S. RDAs are set generously for an "average" adult. They are not intended to assess individual needs, which may vary widely. But they are even less complete than the Dietary Allowances. We know that over forty nutrients are essential in some way; the U.S. RDAs cover only twenty-three. For some we don't know how much we need. Researchers think others are essential but haven't turned up final proof, and no doubt there are some yet to be discovered.

General Eating Guidelines

Because our changed eating habits have been linked to various diseases, the government has developed a set of guidelines called Dietary Goals. (See Resources.) The authors of this book feel that the following list, based on the government's but not exactly following it,* provides good rules for a healthy diet, given what we know today.†

1. Increase the level of complex carbohydrates we eat from 45 to 60 percent of our total calories. These foods include grains, legumes,‡ fruits and vegetables.

2. Decrease refined sugars to no more than 10 percent of our calories. It is now twice that.

3. Decrease fats to 30 percent from about 40 percent. Reduce saturated fats from 20 percent to 10 percent of calories. Saturated fats are fats which are solid at room temperature (about 70 degrees F.): animal fats, hydrogenated (hardened) fats and two vegetable fats, coconut and palm oil. Unsaturated fats are those which are liquid (oils), like corn, safflower or sesame. Those which are monosaturated are liquid at room temperature but solidify easily in the refrigerator, like peanut or olive oil.

*We have added numbers 6, 7 and 8. We have omitted a statement about maintaining an "ideal weight," included in the Dietary Guidelines issued by the USDA. See below and Chapter 1, "Body Image," for a better idea of why we do not include this.

†See Resources and your local library and bookstore for specialized cookbooks to help you eat better. Some give a lot of information about the nutrient content of foods.

‡Legumes are peas and beans like peanuts, split peas, lima beans, chick-peas or garbanzos, kidney beans, lentils, cowpeas, navy beans and pea beans.

NUTRIENTS LOST IN MAKING WHOLE-WHEAT INTO WHITE FLOUR

Nutrients Lost	Nutrients Replaced by Enrichment
88% of cobalt	iron
86% of Vitamin E	niacin
85% of magnesium	riboflavin
85% of manganese	thiamine
80% of riboflavin	
78% of sodium	
78% of zinc	
77% of potassium	
75% of iron	
71% of phosphorus	
70% of Vitamin B_6	
68% of copper	
66% of folic acid	
60% of calcium	
50% of pantothenic acid	
48% of molybdenum	
40% of chromium	
16% of selenium	
biotin (amount unknown)	
fiber (amount unknown)	
inositol (amount unknown)	
niacin (amount unknown)	
para-aminobenzoic acid (amount unknown)	
thiamine (amount unknown)	

4. Reduce cholesterol in foods to 300 milligrams per day, about half of what it is now. Cholesterol is found only in animal products, mostly in egg yolks (one yolk fills the day's limit) and organ meats (liver, brain, etc.).

5. Reduce salt (actually sodium) to three grams per day, one-third of current levels.

6. Cut proteins in half to 10 to 12 percent of the calories you eat, unless you have specific needs. (See Chapter 18, "Pregnancy.")

7. Drink as little caffeine as possible. It is found in coffee, chocolate, black tea, some herb teas such as matte and many soft drinks, especially cola drinks, as well as in others with caffeine listed as an ingredient.

Putting good food into your mouth is only one part of nourishing yourself. You need to be active to help your blood and lymph fluids better deliver the nutrients to your cells where they are used. Exercise probably* plays a crucial role in regulating your metabolism.

*We say "probably" because most of the studies linking exercise with increased metabolism are done on men. Most studies on weight reduction are done on women.

8. If you drink at all, reduce the alcohol you drink to no more than one drink a day. This is one four-ounce glass of wine, a twelve-ounce bottle of beer or one shotglass (one ounce) of hard liquor. (See section on alcoholism in Chapter 3.)

Making Changes

Would you like to see whether you can feel healthier and more energetic by eating differently? First of all, assess why you like the foods that you do and what factors influence your food choices. Do you use lots of sweet, salty and fatty foods as rewards? Do you eat when you're not hungry? Do you always eat certain foods when you are depressed, angry or upset? Are you nostalgic for certain foods you associate with childhood, special holidays or childhood rewards?

Sweets, especially ice cream, were always a treat and a comfort food in my family. I had changed my diet in all kinds of other ways, like eliminating white flour, but I didn't seriously consider cutting out sweets, even though I knew they weren't good for me. I figured I'd always have a sweet tooth. When my asthma acted up, one person suggested I eliminate dairy products and sugar from my diet. I felt so sick I was willing to try anything at that point. It was hard to do, so I took it one day at a time at first.

Now I have stopped craving sweets most of the time. I stopped eating ice cream, which I never thought I could.

Tips to Make the Guidelines Work for You

1. Introduce changes slowly, as they aren't always easy to make. Experiment with one thing at a time so you won't feel overwhelmed. This will help overcome resistance if you are cooking for others and will give your digestive tract a chance to adjust. And if you change too fast, you might find yourself craving what you are used to.

2. Look at what you eat as a whole. One day of high-fat high-sugar foods won't hurt you. (The exception to this is if you have trouble regulating your blood sugar, as with diabetes or hypoglycemia.) Think about what you eat over a one- or two-week period. Don't judge yourself for "indulging" in less-healthy foods. Given time, you will find a balance that's right for you.

3. Try new things when you aren't rushed.

4. Increase the whole foods in your diet. Generally, whole, minimally processed foods have a higher nutrient density than refined, highly processed foods. This means that for every calorie of food you eat you are getting more vitamins, minerals and other important goodies than in a low-nutrient-density food. Vegetables tend to have very high nutrient densities and foods high in fats and/or refined sugar are often low.

5. Change the snacks you keep around the house. Try

Reading Labels

Elizabeth Cole

1. The ingredients are listed in order of amount by weight used in preparation; there's most of the first ingredient and least of the last. If you don't see any ingredients listed it's because the product conforms to minimal ingredients standards set up by the U.S. Food and Drug Administration (FDA). For example, peanut butter need only contain 90 percent peanut butter. A food labeled "imitation" is like the food it substitutes for, but doesn't meet the standard. For example,

mayonnaise must contain a certain percent of fat; imitation mayonnaise usually has less.*

2. "Enriched" means that *some* of the nutrients removed during processing have been replaced by synthetic nutrients (sometimes used by your body the same as naturally occurring ones and sometimes not) to approximately the same levels found in the original food. If flour does not say "enriched" or "whole" or "whole grain," it is the poorest kind of flour you can get. Many bakeries and restaurants still use this. Ask!

3. "Fortified" means that nutrients have been added to foods. These nutrients may not normally be found in the food, as iodine in salt. They may be added in amounts greater than what naturally occurs, such as large amounts of vitamins added to breakfast cereals and to candy bars.

4. Labels must be truthful but may also be literal. For instance, "Beef with Noodles" will have more beef than "Noodles with Beef." The percentage of the named ingredients in the product determines how it is labeled. Or a product may boast that it has "more iron than milk" without also saying that milk is a poor source of iron.

5. On cans, look at how weight is listed. "Net weight" includes any liquid used for packing. "Drained" or "filled" weight tells you what the actual food weighs.

6. Check to see if there is a date listed. This can tell you how fresh the food is.

7. If you need more information about a packaged food, write to the manufacturer or distributor. The name and address must be on the label.

fruits, vegetables, whole-wheat or rice crackers. Popcorn can be made either plain or with seasonings like chili powder. Use nuts, seeds and dried fruit in moderation. (They contain important nutrients but also a lot of fat or sugar.)

6. Gradually reduce the amount of processed foods you buy. These often are "convenience" foods. They tend to be high in salt, sugar and fats, often saturated. They also are more likely to have artificial colors, flavors and other questionable ingredients. You generally get less per dollar for the nutrients in heavily processed foods than in whole foods.

7. Bring your own food as often as possible rather than relying on fast-food restaurants, vending machines and food trucks, for the same reasons as given in number 6. If you eat from them regularly you won't get enough fresh vegetables, fruits or whole grains.

8. Get together with your friends and help each other figure out how to eat healthily away from home.

9. If you eat in restaurants you can request and often get foods prepared just for you. You can also ask about

the method of preparation and the ingredients.

10. Next time you watch TV notice what kinds of foods are advertised and consider how they help or hurt your body. This can be fun to do with children.

11. Sometimes eat food that is just plain delicious whether or not it is nutritious.

Increasing Unrefined Carbohydrates

1. Use whole-wheat pastas instead of white flour ones. Make sure the bread label says "100 percent whole wheat" or "whole grain" and not just "wheat." Caramel and molasses may be added to make white bread look like whole wheat when it isn't.

2. Try eating more kinds of legumes (peas and beans).

3. In baking, substitute pastry or all-purpose wheat

*If you want to know the ingredients, labeling or grading requirements for any food, call or write to your local U.S. FDA office located in the nearest major city. Some helpful grading standards are regulated by the U.S. Department of Agriculture (USDA).

flour for white flour. Whole-wheat pastry flour* is not as widely available as all-purpose whole-wheat flour, but will make lighter-colored and -textured baked goods. Try to get fresh flour and store it at a cool temperature, since it is perishable. When substituting whole-wheat for white flour, start by substituting it for one-third or one-half the total amount. As you get used to the taste you may want to use all whole wheat.

4. Try using some whole grains like brown rice, buckwheat (kasha) or bulgur (a form of cracked wheat). They may take about twice as long to cook (forty minutes for brown rice, compared to twenty for converted white rice), but this is mainly a matter of remembering to start cooking them as soon as you begin to prepare the meal. You can use a pressure cooker to reduce preparation time.

5. For long-cooking foods, make twice as much and either freeze the leftovers or make them into something else the next day. You can buy many beans precooked in cans. Check to see if they have added salt.

Decreasing Refined and Added Sugars

1. Check the sugar content of processed foods, which often have many types of sugar in them, though legally "sugar" means sucrose. The following are all names for different forms of sugar: HFCS (high-fructose corn syrup), invert sugar, molasses, honey (refined by bees), corn sweetener, caramel, corn syrup, sucrose, lactose, maltose, dextrose, levulose, fructose, maple syrup, brown sugar, turbinado, rawkleen sugar, jam, jelly.

2. Drink more water or real fruit juice instead of soda or juice drinks. If you still want something fizzy, add seltzer to real fruit juices.

3. Drink 100 percent juice and not "juice drinks," which have only 35 to 69 percent real juice. "Fruit drinks" have 10 to 34 percent and "fruit flavored" drinks have zero to 10 percent. The rest is water and sugar. "Unsweetened" can have up to 10 percent sugar added. "No sugar added" means just that.

4. Some people find honey, molasses or malt syrup much sweeter than sugar and so use less of these than they would sugar. Blackstrap molasses has some good nutrients, like iron, but is still a highly concentrated sugar. Contrary to popular opinion, honey has no measurable benefits over sugar.†

5. Substitute sweet whole foods or real fruit juices for sugar in recipes. Try mashed cooked sweet potatoes; raisins soaked or boiled in water, then pureed in a blender; or very ripe mashed bananas instead of sugar where they can be substituted. That way you get other vitamins, minerals and fiber with sweetness.

6. If you use cold cereals, choose less sugary ones.

The following are 8 percent or less sugar by weight: Shredded Wheat, Puffed Wheat, Puffed Rice, all flavors of Nutri-Grain, Wheat Chex, Corn Chex, Grape-Nuts, Post Toasties, Rice Krispies, Cheerios, Special K and Corn Flakes. These cereals are moderately processed. Hot cereals, such as regular or quick (not instant) oatmeal, cracked wheat, cornmeal and buckwheat (kasha), take no more than fifteen to twenty minutes to prepare. Wheatena and Maltex are even quicker. They are minimally processed and contain no sugar unless added by you.

7. Use sweet spices and flavorings like cinnamon, ginger, cloves, allspice and vanilla to replace some of the sugar in the food you prepare.

8. Don't use sweets as a reward for kids (or adults!). They fill you up so you don't have room for nutritious foods. Ask relatives and friends to bring love, good stories and fruit for the children. If they persist, suggest they pick up the tab on dental bills.

Decreasing Fats and Changing the Ratio of Fats in Our Diets

1. Check the fats in the foods you buy. Avoid ingredients listed as animal fat, shortening,* tallow, lard, hydrogenated, coconut oil, palm oil or palm kernel oil.

2. Increase your use of fresh fish.

3. Eat more poultry and take the skin off. That's where 25 percent of the fat is.

4. Try some vegetarian main dishes one or more times a week. Use those that rely primarily on grains and beans. (See "Vegetarianism," p. 16.)

5. Substitute low-fat or nonfat milk or buttermilk and low-fat yogurt for some or all of the whole milk you drink.

6. Cut back on red meat, since it is high in saturated fats even if none is visible. About a third of the fat in American diets comes from meat. If your meals don't feel as substantial, remember it's the fat, not the protein, that makes you feel so full after a meat meal.

7. Avoid processed meats like bacon, sausage and cold cuts, which are even higher in fat than fresh or frozen meat. About 80 percent of their calories are from fat.

8. Cut back on the use of hard and processed cheeses if you eat a lot of them.

9. If you fry foods, use small amounts of unsaturated or monosaturated oil. Keep the oil below smoking temperatures and don't reuse it if it has darkened at all. Try broiling, baking, stewing or stir-frying instead.

10. Cut back on the butter, margarine, mayonnaise, cream and salad dressing you add to foods.

11. Reduce the amount of fatty pastries and fried foods you eat. These include pies, doughnuts, Danish, layer cakes, cheesecakes, chocolate bars, potato chips and french fries.

---

*It has less gluten, the wheat protein, than bread or all-purpose whole-wheat flour. Note also that unbleached flour is white flour.

†Honey, however, can be produced locally, aiding diversification in farming and making possible a more ecological agricultural system.

---

*When just the word "shortening" appears, it is animal shortening and should be avoided. Vegetable shortenings are specified as such on the label.

Reducing Salt

1. Reduce or avoid foods cured in salt, most condiments, hard and processed cheeses, salty snack foods including nuts, soy sauce, MSG, ingredients with the word "salt" or "sodium," bouillon and many canned soups. (Look at ingredients in over-the-counter medications also.)

2. Don't add salt to food before tasting it.

3. Some people use less salt when adding it during cooking. Others use less if they cook without salt and add some if necessary at the table. You can see which works better for you. Keep track of how much salt you buy.

4. Don't add water softeners to drinking and cooking water because they add sodium to the water.

5. Check the sodium level of your tapwater. If you are part of a municipal system, the water department will know what it is. If you have a well, you can get the water tested.

6. Substitute plain herbs, spices, onions and garlic for salt. Use oil and vinegar or lemon juice to flavor salad and other vegetables.

7. Some food labels list sodium content.*

VEGETARIANISM

Many of us today are becoming interested in vegetarianism and are eating less meat or none at all. We may do this to reduce our exposure to saturated fats and/or cholesterol, which may reduce our risk of heart disease and certain cancers; to decrease the amount of pesticides or other contaminants we eat, especially if we breastfeed;† to eat more cheaply; to stop killing other living beings; and for other religious reasons.

It is absolutely possible to live a healthy life and never eat any animals.

As a child, I never liked to eat meat, and followed mostly a vegetarian diet with occasional eggs and some dairy. This was before the time when people understood this diet well. I knew that it was right for me, and quickly became labeled stubborn, a fussy eater, etc. But when the household came down with seasonal colds and flus, I was running around quite happy and healthy with an excellent resistance.

Most vegetarians eat both eggs ("ovo") and dairy ("lacto") products. Some eat only one or the other or none ("vegans"). If you are a vegan, it is much more difficult to get protein and certain essential vitamins than if you eat eggs or dairy products. Most children,

*"Sodium free" means less than 5 mg per serving. "Very low sodium" means 35 mg or less per serving. "Low sodium" means 140 mg or less per serving. "Reduced sodium" means processed to reduce the usual level of sodium by 75 percent. "Unsalted" means processed without salt when the food normally is processed with salt.

†This may not actually be the case. See the section on residues, p. 27.

Shopping in a Supermarket

1. Go with a list. Think about *whether you really need* items not on the list. Are they fulfilling a nutritional need or some other need?

2. Don't go when you are hungry or with someone else who is hungry, especially children.

3. Shop the outside aisles first. Most of the less processed foods are there. The specialty or international section may have more whole grains and legumes.

4. If the food is highly processed, read the label so you'll know what you are getting. If you use a lot of processed food, read one new label each time you shop.

5. If your supermarket doesn't carry a food you want, call up the manager to ask for it. Try to get other people to call, too. You can also contact people who shop at other stores which have the foods you want, and go with them or ask them to buy food for you. Use mail order catalogs. Consider starting a food co-op.

6. If you have unit pricing (price per pound) in your area of the country, use it to compare brands and to see if a larger size is really cheaper. Check the total price on the unit price label to see if it is up to date. If you don't have unit pricing, try and organize some friends to pressure your food store to start using it. Failing that, use a calculator to determine the unit price.

7. End-of-aisle display items are not necessarily cheaper than similar items in their regular places. Compare before buying.

pregnant women and nursing mothers need eggs or dairy products in order to get enough protein and perhaps enough calories to stay healthy. However, if you eat soy products and certain fermented foods like tempeh or miso or a supplement to get Vitamin B_{12}, an essential nutrient, you may not need to eat any animal products. Consult a nutritionist familiar with a vegan diet.

In order to stay healthy on a vegetarian diet you must know how your body uses plant proteins. Proteins are made up of amino acids. Some your body cannot make and these must be eaten. You must also eat them in the right proportions to make use of them. Single sources of plant proteins, like most beans, grains and nuts, have the wrong proportions of amino acids for people. It is easy, though, to combine different types of plant foods so that you can get the right balance. These do not necessarily have to be combined in the same meal but should be eaten within three to four hours of each other. For a more complete description of how to combine vegetable proteins and lots of recipes, see Lappe, *Diet for a Small Planet* (revised) and Robertson, et al., *Laurel's Kitchen*. (See Resources.)

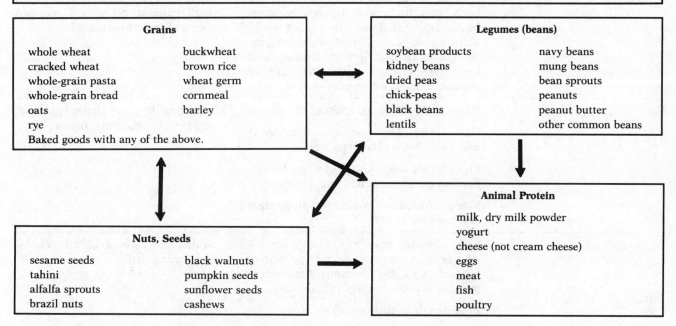

Protein Combination Chart*

To turn nonanimal foods into high-quality protein it is best to combine them with one of the foods pointed to. No arrows point out from the animal foods because they can stand alone but will enhance other groups.

Grains

whole wheat	buckwheat
cracked wheat	brown rice
whole-grain pasta	wheat germ
whole-grain bread	cornmeal
oats	barley
rye	

Baked goods with any of the above.

Legumes (beans)

soybean products	navy beans
kidney beans	mung beans
dried peas	bean sprouts
chick-peas	peanuts
black beans	peanut butter
lentils	other common beans

Nuts, Seeds

sesame seeds	black walnuts
tahini	pumpkin seeds
alfalfa sprouts	sunflower seeds
brazil nuts	cashews

Animal Protein

milk, dry milk powder
yogurt
cheese (not cream cheese)
eggs
meat
fish
poultry

*Chart from Nikki Goldbeck, *As You Eat So Your Baby Grows*, Ceres Press, Box 87, Department D, Woodstock, NY 12498.

SHOULD YOU TAKE SUPPLEMENTS?

The most honest answer is that unless you have an obvious vitamin or mineral deficiency disease, no one really knows. People vary in their ability to absorb and use nutrients. At particular times you are likely to need specific extra vitamins and minerals—from birth through adolescence; when you take birth control pills; when you are pregnant and nursing; and after menopause, when you slowly become less efficient at absorbing nutrients.

In the U.S. today one-fourth of what we eat is often made up of foods which provide calories and not much else, like soda and sugary snacks and alcohol.[2] These "empty calorie" foods, combined with foods stripped of nutrients through processing or for other reasons, may mean we are not getting enough of all the nutrients we need. Government surveys have shown that calcium and iron are two minerals and B_6 is one vitamin often lacking in our diets. Folic acid, a B-vitamin important during pregnancy, is also often lacking. Your specific needs are based on a combination of your unique biochemical inheritance, which currently is difficult to assess; the environmental stresses in your life; and how well you eat.

You may be able to find out if you have a deficiency by experimenting with dietary changes or with nutritional supplements.* *If you feel better the changes are probably what you needed.* We need to pay attention to and trust our bodies to help us find out what our special needs are.

There are particular nutritional stresses that you may be putting yourself under. If you smoke, you need about 120 milligrams of Vitamin C a day, about twice the usual amount. You can get this amount from two oranges or fourteen ounces of baked potato. Many drugs affect vitamin and mineral use. Aspirin affects folic acid absorption and depletes tissues of Vitamin C.

Even though supplements are fast and easy to take and you know exactly what you are getting, they cannot substitute for fresh whole food because we don't yet know all of the nutrients necessary for our health. You can't get some things easily from pills, like fiber. Also, many nutrients are useless or are less effective if taken by themselves.

*Multivitamins sometimes contain more of the cheaper nutrients and less of the expensive ones. To choose a balanced supplement, check to see what percent of the U.S. RDA of each nutrient is contained in the product. (*Laurel's Kitchen* gives you guideline amounts to take so you don't overdose yourself.) Be especially careful with Vitamins A and D. B-vitamins must be balanced. See also *Agricultural Handbook No. 456* for nutrient values in foods (listed in Resources under Adams).

A PARTIAL LIST OF IMPORTANT NUTRIENTS

Nutrient	Chief Functions	Important Sources
Proteins	Provide nitrogen and amino acids for body proteins (in skin tissues, muscles, brain, hair, etc.), for hormones (substances that control body processes), for antibodies (which fight infections), and for enzymes (which control the rates of chemical reactions in our bodies).	Milk, cheese, yogurt, eggs, fish, poultry, meat, beans, tofu, certain vegetable combinations.
Fats	Provide concentrated sources of energy. Carry fat-soluble vitamins (notably A, D and E) and essential fatty acids. Provide insulation and protection for important organs and body structures. Store calories to provide for pregnancy and nursing needs.	Whole milk, most cheeses, butter, margarine, oils, nuts, meats.
Carbohydrates	Keep proteins from being used for energy needs, so they can be used primarily for body-building functions. Also necessary for protein and fat utilization. Provide our main source of energy. Provide the glucose vital for certain brain functions.	Grains and cereals, bread, vegetables, beans, fruits.
Vitamin A (fat-soluble) Toxic in large doses.	Helps prevent infection. Helps eyes adjust to changes from bright to dim light (prevents night blindness). Needed for healthy skin and mucosal tissues, such as the inside of the mouth and lungs, bones and teeth.	Fish liver oil, liver, whole milk, fortified margarine, butter, whole-milk cheeses, egg yolks, dark green, yellow and orange vegetables and fruits.
Vitamin D (fat-soluble) Toxic in large doses.	Regulates calcium and phosphorus absorption necessary for strong bones and teeth.	Sunlight on bare skin, fortified milk, fish liver oil; small amounts in sardines, tuna, salmon, egg yolks.
Vitamin E (fat-soluble) Destroyed by freezing.	Helps preserve some vitamins and unsaturated fatty acids (acts as an antioxidant). Helps stabilize biological membranes.	Vegetable oils (wheat germ, corn and soybean), wheat and rice germ, egg yolks, legumes, corn, almonds.
B-vitamins (water-soluble) including thiamine (B_1), riboflavin (B_2), niacin, pyridoxine, folic acid, cobalamin (B_{12}), choline, etc. Heat, air and sometimes light destroy B- and C-vitamins. Most water-soluble vitamins are *not* stored, so you need some every day.	Needed for steady nerves, alertness, good digestion, energy production, healthy skin and eyes, maintenance of blood, disease resistance. Needed for protein, fat and carbohydrate metabolism.	Whole-grain breads and cereals, liver, wheat germ, nutritional yeast, green vegetables, lean meats, milk, cheese, molasses, peanuts, dried peas and beans, nuts and seeds, eggs, poultry, potatoes, fish.

A PARTIAL LIST OF IMPORTANT NUTRIENTS

Nutrient	Chief Functions	Important Sources
Vitamin C (ascorbic acid) (water-soluble) If you are taking large doses and want to stop, taper off gradually to avoid scurvy.	Needed for healthy collagen (a protein that holds cells together), tendons and bones. Helps wounds to heal. Needed for iron absorption. Spares or protects vitamins A and E and several B-vitamins.	Citrus fruits, sweet peppers, leafy greens, broccoli, cauliflower, tomatoes, fresh potatoes, berries, melons, bean sprouts.
Calcium Too much phosphorus and leafy vegetables that contain oxalic acid (chard, spinach, beet greens) reduce calcium absorption.	Needed for building bones and teeth, for blood clotting, for regulating nerve and muscle activity.	Milk and milk products, leafy greens (except as noted), broccoli, artichokes, blackstrap molasses, ground sesame seeds, canned fish containing bones, tofu made with calcium lactate, soups made from bones plus a little vinegar or lemon juice.
Phosphorus	Needed to metabolize fats and carbohydrates into energy in the body. Makes up part of all the body's cells. Needed with calcium for building bones and teeth.	Milk, cheeses, lean meats, eggs, fish, nuts and seeds, poultry, legumes, whole grains, soft drinks.
Magnesium Large amounts lost in food processing.	Required for carbohydrate metabolism. Helps regulate body temperature, nerve impulses and muscle contractions.	Whole grains, leafy greens, beans, seafood, nuts.
Potassium Sodium	Needed for healthy nerves and muscles. Regulate fluid in cells. Balance between these important.	Potassium: fresh ripe fruits and vegetables (bananas, potatoes, dark leafy greens), legumes (limas, peanut butter), blackstrap molasses, fish, poultry, meat, milk. Sodium: table salt, condiments. (See tips on reducing salt, p. 16).
Iron Daily intake is important.	Makes up an important part of hemoglobin, the compound in blood that carries oxygen from the lungs to the body cells.	Lean meat, liver, egg yolks, leafy greens (dandelions and kale), nutritional yeast, wheat germ, whole-grain and enriched breads and cereals, blackstrap molasses, legumes, oysters, turkey, dried fruit.
Water Most people need 6–7 glasses of fluid a day to keep good water balance in the body.	Not really a nutrient, but an essential part of all tissues. Often supplies important minerals such as calcium and fluorine.	Tapwater, tea, coffee, juice, soups, fruit, vegetables.
Fiber There are two kinds: insoluble, like cellulose; and soluble, like gums and pectins. Both are important.	Also not a nutrient, but important for stimulating the intestinal muscles, encouraging the growth of certain intestinal bacteria and regulating absorption of nutrients.	Fruits, vegetables, whole-grain bread and cereals, legumes.

HELPING KIDS EAT WELL

Mothers often have a lot of conflicts when feeding their kids. Even strangers may condemn us if our kids are "too" fat or skinny, though how we feed them may have little to do with how they look. Since most mothers work outside the home today, we may not be able to supervise our children's eating as much as we'd like. With young children we may have to make sure that the caretaker does not undermine our rules about good foods. Once children are in school, the task of changing the quality of cafeteria food may be bigger than we feel able to take on alone. Changing the food in the school vending machines from sweets to fruit, nuts and yogurt may seem overwhelming when the school football uniforms come out of the money collected and the coach doesn't believe that healthier foods will sell. Our children are under a lot of peer pressure to eat the foods advertised on television or to get a candy bar on the way home from school at the corner store even though they know you disapprove of those choices.

One way to interest kids in eating better is to set an example by eating well ourselves. Children do remember what they eat at home and can learn to make good choices, especially if you explain the reasons for the choices. (This may not seem true if you have teenagers!)

I tell my four-year-old that some foods help him grow better than others, and he wants to grow as fast as he can.

Kids of all ages eat a significant portion of their food in the form of snacks, just like adults. This is fine if the snacks are nutritious. Older kids, especially teenagers, just need a lot of food. Cookies can have wheat germ, whole grains, dried fruit and nuts. Milkshakes can be made from yogurt, banana, crushed ice and vanilla. Stock up on fruits, vegetables, peanut butter and/or wedges of hard cheese. When kids are hungry they'll eat what's there, so make the snacks worth eating and enjoyable.

It's important to let kids decide when they are hungry and when they are full. They eat different amounts at different times depending on how fast they are growing and whether or not they are sick. Helping them to trust themselves in this way teaches them an important lesson they can use in regulating their eating all through life.

Involve children in growing, buying and preparing foods. Have them read the labels for you in the supermarket. Try to find a small space, even if you are in the city, to grow something. Have older kids take their turns at cooking meals. Younger kids usually will be eager helpers. Even a three-year-old can chop soft vegetables for a salad with a table knife, spread nut butters, help mix batters or add ingredients to almost any recipe.

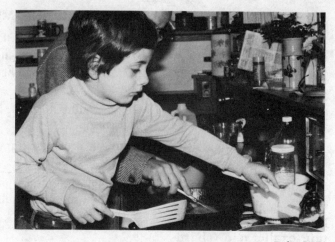

Esther Rome

PROBLEMS ASSOCIATED WITH EATING PATTERNS*

Fear of Fat

Low-Calorie Dieting

Do you find yourself worrying about your weight or thinking all the time about how everything you eat is fattening? Could it be because your lover says you are getting middle-age spread, because you don't look like the fashion models, because the supermarket magazines feature a new diet every month? Everywhere we look we see ads for foods, devices and diet support groups to help us lose weight. We spend over 10 billion dollars a year in the hopes of becoming slimmer. Most of us in the U.S. have been on at least one diet to lose weight and many of us go on several a year. ("Dieting" in this section means low-calorie dieting.) Dieting is medically endorsed as a cure for "obesity" and the diseases doctors think fatness contributes to. (For more on the social consequences of fatness, see Chapter 1, "Body Image.")

But dieting doesn't "cure" fatness. *Over a five-year period 98 to 99 percent of the women who diet regain their weight.*[3] *In fact, 90 percent regain more than they lost.*[4] *Dieting can make you fatter.* Most of us aren't aware that diets don't work in the long run and think that regaining weight is a personal failure rather than a physiological adaptation to stress that our bodies have made to help us survive. After repeated dieting, many of us begin to feel we can never control our eating.

Dieting is debilitating, a form of self-starvation. The World Health Organization defines starvation as a cal-

*See p. 12 ("Disease/Possible Causes from Eating Patterns"); check index to find diseases not covered in this chapter.

20

orie intake of less than 1,000 calories a day; reducing diets in this country commonly restrict calories to 700 to 1,000 a day. The Recommended Dietary Allowance for calories for women is 2,000 calories, with a range from 1,600 to 2,400 calories, depending on size and physical activity. At calorie levels below this you can easily be lacking necessary nutrients, especially if you consume a quarter or more of your calories from alcoholic beverages, sweets and other low-nutrient snacks. When you don't eat enough, your body reacts in specific ways to help you survive. It doesn't matter if you deliberately choose to eat less or if you can't get enough food. Starvation is starvation. The fewer calories you eat, the longer you do it for and the greater the number of times you do it, the more likely you are to permanently damage your body.*

Let's assume you are dieting and getting too few calories. (For some women the common 1,200-calorie diet is too few.) After a few days you are likely to feel physically listless. You may become apathetic, especially if you are on a low-carbohydrate diet. When fat from your body stores is broken down for energy, it doesn't provide any glucose, the fuel the brain normally uses. Your body must break down proteins from food and lean body tissues (muscles and organs, such as your heart) to provide this glucose. Processing the extra nitrogen from the proteins puts a strain on your kidneys. Fat metabolism without adequate carbohydrates leaves waste products called ketones in the blood. If the amount of ketones is too great, the critical acid-base balance of the blood can be upset. Extra blood ketones usually make you feel headachy, lethargic, dizzy, high or possibly lightheaded. Your breath will smell like acetone, somewhat sweet. After a couple of weeks the brain can adjust to using some of the ketones for fuel as a stopgap measure. You may feel irritable, partly because it is harder for you to control your blood-sugar levels without adequate food. You may also find yourself becoming depressed and less interested in sex. You may become obsessed with "quick energy" foods, especially sweets, and devour them uncontrollably as a way of replacing missing calories and glucose for the brain, the most immediate deficits. This carbohydrate craving may be especially severe if more than 10 percent of the diet is from protein. "High protein diets may actually generate cravings for carbohydrates and doom the dieter to periodic calorie-laden binges."[5] One woman describes how she stopped bingeing (and didn't try to be thin).

*Although rats on very low-calorie or protein diets live longer than those on regular laboratory rat rations, according to some recent widely publicized experiments, these rats must have nutritional supplements, because their food does not provide sufficient nutrients for good health. The weight of these rats does not fluctuate as it does with people who diet repeatedly. Human studies do not always corroborate these rat studies. Also, these experiments do not try to assess the role of other kinds of stress or exercise in longevity.

I worked at ignoring the rules and eating whatever I wanted. In the first month of "liberated eating" I craved only sweets. In effect, I was still binging [sic]. However, I chose not to berate myself for eating so much sugar. I reminded myself of all the sweets I'd been denied, and let feelings of nausea and hunger, rather than guilt, determine when I should eat again and what I should eat. At that point nausea and hunger were just about all I could be sure of. A month later, meat and dark green vegetables appealed to me very strongly. I chose a diet very high in protein and vitamins for a while. I think that during this period I was recovering from tissue damage due to previous years of dieting and binging [sic]. In the year that followed my cravings became more subtle and diverse. I ate smaller portions and greater varieties of food in one day.[6]

If you try to follow the often-cited rule that you'll lose one pound of body fat for every 3,500 calories you don't eat, you'll probably be disappointed. First of all, this calculation gives only average weight loss. For each month you continue eating the same low number of calories, your rate of weight loss is usually cut in half.[7] As a way of adjusting to a lower calorie intake, your body becomes more efficient at using and storing calories. Your basal metabolism (the calories you burn to keep your basic body functions going) can slow down by as much as 30 percent.[8] When you stop starving yourself you will probably replace or even exceed your original weight quickly, and mostly in the form of fat.[9] Your body is more efficient now, burning off fewer calories immediately and storing more fat for later use.

Fat often replaces the lean tissue lost from muscles and organs, and you may have done permanent damage. You may have as much as 40 percent more body fat than before you started.[10] On a total fast as much as two-thirds of the weight lost is a result of losing lean body tissue.[11] But usually muscle tissue can be developed again through vigorous exercise. If you continue dieting or adopt a pattern of repeat dieting, you risk amenorrhea, anemia, liver impairment, kidney stones, vitamin and mineral imbalances, gout and elevated blood fats.[12] If you have diverticulitis, tuberculosis, gout, Addison's disease, ulcerative colitis or regional ileitis, weight loss will make you sicker.[13]

> On the average, fat people do not eat more than thin people. Most fat women believe that they eat more than their thin friends but careful studies do not bear this out.[14]

Your general body shape probably resembles your relatives', due perhaps to heredity or to learned eating patterns. If one of your parents was fat, you have a 40 percent chance of being fat; if both were fat, you have an 80 percent chance.[15] We don't really know why people are different shapes and sizes. We do know that people's basal metabolism rates are different and that vigorous exercise may increase the rate. We don't know if fat people's cells (even when the person looks thin after weight loss) act differently from thin people's. Researchers have come up with many theories to account for different body types, from totally psychological to totally physical, but so far none is satisfactory.

Obesity (Fatness)

Ironically, the medical world considers fatness a disease. It is associated with and sometimes said to cause heart disease, high blood pressure, gallstones, diabetes and arthritis. Since doctors assume fat people are eating large amounts of food, a common method of treating many of these diseases is to recommend a severe reducing diet or fast. However, most studies in this country relating disease to fatness are done on people who are chronic dieters. Sudden and repeated weight loss may well be responsible for many of the diseases associated with fatness, but researchers don't consider this when drawing conclusions from their studies.* We have not been able to find any studies to show that over the *long* run thinned-down fat people avoid or are cured of diseases associated with fatness.† Slimming can improve high blood pressure and diabetes, but repeated dieting may make them worse.‡

Even worse than dieting are the various types of surgery medicine offers women labeled obese. They include carving fat off, jaw wiring and various ways to make the stomach and intestines smaller, decreasing a person's ability to eat and thereby absorb nutrients. These operations are performed almost entirely on women, may have a death rate as high as 10 percent and are only moderately effective in achieving the stated goal of weight loss. Doctors performing them really believe they are improving the woman's health, but they actually impair her ability to nourish herself properly. After intestinal tract operations a woman often gets severe diarrhea for several months and is at higher risk for getting gallstones and arthritis, two problems supposedly "cured" by weight loss.[16]

*Fat Liberation was probably the first group to speak about this. See Resources.

†See Resources: Bennett and Gurin, Chapter 5, includes a summary of literature on fatness and disease.

‡A few studies have shown *no* strong correlation between fatness and several diseases usually associated with it. See Bennett and Gurin in Resources as well as two of several studies of heart attacks in Roseto, Pennsylvania: C. Stout et al., "Unusually Low Incidence of Death from Myocardial Infarction: Study of an Italian Community in Pennsylvania," *Journal of the American Medical Association* 188 (June 8, 1964), pp. 845–849; and S. Wolf et al., "Roseto Revisited: Further Data on the Incidence of Myocardial Infarction in Roseto and Neighboring Pennsylvania Communities," *Transactions of the American Clinical and Climatological Association*, Vol. 85 (1973), pp. 100–107.

If You Choose to Diet

Even when we know about the effects of dieting, many of us will continue to diet. These guidelines may help you to avoid the worst problems.

1. Become much more physically active. This may be the single most important change you can make in your life. It will increase your strength and suppleness and probably your self-confidence as well as lifting depression. It may even lead to weight loss without dieting. (See Bennett and Gurin in Resources.)

2. Eat a wide variety of foods and make every bit count nutritionally. Cut out the junk foods. Follow the general eating guidelines previously listed.

3. You are more likely to be successful if you lose weight slowly and if you set your goal within twenty pounds of your present weight.* Do not restrict your calorie intake more than 500 calories a day under what you eat when not on a diet. Even with careful eating, it is virtually impossible to get your major nutrients from food on less than 1,200 calories. You need more to get all your trace nutrients.

4. There are no magic foods or pills to help you lose weight. Most over-the-counter weight-loss pills contain PPA (phenylpropanolamine), which is a relative of amphetamine (speed) and may increase blood pressure or produce agitation and dizziness; it may even set off a stroke or bring on psychosis.[17]

5. Keeping a food diary of exactly what you eat, when you eat it and why you eat it can give you insights into the psychological meanings food has for you, and can help you discover when you get hungry during the day. This can help you change your eating habits *if* they are undesirable.

6. Trust yourself and your body signals. Eat when you begin to get hungry. Don't wait until you are starved. If you feel ill, check what and when you are eating. You definitely should not have any severe symptoms, such as hair loss, shakiness, abnormally dry skin, etc.

7. Don't weigh yourself more than once every one or two weeks if each pound is an obsession. Body water fluctuates daily.

8. Join with other women to discuss dieting, feelings about yourself and your body and societal issues, such as the way ideal body images, both sexual and medical, divert your attention from control over your life and from more productive work.†

*People tend to maintain a fairly stable long-term weight if they do not attempt to modify it by changing caloric intake. However, common short-term weight changes range over ten kilograms (22 pounds). See Garrow in Resources, Chapters 4 and 5, especially p. 70.

†Fat Liberation is one such group. (See Resources and Chapter 1, "Body Image.") This group works to help people with diverse bodies gain physical, psychological, emotional and economic access to the wider world.

Other Eating Problems

Most of us at one time or another have used food to numb or deny our feelings, to comfort ourselves or to put some order into our lives. Who among us hasn't at one time either binged or felt nauseous when scared, angry, depressed, lonely or sad? However, when we let food become the *major* outlet for expressing our feelings, it becomes counterproductive and detrimental to our health. Unfortunately, this way of reacting is becoming more and more common for women, often starting in adolescence. "Figure control is one of the few forms of control that women have been allowed to exercise."[18]

One of the better-known problems is anorexia nervosa, a form of severe and deliberate self-starvation, sometimes leading to death. Another newly labeled syndrome is bulimarexia, or bulimia, which is bingeing and then purging with vomiting or laxatives.* Women can seriously injure their intestines or esophagus, develop severe tooth decay from regurgitated stomach acid and seriously upset their electrolyte balance, which can be life-threatening. You can be both anorexic and bulimarexic. Women with these problems often seem to be acting out the ultimate stereotype of the female role: extreme self-denial, repression of anger and conflict, the desire to remain childlike and conformity to the idea that a woman must be thin. These problems reflect graphically how little control women feel they have over their lives. Two former anorexics recount:

I remember I used to be desperately hungry—but by eating I would be in some way failing.[19]

Just as the worker's ultimate weapon in his negotiation with management is his labor and the threat of its withdrawal, so my body was my ultimate and, to me, only weapon in my bid for autonomy. It was the only thing I owned, the only thing which could not be taken away from me....I had discovered an area of my life over which others had no control....What was going on in my body was as unreal, as devoid of meaning, as were the events in the outside world. The two were part of one whole, a whole of which "I" was no part. "I" had shrunk to a nugget of pure and isolated will whose sole purpose was to triumph over the wills of others and over the chaos ensuing from their conflicting demands.[20]

One woman who has successfully helped many others out of this pattern has found that building self-esteem, developing a sense of control over one's life and receiving support from others are key factors for recovery.[21] In the words of a recovered bulimarexic:

I never "mastered" the urge to binge. The urge to binge disappeared. I'm very glad of that, because fighting it was

*If you have *either* of these problems or know someone who does, contact the American Anorexia Nervosa Association, Inc., 133 Cedar Lane, Teaneck, NJ 07666, or Anorexia Nervosa and Related Eating Disorders, Inc., P.O. Box 5102, Eugene, OR 97405 for the support and information group closest to you.

usually futile and took tremendous amounts of psychic energy which I can now devote to more constructive tasks.[22]

Tooth and Gum Decay

Many of us forget that good teeth and gums are a significant part of good health. Without them we cannot eat many foods which provide important nutrients. Teeth are alive. Your saliva nourishes them through tiny passageways in the tooth. Poor nutrition can cause dental disease just as it causes other diseases of the body. Vitamins A and D, calcium, phosphorus and fluoride are important for tooth development. Reducing sugar in your diet is another way to keep your teeth healthy. Teeth are especially prone to decay in the six-month period after they come through the gums, before they are fully hardened.

Foods containing sugar cause tooth and gum decay in the following way. Certain types of bacteria found in saliva use sugar to make themselves a protective coating. This helps them cling to our teeth as a sticky substance called dental plaque which saliva cannot wash away. These bacteria, tiny organisms known as streptococci, multiply rapidly and produce large amounts of acids, which dissolve the enamel and irritate the gums, causing disease. To remove the plaque and prevent this decay, it's important to brush and floss our teeth daily.

The least cavity-causing way to eat sweets is to have them with meals and not between. The number of times you eat sweets rather than the total amount determines how much acid the bacteria produces. But the amount of sweets influences the quality of your saliva. Avoid, if you can, sticky sweets that stay in your mouth a long time. Also try to brush and floss your teeth after eating sugary foods. Even rinsing your mouth with water is effective. Whenever possible, eat foods with fiber that scrape off plaque, acting as a toothbrush (raw carrot sticks, apples, celery sticks, whole grains, etc.).

Intestinal Problems

Adding fiber to the diet seems to help the intestinal tract. Appendicitis and diverticulitis are practically nonexistent in cultures that eat no refined foods. Different kinds of fiber help with diarrhea and constipation. Soluble fiber like pectin, found in many fruits, absorbs water, thickening the stool, and insoluble fiber like bran from whole grains softens the stool. Some researchers think that by decreasing the time it takes for food to go through the digestive system from one end to the other, fiber indirectly acts to hurry toxins through the system as well as diluting them so that there is less likelihood of developing bowel cancer.

Allergies and Other Reactions

Sometimes it's hard to figure out if you have a food allergy, since it can show up so many different ways. Your symptoms could be caused by many other problems. You may have rashes, hives, joint pains mimicking arthritis, headaches, irritability or depression.

The most common food allergies are to milk, eggs, seafood, wheat, nuts, seeds, chocolate, oranges and tomatoes. Many of these allergies will not develop if these foods are not fed to an infant until her or his intestines mature at around seven months. Breast milk also tends to be protective.

Migraines can be set off by foods containing tryamine, phenathylamine, monosodium glutamate or sodium nitrate. Common foods which contain these are chocolate, aged cheeses, sour cream, red wine, pickled herring, chicken livers, avocados, ripe bananas, cured meats, many Oriental and prepared foods (read the labels!). Some people have been successful in treating their migraines with supplements of B-vitamins, particularly B_6 and niacin.

Children who are hyperactive may benefit from eliminating food additives, especially colorings, and foods high in salicylates from their diets. A few of these are almonds, green peppers, peaches, tea, grapes. This is the diet made popular by Benjamin Feingold. (He has written several books, including *Why Your Child Is Hyperactive*, which you can read if you want to explore this further. Many areas have Feingold Associations. Check your phone book.) Other researchers have had mixed results when testing whether the diet is effective.

Cancer

(See also chapters 7 and 23.)

Certain food substances are likely to *increase* our chances of developing cancer.* They may be natural constituents of our food or may have been added to our foods purposefully by the food industry, or they may be contaminants in our diets. Sodium nitrate is used to cure and preserve meat and fish and to give the food a pinkish color. It doesn't have to be added at all because now there are other less harmful ways to preserve food, such as freezing. The nitrates combine with amines, found in the food or even in our saliva, to form nitrosamines, which are carcinogenic substances. Smoked foods are an additional source of

---

*"Does Everything Cause Cancer?" can be ordered from the Center for Science in the Public Interest (address in Resources). This pamphlet gives more information on methods scientists use to determine what can and cannot cause cancer. For a handy poster of safe and harmful food additives, order "Chemical Cuisine," also from CSPI. The Carcinogen Information Program, Inc., P.O. Box 6057, St. Louis, MO 63139, has a series of low-cost informative fact sheets called the "CIP Bulletin."

---

nitrosamines. Saccharin and many artificial colors derived from coal tar have been linked to cancer or organ damage in animal studies, but are still certified for use by our government because of the food industry pressure.

Naturally occurring carcinogenic contaminants also exist. Aflatoxin is produced by a mold which thrives in damp weather. It most commonly occurs on peanuts, but can also be found on corn, figs, grain sorghum, cottonseed and certain tree nuts. It sometimes gets into cows' milk from the grains the cows eat. Some aflatoxin reaches the marketplace and we eat it, although proper drying and storing of the grains, nuts, etc., can minimize it. Cutbacks in FDA funding will result in contaminants like these being less closely monitored.

A high-fat diet, all too common in this country, is linked with cancers of the breast and colon and probably of the ovary, pancreas and prostate gland. The total fat content of your diet rather than the type of fat you eat seems to be responsible.

Some nutrients and foods seem to protect against cancer, though research on this is not conclusive. Foods high in Vitamin C protect against several types of cancers. Beta-carotene, a form of Vitamin A found in yellow and dark green vegetables and used as a food coloring, protects against lung cancer. Vegetables in the cabbage family as well as spinach, celery, citrus fruit, beans and seeds help the body produce an anticancer enzyme.[23]

WHY EATING WELL DOESN'T COME EASILY

The agriculture and food businesses (agribusiness) are based on making a profit. This is a problem because many of the most immediately profitable methods of producing food deplete the growing ability of the soil and produce less nutritious and more expensive food.

Current planting practices either leave fields bare for periods of time, allowing precious topsoil to wash or blow away, or use large amounts of herbicides to clear them. Widespread use of pesticides, herbicides and inorganic fertilizers destroys the organisms which control the structure of the soil and the balance and availability of nutrients to the plants, and creates poisoning hazards for agricultural workers. Irrigation practices may leave salts poisonous to plants in the soil or use up groundwater faster than it can be replaced.

Business considers the most desirable foods to be those which are as uniform as possible and can withstand the abuse of mechanical harvesting and long-term shipping and storage. The land-grant colleges, supported by tax dollars and run by the states, have for years been responding to agribusiness influence by researching ways to develop complementary foods and labor-saving machines for large farms* while paying little attention to the nutritive qualities of the foods they develop or the needs of the small farmer or consumer. Agricultural research has been partly responsible for the extraordinary decrease in the numbers of types of crops and varieties of seeds grown in the U.S. and elsewhere. Half the wheat acreage is planted in nine varieties out of 20,000 named varieties in the world. If a blight strikes, it strikes across the country, since all the varieties are so similar.†

One product of this system—the mechanically harvested tomato—took twenty-five years to develop. It is designed to be tough and is reputed to withstand a thirteen miles per hour impact without splitting. Normally picked completely green before its full nutritive value has developed, it is then conveniently "de-greened" with gas as stores put in orders for "red" tomatoes. ("Vine-ripened" means that it started to show color before being picked. Then it is either allowed to color up on its own or gassed to hasten the process.) Unfortunately, flavor didn't occur on the same gene with durability. We have a whole generation now that doesn't know what a real tomato tastes like! Fuel-guzzling machines‡ now harvest these tomatoes, compacting the soil so plant roots have difficulty pushing

*For more on the intimate relationship between agribusiness and research at land-grant colleges, see Jim Hightower, *Hard Tomatoes, Hard Times*, Schenkman Publishing Co. (Cambridge, MA), 1978.

†Because we export hybrid seeds along with many industrialized agricultural practices to developing countries, local varieties of foods perfectly suited to the local conditions are being lost forever, so the base of our food supply is really shrinking. (See Cary Fowler, "Plant Patenting: Sowing the Seeds of Destruction," in *Science for the People*, Vol. 12, No. 5, September/October 1980 [897 Main Street, Cambridge, MA 02139].)

‡In 1975, it took ten calories of energy to produce each calorie of food energy; in 1910 it was one for one. In 1980, the equivalent of ninety-five gallons of gasoline was used per *acre* of corn grown. This highly mechanized crop is our largest one.

through it and displacing farmworkers who were never retrained for other jobs.

Our food supply has become more and more centralized. In the last forty years 4.5 million family farms have gone out of business. Farmers grow most food in very few places in the country and ship it far. California supplies 25 percent of the nation's food and half of the nation's year-round domestic fruits and vegetables. New England imports 85 percent of its food. There is a small revival going on in regional agriculture, but it still is hard to say how successful it will be.

Travel time from one part of the country to another can be substantial (an average of five to seven days; up to two weeks for fruits and vegetables to get to New York from California). In that time vegetables lose nutrients: in two days, 34 percent of the Vitamin C in refrigerated broccoli is lost.

The length of time food is stored after arrival and how it is kept during that time are also important. Canned juice loses as much as 70 percent of its total Vitamin C when stored in a hot warehouse, while juice stored at 45 degrees F. keeps most of its Vitamin C.

The Proliferation of Processed Foods

One effective way for agribusiness to multiply profits is to process food as much as possible, which results in the marketing of frozen peas in butter sauce rather than fresh peas; or to synthesize entirely new foods, like nondairy imitation whipped cream. Slight differences from one product to the next also help increase profits. Two cents' worth of vitamins is sprayed onto Wheaties and sold as Total for a substantial price increase. The food industry adds many substances to processed foods to ease manufacture and transportation, reduce manufacturing costs, replace costlier ingredients, improve appearance and texture and increase shelf life (how long the product is good after

General Foods plant, Woburn, Massachusetts

Elizabeth Cole

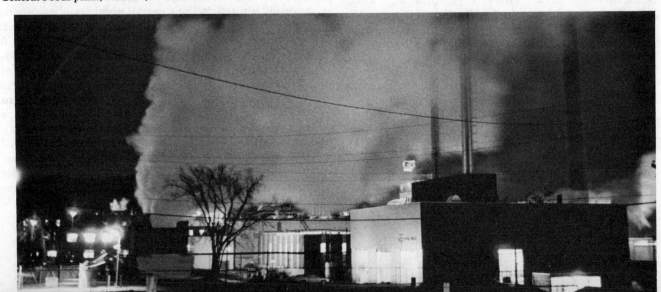

NUTRIENT PROFILE OF TANG AND ORANGE JUICE
% US RDA IN 6 OUNCES OF JUICE OR TANG

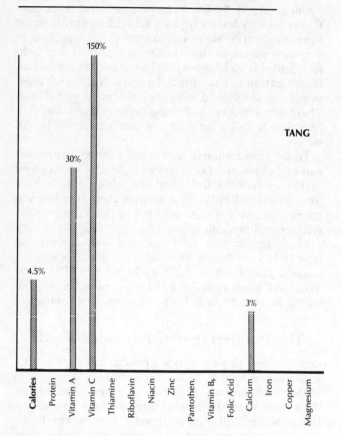

TANG

150%

30%

4.5%

3%

| Calories | Protein | Vitamin A | Vitamin C | Thiamine | Riboflavin | Niacin | Zinc | Pantothen. | Vitamin B₆ | Folic Acid | Calcium | Iron | Copper | Magnesium |

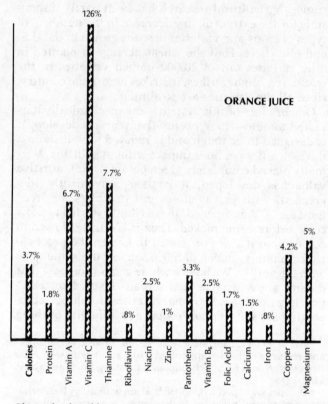

ORANGE JUICE

126%

7.7%

6.7%

3.7%

1.8%

.8%

2.5%

1%

3.3%

2.5%

1.7%

1.5%

.8%

4.2%

5%

| Calories | Protein | Vitamin A | Vitamin C | Thiamine | Riboflavin | Niacin | Zinc | Pantothen. | Vitamin B₆ | Folic Acid | Calcium | Iron | Copper | Magnesium |

Charts developed by Annette Dickinson, artwork by Robbie Pfeufer

picking, processing, etc.). Yellow coloring gives bread the appearance of having eggs in it. Cheaper nonnutritive thickeners like modified foodstarch replace nutritive ones, perhaps eggs, because the parts don't separate as quickly, giving the illusion of a fresher product. Preservatives do the same thing by increasing shelf life, sometimes indefinitely.* We no longer can observe the original color, smell and texture of many foods to help us judge if they are good for us.

Even minimal processing of foods usually involves some nutrient losses. Frozen vegetables have to be blanched first and thereby lose B- and C-vitamins. Vitamin E is reduced by freezing. Sulfur dioxide on dried fruits destroys Vitamin B₁ but reduces losses of A and C. Minerals, unless physically removed from food as

in flour refining, usually are not lost. Canning generally is the least nutritious way to keep vegetables, because they are heated long enough to destroy many nutrients.

More Is Less

Advertisements suggest that the large number of processed foods available represents a wide variety of food choices. In reality, our nutritional choices are severely limited. We see a small number of basic foods transformed into many different forms, none of which are nutritionally equivalent to the original foods. A raw or baked-in-its-skin potato that would make a little under a cup's worth in volume contains 50 percent of the U.S. RDA for Vitamin C. Prepared potato flakes or frozen-mashed-reheated potatoes have 20 percent or less of the original amount. Synthetic potato chips like Pringles, which have been freeze-dried, reconstituted, molded, fried in oil, salted, flavored and packed in a fancy box, contain 10 percent of the U.S. RDA for Vitamin C in a serving. In addition, a pound of Pringles costs ten to fifteen times more than whole potatoes (1982 prices).

*Preservatives can perform a positive function by making more of the food grown available to us, since about one-fifth of the food grown in the world goes bad or is eaten by other animals. They become counterproductive when there is no way to tell if food is a week old or five years old. Generally, the older food gets, the less nourishing it is. Also, some preservatives like salt and sugar are themselves problematic. Another, BHT, has been poorly tested and is known to sometimes cause allergic reactions yet protects Vitamins A and D.

Residues

During food preparation, farmers and processors sometimes add chemicals which they don't intend the food to contain when it is eaten. Vegetable oils are usually chemically dissolved out of the plants that they come from by solvents such as gasoline or carbon tetrachloride. Although the solvent is then boiled off before the oil is bleached chemically and deodorized by heat, chemical traces remain.

Some of the pesticides and herbicides applied in the fields remain on the food at harvest time.* Manufacturers ship abroad chemicals our government bans for agricultural use in this country, and farmers and farmworkers who do not know of their hazardous nature use them freely. Imported foods, including vegetables available in winter and tropical fruits, can contain residues. One examination of coffee beans showed that almost half had pesticide levels higher than U.S. law allows. Antibiotics that farmers use in animal feed to promote growth are a factor in the increasing resistance of microbes to antibiotics. These contaminants are in our foods because the large food corporations' desires strongly influence the regulation of our food supply.

The FDA and USDA

Consumers think the FDA and USDA protect us from contaminated and adulterated food, but they are not nearly as effective as we think they are or wish they would be. The food industry influences how they are run in several ways. There are over eighty-five industry groups which maintain lobbyists in Washington to keep track of and influence pertinent legislation and regulations. Industry proposes most of the regulations and supplies test results when needed for the approval of new substances.† People hop back and forth between working for the FDA or USDA and the businesses they regulate. The people developing and implementing regulations have the industry viewpoint strongly in mind. About one-quarter of the FDA's top officials have worked in regulated businesses before coming to the FDA. Most of the FDA's top people leave to work in the industries they oversaw. This gives the corporations information on where key links exist in the regulatory organizations to help bend them to their purposes. Partly because the industry wants it this way, Congress doesn't allot enough money in the federal budget for the FDA and USDA to be able to do

very much independent testing and to enforce their own regulations very efficiently.

Advertising and Market Share

Through advertising, food companies influence us to buy certain foods, especially the most highly processed, least nutritious foods, because they are the most profitable. Advertising appeals not to our desire for a healthy or reasonably priced meal so much as to our desire for status, reward, popularity, satisfaction, increased fun, increased sexual potency or an illusion of superior quality. One advertising consultant complains: "...the greater insistence on truth and accuracy in commercials also makes selling more difficult."[24] The most pernicious ads are aimed at kids, and emphasize the fun of eating nonnutritious snacks between meals. Some large companies use children by linking sales of a certain brand to some cause that parents usually favor. For instance, large conglomerates—like Campbell—offer a school sports or play equipment if students collect a certain number of labels. If we tally actual costs, usually it's more expensive to buy the national brand than the store brand plus the cost of the equipment.

Corporations use advertising to get a larger market share. "To grow dramatically you have to introduce new products,"[25] says a General Foods executive. Proliferating new products, 90 percent of which fail, requires the company to advertise and to create needs for nonessential products. Food companies also capitalize on trends. An executive of a large food company points out that "People are consuming fewer calories as they watch their weight and that translates to less food tonnage."[26] To keep profits up, companies respond by making food with fewer calories so that people can eat more of it without getting full. They add water and air to whipped products and use artificial sweeteners and other nonnutritive additives.

In order to be able to charge more, companies are now putting brand names on basic produce which otherwise has a low profit margin. Advertising tries to convince the consumer that a brand-name product is superior to unbranded ones. Pioneers in this field are Chiquita and Cabana (Dole bananas), Sun Giant (Tenneco), Bud Antle (Castle and Cook) and Perdue chickens.

In advertising wars, conglomerates win over local companies since they have more resources. Particular strategies include coupon saturation and price cutting.

Large corporations don't limit sales and advertising to this country. Pepsi and Coke are known worldwide and are considered status drinks, even among very poor people. Infant formula is another example. (See p. 614.) In Indonesia processed foods account for 15 to 20 percent of the family food budget, even of the very poor.

---

*To remove some of the pesticide, wash food with dilute dish detergent or soak five minutes in dilute vinegar, then rinse; plain water is often ineffective.

†Companies that do testing for the drug and food industry sometimes falsify or ignore detrimental results. See *Mother Jones*, June 1982 (Vol. 7, No. 5), Douglas Foster and Mark Dowie, "The Illusion of Safety, Part 1."

Food Costs

Concentration in the Food Industry

Increasingly fewer corporations control food production, processing and distribution. Once a small group of companies controls 40 percent or more of the market (called an oligopoly), companies set prices beyond their costs according to what they think they can get for a product. In 1972 the Federal Trade Commission estimated that consumers paid more than 660 million dollars annually because of concentration in the food industry. In another case the FTC said that ready-to-eat cereal manufacturers charge an extra fifteen cents on every dollar spent for cereal products in a year.

Conglomerates buy up companies involved in every link of the food chain, from seed to supermarket shelf. For many commodities the people who plow the fields no longer control farming. To gain more control over raw materials, large corporations own and manage their own farms or hire farmers and specify how and what they grow and for what price, while the farmers assume the risks of financing and growing the crop. Farmers are not getting a share of the increased prices paid in the supermarket. Only 6 percent of the rise in food prices in the past twenty years has gone to the farmer. While we're taught to believe that in farming "bigger is better," the most efficient farms in terms of food produced per acre are family farms big enough to be able to use technology but small enough to run without outside help. But deliberate government policies have encouraged farmers to "get big or get out."

Other Factors Affecting Cost

Some of the other factors in the supermarket price of food include such things as financing, labor, taxes, the world export market, government price supports for some commodities, maintaining the corporate bureaucracy, lobbyists in Washington, and the price of crude oil, which affects fertilizers, pesticides, fuel and transportation costs.

Out of the fifty-nine cents you might pay for a head of iceberg lettuce, nineteen cents goes to the grower, three cents of which is for the farm laborer; three cents is for cooling and refrigeration; fifteen cents is for transportation; and twenty-two cents goes to the wholesaler and retailer.[27]

Packaging increases price, with cans and glass bottles the most expensive containers. In 1979 the can and label on a ten-and-a-half-ounce can of vegetable soup was 27.4 percent of its retail price.

Advertising is expensive, with the food industry spending about fifty dollars per person a year, mostly on processed food and mostly for TV. General Foods, the country's largest advertiser, covers its advertising costs by charging you six cents on each item sold.

Power to control and profits from food production in this country are more concentrated than ever. Fifty years ago 40 percent of the population were farmers. Today 3 percent of the population are farmers but 40 percent of the population works in agriculturally related fields.

WOMEN WORKERS IN THE FOOD SYSTEM[28]

On family farms in the past, women generally were equal partners in decision-making as well as work. As farms become larger and are increasingly mechanized, men are trained to run the machinery and women are pushed out of farmwork. Women are often forced to supplement the farm income with low-paying non-farm jobs like waitressing or factory work. In food factories, it's women who do the repetitive low-paying jobs like disemboweling and dressing turkeys in the assembly line, where it is cold, smelly, noisy and wet. Mechanization will most likely eliminate even these jobs. While more women are attending agricultural school today to go into large-scale farming, it remains to be seen whether we'll get the jobs we want.

Of those who are agricultural workers, migrant women are the hardest hit. Low wages make it difficult to buy sufficient food and other necessities. Most fields do not have toilets or provisions for water, making the women, particularly, more susceptible to many infections. Pesticide and herbicide exposure, harmful to all adults and children, is even more so to pregnant women. When nitrogen from fertilizers leaches into wellwater or reservoirs, it can poison infants who drink formula or other foods prepared with that water. Maternal and infant mortality is more than 100 percent higher among migrants than the national average. At the end of a long, grueling day in the fields, the women are expected to cook and clean and raise their children under the usually squalid circumstances found in migrant labor camps over which they rarely have control. U.S. agribusiness affects women in developing countries as well. (See p. 613.)

CHANGES

We wish we had room to describe some of the projects women and men have organized to take some control back over the sources and quality of our food. See Resources: Weiss, et al., *Community Food Education Handbook*, especially for excellent curriculum materials; Valentine and Lappe, *What Can We Do?*; and the longer bibliography available from our Collective for listings of activist groups and other literature. If you get in touch with one group, you can usually find out about others.

Starting on a personal level, each of us can intentionally work to make our diets more nutritious. Many cities have urban gardening programs through which you can get a plot of land to garden or get help with gardening in your yard or rooftop or porch. (See Resources: "Gardens for All.") If you have no gardening experience at all, try to find someone who has gardened before to help or who is at least willing to look at what you are doing and give advice. Often you can raise all your own vegetables and sometimes fruit in season this way. Not only is it cheaper, but it is also fresher.*

Sometimes a group will have organized a farmers' market near you, or there may be farm stands if you live in a rural area. When you buy at these places, you support local agriculture, benefiting farmers, the land and yourself. Consider preserving some of the foods through freezing, canning or drying. (See Hertzberg, et al., in Resources, and many standard cookbooks like *The Joy of Cooking.*) It is surprisingly quick for some foods.

The next level of activity involves forming or joining a group. On the local level, look for a food co-op or form your own. Find other concerned parents who want to improve the school lunch program or to try to get rid of junk food from the vending machines. Introduce nutritional education in the classroom or workplace. If you are at college, you can work with other students or co-workers to improve the quality and choice in the cafeteria. If you get your foods from vending machines or a truck at work, you can do the same. (See Moyer in Resources.) Work with or support one of many groups advocating and helping small farmers. There are many organic farming and gardening associations. Other groups have set up food banks to collect surplus foods and to distribute them to the poor. There is also one group, Rural American Women, specifically trying to help women.

Then there are political advocacy and information groups, some local or regional and some national. They try to inform the public about what is going on in big business and government, give expert testimony before Congress and sometimes institute lawsuits in the public interest. Groups like these have done important work around such issues as land-use policy, water rights, working conditions of farmworkers or food-processing plantworkers, the effects of tax law on land ownership, ways co-ops help or hinder cooperative behavior, energy use in agriculture and getting food to the hungry.

The food industry is powerful. The only way to challenge it is to work together so we become powerful.

*Beware of problems with heavy metals, such as lead, in the soil. See the Farallones Institute, *Integral Urban House,* listed in Resources, and the Collective's longer bibliography for information on this problem.

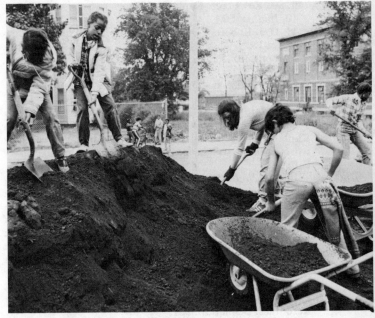

Boston Urban Gardeners/Read D. Brugg

NOTES

1. Robert S. Goodhart and Maurice E. Shils. *Modern Nutrition in Health and Disease.* Philadelphia: Lea and Feibiger, 1980, pp. 990–91.

2. Jane Brody. "Deficiencies of Vitamins," *The New York Times Magazine,* March 29, 1981; "Diets Won't Cure Teenage Obesity," *CNI Weekly Report,* Vol. 10, No. 33 (August 14, 1980), p. 4.

3. Alvan Feinstein. "How Do We Measure Accomplishment in Weight Reduction?" in *Obesity: Causes, Consequences and Treatment,* Louis Lasagna, ed. New York: Medcom Press, 1974, p. 86. Researchers have known for a while that dieting doesn't work for most women.

4. Llewellyn Louderback. *Fat Power.* New York: Hawthorn Books, Inc., 1970, p. 143, quoting Norman G. Jolliffe, M.D., of the New York City Department of Health: "At least 90 percent of all the people who lose weight on a diet gain back more than they have lost." This phenomenon is corroborated by the testimony of many dieters. See also Resources: Kaplan, pp. 50–51.

5. Judith Wurtman, quoted in Jane Brody. "Can Craving for Carbohydrates Be Controlled? Chemical Studies of Brain Point to New Approach," *The New York Times,* September 29, 1981.

6. Vivian Mayer. "Why Liberated Eating?" (ca. 1979), pp. 14–15. Available through Fat Liberator Publications. (See Resources.)

7. S. C. Wooley, O. A. Wooley and S. Dyrenforth. "Theoretical, Practical and Social Issues in Behavior Treatment of Obesity," *Journal of Applied Behavior Analysis,* Vol. 12, No. 1 (Spring 1979), p. 9.

8. H. J. Roberts. "Overlooked Dangers of Weight Reduction," *Medical Counterpoint* (September 1970), p. 15. See Resources: Garrow, pp. 89–90. See Wooley, "Theoretical, Practical and Social Issues," p. 9.

9. See Resources: Kaplan, p. 50.

10. *Ibid.*, p. 50.

11. H. J. Roberts. "Overlooked Dangers of Weight Reduction," p. 15.

12. *Consumer Reports*, Vol. 43, No. 2 (February 1978), pp. 92–95.

13. H. J. Roberts. "Overlooked Dangers of Weight Reduction," p. 17. See Resources: Garrow, pp. 161, 163. See Louderback, *Fat Power*, p. 171.

14. See Resources: Garrow, p. 48, and studies listed in Kaplan, p. 45. This is common knowledge among researchers working in the weight-loss field, although lay people rarely believe it.

15. S. C. Wooley and O. W. Wooley. "Obesity and Women— I. A Closer Look at the Facts," *Women's Studies Int. Quart.*, Vol. 2 (1979), pp. 69–79.

16. See Resources: Garrow, p. 180; and Teis Andersen, Erik Juhl and Flemming Quaade. "Jejunoileal Bypass for Obesity: What Can You Learn from a Literature Study?" in *American Journal of Clinical Nutrition*, Vol. 33 (special supplement on weight-loss surgery) (February 1980), pp. 440–45.

17. Douglas Foster and Mark Dowie. "The Illusion of Safety, Part 1," *Mother Jones*, Vol. 7, No. 5 (June 1982), p. 47; and Resources: Bennett, p. 224.

18. Vivian Mayer. "The Fat Illusion," *Hagborn*, Vol. 1, No. 4 (Winter 1980), pp. 3 ff. Also available through Fat Liberator Publications. (See Resources.)

19. Anonymous. "Self Starvation," *Spare Rib* (June 1979), p. 43.

20. Sheila MacLeod. *The Art of Starvation: A Story of Anorexia and Survival.* New York: Schocken Books, 1981, pp. 56, 66, 98. A perceptive autobiography and analysis of anorexia.

21. Marlene Boskind-White and William White (67 W. Malloryville Road, Freeville, NY 13068) have been working with bulimarexics for many years and have written *The People Pleasers: Women Who Binge and Purge.* New York: W. W. Norton, 1983.

22. Vivian Mayer. "Why Liberated Eating?" pp. 14–15.

23. Jane Brody. *Jane Brody's Nutrition Book.* New York: W. W. Norton and Co., Inc., 1981, p. 442.

24. Fred A. Lemont, quoted in "Trouble for Packaged Goods," *The New York Times*, June 8, 1981.

25. Peter Rosow, general manager of General Foods dessert division, quoted in "Introducing a New Product," *The New York Times*, July 14, 1981.

26. William D. Smithburg, chief executive officer of Quaker Oats Co., quoted in "Quaker Oats Names New Chief Officer," *The New York Times*, July 10, 1981.

27. Bernard Taper. "The Bittersweet American Harvest." Reprinted from *Science 80 Magazine* in *Eastern Review* (February 1981), p. 121.

28. For more, see Sally Hacker. "Farming Out the Home: Women and Agribusiness" in Kaplan. (See Resources.) This article also appeared in *The Second Wave: A Magazine of the New Feminism*, Vol. 5, No. 1 (Spring/Summer 1977) (Box 344, Cambridge, MA 02139), pp. 38–49; and *Science for the People* (March/April 1978) (897 Main Street, Cambridge, MA 02139).

RESOURCES

For a more extensive listing of materials in all these areas we invite you to send to us for a longer bibliography. Mail one dollar with a stamped (37¢), self-addressed business-size envelope to Boston Women's Health Book Collective, P.O. Box 192, W. Somerville, MA 02144.

Nutritional Information

Authors' Note: Most of these books assume that thin is better than fat, and that a reasonable way to achieve thinness is through low-calorie dieting.

Adams, Catherine. "Nutritive Value of American Foods in Common Units." *Agricultural Handbook No. 456.* Washington, DC: USDA, 1975. Order from U.S. Government Printing Office, Washington, DC 20402.

Brody, Jane. *Jane Brody's Nutrition Book.* New York: W. W. Norton and Co., Inc., 1981. Many practical suggestions.

Hausman, Patricia. *Jack Sprat's Legacy: The Science and Politics of Fat and Cholesterol.* New York: Richard Marek Publishers, 1981. Looks at medical evidence and the political machinery suppressing known research.

National Academy of Sciences. "Dietary Allowances," Ninth Ed., 1980. Available from the Office of Publications, National Academy of Sciences, 2101 Constitution Avenue N.W., Washington, DC 20418. The most complete summary of what we know about human nutrition at this time.

U.S. Senate Select Committee on Nutrition and Human Needs. *Eating in America: Dietary Goals for the United States.* Cambridge, MA: The MIT Press, 1977. "First comprehensive statement by any branch of the federal government on risk factors in the American diet" (p. 1). The USDA then issued Dietary Guidelines based on these goals.

Winter, Ruth. *A Consumer's Dictionary of Food Additives.* New York: Crown Publishers, 1978. An excellent resource.

Wurtman, Judith J. *Eating Your Way Through Life.* New York: Raven Press, 1979. Good on practical suggestions.

Vegetarianism

Adams, Carol. "The Inedible Complex: The Political Implications of Vegetarianism," *The Second Wave*, Vol. 4, No. 4 (Summer/Fall 1976). Weaves together vegetarianism and feminism.

Hartbarger, Janie Coulter, and Neil J. Hartbarger. *Eating for the Eighties: A Complete Guide to Vegetarian Nutrition.* Philadelphia: Saunders Press, 1981. A good general reference on vegetarianism. Includes list of several vegetarian cookbooks.

Lappe, Frances Moore. *Diet for a Small Planet.* New York: Ballantine Books, 1975. The popular vegetarian cookbook that explains protein complementarity.

Robertson, Laurel, Carol Flenders and Bronwen Godfrey. *Laurel's Kitchen.* Petuluana, CA: Nilgeri Press, 1976; New York: Bantam Books. A wealth of nutritional information (especially on how to get specific nutrients) as well as recipes. Less reliance on eggs and dairy products than *Diet for a Small Planet.*

Untema, Sharon. *Vegetarian Baby: A Sensible Guide for Parents.* Ithaca, NY: McBooks Press, 1980 (106 N. Aurora Street, Ithaca, NY 14850). An informed guide for feeding child from pregnancy through two years. Includes information on a vegan diet. Recipes.

Vegetarian Information Service, P.O. Box 5888, Washington, DC 20014.

Women and Food

ISIS, *Women in Development*. Philadelphia, PA: New Society Publishers, 1984. Available from NSP, 4722 Baltimore Ave., Philadelphia, PA 19143. Feminist. Additional resources listed.

Jensen, Joan M. *With These Hands: Women Working on the Land*. Old Westbury, NY: The Feminist Press; New York: McGraw-Hill Book Co., 1981. A chronological anthology of short excerpts of conversations with farming women in the U.S. from the days before European settlers arrived to the present. Good introductions for each section.

Leghorn, Lisa, and Mary Roodkowsky. "Who Really Starves? Women and World Hunger." New York: Friendship Press, 1977. Excellent.

Fatness

Bennett, William, and Joel Gurin. *The Dieter's Dilemma: Eating Less and Weighing More*. New York: Basic Books, Inc., 1982. Shows role of exercise in weight reduction may be more important than how much you eat, but still out to get you thin. Draws on many of same scientific sources as Fat Liberation.

Fanlight Productions. *I Don't Have to Hide: A Film About Anorexia and Bulemia*, a 28-minute 16-mm. 1983 color film. Available from Fanlight Productions, 47 Halifax Street, Jamaica Plain, MA 02130. Good for use in high school and college settings.

Fat Liberator Publications., P.O. Box 5227, Coralville, IA 52241 or c/o Judith Stein, 137 Tremont Street, Cambridge, MA 02139. An extensive list of well-researched publications.

Garrow, J. S. *Energy Balance and Obesity in Man*, Second Ed. New York/Amsterdam: Elselvier; North Holland: Biomedical Press, 1978. A careful and critical overview of the scientific literature on obesity.

Kaplan, Jane Rachel. *A Woman's Conflict: The Special Relationship Between Women and Food*. Englewood Cliffs, NJ: Prentice-Hall, 1980. An excellent anthology of issues vital to women. Good section on fatness.

Millman, Marcia. *Such a Pretty Face: Being Fat in America*. New York: Berkley Books, 1980. Explores both social and personal aspects.

Agribusiness and Related Issues

Berry, Wendell. *The Unsettling of America: Culture and Agriculture*. New York: Avon Books, 1977. An important exploration of the impact society and agriculture have on each other.

Burbach, Roger, and Patricia Flynn. *Agribusiness in the Americas*. New York: Monthly Review Press, 1980. Analyzes the workings and impact of agribusiness on an international scale.

Financial pages of any major newspaper, for example, *The New York Times*, *The Wall Street Journal*, keep you current on the workings of agribusiness.

George, Susan. *How the Other Half Dies: The Real Reasons for World Hunger*. Montclair, NJ: Allanheld, Osmun and Co., 1977. A well-documented look at how multinational corporations influence governments here and abroad to channel food to make themselves the most profit, not to feed the hungry.

Hall, Ross Hume. *Food for Naught: The Decline in Nutrition*. New York: Vintage Books, 1976. An excellent discussion of problems resulting from increasing high-technology food production.

Hightower, Jim. *Eat Your Heart Out: Food Profiteering in America*. New York: Vintage Books, 1975. How large food companies charge you more and give you less. Extensively documented.

Lappe, Frances Moore, and Joseph Collins. *Food First: Beyond the Myth of Scarcity*. New York: Ballantine Books, 1978. How food for profit keeps the world hungry. Well documented.

Lerza, Catherine, and Michael Jacobsen. *Food for People, Not for Profit*. New York: Ballantine Books, 1975.

Main World Research Collective. "Agribusiness: How Multinationals Eat Up Your Food Budget." Pamphlet available from MWRC, 19 Howe Street, New Haven, CT 06511.

Rodefeld, Richard D., Jan Flora, Donald Voth, Isao Fujimoto and Jim Converse, eds. *Changes in Rural America: Causes, Consequences and Alternatives*. St. Louis: C. V. Mosby Co., 1978. An anthology with good introductions to each section.

Resources for Change

Agricultural Marketing Project, 2606 Westwood Drive, Nashville, TN 37204. Educational and direct-action group. Good publications. Send for list.

Center for Science in the Public Interest, 1755 S Street N.W., Washington, DC 20009. Publishes *Nutrition Action* magazine and a long list of valuable books and posters. Does research and prods government. Send for publications list.

Earthwork, 3410 19th Street, San Francisco, CA 94110. Agribusiness Accountability Project. Has long film list. Publishes fact sheets and sponsors conferences.

Farallones Institute. *The Integral Urban House*. San Francisco: Sierra Club Books, 1979. Section on food-raising (plants and animals) contains much useful information for urban gardeners. Includes information on lead.

Games for Life, P.O. Box 39222, Cincinnati, OH 45239. Card game called "Soup to Nuts" that can be played with several variations by three-year-olds and up. Cards all have wholesome foods except for Candy Monster.

Gardens for All, The National Association for Gardening, 180 Flynn Avenue, Burlington, VT 05401. National gardening advocacy group. Contact them to find out about gardening groups in your area. Publishes newsletters and other literature.

Harty, Sheila. *Hucksters in the Classroom: A Review of Industry Propaganda in Schools*. Washington, DC: Center for Study of Responsive Law (P.O. Box 19367, Washington, DC 20036), 1979. Excellent section on the food industry.

Hertzberg, Ruth, Beatrice Vaughn and Janet Greene. *Putting Food By*. Brattleboro, VT: The Stephen Greene Press, 1974. Comprehensive. Covers all methods of preservation that can be done at home.

Institute for Food and Development Policy, 2588 Mission Street, San Francisco, CA 94110. Publishes written and audiovisual material about the politics of food distribution and hunger.

Moyer, Ann. *Better Food for Public Places: A Guide for Improving Institutional Food*. Emmaus, PA: Rodale Press, 1977. Documents strategies used. Includes quantity recipes.

National Nutrition Education Clearing House, Society for Nutrition Education, 2140 Shattuck Avenue, Suite 1110, Berkeley, CA 94704 ([415] 548-1363). Has extensive written and audiovisual materials, some in Spanish, for lay and professional persons.

Public Documents Distribution Center, Pueblo, CO 81009. Distributes government pamphlets, including several on food and related topics. Many free. Send for list.

Rodale Press, 33 E. Minor Street, Emmaus, PA 18049. Write for current publications list for books on gardening, self-help and nutrition. Includes classics such as *Encyclopedia of Organic Gardening*. Also sponsors "Cornucopia Project," an education project to help agriculture toward self-sufficiency. Ads and notices in *Organic Gardening* magazine will lead you to other groups.

Rural American Women, 1522 K Street N.W., Suite 700, Washington, DC 20005. Has news journal, support network, advocacy on federal government level.

Valentine, William, and Frances Moore Lappe. *What Can We Do? A Food, Land, Hunger Action Guide.* San Francisco: Institute for Food and Development Policy, 1980. Good resource for action-oriented groups. Has case studies and lists of organizations.

Weiss, Ellen, Harriet Davidson, Laurie Heise and Nance Pettit. *Community Food Education Handbook.* Distributed by The Cooperative Food Education Program, 2606 Westwood Drive, Nashville, TN 37204. Copyright 1980 by Agricultural Marketing Project. Excellent. Good list of resources of groups and all aspects of how to do it. Curriculum materials.

3

ALCOHOL, MOOD-ALTERING DRUGS AND SMOKING

By Marian Sandmaier

As much as we would like it to be otherwise, all of us encounter stress in our daily lives. At one time or another, each of us struggles with work pressures, problems in our relationships, health concerns, loneliness, financial worries. Without thinking too much about it, many of us often respond to these pressures by pouring ourselves a drink, lighting a cigarette or taking a mood-altering pill; whether we're conscious of it or not, in each case we're using a drug to deal with what's bothering us.

Whether we use alcohol, pills or tobacco only occasionally or to the point where we feel dependent on them, we owe it to ourselves to find out more about the substances we're taking in.*

ALCOHOL

More of us are drinking than ever before, with two-thirds of adult women and about 80 percent of teenage girls now using alcohol regularly. Whereas society once frowned upon and even punished women for drinking, alcohol is now available to us—at times even pushed on us—in a dizzying range of social and business situations. Now that more of us are working outside the home, we have both more opportunities to drink and more money of our own to spend on alcohol. The multibillion-dollar alcohol industry has been quick to take advantage of women's changing social and economic status with an aggressive advertising campaign geared to the "female market." In magazines as diverse as *Ms.*, *Woman's Day* and *Glamour*, we can scarcely turn a page without being offered a new kind of drink, and with it the subtle promise of increased status, sophistication or sexiness. It is perhaps not surprising that in the United States alone, more than three million of us experience problems with alcohol use.

You just don't get many messages that say: hey, take this stuff seriously. You look at the beer commercials on TV or just your own social life where you get offered drinks coming and going, and you just see alcohol as

another way to have a good time. No big deal. I think of all the times I got drunk at parties in college, and never once did it occur to me that I was overdosing on a drug. And now I come home from work every day and sit down with my two drinks before dinner, and if I was really honest with myself I would have to admit that in some small way I'm dependent on it.

We often forget that alcohol is a powerful, potentially addictive drug. Whenever we have wine with dinner, a vodka and tonic at a party or a couple of beers with the late movie, we are consuming a central nervous system depressant that slows down all our body's major functions. Taken in small quantities, alcohol has a mildly relaxing effect that under most circumstances is harmless and pleasant. But if we continue to drink, motor coordination, judgment, emotional control and reasoning powers are diminished. In having sex with a man, it is easier to forget protection and risk an unwanted pregnancy. In heavy-drinking situations we also may become more vulnerable to rape or other physical abuse.

Excessive drinking over a period of time not only leads to physical addiction but increases the risk of heart attack, stroke, brain damage, liver disease, muscle disease, pancreatitis, phlebitis and gastrointestinal problems. Alcohol abuse is also associated with cancers of the liver, breast, mouth, larynx, esophagus, stomach, colon, rectum and thyroid gland. Women who both smoke and drink are at particularly high risk for developing cancers of the upper respiratory and digestive tracts.[1] In some cases, an alcohol overdose can be fatal.

Women who drink very heavily during pregnancy—at least six drinks per day—may give birth to babies with "fetal alcohol syndrome," a pattern of irreversible abnormalities that include mental retardation, prenatal and postnatal growth deficiencies and joint defects. As little as two drinks per day during pregnancy has been associated with lesser effects, notably lower birth weight in newborns. At present, no safe level of alcohol use during pregnancy has been established.* [2]

---

*Due to lack of space we will discuss only legal mood-altering drugs.

*Because the federal government has withdrawn plans to place warning labels on alcoholic beverages, public interest groups need to apply pressure to revive these plans.

If You Drink

- It is a good idea to eat something before or while drinking. Sipping drinks, rather than gulping them, also slows down the rate at which the alcohol enters the bloodstream. A woman weighing between 100 and 140 pounds should allow about two hours for her body to metabolize or "burn up" each drink; a woman weighing between 140 and 180 should allow at least one hour between drinks. (A "drink" consists of three to five ounces of wine, twelve ounces of beer, or one ounce of hard liquor. Each contains the same amount of alcohol.)
- If you've been drinking, don't drive. Even small amounts of alcohol seriously interfere with judgment, coordination, vision and reaction time, all of which are crucial for safe driving.
- Avoid using alcohol within a few hours of using *any* other drug, including over-the-counter medications. When taken together, alcohol and many other drugs dangerously multiply each other's effects, with results ranging from headache, nausea and cramps to loss of consciousness and even death. It is particularly dangerous to mix alcohol with another central nervous system depressant, such as a barbiturate or tranquilizer.
- Sometimes the body is especially vulnerable to alcohol. When you're feeling sick or tired, for example, alcohol can affect your system more powerfully than usual. Women may be particularly vulnerable to alcohol's effects just prior to menstruation,[3] so it is a good idea to avoid using alcohol to relieve premenstrual discomfort. And during pregnancy, the safest course is not to drink at all.
- Avoid using alcohol as a problem solver. Many recovering alcoholic women report that they first began drinking heavily to cope with a specific crisis, such as a divorce or job loss, or to relieve chronic depression or anxiety. Such escape drinking keeps us from dealing with our underlying difficulties and tends to make us increasingly dependent upon alcohol—to the point where we can become addicted to it.

In a society which judges women more harshly than men for dependence on alcohol, women tend to hide and deny their alcohol abuse rather than seek the help they need. Internalizing our culture's condemnation, alcoholic women suffer more guilt and anxiety than alcoholic men, have lower self-esteem and attempt suicide more often. Many women with drinking problems also become addicted to mood-altering pills prescribed by physicians who misdiagnose their alcoholism as "nerves" or depression. (See p. 36 for "Getting Help.")

MOOD-ALTERING DRUGS

Unlike alcohol, mood-altering drugs, such as tranquilizers, antidepressants and sedatives, have long been marketed as *medicines*. They also have been primarily aimed at—and used by—women. In the nineteenth century, patent medicines containing dangerously large amounts of opiates were sold to women for relief of "female troubles." Today, physicians prescribe two-thirds of all legal psychoactive (mood-altering) drugs to women. More than one million women report dependence on them.

Prescription psychoactive drugs have justifiable and effective uses in certain short-term crisis situations, for truly disabling depression or anxiety and for some physical ailments. But too often, physicians prescribe these powerful, often addictive drugs to "treat" the ordinary stresses of daily life: boredom on the job, rambunctious children, loneliness, marital difficulties. With older women, the onset of menopause or a husband's death often becomes a reason to prescribe these drugs. Much of this "medicalization" of normal life problems is encouraged by the aggressive American drug industry.[4] (See Chapter 24, "The Politics of Women and Medical Care.") Drug ads in medical and psychiatric journals often suggest that women are particularly unable to withstand the stresses of daily life without chemical relief.

I was in therapy when I got a new job in another state, and I talked with my psychiatrist about how nervous I was about the move and all the changes it would bring. She was very sympathetic about the problems involved in moving and adjusting to a new job. Then I watched as she took out her pad and wrote out prescriptions for a hundred Valium, a hundred Nembutal and a hundred Ritalin. "These might come in handy," she said as she handed me the three slips. At the time it never occurred to me not to get the prescriptions filled—that I might not need three hundred pills to survive the move.

Minor Tranquilizers

The minor tranquilizers (e.g., Valium, Librium, Serax, Equanil, Miltown) are designed to relieve anxiety and tension without significantly interfering with mental or physical functioning. Although their classification as "minor" distinguishes them from the "major" tranquilizers used primarily in the treatment of psychosis, there is nothing minor about the effects of these drugs or their abuse potential. Use of this term, encouraged by the drug industry, confuses both physicians and patients.

By far the most commonly prescribed of the minor tranquilizers are the benzodiazepines, which include Valium (diazepam) and Librium (chlordiazepoxide). Valium, an effective muscle relaxant as well as an antianxiety drug, is one of the most commonly prescribed drugs *of any type* in the United States, with women its primary users.

Although the benzodiazepines have long been considered one of the safest types of depressant drugs, negative effects reported for Valium and Librium include drowsiness, decreased muscular coordination, confusion, skin rashes, nausea, constipation, menstrual irregularities and changes in sexual drive. With Valium, "paradoxical effects" also have been reported, including insomnia, a reduction in REM (dream-producing) sleep, irritability, hostility and even rage. Still more alarming, Valium is the drug most frequently reported in connection with emergency-room visits caused by drug misuse or overdose.

In recent years, the addictive potential of Valium and Librium has become increasingly apparent. The 1979 Senate hearings on problems associated with mood-altering drugs revealed that those who take the benzodiazepines regularly for more than four months are at the highest risk for addiction. In doses of only fifteen to forty milligrams per day, withdrawal symptoms have been reported when Valium has been abruptly discontinued.[5]

New self-help approaches for gradually ending dependence on tranquilizers are being developed, with an emphasis on megavitamin therapy, nutrition, exercise and relaxation techniques. If you want to try this kind of program, be sure to get information about reliable methods* and the support of a knowledgeable person. Never try to kick a tranquilizer habit suddenly—or alone.

Barbiturates

Prescribed by physicians primarily to treat insomnia and anxiety, these depressant drugs include amobarbital (Amytal), butabarbital (Butisol), pentobarbital (Nembutal) and secobarbital (Seconal). Considered the most dangerous central nervous system depressants used in medicine today, barbiturates have a considerably higher potential for addiction and overdose than do the minor tranquilizers. They are also a major factor in many suicides, suicide attempts and accidental drug poisonings.

Although small doses of barbiturates will usually induce sleep, their effectiveness as sleeping pills lasts only about two weeks. At that point physical tolerance begins to develop, which means that it takes increasingly large doses to produce the same effects. Also, even with small doses, barbiturate-induced sleep often leads to grogginess, headache and a decrease in motor performance for several hours.

We cannot emphasize strongly enough the potential hazards of barbiturate use. Once you have developed a physical tolerance, the margin between a sleep-producing dose and a fatal dose is dangerously narrow. Barbiturates are also extremely hazardous in combination with alcohol: as little as two drinks taken with a moderate dose of barbiturates can cause an overdose. Finally, withdrawal from barbiturates must be undertaken gradually and under competent medical supervision, as abrupt discontinuation of these drugs can cause possibly fatal seizures.

Sedative-Hypnotics (Nonbarbiturate)

Among the most commonly prescribed of these sleep-inducing drugs are methaqualone (Quaalude), flurazepam (Dalmane), glutethimide (Doriden) and methyprylon (Noludar). Originally hailed as safer alternatives to the barbiturates, these drugs have been shown to pose many of the same risks of physical tolerance, addiction, dangerous withdrawal symptoms and overdose. Dalmane and Quaalude are among the most frequently named prescription mood-altering drugs in connection with drug-related emergency room visits. Both Quaalude and Doriden are stored in the body's fat tissue and are difficult to expel from the system, so that a person may apparently recover from the adverse effects of one of these drugs only to have the stored drug released into the system later, causing further complications.

Common side effects of these drugs are headache, hangover and dizziness; less often reported effects include nausea, vomiting, blurred vision and paradoxical nervousness and excitement. All these drugs are extremely dangerous in combination with alcohol.

Antidepressants

The most widely prescribed of these drugs are the tricyclic antidepressants, including doxepin (Sinequan), imipramine (Tofranil), amitriptyline (Elavil), desipramine (Norpramine, Pertofran) and nortriptyline (Aventyl). Although they are considered effective for some types of depression, improvement is usually not apparent for several weeks. There is also evidence that antidepressants may not always be the crucial factor in relieving depression: in one study, 60 percent of patients improved after taking Tofranil, while 40 percent improved with a placebo, or sugar pill.[6]

Common side effects of tricyclic antidepressants are dry mouth, constipation, urinary retention, blurred vision, weight gain and drowsiness. When these drugs are stopped abruptly after prolonged use, nausea and headache may result.

Amphetamines

Amphetamines, or "pep pills," are highly addictive stimulant drugs usually prescribed for weight loss,*

*See Resources: *Goodbye, Blues: Breaking the Tranquilizer Habit the Natural Way,* by Bernard Green.

*In 1978 the Food and Drug Administration disapproved the use of amphetamines for weight loss, but many doctors still prescribe them.

Safe Use of Drugs

- Before accepting a prescription for *any* drug, mood-altering or otherwise, ask your doctor: What is this drug for, and what are some non-chemical alternatives to it? Exactly how does this drug work on my body and mind? What are the risks, benefits and possible negative effects? Can I become addicted to this drug? How does it interact with other drugs, with certain foods and with alcohol? What are the specific risks of using this drug during pregnancy? How do I take the drug—when, how often, for how long, with food or not? How do I store the drug?
- If a prescribed drug comes with a patient information brochure, read it and follow instructions carefully. If there is no brochure, ask your doctor or pharmacist to show you the information on prescribing and adverse effects that the government requires drug companies to provide for each drug, or check the Physician's Desk Reference in your library. If any of this information is difficult to understand, ask to have it explained to you in layperson's terms. Be aware that brochures do not always list all side effects.
- Pay attention to your physical and emotional response to *any* drug you take. Even over-the-counter drugs can have unpredictable and hazardous effects and should always be used with caution.
- Although it may seem like a helpful gesture, avoid sharing pills with family members or friends. A drug that is safe for one person may have unpredictable and harmful effects on someone else.
- Never take any mood-altering drug within a few hours of using alcohol or any other drug. A mixture of alcohol and tranquilizers, barbiturates or other sedative drugs can be an especially dangerous, even fatal, combination.
- Avoid taking mood-altering drugs during pregnancy. Minor tranquilizers, barbiturates and amphetamines have been associated with birth defects in newborns.
- When accepting a prescription for any mood-altering drug, make an appointment with your doctor for a reevaluation within one month. At that point, fully discuss with your physician the risks and benefits of the drug before accepting a refilled prescription or an increase in the dosage. Since extended use of many drugs can produce dependence and other harmful effects, it is important to explore nonchemical ways of coping with the stresses you are facing. (See "Stress and Tension," p. 42.)

chronic fatigue and sleep disorders. Common brand names are Benzedrine and Dexedrine. These drugs have such a high potential for abuse and dependence that they are now accompanied by a written warning to physicians: "Should be prescribed or dispensed sparingly." They also have been shown to have so little value in long-term weight reduction that several states have banned their use for this purpose.

Low doses of amphetamines temporarily decrease appetite, relieve drowsiness and increase heart rate, blood pressure and breathing rate. Physical tolerance can develop within a few weeks of regular use, requiring increasingly large doses. With higher doses, some people report feelings of intense excitement and overconfidence; others become irritable and anxious. Common effects include sweating, insomnia, blurred vision, dizziness and diarrhea. Hazards of high doses also include risk of vascular damage or heart failure from a sudden increase in blood pressure, severe appetite loss and resulting malnutrition, and a general weakened condition which invites infection.

Drugs and Alcohol: Getting Help

Our use of alcohol or mood-changing pills can become such a part of our daily lives that sometimes we don't notice when it has become a problem. Here are some questions you can ask yourself.

- Has someone close to you sometimes expressed concern about your drinking or drug use?
- When faced with a problem, do you often turn to alcohol or pills for relief?
- Are you sometimes unable to meet home or work responsibilities because of pills or alcohol?
- Has your drinking or pill use caused any problems in relationships with family, friends or co-workers?
- Do you often take a pill or have a drink to get going in the morning?
- Do you find you have to take increasing amounts of pills or alcohol to achieve the same effects?
- Have you had distressing physical or psychological reactions when you've tried to stop drinking or using drugs?
- Have you—or has anyone else—ever required medical attention as a result of your drinking or pill use?
- Have you often failed to keep the promises you have made to yourself or others about controlling or cutting out your drug use or drinking?
- Do you ever feel guilty about your drinking or pill use or try to conceal it from others?

If you have answered "yes" to any of the above questions, your drinking or pill use is probably interfering with your life in serious ways and you should seek help. You can overcome alcohol and other drug problems, and the sooner you get help, the easier it will be to free yourself from dependence on these substances.

I was positive I didn't have a drinking problem. After all, I only drank beer and wine, I never drank till after five o'clock, I still had my kids and I wasn't on skid row. But I needed alcohol to blot out something—some reality about myself and my life that I couldn't stand to feel. And I could say all I wanted about being "just a social drinker," but the truth of it was I couldn't stop on my own. I needed help.

Few people struggling with alcohol or drug problems can overcome them alone, without the support and help of others who have "been there." Probably the best-known self-help group for recovering alcoholics is Alcoholics Anonymous (AA), which holds group meetings in most communities across the country, including groups for women and for lesbians and/or gay men in some areas. If there is no women's or gay AA group in your community and you would like to be part of one, you can talk to your local AA organization about starting a new group. Two other well-established networks, Al-Anon and Alateen, help the families and friends of problem drinkers. A relatively new but fast-growing organization is Women for Sobriety, a network of local support groups focusing on the special issues and needs of women with drinking problems. (See Resources for more information.)

In addition to these independent self-help groups, most local alcohol and drug treatment programs sponsor their own outpatient therapy and support groups. If you have a serious problem with alcohol or drugs, you may want to participate fully in one of these formal treatment programs, which provide medical care, individual and group therapy and a range of support services. It is important to emphasize that the aim of such treatment is not simply to "get you off drugs" but to help you better understand yourself and create a new life situation in which you won't *need* alcohol or pills to function. If there is a treatment program in your community designed specifically for women and staffed by women, you may find it particularly helpful. Other women may be more likely to understand your situation, your pressures and conflicts, and your practical as well as your physical and emotional needs. Childcare also may be available at some programs.

To find an appropriate treatment program or support group, check your area council on alcoholism, your community mental health center, the social services or health department of your city or county or the employee assistance program of your workplace,* if there is one. (Check the yellow pages of your local phone book under "Alcoholism" or "Drug Abuse.")

---

*Many large companies run assistance programs that include help for drug or alcohol problems. Most of these programs assure anonymity and job security, provided you agree to receive treatment.

After being that wiped out, I want it all. I'm fifty-one years old and I want everything that's due me as a person. I got off drugs to get a new life—and I'm going to have it.

SMOKING

By the time I was twenty years old I was up to two packs a day and a lot of the time I just felt rotten. I had a chronic cough and I would wake up in the middle of the night and cough and gag until sometimes I threw up. I felt my chest was so full of fluid I could almost scoop it out with a ladle. I always felt weak, like I had a cold I could never get rid of. What made me decide to quit was the thought that if I'm this bad off at twenty, what do I have to look forward to later?

More women smoke now than fifty years ago, for many of the same reasons that more of us are drinking. Although smoking has been slowly declining among adult women in recent years—about 28 percent of women currently smoke—those of us who do use cigarettes are more likely to be heavy smokers than in the past. Teenage girls are beginning to smoke at younger ages than ever before, and among young people seventeen to nineteen, more girls than boys are now using cigarettes for the first time in history.[7]

For those of us who smoke, the news is not good. Cigarette smoking now contributes to one-fifth of newly diagnosed cases of cancer and one-fourth of all cancer deaths among women. Women who smoke have an up to five times greater likelihood of developing lung cancer than nonsmoking women. In 1983, the female lung cancer death rate was expected to surpass that for breast cancer[8] (and did so in at least several states), the chief cause of cancer deaths in women for many years.

Compared to nonsmoking women, those who smoke cigarettes are more likely to suffer heart attacks, strokes and other serious cardiovascular disorders. Women who use oral contraceptives and also smoke are *ten times* as likely as female nonsmokers to suffer coronary heart disease. Cigarette smoking in women is also causally associated with cancers of the urinary tract, larynx, oral cavity, esophagus, kidney, pancreas and uterus. Women who smoke are also at greater risk for death from chronic obstructive lung disease, and are more likely than nonsmokers to suffer from chronic bronchitis, emphysema, chronic sinusitis, peptic ulcer disease and severe hypertension. Smoking has also been linked with decreased fertility in women and with early menopause.

There is growing evidence that "passive smoking"—that is, exposure to the cigarette smoke of others—is a serious health risk. One study showed that nonsmoking women exposed to their husbands' cigarette smoke were twice as likely to develop lung cancer as nonsmoking women with nonsmoking husbands.[9] Other studies have shown that children of parents who smoke are at higher risk for respiratory ailments than children of nonsmoking parents.

Smoking during pregnancy poses serious risks for the unborn. Babies of women who smoked cigarettes during pregnancy are likely to be smaller and to weigh less at birth and appear never to catch up. Smoking during pregnancy also increases the risk of bleeding, premature rupture of membranes, miscarriage, premature delivery and neonatal death. Risk of "sudden infant death syndrome" (SIDS) may also be increased by smoking during pregnancy.[10]

I wish some of this information had been around when I was young. I started smoking back in the thirties when I was twelve years old, and I never knew there was anything wrong with it. They did tell us that smoking stunted your growth, but I was tall so I didn't care. I smoked all through my teens, twenties and thirties and not a single person ever suggested that I stop. I remember now that when I was pregnant with my second daughter, I went for a visit to my obstetrician and I must have seemed nervous or something, because halfway through the visit he pulled out a pack of cigarettes and offered me one. And that just reinforced the idea that nothing could be wrong with it.

Kicking the Habit

There is simply no "safe way" to smoke. Although low-tar and -nicotine cigarettes may reduce the risk of lung cancer to some extent, they do not lessen the risk of other lung diseases, heart disease or fetal damage during pregnancy. The safest and healthiest course is simply to stop smoking. Difficult as quitting may be, more of us than ever are successfully freeing ourselves from dependence on tobacco. One out of every three women who has ever smoked has now kicked the habit, and since 1976 the percentage of women who smoke has declined from 33 to 28 percent.

The results are worth it. Even if a woman is a heavy smoker, after quitting her risk of developing lung and laryngeal cancer drops gradually, equaling that of nonsmokers after ten or fifteen years. Although some of us fear that when we stop smoking we will gain unwanted weight, research shows that only one-third of those who stop smoking gain weight, another third report no weight change, and a final third actually *lose* weight, possibly because many women begin exercise programs at the same time. Women who quit report that they have never felt better.

It's a great feeling to be able to do so many of the things that were just out of the question while I was smoking—running around the park, dancing for hours at a time, little things like enjoying the fragrance of my own clean hair. Just knowing that I'm healthier and my kids are probably healthier.

There's a great sense of accomplishment and power that comes from quitting—power to get ahold of your own life. But there's no way it's easy. I still identify with being a smoker. I still smoke in my dreams. If I thought I could go back to cigarettes and only smoke two or three a day, I'd do it in a minute. But I know I can't smoke that way. If I smoked one I'd smoke a pack, and I won't do that to myself anymore.

Studies indicate that the ability to quit smoking successfully depends largely on a strong commitment to stop, the belief that we *can* stop and support from others. There are a number of free or low-cost programs available to those of us who want to stop smoking, including those offered through local chapters of the American Cancer Society, the American Heart Association and the American Lung Association. Some of these programs offer special support groups for women. Other low-cost programs can be found through hospitals, health maintenance organizations, schools, businesses and community groups. Commercial smoking-cessation programs are also available, but they tend to be considerably more expensive.

We can participate in one of the formal programs offered in our community, or we can ask a friend or relative to stop smoking with us. And if we swear off cigarettes, then "slip" at some point along the way, we need to remember that nearly everyone does at one time or another. We need to try again—and again. It *is* hard to stop smoking. But it is also possible—and it is one of the biggest favors we will ever do for ourselves and our health.

NOTES

1. U.S. Department of Health and Human Services. *Fourth Special Report to the U.S. Congress on Alcohol and Health.* Washington, DC: U.S. Government Printing Office, 1981, pp. 47–59.

2. U.S. Department of Health and Human Services. "Surgeon General's Advisory on Alcohol and Pregnancy," *FDA Drug Bulletin,* Vol. 11, No. 2 (July 1981), pp. 9–10.

3. Ben M. Jones and Marilyn K. Jones. "Women and Alcohol: Intoxication, Metabolism and the Menstrual Cycle," *Alcohol Problems in Women and Children,* M. Greenblatt and M.A. Schuckit, eds. New York: Grune and Stratton, 1976, pp. 103–36.

4. Richard Hughes and Robert Brewin. *The Tranquilizing of America.* New York: Harcourt Brace Jovanovich, Inc., 1979, pp. 192–93.

5. David Smith. "Valium Abuse and the Low-Dose Benzodiazepine Withdrawal Syndrome." Unpublished paper, 1980, p. 2.

6. Conan Kornetsky. "Drugs Used in the Treatment of Depression and Anxiety," *Pharmacology: Drugs Affecting Behavior.* New York: John Wiley and Sons, 1976, p. 109.

7. U.S. Department of Health and Human Services. *The Health Consequences of Smoking for Women: A Report of the Surgeon General.* Washington, DC: U.S. Government Printing Office, 1980, p. 275.

8. *Ibid.*, p.8.

9. Takeshi Hirayama. "Non-Smoking Wives of Heavy Smokers Have a Higher Risk of Lung Cancer: A Study from Japan," *British Medical Journal*, 282 (Jan. 17, 1981), pp. 183–85.

10. U.S. Department of Health and Human Services, *The Health Consequences of Smoking for Women*, pp. 10–11.

RESOURCES

Alcohol and Drugs

Readings

Allen, Chaney. *I'm Black and I'm Sober*. Minneapolis: CompCare, 1978. Available from CompCare, Box 27777, Minneapolis, MN 55427.

Christenson, Susan, and G. Ihlenfeld. *Lesbians, Gay Men and Their Alcohol and Other Drug Use: Resources*. Madison, WI: WCAODA, 1980. Available from the Wisconsin Clearinghouse, 1954 E. Washington Avenue, Madison, WI 53704.

Green, Bernard. *Goodbye, Blues: Breaking the Tranquilizer Habit the Natural Way*. New York: McGraw-Hill Book Co., 1981. A step-by-step self-help program for gradually ending dependence on tranquilizers.

Hughes, Richard, and Robert Brewin. *The Tranquilizing of America: Pill Popping and the American Way of Life*. New York: Harcourt Brace Jovanovich, Inc., 1979. A well-researched analysis of the politics and economics of psychoactive drug use and the drug industry.

Sandmaier, Marian. *Helping Women with Alcohol Problems: A Guide for Community Caregivers*. Philadelphia: Women's Health Communications, 1982. Risk factors, interventions, family issues, how to get help, readings and resources. Available for $5.50 from Women's Health Communications, 4512 Springfield Avenue, Philadelphia, PA 19143.

Sandmaier, Marian. *The Invisible Alcoholics: Women and Alcohol Abuse in America*. New York: McGraw-Hill Paperbacks, 1981. Explores why women drink, social attitudes, treatment needs and how and where to get help. Includes in-depth interviews with diverse women.

Audiovisual Materials

The Last to Know, a 45-minute 1981 film or videocassette. Rent $70, sale $685. Available from New Day Films, P.O. Box 315, Franklin Lakes, NJ 07417 ([201] 891-8240). A powerful feminist film on women's experience with alcohol and drug abuse.

Women, Drugs and Alcohol, a 21-minute 1980 film or videocassette. Rent $65. Available from MTI Teleprograms, Inc., 3710 Commercial Avenue, Northbrook, IL 60062 ([800] 323-5343). Discusses the cycle of addiction and recovery.

Organizations

Al-Anon Family Groups, P.O. Box 182, Madison Square Station, New York, NY 10010. Sponsors self-help meetings for spouses and children of alcoholics. For information, literature and groups, contact your local Al-Anon office.

Alcoholics Anonymous, P.O. Box 459, Grand Central Station, New York, NY 10017. A worldwide self-help organization for recovering alcoholic women and men, with local chapters in most communities. Offers pamphlets for women, and for lesbians and gay men, and sponsors meetings for women and gays in some cities. To find meetings, contact AA headquarters or your local AA office. (See phone directory.)

National Association of Gay Alcoholism Professionals, 204 W. 20th Street, New York, NY 10011 ([212] 807-0634). A communication and support network. Publishes newsletter, bibliography and list of treatment resources for gay alcoholics, and provides referrals to gay groups of AA and Al-Anon.

National Clearinghouse for Alcohol Information, Box 2345, Rockville, MD 20852. A federal information service offering free publications on women and alcohol.

National Clearinghouse for Drug Abuse Information, P.O. Box 416, Kensington, MD 20795. A federal service offering free pamphlets and fact sheets on drug abuse for general and professional audience.

National Council on Alcoholism, 733 Third Avenue, New York, NY 10017. A national coordinating organization for local councils on alcoholism with publications on women and families. Local councils provide treatment referrals. (See phone directory.)

State Task Forces on Women and Alcohol, c/o National Women's Congress on Alcohol and Drug Problems, 239 E. Manchester Boulevard, Suite 203, Inglewood, CA 90301. Statewide groups that coordinate efforts to improve treatment, outreach and prevention services. Some publish referral guides and conduct educational programs.

Wisconsin Clearinghouse on Alcohol and Other Drug Abuse, 1954 E. Washington Street, Madison, WI 53704. Offers low-cost, readable materials, including resources for lesbians and materials on fetal alcohol syndrome.

Women for Sobriety, P.O. Box 618, Quakertown, PA 18951. A national self-help organization for recovering alcoholic women. Write for referral to a local group.

Smoking

Readings

American Cancer Society. *When a Woman Smokes*. 1977 6-page leaflet. (Also available in Spanish.) Hazards and suggestions for breaking the habit. Available free from local units of the American Cancer Society.

U.S. Department of Health and Human Services. *Clearing the Air: A Guide to Quitting Smoking*. Washington, DC: U.S. Government Printing Office, 1979. A readable guide with information on smoking-cessation programs. Available free from the Office of Cancer Communications, National Cancer Institute, 7910 Woodmont Avenue, Bethesda, MD 20205.

U.S. Department of Health and Human Services. *The Health Consequences of Smoking for Women: A Report of the Sur-*

geon General. Washington, DC: U.S. Government Printing Office, 1980. A thoroughgoing report. Available free from the Office on Smoking and Health, Park Building, Rockville, MD 20857.

U.S. Department of Health and Human Services. *Smoking and Health: An Annotated Bibliography of Public and Professional Educational Materials.* Washington, DC: U.S. Government Printing Office, 1978. A guide to free educational materials. Available free; see address for *Clearing the Air.*

"Women: Smoking's New Victims." *New Scientist* 21, May 1981.

Audiovisual Materials

The Feminine Mistake, a 22-minute 1977 videocassette. Rent $55, sale $295. Available from Trainex Corporation, P.O. Box 116, Garden Grove, CA 92642 ([800] 854-2485). A straightforward presentation of the dangers of cigarette smoking aimed primarily at young women. Includes an interview with a lung cancer victim.

Organizations

Action on Smoking and Health, 2013 H Street NW, Washington, DC 20006. A citizen's group working for legislation to reduce the health toll of smoking and protect nonsmokers' rights.

American Cancer Society, 777 Third Avenue, New York, NY 10017.

American Heart Association, 7320 Greenville Avenue, Dallas, TX 75231.

American Lung Association, 1740 Broadway, New York, NY 10019.

The above three are national voluntary organizations that provide free or low-cost smoking-cessation programs and publish materials. Contact your local branch for information.

4

WOMEN IN MOTION

By Janet Jones

With special thanks to Pat Lyga, Judith Stein and all the wonderful women who shared their experiences, feelings, thoughts, hard work and dreams, and so made this chapter possible

This chapter in previous editions was written by Janet Jones and Carol McEldowney.

A lot more of us women are out in the world moving around and *it feels good*. We are swimming, walking, dancing, jogging, power lifting, fencing and hiking. We play basketball, softball, soccer, rugby, badminton, racquetball, volleyball, lacrosse. We are bowling, skiing, gardening, canoeing, wrestling, skating, rock climbing. We play tennis, football, ice hockey, golf. We are boxing, surfing, scuba diving, motorcycle racing. We take archery, karate, yoga, judo, aikido, tai chi and gymnastics. We bike, sail, ride horses, race cars, take jazzercise and skydive. Times have changed!

North American women did not always exercise and do sports. The urban woman toiling long hours in factories, the pioneer woman, the slave woman, the poor white fieldworker—the lives of these women in the nineteenth century were so physically demanding that "exercise" as such was meaningless. For the middle-class woman, exercise was for the most part deemed "unladylike." She wore long, heavy dresses that allowed a minimum of movement and corsets which inhibited or impaired every organ in the torso, from lungs to uterus. Today only a few jobs are as physically demanding as those in the nineteenth century. Though many occupations are stressful and emotionally draining, almost none provides all the kinds of movement a healthy body, mind and spirit need.

Most women agree that over the past decade we have grown more active, both because of our increasing awareness of the health benefits of exercise and because the women's movement has brought a consciousness of our right to be vital, strong, confident people. All of us are not out there exercising all the time because there still are obstacles, both external and internal. But we are out there more often.

EXERCISE, SPORTS, PHYSICAL PLAY: WHAT THEY DO FOR US

Living is moving. Even when we lie still, all is in motion inside: the blood flows, the chest expands and contracts as we breathe, we digest food and eliminate wastes. The mind is full of thoughts, ideas, feelings, dreams. It is natural to want to move externally, too. We go to work, to the movies; we visit friends and shop. When we're forced to remain stationary, the urge to move increases. Hospital patients, confined to bed, look forward to the day they will be able to walk up and down the hall; prisoners locked in tiny, overcrowded cells demand the right to yard and exercise

Peter Southwick/Stock Boston

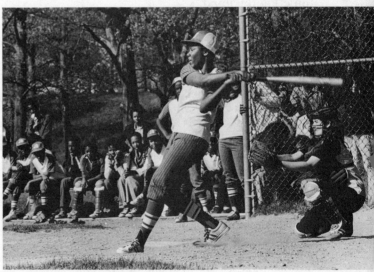

41

privileges; a paraplegic whose specially equipped van is wrecked feels totally cut off from society. Women march in cities and towns every year to protest the violence against women that forces us indoors. Economically and psychologically, we need to be out in the world.

Exercise is good for every system in our bodies. Even women with chronic health problems like asthma or diabetes benefit from exercise.

The Cardiovascular System and Aerobic Exercise

When we move vigorously on a regular basis for twenty or more minutes at a time, the heart (a muscle) gets stronger and more efficient, pumping more blood with fewer strokes. Over time, this kind of "aerobic" exercise—that is, exercise that keeps us breathing hard while our blood is circulating rapidly—increases the actual number and size of blood vessels in our tissues and so increases their blood supply. When we exercise hard, blood circulates faster through these expanded vessels, bringing oxygen and nutrients to every part of us and taking wastes away more quickly. That's why we usually feel refreshed and invigorated afterwards.

The Respiratory System

Exercising makes us breathe more deeply and regularly as more air moves rhythmically in and out of the lungs. The lungs develop a larger capacity, opening the air sacs up to the top and way down to the bottom of each lung for better gas exchange. We end up taking in more oxygen, which is essential for each cell in the body. If we practice rhythmic patterns of inhaling deeply, holding our breath and exhaling all the air slowly, we strengthen the respiratory system while quieting the mind.

The Musculoskeletal System

Muscles increase in size when they are used on a regular basis. Strong back and abdominal muscles are better insurance than Blue Cross/Blue Shield against the lower back pain which plagues so many of us these days. The abdominals also help hold the stomach and intestines in place and are critical to good digestion and elimination. Solid leg muscles get us where we are going and help the heart: when they contract, they squeeze the veins and so push the blood toward the heart, usually against the pull of gravity. Well-developed biceps and triceps muscles in the arms allow us to carry more and to perform everyday tasks with less effort and more independence. For self-defense purposes, the more muscle power we have the better. When all our muscles are firm and flexible, they protect us in many ways from the stresses and strains of living.

When we exercise, our bones get stronger, too. As muscles contract they pull on the bones, which increases bone strength over time. Also the body lays down extra minerals in the bones along the lines of stress. So if you walk or run, for example, the long bones in your legs will be gradually reinforced to meet the added pressure from your feet hitting the ground over and over again.*

The Reproductive System

Far from damaging our "internal organs," as women were taught until recently (it doesn't, for instance, hurt breasts or cause prolapsed uterus), exercise helps them. The more active we are the less the premenstrual syndrome and menstruation interfere with our lives. Exercise eases cramps, so unless you have excessive bleeding, nausea or vomiting, you can go to it as hard as you want during this time of the month.† Exercise during and after pregnancy is highly recommended.

Stress and Tension

Living in a stressful society subjects us to incredible daily assaults. Oppressive working conditions, problems at home, transportation hassles and concern for our physical safety can cause frustration, anxiety, anger and fear. When our minds become tense, our bodies do too.

Backache in North America, for example, has reached epidemic proportions, largely because of so much tension and so little exercise.‡ Tense muscles in the neck can cause splitting headaches; in the leg, charley horses; in the gut, stomachaches. Overcontracted muscles restrict breathing, slow down or even cut off the blood supply in their vicinity by squeezing the vessels shut, and actually limit our strength and sap our energy.§ So if you can answer your boss back, do it. If not, walk or run off the irritation and anger. Punch a pillow till you are exhausted. Boogie until three in the morning. Or let go by relaxing every muscle in your

---

*See also "Exercise and Growing Older," p. 46.

†Those of us who run over thirty miles a week, exercise or train heavily in other ways may find we menstruate less or not at all. Probably one or a combination of factors are responsible: intensity of effort, length of workout, fat loss, emotional stress, etc. In general, there is no cause for alarm. If you cut back on your workouts, you will probably resume your cycles. Note that you can become pregnant during long periods of amenorrhea. See "House Calls," by Joan Ullyot, *Women's Sports*, December 1981, pp. 46–47, and "Athletics Not Cause of Gynecological Concerns," by Dr. Mona Shangold, *New Directions for Women*, January–February 1981. See Chapter 12, "Anatomy and Physiology of Sexuality and Reproduction."

‡See Hans Kraus's excellent book, *Backache, Stress and Tension* (New York, Simon and Schuster, 1965; Pocket Books, 1969).

§Unfortunately, these are only a few of the negative effects of stress on our bodies.

body one after the other, listening to your breathing or imagining yourself in the most beautiful of all beautiful places.

I drink in the sky colors around me, concentrate only on breathing and the feel of my body moving, on the joy of being. The franticness of the day subsides.

While we work to change this oppressive society into a humane one we can all live in, soothing our nerves through physical or mental activity is an important and necessary release, and gives us more energy to work for the changes we need.

Many health practitioners suggest exercise as an actual treatment for depression. Some, looking into what joggers call "runner's high," are beginning to think that "strenuous exercise increases levels of a natural, narcotic-like painkiller in the blood..."* This interest in endorphins may also lead to an explanation of why exercisers get restless and irritable when they are "grounded" due to illness or injury: they are actually suffering withdrawal symptoms! Altogether a very interesting area of investigation and ripe for new discoveries.

You may or may not be "flying" after a workout, but you will almost invariably feel better than you did before: calmer, less tired, most likely refreshed. Maybe it was the one good thing you did with and for yourself in a time of messy problems with no neat solutions. Maybe it was wonderful because you did it with friends or because your basketball team played its best game ever—win or lose. Maybe you took on a real adventure, and the risk was exhilarating—made you feel alive all over. Being physically active builds confidence, independence, greater peace *and* vitality of mind. You connect to your own body and at the same time sense yourself a part of a larger whole. You are one with the energy of the universe.

OVERCOMING OBSTACLES

This all-out pep talk sounds great, *but*—there are real problems which keep us from becoming and staying physically active.

Economics

For every dollar men make, white women make about fifty-seven cents, women of color fifty-three cents and "disabled" women much, much less. Our paychecks go for food, shelter, clothing, transportation, medical care. Who can spend much on recreation? Many women cannot afford the money to join a club or a Y, or the time away from work. Accessibility, too, is a problem.

The facilities I use are pretty far from both my job and my home. It's too hard to get there every day in rush-hour traffic. Plus my best exercise time is other people's, too, so the place can be discouragingly overcrowded.

TV and automobile-induced passivity; hard, dirty streets; heavy traffic; pollution; lack of daylight hours before and after work; and safety factors also take their toll.

The obstacles that confront us are all much more formidable for women of color. During hard times, those of us who have never had much in the way of public facilities will have even less. Carmen, a teenager, remarks:

My mother walks for exercise. There has never been a dime available for her to go to an evening group of any kind.

I try to run around a lot and have fun in gym class because the way everything is getting cut, after-school sports may get dumped. The Y is down the street from my house, but there are too many gang fights so I never go there. Too bad, because I love games, love being a tomboy. It makes me feel I'm as good as anybody.

Last summer I spent hours on the bus every day going to a daycamp that turned out to be racist on top of being miles away. I've already started looking for a better one for next year, but, well, I'm not too hopeful. They keep closing things down.

When we are face to face with survival, any kind of real health care for the body and soul—sufficient and nutritious food, regular exercise and good times—appears to be an extravagance. So the challenge is how we can all join together to fight not just the cutbacks but also the prevailing government attitude which says scraping by is enough. We need bread *and* roses.* Nothing less will do.

Family

If a mother wants to exercise, what happens to the kids? We may not have money for a sitter, or have a husband, lover, friend or relative to leave them with while we go for a workout. Some places offer childcare, but it is usually limited.

Getting Jody to her infant swim, then Michael to preschool gymnastics and later on Mary to her teen dance class takes all my spare time. When do I have time for me? During one of their sessions, if I'm lucky!

Boston Globe article of 3 September 1981 reporting on a study by Daniel B. Carr and others in *The New England Journal of Medicine* of the same date. Others note that being outdoors in the sunlight stimulates the pineal gland in your brain, thus benefiting the whole hormonal system.

*A slogan from a banner carried by young girls in a march during the great Lawrence, Massachusetts, textile mill strike of 1912. "Bread and Roses" was made into a poem by James Oppenheim and set to music by Caroline Kohlsatt.

What We Can Do

We can exercise in the privacy and relative safety of our own homes—it's cheaper and we can do it at the most convenient times for us—alone or with family and friends. If your apartment is small, clear a space so your body doesn't feel hemmed in. Keep whatever equipment you like around for easy use. Hang a chin-up bar over the door opening and buy some dumbbells. Stretching, strengthening exercises, yoga, dance, karate techniques, jumping rope, running in place, stationary bicycling and rowing can all be done in your own living room or bedroom.*

Turn on the music. A steady upbeat makes you want to move; the slower rhythms are good for stretching, where the point is to hold to a count of ten to twenty (repeat at least once) with no bouncing. Stretch in quiet sometimes, though, so you can tune into your own rhythms, get a sense of what your body can and can't do. Visualizing how you want to feel and what you want your body to look like as you move on to more difficult feats is extremely helpful.

Women with older children can do physical things with their kids. Vanessa, a woman in a local black community, used to manage a dance school that her daughters started.

I got a lot of pleasure out of joining those classes. Later I took karate with my boys at the community school night program. Even with a tight schedule, my motto is: you make *time for what is important to you.*

Carla jogs with her kids, especially on weekends, and this works well for them. If you jog with your children (from six years on), be sure it is *fun*; they will run *playfully* for long distances without tiring (miles and miles) and will prefer this to sprinting.

At my son's suggestion, I got a baseball mitt when he was eight, and we've played a lot of catch since then, in addition to the jogging.

Sonya missed her every-other-day run so much when her baby came she decided she couldn't wait six, seven, ten years.

After a few months, I put Charelle in a sturdy stroller and now I jog pushing her along. This way I can keep active and my daughter is getting a feel for movement right from the beginning!

Old Myths and Prejudices

Even with a minimum of obstacles, many of us still don't exercise on a regular basis. This may be because of some old myths and prejudices which we need to throw out once and for all. We know well the long, cold stare and remarks like:

- Big shoulder muscles are really ugly on a woman.
- Hey, fatty, you should get your exercise pushing away from the dinner table.
- You four girls are going to hog this court when we guys need a team practice? No way!
- Don't you know that sweating is unfeminine?
- You're fifty-one and you're taking up—*what*?!
- Keep on pitching like a man, sweetheart—we know you're a dyke!
- What are these crippled women doing here? If I looked like that I wouldn't be caught dead in a bathing suit.

We have internalized many of these negative attitudes about women and exercise.

For my brother, physical fitness is like breathing, but not for me.

Everyone and everything still come first—that old pattern of taking care of ourselves last if at all. Somehow we don't feel entitled to the time, still don't feel we're worth it. Moreover, my husband gives me very little support, and my girlfriend's husband actively discourages her.

An end to these old prejudices! We must start getting the exercise we want and need.

EXERCISE AND DISABILITY

Differently-abled women are finding each other and the programs they need. One very fine adapted yoga program takes place once a week at an urban self-help center.* Linda spends her day in a wheelchair. Her leg muscles cannot hold her up, but her back muscles are okay. If she sits hour after hour with no chance to exercise, her back and abdominal muscles will wither away, and she will become even more disabled. Since several of the women, like Linda, are in wheel-

---

*There is a lot of glamorous (and expensive) exercise equipment on the market that you don't need to buy in order to get fit. Start with what you can do with the basics and then invest later (if at all) when you know what you really want or need.

*People come to the class with a wide variety of disabilities, from multiple sclerosis to cerebral palsy, from angina to sickle cell anemia.

Use bike paths in your area. If you live in the country, get together and make tracks for cross-country skiing, a network of paths to connect your houses.

Since many commercial clubs and health spas are unsatisfactory,* you may want to start an exercise group. For example, after working unhappily in a very competitive club in the city, two women in a suburb of Boston decided to go into business for themselves and set up a "Creative Movement Center." They run a very personal set of classes for women with kids. Mothers bring their babies (four to fourteen months), toddlers (fifteen months to two-and-a-half years) and preschoolers (and later schoolers) in for gym. During the baby class, the mothers exercise with their infants or help them exercise. This routine includes stretching and strengthening exercises, gentle bouncing on the trampoline, rolling the baby downhill on a foam mat, helping her/him hang on a bar or set of rings and other activities that develop self-awareness, balance and coordination. In midmorning, there is an aerobic dance class for the women, while two sitters watch their kids in the adjacent daycare room. The atmosphere is caring and noncompetitive. There is lots of movement and music, and every young participant is treated as a full individual. The equipment is simple: inexpensive foam mats, a wooden bar set between two posts, small and colorful hoops that the kids sit in or dance with.

We need more such groups around the country, perhaps run cooperatively to keep the fees low. With a little money, space and ingenuity women can make them happen. One single mother is planning to do just this for herself and her friends.

I feel so much better when I exercise, but it's tough being motivated alone. I'm sick and tired of funneling my hard-earned money into the local exercise spas when I can do it in my own living room on a thick rug with some weights,* a couple of exercise books or exercise records (even a video), music and common sense. We'll work out the childcare arrangements, taking turns or chipping in for a sitter.

Think about raising money for the facilities, equipment and ongoing political work we need to do by organizing walk-run races, swimathons, exhibition games, a play day. What better way to create an upward spiral? The healthy energy we spend developing our bodies and spirits can help to fund the next cycle of growth for us all.

---

chairs, they are encouraged to walk a number of steps with help and then spend time on mats breathing, stretching and doing visualization exercises. Loretta Levitz, the woman who developed and runs the program, explains:

I want people to stay as active as they can and then start reclaiming the parts of their bodies that the doctors usually consider lost. The group support is very important; so is healthy food.

Tosca, a woman with multiple sclerosis who has been a regular for a long time, explained that when she tries too hard and gets too frustrated, she blocks her own progress.

About a year ago, one of my legs started "tremoring," as it often does. In anger I hit it. Then my other leg began shaking, too, but I decided to pat that one instead. The leg getting the loving treatment stopped its movement almost immediately, while the "abused" leg kept right on shaking.

Relaxation and breathing have helped me expand my physical abilities, given me hope and renewed determination.

Swimming has always been a physical activity for those of us with differing abilities. Women of all ages come to an adapted swim class at one local YWCA with many differences, from blindness to cerebral palsy, and each goes at her own pace. The instructors help their students get over fear of the water and then proceed to teach swimming and water safety skills. It is liberating to be free of the "hardware"—canes, crutches, wheelchairs—and into a medium that buoys you up. The women tell each other about the events of their week with great humor and caring.

Across town at another facility, the pool coordinator and special-needs coordinator have made people of all ages with special mental, emotional and physical needs

---

*Many commercial "figure salons" are making big bucks off women's interest in exercise and obsession with weight. They have little useful equipment and offer pitifully little variety in terms of classes. The ones with more equipment and variety are expensive. Almost all are depressingly "diet" oriented. The women who staff them are usually undertrained and grossly underpaid for the work they do. Too many of us are tricked into worrying about the number of "inches" we are told we should lose when we need to be much more concerned with getting strong and resilient and developing our powers of relaxation, endurance and coordination in ways that challenge us physically and mentally.

*Dumbbells, barbells, ankle weights. For dumbbells you can use sand-filled juice or coffee cans, jugs of water or make beanbags with pellets in them.

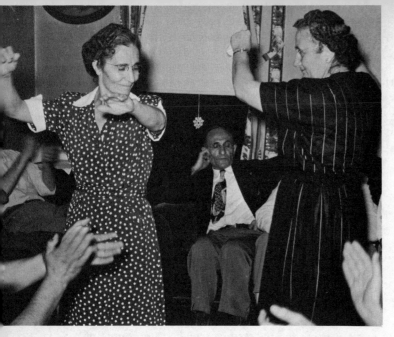

Varkey Sohigian

a priority. Their sessions run for two-and-a-quarter hours twice a week with support group first, then stretch and swim time. All the pool activities there emphasize the *whole* person, not just swim lessons.

Jean, a mentally disabled woman, loves the pool now that she has overcome her fear.

Swimming is great. I like the way the water feels and the fun we have in it.

Unfortunately, the local medical establishment takes faint interest in programs like these, and seems to think that these people might as well accept their limitations and forget it. Society's attitudes and economic priorities cause problems: class cost, odd-hour scheduling, transportation hassles and limited wheelchair accessibility keep more people from coming.

EXERCISE AND FAT

Our access to movement is limited by the prejudice we encounter. (See Chapter 1, "Body Image.") The ridicule, hostility and fear that greet us every time we walk down the street keep a lot of us immobilized in our homes. Learning to move around in public despite the harassment we face, learning to relax and take up all the space our bodies occupy instead of always trying to look smaller—these are victories over the people who want us always to feel ashamed of our size.

Some Guidelines on Movement for Fat Women*

- Choose something that looks like fun. Don't worry about whether it's "good" for you or not, or, if you do, think about improving your circulation and heart tone.

*From Judith Stein, co-founder of Boston Area Fat Liberation.

- Forget about losing weight or "firming flab."
- Find a place where you already see big women exercising, or do it at home.
- Go with a friend. Pick someone about your size or similarly new to the activity. Don't start out with a "jock."
- Give yourself leeway to be good or not so good at something.
- Get together with other fat women to find facilities. (Swimming is great, but locker rooms and bathing suits can be humiliating. A group of women in San Francisco rent a city pool a few hours a week for a fat women's swim, which makes all the difference.)
- Try walking, depending on your neighborhood; bowling, which requires no special clothes; social or ballroom dance classes, where you can have a friend as a partner.
- You have a right to remain physically inactive if you choose.

EXERCISE AND GROWING OLDER

Our need for exercise continues, even increases, as we grow older. Some say it is essential. As our bodies age we can lose flexibility, muscle strength and aerobic power. Joints can become stiffer because the fluid in them can begin to dry up, joint space can narrow and bones weaken.* Muscles may sag more readily, and our minds, taking in all the ageist propaganda, may say, "Well, it's all downhill from here." We mustn't buy that line! Being active (perhaps with a longer warmup period) will keep joints supple, although the first movements at the beginning of a workout may be more painful than in younger years. We can walk, swim, jog, lift weights, take up a new sport. Pay attention to your body; go slow but *don't* let your muscles and bones, heart and lungs deteriorate and your confidence with them. A friend, Woodie, took scuba diving recently to celebrate her fifty-fourth birthday:

Why wait? I said to myself. It's something I've always wanted to do.

Maybe we can't be as undaunted as Ruth Rothfarb, who at eighty ran her first marathon (Ottawa, 1981), but what a role model! At the end of the 26.2-mile course, her legs were tired, but:

It was the greatest day of my life! I worked all my life in a store. I always liked the outdoors and enjoyed long walks, but there was never time for more. Eight or nine years ago I started jogging, and for the last five I have been competing.

*The gradual loss of calcium from the bones is called osteoporosis. (See page 461.)

She runs about ten miles every day, walks a lot and dances, too. The people in her apartment building used to think she was crazy, but now they encourage her with, "Go, Ruthie!" She wishes they would get into it also, but so far very few have. She explains that women of her generation have many fears about their bodies, many don'ts and can'ts. Ruth guards her independence with a determined spirit, doing what feels right to *her*.

I need my sleep. I rest my arthritic leg when it bothers me, but I never miss that daily run.

Those of us in our sixties, seventies, eighties, nineties who are not out running ten miles do not need to let her example make us feel defensive but can let it inspire us to do something at home, at our social center or local Y. For instance, Miriam, living in a complex for the elderly in Pittsburgh, attends an exercise class in one of the lounges several times a week and goes walking regularly.

EXERCISE AND ILLNESS

After surgery or a long illness, we need exercise. Even in hospitals patients are encouraged to get out of bed as soon as possible. When we're ill, exercise gets the blood circulating, prevents painful bedsores and stimulates the respiratory system as well. If you are bedridden, it's important to get help with exercising the moveable parts of your body; even tensing and relaxing your muscles in a methodical way will help. Do some deep breathing at least once every hour.

Those of us who live in institutions would benefit from as much physical activity as possible, although we rarely get a fraction of what we need. Prisons, mental hospitals, nursing homes and similar institutions with their understaffing, heavy reliance on drugs and/or lockups remain inert if not crippling places. As Crystal tells it:

I've been in the nuthouse twice and jail once. If you let out how you feel in a physical way—and believe me, you need to—they just drug your ass, that's it. Or put you in max. I lost my body in there, and my mind.

OPTIONS

There are a lot of possibilities for fitness. Pick an activity that gives you pleasure, one you already enjoy or something new. Suit your exercise to your work. For stultifying jobs with a lot of sitting, pick an activity that excites you and gets your blood moving. If your work is physically exhausting, relax and stretch. Take breaks during the day (or night shift), too—stretch, walk around. A few wise employers provide company space and/or programs for employee fitness.

Many more should be encouraged to do so—for everyone, not just VPs. Watch out for stereotypes: certain races, body types, "disabled" people can't do this or naturally excel at that. Never restrict your options based on other people's say-so. You can set modest health-oriented goals for each week, train seriously or go for a much more spontaneous kind of play—whatever keeps you moving. You may want to pick an aerobic activity first,* then add others according to your interests. Ask someone who has a lot of experience with the activity you choose, or read books to find out what it *is* and *isn't* doing for your body.† Just as walking, biking or running do little to develop our arms, torso and neck, so stretching and weightlifting need a supplementary aerobic exercise. Extra abdominal and back exercises are always in order. Some of us find it reasonably easy to be motivated alone. We turn inward more and prefer performing only for ourselves. Others of us need the push and encouragement of a group or TV show to get going and stay going. Some of us love team activities in which the social aspect—playing together—is very important. And "new games" are fun for everyone.‡

WALKING

Walking is excellent for all women who can use their legs. If you move along briskly, walking will do what running does: improve your circulatory and respiratory systems, increase muscle and bone strength, calm the nerves. It's great in sunshine, but a walk in the rain or snow can be equally terrific when you're dressed for it. Walk to work or, if that's too far, get off the bus two stops away. Go to the store on your feet not on your behind; climb stairs instead of riding the elevator. Carrying a small pack on your back (three to five pounds) adds a lot of benefit to brisk walking. Start slow, build up. After a while, you'll be going for an hour with no tiredness. Set a pace that feels good to

*The government has published an excellent free booklet on the basics called *Exercise and Your Heart*. Write to the National Heart, Lung, and Blood Institute Information Office, Box W, Building 31, Room 4A21, Bethesda, MD 20205, for a copy.

Forms of aerobic exercise include walking, jogging/running, swimming, biking, skipping rope, hiking, cross-country skiing, some forms of dance and group sports like basketball and soccer. For a detailed aerobic program see, for example, *The New Aerobics* by Kenneth H. Cooper (New York: Bantam Books; 1970).

†Like *Sports for Life* by Robert Buxbaum and Lyle J. Micheli, Beacon Press, 1979. As far as we know, a whole popular book on activities and exercises for people with differing abilities has yet to be written, but Glorya Hale's *Source Book for the Disabled*, Bantam Books (also Saunders), 1979, does include a section on physical activity.

‡See *The New Games Book*, Andrew Fluegelman, ed., Garden City, NY: Dolphin, 1976, and *More New Games*, Dolphin, 1981. The new games books are full of new and old games that you can play "their" way or your own way with all ages, groups, and numbers of people—outdoors and in. The energy in the pictures and directions is infectious—it makes you long to head for a wide-open field and romp.

you and develop an easy unbroken rhythm with the right stride for your leg length. Keep your feet pointing straight ahead and let your arms swing naturally at your sides (which means not carrying a pocketbook). Walking, like dancing and running, is primal movement. Women have been doing it for hundreds of thousands of years over fields and deserts, mountain slopes and city streets. It is free and requires no equipment (besides good shoes). Many of us who are older or fat have discovered that walking keeps the body active but does not stress it.

> Unfortunately, physical safety is always a concern for women. Walk or run when and where there are a lot of people. If this isn't possible, go with a friend or a dog. When running or walking alone, assess your surroundings. Act confident. Keep an eye on any man who makes you feel uncomfortable—intuition is often right. Have a plan of action ready if a threatening situation develops. (See "Martial Arts," page 49.)

JOGGING/RUNNING

Jogging and running do for you what walking does, but at a faster pace: your heart, lungs and all your systems get more of a workout. You can run purely for fun, for the good it does you physically, mentally and spiritually. Or you can get into a serious training program for competing in races or marathons.* Some people are bored by running; for others, it is a positive addiction. Mary, who is visually impaired, loves it. On weekends she runs with a friend:

We talk the miles away, getting caught up on each other's news over a five-mile course instead of a coffee cup.

Running does put a great deal of pressure on the weight-bearing parts of the body: feet, ankles, knees,

---

*Women's physiques are built so that we do very well at endurance sports like running. It's ironic that an official tried to literally run Kathy Switzer out of the Boston Marathon in 1967,

> Do warmups and cooldowns with blood-moving exercise and stretches.* Include several varieties: 1. back-of-the-leg, thigh and pelvic stretches that pull out the muscles, tendons and ligaments in these areas, because they tighten up on you as you run; 2. foot and knee circles; and 3. some torso, arm and head stretches, too. Every couple of days do additional muscle-building exercises that develop the major muscle groups. Listen to your body; don't push too far too fast.

hips, spine. For this reason, well-fitted, well-padded running shoes (not sneakers) with good arch supports† are critical; the more protection between you and the ground, the better. Run on earth if it's even, tar-based pavement if necessary, concrete as little as possible. Keep your strides a comfortable length and low enough to the ground so you keep pounding to a minimum. Your feet should hit the ground heel first and roll forward to the toes. (Hitting toe first for any length of time will devastate your calf muscles.) Develop a rhythm but don't let it limit you. Vary your pace and gait from time to time. Think light and lift your torso up off your pelvis and legs as you move along. Let your arms swing easily at your sides, shoulders relaxed, head steady but floating on the neck.

At least twenty minutes of jogging or running a few times a week, *plus* warmups, cooldowns and additional muscle-building exercises, will do it for fitness and keep injuries to a minimum for most people. Beyond this the risks are greater, as with any sport. Know what you are getting into. Look for good information on shoes, beginner's schedules, tips for running in different seasons, training for long-distance and injuries.

SWIMMING

Swimming is probably the most full-body and least physically stressful exercise going, once you know how to do it. Nonswimmers may have to overcome fear of

---

and the Olympic Committee only recently gave women official permission to run in marathons. Our finishing times are improving with every race, and when it comes to the ultramarathons, we hang tough. A woman even finished at the head of the whole pack in one hundred-miler. See Ernst Van Aaken, *Van Aaken Method* (Mountain View, CA: World Publications, 1976) and Joan Ullyot, *Women's Running* (Mountain View, CA: World Publications, 1976).

*A thorough and easy-to-use book on stretches for many different activities is Bob and Joan Anderson's *Stretching* (Shelter Publications, P.O. Box 279, Bolinas, CA, 1980).

†Or even special arch supports (called orthotics) made from a mold of your own foot by a chiropractor or podiatrist.

Sarah Putnam

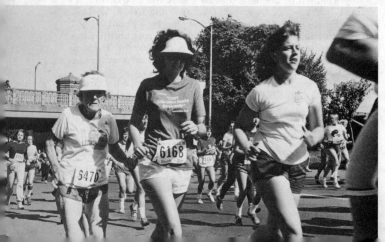

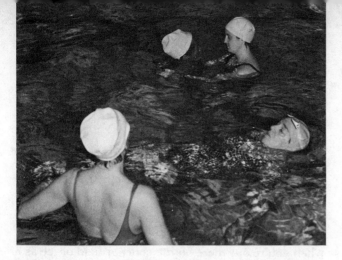

Phyllis Ewen

the water, which is sometimes difficult, but the rewards are great. The water buoys you up, taking weight off aching backs, arthritic hips, bad knees, tired feet, weakened legs. You can do laps (twenty to thirty minutes several times a week) and get an excellent workout for a wide variety of muscles and your cardiovascular system even if you don't swim very fast. A lot of pools now offer aquatic exercises which put you through your paces whether you know how to swim or not.

If people are sensible and pools and beaches well guarded, swimming is a safe activity. While there are disadvantages to pool swimming—such as chlorine, membership or admission fees and crowds—most are well-organized for lap swims at peak times and schedule swim classes to help you improve your skills.

As Lynn tells us:

Water is relaxing and calming for me, and some days very sensuous as well. The noise and distractions of the day just go as I tune into my own body and thoughts.

Water is really irresistible, maybe because our bodies are 70 percent water themselves and because we float in it for nine months before birth. Unless traumatized by some unhappy accident, children take to it fast. Mothers bring their infants as young as two to three weeks to the pool!* Playing in the water is a joy, too—watch how long kids will keep busy, jumping in, sitting on the bottom, racing each other, playing catch, inventing new games all the time.

EASTERN DISCIPLINES

Eastern cultures have long understood that exercise involves body, mind and spirit, and that is why yoga, which means "union," is such an integrating experience. Everything you do as you practice yoga strengthens, stretches and relaxes your whole being. During half an hour to forty-five minutes of many poses you

*Claire Timmermans describes the whole process in *How to Teach Your Baby to Swim* (Briarcliff Manor, NY: Stein and Day, 1976).

can stimulate all the major organs of the body. (For more, see "Yoga," p. 66.)

Tai chi also originates in the East. It involves rhythmic body movements which put you in touch with your energy and the energy around you. You focus on balance and weight distribution. You are strong, not rigid; relaxed, not limp. You begin to heal yourself as you move. With calm and graceful motion you dance. It can also be a method of self-defense.

MARTIAL ARTS

Women continue to train in martial arts schools (run by women and men) at karate, aikido, judo, jujitsu. We develop self-defense skills, and with them confidence, a new physical presence and a mental awareness. We also enjoy the sports aspects. For instance, sparring in karate (controlled fighting with light or no body contact) is tremendously exciting, sometimes scary but often a tension releaser. Certain patterns and moves we learn in martial arts are very satisfying as art form, as fighting dance, as challenging sport, as meditation. Workouts often put a lot of stress on muscles, tendons, ligaments—especially in joint areas. Stretch properly beforehand. Don't get recklessly carried away in the thrill of learning how to strike or throw or in an effort to prove your seriousness to men in the class. Women's schools are or should be supportive of the slow and steady method for everyone—encouraging women with differing abilities to join and helping them to adapt standard techniques to what fits their situations best. These schools also need to help us deal with our feelings about all the violence around us and the political implications of what we are doing. Organizing a women's group inside a male school is useful for the same reasons—it may keep us going when we would otherwise drop out.

DANCE

Turn on the radio or put on your favorite record and move. Don't worry about the latest "steps," don't be shy, just get your body going. Dance for the sheer joy of it or dance off the effects of a long, frustrating day. Do it alone or with friends—at home or out on the town. Take a class in modern, jazz, African, belly, improvisational, ballet or aerobic dance. Or keep right on inventing what gives you pleasure. It's a great way to express emotion and moods physically without words. Stretch well before you start, know your limits and really get into it. Each time your body comes more alive, grows stronger, more coordinated and balanced. No matter what happens, no matter how depressing life becomes or how many hours we put in fighting against the injustices of the times, we must never forget to dance. We can dance (and sing) on the picket line, we can dance as we march and rally, we can dance as we celebrate our victories. Emma Goldman knew it when she proclaimed, "If I can't dance to it, it's not my revolution!"

BIKING, HIKING, SKIING, RACQUETBALL, ETC.

The beat goes on. Biking is terrific—you're outdoors with legs, hearts, lungs pumping hard and a helmet on! More and more people are riding to work. Hiking is excellent, too. In certain areas of the country we can enjoy it all year round while the rest of us switch in the winter to snowshoeing or cross-country skiing—equally great exercise. Racquetball has become a big favorite very fast; often, prime court time (i.e., before and after regular work hours) is at a premium. Gerry, though, signs up ahead of time for courts with reasonable fees, fitting it into her busy schedule.

I love the fast pace, the intensity of the game that wipes out all my problems for an hour—you don't have to excel at racquetball to have a lot of fun.

Tennis needs no introduction—it's a fast, total body sport, but your participation in it can suffer from cost and space factors, too. Badminton can be *much* more than a halfhearted backyard game. The equipment isn't expensive and you do not necessarily need a specially constructed area to play on. Jumping rope can be a super conditioner for lungs, heart, arms, legs.

WEIGHTS

No chapter on women's fitness these days would be complete without a word on pumping iron: weight-lifting, weight training, body building. A male preserve no longer, women are buying weights (barbell and weight set), an instruction book and are doing it at home. Others join a health club, a gym or a Y with a Universal or Nautilus (machines with weights on them). Some of us lift to be fit, feel strong, get to know our bodies, or for the sheer challenge of it; others to be more powerful (and protected from injury) at the sports we play or to be able to handle our jobs with less fatigue and more independence; a growing number to compete in body-building contests. If you start your program with a book, follow *all* the advice. Stretch before you begin heavy lifting and don't overdo it. Before you go the health club route, check out the program thoroughly, especially the instructors—they should be trained in anatomy and physiology as well as in how to use the equipment.

GROUP SPORTS

More and more of us are participating in group sports—practicing more often and developing our skills more seriously than ever before, whether in school or city (town) leagues. Basketball, volleyball and softball have always been and continue to be very popular; soccer, rugby and ice hockey are relatively new and growing. The challenge, excitement and great satisfaction come when you're out there on the court or field or ice as a part of a group with everyone playing hard and you make it all click. There is nothing like it. And who would miss the socializing afterwards—the jokes, the stories about last year and plans for next season.

Make sure you find the right team for you. Some are very competitive—winning is all. Others are more fun-oriented; every woman gets to play in every game, people take turns playing different positions and help each other improve. You might want to check out the coach; she or he often sets the tone for the whole team. While stiff competition can be exhilarating and we are inspired by women who excel, it is more important for women of all races, ages, economic backgrounds and abilities to have a chance to enjoy a game than to produce a female sports elite. Big-money male athletics, with its superaggressive dog-eat-dog approach, reflects the values of our society at large. It need not be our model.

Some team sports give your body a well-rounded workout—some don't. Basketball, soccer, rugby and hockey are great for cardiovascular fitness and general body strength. They are strenuous, so you usually need to build up to them. Softball and volleyball are less rigorous. If you play a sport where you stand around waiting for the ball to come to you, some aerobic activity would be a good adjunct. Pregame warmup for all group sports is essential.

Getting good court or ice time is still hard; in most places the men's teams always get first choice. The same goes for softball—fields are hard to come by, especially in the city, so you usually have to be on a registered team in order to reserve a field for practice. Pickup games with a group of friends on Sunday morning are fast becoming impossible. Fees for joining a league are escalating at an alarming rate and in some communities you pay extra for lights and umpires.

SCHOOL SPORTS: THE POLITICS OF ACCESS

Title 9 of the Educational Amendments Act, 1972, despite its imperfections and late-in-the-day appearance, has been an important piece of civil rights legislation for women in school and college sports. The law applies to all educational institutions that receive federal funds for anything. For athletics its goal is to "secure equal opportunities for men and women while allowing schools and colleges flexibility in determining how best to provide such an opportunity."* The result (of Title 9 and other laws as well) has been that "hundreds of thousands of young women are competing in organized contests under the same circumstances that their fellow male students have [enjoyed] for many years"—with at least better uniforms, equipment, training, medical services, facilities, transportation, publicity, scholarships, awards, excitement and new respect for themselves, from other women and from the men.† There have been negative results, too: males taking over previously all-female teams; merging of programs so women who once ran their own, if meager, show find themselves administrative assistants to male athletic directors; men snatching up jobs coaching the new women's teams because the pay has suddenly become worth their while; and overcrowded facilities. Much controversy still exists over mixed teams—should highly skilled women play on "male" teams if they want to? Should all the guys who ask be allowed to join the girls' volleyball or field hockey teams?‡

Certainly it is imperative that we know our legal rights in this area as in others. Sometimes all you have to do is get to know the male coaches and persuade them to share or remind a male administrator that he is violating the law to end an injustice. Other times filing a grievance with your regional office of the Department of Education (DE), Civil Rights Division, or going to court will be necessary. But we must never rely on government mechanisms to do things for us by themselves. The DE is woefully understaffed, and already Title 9, along with all civil rights legislation and the DE itself, is under serious attack in Washington. Budget cuts (national and local) are starting to take their toll at the elementary, secondary and college levels with the possibility that women's sports programs are going to be cut by the general abandonment of nonprofessional athletics before we ever get where we should have been in the first place. College sports will probably find a way to survive. But what will happen to the undefeated basketball team at an inner-city high school which proudly celebrated with the first female sports banquet in the city? How long will there be money for a coach, equipment, uniforms, transportation? How long can even one young woman

on the team dream of a college athletic scholarship, which was unheard of for any girl a mere ten years ago? If the high school forecast is for heavy clouds, it's downright gloomy for junior high and elementary. We need to support our local school system's sports program, perhaps organize a sports event to highlight the problem.

TAKING CARE OF OURSELVES

Just as you make space to move in, wear clothes that are loose or very flexible for full range of motion—sweatpants and jackets, loose shorts, T-shirts, jerseys or leotards, socks or bare feet.* For activities that make you sweat, cotton next to your skin is good because it's soft and absorbent, and it "transmits perspiration and heat away from the body."†

If you have or suspect any physical limitation, consider some kind of health checkup before beginning a rigorous exercise program.‡ Some physical prob-

---

*You don't need to be seduced by ads for "designer" running outfits. Plain old cotton sweats are the best, the most durable, and can be purchased for very little money.

†Maggie Rollo Nussdorf and Stern B. Nussdorf. *Dress for Health: The New Clothes Consciousness*. Harrisburg, PA: Stackpole, 1980, pp. 62–63.

‡When consulting with any medical or health professional (chiropractor, exercise physiologist, acupuncturist, physical therapist, trainer, phys. ed. teacher, doctor, fitness instructor, etc.), find out what their views on physical activity are and how much they know about it. A negative attitude may result in their being of little use or support to you. Try to do this when you call to make an appointment. "Sports medicine" is becoming more sophisticated at last (and more expensive), but get more than one opinion for anything serious. No matter whose advice you take, *always experiment carefully on your own—you know your body better than they ever will.*

Jean Raisler

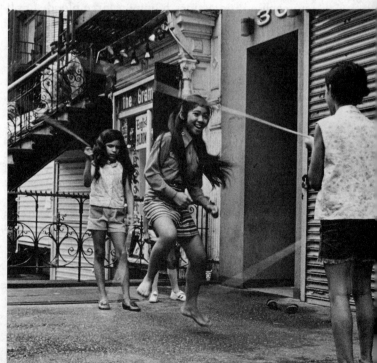

---

*Bonnie Parkhouse and Jackie Lapin. *Women Who Win: Exercising Your Rights in Sports*. Englewood Cliffs, NJ: Prentice-Hall, Inc., 1980, p. 19.

†*Ibid.*, p. 21.

‡Some states, like California, have further refined the rules with a state athletic code which regulates student teams, all-boys teams, all-girls teams and coed teams. (*Ibid.*, pp. 49 and ff.) For more on this and Title 9 in general, see also *Out of the Bleachers*, Stephanie Twin, ed. Old Westbury, NY: Feminist Press, 1979.

lems—heart disease, high blood pressure—may not be symptomatic, and some types of exercise may aggravate them.

For every form of exercise, start slowly and build up, in general and during each session. Muscle growth comes from pushing each muscle involved slightly beyond what you forced it to the previous time. Stretching for flexibility is based on the same principle. Take care. When you're cold, stiff or out of shape you can tear a ligament or tendon (which can take a long time to heal) or permanently damage a muscle by driving it too violently or for too long. If you want to get into an activity that puts a lot of stress on joints, be sure that the surrounding muscles are strong (and coordinated) enough to support them; otherwise there will be trouble. Work up to exercising at least several times a week for at least twenty minutes. A once-in-a-while basketball-shooting spree or fling on the living room rug is of no benefit and could be dangerous. Make sure the equipment you use is in good shape.

Taper off any period of vigorous exercise slowly. Never flop down after an energetic run, for example, without some transitional activity, such as walking. You need time for your heartbeat, breathing and temperature to adjust; you need to keep your blood flowing well in order to remove the wastes that have accumulated in the muscles during the run and bring them fresh supplies of oxygen and glucose. Sudden relaxation may make you dizzy and nauseous.

Don't linger outside if you have been exercising in the cold—that will cause undue stiffness. Put something warm on. A hot bath or shower is ideal (after your circulation has returned to normal): it will relax your body, keep your blood flow up and wash away the sweat. A hot bath before exercising will increase flexibility. In hot weather, be reasonable. Acclimatize yourself and watch out for dehydration.

Don't eat heavily before or after exercising. The stomach and intestines require a large blood supply to digest food, and exercise diverts blood from the digestive tract to the muscles you're using. These organs' attempts to function actively with less blood than they need may cause pain. For most people exercise decreases appetite. Make sure when you do eat to include a variety of healthy foods (see Chapter 2, "Food") to meet the demands of greater physical activity. If you participate in endurance sports, eat more carbohydrates. Don't worry about extra salt unless you eat no animal products of any kind, but be sure to get enough potassium and iron. Drink plenty of water, especially if you are sweating and/or the weather is hot or cold. Cut down on junk food, cigarettes, alcohol and drugs. For women who are using exercise to help lose weight, remember that aerobic activities are the ones that "burn up" the most calories.*

Get enough rest. You may need more when you start working your body harder. Or you may find exercising gives you more energy!

Expect some stiffness. If you're really pushing your muscles they're bound to hurt the following day(s). But don't pamper yourself and stop. The best remedy is moderate exercise: this will increase circulation which will help carry away the accumulated lactic acid causing the stiffness. Moist heat and massage applied to the sore muscle(s) are helpful as relaxants and they also increase blood flow, bringing fresh nutrients and speeding waste removal. As you keep exercising, your body will gradually become accustomed to working harder and the discomfort will disappear. Alternate hard and easy days.

INJURIES

Occasionally you will stretch the ligaments of a joint too far, maybe even tear them (a sprain) or pull a muscle or a tendon in much the same way (a strain). Unless the injury is severe, you can treat it yourself. As we get more in touch with our bodies we are often able to sense what we can heal by ourselves and what needs professional help. For a sprain, elevate and rest the injured part, applying cold immediately and for the next twenty-four to seventy-two hours. This minimizes pain and swelling. At the end of this period you can switch to moist heat. Begin gentle movement as soon as possible; when you are ready to start full-scale exercising again, bind it evenly (not too tight) for support and go easy. If in the meantime you are climbing the walls, be physical with the rest of your body; swimming might be a possibility, for example.

Back trauma is not nearly as easy to deal with. The advice of doctors is so contradictory (they continue to push complete inactivity, drugs and surgery) that women are forming groups to provide emotional support, to figure out where the problem lies, and to share information on how to get relief from pain and on the best ways to promote healing. Back care really means a commitment to overall health through good posture, nutrition, relaxation and sensible but invigorating exercise.

Many headaches and nervous stomachs and much fatigue come from tension, boredom or depression. They can usually be driven off by some exhilarating activity, but any time you are "not yourself," take care. Lack of concentration for physical (a fever or over-tiredness, for example) or psychological (anxiety over

---

*See *Exercise and Your Heart* for a good list of the most com-

mon activities and the calories they consume per hour. (Many exercise books will include this information, too.) Note that these figures are only *averages*—each person is different—and that you should subtract from these numbers the number of calories you would spend doing what you would be doing if you were not exercising.

a personal problem, for example) reasons are injury-prone times.*

CONCLUSION

In the end we must deal with some depressing but up-front questions for the eighties. Will we lose the few decent facilities we've got? Will girls' school sports be budget-cut to death? Will women's competitive moneymaking sports continue to be almost all white? Will we let men convince us again that none of this matters because we've never had what it takes anyway? Will the national and state governments allow big business to pollute the air so badly that we won't be able to play and exercise outdoors? Will the ulti-mate chemical spill in the sky (or on the ground) end it all?

No! Working together we will hold the line and win back what we have lost. We will have a recreation center in every neighborhood where people of both sexes and all races will share the space equally. We will demand that our jobs be restructured in ways that are constructive for us physically and mentally. We will see to it that jogging is safe any time of the day or night. Our kids will grow up healthy with outstanding gym programs in decent public schools. Working together we will help to create a time when the spirit of the land is people before profit. But we must begin now to fight for it with the energy that comes from strong yet relaxed bodies and minds, with love and respect for each other and ourselves.

*What to Do About Athletic Injuries by Thomas Fahey (New York: Butterick, 1974). Both Fahey's and Kraus's book, Backache, Stress and Tension (previously cited), are useful for the prevention and care of injuries.

5

HEALTH AND HEALING: ALTERNATIVES TO MEDICAL CARE

By Pamela Berger and Nancy P. Hawley, with Jane Pincus

With special thanks to Rose Dobosz, Jon Kabat-Zinn, Pamela Pacelli, Billie Pivnik and Susan Reverby

Many women today are excited by a compelling range of alternative healing methods which complement and challenge conventional medicine and broaden our options for health care. Some alternative methods currently practiced, like massage, herbal medicine and visualization, are traditional female healing practices in use for centuries. Women have used them in their simplest forms, soothing and caring for members of their families and communities, applying herb poultices to wounds, assisting one another during labor and birth, attending to people through long illnesses and handing this knowledge down from mother to daughter.[1] In our culture a cool washcloth for a headache, a massage for an aching back or a kiss to a child's bruised knee are simple examples of how we communicate positive healing energy; our confidence that we can "make it better" has a calming effect. The very fact that people think generously and kindly toward others is an important step in the healing process.

I think in terms of chicken soup and ice cubes. As a child I felt so reassured when my mother or grandmother cared for me. I felt so good lying in bed. The power of mother as healer, the oldest mode of care, can't be transformed into the setting of a doctor's office.

MEDICINE

Grandma sleeps with
my sick
        grand-
pa so she
can get him
during the night
medicine
to stop
  the pain

    In
the morning
  clumsily
     I
wake
  them

Her eyes
look at me
from under-
        neath
his withered
arm

  The
medicine
is all
  in
her long
un-
   braided
     hair.

Alice Walker [1968]

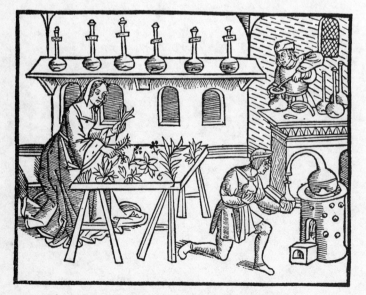

A late Medieval woodcut of an abbess as pharmacist
(from *A History of Women in Medicine*, K.C. Hurd-Mead)

Other alternative healing methods, like acupuncture and yoga, are practices from distant cultures. Some of us are using these methods alone, others in combination with conventional medicine. They can help us stay healthy when we are well, cure some illnesses and enable us to live more comfortably with diseases for which there are no known cures. The alternatives have often helped where the conventional methods of drugs and/or surgery could not. Finding and using these alternative approaches has given us insights into their possibilities, powers and limitations.

We can learn to practice some alternative approaches ourselves with the help of books and knowledgeable friends. We can go further by apprenticing to teachers and practitioners and, in some cases, studying more formally by taking courses and teaching. Or sometimes we find one or two methods helpful at certain times in our lives, use them, and go on without having or wanting to use them again.

UNDERLYING ASSUMPTIONS OF ALTERNATIVE HEALING APPROACHES

Alternative modes have become incorporated into the current practice of "wholistic" health. Wholistic health is based both on the idea that the body, mind and spirit form an integrated whole and on an understanding of the connectedness of the individual to her environment, her community and her world.

Alternative or wholistic approaches to healing are based on certain underlying assumptions: first, that we are healthy when our body/mind/spirit exist in a dynamically balanced state of well-being. Though we are physically made up of cells, tissues, organs, etc., no parts of us can be understood as isolated entities; all interconnected, they are harmoniously related.

Second, we have a great capacity for self-healing. Our cells are always engaged in the process of self-renewal, for our bodies continuously break down and build up structures, with tissues and organs replacing their cells in an ongoing process (with the exception of brain cells). We experience the physical body repairing itself in many ways, as, for instance, when scraped skin heals itself in a few days, or when the eye tears and washes away a foreign particle. In addition, we may consciously use the mind to focus healing energies on those aspects of our being that are hurt or feel unbalanced, or, we can use physical touch, as with massage, to help us relax, release tension and relieve pain. Part of our role in the healing process is to secure the information and support we need to enable us to return to a state of ease.

Third, in the broadest sense, our interactions with our family, community and world affect and shape our health. Positive, loving, supportive relationships with our family and friends help us keep healthy and give us opportunities to nurture and heal others and to receive love and nurturance which strengthen us. Our health also depends on our larger social, economic, political and ecological environment, which affects us through the nutritional content of our foods, the potential dangers of the various products we buy and are exposed to, the energy sources we use, the air we breathe and particularly the financial and educational resources available to us. It is as crucial to try to achieve a balance between the individual and her surroundings as it is to balance body, mind and spirit.*[2]

Implicit in these premises is a particular way of defining healing and of thinking about how healing takes place. Though it is often important and sometimes necessary to seek help from practitioners, they are not responsible for healing us.

"Healing comes from within. Every culture evolves a set of remedies that are given for dis-ease: some are thought to "cure," while others comfort, take away pain, overcome dysfunction or disability....But no remedy, in and of itself, will restore good health."[3]

We ourselves play a significant role in making the treatment work through our willingness to be healed. While sound health practices can promote well-being and be a source of pleasure in their own right, they do not guarantee longevity or freedom from illness.

Though the words "heal" and "cure" are often used interchangeably, they are not synonymous. Sometimes no cures exist for particular diseases, yet people feel "healed," i.e., able to reconcile themselves, accept and live with the effects of asthma, polio or even a terminal illness. Illness can provide opportunities for self-examination, growth and change, as seen in the experiences of the following two women:

I was in my forty-fourth year when I began experiencing what I called "fatigue." Weeks of "good nights' rest" did not change my stiffness and pain on arising. I had a three-year-old daughter, two teenage sons, a husband and a part-time job; I loved them all; I had no time to be sick or feel pain. When I found myself holding the wall as well as the banister to creep down the stairs one step at a time, I had to admit to myself that something was wrong. My wrists and fingers hurt; my elbows, knees and ankles; my back, legs and neck. An orthopedic surgeon told me that I had osteoarthritis.

Now I had to allow myself the luxury of time for ex-

*For example, Joanna Macy, a teacher, meditation instructor and organizer for social change, believes that deep despair about nuclear war keeps many of us from working effectively against it. She runs workshops in which people go through the process of acknowledging this despair with each other and feeling it as fully as possible. As a result, many become reenergized, reconnect with others and are moved to greater commitment and social action.

ercise classes; a regime of exercise and aspirin soon made life more possible. I still only resentfully recognized that I probably would never be completely pain-free again, would never again feel that careless strength and flexibility which so informed my body in my first forty years. And for the last four years serious back problems have prevented my exercising as I used to; now I must more often live with pain. Some days the distance from car to store or bed to bathroom seems the longest and most painful ten miles I could ever walk. Nevertheless, some days are better than others. I have learned to rest on the bad days, and to insist on some daily rest even on the good days. Good physical therapy is helping my back; I may be able to return soon to exercise.

Most important, in seeking to understand why I denied the pain so adamantly when I first felt it, I entered therapy and learned how forcefully I had been denying emotional pain. My life is qualitatively different now—and better, even though lived with pain—as a result of my reevaluation of how I feel about myself, my goals, and my relations with others.

In the words of a woman who has since died of cancer:

A lot of people think dying suddenly in their sleep is a great blessing. I've realized that all I learn while dying is important; dying suddenly would be like reading a good book and leaving out a very important part. I'm not for exaggerating: of course I do take pills to make myself more comfortable...but I don't feel pain is wrong. I don't feel it's out of the flow. It's hard—like childbirth.

Many alternative methods present healing as taking place with the help of some form of energy, coming from a source within ourselves; from both within and without; or from a god or universal being: feeling connected to a "being within and beyond" through prayer, meditation or the laying on of hands can tap a life-enhancing flow of energy which helps the healing process.

As the acute stage of my asthma passes, I relax and further ease my breathing, reduce wheezing by feeling warmth and light flow through me, part of an energy I imagine to be universal energy of which we are all a part. As I am able to breathe fully again, I picture myself giving that energy back into the larger cosmos. In a concrete way this interchange enables me once again to be available to family, friends and co-workers.

I want to pray, but I don't believe in God. I'm going to pray "To whom it may concern"!

SOME PROBLEMS WITH ALTERNATIVE METHODS AND PRACTITIONERS

While the perspective common to many alternative modes of healing would seem to promise us a richer way of practicing health care than does the conventional medical system, alternative practices and practitioners have some of the same drawbacks.

Limited Availability

The majority of the alternatives discussed below are available only to relatively few people. Most can be found only in large cities, and they are often expensive. Insurance companies and government aid, which provide low- and moderate-income people with access to the costly medical system, discriminate against many who choose nonmedical alternatives. Some alternative practices may have started out as informal, low-budget enterprises but often, in the process of making themselves "legitimate" and acceptable to insurance companies, they become more professional, hierarchical and expensive. Insurance companies also require licensing, which means that many compassionate, highly skilled but unlicensed practitioners are excluded from coverage. As a result, many wholistic alternatives are available mainly to middle- and upper-middle-class people.

Risks of Professionalization

Just as with conventional medicine, you can learn a lot from professionals who have crucial information you need to stay well. However, we live in a time of excessive dependence on experts, which means we often turn to professionals for things that they are not trained to do or that we could do better for ourselves. Some alternative practitioners, like conventional doctors, are setting themselves up as experts in such a way that they keep power for themselves, are unwilling to share their knowledge with you and try to get you to keep returning to them for additional services.

Lack of Social and Political Awareness

When wholistic alternatives identify the locus of healing only in the individual, as medical practice does, they disregard political and social factors like poverty and racism as major sources of ill health. For instance, a practitioner might prescribe rest, exercise and change in diet, and not attend to the fact that the problem is caused by a dangerous on-the-job situation. All practitioners should be aware of the social causes of illness.

Blaming the Victim

Implicit in the practice of alternative healing is that you have a certain responsibility for keeping yourself healthy and for helping yourself get better. While trust in our capacity for self-healing is a welcome change from medicine's dependence upon outside intervention, some writers and practitioners of wholistic health place *too much* emphasis on the individual's responsibility for her own sickness and health. They seem to imply that if you get sick or if you don't get well, it's your fault—your "wrong thinking," lack of will, personality defect (i.e., a "cancer personality") or insufficient faith in the practitioner. From several books on wholistic health:

We should not fool ourselves into thinking that disease is caused by an enemy from without. We are responsible for our disease.[4]

Health and happiness *can* be ours if we desire: we can create our personal reality, down to the finest detail.[5]

The only tyrant you face is your own inertia and absence of will—your belief that you are too busy to take your own well-being into your own hands and that the pursuit of self-health through a wellness-promotive lifestyle is too hard, complicated or inconvenient.[6]

This kind of thinking again disregards political and social factors. And sometimes, no matter how much we try to stay healthy, we become ill. It is both cruel and useless to blame ourselves or let others blame us for getting sick.

Sexism

"Alternative" does not automatically mean nonsexist or feminist. Like conventional medicine, these methods originated in male-dominated cultures. At present the leading practitioners in most of these methods are men; both male and female practitioners may treat women disrespectfully, even harmfully.

Possible Ineffectiveness

Sometimes alternatives provide no more help than conventional medicine. They can also be harmful and outright dangerous when practiced by "quacks." Just as the vast majority of medical therapies have not been evaluated in terms of effectiveness and safety, it is also true that few alternatives have been adequately tested in comparison with no treatment.

CHOOSING ALTERNATIVE METHODS AND PRACTITIONERS

Keeping both the advantages and limitations of alternative practices in mind, we can formulate guidelines for choosing and using practices and practitioners.

- Speak to other people who have been helped by a certain practice. Be sure to ask about the particular practitioner they used. Ask about negative as well as positive experiences with both method and practitioner.
- Seek out other women in your community who are also interested in getting information about how to approach and heal a certain illness. Together you may be able to form a research group. Get your local library to order books pertinent to your interests and to subscribe to women's health and wholistic health publications. These resources may help you evaluate the use of a particular method for your health problem.
- Call some of the national boards and information services listed at the end of this chapter. They may be able to tell you whether or not they think their approach is effective for your problem, and they may be able to recommend practitioners in your area.
- Call local practitioners of these approaches to healing. Ask if they treat your specific condition. Ask about free consultations. It's also a good idea to ask them for names of other people with a similar problem whom they have treated.
- It may be important to you to know whether the method you want to use is based in any way on a sexist philosophy; whether it is organized hierarchically, dominated by white males with patriarchal attitudes toward women; whether it excludes or limits women or minority practitioners or clients; whether it is responsive to community needs (e.g., offering free classes, located near public transportation and in a building that is wheelchair accessible).

The best practitioners do not emphasize the "conquest" of disease, but see themselves as facilitating the healing process and helping you maintain your health. It is important to find someone with whom you feel comfortable, who works in partnership with you and whose ideas make sense to you. Ideally you should come away from each and every encounter feeling more confident in your ability to promote the healing process in yourself and supplied with the tools you need to make changes in your life.

- Good practitioners need to listen carefully to you and be interested in the particular ways you present your health concerns. Together, try various possibilities until you hit upon the one which makes you feel better. Expect practitioners to be willing to teach you the skills you need to maintain or improve your health.
- Good practitioners must be well trained in their own healing methods. While a license or training

certificate indicates a certain amount of knowledge and standardized training, no piece of paper ever guarantees a person's ability to heal. The system of licensure itself has drawbacks, among them that licensing requires attendance at expensive professional schools. Many people develop excellent skills by apprenticing to other practitioners.

- If your practitioner is in training, make sure that s/he receives supervision from someone more experienced.
- You may want to look for practitioners who have sliding fee scales or who are willing to barter services. Often practitioners are able to charge less when, as part of a group, they receive a salary (rather than a fee-for-service arrangement) and share expenses with others.
- Practitioners should be knowledgeable about other approaches to healing and willing to refer you to other practitioners if necessary. Beware of practitioners who think their treatment is the only good one.
- You may often want to combine the least invasive of modern medical diagnostic techniques with the best that a healing method has to offer. It's important to look for practitioners who are open to any information you may bring from conventional medicine, and who will evaluate it with you and with any consultants they might need.
- Beware of practitioners who offer miraculous cures. Even though you want definite answers, don't accept promises of magic any more than you would from medical practitioners. Occasionally immediate and dramatic results do occur, but many alternative methods of healing require time and patience.
- Scrupulously avoid practitioners who directly or indirectly blame you for getting sick or not responding to treatment. They may be more concerned with their reputations than your well-being.
- Good practitioners should be especially sensitive to the larger social, political and economic issues which affect women's health.

We need to keep talking with one another, checking out, evaluating and reevaluating methods and practitioners. By doing so, we can make sure that they continue to be viable alternatives for us.

I asked my friends for recommendations for a yoga teacher and several suggested one man. When I went to meet him, a voice inside me told me this man was not the teacher for me. I said to myself, "I really want to do yoga; this teacher has been highly recommended; perhaps it's because I don't get along well with men." But that voice kept saying, "I don't want to." I contemplated the matter by sitting down, closing my eyes and just being quiet. The thought kept rolling through my mind, getting stronger and more persistent: This is not the right teacher for me. I dropped the idea of studying yoga with him.

In general, be as informed and assertive as you can. Balance the isolation of the one-on-one therapeutic encounter by joining or forming self-help groups of women who share your health problem or who want to learn more about the method. Work in whatever ways you can for changes which would make the alternative healing methods available to more people (e.g., suggesting that your practitioner adopt a sliding scale, pressing your insurance company to cover alternatives). There are many sincere, skillful, compassionate alternative practitioners and healers. We must look for them, ask them to share their skills with us, tell our friends about them and find ways of using them without becoming unnecessarily dependent upon them.

ALTERNATIVE METHODS

In this section we describe some alternative healing methods and give information and guidelines so that you can look further on your own. Since so many alternatives exist and since we have to select a sampling of what you might find, we chose those most generally useful, most widely available and most familiar to us.

When you use alternatives for the first time you may have to change habits—the way you eat, the way you move, even the way you think about things. It is best to learn as much as you can about the method you choose. Understanding the terms the practitioner uses—jargon, as in conventional medicine, often is mystifying—can make you a more active participant in your care.

If you are used to going to conventional doctors, it may feel strange to try something new. Family, friends and acquaintances can sometimes make it tougher by telling you that what you are doing is weird.

I tripped on the sidewalk and hurt myself so badly that I couldn't walk or work. I was taken to the hospital and had X-rays. The head orthopedist looked at the X-rays and told me that there was nothing wrong with my foot. But I still couldn't walk. At that point I decided to see a chiropractor. I didn't know anything about chiropractors except that they were an alternative to medical doctors. My sister was the only one I knew who had used a chiropractor.

When I went to the hospital to pick up my X-rays, I told them I was going to visit a certain chiropractor. "Don't go to him; he's a Communist," they said.

"I don't care what his political beliefs are if he can help me," I answered.

I made an appointment and after he adjusted my back and foot I could walk again in comfort.

Doing something new can feel strange.

I went for my first massage to a good friend's house where she did massages in a warm room with a special table. I took off all my clothes and even though I knew her well I felt very naked. I was surprised to feel so exposed.

Many women, not wanting to leave the medical-care system entirely but finding that it does not meet their needs for preventive "whole person" care, are learning to combine alternative approaches with conventional ones.

How do I integrate different health-care models in my life? I go to MDs mostly, but I understand their limits. I've done "talk" therapy and get (and give) massages. I take baths for aching muscles—water relaxes. Once in a while I experiment with herbs. I think about the food I eat, take some vitamins and have done some work with the Alexander Technique, which has helped chronic back and shoulder aches. I take my baby to doctors sooner than I take myself. Mainly I need sleep!

Here are some ways that people we know have combined methods.

- To monitor a child's health: well-baby checkups with a family practitioner, nutritional information from reading, discussions with other parents.
- Chronic back pain: diagnostic X-rays, chiropractic adjustments, appropriate exercise and nutritional supplements, household help and childcare from friends and women's groups.
- For profuse and erratic bleeding around the time of menopause: acupuncture, Vitamin A, figuring out when bleeding occurs (especially at times of stress), endometrial biopsy or D and C.
- Insomnia: diet changes, meditation, more exercise, psychotherapy, massage by friends, tryptophan (an amino acid naturally occurring in milk and certain other proteins), soporific herbal teas, occasional use of sleeping medications.
- Asthma: diet changes, massage, yoga, acupuncture treatments, psychotherapy, meditation, bronchial dilators, talking with family and friends.
- Cancer: diet changes, meditation and visualization, radiation therapy, chemotherapy, surgery, being able to talk about hopes, fears and worries with family and friends.
- Inoperable brain tumor: drugs, diet changes, yoga, meditation, psychotherapy, discussions with family and friends about feelings and treatment, radiation therapy.

Just as there is no one right way to keep healthy, there is no one right way of healing or acceptable path to follow. Bringing ourselves back into balance can mean something as simple as treating a cold by resting or as complex as totally altering our diet and other life habits to cope with severe chronic illness such as hypertension or arthritis. A method may work for one person or health problem but not for another. Some-

times it is possible to figure out which approach helps the most; at other times it is not so clear. We have to evaluate and make decisions about each situation as it comes up; our own experience and intuition and the wisdom of trusted friends, family members, teachers and professionals will be our best guides.

Meditation

Meditation gives us the opportunity to be with ourselves. A simple definition of meditation is "the intentional paying of attention from moment to moment." In the words of a woman who has been meditating and teaching meditation for fifteen years:

Meditation in its essence is different from every other human activity, but its essence is contained in every activity. Meditating, each one of us touches base with our deepest concerns, with the truth of our aliveness.... You could say it is acknowledging the radiant core of our being...our godliness, our buddha nature, or whatever you like to call it—speaking out.

Meditating at its best doesn't remove us from living, numb us to stressful situations or stop us from acting effectively. It puts us in touch with the moment and helps us respond directly. If we have meditated recently we are more likely to be alert and resourceful when we are called upon to help someone.

People begin to meditate for different reasons—because it feels good in itself or because they want to feel calm, to diminish physical or mental stress or pain or to get through a spiritual crisis. You might approach meditation only for practical reasons—to relax or reduce stress—and then discover that something happens that makes you want to go deeper, to attain a different level of consciousness.

Although meditation practices have been directly or indirectly related to healing for millennia,[7] only in the last two decades have health practitioners in this country understood its potential and begun teaching people to use it for a variety of specific conditions. Meditation helps us slow down breathing and heart rate, reduce oxygen consumption, lessen muscular tension, change brain-wave patterns and respond calmly to stressful situations, thereby lowering the risk of having a heart attack or a stroke.[8]

There are many ways to meditate. Though you can meditate while you stand, walk, dance or jog, many people sit or kneel in a quiet environment. You can sit on a cushion with your legs crossed or tucked under you or on a chair with your feet on the ground. Repeating a word or sound over and over again can calm your mind; concentrating on your breathing can help focus your attention. You can meditate at home indoors or outdoors, or in formal settings—churches, synagogues, zendos, ashrams and other places of worship. You can practice alone or with others in a common meeting place.

Like many women, I spent my whole life doing things for others, and looking to others for a definition of who I am. I've been successful in living this way but the price was high—constant anxiety over whether I would succeed or fail not only others but my own exacting standards as well. I turned to meditation as a way to help me feel good. It really helps to be with others in my meditation group who are committed to the same inner journey.

You might feel best learning meditation practice by yourself, or you might want a religious or secular teacher to guide you and discuss your progress and problems with you along the way. However, if you expect to rely on a teacher to provide answers or a group to offer prescriptions for living, you're on the wrong track.

The role model of women was really questionable in the group I belonged to. The hierarchy was composed of men, and the leader set the standards for behavior. Women were expected to play traditional and outdated roles. I objected to the lack of morality and to people not taking responsibility for their actions. For instance, heavy drinking and sexual promiscuity were encouraged, while closeness with one other person was not. Yet the whole meditation practice of being with yourself was inspiring and wonderful.

The group provided a lot of security, especially during times of transition in my life. I felt less alone. But it was a bit of a cop-out because the group presented a single view of the world, one that was unaccepting of other perspectives.

Since I left the group I have felt more balanced and better able to cope with making decisions in my life. While the group dynamics were distressing to me, the experience of meditation has helped me pull my life together.

When properly practiced, meditation can help us pull our lives together.

My early-morning meditation is part silence, part chanting. Sometimes I actively pray while I sit looking out the window at the rising sun. It's important for me to meditate every morning, if only for ten minutes, to touch base with myself. I am continually surprised at how I get upset more easily on the days I don't meditate. Sometimes during the day when I'm silent or alone I find myself automatically feeling the tranquility I experience during meditation. This calmness helps me. Though usually my meditations are rather ordinary, on some days they are profound.

Visualization*

We all create images in our minds, sometimes consciously, sometimes without being aware of it. We picture how we would like a future event to turn out or how we want our relationships to change. Images fill our dreams; some of them last into the next day.

David and I made love last night beautifully, ecstatically, delicately. Then I dreamed about creating a strong, beautiful simple child? Jewel? I held it in my hand. And woke this morning perfectly content. So rare.

Positive images make us happy and carry us through difficult times.

Many women are finding that visualizing a certain symbol, scene or process has a positive healing effect on their bodies. Midwives have long used images and relaxation exercises to help women in labor relax, diminish fear or tension and open up. The earliest records of visualization techniques used in healing date back to Babylonia and Sumeria; other ancient peoples used these techniques as well.[9] In our day, Canadian Eskimos, Navajo Indians and some Hispanic peoples (to mention only a few) use forms of healing based on visualization.[10] Placebos (substances with no known pharmacological action) can profoundly affect the course of a disease. People using a placebo often get better just because they *believe in it*—the pills, charm,

*Though visualization is now being used for everything from decreasing drug dependence to the improvement of athletic ability, we concentrate on visualization used in conjunction with meditation to help heal specific conditions.

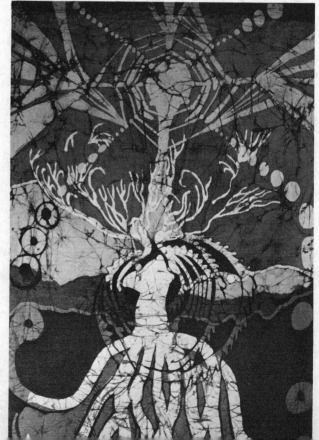

talisman or ritual. Perhaps one way placebos work is by helping the person visualize herself as healing; perhaps the placebo itself represents a visible symbol of healing.

Visualization works in a general way by helping people relax. We can also use visualization techniques to affect the involuntary systems of the body, increasing blood flow to one particular area or slowing down the heartbeat. We can also use visual images to help minimize or control pain.[11] In the words of a scientist who had several operations for cancer:

The two years since I've had the last operation have been the most productive of my life. I've had the opportunity to investigate healing in a way that I never did before. At first, when I felt the pain, I kept looking for an outside figure, a god figure to help me, to care for me, to make it better. Then I said to myself, "Who's the most caring, best mother you know?" And I said, "I am." So I pictured myself cuddling myself. When the pain came, I went to it as a mother would to a child. I said, "How can I help it? How can I go to it?" Now when it comes, I say, "Poor baby." I tried to treat myself in a loving way. The more loving I was to myself, the more healed I felt. Now the pain is mostly gone.

Visualization involves relaxing, feeling at one with the object, scene or process you imagine, letting it expand to fill your consciousness and become the only thing in your awareness. Hold your mind upon it. Sometimes it helps to have someone guide you. Some people must practice this meditative visualization; it is a skill to be learned. Others do it more quickly.

An example of a healing visualization:

Relax and let your attention go to the particular body part causing discomfort or pain, or which does not function as it should. Focus your attention on this place and let yourself experience what it feels like right now. Don't feel pressured to achieve a specific goal. After a while, allow an image related to that area to come to your mind. It may be a detailed picture of what you think that part looks like, or it may be more abstract. Keep your mind focused until you are content with your image. Change it whenever you want. Now begin to visualize something happening within that part of your body to make it work better or start to heal. You might see energy, light or color flowing into it; imagine it becoming warm or cool. A powerful image could help you feel better right away.[12]

If visualization doesn't work, it may mean that you take in information in other ways than by using images—you might do it through your ears, so imagining sounds might be your way of "visualizing"; you might do it in terms of movement or spatial relations or touch. The possibilities are endless.

Autogenic training is the most fully researched and widely applied visualization method used for healing.[13] It uses a series of visualization exercises to en-

able people to regulate their bodies and keep them in balance.[14] To learn this particular visualization method, you need guidance from a knowledgeable practitioner. Once you have learned the exercises, you can practice on your own and teach others as well.

You can do these exercises lying or sitting in a relaxed position with eyes closed. Imagine you are in "mental contact" with the part of your body you are concentrating on, without feeling pressured to achieve a specific goal. In the first exercise, concentrate on a feeling of heaviness in your arms and legs, and repeat to yourself a phrase such as "My right [left] leg [arm] is heavy." After you focus on the specific limb, generalize the heaviness to all limbs and visualize a peaceful scene at the same time. The heaviness exercise can create a state of deep relaxation. In the second exercise, concentrate on the sensation of warmth in your extremities. This exercise is supposed to increase peripheral blood flow and relax blood vessels. In the third exercise, repeat a sentence like "My heartbeat is calm and regular," which can help regulate the beating of the heart. In the fourth exercise, repeat, "My breathing is calm and regular," an exercise intended to promote slow, deep, regular breathing. In the fifth exercise, repeat, "My solar plexus is warm," a sentence which can calm the central nervous sytem, facilitating sleep and increasing blood flow to the abdomen. If, however, you have certain abdominal conditions, such as ulcers, use a more generalized sentence like "My stomach is healed," because increased blood flow to the stomach could possibly make the ulcers worse. In this and other conditions, a practitioner might omit one of the sentences or phrases because focusing on a particular area would produce an undesirable effect; for instance, if you have an irregular heartbeat, the practitioner might not ask you to focus on your heartbeat; or if you are pregnant, the practitioner would have you omit the sentence, "My solar plexus is warm." The last overall calming exercise is the repetition of the words "My forehead is cool" or "The wind is blowing over my forehead."

While autogenic training is widespread in Europe, more and more practitioners, particularly psychologists, are now using it in this country in "stress management" programs or in conjunction with helping people deal with anything from a life crisis such as the death of a family member to problems such as stage fright. In coordination with drugs and surgery, autogenic training can help us heal specific organs, or conditions such as ulcers, gastritis, gallbladder attacks, irritated colon, hemorrhoids, constipation, angina, headaches, asthma, diabetes, arthritis, low back pain, skin conditions and thyroid disease.[15] Results vary with the condition and with the person using the exercises. Anyone using autogenic training for a specific disease must first find a physician to diagnose the condition. Autogenic practitioners should watch whether/how the practice of these visualization exer-

Batik by Jane Pincus. One visual image: a strongly rooted tree

cises changes your disease or affects your particular problem.

Cancer specialists are experimenting with visualization and autogenic training in conjunction with drugs, surgery and radiation,[16] and they are designing visualization exercises to affect the cancer patient's attitude toward living and dying, as well as to alleviate the stress of the disease. Even more exciting, these early experiments suggest that meditation and visualization techniques may help us change the immune system and therefore the body's response to cancer as well.[17]

Biofeedback

Over the last decade lay people and practitioners have begun to use machines to help us monitor the ways we can influence our supposedly involuntary systems. Electronic devices connected to the body through wires and electrodes monitor certain physiological processes such as heart rate, muscle tension or brain waves, and convert them into signals which you observe on a screen or hear as a beep or sustained tone. (Smaller, simpler devices exist which you can hold in your hand and use at home.) The sight or sound of the signal, indicating the rate or intensity of the process, encourages you to control it voluntarily. People use this technique to bring a variety of responses under control: heart rate, blood pressure, hand temperature, muscle tension, brain and sweat gland activity, genital responses, stomach motility, etc.[18] It can help us deal with such diverse conditions as tension or migraine headaches, hypertension, insomnia, rapid heart rate, asthma and pain. For example, if you have Raynaud's disease (excessively cold hands caused by reduced blood flow) and go to a biofeedback session, the practitioner will explain how physiological conditions caused the symptoms, describe how to use the electronic thermometer and suggest general strategies you can use to regulate your internal activity and warm your hands. Suggestions often include relaxation and visualization techniques. In the early sessions s/he will adjust the machinery to register even small changes in the desired direction, indicating success. After you learn how to warm your hands with the machinery, you can practice without it at home. Training sessions take place from once a week to daily, and last from thirty to sixty minutes apiece for periods ranging from one week to three months or more. Insofar as you continue to practice the exercises, you continue to have increased control of the temperature of your hands.

Encouragement and good coaching are important. Be wary of anyone who sticks you in a room, hooks you up to a machine and then leaves you alone; if you have contracted for guided biofeedback therapy, see that you get it. Bring a friend along with you to observe the practitioner and the process. The experience may be useful to her or him as well as to you.

Though some people are put off by machines, biofeedback does convincingly indicate that we can indeed alter specific biological processes. Skilled biofeedback practitioners can teach people eventually to regulate their "involuntary" processes without the use of machines. They warn that overdependence on the machine can actually limit the application of your newly learned control. In other words, the machine simply teaches you a level of self-mastery you didn't have before.

Because of the cost of the machinery, biofeedback clinics and practitioners are usually based in hospitals. Though some physicians have tried to limit this technology to physicians only, well-trained nurses and psychologists can also teach you the skills you need to know.

Massage

Touching is one of the most natural ways we have to communicate and to comfort one another. Whether it's with a simple hug or a complete body rub, we can help one another feel better.

Foot rubs are my favorite kind of massage. They bring back childhood memories of my father rubbing my feet; they feel so good to give and to get. My children often ask me to hold and rub their feet when I go into their rooms to say good night. Some of my friends and I exchange them as a way of being close and helping each other relax.

When done effectively, massage relaxes the body, releases muscle tension, improves joint flexibility, increases circulation and sensation and generally enhances our well-being. We can use many massage

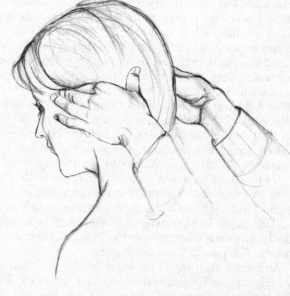

Christine Bondante

techniques on ourselves as well as on others.

When you have the following conditions do not get a massage: phlebitis, skin disease, blood clots, redness or contusions and infections. Skin that has become thin due to burn or injury should not be massaged either.

You don't need any special training to do general massage. Just get into a comfortable position and begin. Hold your friend's foot, head, hand, back, neck, shoulders. Ask her where she wants pressure, whether you are applying too much pressure or not enough. With your thumb or whole hand,* find and rub tender areas or sore spots. Alternate gentle stroking with deep kneading and use visualization, too, if you want to help the person relax even more. Avoid direct pressure on the spinal column; instead, press on either side. Breathe regularly and deeply while giving the massage.

Many people who do massage see themselves as channeling energy through their bodies and hands to heal their family, friends and, if they are masseuses, their clients.

The massage methods most familiar to Westerners are Esalen and Swedish (generally whole-body, sometimes using deep pressure), the more specialized Shiatsu and acupressure. Acupressure practitioners apply pressure with their fingers to energy points along the same meridians (the pathways of "energy" in the body) used for acupuncture treatments; likewise, people who do Shiatsu concentrate on putting pressure on a particular sequence of points on the meridians, relieving tension in specific muscle systems. Most practitioners combine techniques from several methods. Some masseuses incorporate the techniques of polarity therapy[19] or deep breathing and visualization.[20] Others use reflexology points and focus attention on feet[21] or hands. Still others include insights gained from bioenergetics or psychotherapy practices. A masseuse said:

The way *you touch someone is more important than the actual system you use. Whether you see yourself as channeling energy or are concerned with the muscle tone in your body and how you communicate it to someone else, you have to be rooted in your own body and pay attention to what is happening to you all the time you are giving the massage. While I give everyone the same massage in the order of things I attend to, my touch feels different to different people. It was wonderful when a woman told me she not only knew where her body was during the massage, but was aware of mine as well.*

One of my first experiences with emotional healing and massage happened in a small and simple apartment in

Cambridge. I had gone to see the masseuse (who worked at her home) because my body was filled with tension and I wanted some relief. When I arrived, she suggested to me that I might be storing old emotional wounds in my body, as indicated by my posture. I asked her what she meant, a bit defensively. After all, I was doing yoga, walking and eating well. I just had a lot of tension, that's all.

She didn't give a mental explanation. Instead, she asked me to lie down, and she began to massage the vertebrae in my neck. Massage, hold steady, massage, hold steady. At first I felt only the degree of tension in my neck; gradually I experienced a lump forming in my throat, my chest heaving and a bunch of old sensations returning to mind. I began to cry, small jerky sobs at first, like the opening of a faucet that has been shut off for a long time. Then a burst of tears, and finally several minutes of sobbing.

I was both terrified and relieved—terrified to think that there was so much deep emotion behind a stiff neck and relieved to know that it could be unlocked and soothed. At that moment I made a decision to see what else I could learn from this mysterious body that walked around with me all day.

If at some point you decide you want a professional massage or want to take a course or apprentice yourself to someone, get names from friends, your local woman's center, health club, YWCA, or from a wholistic health center if one exists in your area. Carefully select the person you go to for massages; recommendations from friends are often the best kind of referrals. Choose someone who uses techniques you like, and with whom you feel comfortable and can communicate well. Good two-way communication relaxes and energizes the masseuse as well. Masseuses work either in private practices, as part of a group practice or collective or as part of organizations like health clubs.

You may not know what you want or what to expect the first time you make an appointment for a massage.

Some people come in with specific physical complaints or problems with body alignment; others just want a chance to stretch and relax, and others want to do emotional "work" along with the massage. Before we begin I work out an understanding with them about what they want.

Without any words, I begin to realize that my shoulders are getting a lesson in where they should be. The lesson feels very good, very soft and respectful of how they would be if I let go of the tension I begin to notice in them. But the massage is a lesson, not just a pat on the back. . . . The masseuse's hands are really asking my back questions and getting answers. The communication is clear and direct. As the hour comes to an end, I feel very good all over. I feel the connection between my head and my toes,

---

*Massage is usually done with the hands, but sometimes feet are used, as in menstrual massage, illustrated in Chapter 12, "Anatomy and Physiology of Sexuality and Reproduction." Japanese massage is often done entirely or partly with the feet.

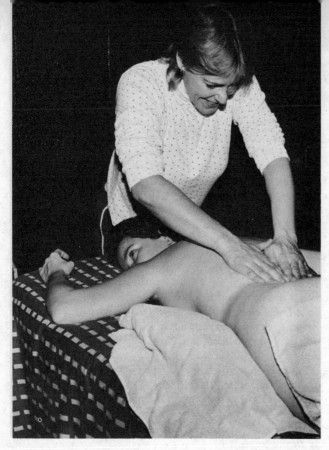

and I feel the connection between body, heart, mind and soul, because I feel touched in all these places. But I find myself missing a touch on my solar plexus, the "center" I feel as the hub of my interconnection. The masseuse's final gesture, ever so slight, is a touch on my solar plexus. "Do you always do that?" I ask her.

"Things come to me sometimes," she says.[22]

Acupuncture

Acupuncture is the healing art central to the practice of traditional Chinese medicine. Developed and used over at least the last 2,000 years, acupuncture is now also accepted in some places in the West as a method for maintaining health and curing disease. In acupuncture the practitioner stimulates specific points on the body by inserting needles, applying heat (thermal therapy), pressing, massaging (acupressure) or by a combination of these.

Chinese medicine, intimately tied to the classical Chinese philosophy of Taoism, aims to maintain or restore balance in the body to insure health. Central to the beliefs of Taoism is the notion that the body has the power to repair and regenerate itself or to restore its own equilibrium. Acupuncture is thought to stimulate or awaken these natural healing powers within the body.[23]

Acupuncturists often state their diagnoses and methods of treatment in terms of Yin and Yang. The terms Yin and Yang denote what the ancient Chinese saw as twin polarities that regulate humans and the universe. Though Taoism describes Yin as "negative" (e.g., earth, moon, coolness, moisture, quiescence, things female) and Yang as "positive" (e.g., heaven, sun, warmth, dryness, movement, things male), the terms are equivalent to modern physicists' calling protons "positive" and electrons "negative."[24] (A proton is not "better" than an electron. They are equally powerful forces.) Practitioners say that the Yin-Yang concept, though it is open to misunderstanding and misuse, does not imply bias against the female.

Unlike Western medical practitioners, the Chinese do not base traditional healing practices on the study of anatomy as we know it. Because Chinese people worshiped their ancestors, the dissection of a cadaver was not permissible. Instead of concentrating on the physiological or material structure of the body (muscles, nerves, bones, etc.), they focused on how we function—the dynamic aspects of the body, the "life force" that keeps the body alive and in healthful balance. They call this life force or vital energy *chi*. According to traditional Chinese medical theory *chi* circulates throughout the body along precise pathways or channels, the acupuncture meridians. The *chi*, which controls the blood, nerves and all organs, must flow freely along the meridians and be of a certain strength and quality if each organ is to function correctly. When the flow of *chi* is impaired, a person becomes susceptible to disease.

Trauma, improper nutrition, stress and many other factors can block or impair the flow of *chi*. In acupuncture, stimulating certain points along the meridians controls the flow of *chi* by attracting energy to a deficient area, dispersing an excess of energy or dissolving a blockage, thereby lessening pain or strengthening the body's ability to maintain health.

A traditional acupuncturist diagnoses the body's imbalance by a variety of techniques: questioning, observing, examining the tongue, listening (to breathing, voice, etc.), reading the pulses.* Often the practitioner takes a complete health history and looks for ways in which changes in diet, exercise, etc., could complement the acupuncture treatments. Many acupuncturists in the U.S. will also ask you to get a diagnosis from a conventional medical practitioner.

In my initial encounter with acupuncture, the acupuncturist was attentive and caring; even before I saw her, when I was just inquiring on the phone, she was taking notes. She sounded interested in my problem (heavy menstrual bleeding). She thought that she could help me

*Reading the pulses is one of the primary diagnostic procedures. Acupuncturists use this method to diagnose the subtle fluctuations in the flow of energy along the meridian circuit. In Chinese medicine, the practitioner takes the pulses at three finger positions on each wrist and at two depths for each finger position. Each of these twelve positions corresponds to a functional organ system of the body. By palpitating these pulses, the experienced practitioner can discover both the energy imbalances within the body at the time of diagnosis and some indication of past conditions as well as potential difficulties.

heal it. I had a good impression of her as a person and a healer.

When I walked into the acupuncturist's office for the first time there was an herb burning that smelled like pot to me, and the first thing that went through my mind was, What am I doing here? These are really "New Age" healers; this is more than I bargained for. I started to feel very nervous. I asked her what the smell was, and she told me that it was an herb called moxa [common mugwort] which they use to heat the needles and which adds to the treatment's effectiveness. I was ready to try something new, but I was also mistrustful.

After I sat down, the acupuncturist asked me a series of questions having to do with digestion, elimination, menstruation, sleep patterns, level of energy, emotional state, pain, other illnesses, diet, lifestyle. This was a lengthy initial question period. Now each time I come she asks me how I've been feeling that week, if there is anything out of the ordinary. She takes my pulse and looks at my tongue, skin, eyes. After gathering all this information, she adjusts the treatment to meet the specific needs I have that week.

During treatments the acupuncturist stimulates the appropriate acupuncture points with sterilized hair-thin stainless steel needles. Needles vary in length from half an inch to several inches for use in different parts of the body. When the needle is inserted, you may feel a slight prick, tingling, numbness, pain or nothing at all.

Part of the initial high of starting acupuncture was that I had expected it to be very painful because my image of it was that they used these big long needles and stuck them into people. When she actually did it, she used very small needles. The prick was quite mild and I got an almost euphoric feeling.

Acupuncture treatments have really minimized my problems with asthma. But I won't deny that the needles hurt as she was putting them in. Once in place, they didn't hurt anymore.

The needles are so small that they do not cause

Elizabeth Cole

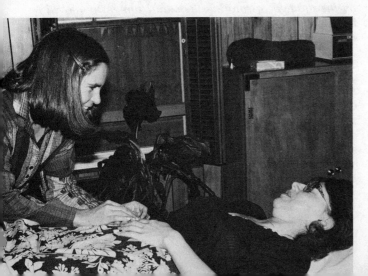

bleeding, though a practitioner may draw as much as three drops of blood from certain points to achieve a special effect. Anywhere from two to fifteen needles can be used. The hands, forearms, lower legs, feet, back, abdomen and ears are the most common places to insert needles. Often the acupuncturist inserts the needle far from the symptomatic area or what you would think of as the site of the disease, because the meridians s/he wishes to affect run the length of the body. S/he can direct the *chi* to bring back balance and harmony within the body from many places on the meridian. For acute ailments few treatments—sometimes just one—are needed. Chronic ailments usually require more treatments, but some people experience relief right away. Others initially feel worse and only begin to experience improvement after many sessions:

I am sixty years old and have severe arthritis, especially in my hands, feet and hips. I had been pushing this pain out of my mind while I was taking care of my husband. He was very sick and if he knew I was in pain he would have wanted to go to the hospital. After he died I was very depressed, and when I went for psychological counseling the counselor suggested that I try acupuncture for the arthritis. He researched it and got me in touch with the acupuncturist. The first few treatments were very painful. I even screamed out. We went through hell together. The acupuncturist told me that chronic pain like mine was deep-seated and harder to take care of. I had to go twice a week for a long time. It was expensive for me, and when after eight treatments I didn't feel any better, I didn't know what to do. Meanwhile, I had been put on a special arthritis diet by a nutritionist who worked with the acupuncturist. I decided I would go on with the acupuncture treatment, and when I got to sixteen treatments I started to feel a little better. By twenty weeks I had found the acupuncture really helped me. Now the treatments have tapered off, one every two or three months, when I start getting sore. So it was definitely worth continuing with them. You either sink or swim, and I didn't feel like sinking.

In the West, acupuncture has been effective in the treatment of menstrual disorders (amenorrhea, excessive bleeding, pain, premenstrual syndrome), conception problems, gastrointestinal disorders, urinary and respiratory problems (asthma, allergies), hemorrhoids, constipation, insomnia. It is also effective in treating osteoarthritis localized in specific joints, muscle contraction and migraine headaches. Various neuralgias and pain related to nerve injury can also be helped. Some acupuncturists will treat patients suffering from anxiety or severe depression, usually when the person is under the care of a psychotherapist as well.

As helpful as acupuncture can be, when not practiced properly it can cause infection or nerve, vessel or organ damage. Make sure that the acupuncturist uses sterilized needles because a number of blood diseases can be transferred by skin puncture, including hepatitis and AIDS. Even though you may have a condition that acupuncture can successfully treat, you may not be able to find a formally trained and experienced acupuncturist. There is as yet no national board for licensing acupuncturists, but certain states do or will soon have a certification procedure. At present, you might try finding out about licensing procedures for acupuncturists in your state through your state board for registry of medicine.

Chiropractic: One Method of Body Alignment and Adjustment

While the extraordinary flexibility of our bodies allows us to move with ease, it also makes it possible for our bodies to become unbalanced. The connective tissues which enclose our muscles and bones and give our body shape can become distorted by the ways in which we habitually sleep, walk or sit, as well as by accidents. We can get into the habit of pushing the head forward as we walk or tightening the knees when we stand. Emotional stress also creates physical tensions which over time change the shape of our bodies. We accommodate to the distortions so that an unbalanced state becomes familiar, even comfortable. The longer we remain out of alignment, however, the more our movement becomes restricted. The resulting chronic muscle tension can affect us emotionally as well as physically; we sometimes lose our range of emotional responsiveness as we lose the flexibility of our physical movements.

Many methods can help us readjust and realign our bodies: chiropractic, Rolfing, The Alexander Technique and the Feldenkrais method are some of them. Space does not permit a discussion of all these methods; we have chosen chiropractic because it is the most widely available.

Chiropractors believe that the human body works at its fullest potential only when the nervous system functions smoothly. The spinal column (the bony vertebral column which covers and protects our brain stem and spinal cord) is the "lifeline of the nervous system."[25] Chiropractors make adjustments (move the vertebrae) in the spine to restore proper nerve function and nerve flow from the brain to muscles and organs of the body, making normal motion possible again. Spinal misalignments result from a number of causes: trauma from car, bike, motorcycle or walking accidents; physical strain from overexertion or from sitting too long in one place; muscle tension from extreme mental stress; even poor diet or overuse of drugs.[26] When proper nerve function is restored to all areas of the body, the organs will function more completely, too. For instance, after adjustments have been made on the specific vertebrae associated with your adrenal glands, allergies connected to adrenal functioning may improve. Chiro-

practors can help with hands and feet. Many women visit chiropractors for preventive health care.

When I was pregnant, I visited my chiropractor once a month to be sure my back was aligned properly as my belly expanded and my weight shifted.

There are two distinct groups of practitioners within chiropractic. Believing that spinal misalignments cause diseases, the "straights" restrict their practice to spinal adjustments alone. The "mixers" have expanded their practice and offer other natural forms of treatment—suggestions about diet, exercise, meditation, visualization—in addition to spinal manipulation. The debate continues between these two groups. Some of these chiropractors use X-rays and some don't.

As with other alternative approaches to healing, women tell a range of stories about their experiences with chiropractors.

I went to see a chiropractor recommended by several friends. He helped me with a specific back injury from running, but after a while I didn't like his attitude. Even though I was no longer having back problems he suggested I keep coming more often than I wanted to. When I asked why, he said, "Well, there is always something to adjust."
"True," I said, "and I often feel better, but I can't afford the money."
So I looked and found another chiropractor who was willing to see me periodically for preventive care and in any crisis, too.

I've seen three different chiropractors over the last twelve years. I've enjoyed seeing each of them and have learned a lot about how to help myself heal. Each visit was not expensive, but you are expected to return regularly. All three chiropractors emphasized how important it is to prevent illness, and to be aware that sometimes slight illnesses, emotional upsets and even changes in seasons can throw your whole body off.

Yoga

I get up in the morning and do the exercise "Salute to the Sun" (actually a series of twelve postures). Whether I have a few minutes or a longer time to practice yoga, I benefit from the fullness of this exercise. I am cheered by the thought of saluting the sun. I am easily moved beyond the awkwardness of my body and the sleepy nature of my mind as I get into the movement of this exercise. After a while I am ready to welcome the day.

The aim of yoga is to renew the body, focus the mind and still the emotions. Yoga is a Sanskrit word which essentially means union. Underlying yoga practice is the belief that "the body and mind are part of the continuum of existence, the mind merely being more subtle than the body."[27]

The basic aspects of yoga practice include *asanas*, *pranayama* and *meditation*. All the exercises empha-

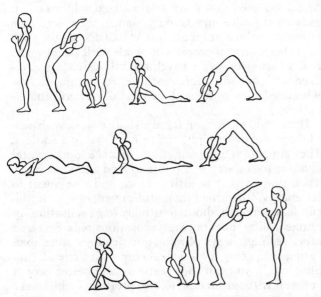

Jane Pincus

size awareness—awareness of the moves and the breathing, of areas of flexibility and tightness, and of applying your mind to the task.

Asanas

Asanas are physical postures which help stretch and limber the body.

Before yoga my main experiences with exercise had been in gym class or in modern dancing. These exercises were a variety of stretches to strengthen or loosen a particular part of my body and were usually done in short repetitive motions. In contrast, when doing yoga postures I was asked to move slowly into the posture, hold it still for some time, and then gradually release. This way of exercising has dramatic effects on my mind. I often begin in some turmoil, filled with the concerns of my day. As I focus my attention on my movements and my breathing, I experience my mind slowing down and relaxing. The practice gives me some distance from my problems. Doing the postures releases new energy, relaxes me and allows for another perspective to emerge.

Pranayama

Pranayama are breathing exercises which increase the flow of oxygen, thereby relaxing your whole being.

The first time I did yoga breathing exercises I was amazed at the capacity of my lungs. I watched my belly fill up, my chest expand, the air move into my shoulders. I realized I never had experienced a complete breath before—and I was in my thirties at the time!

Jana had us breathing deeply after the asanas. "You are light," she'd say, drawing out the word "li-i-ght." "Take the light into your body, down your spine....Be aware ("avare," in her Eastern European accent). We'd hold one nostril shut with one finger and breathe through the other, holding the breath, and then breathe out. It made me feel strong, calm and luminous.

Meditation

While the postures and breathing exercises are valuable in and of themselves, they also prepare you for meditation, or a practice of conscious relaxation that enables you to experience a coming together of the physical, mental and spiritual aspects of yoga. The breathing exercises and meditation are accessible to anyone, and no matter what your physical restrictions, you can do them.

Objective evidence exists about the benefits of yoga. Studies show that it can cause physiological changes such as reduced blood pressure, lowered pulse rates, diminished stress, increased joint movement and improved hormonal functioning.

We can learn yoga on our own by using books, records and tapes. However, there is no substitute for a good teacher who can give us individualized help with the various techniques. Yoga classes are taught in local YWCAs, adult education programs, college extension courses and dance centers. Whether you practice for fifteen minutes a day or for more extended times, it is important to practice regularly.

The problems with yoga are the problems of any healing method applied improperly. Don't push through the pain to complete the exercise no matter what. Be cautious and proceed at your own pace, trusting your limits. In all these practices, you must pay attention to the fine line between simply exerting yourself and pushing beyond your limits—and this is different for everyone. Benefits come from your efforts rather than from reaching a specific goal.

Dance and Movement Therapy

Women have always danced for pleasure and relaxation. You find your own rhythm, experience control over your body and discover the freedom to move in new ways. Movement and dance also can be modes of healing, modes in which women today have a predominant influence. Dance and movement therapy are not recent innovations, though they have become more popular. Using movement rather than words, they treat a variety of physiological and psychological conditions, addressing a person's body, emotions, mental attitudes and relatedness to the world. The therapist, by observing you and moving rhythmically with you, is able to mirror not only your physical movements

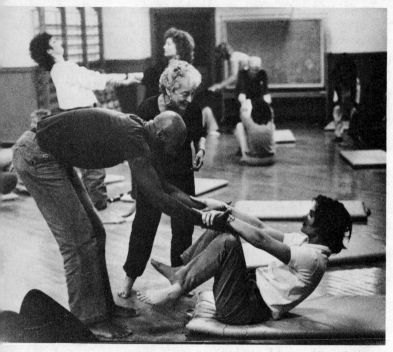

Nona Charleston

but also the *feelings* behind those movements. As you learn to identify certain details of your physical and emotional states while you move, you can learn to alter your movements so that you feel more comfortable with yourself and with the people around you.

I was incredibly timid and anxious, so shy that I had trouble making friends or having any social life at all. I went to a dance therapist who worked with me in her office, just moving, getting rhythms going. We began to breathe together, dance together, reach toward each other and move back. It was a way of communicating without needing to say anything. Once as we were moving I remembered my mother rocking me, and also the way I used to feel when she suddenly put me down to go take care of my brother. That memory released something in me and I started to cry. I never thought I could get such a feeling of release.

The therapist follows the person's lead rather than imposing a rigid set of strictures. S/he teaches exercises and techniques, but except for a few basics, the exercises suggested are natural outgrowths of the person's spontaneous discoveries about her body. Dance and movement therapists also use guided relaxation, role playing, breathing techniques and meditation as part of their treatment.[28] Dance and movement therapists in clinics and hospitals usually work as part of a team. Women often do movement therapy in groups to avoid the isolation characteristic of other modes and to be energized by the group as well as by the therapist. In the 1940s Marion Chace, a dancer, was the first therapist to work within a hospital setting.

She discovered that when traumatized soldiers could express their feelings through dance, they were able to leave the hospital more quickly. Chace set the path for other dance therapists to work with people who had a variety of severe psychiatric illnesses (e.g., children with autism, adults with schizophrenia, etc.) or who needed to counter the effects of powerful medications.[29]

Dance and movement therapists also work with people who feel overweight and/or have eating disorders. They support you in your efforts to make fundamental changes in the way you relate to food and your body. Their emphasis is on using dance and movement to let energy out rather than stuffing energy in. If you can learn enough about your body (e.g., sensations of hunger, differences between sensations of hunger and other feelings, ways of managing feelings other than eating [i.e., going for a walk, being with a friend, running, etc.]), you can then learn to take better care of yourself without turning to diet programs which take a huge toll. (See Chapter 2, "Food," and Chapter 4, "Women in Motion.") In the words of a movement therapist:

As part of an exercise the group was physically lifting up a very large woman. This woman strongly believed that she always had to be supporting other people, but other people could not support her, especially because of her size. So the experience of being lifted up was a turning point for her. After this experience she could believe that she would be supported by people in other ways as well.

"Paranormal" or "Psychic" Healing and Therapeutic Touch

Though rigorous documentation does not exist, there are on record incidents of physical healing which cannot be explained in purely medical, physical or psychological terms.[30] Sometimes when a surprisingly rapid rate of healing or a total reversal of symptoms occurs, people attribute the healing to a nonphysical entity (spirit or deity), a group (prayer group, healing circle, church group), an individual (minister, shaman, psychic) or the person's attendance at a "miraculous" place (such as Lourdes).[31] The techniques and rituals used in association with these incidents include meditation and prayer, touching with the intent to heal and visualization.

Insofar as the healer and the setting promote your belief in the efficacy of a ritual or activity, you may be able to make an extraordinary effort to heal yourself. As the healer communicates her/his concern through compassion, physical touch and a strong "healing" intention, you may be able to relax and let your body's healing energy take over. Like shamans in "primitive" societies and religious or faith healers in Western societies, modern psychic healers can mo-

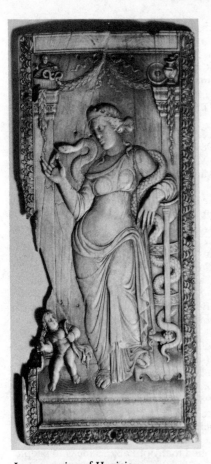

Ivory carving of Hygieia,
ancient deity of health and healing

Merseyside County Museums, Liverpool, England

bilize the body's healing forces. Many healers emphasize the importance of "compassionate love" going from healer to person to be healed. They believe that the energy of compassionate healing love is greater than that of words. Religious healers speak of this "love" as the most potent factor in religious healing. Perhaps the emotional atmosphere these healers create, combined with physical touch and with people's faith in their own healing powers, makes possible any physical healing that takes place.[32]

One noted psychic healer[33] emphasizes that a healer should focus on the whole person, not just on the particular part to be healed. He warns people to be wary of healers who charge money and/or promise a cure, and he cautions against the sleight-of-hand tricks some "healers" use to reinforce their clients' belief in them. He also requires that all his clients be in consultation with a physician.

Therapeutic Touch, studied and taught by Dolores Krieger[34] and Dora Kunz, is another technique for channeling energy through yourself to help the healing process in another person. The practitioner "centers herself" so that she feels peaceful and strong. She then moves her hands a few inches away and along the periphery of another person's body both to disperse blocked energy and to channel her healing energy into the other person's "field." According to Krieger and Kunz, the practitioner's hands, moving in this way, can bring about profound relaxation, relieve pain and facilitate healing. Therapeutic Touch has been effective in relieving stress-related conditions such as rashes, headaches, asthma, colitis, sleep disorders, high blood pressure, palpitations and angina.

From a woman who used Therapeutic Touch for the first time:

I have a long history of migraines. I went into the nurse's office as a migraine was just beginning. While I had heard about Therapeutic Touch, I had never tried it before. When the nurse offered me a choice of decongestants, pain relievers, Therapeutic Touch or some combination, I decided to try Therapeutic Touch. (After all, I knew what the drugs could and couldn't do for me.) After the session my head felt lighter and less congested.

From a nurse who began practicing Therapeutic Touch after twenty-five years of conventional medical nursing:

A woman had been to four or five doctors before she saw me. Her symptoms were back and leg pains with a lot of swelling on her ankles. She was told that she had no disc or circulatory problems, and was sent home with a diuretic for the swelling. "Sometimes middle-aged women develop these problems," one doctor said.

I worked with this woman every three to four weeks for a year. With her energy back, she has returned to leading an active life with no physical restrictions. When she occasionally has pain, she returns for a single treatment.

Practitioners must develop sensitivity through repeated practice and must understand why they want to become healers. Healing is a "power tool," and the healer must be sure s/he works in the best interests of the person being treated.

Check at alternative health centers and therapy organizations or through listings in alternative health journals to find both practitioners and classes. You can also learn and practice techniques in groups of women doing Therapeutic Touch. Once learned, it's a method we can easily use to help each other. Krieger points out:

Since Therapeutic Touch derives from a mode of healing that persons of all cultures since the dawn of documented history have been able to use, *you* too can learn to heal ... there is little I have to teach you that you haven't done before at some point in your life.[35]

69

NOTES

1. Much of this healing work, however, was so taken for granted that little of it has been recorded in historical documents. See Muriel Joy Hughes, *Women Healers in Medieval Life and Literature*, New York: 1943, and Kate Campbell Hurd-Mead, M.D., *A History of Women in Medicine*, Connecticut: Haddam, 1938.

2. Joanna Macy. "Despair Work," *Evolutionary Blues*, Issue No. 1 (available from Evolutionary Blues, Box 4448, Arcata, CA 95521); also, *Despair. Personal Power in the Nuclear Age*. Philadelphia: New Society Publishers, 1983.

3. Mary Howell, M.D., Ph.D. *Healing at Home*. Boston: Beacon Press, 1979, p. 87.

4. N. Muramato. *Healing Ourselves*. New York: Avon Books, 1973, p. 4.

5. E. Bauman. "Introduction to Holistic Health," *The Holistic Health Handbook*, compiled by the Berkeley Holistic Health Center. Berkeley, CA: And/Or Press, 1978, p. 19.

6. D. Ardell. *High-Level Wellness: An Alternative to Doctors, Drugs and Disease*. Emmaus, PA: Rodale Press, 1977, p. 2.

7. Herbert Benson. *The Relaxation Response*. New York: William Morrow and Co., Inc., 1975, pp. 75–98.

8. *Ibid.*, pp. 70–71, Table 2.

9. Mike Samuels, M.D., and Nancy Samuels. *Seeing with the Mind's Eye*. New York: Random House, Inc., 1975.

10. Stanley Krippner and Alberto Villoldo. *Realms of Healing*. Millbrae, CA: Celestial Arts, 1976. See also Krippner's tapes from Healing in Our Times, a conference sponsored by the Sufis in Washington, D.C., November 7 and 8, 1981. Future conferences are being planned. For details about tapes and conferences, contact The Healing Order of the Sufi Order, Rt. 2, Box 166, Leicester, NC 28748. See also Robert T. Trotter, II, and Juan Antonio Chavira, *Curanderismo: Mexican American Folk Healing*. Athens, GA: University of Georgia Press, 1981.

11. Images stored in the cerebral cortex affect the autonomic nervous system, which controls sweating, blushing, blood vessel expansion and contraction and rate and force of heartbeat. The autonomic nervous system is also connected with the pituitary gland and adrenal cortex, which secrete hormones and steroids affecting thyroid and sex glands and metabolic processes. (See Samuels and Samuels, *Seeing with the Mind's Eye*, cited above.)

12. Paraphrased from Dennis T. Jaffe, *Healing from Within*. New York: Alfred A. Knopf, 1980, pp. 241–42.

13. W. Luthe. *Autogenic Therapy*. New York: Guine-Stratton, 1969, Vol. I, p. 1.

14. Exercises developed by Dr. J.H. Schultz in the 1930s and summarized by Samuels and Samuels, *Seeing with the Mind's Eye*, p. 223; by Kenneth Pelletier, *Mind as Healer, Mind as Slayer*, New York: Delta, 1977, pp. 233–62; and E. Peper and E.A. Williams, "Autogenic Therapy," in *Health for the Whole Person*, Boulder, CO: Westview Press, 1980, p. 133.

15. E. Peper and E.A. Williams, "Autogenic Therapy," p. 134.

16. O. Carl Simonton, M.D., Stephanie Matthews-Simonton and James L. Creighton. *Getting Well Together*. New York: Bantam Books, 1978, pp. 183–85.

17. *Ibid.*, pp. 127–48.

18. G.E. Schwartz. "Biofeedback and the Treatment of Dysregulation Disorders," *Ways of Health*, New York: Harcourt Brace Jovanovich, Inc., 1979, pp. 362–68; and J. Kamiya and J.G. Kamiya, "Biofeedback," *Health for the Whole Person*, pp. 115–29.

19. Richard Gordon. *Your Healing Hands: The Polarity Experience*. Santa Cruz, CA: Unity Press, 1978.

20. Margaret Elke and Mel Risman. "Sensitive Massage," *The Holistic Health Handbook*, p. 175.

21. Lew Connor and Linda McKim. "Reflexology," *The Holistic Health Handbook*, p. 183.

22. Christina Robb. "A Sense of Touch," *The Globe Magazine*, November 15, 1981, p. 22.

23. Stephen Chang, M.D., Ph.D. "Acupuncture: A Contemporary Look at an Ancient System," *The Holistic Health Handbook*, p. 48.

24. Fritjof Capra. *The Turning Point*. New York: Simon and Schuster, Inc., 1982, pp. 79–80.

25. G.F. Rickeman, D.D., "Chiropractics," *The Holistic Health Handbook*, p. 173.

26. T.A. Vondarhaar. "Chiropractic in Theory and Practice," *The Holistic Health Handbook*, p. 173.

27. Judith Hanson Lasath. "Yoga: An Ancient Technique for Restoring Health," *The Holistic Health Handbook*, p. 36.

28. Billie Pivnik, M.Ed., DTR. "Dance Movement Therapy at New England Rehabilitation Hospital," *Spokes*, February 1977.

29. Another school of movement therapy is based on the work of Rudolf Laban (see *The Mastery of Movement*, Boston: Plays, Inc., 1971) and elaborated by Irmgard Bartenieff (see *Body Movement: Coping with the Environment*, New York: Gordon and Breach, 1980). (Also see Fritjof Capra, *The Turning Point*, New York: Simon and Schuster, Inc., 1982, pp. 347–48.) Laban believed that we all express ourselves as we move, no matter what we are doing. Bartenieff, a physical therapist, applied many of Laban's ideas to people with physical problems. She works with people who have a variety of chronic illnesses (heart, brain and spinal cord diseases, multiple sclerosis, Parkinson's disease, etc.) and helps them with depression or simply teaches them to have fun.

Judith Kestenberg (see Resources), a psychoanalyst, uses the Laban-Bartenieff system for analyzing movement in her studies of the movement patterns of people through life-cycle changes. Especially interested in facilitating healthy parent-child relationships, she and other dance therapists are now working with bonding between young children and their parents.

30. Here are a few examples: Stanley Krippner, Ph.D., "Psychic Healing," in *Health for the Whole Person*, p. 169, and other references to his work cited in Note 10; Dolores Krieger, Ph.D., R.N., *Therapeutic Touch: How to Use Your Hands to Help or Heal*, Englewood Cliffs, NJ: Prentice-Hall, 1979; Lawrence LeShan, *The Medium, The Mystic and the Physicist*, New York: Ballantine Books, 1982.

31. Stanley Krippner. "Psychic Healing," p. 169.

32. Dolores Krieger. "Theraputic Touch: the Imprimatur of Nursing," *American Journal of Nursing* 75(5) (May 1975), 784–87.

33. Lawrence LeShan. *The Medium, The Mystic and the Physicist*.

34. See Dolores Krieger, *"Therapeutic Touch,"* for a detailed description of her method, philosophy and findings.

35. *Ibid.*, p. 17.

RESOURCES

Books and Articles

Bartenieff, Irmgard. "Dance Therapy: A New Profession on a Rediscovery of an Ancient Role of the Dance?" *Dance Scope* (Fall/Winter 1972/73).

Benson, Herbert, M.D. *The Mind-Body Effect*. New York: Berkeley Publishing Corp., 1979.

———. *The Relaxation Response*. New York: William Morrow and Co., Inc., 1975. A guide for reducing tension and stress for people with high blood pressure.

Berkeley Holistic Health Center. *The Holistic Health Handbook*. Berkeley, CA: And/Or Press, 1978. A useful compilation of articles on various approaches to healing.

———. *The Holistic Lifebook*. Berkeley, CA: And/Or Press, 1981. A sequel to *The Holistic Health Handbook*.

Capra, Fritjof. *The Tao of Physics*. Boulder, CO: Shambala, 1975.

———. *The Turning Point: Science, Society and The Rising Culture*. New York: Simon and Schuster, Inc., 1982. This book shows how the revolution in modern physics foreshadows the new wholistic approaches to health. It provides the philosophical underpinnings for the fundamental changes in our concept of healing.

Cousins, Norman. *Anatomy of an Illness*. New York: W.W. Norton and Co., Inc., 1979.

Crawford, Robert. "Healthism: The Medicalization of Everyday Life," *Journal of Health Services*, Vol. 10, No. 3 (1980), pp. 365–88.

Davis, Martha, ed. *Research Approaches to Movement and Personality*. New York: Arno Press, 1972.

Ehrenreich, Barbara, and Deidre English. *For Her Own Good*. New York: Doubleday and Co., Inc., 1978.

Feldenkreis, Moshe. *Awareness Through Movement*. New York: Harper and Row Publishers, Inc., 1972.

Ferguson, Marilyn. *The Aquarian Conspiracy: Personal and Social Transformation in the 1980s*. Los Angeles: J.P. Tarcher, Inc., 1980.

Gardner, Joy. *Healing Yourself*. P.O. Box 752, Vashon, WA 98070, 1972. $2.50 + $1.00 postage.

Gordon, Richard. *Your Healing Hands: The Polarity Experience*. Santa Cruz, CA: Unity Press, 1978.

Hastings, Arthur C., Ph.D., James Fadiman, Ph.D., James S. Gordon, M.D., eds. *Health for the Whole Person*. Boulder, CO: Westview Press, 1980. Contains good biographies on various topics in wholistic health.

Howell, Mary, M.D., Ph.D. "Curing, Caring and Healing." Address to medical students at Duke University, Autumn 1980.

———. "A Paradigm of Healing." September 15, 1981. Available from the Boston Women's Health Book Collective for $1.00.

Hughes, Muriel Joy. *Women Healers in Medieval Life and Literature*. New York: Kings Crown Press, 1943.

Hurd-Mead, Kate Campbell, M.D. *A History of Women in Medicine*. Connecticut: Haddam, 1938.

Hyatt, Richard. *Chinese Herbal Medicine*. New York: Schocken Books, 1978.

Jaffe, Dennis T., Ph.D. *Healing from Within*. New York: Alfred A. Knopf, Inc., 1980.

Jones, Frank Pierce. *Body Awareness in Action*. New York: Schocken Books, 1976.

Kaptchuk, Ted. J., O.M.D. *The Web That Has No Weaver: Understanding Chinese Medicine*. New York: Langdon and Weed, 1983.

Kestenberg, Judith. *Children and Parents: Psychoanalytic Studies on Development*. New York: Jason Aronson Inc., 1975.

Krieger, Dolores, Ph.D., R.N. *The Therapeutic Touch: How to Use Your Hands to Help or to Heal*. Englewood Cliffs, NJ: Prentice-Hall, Inc., 1979.

Krippner, Stanley, and Alberto Villoldo. *The Realms of Healing*. Millbrae, CA: Celestial Arts, 1976.

LeShan, Lawrence. *The Medium, The Mystic and the Physicist: Toward a General Theory of the Paranormal*. New York: Ballantine Books, Inc., 1982.

———. *You Can Fight for Your Life: Emotional Factors in the Treatment of Cancer*. New York: M. Grans and Co., 1977.

Lucas, Richard. *Nature's Medicines: The Folklore, Romance and Value of Herbal Remedies*. No. Hollywood, CA: Wilshire Book Co., 1973.

MacNutt, Father Francis. *Healing*. New York: Bantam Books, 1974.

Macy, Joanna. *Despair and Personal Power in the Nuclear Age*. Philadelphia: The New Society Publishers, 1983.

———. "Despair Work," *Evolutionary Blues*, No. 1. Available from Evolutionary Blues, Box 4448, Arcata, CA 95521.

North, Marion. *Personality Assessment Through Movement*. London: MacDonald and Evans, 1972.

Pelletier, Kenneth R. *Mind as Healer, Mind as Slayer*. New York: Delta, 1977.

Pivnik, Billie, M.Ed., DTR. "Dance Movement Therapy at New England Rehabilitation Hospital." *Spokes*, February 1977.

Popenoe, Cris. *Wellness*. Washington, DC: Yes!, 1977. A bibliographical guide to books on health and healing.

Samuels, Mike, M.D. and Nancy Samuels. *Seeing with the Mind's Eye*. New York: Random House, Inc., 1975.

Schuster, Karolyn. "Dance Therapy: Moving with the Beat—Toward Health," *The Physician and Sports Medicine*, December 1978.

Simonton, O. Carl, M.D., Stephanie Matthews-Simonton and James L. Creighton. *Getting Well Again*. New York: Bantam Books, 1980. A self-help guide to dealing with the stress of cancer.

Sobel, David S., ed. *Ways of Health: Holistic Approaches to Ancient and Contemporary Medicine*. New York: Harcourt Brace Jovanovich, Inc., 1979. Compilation of well-documented articles on health and healing.

Tennor, Dorothy. *Psychotherapy: The Hazardous Cure*. New York: Abelard-Schuman, 1975.

Tierra, Michael, GA., N.D. *The Way of Herbs: Simple Remedies for Health and Healing*. Santa Cruz, CA: Unity Press, 1980.

Trotter, Robert T., II, and Juan Antonio Chavira. *Curanderismo: Mexican American Folk Healing*. Athens, GA: The University of Georgia Press, 1981.

Verbruege, Martha H. "The Social Meaning of Personal Health: The Ladies' Physiological Institution of Boston and Vicinity in the 1850s," *Health Care in America, Essays in Social History*. Reverby, S. and D. Rosner, eds. Philadelphia: Temple University Press, 1979.

Journals and Guides

Co-Evolution Quarterly. P.O. Box 428, Sausalito, CA 94905, (415)332-1716. $12 per year (4 issues).

East/West Journal. 17 Station Street, Box 1200, Brookline, MA 02147, (617)232-1000. $26 per year (12 issues).

Holistic Health Review. Human Sciences Press, 72 Fifth Avenue, New York, NY 10011.

Human Geologist. 505 North Lake Shore Drive, Chicago, IL 60611. $12 per year (12 issues).

Journal of Health Science. 1238 Hayes, Eugene, OR 97402, (503)484-2311. $10 per year (4 issues).

Let's Live. P.O. Box 74908, Los Angeles, CA 90004, (213)469-3901. $8.50 per year (12 issues).

Madness Network News. P.O. Box 68, San Francisco, CA 94101, (415)548-2980. $5 per year.

Medical Self-Care Magazine. P.O. Box 718, Inverness, CA 94937.

Mothering Magazine. P.O. Box 2046, Albuquerque, NM 87103. $8 per year.

New Age Journal. 244 Brighton Avenue, Allston, MA 02134, (617)254-5400. $15 per year (12 issues).

Prevention Magazine. 33 East Minor Street, Emmaus, PA 18049, (215)967-5171. $12 per year (12 issues).

Well-Being Magazine and Vegetarian Times. 41 East 42nd Street, #921, New York, NY 10017, (212)490-3999.

Whole Life Times. 132 Adams Street, Newton, MA 02158, (617)964-7600. $9.00 per year (6 issues).

Yoga Journal. 2054 University Avenue, Berkeley, CA 94704, (415)841-9200. $11 per year (6 issues).

Associations and Organizations

American Association of Acupuncture and Oriental Medicine, 50 Maple Place, Manhasset, NY 10030.

American Chiropractic Association, 1916 Wilson Boulevard, Arlington, VA 22209.

American Dance Therapy Association, 2000 Century Plaza, Columbia, Maryland.

American Holistic Medical Association, 6932 Little River Turnpike, Annandale, VA 22005, (703)642-5880.

American Holistic Nurses Association, 4106 Bluebonnet, Houston, TX 77025, (713)666-0610.

Holistic Health Practitioners' Association, 396 Euclid Avenue, Oakland, CA 94610, (415)835-5018.

Holistic Health Referrals (Michael Dawson), 1 Brattle Circle, Cambridge, MA 02138, (617)661-3732. Publishes a directory of Holistic Health Referrals in Eastern Massachusetts.

Holistic Psychotherapy and Medical Group, 1749 Vine Street, Berkeley, CA 94703, (415)843-2766.

National Feminist Therapists Association, 5030 Del Monte Avenue, #14, San Diego, CA 92107, (714)233-8984.

Wellness Associates, 42 Miller Avenue, Mill Valley, CA 94941, (415)383-3806.

Conferences

Healing in Our Times. Contact The Healing Order of the Sufi Order, Rt. 2, Box 166, Leicester, NC 28748.

New Medicine Conference. Contact Interface, 230 Central Street, Newton, MA 02166, (617)964-0500.

6

PSYCHOTHERAPY

By Nancy P. Hawley, with Wendy Sanford

With special thanks to Judy Norsigian and Norma Swenson

When we feel depressed, anxious or hopeless or realize that certain problems keep repeating themselves in our lives, it can help immensely to talk about it with supportive friends and family. Sometimes, however, those closest to us are not able or willing to talk about what's wrong, offer too much advice, are too much a part of the problem or can't give us enough time and focused attention. We may then carefully choose a trained psychotherapist who will offer the objectivity, skill and attentiveness necessary to help us deal with emotions and complex problems.

In an ideal therapeutic situation you feel safe talking about the most intimate details of your life. As you and the therapist get to know each other, s/he helps you identify your problems and your strengths and develop the skills you need to uncover your feelings, experiment with solutions to problems, change your life or deal constructively with the unalterable.

One evening, while I was nursing my one-month-old daughter, a friend criticized my character—at length. In fact, she tore me to pieces. That night I had a powerful dream: as I went up a steep hill all my possessions fell away from me. Once at the top, I slid back down, and at the bottom, in a gutter at a crossroads, lay a magazine. It was the story of my life, but it had just a short introduction; the rest of the pages were blank. As I stood there, everything I'd lost miraculously tumbled back down around my feet. I woke up. A few days later I decided to see a therapist, a psychiatrist who had counseled my brother. He seemed "safe," was like a wise turtle. And he already knew something about my family. Therapy turned out to be a revelation. Each session those first four months led to discovery. I sat and faced him; he asked me useful questions. I laid my life out. All those events I'd never thought much about before were brought together, were in fact connected, formed patterns, a whole. I was at the center, the one responsible. This was the beginning of my conscious wish to change myself, and of my belief that I could.

Before consulting a therapist—or while you do—it makes sense to check for physical causes of confusion or depression, such as certain medications like birth control pills, certain combinations of medications (see, in particular, Chapter 22, "Women Growing Older") or exposure to toxic substances at work or in the home. Sometimes an improved diet, more exercise or simply more sleep can make a person feel better emotionally. Often a physician will refer a woman for psychiatric treatment when he or she cannot identify a physical cause or treatment for a problem, or because s/he learned in medical training that many of women's physical problems are "all in their heads." Sometimes therapy is just right; sometimes, despite what doctors or even family and friends tell us, it is not what we need.

Women must approach psychotherapy with caution.[1] Most mental-health professionals, especially male psychiatrists and psychologists, have distorted ideas about women based on their training, their personal experiences with women, inadequate information about women's psychological development as it differs from men's* and the realities of most women's lives. Discussing sex bias in therapy, three women professionals wrote:

Clinical theories of personality specify women's innate nature as passive, dependent, masochistic, and childlike, and psychological treatment has often aimed at reducing her complaints about the quality of her life and promoting adjustment to the existing order.[2]

A well-known study revealed that psychologists see positive adult qualities and "healthy" male qualities as *the same*, while they portray the "healthy" woman in very different terms: for instance, as more submissive, suggestive, emotional and illogical.[3] The many therapists who hold such stereotypes are of little use to women, and can do a lot of harm.

Rarely do mental-health professionals realize how

*See Carol Gilligan's *In A Different Voice: Psychological Theory and Women's Development*. (Listed in Resources.)

women's disadvantaged status is directly damaging to our mental health. They are more likely to see women's emotional problems as internally caused (intrapsychic) than men's, and fail to look at the external reality and stress of women's lives.* Consequently, they are more likely to prescribe psychoactive drugs to women than to men, and women are twice as likely as men to receive electroshock. Practices like these draw many women into a web of inappropriate psychotherapy, drug dependence and reduced self-esteem.

The medical model dominates most psychotherapy today. Most therapists who are not physicians have physicians as their teachers, supervisors or superiors in institutional settings. In the medical model the client is the "patient," who by implication is sick; the therapist is the "doctor," who by implication will "cure" the patient. (A nonmedicalized alternative is to see the client as having the sources of healing, insight and wholeness within her, and the therapist as a facilitator of a process by which s/he uncovers these.) The doctor-patient relationship carries a power imbalance which can work against women in therapy, especially when the therapist is male and/or misuses this power.†

Tragically, in the extreme, this power imbalance can lead therapists to physically and psychologically abuse women. Some have colluded with family members to lock us away in mental institutions (where women are the majority of patients) when we refuse to comply to society's norms for us. Some have molested and raped us in the name of "therapy." Most widely, they have used myths about woman's supposedly passive, masochistic nature to keep us "in our place." Their underlying motivation is often a fear that we will gain and use our full powers. While extremes such as these by no means represent the majority of women's experiences, they illustrate the potential for the misuse of power which occurs with considerable frequency when women consult mental health professionals. By far the greatest damage done to women is accomplished through the subtle ways in which women are encouraged to stay in positions of service to men rather than to realize our fullest potential.

There are approaches to therapy that avoid some of the possible abuses. In Co-counseling (Reevaluation Counseling), people learn counseling techniques in a

*Consider, for example, this observation by an incest survivor: "Therapists buy into their client's denial of incest—if the client doesn't mention it—it never comes up because most therapists are just as afraid to get into it as their client. Either because it threatens them or they are just plain ignorant of the issue. They aren't aware of how certain behavior patterns, responses could indicate an incest experience, so they can't help her bring it to the surface."[4]

†It is difficult to bring complaints against a therapist or to sue for malpractice, because your protests themselves may be misinterpreted as signs of your "mental instability." Other forms of medical malpractice are usually quite visible; it's hard to *prove* you're mentally or emotionally damaged.

teacher-led group, then take turns "counseling" one another as equals, and for no money.

Co-counseling is based on the belief that human beings are born with a tremendous intellectual potential, natural zest and lovingness, but that these qualities have been blocked and obscured as a result of accumulated distressing experiences which begin early in life. The belief is that any person can recover from these hurtful experiences by the natural healing process of emotional discharge—through laughing, crying, trembling, raging, yawning, for example. Co-counselers' basic aim is to assist each other in recovering and in using this natural healing process.

Therapists with a *feminist* approach (whether they name it this or not, because it is the attitude, not the label, that's most important) seek to help us find and use our strengths. They are aware of the power imbalances in the therapy relationship and try to use respectfully the power they do have. They are likely to recognize social, political and economic influences upon our emotional well-being. Often the first to raise mental-health issues which traditional therapists have ignored—incest, rape, wife battering, child abuse, alcoholism—they are also likely to be more understanding of women in their interpretations. (For a discussion of lesbians and therapy, see p. 153.)

I don't fit into a slot, nor does any woman I know. Yet our social structure suggests we all want the same thing, should give the same thing and respect the hierarchical patriarchal authority that limits our different paths. As a feminist therapist I believe it is often helpful and sometimes vital for a woman to unwind herself from these societal expectations. I only know where women come from. Where we are going is a process of unfolding.

By no means is every woman therapist a feminist, and a few male therapists have a feminist approach. Also, women can encounter many of the same problems with their therapist, whether feminist or not. To find a good therapist, talk with friends who have had positive therapy experiences, look in women's newspapers, call a local women's center or the local NOW (National Organization for Women) office.

In choosing a psychotherapist, check the guidelines listed on pp. 57–58 for choosing any practitioner. We suggest that you look for those therapists who are able to go beyond the limitations of conventional medical training or supervision or who do not come out of this tradition at all. It may take a while to find someone with whom you can work well. In the exploratory session, feel free to ask about the therapist's goals, training, fees and attitudes toward women. Shop around if you can. (Cost is a factor here. While therapists at clinics affiliated with prepaid health plans or at community health centers are more reasonably priced, your choice in terms of variety and sometimes quality is more often limited. The more nonconventional therapists may not be covered by insurance.*) It's worth taking the time to find someone whose training, style and personality are suited to what you need.

I've gone to a variety of therapists for shorter and longer periods of my adult life, by myself and with family members. The first time I went, I chose to see a woman, but men have helped me as well. The best of these therapists had these features in common:
They were gentle, friendly and respectful.
They listened well and understood what I was saying.
They accepted the way I presented issues and didn't alter them to fit some theory.
Their own life problems didn't usually get mixed up with mine; when that happened they were able to acknowledge the fact.
They helped me define my problems and see my way to making the changes I wanted to make.
They were open to my criticisms of them.
They cared that I succeeded without claiming responsibility for my success.
Working with the help of therapists who had these qualities, I felt stronger as a person after each session and clearer about my life.

APPENDIX
Different Kinds of Psychotherapists

The most important thing to keep in mind when selecting a therapist is that the particular title someone has earned is no guarantee of the kind of attitudes s/he holds. Each category contains people with a full spectrum of attitudes and beliefs about women. The specifics about different specialists are useful to know, but ultimately you must trust your perceptions and not under- or overestimate the title's meaning.

Counselors

Counseling programs exist in schools of education and psychology. Talented counselors can be extremely helpful. They are often more flexible and less dogmatic than therapists with extensive formal training, though there are also lots of problems they haven't been trained to tackle. They must be willing to refer you to someone else when necessary. Marriage and family counselors and pastoral counselors are particular kinds of counselors many women consult.

*Furthermore, some women have hesitated to use the mental-health benefits included in their individual insurance policies, as employers have misused therapists' notes and evaluations to deny women (and men) jobs because they have psychiatric histories.

Clinical Psychologists

Clinical psychologists hold masters' degrees or doctorates from graduate schools of psychology, education and social science. Although not medically trained, many of them follow the medical model for therapy. A lot of psychological testing is developed and administered by clinical psychologists; these tests set guidelines for "normal" behavior which other therapists often use to evaluate a person's mental health.

Social Workers

Social workers are trained in schools of social work to do either psychiatric, medical or community social work. (Some people with the title of social worker— e.g., in welfare offices and mental hospitals—do not actually have social-work training.) Social workers practice in hospitals and schools or privately, doing casework, group work and community organization. Though they often have a medicalized orientation, they do tend to place emphasis on the entire family rather than just the individual. Unfortunately most social workers are overworked and underpaid; although they can be helpful, caring and insightful, they are often not taken seriously or given power within the medical hierarchy. In the last several years many states have licensed social workers to practice independently, which gives them more control over their work.

Psychiatrists

Psychiatrists have gone through medical school, are licensed physicians and can prescribe drugs. Their special training process prepares them to work with people who are severely disturbed and may require hospitalization. If you need medication or hospitalization, you will need at least to consult with a psychiatrist. However, for most problems which people bring to therapy, it is not accurate to assume that their training makes them better therapists. With rare exceptions, psychiatrists bring a medical bias into therapy work and with it the reinforced sexism and authoritarianism which come with medical training.

Psychoanalysts

Psychoanalysts (almost all in the U.S. are psychiatrists first) receive training in a psychoanalytic institute for a specialized type of individual therapy work which involves many sessions per week and often many years of therapy. This work, which involves slowly taking your personality apart and building it back up again anew, is lengthy and expensive. Make sure that any psychoanalyst you see is fully credentialed and not just a bona fide member of the local psychoanalytic institute. Classical psychoanalytic theory has been the source of most of the distorted ideas about women that pervade all medical training.

Special Approaches

Family therapists (who may have previous degrees as psychiatrists, psychologists, social workers or counselors) attend training programs at the growing number of family therapy institutes across the country. They work with different kinds of family groups, and assume that whatever problems arise result from interactions within the family rather than from the individual alone.

Finally, there are many *specific therapy training programs* which develop their own professional criteria— often in experimental therapies such as Transactional Analysis, Transpersonal Therapy, Gestalt, Psychodrama, Psychosynthesis, Neurolinguistic Programing (NLP), Ericksonian Therapy and the body-oriented therapies, such as Bioenergetics, Psychomotor or Primal Scream.

Some therapists, influenced by feminist and holistic perspectives, are doing exciting new work. Transpersonal therapists are working with meditation; psychotherapists are using biofeedback; psychoanalytically-oriented psychiatrists are studying family therapy and finding it full of possibilities; family therapists are learning hypnosis and visualization. The communication between traditionally trained therapists and alternative therapists has increased greatly in the last fifteen years. We look forward to this trend continuing.

NOTES

1. See Dorothy Tennov, *Psychotherapy, the Hazardous Cure* (New York: Abelard-Schuman, 1975) for an insightful discussion of the effects of psychotherapy on women. See also Phyllis Chesler's *Women and Madness* (New York: Avon Books, 1972), and Jean Baker Miller's *Toward a New Psychology of Women* (Boston: Beacon Press, 1976).

2. Elaine Hilberman Carmen, M.D., Nancy Felipe Russo, Ph.D., and Jean Baker Miller, M.D. "Inequality and Women's Mental Health: An Overview," *Am. Journal of Psychiatry*, 138:10 (October 1981), p. 1324.

3. I.K. Broverman, D.M. Broverman, F.E. Clarkson, P.S. Rosenkrantz and S.R. Vogel. "Sex Role Stereotypes and Clinical Judgments of Mental Health," *Journal of Consulting and Clinical Psychology*, No. 34 (1970), pp. 1–7.

4. From an interview with lesbian incest survivors in *Off Our Backs: A Woman's News Journal* (October 1982), p. 17.

RESOURCES

Black Women's Community Development Foundation. *Mental and Physical Health Problems of Black Women* (Report of Conference, March 1974). 1028 Connecticut Avenue NW, Suite 1010, Washington, DC 20036. ($9.95 including postage).

Brodsky, Annette M. and Rachel Hare-Mustin, eds. *Women and Psychotherapy*. New York: Guilford Press, p. 428.

Brown, Phil, ed. *Radical Psychology*. New York: Colophon Books, Harper and Row Publishers, Inc., 1973.

Chamberlain, Judi. *On Our Own: Patient-Controlled Alternatives to the Mental Health System*. New York: McGraw-Hill, Inc., 1978, p. 236.

Chesler, Phyllis. *Women and Maaness*. New York: Avon Books, 1972, p. 351.

Conrad, Peter, and Joseph W. Schneider. "The Medical Model of Madness: The Emergence of Mental Illness," *Deviance and Medicalization: From Badness to Sickness*. St. Louis, Mo: C.V. Mosby Co., 1980.

Ernst, Sheila, and Lucy Goodison. *In Our Own Hands: A Book of Self-Help Therapy*. Los Angeles: J.P. Tarcher, 1981.

Frank, Kay Portland. *The Anti-Psychiatry Bibliography and Resource Guide*. Press Gang Publishers, 603 Powell Street, Vancouver, B.C., Canada, 1980.

Franks, Violet, and Vasanti Burtle, eds. *New Psychotherapies*. New York: Brunner-Mazel, 1974.

Gilligan, Carol. *In A Different Voice: Psychological Theory and Women's Development*. Cambridge, MA: Harvard University Press, 1982, p. 184.

Greenspan, Miriam. *A New Approach to Women and Therapy*. New York: McGraw-Hill, Inc., 1983, p. 355.

Howell, Elizabeth, and Marjorie Bayes, eds. *Women and Mental Health*. New York: Basic Books, 1981, p. 448.

Kaplan, Alexandra G., and Joan P. Bean, eds. *Beyond Sex-Role Stereotypes: Readings Toward A Psychology of Androgeny*. Boston, MA: Little, Brown and Co., 1976, p. 392.

Light, Donald W., Jr. *Becoming Psychiatrists*. New York: W.W. Norton and Co., Inc., 1980.

Mander, Anica Vesel, and Anne Kent Rush. *Feminism as Therapy*. New York: Random House/Bookworks, 1974, p. 127.

Miller, Jean Baker. *Toward a New Psychology of Women*. Boston, MA: Beacon Press, 1976, p. 143.

Mitchell, Juliet. *Psychoanalysis and Feminism—Freud, Reich, Laing and Women*. New York: Vintage Books, 1975, p. 455.

Notman, Malkah T., M.D., and Carol C. Nadelson, M.D., eds. *The Woman Patient: Medical and Psychological Interfaces*. New York: Plenum Publishing Corp. (Vol. 2: *Concepts of Femininity and The Life Cycle*, 1982, p. 206; Vol. 3: *Aggression, Adaptation and Psychotherapy*, 1982, p. 314).

Scarf, Maggie. *Unfinished Business: Pressure Points in the Lives of Women*. New York: Ballantine Books, Inc., 1980, p. 623.

Sheehy, Gail. *Passages*. New York: Bantam Books, 1976, p. 564.

Smith, Dorothy E., and Sara J. Davis, eds. *Women Look at Psychiatry*. Vancouver, B.C., Canada: Press Gang Publishers, 1975.

Szasz, Thomas. *The Manufacture of Madness*. New York: Harper and Row Publishers, Inc., 1970.

Task Force on Consumer Issues in Psychotherapy of The Association for Women in Psychology and The Division of The Psychology of Women of The American Psychological Association. *Women and Psychotherapy: A Consumer Handbook*. Federation of Organizations for Professional Women, 2000 P Street NW, Suite 403, Washington, DC 20036 ($3.75 plus $1.00 for postage and handling).

Tennov, Dorothy. *Psychotherapy, The Hazardous Cure*. New York: Abelard-Schuman, 1975.

7

ENVIRONMENTAL AND OCCUPATIONAL HEALTH

Environmental Health by Patricia Logan
Occupational Health by Letitia Davis, Marian Marbury, Laura Punnett, Margaret Quinn, Cathy Schwartz and Susan Woskie (all are members of Mass COSH Women's Committee)

With special thanks to Judy Norsigian, the Shalan Foundation and the thousands of women around the country working in community groups and fighting toxics

We live in a small town. One morning a neighbor came over and said, "Don't drink the water," just after my husband and I drank two cups of coffee made from tap-water.

We had been drinking it for years, and we didn't know how long it had been contaminated. Then our neighbor said just how bad it was, how many milligrams of the chemicals were in it. No one knows where it came from or who caused it. I felt very angry. You pay your taxes— they get higher every year—and you've got people sitting down there in their offices letting things get that bad.

Everybody should have pure, clean water to drink. But what could I do about it? I don't know enough. And anyway, what about everything else? When you eat your chicken, how do you know if you get pure meat? Or what's in your vegetables? Or what's in your bottled water?

Where and how we live and work affects our health in some obvious and not so obvious ways all the time. Sixty to 90 percent of all human cancers and high percentages of other lung, heart, nerve and kidney disease as well as reproductive problems, birth defects and even behavioral disorders are now thought to be environmentally caused.[1] (Environment here includes our diet and living habits.) Environmental hazards have increased tremendously in the last forty years. To the accidents, stress and disease which people have always encountered, twentieth-century society has added toxic chemical and radioactive substances. Through their manufacture, processing, distribution, use and disposal, these substances create a severe and unreasonable risk of injury to our environment and to our health.

CHEMICALS

Between 50,000 and 75,000 chemical substances are in common commercial use in this country, especially in farming, forestry and the chemical, drug and manufacturing industries. About a thousand new chemicals appear each year. The vast majority of these chemicals has not been tested for their potential ill effects, yet they are in our food, water, air, clothing, homes and workplaces. American industry generates 96 billion pounds of hazardous chemical wastes each year, and disposes of 90 percent of these in unsafe ways.[2]

Our sewers are loaded with acid and chemicals. You can see them cooking in there, coming right up in my cellar. I called the city officials and they said they have nothing to do with it anymore. It's up to the state. The state people came and took samples from the sewer. I have yet to hear the results. That was five months ago.
I have been going to the doctor for the past 30 years. I've got breathing problems, kidney and bladder trouble, my kid has a heart condition, my husband can't breathe. Every morning I get up I know I am going to get that "sweet air" from the sewer disposal, and then I say, what's going to be next?[3]

RADIATION

Available evidence suggests that low-level radiation from normally functioning nuclear power plants and weapons facilities and testing contaminates our environment and our bodies in slow stages. Mining of uranium and disposing of the milling wastes (called tailings) and the spent fuel create even more hazards. Waste from a nuclear reactor or weapons plant remains radioactive for as long as 250 centuries.

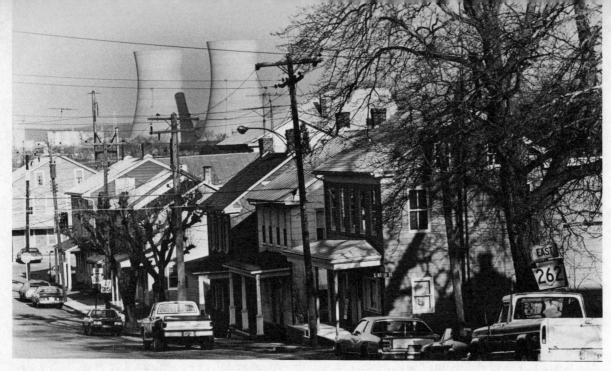

Lionel J-M Delevingne/Stock Boston

Our immediate community has been threatened by the effluent from one of the largest uranium mines in this hemisphere. For many months this effluent contaminated our public water supply—our people drank, cooked with, and bathed in this water, which had radiation in excess of recommended exposures. It took litigation and thousands of dollars of taxpayers' money to remove this community from that contaminated water supply.

In 1978 I lost a very good friend and neighbor of twenty-five years to pancreatic cancer. I had maintained an almost bedside vigil for six months prior to her death. During her final weeks we spoke of the many people in our neighborhood who had succumbed to the ravages of cancer. We wondered if the number of deaths was unusually high, even though cancer is proclaimed the number-two killer.

Only time will tell, I guess, and then the burden of proof will be on whom?

In the ultimate accident at a nuclear power plant, a meltdown, thousands would die immediately of lethal radiation exposure; tens of thousands would die within two or three weeks of acute radiation sickness; hundreds of thousands of cancers would occur five to thirty years afterwards. And of course, nuclear war itself is the ultimate environmental hazard. The U.S. alone has over 30,000 nuclear warheads and can kill every human being on earth twelve times over.

Today environmental hazards are so widespread that none of us can totally avoid them. Even snow in Antarctica carries residues of PCBs, DDT and lead.*[4] Human breast milk contains high levels of some toxins and human sperm samples contain PCBs.

*Polychlorinated biphenyls, once widely used in adhesives, paints, lubricants, electric insulators and printing inks, can cause everything from skin discoloration to liver disorders to cancer; DDT causes cancer and endangers wildlife; lead damages the nervous system.

Although we encounter the most concentrated and dangerous hazards in the workplace, our general environment creates a toxic burden for everyone and an added burden for workers.

- Lead and gases from car exhaust; particles, ash and smoke from factories; emissions from chemical and nuclear plants; and drift from pesticide spraying contaminate our air.
- Pesticides applied to crops, herbicides sprayed on forests and industrial chemicals flushed from factories and leaking from dumps contaminate our water.
- Pesticides, fertilizers, preservatives and additives pollute our food. Lead can concentrate in food grown near roadways. Hormones and antibiotics added to cattle feed, pesticides sprayed on rangeland and low-level radiation accumulate in animal fats to be passed up the food chain to people who eat animal products.
- Typical household cleaners and appliances can produce toxic fumes and dusts. With the energy crisis, increased weatherproofing of homes traps and concentrates toxics like radioactive radon gas (from concrete foundations containing uranium tailings) and the fumes from formaldehyde (used in products like permanent-press fabrics, foam insulation, carpets, drapes and plywood). Even low levels of formaldehyde vapors, carbon monoxide and other air pollutants in the home may disrupt moods and impair mental abilities.

We are involuntarily exposed to some environmental health hazards no matter who or where we are. Toxics don't discriminate—they cross regional, sex, class and racial lines. In these cases economic power determines how much we can protect ourselves. Some people can afford to move away from a chemical dump or nuclear power plant; some can buy bottled water or food without additives or get better health care.

Others at this point in our country's history cannot. Many people of color are forced into the most dangerous and low-paying jobs and live in the more polluted inner cities. As a result they carry a heavier toxic burden. Among black people in the United States the number of cancers and cancer deaths has risen since 1955.[5] And exposure to heavy metals, particularly lead, causes nervous system damage resulting in everything from distraction to learning disabilities, numbness, miscarriages, paralysis and death. Recent work shows that 2 percent of white children, 12 percent of black children and 19 percent of inner city black children have lead levels high enough to require treatment.[6]

Nor are environmental health hazards simply an urban problem. Rural people face heavy exposure to pesticides and herbicides, especially since agribusiness has taken over food production. Native Americans live with persistent low-level radiation from the uranium mining that has taken over more and more of their land. Some companies have targeted their reservations for toxic-waste dump sites.[7]

In addition, pesticides, drugs and industrial chemicals and processes banned as too dangerous in the U.S. are exported for manufacture or use in developing countries where regulations are nonexistent or not enforced. Some industries and chemical companies are even eyeing Third World countries as easy, unregulated sites for hazardous wastes as community resistance to dumps here grows.[8]

Women have had little to say about what we need or want. We have been targeted by industry and advertising as the consumers, not the producers, of the new technology that creates environmental hazards.

Marg Deutsch

Yet women have also been instrumental in many struggles to curb hazards.

Official government and business statements about environmental hazards are almost universally reassuring. "Don't worry, no long-term dangers have been scientifically proved." They put profit and prestige before people's health. Today we face the tragic consequences of trusting the reassurances of earlier decades—about DDT, for instance, or atomic testing. We who are writing this chapter believe that we *must* be concerned about environmental hazards whether or not they are at present conclusively "proven" dangerous. We don't want ourselves, our loved ones or anyone anywhere in the world used as guinea pigs in long-term safety experiments. We know our bodies, our workplaces and our communities better than any scientist does.

THE HEALTH EFFECTS OF ENVIRONMENTAL HAZARDS

At Love Canal* they told us to go home and tend our gardens. But women are no longer at home tending their gardens because both have become unsafe.

There are many effects of Love Canal chemicals, like central nervous system disease, including nervous breakdowns, migraine headaches and epilepsy. We have not conducted a survey on cancer to see if the rate is abnormally high here, but we have found many women throughout the neighborhood with breast and uterine cancer. There are many cancers, and they are not just in middle-aged women. One twelve-year-old child had a hysterectomy. We have many people with urinary problems, brain damage, and the list goes on. We have to wonder what the future holds: cancers and other diseases may not surface for years.

To understand environmental health, we must understand that *everything* is connected—our body systems and organs, our life habits, our work and our wider environment. Environmental hazards can attack a particular organ or body system, directly damaging it and/or leading to further complications. While scientists generally test substances in labs one at a time, in real life our bodies always deal with more than one hazard at once. The combined interaction of two or more hazards to produce an effect greater than

*From the 1920s to the 1950s, the Hooker Chemical Company buried metal drums filled with tons of chemical wastes in the excavations in the Love Canal neighborhood of Niagara Falls, New York. In 1953 they covered the dump and sold the land to the Board of Education, which built a school on the site. Over the years the drums rusted and chemicals seeped, mixed and were spread by flooding and underground streams. Toxics killed plants, grass and wildlife, sickened local residents and caused birth defects and spontaneous abortions. In August 1978, the government declared Love Canal a national emergency area.

that of either one alone is called *synergism*. The amount of exposure, route of exposure and the toxic substance(s) we are exposed to determine whether we will feel acute or chronic effects.

An *acute effect* is a severe immediate reaction, usually after a single, large exposure—like the nausea and dizziness of pesticide poisoning or the pulmonary edema (a blistering of the air sacs in the lungs) from the burns of toxic gases like ammonia or chlorine. A *chronic effect* is a recurrent or constant reaction usually after repeated smaller exposures. Chronic effects can take years—the *latency period*—to develop. For instance, exposure to asbestos causes lung disease years later, and most cancers and progressive liver diseases develop only after fifteen to forty years. Many scientists think we will see more and more problems as the toxics introduced after World War Two "come of age."

We can absorb toxic substances in three ways: through the skin, through the digestive system (eating or drinking) or through the lungs. Often toxics cause damage on first contact—burns, rashes, stomach pain, for example. Once in the bloodstream, they can damage many internal organs and systems.

In general, toxics affect women and men in the same ways: anyone can have an allergic reaction or liver damage, chronic headaches or respiratory problems, mental retardation or lung cancer. Environmental hazards put extra stress on our bodies and compound any other health problems that we might have.

Environmental Health Terms

Carcinogen (car-*sin*-o-jen) — A substance or agent that causes cancer, a condition characterized by usually rapidly spreading abnormal cell growth.

Mutagen (*mew*-ta-jen) — A substance or agent that causes changes (mutations) in the genetic material of living cells. When a mutation occurs in the egg or sperm (germ cells), it can be passed on to future generations. Recent research suggests that since genetic material controls the growth of cells, mutagens may either immediately or after a latency period cause abnormal cell growth, which becomes cancer.

Teratogen (teh-*ra*-to-jen) — A substance or agent that can cross the placenta of a pregnant woman and can cause a spontaneous abortion or birth defects and developmental abnormalities in the fetus.

All carcinogens are mutagens. Most mutagens are carcinogens. Many mutagens are also teratogens.

ENVIRONMENTAL HAZARDS AND OUR BODY SYSTEMS*

Body System/Function	Acute and Chronic Effects	Some Common Causes
Skin—Body's first line of protection from the environment. Can be initiated directly. Toxics can also penetrate skin to enter bloodstream.	Redness, dryness, itching	Solvents, plastics, epoxies, metals
	Redness, burns, blisters	Ultraviolet and infrared radiation, acids
	Severe acne (chloracne)	PCBs, dioxin
	Skin cancer	Mineral oils, ultraviolet radiation, X-rays, arsenic
Respiratory system (nose, throat, lungs)—Transfers oxygen to the blood. Lungs, nose, throat can be burned or scarred directly. Toxics can also be absorbed from lungs into bloodstream.	Sneezing, coughing, sore throat, wheezing, congestion	Gases, ammonia, solvents, formaldehyde, cotton and mineral dusts, beryllium, metal oxide
	Burning, fluid build-up (pulmonary edema)	Ammonia, nitrogen oxides, sulfur dioxide, chlorine, kerosene
	Chronic lung disease (bronchitis, emphysema)	Asbestos dust, soft coal dust
	Lung cancer	Mineral oils, chromium, asbestos, cigarettes

*Compiled from *Work Is Dangerous to Your Health*, Jeanne Stellman and Susan Davis (Vintage, 1971), and *We're Tired of Being Guinea Pigs*, Maxine Henry, Juliet Memfield, *et al.*, Highlander Research and Education Center, 1980.

Body System/Function	Acute and Chronic Effects	Some Common Causes
Cardiovascular system (heart and blood vessels)—Pumps and carries blood throughout the body. Damaged when deprived of oxygen.	Irregular heartbeat Arteriosclerosis Coronary heart disease	Carbon monoxide, barium, organophosphates, glues and solvents, heat and cold, carbon disulfide, cigarettes
Gastrointestinal system (stomach, intestines)—Digests ingested toxics either breaking them down or passing them on to the bloodstream.	Nausea, vomiting, diarrhea, constipation	Pesticides, chloroform, cyanide, fluonide, solvents, lead
Liver and kidneys—Toxics pass into the blood from the digestive system and are carried to the liver and kidneys, which work to break them down and pass them from the body. They can be inflamed, scarred or even poisoned in the process.	Jaundice Hepatitis (inflammation of liver) Acute kidney disease Chronic kidney disease	Carbon tetrachloride, vinyl chloride Tetrachlorethane, chlorinated hydrocarbons, anesthesia Lead, mercury, carbon monoxide, arsenic, high voltage electricity Lead, carbon disulfide, alcohol
Central nervous system (brain, nerves)—Toxics can reduce oxygen to the brain and interfere with communication between nerves and other body systems, causing disorders.	Behavioral disorders, confusion, lethargy, depression, anxiety, headache, irritability Learning disability or impairment, depression of central nervous system Oxygen deprivation, brain damage Nerve function disorders	Noise, metal poisoning (lead, mercury), stress, kepone, carbone disulfide, pesticides Acetates, brominated/chlorinated chemicals Asphyxiating gases, carbon monoxide Organophosphate pesticides, mercury, lead, arsenic, manganese
Immune system—Minimum exposures to toxics can tax and suppress the body's ability to fight disease or poisons. Some believe dysfunction of the immune system allows cancer to develop.	Burning, nausea, headaches, psychosis, allergic reactions	Epoxy resins and plastics, hexachlorophene, nickel compounds, mercury compounds, formaldehyde
Circulatory system (blood)—Absorbs toxics from digestive system, lungs or skin and carries them to other organs.	Anemia Leukemia	Lead Benzene, ionizing radiation
Reproductive system—Toxics can harm the reproductive organs themselves, cause direct damage to eggs, sperm or a developing fetus, or cause mutations in eggs and sperm that can be passed on to later generations.	Infertility or reduced fertility Decreased libido Menstrual changes Birth defects	Lead, carbon disulfide, ionizing radiation Carbon disulfide, estrogens (in men) Carbon disulfide, estrogens, lead, PCBs Anesthetic gases, mercury, lead, DDT

Reproductive Health Hazards

A reproductive hazard is any agent that has harmful effects on the male or female reproductive system and/or the development of a fetus. These hazards can be chemicals (like pesticides), physical agents (like X-rays) or work practices (like heavy lifting).

Reproductive health hazards are probably the most controversial issues in environmental health. Because women bear children, reproductive hazards are too often considered "a woman's problem" involving pregnancy alone. This view ignores two important facts: that men are also affected by reproductive hazards, and that reproductive health means more than having healthy babies. All through life, men and women need healthy sexual and reproductive systems. As it is, reproductive hazards are often used as excuses to penalize women workers and permit management to avoid cleaning up the workplace.

Infertility in either sex, a spontaneous abortion early in pregnancy or a baby with birth defects can all be early signs of a toxic environment. These can be important signals that something is wrong, since other signs like cancer can take a fifteen- to forty-year latency period to develop.

How Reproductive Hazards Affect Men

A recent government study found PCBs in every human sperm sample tested.[9] Environmental toxics can disrupt the production of male hormones in the testes, causing loss of sex drive and impotence. They can also cause problems with sperm production. A toxic agent can disturb sperm cells at any one of several stages of rapid growth, causing problems with fertility through a total lack of sperm, low sperm production or malformed sperm. Toxics may be causing an overall decline in sperm counts in American men.[10]

In addition, some reproductive hazards are mutagens. When a mutation occurs in sperm cells, men can pass damaged genes on to future generations, which can result in spontaneous abortions or inherited birth defects.

- Men exposed to lead have decreased fertility and malformed sperm.[11]
- Higher rates of birth defects are showing up in the children of Vietnam veterans exposed to Agent Orange. This herbicide was contaminated with dioxin, considered the most toxic man-made substance. It can concentrate in the food chain and accumulate in human fat; it can also pass through the skin.*[12]
- DBCP (dibromochloropropane), a pesticide, was found to cause dramatically decreased sperm counts in men who work with it or in its manufacture. The

*For report of a major epidemiological study by Colin Norman, see "Vietnam's Herbicide Legacy," in *Science*, Vol. 219, March 11, 1983, pp. 1196–97.

men in one California factory noticed that none of them had fathered children since they started working there, and demanded fertility tests. Many were found sterile.[13]

How Reproductive Hazards Affect Women

When toxic substances disrupt the reproductive hormones, they can cause menstrual disorders, sterility or loss of sexual drive.[14] Toxic substances may also directly damage the ovaries, eventually resulting in early menopause or ovarian disease. And, as with sperm cells, environmental mutagens can damage the genetic material in a woman's eggs, with the same effects—spontaneous abortion or birth defects. Recent animal studies show ovary damage from polycyclic hydrocarbons (used in the petrochemical industry), alkylating agents (used in cancer treatment) and ionizing radiation. Exposure to lead, PCBs and vinyl chloride can cause menstrual changes.

The Developing Fetus and Young Children

The fertilized egg and the fetus can react to toxics that do not apparently harm an adult.

Teratogens (see p. 80) are particularly dangerous during the first three months of pregnancy, so early that the woman may not be aware she is pregnant. During the first two weeks, the fertilized egg is so sensitive that an environmental hazard powerful enough to damage it will also destroy it. From the fifteenth to the sixtieth day of a pregnancy, the cells of the fetus multiply and differentiate into specific organs and systems. A toxin can disrupt this process, and there is no second chance for the system to establish itself. If the teratogen is very strong, the pregnancy often ends in a spontaneous abortion (miscarriage). If the fetus survives, the child may have a low birth weight or physical, developmental or behavioral defects, some of which may not show up until years later.

The most common way that a fetus is exposed to toxics in the environment or workplace is through the mother's direct exposure. However, since semen is one place where toxics accumulate, having intercourse during pregnancy may expose a fetus to concentrations of toxics that can cause birth defects.[15] (Pregnant couples might consider ways of making love other than intercourse; men exposed to environmental hazards can use condoms.)

The developing fetus and young children are particularly susceptible to environmental hazards because their cells are dividing and growing rapidly. This is why pregnant women and young children were evacuated first from both Love Canal and from the area near the disabled nuclear reactor at Three Mile Island during the 1979 incident. Yet the government still sets standards for "safety" levels of toxics based on effects on adults.

Certain toxics concentrate in human breast milk, to be passed along to newborns. According to an EPA study, 99 percent of all American women have enough PCBs in their breast milk to show up in tests.[16] (A study by the Environmental Defense Fund concluded that nursing infants get almost a hundred times the amount of toxics ingested by adults in proportion to body weight.) Yet breastfeeding is so beneficial to babies that unless you live in an area where there's known excessive pollution, the benefits outweigh the risks.[17] Unless a new mother knows she has been exposed to particular toxics, in most cases the benefits of breastfeeding seem to outweigh the risks.

Other Effects

Environmental mutagens also pose dangers for the entire human species. Damaged genetic material, whether it causes visible damage or not, contributes its permanent changes to the total human gene pool. A mutation rate increased by the effects of chemical and radioactive toxins could not only produce a general decline in human genetic health, it could threaten human existence.

TACKLING THE ENVIRONMENTAL HEALTH CRISIS

As women we are learning both to be more aware of environmentally caused problems and more confident about the power of such awareness. Often in the past we have just "accepted" a miscarriage or infertility or a chronically sick child. Now, instead of accepting, we're investigating. And when we do, we often find that the problems are environmentally caused. It's important not to just accept physicians' statements that "this is normal" or that we are "just being emotional." Environmental damage is often hard to prove. Persist. Don't just remain frustrated with the doctor. Find a new one. Find someone you can talk to about it.

And keep on learning to be more alert to things that can go wrong with your body because of environmental exposures. Don't discount your own knowledge of yourself, your own power.

We can begin to minimize the effects of some environmental hazards by avoiding voluntary exposures* and staying as healthy as we can. Yet the larger

problems with environmental hazards can seem overwhelming and confusing. Taking action often seems too complicated—there is too much bureaucracy, too much chemistry and biology to learn and the polluters have too much power. "Surely someone is taking care of it all," we say. No one is. "It's all too impossible to deal with," we say. It's not.

Environmental health is basically a community issue, one we cannot fight alone. Luckily, we don't have to. A Harris survey from the summer of 1981 shows that 93 percent of the American public wants to see stricter government standards for hazardous waste disposal. Eighty-six percent opposed weakening of air quality laws, and 93 percent opposed weakening of water quality laws. People don't want hazards in their backyards, and they're saying so. But the manufacturing and agricultural industries will not regulate themselves, and government cannot do it all.* It's up to citizens, supporting national laws and acting locally, to take on the work.

Strategies

Citizen action against environmental health hazards can take many routes. (See Resources for more information.) Experienced activists agree on some basic points:

1. The first step is education. What hazards are manufactured, used, stored or transported in your community and how do they harm people? Where do they come from? Become familiar with what's in use in your area and what the effects are. Pass on what you learn. Try working with existing community groups, bring in speakers, write letters to newspapers, show films, set up information tables.

2. Keep a log of any changes in your health and try to correlate them with what industries are doing in your area.

3. Talk to your neighbors. Work with other people. Many citizens' groups get going when people realize that they're not alone, that others are also being affected. Do a citizens' health survey.

4. Monitor your own "backyard." Watch for odd smells, bubbles or oozes in the air, land or water. Watch for sick and dying wildlife and pets. Watch for oil drums abandoned in fields or trucks dumping at night. Watch for "invisible" hazards, too: radiation can't be seen, but the industries manufacturing it can be. Pay attention to reproductive patterns in your community. Government agencies may try to dismiss your results as "nonscientific," but this information can be very

---

*For example, avoid unnecessary X-rays, especially during pregnancy. Drugs, including lotions containing hormones; douches; nosedrops; and other self-prescribed medications are the chemicals most implicated as teratogens. Hair dyes have been shown to be mutagenic and carcinogenic. The coal-tar food

dyes cause allergic reactions. Processed vegetables can have high concentrations of lead from the soldering on the cans. Caffeine is suspected of reducing fertility and causing birth defects. Eat carefully washed fresh foods rather than the dairy and meat products in which chemicals and radioactivity concentrate.

*Especially with the budget cuts imposed by conservative governments at every level.

helpful in showing patterns, establishing that there is a problem, keeping facts and history clear, activating citizens and helping health professionals know—later—what to focus their studies on.

5. When industry or government presents you or your group with information, statistics or data on a substance and its effects, always ask who paid for the study. The answer should help you to evaluate the data. Demand that information be presented in terms you can understand, not in the jargon of "experts."

6. Use the consumers' tool: the boycott. Find out where pollutants come from and what products they're used in, and refuse to buy them. Women especially have enormous power as consumers.

The Delaware Valley Toxics Coalition (DVTC) and the Philadelphia Project on Occupational Safety and Health (PhilaPOSH) offer citizens organizing around environmental hazards a strong and successful model to follow. Starting in the summer of 1979, they built a coalition of labor, community, environmental and health groups to work for the first "right-to-know" legislation for communities. A Philadelphia ordinance, passed in January 1981, requires all businesses in Philadelphia to make available to workers and community residents the names and health effects of selected toxics they use, store, manufacture or vent into the air.

Women's Activism

Women have always been active in exposing and working to eliminate environmental health hazards.

- Ellen Swallow, the first woman student admitted to MIT, created the interdisciplinary study of nutrition, air and water pollution, architecture, waste disposal and occupational health and safety. In 1892 she named this study "ecology."
- Rachel Carson, in 1962, wrote *Silent Spring*, the book that exposed the widespread use and dangers of pesticides in our environment. Her work brought this problem to public attention, led to the ban on DDT in the U.S., and marked the beginning of the American environmental movement.
- Lois Gibbs organized the Love Canal Homeowners' Association and, with the women of Love Canal, forced the state of New York to recognize the problems. They signed petitions, did health surveys, embarrassed government and industry officials, picketed, blocked buses and testified in Washington. Because of their work, the government evacuated 1,000 families, purchased their homes, and established a safety plan for the workers on site, a retroactive tax break and a health fund to cover future problems.
- Bonnie Hill and seven other women correlated their miscarriages with the spraying of 2,4,5-T, a herbicide, near their homes in rural Alsea, Oregon. Their protests to the EPA led to the emergency ban in 1979 on the chemical for most uses in the U.S.

- Polly Heran, a member of the local water board of Rocky Flats, Colorado, discovered that the water supply had double the normal amount of uranium. The community is near a uranium mine and a nuclear weapons facility. Ms. Heran, along with a group of housewives, studied the issue. When they could not get the local authorities to act because there was no "conclusive" information on the radioactive effect of the uranium, they threatened to boycott and bankrupt the water department. They proved the toxicity of the uranium as a heavy metal rather than as a radioactive element, forcing the local government to take action.
- On Earth Day 1980, the Chemical Control Company dump exploded in Elizabeth, New Jersey, forcing people from Elizabeth east to Staten Island to stay indoors while the chemicals burned. For years before this, residents had complained of respiratory and other health problems, suspecting the heavy concentrations of chemical manufacturers and the chemical dump as the cause. A citizens' group, led by Sister Jacinta Fernandes and other community women, had conducted health surveys, marched and held speakouts. Their pressure had forced cleanup of the worst chemicals from the dump *before* it exploded. Without their work, the fire would have been even more devastating.

As the women's health movement has shown, we must take charge of our bodies, our health, our environment and our lives.

Any average man or woman can do what we did. You can write press releases, push government, get things done. If you keep hammering the nail, eventually it's going to go in. I was "just a housewife." I'm proof that you don't need special talent or experience. I don't think people understand that. If I can get up and address five hundred people, believe me, anyone can. If something has to be done, there are ways to do it. You don't need a college education—just determination.

WORK CAN BE HAZARDOUS TO OUR HEALTH

The work we do affects our health not only while we are working but throughout the rest of the day, on weekends and vacations and even in the years after we have left the job. The consequences of hazardous working conditions are severe. More than 100,000 workers die each year from known job-related diseases, and more suffer from other diseases not yet recognized as resulting from exposures on the job. Over 16,000 American workers are killed every year in workplace accidents, and thousands more are disabled. We cannot take poor working conditions for granted as "just part of the job." We have to think

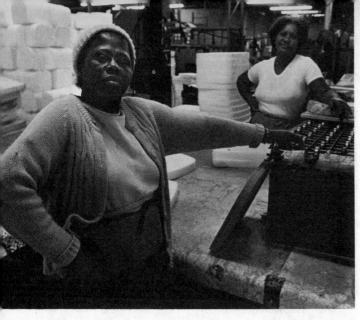

about them—why they exist, what they might be doing to us and how they can be changed.

Workplace safety and health are usually associated with traditional "men's work," like mining, construction and heavy manufacturing. Women in the paid labor force have tended to be concentrated in "women's work," such as cleaning, nursing, teaching, garment making, clerical and "service" work. These jobs are not so safe either.

I had worked at the hospital for four years as a housekeeper when I got sick with hepatitis. I found out that a patient on my floor had hepatitis and nobody had bothered to tell me what precautions to take. I filed a claim for worker's compensation and the hospital fought my claim! I never thought that a thing like that could happen. I was working in a place that was supposed to care about people's health and they never told me anything about protecting my health.

The growing number of women in heavy industry and construction jobs generally face the same, often dangerous conditions that men face. But women often feel pressure to prove that they are "as good as" the men they work with, and when they speak up about health and safety they're seen as "too weak to take it." Yet the problems we are concerned about also affect men, and women's vocal presence in these traditionally male workplaces is bringing a change in the way people think about health and safety issues.

Women have special concerns because of our social and economic situations. Sexist job discrimination puts a large majority of women into low-paying and stressful occupations. Many women carry the double duty of paid work *and* responsibilities at home, which makes it more difficult to get involved in after-work meetings about working conditions. Women often have low seniority, or jobs that place them in caretaking roles or require close working relationships with their bosses, making them hesitant to bring up complaints about hazards. In addition, only 16 percent of women work-

ers belong to unions, which makes organizing more difficult.

Minority women are more often stuck with dead-end, "no transfer" jobs that expose them to more dangerous conditions for longer periods of time than their white counterparts. Black workers have a 37 percent greater chance than whites of suffering an occupational injury or disease.[18]

I worked in a parts plant in Detroit. The worst job in the place was packing ball bearings in lithium grease— all day long. There were about twenty-five women who did that—and they were all black. There never was a white woman assigned to that job.

Seventy percent of all migrant farmworkers are black and Latino. These workers face appalling working conditions, including exposure to pesticides that have well-documented harmful health effects.

Did You Know?

54% of all women in the U.S. are in the paid labor force.
43% of the paid work force is women.

Where Women Work

White collar work: 66%
   clerical: 35%
   sales: 7%
   professional and technical: 17%
   management and administration: 7%
Blue collar work: 14%
Service work: 19%
Farmwork: 1%

Bureau of Labor Statistics
April 1981

Recognizing Hazards in the Workplace

Management is supposed to provide a safe workplace, but this task is frequently low on its priority list. Improving conditions often costs money, and in addition management may be afraid of giving up, or appearing to give up, control. Who controls the workplace is often an important, if unstated, issue in workplace health and safety struggles. If workers become knowledgeable about work processes and practices in order to make them safer, we are then more likely to question in general why and how things are done.

Recognition is the first step in eliminating hazards. You don't have to be an expert, but you do have to be persistent and thorough. A good way to begin is by talking with the people you work with. You and your co-workers are the best qualified to identify what the hazards and dangerous jobs are.

Some hazards are obvious. Just using your eyes, ears and nose will help you pick out safety hazards such as obvious dust or fumes and excessive noise. Recognizing hidden hazards is often more difficult. See if there is any pattern in who gets sick in your workplace. Talk to people or use a simple questionnaire to ask about mild symptoms, headaches, frequent illnesses, coughs, etc. These activities will not only help identify problems, they will also help to build awareness and interest among fellow workers about job conditions.

Learn about the chemicals and other substances you work with. A trade name such as Wite Out is not useful; you need to know the names of the actual chemicals in the product (in this case, trichlorethylene) because almost all information on chemicals is organized by the scientific chemical name. It's hard to believe that in most places we still don't have the legal right to know the name of the chemicals we work with. In many areas workers and environmental groups have

SOME COMMON WORKPLACE HAZARDS

Potential Safety Hazards	Potential Health Hazards
No machine guards Faulty switches, exposed wiring Dangerous floors, doors, exits, aisles, stairs Cranes, lifts, hoists Poor lighting Explosives No fire extinguishers No protective gear for emergencies Poor maintenance of equipment Lack of training in safe work practices and first aid Speedup No first aid equipment	Dusts, mists, gases, vapors, smoke Heat, cold, dampness Radiation Noise, vibration Stress

COMMON HAZARDS IN WOMEN'S OCCUPATIONS

Type of Work	Common Hazards	Health Effects
Household workers: over 1 million	Cleaning substances (drain and oven cleaners, bleach, aerosol sprays, waxes), pesticides Lifting, falls, infections from children, electrical shock, noise	Irritation or burns of skin, eyes or lungs, allergies Muscle soreness, slipped disc, torn ligaments, bursitis
Clerical workers: over 14.5 million	Stress, VDTs (video display terminals) Poor air quality and ventilation, toxic substances from photocopy, duplicators, correction fluids Noise Poor lighting and chair design	Headache, heart disease, eyestrain, neck and back pain Nausea, colds, respiratory problems, eye, nose and throat irritation Anxiety, hearing damage Varicose veins, neck and back pain, eyestrain
Hospital workers: 4.1 million	Infections Lifting and falls Radiation Chemical hazards (sterilizing gases, anesthetic gases, drugs) Stress, electric shock	Infection from patients, utensils, specimens Back strain, slipped disc, torn ligaments Tissue damage, genetic changes from X-rays Skin and respiratory irritation, liver, kidney, nervous system damage, cancer, reproductive problems Headaches, heart disease, gastrointestinal problems
Retail salespersons: 1.7 million	Standing, lifting, stress Safety hazards (blocked aisles, exits; poorly designed equipment) Poor ventilation Infection	Leg pain, varicose veins, back and shoulder pain, headaches, irritability, high blood pressure Accidents Colds, respiratory problems, eye, nose and throat irritation Communicable diseases

ENVIRONMENTAL AND OCCUPATIONAL HEALTH

Type of Work	Common Hazards	Health Effects
Sewers and stitchers: 773,000 Textile operatives (number unknown)	Chemicals (fabric treatment, dyes, cleaning solvents)	Skin and lung irritation, damage to liver, kidney and nervous system; dermatitis
	Synthetic fiber and cotton dust	Asthma, respiratory disease
	Noise	Hearing loss
	Vibration	Wrist and hand inflammation
	Heat, cold, poor ventilation	Heat stress, colds
	Unsafe equipment	Accidents, electric shock
	Lifting, standing, sitting	Back and shoulder strain, varicose veins
	Stress	High blood pressure, headaches, anxiety
Artists: 96,000	Solvents	Dizziness, dermatitis, damage to liver, kidneys, nervous system
	Paints, solder	Heavy metals can damage kidney, liver, lungs, reproductive system
	Clays, glazes, welding fumes, fumes from firing	Lung damage
	Poor equipment maintenance; poor ventilation	Accidents, fire
Lab workers: 221,000	Handling biological specimens or animals	Infection
	Toxic chemicals, including carcinogens	Organ damage, changes in genetic material, reproductive problems, cancer
	Radiation in specimens, radioisotopes, machinery using radiation	Tissue changes or genetic changes, reproductive problems
Electronics workers (number unknown)	Solvents	Dermatitis, dizziness, damage to nervous system and organs such as liver
	Acids	Skin burns and irritation
	Sitting and standing, fine work under microscope, repetitive work	Back and shoulder pain, varicose veins, headaches
	Stress	Heart disease, gastrointestinal problems
	Solder fumes, poor ventilation	Eye, nose and throat irritation, lung disease
Meat wrappers: 75,000	Lifting	Shoulder and back strain
	Standing	Low back pain, varicose veins
	Repetitive motion	Swelling and inflammation of the hands
	Plastic wrap fumes	Asthma, eye, nose and throat irritation, nausea, flulike symptoms
	Cold, cuts, slips, falls	Numbness, circulation problems
Hairdressers and beauticians: 482,000	Standing	Low back pain and varicose veins
	Chemicals (hair sprays and dyes, aerosol sprays, cosmetics and other preparations)	Lung disease, reproductive effects, cancer, allergies, skin irritation
Laundry and dry cleaners: 118,000	Laundry: soaps, bleaches, acids	Irritation or burns on hands, irritation of eyes, nose or throat
	Dry cleaning: solvents	Dermatitis, dizziness, damage to nervous system or liver
	Both: lifting	Back injuries, strains, hernias
	Heat	Heart disease
	Contamination	Exposure to whatever chemicals or biological materials are on clothes

Methods for Controlling Workplace Hazards

1. *Substitute.*
   Can a different substance or equipment (chemical or process) be used that will be safer?
   Clerical workers can use a water-based correction fluid to correct typing instead of a solvent-based fluid.

2. *Change the process.*
   Can the job be done in a completely different and safer way?
   Retail salesworkers are usually required to stand for most of the workday. This can lead to leg pain and varicose veins. If stools are provided and clerks encouraged to rotate sitting and standing, this stress will be reduced.

3. *Mechanize the process.*
   Is automating an operation the best answer to a dangerous job?
   Garment workers often have to lift large bundles of material and bins of finished products. If mechanical lifting devices are provided and used, the back and shoulder strain caused by manual lifting will be avoided.

4. *Isolate or enclose the process.*
   Can the hazardous job be removed to a different area or time where fewer people would be exposed? Can the worker be isolated from the operation or can the process be completely enclosed?
   Hospital workers are often exposed to irritating fumes when soldering parts. If ventilating hoods are installed, the fumes will be exhausted away from the breathing zone of the worker.

5. *Improve housekeeping.*
   In many operations strict housekeeping is essential to keep toxic materials from being reintroduced into the air or to prevent safety hazards.
   Textile workers can be exposed to cotton dust that causes brown lung disease. Strict housekeeping can keep dust levels down and keep obstacles out of the work areas and exits to prevent accidents.

6. *Improve maintenance.*
   Is equipment regularly serviced and repaired?
   Teachers and clerical workers often use photocopy machines. If poorly maintained these machines can give off irritating ozone gas.

7. *Provide personal protective equipment.*
   When other methods fail, or as a backup, can respirators, gloves, aprons or other protective clothing be used?
   Household workers often use toxic chemicals, such as drain cleaners, oven cleaners, pesticides and detergents, for example. Rubber gloves can protect the hands and arms from irritation and prevent the chemicals from being absorbed into the blood by the skin.

8. *Institute administrative controls.*
   When other methods don't work, can people be rotated through stressful or dangerous jobs to minimize their exposure?
   Clerical workers often work with VDTs (video display terminals). Considerable back, neck and eye strain can occur. With frequent rest breaks and job rotation, some stress can be relieved.

been fighting hard for people's "right to know." (See p. 84.) Ways to get information about substances in your workplace include:

- Asking management. If necessary you could force the information through contract grievances or National Labor Relations Board complaints if you have a union. Or you can use direct action such as slowdowns and walkouts, publicity efforts or other creative strategies.
- Writing to the manufacturer of the chemical or product and asking for the Material Safety Data Sheet. These sheets should list the chemicals in the product, the acute and chronic effects and safe handling procedures.
- Asking fellow workers in the supply departments. Often when barrels of chemicals are delivered, they are labeled with the scientific names of the chemicals.
- Calling COSH groups (Committees on Occupational Safety and Health), OSHA (Occupational Safety and Health Administration), NIOSH (National Institute of Occupational Safety and Health) or the health and safety department of your international union.

If the chemical has been tested for its effects (which many have not been), you should be able to find out more information from books or organizations listed in Resources.

Work and Stress

In the garment shop where I work, a lot of us who've been sewing there for a while have been having pains in our hands or our legs. The union is collecting information to see if some jobs are worse than others (like hemming or making linings). We're hoping that we can find out whether there are any changes that would help, like changing the height of the tables or the angle of the machines. Anything that would make the job more comfortable would help my general level of tension! Between the noise from the steam pressers, working fast enough to make a good rate and bending over the machine all day without enough light, I'm lucky if I get out of there without my shoulders all bunched up and *a splitting headache at the end of the day.*

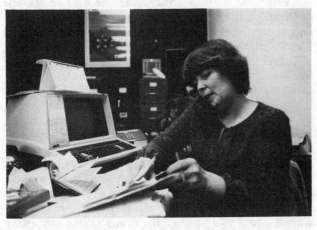

Ellen Shub

Management often tells us that stress is our fault, that we shouldn't bring our personal problems to work. But work conditions can *create* stress, which goes home with us and affects our personal lives, too.

Stress can result from physical factors, such as repetitive hand motions, poor seating conditions, excessive noise, heat or cold, eyestrain or general work overload. Other causes of stress range from relations with the boss and our co-workers, to sexual harassment, to worry about safety and health hazards. Many women have jobs with low pay and no chance of promotion or retraining because of sexual and racial discrimination in employment and limited educational opportunities. Women who have children or want to must worry about maternity leave, childcare and loss of seniority.

Most women in jobs traditionally held by men have to deal with not being very welcome or accepted at the workplace, at least at the beginning. A black woman who works as a union carpenter's apprentice said:

It's difficult not to become paranoid that every insult or putdown comes from people's racist or sexist attitudes, even when you know that all apprentices get dumped on a lot.[19]

Stress can cause serious medical problems. (See p. 88.) We won't end stress on the job as long as job exploitation or racial oppression continue, but we can win some improvements, such as increasing the availability of information about the substances we work with, obtaining adequate staffing and securing a say in decisions that affect our work conditions.

One of the most stressful things about our job at the phone company was the "clacker" that would start going CLACK CLACK CLACK whenever all the incoming lines were busy. The idea was to make us work faster. But it would make my stomach tie into knots and my hands get sweaty whenever I heard that thing. So one day I got a big group of us to go in to the supervisor and say that we just couldn't work like that. There were so many of us that he had to give in.[20]

Though today many companies have "stress management" programs for employees, these programs define stress as an individual problem and allow the company to avoid changing the conditions that cause stress on the job.

"Protecting" Women Out of the Workplace

The distinction between protection and discrimination is often a fine one. For example, some states passed legislation after World War Two limiting the number of pounds a woman could lift or the number of hours she could work on the job. While these laws were supposed to protect women from undue stress, the result was that women lost their jobs to returning servicemen.

Currently an increasing number of companies are instituting policies which prohibit women of childbearing potential from working in areas where they might be exposed to chemicals that would be harmful to fetuses. The reason given for these policies is the need to "protect the unborn child"; the result is that women have lost access to jobs that were only recently opened to them. It is no coincidence that such policies do not exist in companies or institutions which employ a largely female labor force, such as hospitals or the electronics industry. When studies found that anesthetic gases cause spontaneous abortions, hospitals didn't ban women workers from operating rooms. Instead they installed devices that eliminated the problem.

Exclusionary policies ignore the fact that women are not pregnant most of their lives and that many exposures which may be harmful to a fetus are also

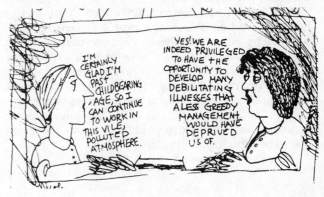

Nicole Hollander

harmful to an adult. Barring women from jobs instead of cleaning up the workplace diverts energy and attention from the real issue: the need to protect all workers from reproductive and other health hazards. Women's presence on the job may in fact raise awareness about hazards.

On my job as a field service technician, three women have become pregnant during the last year and were immediately transferred to other jobs within the company for the duration of their pregnancies. Their doctors, three different doctors, recommended this precaution because of the strong cleaning solvents which we use. Their situation has drawn everyone's attention to the possible dangers which we face on our jobs. Both men and women have been discussing symptoms they believe to be job-related. This is the first time in the nine years that I have been here that the issue has become a major and universal concern, and I believe that it is the pregnancies of our women workers which has brought it to the fore.

If you are barred from a job where reproductive hazards are thought to exist, your legal rights are uncertain. You can file a complaint with the EEOC (Equal Employment Opportunity Commission). You can also fight the case through your union if you have one. Various reproductive-rights organizations may be able to give you additional help and suggestions.

If you are pregnant, it becomes more urgent to remove yourself from possible hazards. One possibility is to request a transfer to a safe job with the same pay, benefits and seniority. If you have a union this should be written into your contract. You may need to leave the workplace if there are no jobs without hazardous exposures available. Management will usually want you to leave without pay, but you may have certain rights to job transfer or paid leave under the pregnancy disability amendment to the Federal Civil Rights Act. Under this law, women "disabled by pregnancy" must be treated the same as other temporarily disabled workers, like those who have had heart attacks or accidents. ("Disabled" is a legal term meaning that one is unable to work.) Some states also have pregnancy disability acts.

Male co-workers often think that reproductive hazards are just a woman's problem. Getting their support by educating them to realize that this isn't true is an essential task. Women are not expendable in the workplace, just as men are not expendable in the family. Job conditions which enable us to be both working people and parents are important for everyone. The United States is one of the few industrialized countries that fails to provide leave and monetary compensation for childbirth.

Legal Rights to a Safe Workplace

The major law dealing with workplace hazards is the federal Occupational Safety and Health Act, which requires employers to make their workplaces safe and free of health hazards "as far as possible." The law (first passed in 1970) established the Occupational Safety and Health Administration (OSHA), which sets standards for workplace conditions and inspects workplaces to see if the standards are being met. OSHA can impose fines on employers who violate standards and order them to clean up. Workers have a right to file complaints with OSHA calling for inspections.

Although the passage of the act was a victory for working people, OSHA alone unfortunately cannot solve all our problems. For example, few OSHA standards cover hazards found in jobs traditionally held by women, and OSHA has seldom inspected offices, hospitals or other predominantly female workplaces.

Up to this time, the Reagan Administration has generally opposed the government regulation of industry and made OSHA even weaker. Yet some workers have been able to use OSHA effectively as a legal tool to win health and safety improvements. We must keep working to protect our rights under OSHA and make them even stronger.

Here are several other laws you should know about:

- *State Workers' Compensation laws*: All states have workers' compensation laws which cover workers who are injured on the job or become ill as a result of work. These laws provide for the payment of medical expenses and part of lost wages.
- *State Health and Safety laws*: Some states have their own health and safety laws which are particularly relevant to state and local government workers who are *not* covered under OSHA.
- *State and local Right-to-Know laws*: In some areas laws have been passed which give workers the right to know the chemical names of the substances they work with.
- *Civil Rights Act*: Gives women "disabled" by pregnancy the same rights as other temporarily disabled workers, and possibly offers some protection against policies excluding women from jobs on the basis of "protecting their health."
- *National Labor Relations Act*: Provides some legal protection for concerted worker protests or job actions against unsafe working conditions. The act covers both unionized and nonunionized workers.

Women Taking Action

The Lowell millgirls struggled against hazardous conditions in the 1840s. In 1909, thousands of women in the garment industry in New York City went on strike to protest "sweatshop" working conditions and low wages. In 1943, 200 black women "sat down" at their machines in a tobacco plant in North Carolina in re-

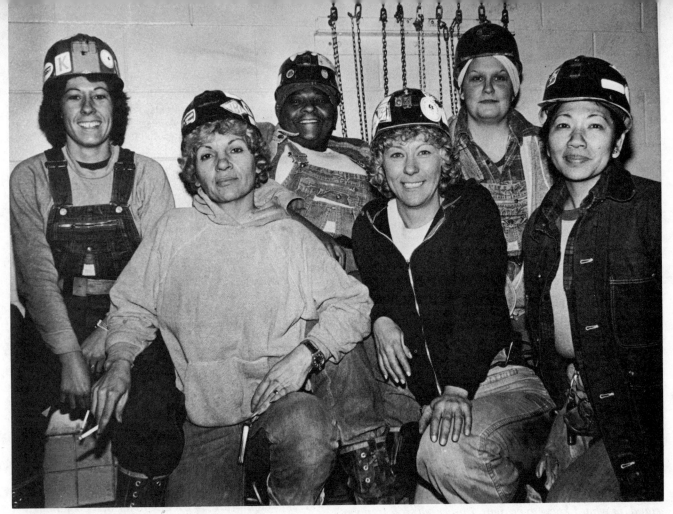

Marat Moore

sponse to the death of a co-worker on the job, which the women saw as being the result of years of exposure to excessive heat, dust and noise. In 1979, women led a strike to improve health and safety conditions and end sexual harassment at a poultry farm in Mississippi. With a long history behind us, we continue to take action.

The process of workers coming together over a particular health and safety problem often starts informally. A woman who worked as a word processor at a major Boston bank contacted 9 TO 5 (an affiliate of Working Women) with concerns about her equipment, specifically the noise from the printers. She and her six co-workers met and discussed the problem with 9 TO 5 and came up with some reasonable solutions. The women met with their supervisor and presented these solutions to him. At first he stalled, but they kept insisting, and eventually the company bought printer covers to reduce the noise. As one woman said, "While this may seem small, it is a big step for us. We've begun to talk together about our common concerns and now our supervisor is nervous that we may get together again on other issues."

I work as a printer, the only woman with six men. One of the men developed sore, red, cracked hands and arms. We all knew it was from the chemical he had to use on the job, and that there was an inexpensive piece of equip-

ment that could be used so that the work wouldn't have to be done by hand. But he was being "macho man" and didn't want to complain. I encouraged him to speak up because I knew that sometime someone else might have to do that job. I got a book about chemicals from a COSH group and brought it to work. We looked up the chemical he was using. We found it does cause dermatitis, and serious liver damage if exposure is great enough. So he complained, but he didn't get anywhere. When he came back we were so mad we stopped working and gathered together reading the book again. The boss saw us and the next day told us he ordered the equipment we wanted. It was very exciting to do something together about a work problem for the first time.

Whenever possible it is most effective to form an ongoing workers' health and safety committee. Instead of just responding to emergencies, a committee can work preventively, uncovering potential problems before anyone gets hurt. A committee will have the task of approaching management, and there are lots of ways to get management's attention even when they don't want to listen.

I was working in a supermarket as a meat wrapper. You know, behind the windows at the meat counter. We take the cut-up meat and wrap it in plastic. The plastic comes off a big roll that we cut to size by pulling it against

91

a hot wire. A bunch of us were having asthma attacks and getting acne real bad. The health and safety committee met and decided that it was from the fumes of the plastic when it melted. We talked to our supervisor and he basically said, "Don't worry, ladies, it's all in your head." So we got mad and decided to try a new approach. We planned it so on one busy Saturday we all came to work with respirators on. After about an hour behind the meat counter with the customers staring at us in shock, the manager decided we were serious and agreed to meet with us and discuss what could be done.

Committees can gather information, educate themselves and their co-workers, help set priorities and provide leadership and persistence to get things changed. Also, in groups we are less likely to be singled out as "troublemakers" and subjected to special harassment or even fired. A health and safety committee is most effective as part of a union. When you have a union, the company *has to*, by law, talk to the union—negotiate—about health and safety.

Our work has more impact on our physical and mental health than we often acknowledge. Getting involved in improving working conditions is one more way that we as women can take control of our lives.

One of the best periods of my life was when we were on strike. We were all like one big family. Once I took a stand on what I knew to be right, I never felt freer in my life.

NOTES

1. The Environmental Defense Fund and Robert H. Boyle. *Malignant Neglect*. New York: Vintage Books, 1980, p. 5. See also Erik P. Eckholm. *The Picture of Health: Environmental Sources of Disease*. New York: W.W. Norton and Co., Inc., 1977, p. 90.

2. *Federal Register*, Volume 45, 1980, p. 33072; Council on Environmental Quality. *The 11th Annual Report of the Council on Environmental Quality*. Washington, DC: U.S. Government Printing Office, December 1980, p. 218. For copies, write to: Superintendent of Documents, U.S. Government Printing Office, Washington, DC, 20402. See also Robert Richter. *A Plague on Our Children*. Boston: WGBH Educational Foundation, 1979, p. 39 (transcript of a television documentary, available from WGBH Transcripts, 125 Western Avenue, Boston, MA 02134).

3. "Citizens Spoke Out on Chemical Control," *On CUE*, Vol. 4, No. 6 (July 1980), p. 1. (*On CUE* is the newsletter of the Coalition for a United Elizabeth, 135 Madison Avenue, Elizabeth, NJ 07201.)

4. Carol Sue Davidson. "Antarctic Lore," *The Cousteau Almanac: An Inventory of Life on Our Water Planet*. New York: Doubleday, 1981, p. 285; Tom Conry. "Chemical of the Month: Lead," *Exposure*, No. 13 (December 1981), p. 6.

5. Jack E. White, John P. Enterline, Zahur Alam and Roscoe Moore, Jr. "Cancer Among Blacks in the United States—Recognizing the Problem," *Proceedings of the International Conference on Cancer Among Black Populations* (May 1980), pp. 5 and 10.

6. Joanne Omang. "Chemicals' Wider Effects on Humans Described." *The Washington Post*, January 9, 1982, p. A4. (Based on a study by the National Center for Health Statistics.)

7. Daniel Bomberry. "Toxic Waste Firm Targets Reservations," *Native Self-Sufficiency*, Vol. 5, No. 1 (May 1982), p. 1.

8. *Exposure*, No. 9, July 1981, p. 1.

9. Robert Richter. *A Plague on Our Children*, p. 39.

10. Jane E. Brody. "Sperm Found Especially Vulnerable to Environment," *The New York Times*, March 10, 1981; Michael Castleman. "Why Johnny Can't Have Kids," *Mother Jones*, April 1982, pp. 14–18.

11. Vilma Hunt. *Work and the Health of Women*. Boca Raton, FL: CRC Press, 1979, p. 155.

12. Constance Holden. "Agent Orange Furor Continues to Build," *Science*, Vol. 205 (August 24, 1979), pp. 770–72. See also Clifford Linedecker with Michael and Maureen Ryan. *Kerry: Agent Orange and the American Family*. New York: St. Martin's Press, 1982.

13. Daniel Ben-Horin. "The Sterility Scandal," *Mother Jones*, May 1979, p. 61.

14. M. Donald Whorton et al. "Reproductive Hazards." Chapter 20 in *Occupational Health: Recognizing and Preventing Work Related Disease*, Barry S. Levy and David H. Wegman, eds. Boston: Little, Brown & Co., 1983.

15. Jane E. Brody. "Sperm Found Especially Vulnerable to Environment."

16. Deborah Baldwin. "The All-Natural Diet Isn't," *Environmental Action*, Vol. 9, No. 15 (December 3, 1977), p. 5.

17. Mason Barr, Jr., M.D. "Environmental Contamination of Human Breastmilk," *American Journal of Public Health*, Vol. 71, No. 2 (February 1981), p. 124. See also "PCBs and Breastmilk," *Nutrition Action*, November 1980.

18. *Taking Back Our Health: A Training Manual on Job Safety and Health for Black and Latino Workers*. Urban Environment Conference, 1314 14th Street NW, Washington, DC 20005, p. 1.

19. *Connections*, Network of Women in Trade and Technical Jobs, 1225 Boylston Street, Boston, MA, February 1982.

20. "Women at Work—Their Dual Role." Women's Occupational Resource Center.

RESOURCES
ENVIRONMENTAL HEALTH

Readings

General

Brand, Stewart. "Human Harm to Human DNA," *The Co-Evolution Quarterly* (Spring 1979), pp. 4–21. Shows links between environmental carcinogens, mutagens and teratogens, including potential effects on the human gene pool. This issue also includes articles on herbicides and "voluntary" exposures to be avoided, along with a resource list of organizations and publications focusing on biohazards.

Cousteau, Jacques-Yves, and the staff of the Cousteau Society. *The Cousteau Almanac*. New York: Doubleday and

Co., Inc., 1981. $15.95. Good political and economic background on local and global environmental pollution; many articles focus on specific incidents.

The Data Center (a nonprofit library and research center). *Toxic Nightmare—Environmental Perspectives.* Three volumes of selected magazine and newspaper articles crucial to environmental activists, researchers, journalists and other concerned citizens. Data Center, 464 19th Street, Oakland, CA 94612.

Eckholm, Erik P. *The Picture of Health, Environmental Sources of Disease.* New York: W.W. Norton and Co., Inc., 1977 (paper). $3.95. A global survey of environmental effects on health, including diet and population as well as toxic hazards.

Epstein, Samuel S. *The Politics of Cancer.* San Francisco: Sierra Club Books, 1978 (paper). $12.50. A comprehensive study of environmental carcinogens and how government has and has not regulated them; includes thirteen case studies.

Highland, Joseph, Marcia E. Fine, Robert H. Harris, Jacqueline M. Warren, Robert J. Rauch, Anita Johnson and Robert H. Boyle. *Malignant Neglect.* New York: Random House, Inc., 1979 (paper). $3.95. A thorough study of human exposure to carcinogens, including industrial chemicals, pesticides, consumer products, diet, radiation. Sections on children and cancer and the biology of cancer. Extensive bibliography.

New Jersey Public Interest Research Group. *Toxic Substances: A Brief Overview of the Issues Involved.* Washington, DC: Environmental Protection Agency, 1980 (paper). Free.

Norwood, Christopher. *At Highest Risk: Environmental Hazards to Young and Unborn Children.* New York: McGraw Hill, Inc., 1980. $10.95. A readable and inclusive overview on how environmental hazards are even more toxic to the developing fetus and to young children. Covers chemicals and radiation and includes a list of recommended readings and a glossary.

Samuels, Mike, M.D., and Hal Zina Bennett, *Well Body, Well Earth*, San Francisco: Sierra Club Books, 1983. $12.95 (paper). Layperson's overview on the environment, how it affects human health, and a wholistic program for dealing with radiation and chemical hazards.

Task Force on Research Planning in Environmental Health Science. *Basic Concepts of Environmental Health.* Washington, DC: NIH Publications (#80–1254), 1980 (paper). Free. A useful but somewhat technical overview, particularly good on what research has been done and what is still necessary. (Write to National Institute for Environmental Health Sciences, P.O. Box 12233, Research Triangle Park, NC 27709.)

Urban Environment Conference. "Environmental Cancer: Causes, Victims, Solutions." Washington, DC: UEC, 1980 (paper). $1.50. Pamphlet includes overview, case studies and politics. Each article has bibliography.

Urban Environment Conference. *Inner City Health in America.* Washington, DC: UEC, 1979 (paper). How inner city residents suffer most from environmental pollution.

Waldbott, George L. *The Environmental Effects of Environmental Pollutants.* St. Louis: C.V. Mosby Co., 1973/1978. Packed with information, somewhat technical, on a range of pollutants.

Chemicals

Waste and Toxic Substances Project. *Waste and Toxic Substances Resource Guide.* Washington, DC: Environmental Action Foundation, 1981 (paper). $2.00. The best and most thorough annotated bibliography on toxics, covering books, articles, periodicals and audiovisual materials. Start here.

Brown, Michael. *Laying Waste: The Poisoning of America by Toxic Chemicals.* New York: Pantheon Books, 1980 (paper).

California Department of Consumer Affairs. *Clean Your Room! A Compendium on Indoor Air Pollutants.* Sacramento, CA: Department of Consumer Affairs, 1982. $15.00. The most thorough, recent information. Write to DCA, P.O. Box 310, Sacramento, CA 95802.

Council on Environmental Quality. *Chemical Hazards to Human Reproduction.* Washington, DC: Government Printing Office, 1981. (Publication #1981–337–130/8008.) Fairly clinical report describes what is currently known, what research needs to be done and what policies should be enacted. Includes detailed scientific bibliography and tables of chemicals and drugs.

Davis, Earon, and Valerie Wilk. *Toxic Chemicals: The Interface Between Law and Science.* Washington, DC: Farmworkers' Justice Fund, Inc., 1982. (806 15th Street, Suite 600, Washington, DC 20006.)

Epstein, Samuel S., Lester O. Brown and Carl Pope. *Hazardous Waste in America.* San Francisco, CA: Sierra Club Books, 1982. $27.50. Order from 530 Bush Street, San Francisco, CA 94108. A comprehensive book which surveys the sources and dangers of hazardous waste, including case studies, laws, a directory of 8,000 dumps, how to locate undisclosed dumps and solutions to the problem.

Freedberg, Louis. *America's Poisoned Playgrounds: Children and Toxic Chemicals.* Washington, DC: Youth News and the Conference on Alternative State and Local Policies, 1983. $5.95 + $1.00 postage.

League of Women Voters Education Fund. "A Toxics Primer." Washington, DC: League of Women Voters, 1979 (paper). $.40 each. A handy pamphlet that can be distributed at meetings. Write to LWV, 1730 M Street NW, Washington, DC 20036.

Nader, Ralph, Ronald Brownstein and John Richards, eds. *Who's Poisoning America: Corporate Polluters and Their Victims in the Chemical Age.* New York: Charles Scribner's Sons, Inc., 1981.

Regenstein, Lewis. *America the Poisoned: How Deadly Chemicals Are Destroying Our Environment, Our Wildlife, and Ourselves—and How We Can Survive!* Washington, DC: Acropolis Books, Ltd., 1982.

Citizen Action

Chess, Caron. *Winning the Right to Know: A Handbook for Toxics Activists.* Washington, DC: Conference on Alternative State and Local Policies and the Delaware Valley Toxics Coalition, 1983. $7.95 + $1.00 postage.

Gibbs, Lois, with Murray Levine. *Love Canal: My Story.* Albany, NY: State University of New York, 1982. How "just a housewife" took on the local, state and federal government—and won. Great for inspiration and ideas.

Highlander Research and Education Center. *We're Tired of Being Guinea Pigs!* New Market, TN: Highlander Research and Education Center, 1980 (paper). $6.00. Geared specifically to Appalachian areas, but adaptable to other locales.

Excellent how-to manual for organizing around toxics. (Write to HREC, Route 3, Box 370, New Market, TN 37820.)

National Wildlife Federation. *The Toxic Substances Dilemma: A Plan for Citizen Action*. Washington, DC: NWF, 1981 (paper). An accessible guide that includes effects of chemical pollutants on people.

Sierra Club. *Training Materials on Toxic Substances: Tools for Effective Action*. San Francisco: Sierra Club Books, 1981 (paper). Divided into two handbooks that cover the full range of toxics issues and what citizens can do about them. Offers a complete curriculum for citizen education, including backup reading. Full of ideas and particularly good for locating government information that is available inexpensively.

Consumer Products

Center for Science in the Public Interest. *The Household Pollutants Guide*. New York: Doubleday and Co., Inc., 1978 (paper). $3.50. An A–Z list and discussion of health hazards in the home.

Conry, Tom, and the Science Action Coalition. *Consumer's Guide to Cosmetics*. New York: Doubleday and Co., Inc., 1980 (paper). $3.95. Includes the politics and the products, as well as information on reporting a problem.

Dadd, Debra Lynn and Alan S. Levin, M.D. *A Consumer Guide for the Chemically Sensitive*, August 1982. $17.00 from Non-Toxic Lifestyles, 450 Sutter Street, Suite 1138, San Francisco, CA 94108.

Pim, Linda R. *The Invisible Additives: Environmental Contaminants in Our Food*. Toronto: Doubleday and Co., Inc., 1981.

Pesticides

Boraiko, Allen A. "The Pesticide Dilemma," *National Geographic*, Vol. 57, No. 2 (February 1980), pp. 145–83. A good overview of the development, history and effects of pesticide use in the U.S.

Carson, Rachel. *Silent Spring*. Greenwich, CT: Fawcett Crest, 1962 (paper). $1.95. The book that started it all by explaining the effects of DDT.

Van Strum, Carol. *A Bitter Fog: Herbicides and Human Rights*. San Francisco: Sierra Club Books, May 1983. $14.95. Tells the story of Van Strum's struggles as a mother-turned-activist to confront the agribusiness interests which want to tame forests while poisoning the people.

Weir, David, and Mark Schapiro. *Circle of Poison: Pesticides and People in a Hungry World*. San Francisco: Institute for Food and Development Policy, 1981 (paper).

Whiteside, Thomas. *Defoliation: What Are Herbicides Doing to Us*? New York: Ballantine Books, Inc., and Friends of the Earth, 1970 (paper). One of the first popular accounts of the phenoxy herbicides and their effects. Appendices include extensive reprints of government reports and statements.

Radiation

Brodeur, Paul. *The Zapping of America: Microwaves, Their Deadly Risk, and the Cover-Up*. New York: W.W. Norton and Co., Inc., 1977. The bad news on another invisible hazard that has not been thoroughly enough explored. It's interesting to note that the Soviets have set a permissible level of exposure to microwaves a thousand times lower than that in the U.S.

Caldicott, Helen. *Nuclear Madness: What You Can Do*. Brookline, MA: Autumn Press, Inc., 1978 (paper). $3.95. A fervent, moving account of dangers and health effects of nuclear weapons production and nuclear war. Extensive bibliography.

Gofman, John W. *Radiation and Human Health*. New York: Pantheon Books, 1983. Exhaustive examination of the effects of radiation hazards. Club Books, 1981.

Gyorgy, Anna, and friends. *No Nukes: Everyone's Guide to Nuclear Power*. Boston: South End Press, 1979 (paper). $10.00 A thorough look at the issue. Each chapter includes a resource list.

Koen, Susan, and Nina Swaim. *Ain't Nowhere We Can Run: A Handbook for Women on the Nuclear Mentality*. Norwich, VT: Women Against Nuclear Development, 1979 (paper). $2.00 plus $.50 postage. Explains specific health effects of radiation on women. Includes a more philosophical/political resource list of books, periodicals and organizations. (Write to WAND, Box 421, Norwich, VT 05055.)

Nuclear Information and Resource Service. *Radiation Packet*. Washington, DC: NIRS, 1981. Explains what radiation is, where it comes from and health effects. Includes bibliography and resources.

Physicians for Social Responsibility, Inc. *Medical Hazards of Radiation Packet*. Watertown, MA: PSR, 1981 (paper). $3.00. A collection of xeroxed articles on radiation and health. (Write to PSR, P.O. Box 144, Watertown, MA 02172.)

Wasserman, Harvey, and Norman Solomon. *Killing Our Own: The Disaster of America's Experience with Atomic Radiation*. New York: Delacorte Press, 1982.

Technical References

Casarett, Louis J., and John Doull. *Toxicology: The Basic Science of Poisons*, 2nd ed. New York: Macmillan Publishing Co., Inc., 1980.

Clayton, George D., and Florence E. Clayton, eds. *Patty's Industrial Hygiene and Toxicology*, 3rd rev. ed. New York: Wiley Interscience, 1978.

Sax, N. Irving. *Dangerous Properties of Industrial Materials*, 4th ed. New York: Van Nostrand Reinhold Co., Inc., 1975.

Shepherd, Thomas H. *Catalog of Teratogenic Agents*, 3rd ed. Baltimore: Johns Hopkins University Press, 1980.

Vander, Arthur J., James H. Sherman and Dorothy S. Luciano. *Human Physiology: The Mechanisms of Body Function*, 2nd ed. New York: McGraw-Hill, Inc., 1975.

Women and the Environment

Gray, Elizabeth Dodson. *Green Paradise Lost*. Wellesley, MA: Roundtable Press, 1979 (paper). A theological and philosophical exploration of connections between feminism and ecology.

Griffin, Susan. *Woman and Nature: The Roaring Inside Her*. New York: Harper and Row Publishers, Inc., 1978 (paper). An extensively documented, lyrical account of connections between women and nature and how they have been shaped by the patriarchy. Good political context.

Merchant, Carolyn. *The Death of Nature: Women, Ecology, and the Scientific Revolution*. San Francisco: Harper and

Row Publishers, Inc., 1980. An academic, historical account of the rise of science from a feminist perspective.

Smith, Judy. "Something Old, Something New, Something Borrowed, Something Due: Women and Appropriate Technology." Butte, MT: National Center for Appropriate Technology, 1978 (paper). A pamphlet that explores connections between feminism and environmentalism: does AT offer us anything new? Extensive resource list. (Write to NCAT, P.O. Box 3838, Butte, MT 59701.)

Women's Resource Center. *Women and Technology: Deciding What's Appropriate*. Missoula, MT: WRC, 1979 (paper). Raises tough and important questions and talks about health technology and potentially hazardous technology. (Write to Women's Resource Center, 315 S. 4th E., Missoula, MT 59801.)

Zimmerman, Jan, ed. *Future, Technology, and Women: Proceedings of a Conference*. San Diego, CA: San Diego State University, 1981 (paper). $6.50 plus $1.00 for postage. A provoking collection of ideas, some specifically on environmental and women's health. (Write to Women's Studies Department, SDSU, San Diego, CA 92182.)

Audiovisual Materials

For Export Only: Pesticides and Pills. Richter Productions, 330 W. 42nd Street, New York, NY 10036.

In Our Own Backyards: Uranium Mining in the United States. Bullfrog Films, Oley, PA 19547.

In Our Water. The story of well-water contamination in New Jersey. New Day Films, Box 315, Franklin Lakes, NJ 07417, or Meg Switzgable, Foresight Films, 18 2nd Place, Brooklyn, NY 11231.

The Killing Ground. The story of improper chemical-waste dumping. ABC Learning Resources, 1330 Avenue of the Americas, New York, NY 10019.

Medical Implications of Nuclear Energy. With Dr. Helen Caldicott. Earth Energy Media, Box 188, Santa Barbara, CA 93102.

Medical Implications of Nuclear Power and Weapons (slideshow). With Dr. Helen Caldicott. Packard Manse Media Project, Box 450, Stoughton, MA 02072.

Our Hidden National Product. The siting of a hazardous waste facility. Durrin Films, Inc., 4926 Sedgewick Street NW, Washington, DC 20016.

A Plague on Our Children. Two-part film on 2,4,5-T, PCBs, DDT and Love Canal. Time/Life Multimedia, Time and Life Building, Room 32–48, New York, NY 10020.

Women and Power in the Nuclear Age. With Dr. Helen Caldicott on how to get the system to work. High Hopes Media, 233 Summit Avenue E., Seattle, WA 98102.

For audiovisual lists on environmental issues, contact:

Green Mountain Post Films
Box 229
Turners Falls, MA 01376

Third Eye Films
12 Arrow Street
Cambridge, MA 02138

Organizations

All of the following organizations provide information on issues involving environmental health. Many, as noted, provide newsletters. Usually the focus or constituency is obvious from the name; we've included additional information where necessary or useful.

Citizens' Clearinghouse for Hazardous Wastes, Inc.
P.O. Box 926
Arlington, VA 22216
(703)532-6816
Founded by Lois Gibbs, this group provides technical and organizing assistance to citizens facing a hazardous waste problem.
Newsletter: *Everyone's Backyard*

Delaware Valley Toxics Coalition
1315 Walnut Street, Rm 1632
Philadelphia, PA 19107
Coalition of labor and community groups that passed the first community and worker right-to-know legislation in the country.
Publishes *Winning the Right to Know: A Handbook for Activists* (Fall 1983). ($7.00)

Environmental Action Foundation
Waste and Toxic Substances Project
724 Dupont Circle Building
Washington, DC 20036
Information packets, fact sheets, referrals for citizens' groups, particularly good for information on laws and regulations.
Newsletter: *Exposure* (bimonthly)

Environmental Defense Fund
475 Park Avenue South
New York, NY 10016
1525 18th Street NW
Washington, DC 20036
Litigation on environmental issues, including environmental health and consumer welfare. Bimonthly newsletter.

Friends of the Earth
1045 Sansome Street
San Francisco, CA 94111
National lobbying group on environmental issues.
Newsletter: *Not Man Apart* (monthly)

Hazard Evaluation System and Information Service (HESIS)
State of California Department of Health Services
2151 Berkeley Way
Berkeley, CA 94704
Detailed information on toxics in laypeople's terms.

National Coalition Against the Misuse of Pesticides
530 7th Street SE
Washington, DC 20003
Health, environmental, legal and community groups lobbying and educating on pesticides. Newsletter.

Nuclear Information and Resource Service
1346 Connecticut Avenue NW, Suite 405
Washington, DC 20036
Resource guides, fact sheets, referrals on radiation and health.
Newsletter: *Groundswell* (bimonthly)

Sierra Club
530 Bush Street
San Francisco, CA 94108
One of the oldest environmental groups; periodicals and books.
Magazine: *Sierra Club Bulletin* (ten issues yearly)

Urban Environment Conference
1314 14th Street NW
Washington, DC 20005
Focuses on urban environmental health, particularly among black and Latino people.

Worldwatch Institute
1776 Massachusetts Avenue NW
Washington, DC 20036
Papers on environmental health with a global perspective.

Government Agencies Regulating Toxic Substances

Consumer Product Safety Commission
Washington, DC 20207
(800)638-8326 (toll-free hotline for information on product safety)
(301)492-6800 (hotline number for DC area)
Consumer goods, particularly household items.

Environmental Protection Agency
Public Information Center
401 M Street NW
Washington, DC 20460
(202)755-0707
Chemical and nuclear hazards in the general environment.

Food and Drug Administration
Office of Consumer Affairs and Inquiries
5600 Fishers Lane
Rockville, MD 20857
(301)443-3170
Food additives, cosmetics and the drug industry.

Nuclear Regulatory Commission
Washington, DC 20555
(202)492-7000
Public Affairs Office: (202)492-7715
Regulating and licensing of nuclear facilities.

Occupational Safety and Health Administration
Office of Information and Consumer Affairs
Room N3637
3rd and Constitution Avenue NW
Washington, DC 20210
(202)523-8151
Chemical and nuclear hazards in the workplace.

U.S. Department of Energy
Washington, DC 20585
(202)252-5000
High level waste management and weapons production.

U.S. Department of Transportation
400 7th Street SW
Washington, DC 20590
(202)426-4321
Transportation of toxic substances.

RESOURCES
OCCUPATIONAL HEALTH

Some Basics

American College of Obstetrics and Gynecology. *Guidelines on Pregnancy and Work*. NIOSH Publication 78–118. Superintendent of Documents, U.S. Government Printing Office, Washington, DC 20402, 1978.

Boston Women's Health Book Collective and Massachusetts Coalition for Occupational Safety and Health. *Our Jobs, Our Health*. Order from BWHBC, Dept. OH, 465 Mt. Auburn Street, Watertown, MA 02172. Single copies: institutions and professionals $6.00; unions, nonprofit organizations and individuals $4.00; bulk rate for 50 or more $3.00 each; $1.00 per book (25¢ for each additional book) for shipping and handling.

Coalition for the Reproductive Rights of Workers. *Reproductive Hazards in the Workplace—A Resource Guide*. 1917 I Street NW, Washington, DC 20006, 1980.

Hricko, A., and M. Brunt. *Working for Your Life: A Woman's Guide to Job Health Hazards*. LOHP, University of California, 1976.

Hunt, V. *Work and the Health of Women*. CRC Press, 1979.

9 TO 5. *Race Against Time: Automation of the Office*. Report by 9 TO 5, National Association of Working Women, 1224 Huron Road, Cleveland, OH 44115, 1980. Analyzes the impact on the office workforce and management of trends in office automation, and includes references and proposals for government action.

NIOSH. *Occupational Diseases, A Guide to Their Recognition*. NIOSH Publication 77–181. $5.25. A very informative guide to work-related disease. Describes the wide range of occupational health hazards, their harmful effects and their legally permissible exposure limits. Superintendent of Documents, U.S. Government Printing Office, Washington, DC 20402. #017–033–00266–5.

Ontario Federation of Labor. *Occupational Health and Safety: A Training Manual*. Clark Pitman, Toronto, 1982.

Procter and Hughes. *Chemical Hazards of the Workplace*. Lippincott, 1978. This paperback contains several chapters on industrial health problems and an extensive list of health effects for many chemicals.

Sax, I. *Cancer Causing Chemicals*. Van Nostrand Reinhold Co., Inc. This volume contains information on many known and suspected carcinogens.

———. *Dangerous Properties of Industrial Materials*. Van Nostrand Reinhold Co., Inc., 1979. This book is similar to the one by Procter and Hughes (above) but may have information on more materials. It contains information on health effects and also fire and explosion hazards.

Society for Occupational and Environmental Health. *Proceedings on the Conference on Women in the Workplace*. 1717 Massachusetts Avenue, Washington, DC 20036, 1977.

Stellman, J. *Women's Work—Women's Health, Myths and Realities*. Pantheon Books, 1977.

——— and S. Daum. *Work Is Dangerous to Your Health*. Vintage Books, 1973. A readable guide to health hazards in the workplace and what you can do about them. Contains a useful description of how the body works and lists health hazards by occupation as well as by substance. Has clear descriptions of noise, stress and occupational disease.

Urban Environment Conference. *Taking Back Our Health—A Training Manual on Job Safety and Health for Black and Latino Workers.*

Winter, Ruth. *Cancer Causing Agents—A Preventive Guide.* Crown Publishers, Inc., 1979. This popular book is a readable guide to 250 substances that may cause cancer.

Bibliographies

Chavkin, W., and L. Welch. *Occupational Hazards to Reproduction: An Annotated Bibliography.* The Program in Occupational Medicine, Department of Social Medicine, Montefiore Hospital, 111 E. 210 Street, Bronx, NY 10467, 1981.

Hunt, V. *The Health of Women at Work, A Bibliography.* Northwestern University Occasional Papers, No. 2, The Program on Women, Northwestern University, 619 Emerson Street, Evanston, IL 60201, 1977.

Ives, J. *International Safety and Health Resource Catalogue.* Praeger Publishers, 1981.

NIOSH. *A Resource Guide to Worker Education Materials in Occupational Safety and Health.* Publications Dissemination, 4676 Columbia Parkway, Cincinnati, OH 45226, 1982.

———. *NIOSH Publications Catalogue.* Publications Dissemination, 4676 Columbia Parkway, Cincinnati, OH 45226, 1980.

Resource Groups

Congreso de Trabajadores y Consumidores de Puerto Rico (CO-TACO): Box 10646, Capara Heights Station, Puerto Rico 00922. A group that works with unions, workers and the community around health and safety issues.

COSH Groups: Coalitions or Committees for Occupational Safety and Health. COSH groups are made up of union locals, workers and prolabor health and safety professionals and lawyers. They can provide technical assistance, informational fact sheets and worker education. They have experience in working with unions and other worker groups setting up health and safety committees at the workplace. There are many COSH groups around the country, and they will be very responsive to your request for information and other help. In addition, some COSH groups are in touch with similar groups in other countries. For information about COSH groups nearest you, contact:

MassCOSH
718 Huntington Avenue
Boston, MA 02115

Urban Environment Conference
13 14th Street NW
Washington, DC 20005

WOSH
824 Tecumsah Road E.
Windsor, Ontario N8X2

"New Directions" Grantees: These are unions, COSH groups, public interest groups, labor unions which have received grants from OSHA to do health and safety programs. To obtain a list of grantees, write: OSHA New Directions Office, Room N3419, Department of Labor, 200 Constitution Avenue NW, Washington, DC 20210.

Unions: Many unions have health and safety departments, both within local unions and the national office. If you are in a union, find out if your union has one. They can provide much information and assistance. The AFL-CIO has a health and safety department located at 815 16th Street NW, Washington, DC 20006. Telephone: (202)637-5000. They may be able to help you find other resources close to you.

Many unions publish health and safety materials that deal with hazards faced by their members and with how to get changes made.

Women's Occupational Health Resource Center (WOHRC): A national clearinghouse focusing on the occupational health concerns of women workers. Has a newsletter and many informational fact sheets and packets on the hazards in occupations dominated by women. WOHRC, Columbia University School of Public Health, 60 Haven Avenue, B-1 New York, NY 10032.

The following is a list of some groups that have been involved in health and safety as part of their work:

Coalition of Trade Union Women (CLUW)
15 Union Square
New York, NY 10003

Household Employment Project of the National Urban League for Household Workers
500 East 62nd Street
New York, NY 10021

Labor Council for Latin American Advancement—Health and Safety Department
Suite 707, AFL-CIO Building
815 16th Street NW
Washington, DC 20006
(202)347-4223

Working Women
1224 Huron Road
Cleveland, OH 10003

There are many short, easy-to-read publications about particular hazards that are published by many different groups. They tend to be inexpensive. Some examples are:

Low Level Radiation Project, Coalition for the Medical Rights of Women. *Radiation on the Job, A Manual for Health Care Workers on Ionizing Radiation.* Coalition for the Medical Rights of Women, 1638 Haight Street, San Francisco, CA 94117. $2.00.

NYCOSH. *Health Protection for Operators of VDT's/CRT's.* NYCOSH, 32 Union Square, Room 404, New York, NY 10003. $1.00.

United Auto Workers. *The Case of Workplace Killers: A Manual for Cancer Detectives on the Job.* UAW Purchase and Supply Department, 8000 E. Jefferson, Detroit, MI 48214. $1.00.

Legal Resources Agencies

Bargaining for Equality. A guide to legal and collective bargaining solutions for workplace problems that particularly affect women. Has a health and safety section. From The Women's Law Project, P.O. Box 6250, San Francisco, CA 94101.

Equal Employment Opportunity Commission (EEOC). En-

TAKING CARE OF OURSELVES

forces the Federal Civil Rights Act, including the pregnancy disability amendment. For the office nearest you, look under "EEOC" in the federal-government listings of the phone book.

National Labor Relations Board (NLRB). Handles unfair-labor-practice charges of discipline or discharge of workers for engaging in activities around health and safety at work. For the office nearest you, look in the phone book under "Federal Agencies." If it's not there, contact NLRB, 1717 Pennsylvania Avenue NW, Washington, DC 20570, for information.

   If you are not covered by the NLRB (if you are a public employee, for example) you will be covered by a state agency. Call your state department of labor to find out.

NIOSH (National Institute for Occupational Safety and Health). 4676 Columbia Parkway, Cincinnati, OH 45226. NIOSH is the "research partner" of OSHA. It publishes criteria documents for many chemicals, and other useful documents. It may recommend standards to OSHA and conduct health hazard evaluations at workplaces.

OSHA (Occupational Safety and Health Administration). U.S. Department of Labor, 200 Constitution Avenue NW, Washington, DC 20210. The federal agency responsible for setting workplace standards and enforcing them. The agency inspects workplaces, responds to worker complaints and has the power to fine companies that are in violation of the law and to require correction of the violation. Some states have "state OSHAs" that are administered by state government rather than federal government. Public work-

ers are not covered by OSHA. Your state department of labor can tell you where the OSHA office closest to you is, and where to go for help if you are not covered by OSHA. You can get a free copy of the OSHA standards by requesting one.

Workers' Compensation. Each state has an agency responsible for handling workers' compensation claims. Look in the state government section of the phone book under "Workers' Compensation" or "Industrial Accidents." If you don't find it there, try calling your state department of labor and asking for the name of the agency responsible.

Right to Know

To obtain a packet about state and local "right to know" legislation, contact AFL-CIO Health and Safety Department, 815 16th Street, Washington, DC 20006.

NLRB Decisions. Several NLRB decisions have come down enforcing unions' rights to health and safety information from the company and enforcing unions' rights to take experts into the plant to do inspections.

OSHA Rules on Access to Employee Exposure and Medical Records. Guarantees access of employees and unions to certain company records regarding exposure and medical records. For a free copy of this OSHA standard, call your local OSHA office or write for a copy (29CFR 1920.20) to OSHA Office of Information, 200 Constitution Avenue NW, Washington, DC 20210. Telephone: (202)523-8151.

8

VIOLENCE AGAINST WOMEN

By Dina Carbonell, Lois Glass, Suzanne Gosselin, Carol Mamber and Jill Stanzler (all members of Boston Area Rape Crisis Center, who wrote sections on rape, battering, incest and child abuse); Alice Friedman, Margaret Lazarus, Lynn Rubinett, Lena Sorensen, Denise Wells and Nancy Wilbur (all members of Alliance Against Sexual Coercion, who wrote the introduction, sexual harassment and activism box); Terrie Antico (self-defense); Wendy Sanford (prostitution)

With special thanks to Freada Klein, Boston Area Rape Crisis Center and Andrea Fischgrund

This chapter is an expansion of previous chapters on rape, written by Gene Bishop, Roxanne Hynek and Judy Norsigian; and self-defense, written by Janet Jones and Carol McEldowney.

In this society violence against women occurs with shocking frequency.*

- FBI statistics indicate that every eighteen seconds a man batters a woman in her home.[1]
- One out of three women will be raped (forced to have sex without her consent) during her lifetime.[2] This means a woman is as likely to be raped as to be divorced.
- Forty-two percent of women working for the federal government during a two-year period reported some form of sexual harassment.[3]
- By age eighteen, 25 percent of girls will have experienced sexual abuse, probably by a family member.[4]

Every day we see real and imagined violence against women in the news, TV shows and movies, in advertising, in our homes and workplaces. It becomes a fact of life.

*This chapter focuses on male violence toward women. While there are instances of female-to-male and female-to-female violence, they are relatively rare, and factual information is hard to obtain. In battering cases involving women assaulting men, the usual pattern is for a woman to act in self-defense or to strike out after having endured chronic abuse, often for years.

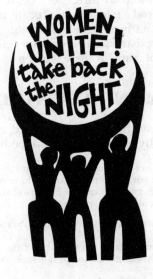

Bonnie Acker

I have never been free of the fear of rape. From a very early age I, like most women, have thought of rape as part of my natural environment—something to be feared and prayed against like fire or lightning. I never asked why men raped; I simply thought it one of the many mysteries of human nature.[5]

In the broadest sense, violence against women is any violation of a woman's personhood, mental or physical integrity or freedom of movement, and includes all the ways our society objectifies and oppresses women. Over the past decade, activists have made the definition more specific in order to facilitate organizing efforts around certain forms of violence. They have identified at least thirty specific forms of violence against women, ranging from sterilization abuse to prescription-drug abuse to pornography to violence against women in prisons, from self-hatred to economic and class oppression.*

Every form of violence threatens women with physical or psychological violation and limits our ability to make choices about our lives. Sexual violence is particularly insidious because sexual acts are ordinarily and rightly a source of pleasure and communication. It is often unclear whether a sexual violation was done out of sexual desire or violent intent, or whether these motivations are even distinguishable, since violence itself has become eroticized in this culture.

Twenty years ago, most forms of violence against women were hidden under a cloak of silence or tacit acceptance. As more and more women talked with each other in the recent wave of the women's movement, it became apparent that violence against us occurs on a massive scale, that no woman is immune, and that family, friends and public institutions have been cruelly insensitive about it. Over the past fifteen years, women in communities throughout the country have mobilized to offer direct services to women who have encountered violence, to educate people about the range and nature of the violence and to develop strategies for resistance. This chapter reflects the important work of some of these women.

BLAMING THE VICTIM

Women who have been raped, battered, sexually harassed or sexually assaulted in childhood report these

*We do not address the subject of pornography primarily because we disagree with one another and/or have not come to any clear positions yet on some crucial aspects of this issue. However, a few things all of us agree upon:

- we abhor all pornography which we find violent or degrading to women;
- we believe it important to protest the existence of this type of pornography, though we would not seek government censorship;
- we protest the fact that a huge pornography industry is making billions of dollars by objectifying, degrading and dehumanizing women, children and sometimes men. The work women are doing to expose this industry is central to our understanding of violence against women in cultures throughout the world.

We recognize that some of us will find offensive what others view as erotica, and vice versa; that not all pornography represents "violence against women." But this need not keep us from speaking out against what we believe is degrading to women, and, ultimately, everyone.

emotions most frequently: guilt, fear, powerlessness, shame, betrayal, anger, denial. Guilt is often the first and deepest response. Anger often comes only later, which is not surprising since our socialization as women allows us so little sense of a right not to be violated.

We feel guilty about violence done to us because society tells us that we caused it or brought it on ourselves in some way—a clear case of "blaming the victim." Most of us heard from our parents, "Boys will be boys, so girls must take care," the message being that we can avoid unwanted male attention provided *we* are careful enough. If anything goes wrong, it's *our* fault. Blaming the victim releases the man who commits sexual violence from the responsibility for what *he* has done. By making us feel guilty, it discourages us from fighting back. *WOMEN ARE NOT GUILTY FOR VIOLENCE COMMITTED BY MEN ON OUR BODY, MIND AND SPIRIT. THIS VIOLENCE HAPPENS BECAUSE OF MEN'S GREATER POWER AND THEIR MISUSE OF THAT POWER.* As one battered woman wrote of her husband's violence, "I may be his excuse, but I have never been his reason."

MEN, WOMEN AND POWER: WHAT VIOLENCE AGAINST WOMEN REALLY DOES TO US

One man's violence against one woman may *seem* to result from his individual psychological problems, sexual frustration, unbearable life pressures or some innate urge toward aggression. Though each of these "reasons" has been used to explain and even justify male violence, they hide the truth. *Men use violence against women to exert and maintain their power and control over us.* When a battering husband uses beatings to confine his wife to the home and prevent her from seeing friends and family or pursuing outside work, he exerts dominance, hostility and control. When a boss sexually harasses his employee, he exerts his power to restrict her freedom to work and improve her position. When men rape women, they act out of a wish to punish or dominate, a desire that is often eroticized.

Whether or not an individual man who commits an act of violence views it as an expression of power is not the point. The fact that so many individual men feel entitled to express their frustration or anger by being violent to so many individual women illustrates the power men as a group hold over women as a group. In this distorted way even the most powerless men benefit from sexism.

Thousands of daily acts of violence throughout the country create a climate of fear and powerlessness which limits women's freedom of action and controls many of the movements of our lives.[6]

I learned not to walk on dark streets, not to talk to strangers or get into strange cars, to lock doors and to be modest.

I came to the vocational school instead of the regular high school because I thought I'd like the electronics shop. But during orientation I met the two girls who are now in electronics and heard how they get teased and harassed. I'm taking cosmetology. It's all right, I guess.

The threat of male violence continues to keep us from stepping out from behind traditional roles and boundaries. It literally "keeps us in our place."

RACE, CLASS AND VIOLENCE AGAINST WOMEN

Public violence—rape and sexual harassment in particular—serves as a tool for keeping down or punishing women deprived of power by racism and other forms of discrimination. White men often use sexual violence as a means of asserting racial dominance over women of color. A married black woman who was fired for refusing to sleep with her supervisor said:

On many occasions Mr. —— said to me, "For a colored girl, you are intelligent." I told him that if he has to refer to a color or race concerning me, I considered myself "black." He replied, "I don't believe in black or all that stuff. To me you're colored, and that's it." One day he made a comment concerning my, as he called it, "voluptuous" shape. When I asked him politely to discontinue making such comments that include sexual overtures, he replied, "Why not? For a colored, you're very stacked, light-skinned and pretty."

It can be difficult for a woman of color to tell whether violence or harassment is prompted by her sex or race or both. In rape, the double jeopardy is even worse.

The man who raped me was white, and the cops here are all white. I didn't report it. I just told a few people I trusted. It helped, but I still feel scared, knowing he's out there and that nobody would do anything about it.

People in positions of power (usually white, affluent men) dismiss violence done to women of color as insignificant.[7] In addition, a woman of color in the U.S. faces a heightened vulnerability if she is not fluent in English or not a citizen, because it is easier for men to take advantage of her and harder for her to get help.

Other forms of discrimination create other special vulnerabilities. People rarely take acts of violence as seriously if the woman is poor, old, a prostitute, a lesbian, a woman with physical or intellectual limitations or institutionalized. This is true for all women

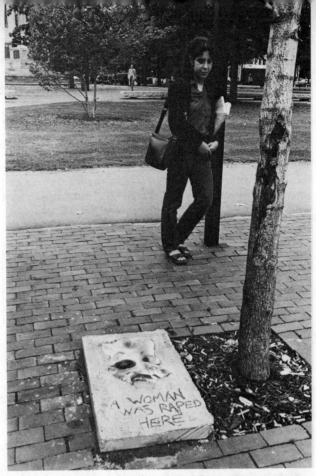

Ellen Shub

whose "male protectors" are nonexistent, invisible or socially less powerful than other men. Open lesbians have been raped by men or groups of men angry at their social independence. ("All she needs is a good fuck.") Older women have less freedom to fight sexual harassment at their jobs or to leave a battering husband, because age discrimination means they won't easily find other ways of supporting themselves. Older women and disabled women are frequently raped.

RESISTING VIOLENCE: PREVENTION VS. AWARENESS

Most safety advice offered to women is based on the "blame the victim" mentality: "Don't go out alone at night."..."Don't wear sexy clothes."..."Don't be friendly to strangers."..."Stay out of risky situations." As if what *we* do is decisive. The argument goes: because it is women's behavior—our seductiveness or carelessness—which "invites" violence or allows it to happen, then it is up to us, by changing our behavior, to prevent it. Women sometimes tend to accept this view because it offers a false but desperately wanted sense of security. We think we can perhaps avoid violence by staying in or by being accommodating to an angry mate. We pay close attention to every detail about a woman who was raped and try not to be like her. Protective measures like self-defense may help individual women (see p. 111). However, what we do doesn't decrease the incidence of men's violent acts.

101

When we take steps to protect ourselves, we want it to be with full awareness that the true responsibility for preventing and eradicating violence belongs to men. *Men must stop committing violence against women, stop each other from doing it, stop condoning it in others and stop blaming women for it.* This is the most important and appropriate form of prevention.

> Golda Meir said, when legislators in Israel proposed a curfew on women in an attempt to lower the incidence of rape: "But it is the *men* who are attacking women. If there is to be a curfew, let the *men* stay home."

THE LEGAL SYSTEM

As women have brought each form of violence against women to public attention, reform in laws and protocol has been one important goal. There have been a few gains: see pages 111–13 for specific accomplishments in legal reform. It may now be slightly easier to report and prosecute rape, battering and cases of sexual assault against children; court and police personnel have been sensitized in some areas, and women and children are less often blamed; rape convictions have risen somewhat; emergency protection for battered women is more often available; some women who were sexually harassed have won back pay, damages and changed policies. Changing the laws has educated the public and made it possible for women to say, "I was violated and I want the assailant held accountable." Yet turning to the legal system is time-consuming, risky, expensive and traumatic, and it is available only *after* sexual violence has been committed. We have no idea whether or not better laws deter men from assaulting women. Furthermore, the legal system doesn't work the same for everyone. Women of color, poor women, divorced women and lesbians, for example, are believed and respected even less than white, financially stable, married, heterosexual women in court. White, married, middle-class (respectable) men are rarely prosecuted. Because of the limitations of the legal system, every woman must make her own decision to report or prosecute her case.

SUMMARY OF MYTHS THAT SUPPORT VIOLENCE AGAINST WOMEN

| Type of myth | How the myth gets applied to each specific form of violence | | | |
	Rape	Battering	Sexual harassment	Child sexual assault
Victim-blaming.	Women invite by their dress or behavior; women lead men too far; women want it and/or enjoy being raped.	Women invite by their behavior; women pick violent partners; women stay so they must like it.	Women invite by their dress or behavior; women sleep their way to the top or for good grades.	Little girls are seductive; mothers set up incestuous relationships by their own failure as sexual partners.
Not a common problem or not a real issue.	It's only done by perverts leaping from bushes.	Wives are violent, too.	It's just mutual attraction.	It isn't harmful to girls.
Male perpetrator isn't responsible for his actions.	Rapists are psychopaths; rapists are provoked.	Batterers are alienated at work or unemployed or grew up in violent homes, or are alcoholic.	Most harassers don't intend harm; they're just complimenting women.	Male relatives had no choice because their sexual needs were unmet by their wives, or they're psychopaths.
Racist assumptions.	Black men rape white women; black women are looser about their sexuality; Hispanic women are hot lovers.	Black and Hispanic families condone violence.	Black women are looser; Hispanic women are hot lovers.	Black and Hispanic families condone sexual activity between adults and children.

Copyright 1981, Freada Klein. Use with permission only.

RAPE

Rape is any kind of sexual activity committed against a woman's will. Whether the rapist uses force or threats of force is irrelevant. Men use different kinds of force against women, from pressuring us for a "good night kiss," to withdrawal of economic support from wives, to using weapons. Rape is always traumatic. When we are raped, survival is our primary instinct and we protect ourselves as best we can. Some women choose to fight back; others do not feel it is an option. If you were raped and are now reading this chapter, you did the "right" thing because you are alive.

Here are several facts which disprove common myths about rape. Rape is more likely to be committed by someone we know than by a stranger ("acquaintance" rape and marital rape). Two-thirds of reported rapes are planned and more than half occur indoors, usually in the woman's own home. Nine out of ten rapes occur between members of the same racial group. Most rapists lead everyday lives, go to school, work, have family and friends.

Emotional Reactions to Rape*

Rape hurts in every way. No two rapes are exactly alike, and no two women respond with exactly the same reactions in the same sequence. Differences in our culture, ages, personalities and the responses we get from others will influence how we respond.

Initial Responses

Immediate responses can range from numbness and disbelief, causing a woman to appear calm and rational, to extreme anxiety, fear and disorganization.

When he left, I fell into a deep sleep. As I was falling asleep, I told myself that when I got up in the morning I would have trouble remembering what happened to me.

I just sat on the floor and cried. When my husband came home, he asked me what was wrong. I was so upset I couldn't answer.

I called up a friend and in a real calm voice asked her if she could come over. I was fine till she got here, and then I broke down and cried.

You deserve support for however you respond to rape. What is important is that you do what you feel

*Other forms of violence provoke many of the same emotions as rape does. We do not have room to discuss emotional reactions fully in each part of the chapter, and hope that going into some detail here will be helpful to readers looking for support and understanding after being submitted to other kinds of violence as well.

you have to do and then, once you're ready, go to a hospital or doctor for care.

How people treat you when you seek medical care or report a rape makes a big difference in how you will feel. Medical providers and police are often insensitive and blaming.

I was telling the doctor about what had happened. He seemed kind and concerned, but after the exam was over, he asked what I was doing out so late at night by myself.

The officer I spoke to didn't seem to trust me because I was acting so "emotional," as he said. His rough questions felt almost like being raped again.

As a woman of color I was not able to allow myself to feel and express my reactions to the rape because I didn't feel safe from racist responses at the hospital, the police station, the counseling center.

Two major goals of feminists organizing around rape have been to get training programs into hospitals and police departments to teach personnel to respond more sensitively, and to make sure women going for care after a rape have the company of an advocate—a woman who is there specifically to give you support and get you fair treatment. If there are no such programs in your area (and even if there are), bring a friend with you if you possibly can. If anyone tries to make you feel guilty about the rape, s/he is buying into the myths which say that being raped is the woman's fault.

Second Phase

Once you are in a safe environment, you will often allow yourself to feel the full impact of what has just happened. You may be in physical pain from bruises, genital lesions, nausea or stomachaches. You are also likely to feel depressed, angry, afraid, humiliated and unable to sleep.

The responses we receive from loved ones can influence us during this time. Culture has a strong influence. If we are black we may not receive the respect we deserve, because black women are stereotypically seen as personifying sexual freedom and abandon. Cultures with strong religious prohibitions against nonmarital sex may ostracize us. If we are Latina, we may find that our loved ones judge us as dishonored, because of a strong emphasis on virginity; we may therefore find it hard to speak about the rape. It's hard not to feel both worthless and at fault when those close to us tell us we are.

During this time, try to find friends, family or counselors who can support you as you discuss the feelings that you are experiencing.

Third Phase

In the third phase you may go through a period of "calm before the storm." It may last for weeks, months or years. You may feel as if the trauma has passed. Unfortunately, this is usually a temporary period of apparently calm readjustment. One woman stated, "I thought it was all over; then I saw a man who looked like the rapist. Again I have begun to think about it, but this time I was obsessed with it."

During this calm period, we forget. Then something happens—a joke about rape, a pregnancy test or a court appearance. Again we feel that we lack control over our lives, just as we felt when we were raped.

Fourth/Final Phase

Finally we may be able to discuss our deeper feelings with others. Many women who speak to someone during the initial crisis choose to discuss the rape again at this time. Many women join support groups to meet with other women who are also trying to understand this experience. To get rid of guilt feelings and regain a strong self-image, we must direct our anger outward at the rapist and at a society that not only allows rape to continue but also blames women for its occurrence. After a rape we may lose faith in our environment as a safe and predictable one, but we *can* regain a strong sense of ourselves in the world.

Medical Considerations

If you have been raped, the first thing you may want to do is take a shower or bath and try to forget what happened. Do whatever feels most comfortable, but consider two things. First, it is very important both physically and emotionally that you receive medical attention as soon as possible, even if you have no obvious injuries. Second, don't bathe or shower if you think you may later decide to prosecute, as you will wash away evidence that may be crucial to your case.

If possible, call a friend, relative or local rape crisis counselor who can give you comfort, support, and act as an advocate on your behalf in the hospital. If you feel reluctant to go because you may not be able to afford it, be aware that a hospital emergency room cannot turn you away because you can't pay.

At the hospital, you have two basic concerns: medical care, and the gathering of evidence for a possible prosecution (you can refuse to be examined for evidence if you are absolutely sure that you will not want to prosecute). Physical injuries to *any* part of the body can result from a rape; therefore, a thorough examination is necessary. That examination should include and/or result in:

1. *A pelvic exam.* (If you are raped vaginally; see p. 477 for a pelvic exam description. You will get a rectal exam if you were raped anally). In collecting evidence, the doctor will look for the presence of semen. (*It is also possible to be raped vaginally with no semen or sperm present.*) S/he will also comb your pubic hair for the possible presence of the man's pubic hair, ask you to describe your physical and emotional condition, and may take your clothing, so take an extra set with you.

All this medical evidence will be available to others, including the police, only with your written permission. You or the person with you at the hospital should check the record for accuracy and objectivity as soon as possible after the exam, while the doctor is still present.

2. *Examination and treatment of any external injuries.*

3. *Treatment for the prevention of sexually transmitted disease (STD).* The doctor will give you two shots of penicillin in your buttocks. If you don't want this, be sure to say so. (Some women may not want to be given an antibiotic without a sexually transmitted disease being diagnosed; however, it is used as a preventive measure.)

4. *Treatment for the prevention of pregnancy.* If you suspect that you will become pregnant as a result of the rape, the doctor or nurses may offer you DES (the "morning-after pill"). This drug has serious effects, so before deciding to take it, read about its dangers and ineffectiveness on p. 248. A pregnancy or STD resulting from rape cannot be detected until six weeks later.* Although you may feel physically recovered shortly after the rape, making a follow-up visit, which would include tests and treatment for STD and a pregnancy test if indicated, would assure you that you are taking care of yourself. If you find that you are pregnant and are considering abortion, see Chapter 16.

Legal Considerations

It is never easy to decide whether to prosecute a rapist. Of the 10 percent or less of rapes that are reported, fewer still are prosecuted. In some states you can report a rape anonymously or without prosecuting (for police records). Whether you report it or not, write down everything that you can remember, so that if you do report or prosecute later your statement will be accurate.

As you are deciding whether to prosecute, here are several things to keep in mind:

1. The police and the legal system very often make prosecuting a rapist a more difficult, painful experience for the woman than it should be. It will help tremendously to have a friend or rape crisis counselor with you throughout the process.

---

*Even though some pregnancy tests are accurate within seven days, some STDs are not detectable until six weeks later, so it is a good idea to return for a six-week checkup.

Protecting Ourselves and Each Other from Rape

Authors' Note: Listing these tips reminds us how angry we are that we have to protect ourselves from men's actions. Yet until men stop or are forced to stop raping women, we will need to take precautions. (The following are much more useful against a stranger than against an acquaintance or husband.)

When possible, *the most effective protection comes from being with other women.* Arrange to walk home together, set up a greenlight or safehouse program in your neighborhood (see p. 112), get to know each other on a street or in an apartment building.

Where You Live

Keep lights in all the entrances; keep the windows locked and in place; have strong locks on every door; be aware of places where men might hide; don't put your full name on your mailbox; know which neighbors you can trust in an emergency; find out who is at your door before opening; say, "I'll get the door, Bill!" when going to the door.

On the Street

Be aware of what is going on around you. Walk with a steady pace; look as if you know where you are going; don't carry a lot of stuff; dress so you can move and run easily; walk in the middle of the street; don't walk through dark places or a group of men; if you fear danger, yell "Fire," not "Help" or "Rape"; carry a whistle around your wrist.

Transportation

Always check the backseat of your car before getting in; while driving, keep doors locked; don't stand near groups of men on public transportation; look aware and don't fall asleep; if you don't know where you are going, ask the driver and sit near the front.

"Legal Weapons" as Protection

A lighted cigarette, a plastic lemon or spray can filled with ammonia, a cheap heavy ring worn on the inside of your hand, a hatpin, an umbrella are all useful.

Body Basics

Use your elbows; if using fists, aim for his face; use your voice in his ear; use your teeth; if you kick, aim at his knees or genitals; pull his hair and clap your hands over his ears; keep your hands and arms close to you.

Hitchhiking

Don't hitchhike if you can possibly avoid it; it is just too dangerous. If you do, check the door handle, keep the window open and never ride with more than one man.

These tactics can help you but they are not foolproof. Practice tactics for the situations which make you feel most at risk and least powerful. Try to remain calm and to act as confident and strong as you can.

Adapted from *How to Start a Rape Crisis Center* (1972) by the Rape Crisis Center of Washington, D.C.

2. Chances of conviction are low: 20 to 40 percent in most states.

3. A trial can last from six months to two years, so you need to be prepared to continue thinking and talking about the rape for a long time, including giving an account of the event over and over while people judge whether you are telling the truth.

4. You will have to prove that you were sexually assaulted against your will and that the man used force or threatened force against you.

5. Rape is considered a crime against the state, so you will be a state's witness for the district attorney's office. You will not have a private lawyer unless you arrange for one to advise you and consult with the district attorney assigned to you. (For more on the legal process in your state, call a rape crisis center or the district attorney's office.)

WOMAN ABUSE

Woman abuse, often referred to as battering, is the most common and least reported crime in the United States.[8] Battering happens to women of every age, color, class and nationality. It is done by the men we married who beat us, by our sons and nephews who bully us and slap us around and by male relatives who verbally harass and degrade us. Twenty-five percent of American families have a history of woman abuse.[9]

Examples

Battering takes many forms. The majority of women who are battered are abused repeatedly by the same person. As time passes, these beatings often increase in frequency and severity.

I have had glasses thrown at me. I have been kicked in the abdomen, kicked off the bed and hit while laying on the floor—while I was pregnant. I have been whipped, kicked and thrown, picked up and thrown down again. I have been punched and kicked in the head, chest, face and abdomen on numerous occasions.

I have been slapped for saying something about politics, having a different view about religion, for swearing, for crying, for wanting to have intercourse.

I have been threatened when I wouldn't do something I was told to do.

I have been threatened when he's had a bad day—when he's had a good day.[10]

Other women are abused less regularly, yet the abuse still affects our self-esteem and our children.

My very upper-middle-class, WASP father hit my mother drunkenly on an occasional Saturday night. Sunday morning she would explain away her bruises. I lived my whole childhood under this shadow—the possibility of violence, the sounds in the night and the toll it took on me that she put up with it.

Some of us have listened to verbal abuse for years and have begun to believe the degrading lies we hear.

Researchers have attempted to understand why violence within families is so prevalent. It is clear that men receive "permission" from law courts, police and other men to batter.

The fact that men all around the world, of every conceivable class, color, religion and ethnic group beat their wives shows that something more is sick than these individuals. Something has got to be wrong with the societies these men live in that they are *allowed* to beat women....How can we explain former Prime Minister of Japan Sato having been given the Nobel Prize for Peace although his wife has publicly declared that he beat her?[11]

Many men learn violence at home; many men who batter saw their fathers abuse their mothers and many women who are abused have grown up in families where male power was never questioned and physical punishment "in the name of love" was accepted. When our families teach us to accept male power in all its forms, the message is difficult to defy.

What makes the problem so complex is that the men who do the battering are the people with whom we have been close or intimate, perhaps the fathers of our children. We may still be bound by love and loyalty. We remain at home not only because the men won't let us leave or make it as difficult as possible, but also because we hope that this episode will be the last one, that things will get better, that our men will change. We make excuses for their behavior.

Before I left I used to say, "Yeah, he punched and kicked me, but I'd said something to make him mad." Or "He only hits me when I argue." Now I see that everyone has a right to get angry—it's natural—but he had no right to express his anger so violently, to hurt me.

We don't leave home because what will we do with the children? How will we live and support ourselves? Where will we go?

We rarely get adequate protection from clergy, courts or police, who often do not take us seriously.

I went early in our marriage to a clergyman, who after a few visits told me that my husband meant no real harm, he was just confused and felt insecure.

Things continued. I turned this time to a doctor. I was given little pills to relax me and told to take things easier. I was "just too nervous."

I turned to a friend, and when her husband found out, he accused me of either making things up or exaggerating the situation. She was told to stay away from me.[12]

Many battered women have had similar experiences of being challenged, patronized or told that our problems are insignificant. In the face of such inexcusable treatment we must remember that *no woman deserves to be verbally abused or beaten. Every woman deserves to have her story taken seriously.*

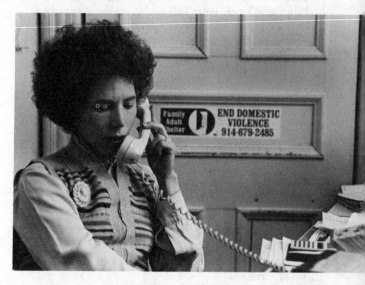

Mark Antman/Stock Boston

What to Do[13]

Try to stay calm during an attack; save your anger for a time when you are safe from physical attack. Remember, no matter what he says to you, that you are a valuable and worthwhile person.

- Defend and protect yourself, especially your head and stomach.
- Fight back only if you judge that it won't make him hurt you more.
- Call for help. Scream or, if you can get away, run to the nearest person or home, say you are being hurt and that you need help.
- Call the police, or have someone else do it; the police have a responsibility to protect you.

- Call your local crisis hotline to find out about a battered woman's shelter in your area.
- Get away. If it is unsafe to stay at home, call a neighbor, friend or a cab. Find shelter and take your children with you, either then or, if it would be safer, the next day. Your personal safety and your children's welfare are primary; you can handle custody and property matters after you leave.

Here are some things that battered women and their children need most frequently: emergency food, shelter, clothing; economic assistance and job training; advocacy with the legal, medical, police and welfare systems; school transportation, childcare by caring adults; safety plans; a chance to think and get advice about separation, divorce, child support, child custody, housing, other relationships, choosing a lawyer; support of other women, often in a group run by a shelter, hotline or community center.

There *are* alternatives to staying in a battering situation. More and more women are leaving men who batter, and finding help in making a new life despite economic hardships. Over the last decade, women in every state have been organizing to help women leave abusive situations, to provide shelter and a more responsive legal system. Women have found the courage to tell their stories publicly. *We are not helpless, and we are not alone.*

SEXUAL HARASSMENT

Sexual harassment is any *unwanted* sexual attention a woman experiences. It includes leering, pinching, patting, repeated comments, subtle suggestions of a sexual nature and pressure for dates. It can also take the form of attempted or actual rape. Sexual harassment can occur in any situation where men have power over women—welfare workers with clients, doctors with patients, policemen with women drivers, teachers with students.* This section focuses on workplace harassment because it has been the most widely studied so far.

In the workplace, the harasser may be an employer, supervisor, co-worker, client or customer. Any unwanted sexual attention causes anxiety and embarrassment, but when it occurs at work, our jobs are threatened.

*Sexual harassment in schools and universities has recently been defined as a form of sex discrimination under Title 9 of the Education Amendments of 1972. Teachers or administrators "barter" for sexual favors with grades, scholarships and recommendations for college or graduate school. Students use sexual harassment to force women out of courses or majors like auto mechanics in high school and engineering in college.

Recent surveys reveal that the majority of women will experience workplace sexual harassment at some point during their working lives. Eighty-eight percent of the 9,000 women answering *Redbook* magazine's questionnaire in 1976 had received unwanted sexual attention on the job. A 1981 survey of federal employees indicated that 42 percent of the women and 15 percent of the men had experienced sexual harassment (by men and by women) in a two-year period. In addition, both studies confirm that no one is immune from sexual harassment—women of all ages and races and holding all types of jobs were affected.

Joan is a forty-three-year-old black woman who works as a waitress in a bar and restaurant. She likes her job because it's close to home and it gives her a steady income to support her children. She often feels isolated, though, as many of her co-workers are white and have racist attitudes.

A customer who comes in every day during the lunch rush begins to flirt with Joan, making suggestive comments about her clothing and physical appearance. Unnerved by his comments, she tries not to show it because she doesn't want to lose any tip money. Often he grabs at her and touches her when she walks by.

After several weeks of this treatment, Joan can't take it anymore. She feels so anxious at work that her stomach hurts, and she starts to call in sick more and more. She knows she needs to figure something out or she'll eventually lose her job. She's afraid if she complains she'll get blamed because she's friendly and attractive-looking.

Chris is a thirty-four-year-old Latina who works as a secretary in a large hospital. Chris has excellent organizational skills and is proud of her ability to take initiative and keep her office running smoothly.

Chris's boss depends on her a lot to take care of business, and is appreciative of her work. He begins asking Chris out to lunch or for drinks after work as a way to thank her. Chris is uncomfortable with these invitations, but doesn't feel able to say no. The other secretaries begin to wonder why Chris is spending her lunch hour with the boss and feel angry about it.

One evening as Chris is getting ready to leave, her boss comes in and asks her to have a drink with him. Chris finally tells him that it makes her uncomfortable to socialize with him outside the office, that it does not seem appropriate to her. He tells Chris that he thinks she is too impressed with herself and it is inappropriate for her to tell him what she will or won't do.

Theresa is an eighteen-year-old white woman who works as an assembler at a big electronics company in her town. It's her first full-time job after graduating from high school, and she's happy because the pay is pretty good since the company is unionized.

Soon after she begins work, one of the men who work near her starts to ask her a lot of questions about her

What You Can Do If You Are Sexually Harassed

Authors' Note: It's crucial to realize that every situation is different. What kind of strategy you choose will depend on many factors, including how much you can afford to risk losing your job and whether you feel you can get support from your co-workers. (Race and class differences sometimes isolate workers from each other, for instance.)

1. Remember that you are not to blame. Sexual harassment is *imposed* sexual attention. No matter how complicated the situation is, the harasser is responsible for the abuse.

2. Document what happens. Keep a diary; save any notes or pictures from the harasser—don't throw them away in anger. Write down specific dates, times, places, kinds of incidents, your responses, his answers, any witnesses.

3. *Generate support for yourself before you take action*: break the silence, talk with others at your workplace or school and outside, ask for help in working out a response. They may feel more responsible then for backing you up if your response to the harasser fails.

4. Investigate your workplace's or school's policy and grievance procedure for sexual harassment cases. Know its overall records before you act. If possible, know the record of particular administrators, managers, union stewards or officials, personnel or equal-opportunity counselors, or others you may need to involve to get your complaint heard.

5. You may discover others who have been harassed who can act with you. Collective action and joint complaints strengthen your position. Some who have not been harassed may join in collective action. Try to use organizations that already exist, such as your union or employee organization, a local rape crisis center or women's organization, or an advocacy organization for your particular racial or ethnic group to help you strategize and carry out a collective response.

6. Let the harasser know as clearly, directly, explicitly as possible that you are not interested in his attentions. If you do this in writing, keep a copy of your letter.

7. Evaluate your options. What do you want from any action you take? What are your primary concerns and goals? What courses of action are available to you? What are the possible outcomes, including the risks of each course of action?

8. First consider taking actions *within* your workplace or school, strategizing with others to be as creative as possible; think about lawsuits only as a last resort.* But remember that sexual harassment is illegal because you may be able to use that fact to strengthen your position.

---

personal life: what she does after work, if she has a boyfriend, where she lives, etc. Theresa doesn't want to talk to him about these things, but she wants to be friendly and sociable with people at work. Soon his questions become even more personal, and he starts to talk with her about his sexual relations with women. When Theresa tells him that she feels uneasy and asks him to stop, he laughs and says that if she can't handle a little friendly conversation, then she isn't ready for the working world.

Sexual harassment is another powerful way for men to undermine and control us. There is an implicit (and sometimes explicit) message that our refusal to comply with the harasser's demands will lead to work-related reprisals. These can include escalation of harassment; poor work assignments; sabotaging of projects; denial of raises, benefits or promotion; and sometimes the loss of the job with only a poor reference to show for it. Harassment can drive women out of a particular job or out of the workplace altogether.

Socializing at work often includes flirting or joking about sex. While it may be a pleasant relief from routine or a way to communicate with someone we are "interested in," this banter can become insulting or demeaning. We have had little power to define this line for ourselves. It becomes sexual harassment when it creates a hostile, intimidating or pressured working environment.

There is such a taboo in many workplaces against identifying sexual harassment for what it is that many of us who experience it are at first aware only of feeling stressed. Headaches, anxieties, resistance to going to work in the morning—it often takes us a while to realize these symptoms may come from being sexually harassed. Sexual harassment can make us question our right to work, our competence, our appearance or attractiveness, our right to look and dress as we please or to go out with whomever we choose. We often respond by feeling isolated and powerless, afraid to say no or to speak out because we fear either that we some-

*The specific legal options for sexual harassment include filing charges of sex discrimination with your state's Human Rights Commission or the Federal Equal Employment Opportunity Commission. In addition, women have used unemployment compensation, civil or criminal assault, rape laws, union grievance procedures and worker compensation. Students have used the federal law, Title 9 of the Education Amendments of 1972. See p. 104, "Legal Considerations," for the problems and limits of legal strategies.

how are responsible or that we won't receive help in facing possible retaliation. But when we take the risk and talk with other women, we often find that they are being harassed, too (or have been), and have had similar responses to ours.

INCEST AND SEXUAL ABUSE OF CHILDREN

Traditionally, incest has been defined as sexual contact which occurs between family members.* Most incest occurs between older male relatives and younger female children in families of every class and color. Because it happens within the family context, an incestuous relationship is one over which a child or young woman has no control. A trusted family member uses his power—as well as our love and dependence—to initiate sexual contact, and to insure also that the relationship continues and remains secret.

My barter with my brother was that he could do sex on me to practice for his girlfriends. I consented not because I enjoyed it but because I was afraid to be alone when my parents went out....I never even thought of talking about it. That just couldn't be done.

Sexual abuse of children is most often committed by family friends who have access to children within their family setting. Abuse is also perpetrated by people normally trusted by parents—doctors, dentists, teachers and babysitters. Despite popular myths, "stranger danger" poses much less threat to boys and girls. Yet parents teach us to expect danger from strangers, not from trusted authority figures, and the violation of this trust is often frightening and confusing.

Incest and sexual abuse of children take many forms and may include sexually suggestive language; prolonged kissing, looking and petting; vaginal and/or anal intercourse and oral sex. Since sexual contact is often achieved without force, you may not show signs of physical abuse. If you were very young when the abuse occurred, you may have scars from vaginal or anal lacerations. You may remember chronic sore throats and stomach pain if the abuse involved oral sex. Some of us became pregnant or contracted a sexually transmitted disease.

It is difficult to talk about incest or sexual abuse of children. Some of us may never have told anyone, though the abuse may have continued for years. We never mentioned how we dreaded family gatherings, where a particular uncle or family friend would come after us. For some of us, exploring our bodies with an older brother turned into a sexual encounter, and we ended feeling oddly abused. Sometimes a father, uncle or teacher abused our sisters and we didn't find out for years, because our sisters were also afraid to tell. Every survivor has her own story. Many of us have kept our stories secret for years.

Feminist Insights

For many years "experts" wrote quantities of nonfeminist material on incest and child abuse. They blamed mothers for "abandoning" their children to sexually deprived husbands and accused young girls of being "seductive" or of fantasizing about a sexual relationship with a male relative. Feminists have challenged these victim-blaming views: incest and child abuse occur primarily because men have power and women and children do not. They are means by which fathers, uncles and significant family contacts bolster their low self-image by taking advantage of the powerlessness of children. Men can put these motives into action because family structures allow them to misuse their power.

Incest Survivors

Those of us who are incest survivors know that the effects of this abuse are lifelong. We often blame ourselves long after the abuse has ended—for not saying no, for not fighting back, for telling or not telling, for having been "seductive," for having trusted the abuser. Often there was no one to confirm that someone treated us cruelly and that this abuse was truly terrible.

For the next twenty years I will probably continue to walk around and ask other women, "What was your childhood like?" Hearing women say that no one touched them sexually at that young an age helps me realize that something in my childhood was really wrong.

Many of us have difficulty with sexually intimate relationships because of the memories they revive. Many of us desire sexual intimacy yet have difficulty trusting. Some incest survivors feel comfortable with sex yet know that something is vaguely wrong.

It's been really hard to figure out how this has affected me with men. I've had a hard time figuring out who is safe and who isn't. Now the only way I will sleep with someone is if I can have complete control. I need permission to feel uncomfortable with certain sexual acts.

Sometimes blaming ourselves takes other forms. Many teenagers with a history of incest "sleep around" to feel accepted, or run away. Many teenage and adult survivors feel depressed and don't know why, and/or turn to drugs and alcohol to mask the pain. Some of us feel worthless.

---

*Each state defines incest differently. In this chapter, we will be discussing *social* attitudes and definitions regarding incest and sexual abuse of children, not legal ones.

I often feel hopeless and suicidal. My father treated me with such violence that this is the only way I know to treat myself. I'm learning better ways now, but it's difficult.

I have been a drug addict. I have been anorexic. I have been a compulsive eater. Food was the only thing I could control and trust when people in my life failed me.

Getting Help

To heal the emotional scars of incest or early sexual abuse, we need to tell our stories to people who understand deeply what we have experienced. Talking with others in counseling or support groups for women with a history of incest breaks the silence, helps us to gain perspective and know we are not alone and eases the pain. Women who have taken advantage of these tools feel healthier and stronger.

I now have a lot of compassion for myself, because I know the implications of the abuse that occurred in my life. I owe myself all the understanding, patience and acceptance I can find—a ton of it.

Some women find that they need to confront the family member who abused them. This is a frightening task, but may also be rewarding:

I feel empowered by letting him know I am aware that the incest occurred. I feel empowered by the fact that I didn't ask him if he remembered, I just told him. I knew he would deny it. I just wanted to say, "This happened." I did not expect results. Telling him was the total opposite of all that happened—what was invisible is now out in the open.

Those of us with a history of incest need to know that whatever we do or don't do, we have done okay because we have survived a childhood that wasn't like a childhood at all.*

SELF-DEFENSE

As much as self-defense may help in certain situations, the most important step in ending violence against women is to stop men from doing the violence and allowing it to be done.

In recent years the experiences of women who have been practicing self-defense have changed our ideas about what self-defense is and how we can use its techniques. We have discovered that self-defense study actually includes any activity—assertiveness training, exercise, sports—which promotes self-confidence,

*See especially Judith Herman's *Father-Daughter Incest*, listed in Resources.

self-knowledge or self-reliance. We have also discovered that skills we once associated almost exclusively with self-defense can benefit other areas of our lives. Self-defense classes teach us to shift our self-awareness so that we remember that we are the sources of our own energy and the initiators of our own actions. Instead of freezing in the face of assault, we learn to mobilize our thoughts, assess the situation, make a judgment about the level of danger, choose the response we wish to make and then make it. We can use this self-awareness in other common life situations when it may seem that someone else is in control; medical examinations, job interviews, confrontations with authority, communication with a difficult person. One woman states:

I have experienced such profound changes in my self-image and in the way that I see the world and relate to people that I really can't separate my study of self-defense from the rest of my life.

Inner and Outer Obstacles

Several myths can prevent us from defending ourselves effectively against a physical assault: that the assailant is invulnerable, that greater physical strength will decide who is to win in an assault situation, that we don't know how to defend ourselves. Yet women have defended themselves against attack in many instances. One woman frightened off three adolescent males who were following her along a city street by turning quickly and letting out a bloodcurdling yell. Another stopped a would-be assailant with a kick to the midsection. A young girl sitting on the train found a wayward hand on her knee. She took the man's wrist in her grasp, raised his hand high in the air and said loudly enough for the entire car to hear, "Who does this belong to?" He got off at the next stop. There are hundreds of such stories. We don't see them on TV, we don't read them in the newspapers, but stop in at any self-defense class run by and for women and you'll hear them. We often attribute such escapes to luck or

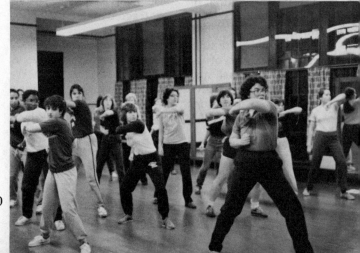

June Austin

Guidelines for Self-Defense Training

I. **Finding a self-defense class:** Check YWCAs, community schools, adult education programs, women's publications, women's centers.

II. **Choosing a class:**
   A. Observe a class.
   B. After class, question the instructor about hypothetical defense situations, particularly those which you fear most.
   C. Talk to the women students in the class, presenting the same hypothetical situations to them; steps B and C will indicate whether or not the instructor teaches application of techniques to situations that women face.
   D. When talking to the instructor and the students, try to determine how much awareness there is about issues of violence against women and about other safety resources in the area; try to find a really complete approach to women's safety.

III. **Training without a teacher:**
   A. Read books on the subject; many written by women provide good guidelines for building self-confidence.
   B. Strengthen your body with good nutrition and regular exercise, preferably with some combination of aerobics and weight training.
   C. Working with friends to give feedback or in front of a mirror:
      1. practice walking with strong, even strides, looking as if you know where you're going;
      2. practice loud yelling, accompanied by ferocious facial expressions;
      3. tell someone to take his hands off you, giving a coherent message through a combination of words, tone of voice and facial expression;
      4. act out "what if" situations, discuss various responses and drill the best ones.

There are people around us, particularly the men in our lives, who may consciously or unconsciously seek to discourage us from learning self-defense. As we begin to learn physical techniques, we feel the stirrings of a fledgling self-confidence. We know how to break a hold, to avoid a grasp, to stay on our feet and keep our emotional and physical balance. Yet when we practice these techniques on men we know, we often fail, both because we have eliminated the element of surprise and because their resistance to our new skills undermines us. It is important to practice with people who support our efforts to become stronger.

We need to be on guard against the ideas that "a little knowledge is a dangerous thing," and that fighting back only makes matters worse. Although compliance is sometimes a prudent response to assault, it does not guarantee that a situation will not get worse. *In fact, studies have shown that women who use active resistance and who act quickly are more likely to avoid rape than those who use passive or no resistance.*

Up to this point we have had little experience in the uses of self-defense by battered women. Street techniques, which depend upon surprise and causing damage, don't work so well against repeated assault by men we live with. Yet other skills developed in the practice of self-defense may be useful, such as learning to overcome the inner obstacles that come up when we are faced with a violent situation. If we feel more self-confident, we may begin to think about resisting the battering situation in some way, about fighting back or leaving it.

We need to develop guidelines for adapting physical techniques for use by women with different physical capabilities: elder women, physically challenged women, injured women, women who are pregnant and others. Furthermore, we need to support the work of safehouse networks, temporary shelters, rape crisis centers and other organizations committed to our safety, because without them, self-defense is a piecemeal approach to women's security.

TODAY AND TOMORROW*

NO WOMAN IS SAFE UNTIL ALL OF US ARE SAFE

Over the past fifteen years, we have directed our collective anger into many kinds of action opposing violence against women.

- We organized consciousness-raising groups and discovered that our experiences of dominance by men were common and shared.

*Throughout history women have protected themselves and each other from men's violence by fighting back, offering shelter, nursing and caring for each other. Unfortunately this chapter has no room for this proud history. Please check the Resources section.

good fortune, and we don't take credit for our own courage and resourcefulness. It is important to our self-confidence to reclaim those successes.

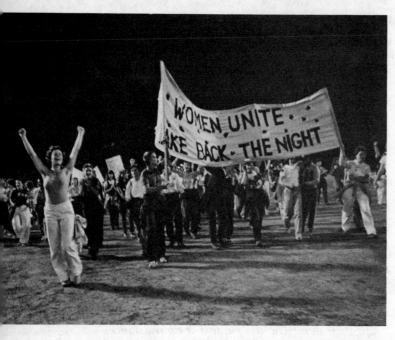

Bonnie Burt

- We demanded that the public listen to us by demonstrating in large groups, holding public speakouts, creating films, radio and TV shows, street theater, dramatic productions, books, pamphlets, newspapers and articles.
- We set up educational programs for thousands of law enforcement and health professionals.
- We took on particular offenders. Women Against Violence Against Women (WAVAW) organized a national boycott of Warner-Atlantic-Electra (a record company) and created a slide show to educate teenagers and adults about ways in which companies profit from depicting violence toward women. After years of sustained pressure, WAVAW won an agreement from Warner to adopt guidelines on the depiction of violence against women and children on record jackets.
- Women defaced billboards advertising a moisturizer called "Self-Defense" because it made a mockery of work against violence through its slogan, "A pretty face isn't safe in the city." Ads were quickly withdrawn from the market.
- Women have supported each other through the process of taking offenders to court.
- For the first time in recent history women organized in support of women of color assaulted by white men. Women held benefits for the legal defense of JoAnne Little, a black woman, and Inez Garcia, a Latina, who killed the men who raped them, and Yvonne Wanrow, a Native American who killed a known child-molester when he came after her and her children.
- Women of color formed organizations such as the Committee to End Sterilization Abuse and worked with white women, winning new regulations to attempt to control sterilization abuse.

- By 1979 as many as a thousand organizations were providing services around the country to assist women who had been raped. Some of these were autonomous rape crisis centers created and staffed by women.
- In 1974 a group of feminists doing legal-aid work in St. Paul, Minnesota, opened Women's House, the first U.S. refuge for battered women and their children. Current estimates suggest there are more than a thousand hotlines, shelters and programs for battered women. The National Coalition Against Domestic Violence, launched in 1977, now attracts over 600 service providers and activists to its conferences. Parallel coalitions of service groups exist in more than thirty-five states.
- Neighborhood groups have formed networks of refuges, called "safehouse" or "greenlight" programs because participating homes are identified by green lights, where women harassed or attacked in the streets can find safety.
- We have worked for legal reform on many fronts. Since 1974, forty-nine states have revised their rape laws in order to make it easier for women to report the crimes and obtain convictions. (Mississippi is the lone holdout.) By mid-1982, eleven states treated rape by a husband or cohabitor (marital rape) the same as rape by a stranger. Some thirty states permit marital rape charges under some circumstances—for instance, in some states the pair must be legally separated. Forty-nine states have now revised their statutes covering battering; thirty-six of these specifically include protective orders for victims. Legislation has been used creatively: fourteen states impose taxes (usually on marriage licenses or divorce filings) whose revenues are earmarked to fund services for battered women. Unfortunately these may not hold up in federal court as constitutional.
- We learned from feminists in other countries. The 1976 Tribunal of Crimes Against Women, held in Brussels and attended by women from all over the world, expanded the definition of violence against women to include dowry murders* and genital mutilation. European feminists inspired both safehouses and "Take Back the Night" marches, which rally thousands of women yearly in cities across the U.S. to protest violence against women.
- Some men have participated in this movement. Men have formed a few groups in which men help batterers to deal with their violence (for example, Emerge, in Boston). Other men have worked for legislation, written articles or made films. Some men have begun to hold each other accountable, legally and socially, for their violence, recognizing that men who do not take action support the system which

*Men marry women for their dowries and then kill them. This happens often in India.

promotes violence against women. They talk about their socialization in relation to women, question the extent and consequences of male dominance, listen to and respect the women around them.

Presently there is a backlash against the very actions which have helped and strengthened so many women. Conservative pressure groups claim that measures to protect women of all ages and to stop male violence undermine "traditional family values." Funding is increasingly harder to get—especially since current budget priorities do not favor social services. Many shelters, rape crisis centers and other services are being forced to close for lack of funding.

We must continue to express our outrage loud and clear by keeping alive all the services to women, and by continuing to speak out. We will continue to teach our daughters to demand equality for themselves and others, and our sons to question sexism and violence, to respect women as equals and fight all forms of dominance. We will continue to support one another in protecting ourselves with ingenuity, strength and pride. We applaud women who say no to male violence, who offer support to a friend, who protect each other, who fight back, who survive.

APPENDIX: PROSTITUTION

About 1.3 million women in this country earn all or part of their living as prostitutes. Contrary to the ugly stereotypes of prostitutes as fallen women, dope addicts or disease carriers,* prostitutes are women at work—supporting children as single parents, trying to save money to go to school, surviving economically in a job market which underpays women at every economic level. Many are housewives or secretaries moonlighting as prostitutes to make ends meet.

Once politically voiceless and isolated from other women, over the past ten years prostitutes have organized for support and political action.† As they speak out and write about their lives,‡ they expose the many forms of violence which prostitutes experience:

1. The poverty which forces women—especially poor women, women of color and runaway teenagers—into work as hookers (many women have no access to other jobs); the sexist job discrimination which means that even middle- and upper-class women can earn more

in prostitution than in other jobs available to them; the fact that a great number of incest victims become prostitutes.

2. Police harassment.

3. Intimidation and beatings by pimps, to whom many prostitutes must give their earnings in return for protection. Many of them fear for their lives.

4. Lack of police protection against other crimes: streetwalkers especially, those women without jobs in safer massage parlors or houses, who are often raped, beaten and left unpaid.

5. The arrest and prosecution of prostitutes while clients (most of whom are white, middle-aged, middle-class married men) go free.

6. The racism and class bias which leads to the arrest and imprisonment of far more prostitutes of color and poor women than white women, even though the invisible majority of hookers are white and middle class.

*As a middle-class white woman, trained as a registered nurse, I could work in a private call business instead of hitting the streets. I was arrested but never did time in prison; the system isn't aimed at putting me in jail. Women of color have less easy access to places like upper-class hotels, where if you're black and alone you're automatically tagged as a hooker. So they're in the streets and in the bars, where they are more visible and more vulnerable to exploitation and arrest—and they're the ones who end up in jail.**

Some feminists have been critical of prostitutes for "reinforcing sex-role stereotypes" by allowing themselves to be sex objects. Prostitutes point out that they are no different from most women in having to sell their services to men. In the words of an ex-prostitute:

I've worked in straight jobs where I've felt more like I was prostituting my being than in prostitution. I had less control over my life, and the powerlessness wasn't even up front. People didn't see me as selling myself, but with the minimum wage so little and my boss so insulting, I felt like I was selling my soul.

In a world where women have so little power, nearly all women depend in some way on men's money, protection, favor. Many who are not hookers, for example, feel they must have sex when their man wants to because he provides financial or emotional security. From feminist Karen Lindsey:

The question of whether or not to sell ourselves to men is a false one: the real question is *how* to sell ourselves in the way that is least destructive to ourselves and our sisters. That is not a decision any one of us can make for any of the

---

*Only about 5 percent of sexually transmitted disease in the United States is spread by prostitutes.

†Examples of such groups are COYOTE (Call Off Your Old Tired Ethics) in San Francisco, and PUMA (Prostitutes Union of Massachusetts). For more information, contact the National Task Force on Prostitution, P.O. Box 26354, San Francisco, CA 94126. Ask for their newsletter, "Coyote Howls."

‡See, for instance, *Prostitutes: Our Life*, edited by Claude Jaget (Falling Wall Press, 9 Lawford Street, Old Market, Bristol, England).

*Prison life in itself is brutal. This, combined with the lack of job opportunities once a woman gets out, makes prison hard to avoid again for many women. Seventy percent of women in prison today were first jailed for prostitution.

others....Prostitutes don't need our condescension. What they need is our alliance. And we need theirs.*

Prostitutes have organized in this country and Europe (including the famous French Prostitutes Strike in 1975) to demand *decriminalization*, the abolition of all laws against prostitution. (Legalizing prostitution isn't enough. In West Germany, where women work in government-run houses, prostitutes feel they have traded illegal pimps for a legal one: they have little control over their working conditions and still turn over a big part of their income in fees.) With decriminalization, prostitutes would have more control over their work and the money they earn. Most of all, they would no longer go to jail for providing a service which society itself puts in such high demand, and for choosing the highest-paying work available to them. A longer-range goal is, in the words of a PUMA member, that "No woman should have to be a prostitute because she has no alternatives." From a British prostitute: "The end of women's poverty is the end of prostitution."†

NOTES

1. This is a popular statistic credited to the FBI. Others have projected that battering occurs in anywhere from one-quarter to one-half of all marriages or male/female cohabiting relationships. National Clearinghouse on Domestic Violence. *Battered Women—A National Concern*. Rockville, MD, 1980.

2. This figure comes from a study by the Los Angeles Commission on Assaults Against Women; it also comes from statistical calculations combining FBI figures as modified with a projection of rising rape rates through the year 2000, using the increase in reported rapes from 1960–1975 as a base. See work of Freada Klein in Resources. Included as "rape" in deriving this figure are marital rape and *any* case of being forced to have sexual intercourse against your will.

3. Merit Systems Protection Board. *Sexual Harassment in the Federal Workplace: Is It a Problem?* Washington, DC: U.S. Government Printing Office, 1981.

4. Linda Tschirhart Sanford. *Silent Children—A Book for Parents About the Prevention of Child Sexual Abuse*. Garden City, NY: Anchor Press/Doubleday, 1980.

5. Susan Griffin. *Rape—The Power of Consciousness*. San Francisco: Harper & Row, 1979, p. 3.

6. A study reported in 1981 revealed that women far more than men report that fear curtails their daily activities. The most fearful women are the elderly, the poor and members of racial/ethnic minorities. Stephanie Riger and Margaret Gordon. "The Fear of Rape: A Study in Social Control." *Journal of Social Issues* 37 (1981), pp. 71–92.

7. A study in 1980 found that black women were less likely to have their rape cases come to trial and to result in conviction than white women. G.D. LaFree. "Variables Affecting Guilty Pleas and Convictions in Rape Cases—Toward a Social Theory of Rape Processing," *Social Forces* 58 (1980), pp. 833–50.

8. "Breaking the Cycle," *Newsletter of the Vermont Governor's Commission on the Status of Women*, September–October 1980.

9. Mildred Daley Pagelow. "Factors Affecting Women's Decisions to Leave Violent Relationships," *Journal of Family Issues*, 2, No. 4 (December 1981).

10. "Letter from a Battered Woman," *For Shelter and Beyond*. Boston, MA: Massachusetts Coalition of Battered Women Service Groups, 1981, p. 6.

11. Lisa Leghorn. "Social Responses to Battered Women." Paper presented at the Wisconsin Conference on Battered Women, October 2, 1976.

12. "Letter from a Battered Woman."

13. Several of the "during an attack" suggestions have been adapted from Milwaukee Task Force on Battered Women, *Battered Women: A Handbook for Survival*, rev. ed., 1978; and from Jennifer Baker Fleming, *Stopping Wife Abuse*. Garden City, NY: Anchor Press/Doubleday, 1979, pp. 32–33.

RESOURCES

General Readings

Aegis: Magazine on Ending Violence Against Women. Feminist Alliance Against Rape (FAAR), P.O. Box 21033, Washington, DC 20009. Subscriptions: $10.50 per year individuals; $25.00 institutions. An excellent quarterly publication which includes analytical articles on all forms of violence against women, discussions of strategies and practical information and resources for organizers and direct-service providers.

Barry, Kathleen. *Female Sexual Slavery*. New Jersey: Prentice-Hall, Inc., 1979. In this powerful work, the concept of female sexual slavery is used to cover "...ALL situations where women or girls cannot change the immediate conditions of their existence; where...they cannot get out; and where they are subject to sexual violence and exploitation" (p. 40). Cross-cultural evidence documents the international slave trade connected to prostitution, genital mutilation, rape, battering, incest and pornography.

Delacoste, Frederique, and Felice Newman, eds. *Fight Back! Feminist Resistance to Male Violence*. Minneapolis: Cleis Press, P.O. Box 8281, Minneapolis, MN 55408. An inspiring compendium of analyses of trends in the movement against violence against women, the interconnections of racism and sexual violence, tales of individuals who fought back and descriptions of group actions to challenge images and practices of sexual violence. A lengthy state-by-state directory of rape crisis centers, battered women's shelters and women's political organizations is also included. $13.95.

Rape

Readings

Columbus Women Against Rape, P.O. Box 02084, Columbus, OH 43202. Several publications are available on primary

---

*Karen Lindsey, "Beginning to Demystify the Oldest Profession," *The Second Wave*, Summer 1976.

†From *Prostitutes: Our Life*, p. 31.

rape prevention, including "Freeing Our Lives," which discusses short-term and long-term prevention strategies ($1.00); "Fighting Back," covering practical safety tips ($.50); and *Rape Prevention Workshops: A Leader's Guide*, designed to teach individuals and organizations how to present workshops on rape prevention ($10.00).

Davis, Angela. "The Dialectics of Rape," *Ms.*, June 1975, 74ff. The author relates the case of JoAnne Little to the history of rape and racism in the United States.

Friedman, Deb. "Rape, Racism—and Reality," *FAAR and NCN Newsletter*, July–August 1978, pp. 17–26. In this well-written article, Friedman includes a historical summary of the issues and discusses black women's critiques of Susan Brownmiller's *Against Our Will*. The publication in which this article appeared has changed its name to *Aegis: Magazine on Ending Violence Against Women* (c.o. FAAR, P.O. Box 21033, Washington, DC 20009).

National Center for the Prevention and Control of Rape, NIMH, #13A–44 Park Lawn Building, 5600 Fishers Lane, Rockville, MD 20857. Since the mid-1970s, the Center has funded a range of research and demonstration projects on rape. Bibliographies, monographs and final reports are available at various prices.

"The Rape of Black Women as a Weapon of Terror," *Black Women in White America: A Documentary History*. Edited by Gerda Lerner. New York: Vintage Books, 1972, pp. 172–93.

Rodriquez, Alvarado M. "Rape and Virginity Among Puerto Rican Women," *Aegis: Magazine on Ending Violence Against Women*, March/April 1979. See above for address. $3.25 per copy.

Audiovisual Materials

The "Acquaintance Rape Prevention" film series has been widely used and well received. It consists of four short films focusing on rape by someone the victim knows. Available from ODN Productions, Inc., 74 Varick Street, Room 304, New York, NY 10013; and 1454 Sixth Street, Berkeley, CA 94710. A version for the hearing-impaired is also available.

Rape Culture, a 33-minute 1975 color film, available from Cambridge Documentary Films, P.O. Box 385, Cambridge, MA 02139. Uses excerpts from popular Hollywood movies and interviews with feminists and convicted rapists to illustrate the role of societal forces in promoting rape. Widely used. Rental $46.00.

Organizations

Community Program Against Sexual Assault (CPASA), 100 Warren Street, Roxbury, MA 02119. One of the too few rape crisis centers run by women of color to provide services to victims and community education and prevention programs.

National Coalition Against Sexual Assault (NCASA), Sharon Sayles, President, Minnesota Program for Victims of Sexual Assault, 430 Metro Building, Minneapolis, MN 55105. A national membership organization, NCASA sponsors annual conferences and publishes a newsletter. Regional representatives facilitate the exchange of information and

resources. Annual dues: $15.00 for individuals; $25.00 for organizations.

Washington, D.C., Rape Crisis Center, P.O. Box 21005, Washington, DC 20009. As one of the first rape crisis centers in the U.S., this center played an important role in fostering communications between projects. They recently sponsored the first national conference on Third World Women and Violence, and publish *How to Start a Rape Crisis Center*, an excellent resource for new programs ($5.00).

Woman-Battering

Readings

Massachusetts Coalition of Battered Women's Service Groups. *For Shelter and Beyond: An Educational Manual for Working with Women Who Are Battered*. Provides practical information on counseling and advocacy, and covers a range of issues that confront service providers in shelters. Available from MCBWSG, 25 West Street, Boston, MA 02116. $5.00.

Schechter, Susan. *Women and Male Violence: The Struggles of the Battered Women's Movement*. Boston: South End Press, 1982. A description of the origins and evolution of the contemporary battered-women's movement, and a critical analysis of major developments. This book is particularly useful to organizations and coalitions in designing future strategies.

Warrior, Betsy. *Working on Wife Abuse*. 46 Pleasant Street, Cambridge, MA 02139. Continually updated since the mid-1970s, this directory is an extensive resource list of organizations and individuals working against battering. Other practical materials, such as sample forms and policies of shelters, are also included.

ODN Productions, Inc., 74 Varick Street, Room 304, New York, NY 10013; and 1454 Sixth Street, Berkeley, CA 94710. Various films, including the "Spouse Abuse Prevention" series, three short films and a guidebook focusing on men who batter, the effects of their actions and alternatives to violence; and "In Need of Special Attention," a 17-minute color film, with training manual, designed to assist emergency room staff in establishing protocol for battered women.

We Will Not Be Beaten, available from Transition House Films, 25 West Street, Boston, MA 02116. Features interviews with staff and residents of a shelter. It is a powerful analysis of the dynamics of battering, institutional response and the role of shelters. In black and white, it is available in two versions of different lengths on film or video. Rental $40.00.

Organizations

Emerge, 25 Huntington Avenue, Room 324, Boston, MA 02116. As the first men's group working with batterers, this organization's efforts have provided battered-women's shelters with an important referral and useful information on the dynamics of battering. They have written a monograph, "Working with Men Who Batter," and produced a film, *To Have and to Hold* which features interviews with men who have been Emerge's counselors and clients. Rental fee for *To Have and to Hold*: $35.00 plus $5.00 shipping.

Marital Rape

Audiovisual Materials

National Clearinghouse on Marital Rape (NCOMR), Women's History Research Center, Inc., 2325 Oak Street, Berkeley, CA 94708. The clearinghouse has published a pamphlet on the Greta Rideout Case in Oregon ($1.00) and a marital rape brochure. Send a self-addressed, stamped envelope for materials and for information about membership in the clearinghouse.

Sexual Harassment

Readings

Alliance Against Sexual Coercion (AASC), the first organization in the U.S. to provide a comprehensive approach to the problem of sexual harassment, has written *Fighting Sexual Harassment: An Advocacy Handbook* ($3.50), available from Alyson Publications, P.O. Box 2783, Boston, MA 02208.

Association of American Colleges, Project on the Status and Education of Women, 1818 R Street NW, Washington, DC 20009. Since 1971 the Project has provided a wealth of information on women in higher education. A packet of articles on rape and sexual harassment is available. Send stamped, self-addressed envelope for order form.

Backhouse, Constance, and Leah Cohen. *Sexual Harassment on the Job*. Englewood Cliffs, NJ: Prentice-Hall, Inc., 1981. Originally published in Canada in 1978, this book is an excellent, quite readable overview of the issue. Case studies, history, analysis of the problem and action plans for management and unions are covered. $5.95, paper.

Farley, Lin. *Sexual Shakedown: The Sexual Harassment of Women on the Job*. New York: McGraw-Hill Co., Inc., 1978. An analysis of the origins of sexual harassment in the economic system and in women's subordinate status within society. Includes case histories.

MacKinnon, Catharine. *Sexual Harassment of Working Women: A Case of Sex Discrimination*. New Haven: Yale University Press, 1978. A sophisticated legal and theoretical analysis of sexual harassment as a form of sex discrimination. Victims' experiences, patterns of women's workforce participation and an analysis of two theories of sex discrimination—as sex differences and as sex inequality—are explored. $5.95.

Audiovisual Materials

The Workplace Hustle, a 30-minute color film, available from Clark Communications, 943 Howard Street, San Francisco, CA 94103. Provides an introduction to sexual harassment on the job. Narrated by Ed Asner, it features interviews with women who have experienced harassment and with Lin Farley (see above), and groups of men and women discussing the topic. It does not include women in nontraditional occupations.

Organizations

Working Women's Institute, 593 Park Avenue, New York, NY 10021. The Institute provides direct service and education and operates a legal backup center for sexual harassment cases and a research clearinghouse. Numerous original publications and reprints are available, including research reports and law review articles. Send a stamped, self-addressed envelope for publication lists.

Sexual Abuse of Children

Readings

Herman, Judith L. *Father-Daughter Incest*. Cambridge, MA, and London, Harvard University Press, 1981.

Rush, Florence. *The Best Kept Secret: Sexual Abuse of Children*. Englewood Cliffs, NJ: Prentice-Hall, Inc., 1980. Rush documents the history of the sexual abuse of children by reviewing the Bible, myths, fairy tales and popular literature. She looks at the role of legal institutions, psychology and "kiddie porn" in perpetuating the victimization of children. $5.95.

Sanford, Linda Tschirhart. *Silent Children—A Book for Parents about the Prevention of Sexual Abuse*. Garden City, NY: Anchor Press/Doubleday, 1980.

Organizations

Child Sexual Abuse Prevention Project, Office of the County Attorney, 2000-C Hennepin Government Center, Minneapolis, MN 55487. Prevention materials aimed at designing programs for children have been developed and used in a variety of settings. Write for more information.

Montana Incest Prevention Coalition, 315 South 4th Street E., Missoula, MT 59801. An innovative conference bringing together feminist activists, incest survivors and human-service workers was held in 1982. Materials produced and collected for the conference are available, both print and nonprint. Write for prices and information.

National Center on Child Abuse and Neglect, U.S. Department of Health and Human Services, Washington, DC 20013. The Center has funded research and has volumes of reports and literature available, including bibliographies. Especially recommended is Kee MacFarle, et al., "Sexual Abuse of Children: Selected Readings," publication #OHDS 78-30161, November 1980.

Pornography

Audiovisual Materials

"Not A Love Story," a 69-minute 1981 color film about the content of pornography and its relationship to physical acts of violence. Available from the National Film Board of Canada, 1251 Avenue of the Americas, New York, NY 10010.

Organizations

Women Against Pornography (WAP), 358 West 47th Street, New York, NY 10036. WAP initiated tours of pornography shops to encourage women to understand the messages conveyed by books, films and peep shows. A membership organization, WAP produces a bimonthly newsletter, *Newsreport*. Their slide show in adult or high school versions is available for purchase or rental. Write for membership and slide show information, and to request their educational fliers.

Women Against Violence Against Women (WAVAW), 543 North Fairfax Avenue, Los Angeles, CA 90036. WAVAW began in 1975 to protest the sexual violence in record album advertising. Their boycott of record companies has, in some instances, brought changes in company policy.

They are a national membership organization with chapters across the country. WAVAW's slide show has, over the years, been broadened to cover other forms of media violence. Write for the address of a local chapter, and information on their newsletter, slide show and other materials.

Women Against Violence in Pornography and Media (WAVPM), P.O. Box 14635, San Francisco, CA 94114. WAVPM sponsors pornography shop tours, pickets of abusive films and other public events. Their monthly newsletter, *Newspage*, has featured bibliographies, an international directory of groups working against media violence and articles on numerous other topics. They have produced a slide show and a media protest packet, "Write Back! Fight Back!" ($3.50). Write for order form and price list.

II
RELATIONSHIPS
AND
SEXUALITY

INTRODUCTION

By Wendy Sanford, with Paula Brown Doress

Loving is essential to our lives. Most of the people we love we are not sexually involved with; some we are. Sexual relationships are intense, puzzling, frustrating, energizing, potentially oppressive and potentially freeing. They enable us to learn about ourselves and our lovers and to get close in ways we never expected. They raise issues of power and vulnerability, commitment and risk. Sexual relationships can be painful; a long-time union breaks up, a love affair promises much and then fizzles, a lover dies, a marriage turns abusive. Yet most of us want and need intimacy, so that we usually recover from the hurt and try again.

This unit looks closely at our sexual relationships. What do they give us? How can we make them more what we want? What is unique to sexual relationships with men? With women? How can we understand our sexuality better and enjoy it more? How can we change the social structures and attitudes—about age, disability, sex roles, sexual preference—which keep us from freely loving others and ourselves?

New Face

I have learned not to worry about love;
but to honor its coming
with all my heart.
To examine the dark mysteries
of the blood
with headless heed and
swirl,
to know the rush of feelings
swift and flowing
as water.
The source appears to be
some inexhaustible
spring
within our twin and triple
selves;
the new face I turn up
to you
no one else on earth
has ever
seen.

Alice Walker

PROLOGUE: RETHINKING SEXUAL PREFERENCE

Over the past two decades more and more women have spoken openly about their choice as lesbians of women lovers and partners. Encouraged by the women's movement to be more open about sexuality, many women who are deeply involved with men have also begun to speak of their sexual feelings or fantasies about women. That every woman is "innately heterosexual" is a myth.

More than twenty years ago, research by Kinsey showed that most people have both heterosexual and homosexual feelings. A woman might have played around sexually with girls and boys in her childhood or fallen in love with her best girlfriend in high school, then married a man. Another who had been involved with men for thirty years may find herself choosing women at fifty. Some women are sexually and emotionally intimate with both women and men through their lives.

As we come to understand that most people have some homosexual feelings, we begin to accept a lot of things we were taught to fear. In our families and schools people either didn't mention lesbians or gay men at all, or joked cruelly about them; they made us feel hesitant about some of our closest female friendships.

When I was seven or eight, I had this best friend, Susan. We loved each other and walked around with our arms around each other. Her older sister told us not to do that anymore because we looked like lesies. So we held hands instead.

We became aware that society penalizes lesbians through job discrimination and violence. In these and other ways, our culture teaches us an irrational fear and hatred of homosexuality in ourselves and others (*homophobia*). Homophobia insults those of us who are lesbian and bisexual and makes our lives unnecessarily difficult. It also hurts those of us who are heterosexual. Fear and prejudice turn us against lesbian friends and family members, depriving us of important relationships. Homophobia makes us fear and dislike aspects of our own personality and looks which are not "feminine" enough (assertiveness, muscular

121

build, body hair, deep voice). It causes us to deny attractions which are natural to us and may prevent us from choosing the sexual partners who are right for us. And it divides us from each other as women.*

With time, familiarity and friendship we can unlearn homophobia.

The main thing that finally helped me start letting go of my homophobia was getting to know a few lesbian women. As we became friends, the myths I'd heard about lesbians—that they are mannish, oversexed, undersexed or out to seduce straight women—fell away. They were just like everyone else.

Once I admitted to myself that I do have sexual feelings for women, I didn't feel so alarmed by lesbians anymore. It was as if they had represented something in myself I was scared of.

Even after I became a lesbian at thirty-five, I found that I had big doses of homophobia inside me. Sometimes I'd wake up after having sex with a woman I loved and have an attack of thinking that the wonderful thing we'd done was "queer." Or I'd get upset when other dykes seemed "too obvious" in public. Slowly I've become prouder and more deeply affirming of lesbians and lesbianism—that is, of myself.

Many heterosexual women believe they know no lesbians personally. However, chances are we all know a number of lesbians who simply don't feel safe being open about it.

OPENING UP HETEROSEXUALITY TO "CHOICE"

Some lesbians today are asking their heterosexual sisters to reconsider the "naturalness" of heterosexual preference. Can heterosexuality be a free choice when we are taught such a deep fear of loving women? Can we comfortably assume that women are "naturally" drawn to men when we consider the many cruelties which drive us to seek protection from men and punish

us for being alone: rape and sexual harassment, consistently lower pay for women workers, the lack of economic protection for widows, the derision of "old maids," the fact that prostitution is often the only available work which pays enough to support a family? If it is unsafe anywhere to be a woman without a man, then heterosexuality is not so much natural as *compulsory*.*

Compulsory heterosexuality may make us feel desperate when we're not with a man, and cause us to jump into the arms of men who are available but not good for us. It means we never have a chance to make a real choice, to ask ourselves whether we would be happier with a man, a woman or alone. Free to ask these questions, we might well end up choosing to be with men, but we would be responding to what we genuinely want and not to what society tells us we ought to want.†

FEAR OF LESBIANS AND OUR UNITY AS WOMEN

Some women hesitate to join feminist projects because friends and family assume that being a feminist means one is a lesbian. Ultraconservative political and religious groups play on these fears by portraying all feminists as man-haters, "bra-burners" and actual or would-be lesbians. Using homophobia as a tool to divide us and turn us against each other, they rob us of our energy and unity as a movement of women trying to build a more just society for everyone. On the other hand, some lesbians struggling for legitimacy and acceptance suggest that "straight" women are less feminist than lesbians or that "true" feminists wouldn't ally themselves with men in any way. As a collective of heterosexual and lesbian women, we hope all women will feel safe enough in this society to become less condemning of each others' choices. We urge more heterosexual women who share feminist goals and visions to identify themselves openly as feminists. The women's movement will become a stronger force for social change when women of all sexual orientations can find friendship, growth and power within it.

*See Adrienne Rich's important and challenging article, "Compulsory Heterosexuality and Lesbian Existence," *Signs: Journal of Women in Culture and Society*, Vol. 5, No. 4 (1980).
†Chapter 11, "Sexuality," seeks to break down false separations by including experiences with both men and women. We wrote two separate chapters on relationships because it first seemed to us that lesbians and heterosexual women encounter different pressures and possibilities. But we learned from each other that we face many similar issues, whether our partners are women or men.

*Homophobia is politically useful for those who want to preserve the traditional forms of family life and to suppress any alternatives.

9

WORKING TOWARD MUTUALITY: OUR RELATIONSHIPS WITH MEN

By Paula Brown Doress
and Peggy Nelson Wegman

With special thanks to Catherine Cobb Morocco, Sandy Rosenthal and Elizabeth Matz

This chapter in previous editions was called "Living with Ourselves and Others—Our Sexual Relationships," by Paula Brown Doress and Nancy P. Hawley.

What do we value about our relationships? Some women's voices:*

The best thing is that we have a long, intimate history together and still feel connected to and admiring and turned on to each other. I consider it a minor miracle as I look around me. I have learned that my husband has many of the same weak feelings—fragile feelings— that I used to think were female—just as he has learned that I have certain kinds of strengths that he doesn't have. The crucial thing is to take time to build up confidence and trust and comfort and kindness. [forty, married twenty years]

Even with all my wonderful friends and my job, which I love, and my dancing and my cat and everything else, life used to be very lonely. Simple little details could suddenly seem so hard...like finding someone to go to the laundromat with. Now that I love Mark I really don't live much differently than I did before, but life feels quite different. We are committed to each other in a way that transcends the little daily ups and downs. Having him there, even with all the fights and issues we have yet to resolve, is like a big, soft cushion between me and the roughness of life. [single, mid-twenties]

The hard thing about widowhood is that I have lost the person I held hands with in life. I was extremely important to my husband....When I was unhappy I could always go to him and talk to him, and when I was happy he had a smile from ear to ear. He gave me unlimited support throughout my whole married life. I don't have that anymore. That's a very, very important loss.

*This chapter is one of the chapters most based on our experiences as white middle-class women. We hope you will find it useful and provocative as you think about your relationships with men, but we don't pretend to speak to or for women with very different kinds of experiences.

I've made up for it by relying more on other close people in my life. I have a close friend that I can call at the drop of a hat and say, "Something is bothering me and I have to talk to you about it," and I'm extremely close with my children. I need about a dozen close people to fill in for the loss of that one special relationship. [sixty-eight, widowed three years]

He has a deep, keen interest in what I do, in my work and my interests, that no other man I've been involved with has ever had. It's absolutely essential that the man I love be tuned in to feminism and able to live that out in a day-to-day way. The mutuality, the give and take and the constant questioning of gender stereotype is critical. And it's not just on an intellectual plane, either; it's also about the mundane stuff like taking care of the house and doing the dishes, not just who does things but who thinks about what has to be done. [thirties, married one year]

The best thing about my marriage is that I have a real friend. When you've done a lot of things together you have a commonality of ethics, a way of looking at the world which is terribly important, so I trust my husband a lot. [sixties, married thirty-nine years]

THE PERSONAL IS POLITICAL

We want to be close to other people—to matter to them, to know that they will be there when we need them, to feel safe, loving and loved—this closeness is essential to our well-being. Most women seek to fulfill much of this need for closeness through intimate sexual relationships with men. As we grew up, we learned one pattern or model for these relationships: our families and communities expected us to marry and have children; men would earn the most money, have the most important jobs and be more logical, while we would cook and "keep house" and be more aware of feelings and relationships. This was the way things had to be, and when our lives fit this pattern we would automatically be happy.

But during the past fifteen years, with the recent wave of the feminist movement, we began to question these assumptions and affirm one of the basic principles of the feminist movement—that our lives, work, ideas, perceptions and wishes are important, as important as those of men, and that society should be reorganized to reflect and support this belief. We saw that most heterosexual relationships in this culture reflect those old assumptions about women and men. In talking with each other, at first tentatively, about our lives, our dissatisfactions, frustrations and sometimes anger began to crystalize and became newly articulated feelings which affected each of our lives differently: some of us worked with our husbands or lovers at changing what went on between us; long-standing relationships which just couldn't change in response to our new visions broke up. Some of us lived with each other in communal living situations, decided not to marry or chose to live only with women. Although our examination of male-female relationships led to a variety of "solutions," some women came to equate feminism with hating men and rejecting marriage and family, and many of these women became reluctant to identify with the women's movement.

However, many of us were committed to finding ways to live out our feminist beliefs without having to give up intimate relationships with men. Frustration and anger don't mean that we want to end these relationships; instead, they make us determined to change them.

When I work on women's issues I have an appropriate outlet for my angry feelings, and I direct my anger at the source of what oppresses women and not only at individual men in my life. Often I am less angry toward men than a lot of women who shy away from being associated with feminism.

We are not proposing any fixed model of "The Ideal Couple Relationship." How we talk together, how we play and fight and work and make love grow not from any external prescription but from who we are. We do propose that the price of the intimacy we build together should not be our own richness as individuals; that we see each other not simply as two halves of a whole, each with our own immutable territory, but as two separate, whole people who have chosen to touch closely, to build something together, to intertwine—enriching one another, rather than detracting from the potential ways that each may grow. Working toward an egalitarian relationship is not a matter of creating a one-time "grand design" that will guide us

for years to come, but a slow and continuing process of negotiation, compromise and renegotiation.

Changes will occur, for the most part, slowly and in very small steps. In an efficiency-minded, goal-oriented culture heavily influenced by technology, these small, slow processes of fixing and adjusting are neither taught nor valued. We live in a disposable age: when it breaks, throw it out and get a new one. When *we* speak of commitment, we don't mean the traditional pressure to be "committed" to a relationship at all costs, which has often meant letting go of our needs or putting up with an empty or abusive relationship. We have in mind a true commitment to a process of working on the relationship, which may make things harder for a time as we attempt to make them better. It involves risk-taking, constant questioning and not always waiting for the "right" moment to bring up a problem. It also means being willing to change as we are asking our men to change. We cannot always be sure how things will evolve; despite our most valiant efforts the relationship may end, and sometimes that may be for the best. While there may be many other sources of tension between a woman and a man— personality differences, family history, ethnic and class differences, illness, economic hardship—this chapter focuses on the tension which comes from living in a culture based on inequality and limiting role definitions between the sexes. When we work toward an equal relationship we are, in effect, swimming against the tide.

Our culture stresses the importance of the individual rather than of the group, and teaches us to believe that our personal circumstances and problems arise from qualities within us, from our own individual histories, our personalities and our conscious choices. As a result, most of us tend not to see the ways in which gender, race and class affect personal "choices." The feminist insight that "the personal is political" expresses our belief—that what seem like "personal" problems are often symptoms of larger social problems.

This chapter is about our vision, and about how our culture's values, expectations and structures affect our intimate relationships with men. In earlier editions of *Our Bodies, Ourselves* we focused on alternatives to couple relationships. In this edition we look at what goes on *within* heterosexual couple relationships because that is still the way so many women live.

Being Single

Some women prefer being single, either fitting lovers into our lives without living with them and settling down together, or living with no romantic attachments at all. For those of us who want to make a major commitment to work, who have finished grieving the end of a relationship or who have already raised families, being single can be positive, creative and peaceful.

I simply don't plan my life around a man even when I am in love. There are so many other things that I want to do, too. I've had two husbands. I also have three grown kids. Naturally I still think about them, but not like when they were little. I can really focus on what I want to do now.

Now *Alone* is a Bed Partner

Now *Alone* is a bed partner, is a
precious gem,
is a bandit she wants, is a woman with
silver hair,
is better than a man.

Alone was a gift she didn't recognize
when it first
arrived. She locked it in the bedroom
and stayed
downstairs. She wouldn't let it come
to meals.

She knew the sweet faces of her friends,
she didn't
trust *Alone* who slept in her mirror, in
her voice,
in the hollow where her hands covered
her eyes.

Alone was patient and when she took its
hand, it gave her
songs and poems, drawings and slow
breath, a peace
larger than sunset. Everyone felt it.
The children

drew around her as if she were the
hearth.
Alone moved in as no one else could,
unpossessive,
leaving space for women and men to
interact with her. Now

Alone is there in the morning and
welcomes her home
and wants nothing from her and gives all
of itself
to her and never turns her away.

Judith W. Steinbergh

However, being single can be hard because in our society, couples are the norm.

...A single woman...is not buttressed by a family and the responsibilities of a family....She has made a choice that cuts her off from a lot of things most people consider life, for the sake of something else, something both chancy and intangible. No wonder anxiety is the constant attendant of such a one!*

A recent survey of single women and men in thirty-six states found that the best aspect of being single was freedom and the worst, loneliness. Men and women who wrote comments for the survey agreed that being single is more difficult for a woman than a man because:

- women have less sexual and social freedom;
- divorced women more often have responsibility for children;
- women are more vulnerable to physical abuse;
- women earn less money and have less social mobility;
- women have been socialized to feel stigmatized by not being attached to a man.

Only one-third of single men and one-fifth of single women in the study liked or desired the single life. The rest regarded it as a waiting period, a special, limited time to do things they'd never done or a time to look for a new partner.*

There are powerful social pressures to "be in a couple," especially one kind of couple—married, heterosexual, racially alike. The pressure starts early. Storybooks and movies of our girlhoods ended with romantic marriage and perpetual bliss. Relatives asked us at age three or four who our boyfriends were and, at twenty, when we were going to marry and have children. Recently it has become more socially acceptable not to marry and not to have children, but the pressure to be part of a couple persists. Indeed, the idea of the "relationship" has taken on some of the mystique formerly reserved for marriage and the nuclear family. Even after divorce or the death of a partner, friends assume we are seeking another relationship. Lesbians and heterosexual women alike often believe that we have to be in a couple to be fulfilled.

When I think of the hours I've spent in bars and at parties trying to meet someone, I am bitter about such wasted energy. I could have started my own business or earned a degree in that time.

Our communities are organized on the premise that the family will meet nearly all our needs for intimacy and continuity. Close friends may organize their social life only around couples.

When I got divorced, I kept all my women friends, but I noticed they would only invite me to lunch. At dinner when their husbands were home they had couples over. It was as if at night I became another species altogether.

There are economic pressures to be in a couple. Women experience severe wage and salary discrimination and are often financially insecure and overworked.

I am part of a circle of friends who have been single for most of the past ten years. We moved fairly easily in

---

*May Sarton. *Plant Dreaming Deep.* New York: W.W. Norton and Co., Inc., 1983, p. 91.

*See Jacqueline Simenauer and David Carroll, *Singles: The New Americans*, New York: New American Library, 1982.

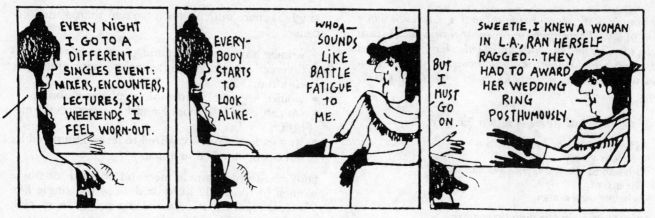

from "Sylvia" by Nicole Hollander

and out of relationships or were involved in several at a time. Now all of a sudden everyone is coupling off. You know, I think it's the economy and the state of the world. Many of my friends are teachers and social-service workers who are being laid off and losing their pensions and health insurance, too. When people are scared they want to be with someone else.

It can be hard to imagine being older and single.

I love my life the way it is now—the freedom to be with different partners or not with any, living by my own rhythms, feeling strong and happy with myself. But sometimes when I wake up in the middle of the night I see myself old and alone, and it is terribly scary and empty.

Ageism makes us fear growing older, because we assume that old people don't have friends or community, that someone who's not with a partner will be totally alone. For many of us it is literally dangerous to be alone because of violence and sexual harassment.

Afraid to be alone, we often jump into relationships only to discover that we have chosen too quickly: our partners aren't good for us; we have given up too much of what we really wanted and our very neediness lessens our relative power within the relationship.

Community is especially important to us as single women. We can develop strong, intimate friendships which stay with us throughout life and make being alone and growing old much less frightening.

I hope I'll be growing old together with Dan, but since he is considerably older [eighteen years] than me it is possible that he will die before me. Then I imagine growing old with Margie, who has been my best friend for the past fifteen years. I like thinking of us as old women together.

We live in a time when it is acceptable for women to work and live in more varied ways than ever before.

It is important to acknowledge that many women feel lonely, and for us to give one another support both for our lives as single women and for our efforts to find a partner. While we don't want to be pressured to find someone and get married, neither do we want friends to assume that we love being single. It is up to us to let people know if we *are* interested in meeting someone. Loving ourselves more when our community values us, we are more likely, when and if we go out looking for a partner, to find a person who will be right for us. Surrounded by the affection and caring of friends and family, we become less vulnerable to exploitative relationships, more able to resist the emphasis on being or becoming part of a couple.

When I broke up with my lover I luckily had a circle of warm affectionate friends who would give me a hug or a pat on the back. Yet I felt the lack of that very intimate whole-body contact. I didn't want to rush precipitously into a new relationship just because I felt so hungry to be touched. One answer was to get a massage every other week for several months.

When my younger sister got engaged my parents bought each of us a beautiful set of cookware. They said they loved us both and wanted to support the life choices that each of us was making by getting us each something for our homes. I felt so affirmed because I understood they were saying, "This is your life, and we value you and your choices."

Here

is what she loves deeply
  her work she drives into with the sun
  polishing wet roads to chrome,
  her son who waits, feigning sleep
  in his crib until he can caress her face,
  her golden-haired, blue-eyed, hell-bent,
  anti-authoritarian daughter who says
  shit at the right time,
  her husband who has left her

126

here is what she loves, but once removed
her men with tongues, who put their mouths on hers,
who make her laugh deeply into the night, who take her
to bed during sesame street, who take her children
to school, or haven't met her children, or never
met a child at all, her men who juggle, who paint
day after day landscapes that have never left the mind,
who walk her on winter beaches, and fly her into
the chambers of coral reefs

here is what she likes with an embarrassing relish
the luminescent stars and comets she's stuck on her
ceiling, the thought of toads in her husband's lover's
bed, her bell bird clanging a pottery sea bell sound,
her shells, colored powders, beach stones, sheep bones,
ropes of feathers, long Indian skirts, filmy violet scarves,
snow over the lakes to ski on, her children's bare bodies,
summer with a wind in the moors, the stitching of night
with the loon's pointed sound

here is what she needs and keeps her
a net of women so strong that when she falls
from the tightrope she walks day after day
sometimes with easy precision, sometimes
with wire cutting her feet into bands,
sometimes with a fatigue so great
her dreams have to hold her, that when she falls,
her women friends tighten their almost
invisible web, and she bounces and breathes,
bounces and weaves every fiber of their strength
into her own body, bounces and is free in a way
that will let her bounce against them again,
she bounces and soars, a dark bird
against the stadium lights, swoops to the crowd
and is off, a speck in the cranberry dawn.

Judith W. Steinbergh

EXPLORING MAJOR AREAS OF TENSION IN HETEROSEXUAL RELATIONSHIPS

Toward Shared Power in Relationships

All kinds of power come into play in our relationships—personal, physical, spiritual, social, economic and political.* However, women and men belong to groups which have different degrees of power. The resulting imbalance inevitably influences the way we think, act and relate to each other. How people perceive and treat us outside our relationships inevitably affects how we feel within them. The conventional heterosexual relationship has been a marriage in which a man agrees to support a woman economically and share his status with her. In return she is responsible for the personal and household services which enable him to perform his role in society without such "men-

*A crucial part of our personal/political power is having control over our bodies and our lives through reproductive and sexual choice. See p. 612.

ial" distractions. In the relationship we envision, each partner supports the other, so both play a role in the world outside the home as well as in the home, and one partner does not gain power at the expense of the other.

Social and Economic Power

We think of politics as having to do with power relationships among large-scale groups and nations, but there is a politics of intimate relationships as well. However strong our commitments to each other and to treating one another as equals may be, it is naive to think that widely held social attitudes and pervasive institutional practices will not affect what goes on between us. For example, a conflict within a heterosexual relationship is not simply a conflict between two persons who are everywhere regarded as social equals, but between two people who have different standing before the law (especially if married) and different rights and privileges.* Most societal institutions are thoroughly permeated with the assumption that the rights of men should take precedence over the rights of women. Since money is the most common source of power in this society and frequently symbolizes social power, it is not surprising that the person who brings economic resources into a family or a relationship has increased power.†

This society values and rewards men's work a great deal more than women's work. Most women cannot bring in an equal amount of money, for we earn on the average only 57 percent of what men earn.‡

Men automatically hold the power in a relationship because they usually earn more money. If a man abuses this power imbalance, he may show it during the early stages of a relationship by making a woman feel indebtedness to him and implying that she should "repay" him with sexual favors. If he does this, watch out. In the words of a forty-year-old divorced woman:

A man took me out, and on the second or third date he wanted to sleep with me. So I told him I didn't want to be that intimate on so short an acquaintance. And he grumbled and said, "I just want to know if there's a pot of gold at the end of the rainbow."

Some men imply that paying for dates is burdensome, but may be reluctant to give up the control that goes with paying when offered a chance to share ex-

*We still need the Equal Rights Amendment to be equal before the law.
†In a study of married couples, wives who worked in paid employment were found to have greater power in family decision-making than nonearning wives. (R.O. Blood and D.M. Wolfe, *Husbands and Wives: The Dynamics of Married Living*, New York: Free Press, 1960.)
‡U.S. Department of Labor, *The Earnings Gap Between Women and Men*, 1976.

penses. Others may be more flexible. A single woman in her twenties told us:

I believe in paying my share when I go out with a man. The man I'm involved with now earns a lot more money than I do, and he enjoys spending it on things that are fun. We often end up arguing about what kinds of things both of us can afford, which he feels limits us to what I can afford. Sometimes we compromise and he treats so we can do something special.

It is important to most people to be economically independent. As women we are socialized to see paid work as secondary to our job as wives and mothers, and believe that work and parenting are mutually exclusive choices. Or else we find work which we can balance with childcare, usually low-paid "women's occupations," e.g., elementary-school teaching, nursing, secretarial work, waitressing, etc., which pay far less than "men's" jobs.* When a woman cannot earn as much as a man, she (and he) are more likely to see her work as less important, more dispensable when children come, less important when a move is contemplated, less worth disrupting the family routine for. Even in couples which start out with egalitarian ideals and plans, the woman usually adapts more and more to the man. Because of this economic imbalance, a man may simply assume that it is his right to take charge. If a woman wants to make changes, she has to change his ideas as well as this conventional pattern. From a woman in her thirties:

When I buy something, even if it's for the house, I'm often afraid to tell Ron. He gets upset and says, "We can't afford it." But what he really means is that I shouldn't have bought it without consulting him. I get afraid to tell him because I think that since he earned the money, it's not really mine, even though he couldn't be out earning it if I weren't here running the house and taking care of the kids.

Sometimes I think getting a job and earning some money myself is the only thing that will resolve the conflict. But I get a strong message from Ron that he doesn't want me to work even though we could use the extra income. He's afraid that then he would have to deal with me differently.

This is not a simple disagreement about *how* to spend money, but raises the issue of decision-making power within the family.

When we were first married, I earned much less than Zach but enough to support myself. But from the time when our first child was born seven years ago, I have worked only part time and my salary is very low. We could not find part-time work for both of us that paid well enough to support us. Neither of us wanted to have the children in full-time daycare when they were young. Now that the children are both in school, I want to earn a living again. All along, Zach has regarded my work as equally important to his own but, in truth, I have more often left work to stay home with a sick child than he has, and while his identity comes largely from work, mine comes primarily from being a mother. I want to change this now and get on an equal footing.

It's going to be a long time before women get equal pay *or* equal work. Meanwhile we must insist in our relationships that the contribution of both people be equally valued.

Developing Our Personal Power

By "personal power" we mean self-reliance, assertiveness, the ability to earn a living, independence, self-confidence; many of us were taught to find a man with these qualities and literally attach ourselves to him ("If you can't be one, marry one"). In this way, we would become complete. Creating an intimate relationship with a man was not to be simply a way to enrich our lives but the foundation of our identities as whole adult people. Whom we are close to became confused with who we are. And so we faced a paradox: to feel stronger, many of us followed the best-traveled route and found a man, yet we were stepping into a role which only served to undermine our inner strength.

And what of physical strength? Many women have been taught that to be physically strong is "unfeminine," and a man's greater physical strength can pose an unspoken threat of intimidation which causes all sorts of problems, from feeling overpowered in a sexual encounter to being intimidated in an argument. Because we live in a society where violence or the threat of violence is ever present, it is not surprising that we have such feelings. When we refuse to accept the cultural image of women as lacking in physical strength and competence, learn new skills and become physically stronger, our self-esteem grows.

One of the things I plunged myself into at age fifty-four was to take Tae Kwon Do (a Korean martial art). I had always been fascinated by martial arts but never had enough nerve to try it. I was stirring up long years of status quo; one more unorthodoxy didn't matter, I reasoned. All through our marriage I was never able to stand up to my husband, and I felt taking a martial art might perhaps help me to become more assertive. My husband was totally put off by my taking up such a "masculine" activity. But I have persisted.

*Because of a combination of sex discrimination and sex-role socialization, 40 percent of all women in the workforce are segregated into ten "women's occupations." These are so poorly paid—even nursing and teaching—that a woman supporting even one child and herself on the *average* salary of these occupations would be living below the poverty level.

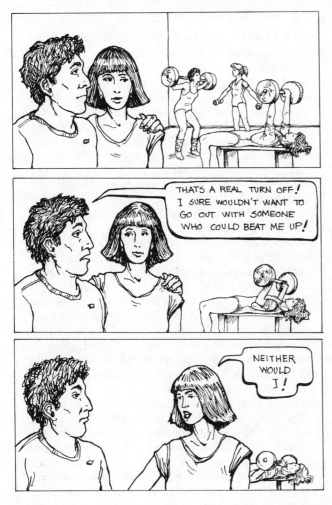

Greg Wenzel

Women are often tentative, prefacing statements with a little laugh and apologies about how little we know about the subject under discussion, while men learn to present their strongest points and to remain silent about their reservations.

One of the hardest things for me to do is to hold my own at points when we really disagree about something. I might start out knowing just what I think but then, the more I listen to William argue his point (he is always so sure of himself), the less sure I feel of mine and the more confused I get about what is true. Sometimes I wind up crying when what I really want to do is fight for myself. Then, later on, I feel angry; a sort of smoldering resentment sets in, and I don't even want to sleep with William at those times. It's because I still feel angry about not being able to hold my own in the fight and I know I can hurt him by withholding sex.

While physicians and mental-health professionals in conventional sex and marriage books often "scold"

women for withholding sex when we are angry about something else, they fail to recognize that it is often the best indirect way of exercising power when more direct ways are blocked.

Women are taught to be uncomfortable with the idea of having power. (It is as unladylike as being physically strong!) Often when we "do what is expected of us" we abdicate our power almost entirely.

I always arranged my life around Larry. When we were first together I was beginning a career in teaching. But soon he got a job offer in another city, and so we moved there. Then he wanted to have children, which I didn't really care about. But he wanted them badly, so it seemed all right to me. Then we moved again, this time to a fancy house in a fancy suburb, but I had no car—he took it—and I was quite lonely. The children became the center of my life, and I loved them and my husband deeply. Several times I thought of returning to school part time to get my certificate. But Larry was not willing for me to do that; he did not want the responsibilities for the house and the children to fall on his shoulders. And he said he was glad to support us, which I think he really was. Then, one day when the children were still quite young (our son was not even a year old), I learned something that terrified me... that for more than a year Larry had been having affairs with other women. They were all women whom he met in his job as a supervisor, professional women, very bright and competent and unattached and ten years younger than I was.

When I confronted him, he said that he found me dull, always talking about the house and the children—of course, since that was my world!—and that these other women were far more interesting, as they had professional lives and were more worldly and more knowledgeable than I was about things which interested him in his work. He did not say, but I think it is true, that he also hated my asking him to be more involved with the children and the house. He ran to these women whenever I criticized him, looking for the things in them which he discouraged me from developing in myself. When I was younger, I did not see any problem with my shaping my life around Larry. Now I know I have paid a very high price.

George Malave/Stock Boston

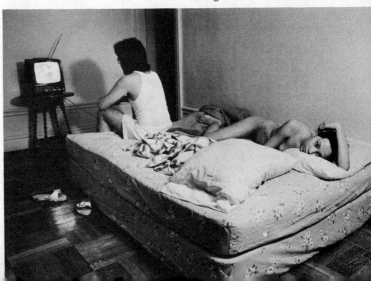

When I started working on my graduate degree I was ambitious to become really well known in my field and fantasized being an adviser to members of Congress or even the President. Then I got involved with Dave and began to spend more and more time with him. He wanted total support for his work and since we were in the same field I could help him a lot and be learning at the same time. But I definitely put my own ambitions on the back burner for about two years. I began to be more attached to the idea of staying in the city when I finished school so I wouldn't have to leave Dave, and I even began to fantasize about a less demanding job, maybe even just three days a week.

When we broke up all my options opened up again and I could reconsider my early ambitions. It was scary to consider the possibility of being as successful as my fantasies.

Traditional Roles and Getting Beyond Them

Roles are like parts in a play. We learn how to be a sexual partner, a wife or a mother by following scripts that we learned as children. The scripts save us the trouble of creating our lives from scratch each and every day, but they may also lead us to drift into rigid roles without questioning them.

Certain qualities are usually reinforced as being appropriate to women or to men. When our behavior varies from the stereotype we may be punished: while a male's assertive behavior is called "leadership," in a female it is called "aggressiveness." Nurturing may be labeled "warmth" in a woman and "weakness" in a man.*

Each partner begins a relationship with a set of experiences and beliefs which shape her/his notions about masculine and feminine roles. Many of us grew up in families which followed conventional patterns. Others of us may have grown up in situations where death, divorce, emigration of one parent, war or a period of unemployment occurred and roles had to be shared or varied in nonconventional ways.

When I was growing up my father was away fighting in the war, and so my mother and I moved in with my grandmother and aunts. I grew up seeing women managing by themselves without men for years at a time.

*One study of mental-health professionals' attitudes found that when they were asked to list the traits of a healthy adult, a healthy man and a healthy woman, they equated traits listed for males with those for healthy adults; but the traits for a "healthy" woman differed from and often contradicted those for a healthy adult (Broverman, I.K., et al. "Sex-Role Stereotypes and Clinical Judgments of Mental Health," *Journal of Consulting and Clinical Psychology*, 34 (1970), pp. 1–7). No wonder that women experience so much role conflict and difficulty reconciling contradictory expectations. (Thanks in great part to the women's movement, these attitudes and limitations are changing, but slowly.)

Some Consequences of Accepting These Roles

The conventional role structure, in which the woman functions as a support system for the man, while receiving no support to earn a living and/or to develop herself, leaves us too vulnerable emotionally and economically. Thousands of displaced homemakers,* after nurturing others most of their lives, are then left without resources or marketable skills. (Most do have skills, unrecognized because of a combination of age and sex discrimination, and because household skills are devalued when in fact they are similar to professional and management skills.) In today's world, where the divorce rate is one in three and where alimony has virtually disappeared (although the income gap remains), where women outlive their male partners, often by a decade or two (80 percent of surviving spouses are women) and where the inflation rate makes the old pattern of one salary supporting two adults and children an alternative available only to a small elite (only 7 percent of families conform to the old norm of husband as sole breadwinner), the traditional role of woman as support system to the man exists only at great risk to women.

From a very first meeting with a man, we may play roles. If we want to pursue the relationship, continue to see one another and spend time together, live together or get married and have children together, each step toward permanence, commitment and formalization of the relationship increases the pressures to assume conventional roles. Structures and arrangements which may have worked well for years can be challenged or shattered by having children.

If we leave our paid work, we lose not only our independent income but our status as a paid worker and our community of work friends. We lose our source of outside validation; we may feel less competent and respected, and become almost completely dependent on our partner and our child(ren). Even when we want to share work and childcare equally, the shortage of good childcare services, the lack of well-paid part-time work and the severe sex discrimination limiting our earning power as women all contribute to a gradual drift back toward conventional arrangements during the early parenting years.

We believe that as long as women do most of the childcare, this will have a fundamental impact on our lives and opportunities and thus influence subsequent generations and *their* choices.

*See Laurie Shields, *Displaced Homemakers*, New York: McGraw-Hill, 1981.

Some parents mistakenly believed they were teaching us that we could do everything boys could do, but they really gave us a mixed message.

I grew up in a household where we believed there were no distinctions between boys and girls. We were always told that girls were equal and the five of us had exciting, far-reaching discussions and no-holds-barred, stimulating, intellectual arguments over dinner. But later I realized that while my father held court with us, my mother was clearing the table. At some point he would call for his coffee to be brought to him. This affected my marriage. I feel intellectually equal or superior to Steven, but it's hard for me to feel okay about doing anything for my own work which demands or requires any adaptation by my family.

We are not taught gender roles simply out of sentiment and tradition, but because they fit us into existing social forms. As we struggle to change our relationships we must at the same time work to end sex discrimination at our workplaces, establish childcare in our communities and end the legal inequities women still face. In this transitional time we have the task of fitting the kinds of relationships we want into a society which may not only fail to support our vision but often actively oppose it.

Making Changes

We can begin to take small steps to change fixed roles. We can devise an "affirmative action" plan, taking time for ourselves to build up our work skills, to work on something which interests us and which brings in some income. We don't have to say no automatically to opportunities that require travel. We can leave an unsatisfactory relationship or work hard toward changing our partner's attitudes and the structure of the relationship.

The change began for me as I prepared for a full-time job when all the kids were finally old enough to take some responsibility. I knew then I had to have Matthew as an active partner, though he preferred being passive and having everything done for him. My therapist told me to make a list of all the jobs that a family required in order to run. It was pages long; it just grew and grew. When I got it all written out after several weeks, it was clear that I did about 95 percent of it. And then I got very angry that I was the one who kept everything working around here. I basically decided I was going to go on strike. We began slowly and painfully to work out a more equitable system in the distribution of housework and cooking and parenting. Matt...felt that he "couldn't" do things that he didn't want to do, so it was painful. But I told myself it was worth it because it was the beginning. I was getting ready to start business school.

In the six months before I started school, I determined that I would teach the kids how to run the washer and dryer, to cook simple meals, to scrub the kitchen floor, to clean a bathroom. We set up job lists and everybody had to do one thing a week: they would cook, and I would just be here if they needed help. And then I started business school full time, and I was immediately overwhelmed. I was struggling. It was far more competitive than I had thought it was going to be....I wasn't home after school, I had study groups late at night and on Saturday and Sunday. Things started to fall apart. Nobody liked it. The kids would grumble because other mothers didn't make their children do so much. We all need order in our lives, and it was chaotic for a while. By the time the first year had gone by, our job system was pretty well in place. This is really my break away from the house. I am no longer going to be here the way I have always been.

To create mutually supportive relationships rather than one in which one partner functions only as the support system for the other, we must realize that there is a difference between sharing *tasks* (taking turns calling for babysitters or paying the bills) and sharing planning (the "overview"—being *aware* of when sitters are needed, when a child needs to go to the doctor and what the long-term financial plans are).

Even when a woman and man both work, they fall into the pattern of the man doing long-term planning, because women until recently have not been in the habit of doing so and believe that men are better at it. Women develop skill at saving small amounts of money by couponing, saving pennies day by day but often not dealing with the larger question of their future economic security. Middle-class women are brought up with the assumption that there will always be someone there to take care of us, while women from working-class backgrounds often learn to be more self-sufficient, providing for themselves. But most women's incomes are so marginal that we can't put any money aside for the future. Middle-class women often find it hard to assume responsibility for planning because they can't envision a time when the coffers may be empty, and it is tempting to let someone else worry, just as our parents once did. When we try to take more responsibility, some in-laws, parents—perhaps even therapists—may accuse us of being emasculating. But many of us have found that when we take more responsibility for money matters, not only do our partners appreciate it but we have more control over our lives.

Understanding Some of the Barriers to Intimacy Between Women and Men

Intimacy is having someone in my life who I can get to know really deeply over time, who can get to know me and who I can be the best and worst of myself with.

131

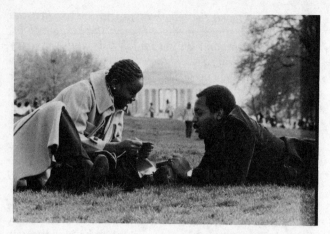

Owen Franken/Stock Boston

There are many different facets to knowing each other well and communicating on a deep level, letting our vulnerabilities show and our secrets be known, trusting enough to depend on someone and to allow them to depend on us.

The quality of our intimacy is exquisite. It's like a river that runs between us, and we can tap into it whenever we want. To me it's a rich and wonderful thing that someone can be intimate with you in so many ways...as a lover, as a friend.

Commitment means working on the relationship even when the early passion and urgency have evolved into a deeper if less dramatic kind of loving, and sticking through the hard, awful, painful, lousy and deadening times (which can be dramatic in its own way!).

I'm still drawn to that rush of passion that I get early in a relationship, but now I'm old enough and I've been through enough with men to know that the rush doesn't last. We can rekindle it; there are times when I feel that passion with Don that always exists at the beginning, but I sure don't feel it twenty-four hours a day every day. It takes a lot of work and creativity to keep things sparking in a relationship. Sometimes I'm attracted to other men, but I think this has mostly to do with my fears about intimacy and with wanting the rush...and trying to disperse some of the intensity of being with one person. As I get older, I'm more interested in whether this person is going to be with me. If the passion isn't there every night, it's okay.

Fearing Intimacy

We are all too often *expected* to merge our identities with our men's, taking *their* names, moving to where *their* jobs are, and so on. We may fear too much closeness if in previous relationships we merged our own wishes, aspirations and identities with those of our partners to such an extent that we lost sight of what we wanted for ourselves.

I wanted to be a satellite to him, revolving around him in his world...to let his life, his work, his friends, his energy pull me along. I was so relieved not to have to work anymore to build my own identity. This is what ultimately suffocated him and me and the marriage.

Often we experience conflicts between dependency and self-sufficiency, between the security of being in a good relationship and our need to remain separate.

One thing that's clear about my second marriage is that, because I'm older and because of who Rob is, I am much closer to him than I was to my first husband. I am able to care for him much more deeply. And there are moments when he's away even overnight that are very painful to me. It's not "Oh, my God, I couldn't take care of myself," because I have and I can—but it's deeply, passionately missing somebody. And it's ironic because I had so strongly identified with the women's movement's "superwomen agenda" of being self-sufficient. Yet it's come home to me just how painful it would be if something were to happen to Rob, how empty life would be. Not because my life isn't full in addition to him, but because I risked having a certain depth of commitment and feeling.

This society, which assigns active and dominant roles to men and passive or subordinate roles to women, exaggerates these conflicts. When we become conscious of men's greater power and prestige, we may fear the vulnerability that naturally comes with intimacy.

My work is lecturing and writing about pornography, child sexual abuse in battering situations and other areas of female sexual slavery. I live two truths all the time: I live in a male-supremist culture, yet I have a relationship with a man who is not a sexist. I used to feel that to be a totally strong woman and a feminist I should be alone, and I would feel guilty for having this real partner who loves me and helps me, whom I love and trust and depend on. But now I think, Why not just enjoy the special life I have and not worry about how I "should" be?

The stronger and more confident I feel about myself, the more able I am to be close to someone without fearing I'll lose myself.

We Learn Different Styles of Intimacy

Frequently women value talking as a way of being close, while many men express intimacy mainly through physical activity or sexual closeness.

My idea about being intimate, more than making love, is having long, deep conversations. My fantasies of love affairs are about conversations like that. You just keep on talking and every once in a while something important or interesting will get said. John's idea is that you don't talk until you have something to say. I want to talk about everything from every possible angle. He considers that gossipy, repetitive and intrusive. He's not secretive, but he wants to work things out for himself. His idea of intimacy is doing something together, like camping or canoeing. I sometimes think that John does not really know the part of me that I cherish most, and vice versa.

Society holds up "the strong, silent type" as a masculine ideal. Many men find self-disclosure very threatening;* showing one's softer side is not considered masculine. While over the past several years some men have been trying to be more emotionally open, the male world continues to expect them to be goal-oriented and to keep feelings concealed, and does not reward openness. Since our sexist culture does not value a personal, "feminine" style of relating to others, most men are not motivated to learn it.

A man I almost married said to me, "I'll bring home the money and you can do the rest," by which he meant all the childcare, the housework, the endless small tasks and, most importantly, I came to understand, all the emotional work.

This arrangement has cost men dearly: many otherwise "successful" men are emotionally impoverished. It costs the women as well, who turn to these men for intimacy and find them seriously lacking. Very often women are responsible for the emotional climate in which a couple exists and also, since many men have no or few intimate friends except for the women they are involved with, we end up having to give them a huge amount of emotional support. Again, a woman winds up doing "invisible" work. Her energy is sometimes so taken up with maintaining a relationship that she is diverted from her own personal achievement and development.

Most men have not yet caught up with women in terms of personal growth, knowing how to work on a relationship or knowing how to be a good friend. Some men have begun to meet together in groups to talk about these issues, to develop the skills necessary for intimate personal relationships and to learn how to pay more attention to their relationships with children, wives or lovers and friends, even though nothing in our society encourages them to do so.

When it works, intimacy makes us feel so good that it enriches other parts of our lives and contributes to our energy and creativity.

*Sidney Jourard. *The Transparent Self: Self-Disclosure and Well-Being,* 2nd ed. New York, Van Nostrand, 1971.

MAKING IT WORK

In any long-term relationship with a man, problems and painful issues come up regardless of how "right" we are for each other, of how hard we have worked to build the relationship and even of how stable and solid we feel together. It can be frightening to look squarely at what is difficult and hurtful, for we want to believe that we chose a good partner, that we have made wise decisions; to become aware of aspects we were afraid to face, to admit deep conflicts may mean that we have made a major error. Sometimes, as we begin to get angry, we become afraid that if we do not immediately squelch this anger it will rage out of control and lead us inevitably to the end of the relationship.

Yet avoiding confrontation is more likely to result in stagnation and resentment than in keeping the peace or making things better. *Conflict can be part of a creative process of working things out.* As a start we can identify the social aspects of our conflicts and avoid the common pitfall of blaming one another or blaming ourselves for everything that goes wrong.

Constantly Questioning Our Assumptions

We need to make a conscious and continuing effort to articulate what we really want in our intimate relationships with men, or the conventions of society will inevitably take over. One way to begin changing our relationships is to reconsider the kind of man we (think we) are looking for and our patterns of relating to men when we first meet them. Making changes at the beginning of a relationship may help us to shift the balance that gets set up in our future relationships.

I thought I was marrying this very exciting man, and I didn't see that his dynamism was an expression of the control he needed to have. I just saw the excitement, the energy. I didn't realize that it would make me feel smaller in the process. I learned that it's not just how "wonderful" the other person is but how they make you feel. Now I pay a lot of attention to how I feel with someone at the beginning of a relationship. If I feel distinctly less wonderful in a man's presence, I don't care how sparkling or brilliant he is—I'm not interested.

My wish in my yearbook was to marry a Marlboro man. I grew up in a family of Marlboro men. But I figured out eventually that I didn't want that anymore. Max is very intense and verbal. He is about my height and weight. From the back we even look alike. He's very emotionally accessible—and vulnerable. We have a great deal of fun together. And it's very easy to talk to him. But sometimes I look at him and think, You're so much a friend and a peer...I wonder if you are strong enough for me to lean on.

133

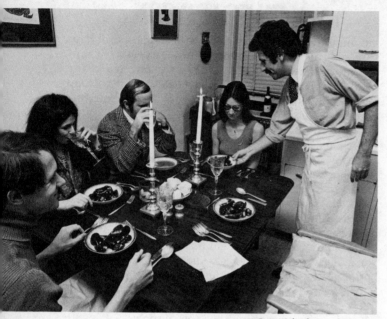

Cary Wolinsky/Stock Boston

Many of us want our partners to be friends and peers. The men's liberation movement has been an important ally in building this consciousness among men.

Only in the feminist men's movement did I finally find men with a commitment to grapple with sex roles, and it has made an immeasurable difference. Yes, in the past I did find other men willing to change to make our relationship work, but only after arguing and buttressing the points over and over from ground zero. After a while, you just want to be with someone who truly has the same values you do and not have to fight that war at home.

As a relationship develops we must continue to be aware of our assumptions. The danger in taking small things for granted is that they are often attached to larger issues. A seemingly small gesture, like choosing a last name when we decide to get married, can serve as a statement right from the start that we want to have a different kind of connection to a husband than that implied when a woman automatically takes his last name as her own.

I had been married once before, had changed my name and then changed it back, and I knew I didn't want to go through that again. I gave up an important part of myself, which didn't feel like a comfortable way to begin a relationship of equals. When Sam and I decided to get married, we wanted a new beginning. We thought about somehow combining our last names, but we couldn't come up with one that we liked. The decision to choose an entirely new name has had a lot of meaning for both of us. The name itself is rich in meaning for me. . . . It is from the language that our grandparents spoke, and it means "rebirth" or "renewal." . . . The process of choosing

it was very moving. I didn't stop using my original name. I still use it as a middle name, and I like it to be very visible. People often ask about our name, and when I tell them how and why we did it, it's like offering them a new option, a new way to deal with old assumptions. This name is a gift.

But many of our relationships began on a very different footing. We didn't question them until years after patterns were set. We may be scared to change or to have our partners change. If we were raised to believe that men should be strong and silent, we may feel uneasy when our partners express vulnerability, even though we have been asking them to talk about their feelings. We may want them to share caretaking chores but fear that they will encroach on our role, neglecting their paid work or being "unmasculine."

After fifteen years of being a full-time homemaker, I decided to go to school. My husband and I divided up all the jobs and responsibilities so I could finish school and work at a fairly demanding job full time. Everything was working out fine, I thought, until one day Jim made some passing remark about one of our daughters and some problem she was having with her boyfriend. I was shocked to realize that something was going on I knew nothing about. I was no longer the "nerve center" of the family. That was a loss, because for many years knowing all those details had been my source of power within the family. Yet on balance the change has been good for all of us. Being the nerve center was holding me back from developing other parts of myself, and as I moved out into the world, Jim grew a great deal closer to the kids.

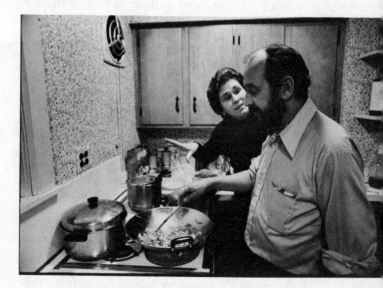

Owen Franken/Stock Boston

134

And we renegotiate these arrangements as time goes on.

We have been married forty-one years, but because of the women's movement there have been some recent changes in our relationship. My husband is a great theoretician. He may have read a hell of a lot more about the women's movement than I have, but to get him to cook dinner is a struggle!

By now we have struggled through the business about making dinner five or six times—different times at which decisions were made and they're acted on for a time, then something happens like he goes away for three weeks, and when he comes back he's tired and he doesn't take the thing up again. So we have to negotiate the whole thing over again. At one point he said, "You know, the truth is I'm just lazy. It's just so much more comfortable not to have to do it." He can recognize that, but it doesn't prevent it from happening again. But the thing that makes it work is that he's open to being challenged about it. And from what I've heard and read about it, an awful lot of men are not.

Paying Attention to Each Other

So many things vie for our attention: work, friends, children, our various activities and chores. A new love eclipses almost everything else, but before too long the balance changes and it gets squeezed in between the children's needs, the laundry, the car's transmission and evening meetings.

An intimate relationship, while often background and sustenance to the rest of our lives, must at times have our full attention.

Several evenings a week since we married eleven years ago, we sit in the living room, each of us in our own favorite chair, and we have a glass of wine after the kids are in bed. And we talk...about the day, about ridiculous details of what happened at work, about some problem we've been having, or whatever. Sometimes it's hard to take the time...the dishes need washing or there is a good show on TV or I just don't feel like it. But this, more than any other single thing, has kept us from getting too far apart without touching base.

We have long dry spells between us....Sometimes I look at him, especially when he's upset about something and very silent and withdrawn, and it feels like I forget what I was ever drawn to in this man. And then we take a morning off from work or we stay up until two A.M. trying to work out some big crisis, and then we might end up making passionate love, and then I remember, Oh! So this is what I love about you! But it's not the lovemaking so much as really talking about something other than whether today is garbage collection day or which check I forgot to enter in the checkbook. It's seeing "into his soul," into the person I am so close to.

While raising children can bring us closer, often their presence distracts us, or just cuts into the time we have alone together.

One of the hardest things for us since having kids is just getting enough time alone together. When I can't get a sitter Bob feels neglected, and I'm sure I've failed, even though I know there's no reason why it should just be up to me to arrange our time alone. When we do have a sitter, the kids complain. Both of us come from working-class families where the kids were always included in everything, so it's easy for us to feel guilty when we do something by ourselves.

What we do when we want to be alone together is get in the car. We go for long drives without the radio on, and we talk. That's a way that we can relax, something we enjoyed doing even when we were eighteen years old. But we have to work at it. The kids take up an enormous amount of time and energy that we used to have just for ourselves. Both of us realize that now that I have a career, too, it would be easy for us to drift into our careers as the kids leave home, and to have nothing left between

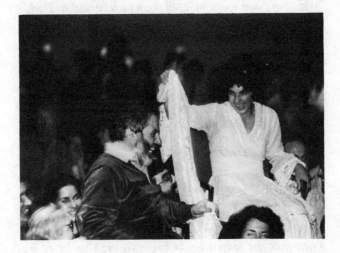

Cheryl Boudreaux

the two of us. It's a danger that we have to pay attention to. In thinking about our future years together, we have considered buying a shack or a beachhouse, something that we could afford, and we would go there on weekends and work on it together. It's relaxing, it's being outdoors and it's doing something we enjoy doing together. And we know from past experience that this is how we can stay close.

Some couples have an annual celebration to affirm their commitment, to review their contract and renew their vows.

There is no one "right" way to nurture a relationship; each of us must find what works best for us.

135

Enjoying Separateness

When partners in a couple go on separate vacations or see separate friends, other people often take it as a sign that something is wrong. Sometimes one member of a couple may be threatened when a partner's life excludes him or her in some way.

I have been seeing a man for almost a year now. I like him a great deal, but he is unable to understand my way of life. He is retired and enjoys just sitting with his feet up for the first time in his life. But I have a new volunteer job, and so I have a number of activities which to me are really stimulating. And these very things, which I've always wanted to do, make it seem to him like I can't stay home and am always running around.

I remember years ago wanting so badly to go to a party we were invited to. But Carl really couldn't stand those people; he refused to go. What I really wanted was to go alone, and I would have had a grand old time, but in those days if you did such a thing people would surely have gossiped that you were on the brink of divorce! Several years ago our college-age daughter said to me, "Well, why don't you just tell them next time that Daddy really doesn't enjoy parties very much, but that you'd love to come!" I have done this several times now; recently I even went out to dinner alone with a couple I particularly like. It's so much better than missing the parties and resenting Carl, or dragging him along and having him sulk and then having to leave earlier than I want to. I resent it far less now when he watches sports on TV, which I dislike. I think that I wasted many years not doing what I enjoyed because sometimes it was different from what we enjoyed.

Martin and I have been together for thirteen years. By together I don't mean married; it has always seemed sort of ridiculous to me to have the state involved in what is really a personal contract. And beyond that, I think that when you get married you begin to make a lot of assumptions and you don't even realize you're doing it. I use my relationship with Martin as a solid base to move out from....I have a very active life independent of him...work and political meetings and seeing my friends. He and they are equally important to me—neither alone would be as good.

While some women think that avoiding legal marriage is a safeguard against falling into conventional roles, most want the commitment that marriage symbolizes.

Sometimes when we are involved with a man we fail to develop certain of our abilities. We may be lulled into thinking that there will always be a man to take care of us. We avoid learning skills like money man-

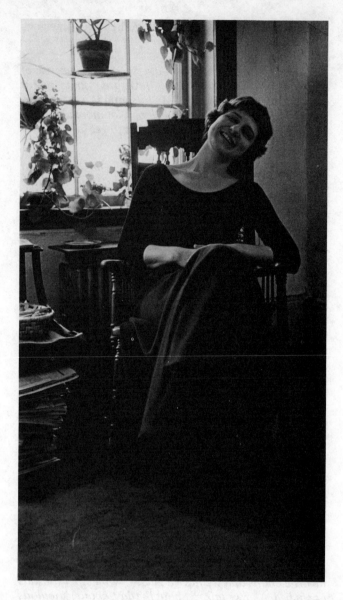

Vaughn Sills

agement, home repairs, strenuous physical tasks.* As a result we may think of ourselves as weaker or less competent than we really are.

I know that I've gotten through the worst times as a single parent, and I've survived and flourished. Being alone and having to learn certain skills, like putting up a Christmas tree alone when your husband used to do

*Many men in turn look to women for the kinds of caretaking they may associate with mothering, like the provision of balanced meals, day-to-day household management and the maintenance of general emotional well-being. The difficulty men have in coping without a woman to take care of them in these ways is suggested by their much higher and earlier remarriage rate after divorce or widowhood, and also by their higher mortality and morbidity rates after these same life crises.

it, wasn't something that gave me so much pleasure, but the fact that I did it was another small incident that showed I could manage, and there's a certain satisfaction in just being able to manage your life. Being able to manage your house and raise kids and work outside the house—it's a sense of accomplishment. Learning new skills, like putting up storm windows, taking the car to the mechanic and negotiating with him, managing your finances, deciding where you're going to have a vacation and with whom—it's all just learning to rely on your own strengths.

Keeping some distinct turf for ourselves, whether it's separate checkbooks or separate vacations, separate friends or not rushing into living together, does not have to threaten our relationship. In fact, it can be renewing to us and contribute to the vitality and growth of what goes on between us.

One of the reasons we have lasted together is that we have always lived in places where each of us could really build a whole life for ourselves—in terms of friends, work, interests—and not have to depend on each other for more than the other could give.

Having Other Friendships

Sometimes couples tend to close in on themselves. We may come to attach less importance to other friendships and let them drop. Yet it is unrealistic to expect that one person can meet all our needs. Other friendships are crucial to our emotional well-being, our happiness, our growth.

Having deep friendships with other people creates a garden in which all of our potential can grow and flourish. We get a broader idea about who we are or can be, and call upon different strengths. We are richer, more complex. What we learn through our intense friendships with others—about how to be close, how we seem to other people, how to fight constructively, what we enjoy—we can then weave back into our lives with our partners. Sometimes we have deep friendships with men, but more often with women. By expanding our intimate circles we relieve some of the pressure on our main relationships, and when times are hard other people can then give us support, nurturance and understanding. We don't have to depend only on our partners.

It's so much easier for me living communally because there are other people one can turn to and I'm not Ed's only source of support. When you live alone with someone, you tend to get locked into roles, to divide the work in half and each take part, and there's far less fluidity than you have in a group. And also, when I've lived in a group there's always been an observer to say, "Hey, I see this going on," which helps us to stop the argument we're in and to look at it.

Sometimes Robert falls completely apart. He drags around the house in his bathrobe, doesn't shave, feels sick and talks endlessly about it and generally comes unglued. This almost invariably happens when I am under the most pressure at work, or when the kids are in shreds and demanding extra attention. I get so enraged at Rob for getting weak just when I need him that I yell and scream and berate him…just what he doesn't need— to be kicked when he's down. What I generally do is call up a friend I really love and trust. She has known me for six years, and knows how to help me talk about things so that I get a better perspective on them. Having her to lean on when I feel overwhelmed or down also helps me to be less angry at Rob for falling apart at those times. I can go back to him able to say what I want to say much more clearly, having talked about it with Marie.

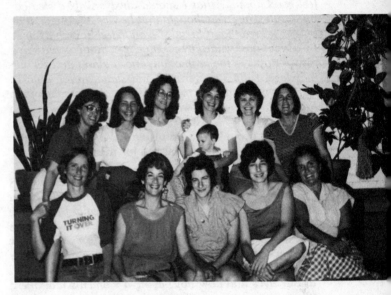

Gina Hawley

Many women have developed strong friendships with other women in the support and consciousness-raising groups which have proliferated over the past fourteen years. Women have always gotten together to talk with each other about the details of their personal lives. Though both women and men have considered these gatherings to be idle and unimportant, trivial "chatting," what we are really talking about is the fabric of our lives. By spending time with other women, we see the potential power of articulating and clarifying what is going on in our lives. We learn that many of the issues we struggle with in loving and living with men are not unique to us.

The six of us have been meeting every week, or sometimes every other week, for almost five years. Many times I've gone to a meeting with one perspective and come out with another…we talk about work and children, lovers and husbands, friendships, our parents and any-

thing else that is important to us. My husband said once that he thought he owed the fact that our marriage was still in existence to my group. In fact, he's right, even though this goes directly against the stereotype some people have that the main activity of women's groups is to go around busting up marriages. Our group helped me work for what I really wanted. I had spent years treading on eggshells. He felt very insecure professionally and really couldn't get his act together at work. I was doing better, and at one point, when I had the chance to get a major promotion which would have made my salary much higher than his, he threatened to leave the relationship if I took it. I was frightened. I wanted to preserve the marriage rather than get ahead professionally. The women in my group knew that my career was important to me, and that I was very, very good at it. They helped me to look hard at whether those were terms I could ultimately feel good about...that I should always walk a step behind him. They also thought that he was bluffing...that he was scared that if I really began to feel how competent I was and how valued by other people, that I would leave him. I did take the promotion, and it didn't destroy our marriage. I am stronger now and stand up for what is good for me, and I say to him, "This does not mean that I don't love you, but I won't buy into your fear."

Support groups are helpful at all ages. Sheila is sixty years old and has been married for thirty-seven years.

I've been a member of a women's group for seven years now, and I think we came together out of a feeling that here we were, middle-aged. We didn't really fit into the women's movement totally. And yet there were things we wanted to talk about, and that was the only place they were getting talked about. We could recognize many of the things these women were talking about. And we looked at our lives and how not having a women's movement when we were younger had made an impact on our lives.

Some men, seeing the value of these groups, have set up their own. Other support groups include both men and women, such as single-parent, postdivorce and widow/widower groups, and groups which deal with a particular problem, such as alcoholism or drug abuse.

Getting Help

When problems are very resistant to change and talking to each other and to friends gets us nowhere, when we feel that we've gone around and around on the same issues with no improvement and are completely overwhelmed, then we may believe that our problems are much worse than they ever were. But often it is simply that we get to a point where we are no longer willing or able to put up with a situation which has been going on for a long time. Profound changes can grow from these most desperate moments.

A few months ago things got to the point where, even though I loved Richard a lot, I just couldn't go on with this marriage the way it was set up. Richard refused to go to a therapist with me. In desperation I talked to two friends, each of whom has known us a real long time. And those conversations led to a mind-blowing realization that everything we did in our marriage had been set in the first six months of our relationship. I knew that I couldn't go on that way, so I told Richard how I felt. We stayed up all night talking and crying, then we slept and in the morning we cried again. He said he didn't want to lose everything he had ever loved and that he would try to change, and I said I would try but I couldn't promise and we would see. Right now things are much better between us and we are really trying to make it work.

But sometimes we get stuck in patterns which make it difficult for the two of us alone to make changes, or sometimes we just don't know how. Talking with friends may not always help enough. At this point, we may turn to therapy for help in understanding our own feelings and changing our behavior.

Therapy has helped me to focus on things I do over and over with men which result in my not getting what I need. For example, when I started therapy, I didn't realize how hard it was for me to ask for certain things. I didn't feel strong enough or confident enough to fight for myself. I found it hard to feel close, and I didn't understand how learning to get what I wanted would make me feel closer. It was a circle....Now that I feel confident enough and aware enough of this pattern, it has changed.

We can use therapy to help improve communication about painful issues.

He didn't feel totally comfortable with my handicap, and he would say so, and that made me terribly angry. I couldn't look at my anger at all, which made him very upset, and then he would clam up. I needed a place to feel safe to deal with all this. So we decided to go into couples' therapy. It helped for me to be able to relax and to hear what he was saying to me. He would say to me, "I love you, but I don't like how that part of your body looks." And a lot of it was really my feeling, that I didn't like how it looked either.

But therapy for women can be a double-edged sword. Most often the woman initiates the move to see a therapist, while the man may resist or refuse to go. But if we accept the cultural conditioning which teaches us that our job is to maintain emotional relationships, to take care of and give to other people, to be sensitive and work out problems, then turning to a therapist implies that we have "failed" at our role. Tragically, traditional therapy has often reinforced this perception.* It is important to find a therapist whose definitions of health and normalcy are based on a world view which sees women as having a full range of options, not on the premise that women's only or main role is to "service" men and take care of children.

After the first few months of couples' therapy, the therapist said to Matt, "So, you think the problem is that Anna is crazy just because she wants to go back to school, and if she would get 'better,' things would be okay again? Well, let me show you how you fit into Anna's problem." Then we began to look into Matt's part of it, how he wouldn't help take care of our four kids, how he needed to change for us to be able to work things out. For me that was enormously freeing. For the first time I saw that I wasn't the "crazy" one. And I began to feel that I could stay in my marriage and still grow and change in the ways I wanted to.

Not all relationships survive these profound changes. When a break-up seems likely, we have to ask ourselves which is more acceptable to us: the cost of leaving things as they are, or the risk that, in trying to improve the relationship, we may lose it.

Knowing When to Leave

Many of us struggle along for years in relationships that are not rewarding or affirming, wanting to make them better but not succeeding, and not yet convinced that we would be better off if we left. We may come again and again to the brink of leaving, and then back off. This is not because things are not quite "bad enough"; even women whose men are violent toward them† or are alcoholics or drug abusers or have incapacitating emotional problems often find themselves staying or struggling with whether or not to leave, or how to leave. What holds us back? We may, even with all the problems, still love our partner and be reluctant to lose him; we may feel loyal to him and perhaps not want to hurt him. Perhaps we think that breaking our commitment is a great personal failure, that we will be harshly judged by friends and family. We may try to stay together "for the good of the children" or may dread the prospect of being alone. And there is often the very real fear that we will not be able to support ourselves, and perhaps our children, financially. Yet many women do ultimately decide that they want to end their relationships.

At first Phil seemed to revel in my accomplishments, my growing self-confidence. But I also grew more able to challenge him where he didn't want to be challenged. I have wanted more from him: more involvement with the children, more sharing of paid jobs and housework. I want him to value my strength as I have come to value myself more. His response has been to have a string of affairs, all with women who are much younger than I am and, as you might guess, totally undemanding, unthreatening, willing to accept him precisely as he is.

My relationship with Greg ended when I said that it was no longer working for us and that nothing we were doing was making it any better. He was not a person with whom I could fully engage. We never really learned to fight well together...not just having arguments but learning to compromise well. I felt turned off sexually, attracted to others, and the pleasure of being with him was gone. I would come home and not want to tell him what was exciting that day....I preferred to tell other people who seemed more "simpatico." What was hardest about the divorce was that the family part of our relationship was good....It was painful to let go of the father of my kids. It was scary to give my own needs so much weight.

The man I was living with began to undercut everything I did—to devalue my work, to be jealous of my friends and my small successes. When I got bogged down in a project, rather than encouraging me he would point out how the project was probably ill-conceived and not of much use anyway. The longer things went on, the more of my good creative energy went into trying to make the relationship work, and the less energy I had for my work and the rest of my life.

When I was first thinking about getting out of my marriage, I would think, Well, I get a lot of satisfaction out of being a parent and I'm very close to my kids. I get a lot of satisfaction from my friendships and I have a really good work situation. My relationship isn't so good, but maybe you just can't have everything. My husband had some serious problems, so I felt I couldn't blame him or just leave him. I never stopped to consider what it was doing to me to be spending years of my life with someone who was giving me so little. After a while I built up so much resentment that I just wasn't able to treat him in a loving way. And I began to be afraid that I would lose my capacity to love someone. I knew that I had a potential for loving that wasn't getting expressed. Yet it was a leap to assume that getting out of our marriage meant that I would have a good relationship again.

If you wind up just accommodating your partner to prevent fights rather than having some hope that it's worth sitting down and trying to work things out; if your relationship is based on evasiveness, deception and withholding; if it is characterized by stagnation and a lack of room for change and growth; or if it just doesn't seem that your life is better in the relationship than it would be out of it, then it is time to consider ending it. You don't need to do this in isolation. There

---

*See Chapter 6, "Psychotherapy."

†See Chapter 8, "Violence Against Women," for a fuller discussion of domestic abuse.

are good books on the subject (see Resources, below). Turning to friends, particularly ones who are willing to talk openly about their divorces or hard times with their partners, can be an excellent source of support and insight. Individual or group therapy can help, as can support groups. Much as we know it is important to work very hard to build a relationship, it is also important to leave before we are damaged by it.

Though it may seem to be contradictory to advocate paying attention to our relationships and at the same time trying to be a separate person and seek other friendships, these multiple aspects of our lives can and do enrich rather than detract from one another. They also provide a balance which stimulates our growth and promotes our joy and well-being—our capacity for independence along with our capacity for intimacy.

We have been married for thirteen years....Daniel is not my best friend. We are quite different in many ways, have different friends, interests and so on. There are ways in which I'm not even as intimate with him as I am with some of my women friends. But ever since I met him, I have not felt the excruciating loneliness which was the core of my life for twenty-six years. Being with him, knowing that we are partners in life, has permitted me to grow from an extremely unhappy, lonely person with little self-esteem and a lot of self-hatred into a happy, fulfilled and self-loving woman. My identity is not derived from him, but being with him has enabled me to create a major transformation in myself.

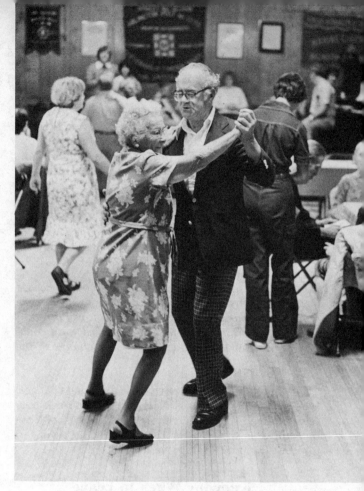

Patricia Hollander Gross/Stock Boston

RESOURCES

Bernard, Jessie. *The Future of Marriage.* New York: Bantam Books, 1972.

Crawford, Linda, and Lee Lanning. *Loving: Women Talk About Their Love Relationships.* Minneapolis: Midwest Health Center for Women, 1981. (155 pages, $6.95)

Ehrenreich, Barbara. *The Hearts of Men: American Dreams and the Flight from Commitment.* Garden City, NY: Anchor Press/Doubleday, 1983.

Fleming, Jennifer Baker, and Carolyn Kott Washburne. *For Better, For Worse: A Feminist Handbook on Marriage and Other Options.* New York: Charles Scribner's Sons, Inc., 1977.

Gettleman, Susan, and Janet Markowitz. *The Courage to Divorce.* New York: Simon and Schuster, 1974.

Gilligan, Carol. *In a Different Voice.* Cambridge: Harvard University Press, 1982.

Hailey, Elizabeth Forsythe. *A Woman of Independent Means.* New York: Avon Books, 1979. Fictionalized account of a strong woman told through her letters.

Lear, Martha Weinman. *Heartsounds.* New York: Pocket Books, 1980. Autobiographical account of a woman's relationship with a husband who is suffering from a serious and eventually fatal heart condition.

Lindsey, Karen. *Friends as Family.* Boston: Beacon Press, 1981.

Malos, Ellen, ed. *The Politics of Housework.* New York: Schocken Books, 1980. Anthology includes the groundbreaking article of that same title by Pat Mainardi.

Miller, Jean Baker. *Toward a New Psychology of Women.* Boston: Beacon Press, 1976.

Miller, Stuart. *Men and Friendship.* Boston: Houghton Mifflin Co., 1983.

Peterson, Nancy L. *Our Lives for Ourselves: Women Who Have Never Married.* New York: G.P. Putnam's Sons, 1981.

Rich, Adrienne. *On Lies, Secrets and Silence.* New York: W.W. Norton and Co., Inc., 1979.

Rubin, Lillian. *Intimate Strangers.* New York: Harper and Row Publishers, Inc., 1983.

Simenauer, Jacqueline, and David Carroll. *Singles: The New Americans.* New York: New American Library, 1982.

Stack, Carol B. *All Our Kin: Strategies for Survival in a Black Community.* New York: Harper and Row Publishers, Inc., 1974.

Steinbergh, Judith W. *Lillian Bloom: A Separation.* Hot Mama Poetry Collective/ Wampeter Press, Box 512, Green Harbor, MA 02041, 1980. ($4.95) These fine poems chronicle a woman's separation from her husband, her pain and anger, and her growing sense of competence and joy as a woman and a mother.

Triere, Lynette, with Richard Peacock. *Learning to Leave: A Woman's Guide.* New York: Warner Books, Inc., 1982.

Women in Transition, Inc., *Women in Transition: A Feminist Handbook on Separation and Divorce.* New York: Charles Scribner's Sons, Inc., 1975.

10

LOVING WOMEN:
LESBIAN LIFE AND RELATIONSHIPS*

By the Lesbians Revisions Groups, including Barbara A. Burg, Loly Carrillo, Sasha Curran, J. W. Duncan, Buffy Dunker, Deanna Forist, D. Hamer, B. J. Louison, Judy Norris, Gwendolyn Parker, Mariana Romo-Carmona, Lynn Scott, Ann Shepardson, and several women who must, with sadness and anger, remain anonymous to protect our jobs, family relations, living situations or parenthood

With special thanks to the Cambridge Women's Center for use of their archives, Jill Wolhandler, the Lesbian Mothers Group (at the Cambridge Women's Center), and to the hundreds of lesbian women who wrote letters in response to the previous lesbian chapter

This chapter in previous editions was called "In Amerika They Call Us Dykes" and was written by a Boston Gay Collective.

Being a lesbian for me is about the joy and wonder of loving women. It means being woman-identified, making women my priority. It is a way of life, so much more than a matter of who I want to sleep with.

In many communities, a lot of the activist work that is being done to free all women from oppression is being done by lesbians. Not having this big emotional or economic dependence on men makes us able to do that. If you're not trying to get so much from men, you can often be more objective, assertive and powerful. That's the freedom we have to shape the world.

Sometimes when I talk positively about being a lesbian, heterosexual friends say they hear me criticizing their choice to be with men. That's not true. For me, part of what's essential in being a lesbian is caring for other women, and this includes women who have made choices other than mine.

The chapter on lesbians in the original *Our Bodies, Ourselves* drew letters from women all over the country telling about their experiences and asking for advice, news, contacts, support. So much has happened for lesbians since that original chapter appeared that

several lesbians decided to work together in bringing the chapter up to date. Ranging in age from twenty-four to seventy-six, we come from diverse backgrounds and experiences.

In revising the chapter we want especially to reach out with information and support to women who are newly exploring their lesbian identity and to lesbians who find themselves isolated from other lesbians, geographically or otherwise. We also want to give heterosexual women a clearer picture of our lives.*

In the past ten years the U.S. lesbian community has grown and flourished. Lesbians are numerous in every ethnic group, economic class and political persuasion. We are factory workers, teachers, translators, doctors, high school and college students, clergy, shopkeepers, flight attendants, politicians, labor leaders, athletes. Some of us have physical disabilities, some have or plan to have children, some are sure we don't want children and find this a freeing choice, some have relationships which last a lifetime, some are celibate. Some of us are married to men and cannot easily leave

*Although this edition of *Our Bodies, Ourselves* includes lesbian voices throughout, the Collective decided also to have a separate chapter for a more careful focus on issues and information which specifically affect lesbians.

*None of the present writers worked on the 1973 chapter, "In Amerika They Call Us Dykes." In fact, it provided crucial support and inspiration for several of us when we first came out as lesbians. We have written a chapter quite different in focus and tone from the original one, which had many long, detailed and powerful personal stories. This time we have used briefer stories so as to make room for more topics. Please check the Resources section for some of the many recent books in which lesbians talk personally at greater length.

our marriages, yet we identify ourselves as lesbian and even make primary commitments to women.

Although most historical records leave lesbians invisible, research is uncovering a lesbian culture dating back to ancient times. We have been present, out and struggling for centuries. Despite periods of intense persecution, we have continued to choose and to love one another, and to challenge patriarchy by the very fact of our emotional independence from men.

We who are writing this chapter are excited by this heritage. While we are grateful to live in a time and place where lesbians can love and live somewhat openly, prejudice and oppression are still a daily fact of our lives. We hope the chapter will help other lesbians—our sisters—grow in understanding, pride and power.

COMING OUT

Coming out is the process of coming to accept and affirm our lesbian identity and choosing how open we want to be about it. It can involve many stages—ad-

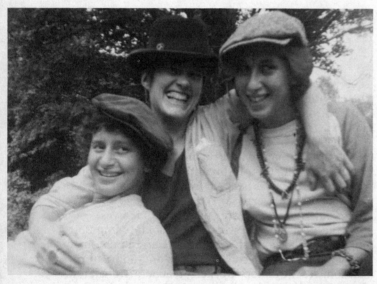

Shay Ogelsby

mitting to ourselves that we are lesbian, getting to know other lesbians, telling friends and family, marching in a gay-rights demonstration, being open at school or work. Many of us will never be free to do all these. We spend a lot of energy deciding whether, when, how and to whom we want to come out. When/if our society one day freely accepts lesbians, we will be able to use that energy in many other ways.

Coming Out to Ourselves

Each of us has her own story of growing lesbian awareness. Since we grow up in a culture which assumes

everyone to be heterosexual, becoming aware of our identity and accepting it is often a gradual process. Coming out to ourselves can happen at any age or stage in life.

At fourteen I already knew I was different. All my girlfriends talked about was boys, and I wasn't interested. I dated a few guys but mostly I skipped the social events. I picked out any strong women I could find and hung around with my coaches a lot. I was in trouble all the time—fighting with my parents, dealing drugs, drinking. I see now it was because I realized I was different and didn't know what to do about it.

I didn't think about becoming a lesbian until at twenty-five I just fell in love with a woman and had to deal with it. As long as I was with her it was pretty simple, but when we broke up three years later, I finally had to ask myself, "Am I really a lesbian?"

I think I was always gay, but it took me seventy years to realize it.

After my divorce I dated men and even slept with a few, but something was missing. I was celibate on and off for five years, mostly glad of the clear space and solitude, but at times in despair that I'd never let anyone really close. I felt a strong political and personal commitment to women and a fascination for lesbians, but it scared me to think that maybe I wanted to love a woman—my parents would explode, my ex-husband would try to get custody of our kids, my friends might think I was out to seduce them. I was also afraid it would be a choice against men instead of for women. Slowly I worked through all this and finally one day I said to myself, "For now, I am a lesbian," and some important piece of my identity clicked into place. I'm glad I chose to be a lesbian before I had a woman lover.

When I went to college there were only two other black students on the entire campus, and they came from comfortable middle-class families. I felt as out of place with them as I did with the middle-class white students. It was about this time that I began to become aware of an attraction to women, which I kept trying to suppress. Since I was out of my element socially, I always came on as tough and aggressive to cover up, and people started accusing me of being a dyke. I was terrified that my fantasies were showing in some way, and I began dating to cover up, to show that I wasn't "like that." Now I realize that the accusations were intended to bring me into line and make me behave "like a lady," and it worked. I knew that being a black woman gave everyone the right to walk on me (or try to, anyway), and I thought that being a black lesbian was some sort of capital crime. It was this more than anything else that made me steer clear of women who showed an interest in me.

The women's movement came along about the time I

finished college. The movement gave me support because I could see other women having the courage to change their lives. Their example gave me the courage to see that I was cheating myself by pretending to be straight. I finally did come out sexually with a black woman I met at work. I reasoned that if a racist society wanted my head, they'd get it because I was black, and being gay wasn't going to make all that much difference. My life has been much fuller since then and a lot happier.

Many of us try to deny our lesbianism at first. It contradicts all the expectations our families and society have for us—and, often, the expectations we have had for ourselves. All we've ever heard about lesbians is negative. We may not even know any open lesbians.

In my little town in upstate New York I didn't know there were other dykes around at all. When I fell in love with a woman and became lovers with her at sixteen, she was the only person I knew who was gay. It was hard to say to myself, "I am a lesbian," when I didn't know any.

Stereotypes of lesbians may scare us away.

I was fascinated by the idea of loving a woman, but totally turned off by what I thought lesbians were supposed to be like. I didn't want to be a man or look like one.

We may want to reject our lesbianism because our sexist upbringing has taught us that women are inferior, or because we know life will be hard or complicated for us as lesbians in certain ways, though satisfying in others.

Many of us have painful memories of trying to deny our feelings for women—dating men, getting married, consulting psychiatrists who tried to "cure" us, becoming dependent on alcohol or other drugs.

I was afraid that if I touched other girls I would like it and keep on touching them. So I became repulsed at the idea. I'm angry that I held the feelings down for so long that now I have a hard time just relaxing and touching someone I love.

Coming out to ourselves means primarily letting go of the guilt, self-hatred and fear learned from living in a homophobic society. (Homophobia is the irrational fear and hatred of homosexuality in ourselves and others.) Coming out means loving ourselves as women and as lesbians.

When you first come out, it's like you're telling yourself something you don't want to believe. "You kissed that girl, didn't you? It felt good, didn't it? So what's wrong with it?" You finally begin to be honest with yourself. After that the rest of your life opens up.

A month after I said to myself, "Okay, I'm a lesbian," and had my first female lover, I suddenly started to go dancing a whole lot, to take bubble baths, swim nude at night, wear soft, slinky shirts.

When I came out, I didn't know any Asian lesbians in my city. It was like juggling three worlds. I was raised in a very traditional Chinese family. I didn't know I was an American citizen until all of a sudden at eighteen I realized I was here to stay, and had to deal with this country as a reality. A few years later I realized my sexual preference was for women, despite all the traditional Chinese expectations and the extreme homophobia of Chinese culture, along with all the other social expectations out there in American society.

I gradually began to integrate all the three together: I tried to maintain my Chinese identity and to integrate that with feeling strong as a woman, tracing it basically through feelings of closeness with my grandmother, who was the matriarch of the family. I tried to pick out strong women in my personal past and to combine the traditions there that could help me to be strong as a woman and help me be able to feel strong about being a lesbian. So although I am not out to my family, I don't feel like I'm going to be put out on the mountain to die.

Coming Out to Friends and Family

Letting other people know we are lesbians is usually more problematic. If we decide to be openly lesbian we become visible targets for physical and psychological harassment. We may be labeled sick, kept away from children, fired from our jobs. Yet if we keep our lesbianism hidden we face insults and embarrassment when people assume we are heterosexual: gynecologists want us to use birth control, friends want to "fix us up" with men, men make passes at us. We live with the fear that others will find out. We feel cut off from many of the people we love.

I want my family and friends to know I'm a lesbian because I want to be honest with them. I don't want to be hiding something from them, especially something so central to my life, something I'm glad about and proud of.

Many of us come out to friends first, choosing the ones who seem likely to be the most accepting.

One friend I came out to said, "I'm happy that you're in love. But I also feel that it's wrong, that you should have those feelings for a man." Once she said the negative part she seemed to let it go. From then on I asked my friends for their negative as well as positive responses, so they wouldn't try to be good "liberal" friends and hide the homophobic feelings that most everyone has somewhere.

My best friend for thirteen years broke off our friendship several months after I told her, and I haven't heard from her in ten years. No matter how well you know someone, you can never know exactly what to expect from them when you come out.

Not being out to family is often particularly painful.

It's hard at family events when everyone is very heterosexual and brings their families and I'm not able to bring my lover. My aunts all ask when I'm going to marry.

Most parents have a hard time with the news.

I look at my parents as being totally isolated. Who can they talk to about their daughter being lesbian? In this society people make very harsh judgments about gay people, and a judgment about a kid is taken as a judgment about the parents. My parents feel that they are responsible for the person I am, and they can get into guilt trips about what they "did wrong."

Thinking lesbianism is something "wrong" and that it has a "cause," parents may blame themselves.* Many react at least at first with anger, guilt, shame, hurt, fear. Some react with violence: they send lesbian daughters into therapy for a "cure," put them into mental institutions, kidnap and send them for "deprogramming," disown them. Others don't take their daughter's choice seriously, and keep hoping she'll meet a nice man and *really* fall in love. Some are more accepting.

My mother's reaction was exceptional. She said, "I don't understand it at all, but I'm glad you're happy."

Coming out to family is usually a process which takes several years. Some parents do come to an understanding, even if they refuse any contact at first; some do not. Coming out makes family relationships more honest and sometimes more close than they would be if we kept living a lie. We may even be pleasantly surprised, as a lesbian grandmother reported: "One of my nineteen grandchildren said, 'I love telling my friends about my gay granny.'"

Beyond Friends and Family

Coming out publicly—to our employers, doctors, therapists, supervisors, teachers or clergy—is risky. These people have the power to make our lives extremely difficult. Job discrimination, a problem for all women,

---

*A recent Kinsey study concluded there is *no* "cause" for homosexuality, neither heredity nor environment (including parents' actions). Looking for a cause usually implies the homophobic assumption that there is something wrong with being lesbian or gay. Who looks for "causes" of heterosexual orientation?

hits lesbians hard. If we are openly lesbian, we are likely to be the last hired and the first fired. And if we hide our lesbianism in order to find a job, we fear being found out. Many lesbians keep totally "closeted" in the public eye, living a scrupulously careful double life.

Yet an increasing number of lesbians today are more open at work about their lesbianism. In certain parts of the country (California, for example) lesbians and gay men have fought against job discrimination and won. Employers in all fields need to learn that we'll work better at our jobs when we can be honest about who we are.

The more that lesbians are able to be visible, the more of a chance people have to see us realistically, to notice our support of each other and to feel our strength. Our increasing visibility in numbers enables us to work more effectively against job discrimination and other kinds of oppression which have made many lesbians keep hidden.

I want us all to announce, "We're Lesbians!" all at the same time. People would be shocked to discover they know lots of lesbians, that they like us, respect us. If people were really aware of how many of us there are, they'd have a much harder time seeing us as abnormal.

I don't think I'm an alarmist when I say that I find it is more often not safe to be obviously out. In my experience homophobia is as intense and pervasive as racial and sexual prejudice, plus it is still legally and socially reinforced. I don't think the answer is to act closeted. I think it is to be aware of the risks, evaluate them, prepare for them and then take them.

FINDING OUR COMMUNITY

Contact with other lesbians is crucial but often difficult to achieve.

My friend and I have been together for five years. We have not "come out" as gay. We have always felt that all we need is each other, but now we are beginning to feel very alone and isolated. When you constantly live a secret, you begin to feel as if you are not real. We need contact with other gays so we can say to someone, "Look! We love each other and we do exist!"

I didn't think there were any older lesbians in the whole city. Then two friends of mine gave a party and invited all the lesbians they knew over forty years old. It made me feel entirely different to look around that room and see how many we were. Now we meet every month.

As late as the 1950s most lesbians were extremely isolated from each other.

Unless you knew someone who knew someone else, the only place to meet lesbians was in the bars, and maybe you didn't like the bar scene. There were few books except lurid novels where lesbians were miserable and usually died unhappily, no newspapers that I knew of, no groups to go to. I was hungry for contact.

Thanks to the many lesbians and gay men who have struggled for our right to live and love openly and with pride, we now have many networks and organizing tools for reaching out to one another. Although the bars offer a place for some lesbians to meet openly and relax together, it has been important to create gathering places which are not built around alcohol and night life, and which reflect all the different interests lesbians have. Daughters of Bilitis (DOB), founded in the 1950s, was the first to provide a place for lesbian women to get together for sociability and discussion. Later, organizations such as Lesbian Liberation and Radicalesbians focused on the politics of lesbianism and feminism. Some cities now have groups for young lesbians and gays, for lesbians of color, for older lesbians, for lesbians with disabilities and for lesbian mothers. The National Gay Task Force and the Lesbian Legal Defense Fund focus on the struggle to challenge the courts and change the laws and social mores which oppress us. The Lesbian and Gay Media Advocates monitors video and print media and the presentation (or lack of presentation) of lesbian and gay images and issues. We have newspapers, independent publishing houses, record companies, bookstores, restaurants, professional and religious organizations, cultural organizations and centers. (See the Resources section at the end of this chapter.) Festivals and dances reach the larger lesbian and gay community. Every summer in cities throughout the country lesbian and gay-pride marches commemorate the anniversary of the Stonewall Riots of 1969.*

Groups and events like these offer chances to take that first step in getting to know other lesbians. Even so, many of us have felt shy or hesitant about walking into a lesbian gathering for the first time.

*After gay men fought back during a 1969 police invasion of the Stonewall Inn bar in New York's Greenwich Village, gay activists started the Lesbian and Gay-Liberation movement.

Ellen Shub

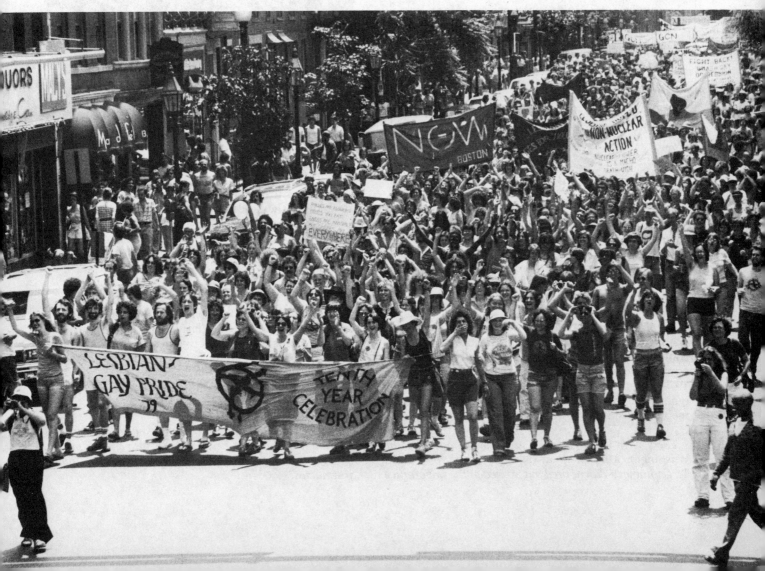

Rural Lesbians

Meeting other lesbians in a small town or rural area can be very hard.

This is one section of the country where nothing different is accepted. It is a backwoods area. There aren't a lot of gay women here. If there are more, they are well hidden from the rest of us.

Some suggestions:

1. Read books and/or listen to records by and about lesbians. (See Resources for mail-order women's bookstores.) They can make you feel good about being a lesbian.

2. Contact the nearest lesbian or gay organization (no matter how far away!). Check guides such as *Gaia's Guide* or *Places of Interest to Women*, or contact national lesbian and gay groups. (See Resources.) Organizations not near you may be able to tell you about nearby groups or give you the name of a woman who could put you in touch with other lesbians in your area.

3. Become involved in women's political activities. Is there a women's center near you, maybe in a university? Any feminist groups? Many lesbians are politically active and most women's groups have lesbian members.

4. Go to women's events such as concerts, conferences and festivals. Many women's music festivals are held in the summertime in rural areas. Listings of upcoming festivals appear in women's and gay newspapers. Even if these events are not close to you, you might meet other lesbians from your area there, or someone who knows someone.

Remember, you are not alone.

The first time I headed for the lesbian support group at the Women's Center I walked around the block four times and went home. I was scared to come out to a whole new group of people. The next month my need for friendship and support won out over my fears, and I went in.

Despite and perhaps even because of our increased visibility, attacks upon us and efforts to silence us continue. In July 1982, arson destroyed the offices of a major weekly newspaper, *Gay Community News*. In 1979, the media chose to play down or completely ignore the historic march by 200,000 lesbians and gay men on Washington, D.C.

There were hundreds, thousands of us, covering the Washington Monument lawns—everywhere you looked. To get home at dawn, tired but excited at the importance

of that day—and turn on the radio to hear nothing! We scanned news broadcasts and papers all the next day—only a small paragraph in one paper. One station gave several minutes' coverage to a local event which only had ten participants—it was absurd. They were telling us it had never happened, that we had never been there, that we did not exist!

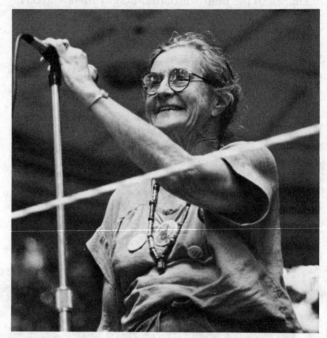

Ellen Shub

RELATIONSHIPS

Knowing that we love women and acting on that is usually an exhilarating experience. Being outside the dominant culture can give lesbians a certain freedom in shaping the kinds of relationships we want. Some of the choices, dilemmas and possibilities which come up parallel those of our heterosexual sisters; some do not.

Pressure to Be in a Couple

This society expects women above all else to find, fall in love with and have a relationship with a man. Lesbians look instead for a woman lover, often maintaining a tremendous emphasis on being part of a couple.

We're so conditioned to think we're only half a person without somebody else.

The only thing that we have in our heads is: you meet a woman, you feel for her, you enter into a relationship, you relate only to her. It's been the downfall of many intimacies.

Often we have to struggle to feel okay if we're not in a couple.

When I'm around lesbian couples for any length of time I feel this sense of creeping desperation, like something's wrong with me because I'm not in a relationship. The pressure makes you latch on to anybody instead of thinking the thing through.

Choosing Not to Be in One Major Relationship

Some lesbians choose to be single—to have many lovers or none, but not one primary lover.

Being on my own lets me find out what my needs are, and find out who I am and just get a better sense of myself.

I like not being answerable to anybody. One reason to be single or celibate is to have clarity about what you want in your life. You make emotional and physical space. What you want is not dependent on what somebody else wants.

When I was in a couple we had to spend so much time hassling out all the little details of everything. Everything had to be a compromise—everything, from the most minute detail to the biggest thing—and it seemed like such a waste of energy most of the time.

When I'm on my own, my security comes from myself and the connections I have with different people. In a relationship, my security depends so much on that relationship and on that one other woman.

It's amazing how much energy it frees up for me. I feel great; I feel a real surge of power!

Not being in a relationship has given me time to reconnect with my friends in a really intimate way.

There are so many more women in my life now, so much room for so many more women.

I found I can get a good deal more work done and am more creative.

I like the feeling of trying to create something new.

In choosing not to be in a couple, we do not distance ourselves from others. We still want, and have, intimate friendships. Some are sexually intimate with friends.

It's very hard for me to draw the line between friends and lovers, so I sleep with some of my very close friends.

I find that really satisfying. A lot of the time I sleep with very close friends without having sex, which I find equally satisfying.

We may choose intimacy without sex because we like our friendships as they are and don't want to change them.

The lesbian community has completely copied the heterosexual community in thinking that relationships, to be really intimate, to be really close and to supply the affection that's needed in a person's life, have to be sexual. I don't think that's true. I think you can have really good relationships, intimate and the most binding, without sex. Bringing sex into a relationship does not necessarily improve it.

How well being single works for us depends on our ability to avoid slipping into feeling dependent on particular people for our feeling of well-being. We often look for the happiness of somebody else liking us, valuing us, and we would do well to find that satisfaction in liking ourselves.

Having One Primary Lover

Many of us choose to be in an intimate sexual relationship with one other woman, whether or not we live together and even if we sleep with other women from time to time. We build a relationship—planning our work and play so we can count on spending time together, helping each other through personal changes and difficulties, working through conflicts. We might stay together as lovers for a few months, a few years or a lifetime.

I like being with someone who follows all the threads of my life, even the most mundane.

It's like having my childhood magical playmate come to life—my best friend who is family to me.

When I hear another lesbian talking about being involved as lovers and friends with lots of women, it excites me. I know that by choosing to be with one woman I am missing out on a certain kind of emotional adventure. But for my lover and me there is a kind of adventure I prefer at this point. Finally, after a year and a half, we are able to say to each other, "I need you," and know what that means. It doesn't mean, "I'm hopeless on my own—I can't let you go," but does mean risking a certain kind of interdependence that I haven't known before.

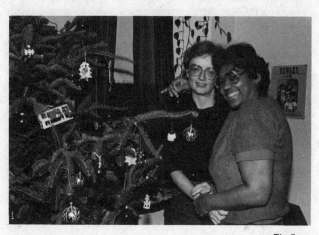

Tia Cross

Intimacy

Models

Whatever kinds of relationships we are in, our families and the media offer us only heterosexual models for intimacy, and limited ones at that. While it is freeing to be without models and sexist role stereotypes, there can also be a lot of uncertainty about how to proceed.

When I was married at nineteen, I knew exactly what I was supposed to do forever. I didn't have to think about it. When I entered into my first lesbian relationship I didn't have any idea. It's scary. I don't know where I'm going half the time; there's no one to turn to and ask, "Is this right?" because nobody knows—there isn't any "right." Without role models, how we live has to come from our gut, and mostly I like it that way.

Family Patterns

Many of the issues in lesbian friendships and sexual relationships have more to do with the ups and downs of intimacy than with the fact that we are lesbians.

In my family no one ever got outwardly angry. There were no fights, only "discussions." So when a lover or close friend blows up at me my first reaction is panic. I know I want to fight more openly and not get so quiet with my anger, but it's hard.

My parents lived and worked together twenty-four hours a day until they died. My lover Lou's family was more traditional; her father was away all day working or being with his male friends and his wife spent a lot of time with her sisters. Lou saw her parents enjoying separate time, and she needed that. I had trouble accepting that she wanted to be without me sometimes. We struggled

over these differences until we could help each other feel safe doing things differently from how our families did.

I went from a mother who spoiled me to a classic butch role where I had no responsibility for any housework. About ten years into living with my lover Roz I realized I had a lot of growing up to do. I saw I was no different from any male if Roz was the one who did all the work around the house.

Separateness

Every one of us who loves another woman has grown up in a sexist society which devalues women and fails to give us a strong sense of identity. Women's "role" in relationships has traditionally been to give in, give over, bend, care for our loved ones. While there are endless differences between any two women, there is a certain closeness that comes from being the same sex—similar body, similar socialization. We can slip into being so close that there isn't enough breathing room. We may have to work to find a healthy balance between closeness and distance, to define ourselves assertively and to encourage each other to grow as individuals.

It's critical that my lover and I really understand our boundaries, where we want to say no and where we want to say yes. If I don't build my own privacy right away into a relationship, then the next thing I know I'm either spacing out or leaving.

If you get involved with a woman who lives far away or has to move for a job, you can't either of you assume the other is going to give up her home, friends or job so you can be together. You both know how important all these are. My lover right now lives in another state. I hate the separation but I value her independence as I value my own.

Monogamy/Nonmonogamy

Some lesbians are excited at the possibility of relationships which are free of sexual exclusivity. Others are more cautious.

Being lesbian gives me a chance to do things differently from the heterosexual couples I've seen. I'd like to be less possessive than they often are. But when it comes down to my lover being sexually involved with another woman (or a man), it hurts. It could even split us up. I've decided that I've got to be up front about my need for sexual dependability; while it may not in some circles be "politically correct," it is very human.

Some of us are clear that we do or do not want to be monogamous. Some of us wrestle with this issue over and over.

Butch-Femme

Many lesbians out and active during the fifties and before followed a strict dress and behavior code, especially in social situations; they chose either a butch role (masculine, aggressive) or a femme role (feminine, receptive). Butches were supposed to initiate sexual relationships, and femmes were supposed to continue their passivity even in bed, allowing butches to make love to them but not reciprocating. Feminist lesbians sometimes criticize butch-femme lesbians for imitating heterosexual models and perpetuating sexism. Others have responded:

I was a femme, a woman who loved and wanted to nurture the butch strength in other women. Although I have been a lesbian for over twenty years and embrace feminism as a world view, I can spot a butch fifty feet away and still feel the thrill of her power. Contrary to belief, this power is not bought at the expense of the femme's identity. Butch-femme relationships, as I experienced them, were complex erotic statements, not phony heterosexual replicas. They were filled with a deeply lesbian language of stance, dress, gesture, loving, courage and autonomy.... Butch-femme was an erotic partnership, serving both as a conspicuous flag of rebellion and as an intimate exploration of women's sexuality.[1]

Some women say that butch-femme is a thing of the past, but many lesbians have spoken up recently to say this isn't true. Although the codes are less strict nowadays, in one way or another many lesbians continue to explore the butch-femme evocation of assertiveness and receptivity, its celebration of "difference in women's textures"[2] and its particular forms of courageous eroticism.

Oppression and Support

Heterosexuals can hold hands in public, go anywhere together, be welcomed as a couple by their families and at religious services, celebrate their relationships openly, make decisions for each other in times of sickness and provide for each other's material well-being in case of death. Lesbians can take none of these commonplace things for granted.

In the faculty room where I work, I hear the other teachers talking about their relationships... nothing real heavy, but they do give each other a lot of support. Since being out to them would mean losing my job, I can't let off steam all day; if Ann's sick and I'm worried about her I can't get any comfort at work. If we have a big decision to make, I can't ask for help in sorting it out. All this makes our lesbian friends terribly important, especially the ones who talk with us about our relationship.

Throughout all eras lesbians have supported each other's relationships despite oppression. Today in simple daily ways we can ask our friends how their relationships are going, give each other a chance to talk about fights, commitment, jealousy, work, housework and all the other things people need to talk about. And many of us are creating our own rituals, where friends and family (sometimes blood relatives, sometimes alternative families) come together to celebrate important events: to affirm our identities as women and lesbians, to honor commitments between women.* We could also gather around each other on other occasions: to mark our children's comings and goings or the endings as well as beginnings of relationships.

Loving each other—as friends, lovers and family— is a source of power, joy, struggle and growth. We look forward to loving more openly, more bravely, more outrageously and more deeply, in as many ways as we can create.

SEXUALITY†

Part of loving women is feeling sexually attracted to women. What we do with this attraction is as varied as we are. Through sex we may express love, friendship, lust, nurturance, need, a sense of adventure, delight in our own bodies. We may kiss and hug a lot, caress our lover's body for hours or have a "quickie." We may play with her nipples or clitoris, explore her vagina with our fingers or our tongues, touch our own bodies, too. We may have orgasms, not have orgasms, use erotic pictures, share fantasies, play sex games, laugh while making love, sleep together without genital sex. There is no one way to be sexual as a lesbian, and no "right" way.

Books and movies always show men and women being sexual together, with certain roles that everyone expects. For lesbians, even what "having sex" means isn't so clearly defined. For me and my lovers it's always been teaching each other, learning together, making it up as we go along. That's how I like it. I feel like anything is possible.

Sex with my male lovers was always okay. But with Paula I'm amazed at the intensity. I want to touch and be touched, make love all the time, be rough, be gentle, penetrate her, feel her moving on me. I think I'm finally

---

*Lesbians are also pushing religious groups to become more open to celebrating lesbian relationships and life events. The Metropolitan Community Church, which has congregations in many parts of the country, has a unique ministry to lesbians and gay men, and some lesbians have married in a "holy union" of that church.

†Please read this section in conjunction with Chapter 11, "Sexuality," which covers more of the specifics about women and sex.

feeling the fullness and depth of my sexuality. I had always suspected there must be more to it, but hadn't figured out how to find it.

In finding out what turns my lover on, exploring her body, tasting her, learning her odors and textures, I am growing to love myself more, too.

It's wonderful not having to think about birth control!

There are also problems, of course, one of which is the myth that lesbian sex is problem-free. We can run into trouble by expecting sex with women to be "blissful, intuitive, spontaneous, and never dull."[3]

Making love with a woman for the first time usually involves a lot more than what happens sexually. We may feel suddenly freed as sexual beings. We may feel exhilarated and joyful and terrified out of our skins. It can take months and even years to learn about our shifting patterns in sex, what we like and what our particular stumbling blocks are.

Making love with a woman, we have at least a basic idea of what would feel good to her. However, we may wrongly expect that because she has a body like ours, we should know what pleases her.

The more women I sleep with, the more I realize you can't assume what you like is what she likes. There are tremendous differences. All kinds of stuff needs to be talked about and often isn't.

I have a real hard time getting started in sex, but once I'm started I have an easy time coming. My lover loves to get started but has a hard time coming and gets real frustrated. We have trouble talking about it.

We had a wildly passionate sex life for a year and a half. When we moved in together, sexuality suddenly became an issue. It turned out our patterns were very different. My lover needs to talk, to feel intimate in conversation, to relax completely before she can feel sexual. I need to touch and to make a physical connection first before I feel relaxed enough to talk intimately. I'd reach out for her as we went into the bedroom and she'd freeze. We battled it out for months, both feeling terrible, before we figured out what was going on.

Back when I was married I used to have sex pretty often when I didn't want to, so when I moved in with Rita I did the same thing. She'd identified as a lesbian since she was a kid. Here I was with a "real live lesbian," and I wanted to live up to her expectations, or what I thought they were. Finally, after two years I started saying, "Wait a minute, I don't want to have sex now." I felt a lot better.

Because women are so deeply socialized not to be sexually assertive or to seek pleasure openly, it can be a revelation to learn with a lesbian lover how to talk freely about what you both want in sex.

When I make love with a woman, the challenge is to be honest more often; to say what I am really feeling; to explore when I'm not feeling present instead of pretending that I am; if I am spacing out, to ask what's the fear.

"We can come to lesbian sex with . . . a legacy of heterosexual role models harmful to women. Whether we have been heterosexual or not, those ideas creep in anyway."[4] We may bring to lovemaking:

- the belief that we don't like sex much and are perhaps undersexed or "frigid";
- the feeling that sex is okay but not very profound;
- the assumption that we owe it to our lovers to have sex when they want to;
- distrust of our sexual responses—the conviction that we can't orgasm in sex with a partner;
- little experience in being assertive or taking the lead in sex;
- shyness about touching ourselves in sex because we think (or we think our partner thinks) she should do it all;
- a focus on performance in lovemaking, including orgasm as a goal every time;
- emotional scars from having had our bodies used or abused sexually.

Some of us may suspect our own impulses and preferences when they seem to follow a male model. We may feel uncomfortable with lust, for instance, or with acting aggressively, having fantasies of dominance or using erotic materials. Yet these may be aspects of sexuality which we would enjoy. A dildo, for instance, is not necessarily a "penis substitute"; it gives us pleasure if we enjoy being penetrated in sex. As lesbians we have a chance to move away from male-defined sexuality, and to reclaim all the dimensions of sexuality which deepen our intimacy, pleasure and love.

Joy Schneider Kendra

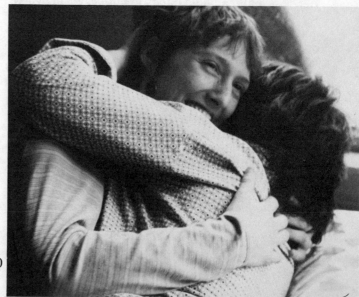

Finding time and energy for sex, if we want it, isn't always easy.

It's all there: how are you feeling about your work? How are you feeling about the people you work with? How are you feeling about the fact that the house hasn't been vacuumed in two weeks? And the fact that the car needs something done to it? Gosh, it really would be nice to have a little time for sex now and then.

I was with a group of five lesbian couples last summer, all close friends. Ten women, and we all wish we made love more frequently than we do. Does it have to do with having kids (some of us are mothers), or that the excitement has gone from the relationship, or are we taking in negative stuff from what society thinks of lesbians?

I go for long periods without feeling my erotic energy at all because it's too scary to let myself feel turned on when I have so much work to do. My fear, I guess, is that it will take me over. Sometimes I don't see how I can have room for both.

We need to feel free to be sexual, whatever form that takes for us. We are learning as women to balance what we give to others by taking time for ourselves: maybe we also have to affirm the need for taking time for sexual pleasure.

If you or you and your lover(s) have problems with sex, you may want to join a lesbian discussion group or seek counseling. (See the appendix in Chapter 11, "Sexuality.") Most important, we can probably help each other as friends more than we do now, by bringing sexual problems and issues into our conversations. "How's your sex life?" may be a timely, kind and enormously helpful question to ask.

LEGAL ISSUES

As lesbians, we struggle—along with other minority groups—for the legal rights and protections we deserve. This dilemma is compounded for poor lesbians, lesbians of color, lesbians in prisons. Most legislators, judges and lawyers in the American judicial system are white heterosexual men who exercise this society's bias against lesbians and other peoples different from themselves.

During the last twenty years there has been some improvement for lesbians in the legislatures and the courts. In some places, especially where lesbians and gay men vote as a bloc, they have won political struggles for lesbian and gay rights. Lesbians have won a small but growing number of child custody and job discrimination cases. Some judges and lawyers are becoming less biased—a few are even open lesbians.

Our increased visibility and openness help to bring these changes.

Lesbians face many legal issues beyond those which are addressed in this chapter, such as protection of the rights of lesbians in prison, legal defense after police raids of bars and public gathering places, protection from housing discrimination, recourse for lesbians committed to mental institutions by homophobic relatives. (See Resources for groups and books which may be helpful.)

Relationship Rights and Contracts

Because relationship laws are oriented toward marriage, lesbian lovers are in a legal vacuum in defining our rights and responsibilities to each other.* Lesbians today are exploring various ways of establishing and protecting our relationships.

If you are in or entering into a relationship which you think will last for some time, you and your lover can protect yourselves by working out a formal written agreement or contract about expenses, purchases, work and so on. (See Resources: *A Legal Guide for Lesbian and Gay Couples*.)

Where property is involved (unlike matters involving children), courts may well consider a notarized contract binding. However, court proceedings are painful and costly, and the outcome in lesbian and gay cases is not predictable. If you wish to separate and cannot resolve property disputes, consider couples therapy or mediation first, as they often help you to continue to treat each other more decently.

Many of us who are lesbian lawyers encourage women to agree in their contract to community arbitration, thus avoiding the sexist, homophobic legal system.

Medical Rights

In time of sickness or death, the law will automatically entrust your nearest blood relative with decisions and leave your lover powerless to choose a course of treatment or a burial site or dispose of your property. Your family may listen to your lover, but they are not obligated to do so. You and your lover can try to guarantee each other control in medical situations by giving each other power of attorney (see Resources; *A Legal Guide for Lesbian and Gay Couples*), by setting up a guardianship to take effect in case of incapacity, and/or by writing each other into your wills.

*Whether or not "marriage" is what we would want, there are some important legal and financial benefits not available to us because we can't legally marry: we can't get health insurance coverage on each other's policies, for instance, or provide for each other in sickness or death through Social Security or death and disability benefits.

Parenthood

Court proceedings are both more necessary and far less predictable in situations involving children, be they children from a heterosexual marriage which has ended, or adopted or born to us as single mothers or as lesbian partners. The court can step in at any time to do whatever it thinks is in the best interest of a minor child, even despite previous court orders or written agreements.

Custody

Some lesbians have fought successfully for custody of their children in the past few years, often with the legal and emotional backing of other lesbians. In many states now, homosexuality alone is not supposed to be used to determine one's fitness as a parent. But winning custody as a known lesbian is still difficult or impossible in many communities. (See below, "Seeking Custody," for some guidelines.)

Sharing Parenthood with a Lover

It is a good idea for two lovers who have or adopt a child (or if one lover "adopts" her partner's child) to write up a contract stating each partner's responsibilities and intentions, particularly with regard to custody and visitation rights after separation or the biological mother's death. Put provisions in each of your wills for your lover to be the child's guardian. The courts do not have to honor your contract or will, but such documents will nevertheless demonstrate a social-psychological basis for your partnership and establish your clear intent to parent together.

Artificial Insemination*

Many lesbians are turning to artificial insemination as a form of conception that doesn't require having sex with a man. Chapter 17, "New Reproductive Technologies," mentions the legal considerations which may arise, and describes insemination techniques.

MEDICAL CARE†

Perhaps the most serious health issue for lesbians is that too often we don't feel comfortable or safe seeking

*The Sperm Bank of Northern California is a program offered at the Oakland Feminist Women's Health Center, a nonprofit organization. The sperm bank features routine sperm counts and semen analysis, a donor-insemination program, donor screening, and private semen storage for men facing infertility due to cancer treatment, surgery or vasectomy. This program is accessible to all men and women regardless of marital status, sexual preference, race, income, and geographical or national residence. The phone number is (415) 444–2014.

†Particular health and medical problems as they affect lesbians appear throughout the book.

Seeking Custody

Even if you think you may want your children to live with their father, it is often wise to establish custody at first so that you can retain control over that choice. If you do not want to live with your children but would like the option of spending time with them periodically, be sure the divorce/custody agreement includes specified visitation rights. If visits are left up to the children's choice, their father may pressure them into staying away from you.

It is invaluable to have a sympathetic lawyer, even if you don't expect that your sexual orientation will be an issue in the divorce and custody negotiations. Try if at all possible to find a lawyer who accepts lesbianism, has experience in custody cases (preferably with lesbian mothers) and is known and respected by the local court. Such an ideal person is often not available, but worth looking hard for. Lesbians with limited financial resources and/or who live in nonurban areas may get some advice and assistance from the Lesbian Mothers' National Defense Fund or another lesbian organization. (See Resources.)

Prepare for a custody case with extreme care. You must demonstrate to the court as conclusively as possible that you are a competent, caring and dependable mother. A social worker may assess your mothering and present evidence at the hearing. You must seem reasonable, friendly and cooperative to the social worker no matter what you are feeling. Keep records of events which will document your concern for your children: medical and dental care, school conferences and reports, clothing and food expenditures. Record your interactions. Gather as much support from friends around you as you can during this stressful time, but if you have a lover, much as you want to, it is best not to move in together now. If things look bleak, you may think of taking your children to another state, but the recent Uniform Child Custody Act makes it difficult to escape court involvement, and an attempt to take them away will reflect unfavorably on your case. Finally, expert witnesses like child psychologists are expensive but may be essential in case the opposition brings in its own "experts."

care when we need it (until an emergency arises) because of the ignorance, antiwoman and antilesbian attitudes we encounter in most of the medical system. As a result of the women's and gay liberation movements, a few more enlightened and unprejudiced providers are available—usually nurses, occasionally physicians, most often in urban areas where large lesbian communities exist and especially in women-controlled health centers. But most of us are dependent on medical care providers who know little about our special issues, such as which sexually transmitted diseases (STDs) we are most likely to catch.

I went to the clinic hemorrhaging badly. The doctor, who knew I was a lesbian and not trying to get pregnant, insisted I was having a miscarriage.

Practitioners who don't know we are lesbian can put us into all kinds of uncomfortable situations. Gynecologists pose a special problem, with their inevitable questions about sex, "intercourse" and what kind of birth control we want. Yet if we tell them we are lesbian we may get lectures, snide remarks and voyeuristic questions. ("What do lesbians do in bed anyway?") Our lesbianism may become the focus of the visit, and our medical problems may never be seriously addressed. We also risk having our lesbianism documented in our medical records, which are supposed to be confidential but are not always kept that way.*

I would not come out in a medical situation unless there were compelling reasons to do so, because in the "patient" role I have so little power and am especially vulnerable to harassment. So I practice in advance how to maintain my privacy and still get the care I need— ways of refusing to answer offensive or unnecessary inquiries, and of asking direct, specific questions about what I need to know. For instance, if a practitioner says, "No sex for a month," I can ask whether I should avoid sexual arousal itself or just vaginal penetration. The book Lesbian Health Matters! *[see Resources] has helped me invaluably in dealing with medical visits.*

Alcoholism

Because oppression creates extra stress in our lives, and because often bars are the only public places where we can get together openly with other lesbians, a lot of lesbians drink. Drinking becomes a problem for anyone who can't control when and/or how much she drinks. If this seems true for you or a friend, please consult Chapter 3, "Alcohol, Mood-Altering Drugs and Smoking." A growing number of alcoholic support and recovery programs are willing to deal openly with lesbians, and the more progressive ones respect lovers as family members. Many chapters of Alcoholics Anonymous and Alanon have lesbian meetings. Within the lesbian community we can all become more conscious about alcoholism. We can create drug-free spaces and serve inexpensive nonalcoholic drinks at the bars to

support recovering women and others who have problems with drinking.

Lesbians and Mental Health

Almost everyone runs into times of emotional confusion, and a lesbian in this society faces extra emotional stress. We may get help by turning to friends who listen well; by being in a women's or lesbian support group,* by asking an objective third person to mediate between us and a lover, co-worker or housemate; by trying to take better care of ourselves physically. When these sources of help aren't enough, we may choose to work for a time with a trained psychotherapist.

Good therapy can be a tremendous help. *Finding* good therapy, however, is not always an easy job for any woman. Historically, psychiatry has been sexist, antihomosexual and male-dominated. Its goal for women has been that we adapt ourselves to our "role" in society. In 1973, the American Psychiatric Association removed homosexuality from its list of illnesses to be "cured," but many conservative therapists still consider it abnormal. Be wary of a therapist who sees your sexual preference as the source of your problems, and therefore fails to take your real problems seriously.

Fortunately today there are more openly lesbian therapists (mostly in urban areas so far) and more heterosexual therapists who are feminist and/or see lesbianism as a valid way of life. To find someone, check with friends, a women's center, the YWCA or in women's journals and newspapers. Sometimes it's important to see a lesbian, who will be more likely to understand your experiences from the "inside." A lesbian therapist said, however:

I don't care who my therapist sleeps with as long as she or he doesn't think sleeping with women is sick. Just because a therapist is a woman or even a lesbian doesn't mean she'd be the best one for you to work with.

In your first interview, don't hesitate to ask about the therapist's views, training and beliefs. You can ask yourself: do I feel comfortable talking to this person? Does s/he listen to me? Is the therapist willing to recognize the importance of political and social factors, like sexism and homophobia? Does s/he have a merely "tolerant" attitude toward lesbians or is s/he genuinely positive and affirming?† It's worth putting energy into finding someone you can work well with. If as the

---

*In many states you do not have a legal right to a copy of your medical records, and nowhere can you change what is in them. In some cases courts, insurance companies, researchers or other medical facilities have gained legal access to medical records.

*See *In Our Own Hands: A Women's Book of Self-Help Therapy* (Los Angeles: J. P. Tarcher, Inc., distributed by Houghton Mifflin, 1981).

†See Chapter 6, "Psychotherapy," p. 75, for general guidelines in choosing a therapist. See also *Getting Help, a Woman's Guide to Therapy*, by Elizabeth Robson and Gwenyth Edwards (New York: E. P. Dutton, 1980).

therapy progresses it feels oppressive in any way, bring this up with the therapist, and if you can't work it out together, leave.

Sometimes frightened or angry parents pressure or force a young lesbian into therapy—or, worse, into a mental institution—in hopes of changing her sexual preference. A young rural lesbian said, "My parents stopped giving me money for school when I came out to them. They said, 'We'll pay for a psychiatrist but nothing else.'" Obviously therapy in such a situation is a mockery and a punishment.

WE ARE EVERYWHERE

Lesbians *are* everywhere. In every possible ethnic group, occupation and geographical location, we are beginning to identify ourselves more openly and to discover our common issues. To conclude this chapter, lesbians in four different kinds of groups have spoken of their special experiences and concerns.

Older Lesbians

A forty-five-year-old woman in her first lesbian relationship said:

I have a whole different feeling about aging since I met Ruth. Partly it's loving her and feeling so loved and so fully known for the first time. Also, as she and other lesbians teach me about being strong, being your own person, I feel more optimistic about growing older.

A lesbian in her seventies said:

Many women have a false security. A woman will say, "I'll always have my husband to take care of me." No, she won't. There's no security for any animal, any organism in the natural world. But lesbians are accustomed to the reality of life. That keeps them flexible and more prepared for the later years. It's partly the rigidity that people nurture within themselves that makes their old age hard for them. Most lesbians don't have the luxury of being rigid.*

When asked about the disadvantages of being lesbian and old, this woman said, "You've asked the wrong person. For me there are no negative aspects to it at all."

Like most older women, lesbians resent the various stereotypes about aging. We object to the patronizing way the young often assume that we are weak and helpless. We also object to being seen as wise, serene, above the passions of youth. People generally don't want to think of older women as sexual beings; an old lesbian, with the sexual connotations of the word, is considered even more unacceptable. We are still quite human, emotionally alive and sexually active, and proud of that.

Any older woman can find herself isolated and unable to find satisfying, sustaining work. This is even more true for older lesbians, because homophobia operates in addition to ageism and sexism. Therefore, it's necessary for us to find and develop a family—if not our own, a family of friends, homosexual and heterosexual, old and young, with whom we can share, care, love and encourage. This is especially important for older lesbians who are single, have lost a lover or live in remote areas where it's hard to find support.

For some single older lesbians who feel that there isn't much time left, a scary question is "Can I ever find a lover?" It takes courage and initiative.* If a lover is considerably younger, age difference can be an issue. Some women feel that wide age differences are inappropriate ("I should act my age" or "I won't be able to keep up with her"); others feel that age doesn't matter.

Alice and I grew up in different worlds—she in the fifties and I in the twenties. So much has changed, especially for women. What she wants for her life is not what I ever wanted or expected for mine. As long as both of us notice, respect and understand these differences, we do well together. In a way, the age span is good—it makes us see that we can't be everything for each other, that we need friends our own age.

Older lesbian couples need to be prepared for some special situations. See "Legal Issues" (p. 151) for strategies to make sure that close relationships are honored in times of sickness or death. We must face the inevitability of death, and talk together about dying, loneliness and pain. See Chapter 23, "Women Growing Older," for more on this, and on taking control of our death.

An older lesbian who is out, strong, independent and unafraid, can find support from younger women who may welcome such a role model. But we also need support for our fears, dependencies and weaknesses.

It's good to mix older and younger lesbians. When younger people get together more often with older lesbians and see that they're not doddering and so on, they'll be aware that there's not that much difference, and perhaps it will make it easier for them as they grow older.

---

*Poverty, ageism and racism are probably the most significant factors in making old age hard for many women. (See Chapter 22, "Women Growing Older.")

*An unusual resource for finding a lesbian friend is The Wishing Well, Box 1328, Novato, CA 94948. This is a quarterly publication with self-descriptions (by code number) of lesbian women wishing to meet others, as well as letters, ads, resources, etc.

Lesbians of Color—Our Rich Variety

The fabric of our lives as lesbians of color is as dense as a tapestry, woven of the hundred shades and hues of our variety. It is difficult to tease out a thread and let it stand for the whole. For some of us, the brilliance of our color is the tapestry's dominant theme.

I was with two friends of mine one morning—one is Dominican and the other is from the Philippines. We were all in the bathroom getting ready for work and we each touched the others' hair. One thick, one wavy, one kinky. I kept smiling during the day when I thought about it.

Sometimes I get almost a physical charge from being black. I hear a beautiful black woman singing, and I feel like jumping up and down for joy. I think, How powerful, that's me.

The Women of Our Tradition

Our eyes are often drawn to the images of the renegade women we have known, women who haven't "fit" our culture's ideal for women—an aunt, a cousin, an old friend of the family. Often, despite their differences, these women were (and are) not cast out of their community; as part of an oppressed culture in the U.S., our friends and families may rely on each other too much not to encourage and accept anyone—regardless of gender—who is spirited. Some of us, however, draw more pain than strength from these outsiders in our culture, some of whom must have been lesbian. Although they might have lived with a sister or a friend, their lives were still seen in terms of their role within the family. Mother, father or brother had a considerable say over what they did. The silence which veiled whatever intimate relationships they enjoyed obscures our heritage as lesbians of color.

Our Particular Oppression

Homophobia, woman-hating and distortion of our self-image as women are woven into our lives and cultures. The stark fact of our oppression as lesbians and as women may not differ from what our white sisters experience. But the expression, the contradictions, the meanings and contexts may all be vastly different, both from our white sisters and among ourselves.

Coming to womanhood as a Third World woman, regardless of your sexual preference, you have to deal with certain stereotypical images of Third World women that are prevalent in this society. If you're a lesbian, it's even more difficult to struggle against these images. For a black woman, the images of the strong black woman who can carry everybody on her back or the earthy, sexy vamp are hard to fight against. Those images are unreal, con-fining and racist, to say the least. Many people expect you to fit into some preconceived idea they have about what a black woman is supposed to be. They deny whole sides of you as a woman.

I remember the sting of words like maricón *[fag] and* tortillera *[lesbian]. I began to realize these words had something to do with me. But they didn't speak for me, for my feelings as a human being. The Catholic Church had placed me in all-girl schools all my life and taught me to love others. Now it was wrong. This was a time of incredible contradictions.*

Coming out to my family meant I risked losing not only them as loved ones but a whole safety net, a barrier between me and a hostile world. It made it more frightening, but the need I had for my family made the desire to be honest more pressing as well.

Creating Ourselves

As lesbians of color, we are women moving between two or more cultures or value systems, none of which fully sees or accepts us. As Afro-American, Latin, Asian or American Indian women, we each carry within us the traditional expectation of womanhood in our culture. At the same time, we live within the greater Anglo-American society, which through its schools, mass media and political and economic systems teaches us another brand of ideal womanhood. Both images are predominantly heterosexual. We must face this denial of our love for women in a society where the color of our skin and the language of our people as well as our identity as women who love other women are all strikes against us, tools used to separate us from one another.

Our struggle to survive and grow as lesbians of color becomes the difficult task of always balancing all the elements of who we are and who we choose to become. We can explore our past and our diverse cultures and draw from each those qualities and traditions which will most enrich and strengthen our lives.

As women, and especially as Latina women, we have been programmed to be caretakers. Especially as lesbians, because we have never married, we often have to take care of everybody else, everybody else's family, everyone's needs. I'm taking care of myself now, too. I am affirming my life.

Our Experience in a White Community of Women

As lesbians we are drawn to the growing lesbian community and culture of women in this country—to bars, concerts, support and political groups. Many white sisters reading this can share the feeling of excitement we've had entering these places, where it's safe to be open in our love and care for other women.

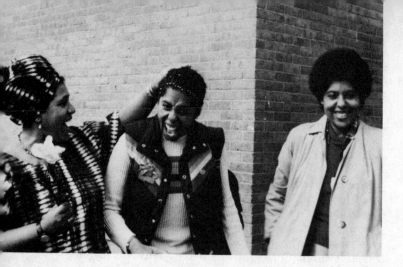

Yet there is a painful contradiction. It is in these, the places where we expect to feel most accepted and supported, that we often meet with barriers of misunderstanding and ignorance from white sisters unfamiliar with our lives and needs as women of color. Much of the structure of the women's community excludes us and makes us invisible. The language and approach are largely those of a white culture, not our own.

I was doing some volunteer legal work for a women's music-archives group. Almost all the music in the collection was by white women. I'd name women of color whose music I loved, and they kept saying their collection was "feminist." I said I questioned how they defined "feminist," since in reality it kept translating to "white."

Some people in the women's community give me a hard time about my nails—the length and color. My feelings about color and adornment are wholly different from theirs.

At a drumming concert a lot of the women began beating time (not even on the beat, mind you) on their knees. I know they wouldn't presume to sing along unless asked to with, say, Holly Near. It's a subtle thing but spoke clearly to me about a lack of respect for a culture.

Many of us feel that as soon as we stop talking with white women about our experiences as women of color or about racism, that part of us ceases to be in their eyes. It can be lonely, disheartening and infuriating. A sharing of the load is welcome.

A white friend of mine broke into a conversation I was having with two other women about racism among lesbians. She defended what I was saying. When we talked later, I said what an easing it was not to have to struggle alone. A patch on her face that turns red when she's excited blazed bright. "You shouldn't have to fight. We should do it. We should do it!" Tears came to my eyes with the relief I felt.

We need to talk, to be unafraid to confront each other about our misperceptions and our fears. The con-

versation must be not only between us and our white sisters but among ourselves as well. As members of oppressed groups, we have been divided by suspicion and ignorance about other peoples of color and even about our own. Sometimes when we look at another woman of color we see reflected in her the oppression of our culture, our language, our ways, and we experience a fear of looking at ourselves.

Whenever I saw other Asian women on the street or at a gathering, we wouldn't look at each other directly and would actually be embarrassed, as though we weren't supposed to be there. It showed me how effective racism is in destroying bonds between people.

Those of us who are or have been involved in interracial relationships and friendships are sometimes torn by the pressure to separate, by the fears that have always divided our peoples. When we talk openly with other women who are different from us, we see the common patterns of gender, class and racial oppression, and can begin to find our unity.

We are reclaiming our right to join as women and lesbians of color, celebrating our heritage and our rich tradition. At the same time, we recognize the importance of a common struggle waged by all women, particularly lesbians. We must remember that our common roots span continents, races and languages. Our conversation has just begun.

Lesbians with Physical Disabilities

Disabled lesbians are a large and growing group which the lesbian community acknowledges but doesn't yet fully embrace. We are all colors and races, all cultures, shapes, sizes and ages. Some of our disabilities are hidden, some are very visible. Some of us are born differently-abled; some of us acquire a disability suddenly and unexpectedly, or over time.

For a long time we have been isolated from each other in our dual identity as lesbians and disabled women.

From my perceptions and from other disabled dykes I've talked to, there are lots of reasons differently-abled dykes hesitate to come out as lesbians. Being someone who is physically different in appearance leaves me already open to ridicule and stares. Lesbians are attacked all the time for being different. Why choose to get hurt twice if you can avoid it? Also, people think disabled women are sexless. If I came out at work I don't know if they'd be upset or just laugh. They'd say, "How can you be a lesbian if you have no sex?"

Today more and more of us are coming out, and our networking is working. At the Michigan Women's Music Festival in the late seventies, some of us exchanged names and started a mailing list. The Disabled Lesbian Alliance (see Resources) helps us keep in touch. There is also the National Rainbow Alliance of the Deaf, for lesbians and gay men, which has chapters all over the U.S.

Loving women is sometimes part of coming to accept ourselves as women, which can be hard to do if we don't fit the description of what a woman is "supposed" to look like.

I was disabled by an accident before I became a lesbian. As a woman in a wheelchair I felt something less than a person. But my nurse, who is a lesbian, told me I could have a strong self-image. She said that we are taught to hate ourselves because we are women, and that we can love ourselves instead. I started spending time with lesbians. The closer I came to lesbianism the more I began to like myself.

Lesbians are often more accepting of us and our bodies than men are. But even lesbians often hold us at a distance.

Some women are uncomfortable just being around a disabled woman; others are comfortable with being a friend but can't consider a sexual relationship. I feel like my sexuality is taboo.

Sexually we are often stereotyped as sexless or overly needy.

When I tell people Janet is my lover they look at her like they're thinking, Poor thing! or, She must be a nurse! or, Maybe she's a pervert who gets off on sex with a disabled woman. They can't imagine that she loves me and the disability is only one thing about me.

Though it is common for those of us who spend time in institutions or hospitals or with daily attendants to have sexual relationships with our primary caretakers, it isn't necessarily a "nursing" relationship. Our lovers take care of us no more than we take care of them. We may have to make special arrangements for sex or give our lover certain information about our sexuality, but every sexual relationship in the world is shaped by both individuals' wants, needs and capabilities.

I felt weird because I had to explain what my sexual needs were to anyone I wanted to sleep with until I realized that everyone has to explain what their needs are in order to get them met. I don't have sensation in my pubic area, but since there is no set standard to what lesbian lovemaking is, it leaves a whole world of sexuality and sensuality open to explore.

Once we have accepted our dual identity, we would like to be able to live it more easily. But many people we meet have a hard time with it.

People on the street will deal with my disability sometimes, but no matter how butch I am or what buttons I have on, they won't deal with me as a lesbian.

In health care, heterosexual physicians will look at our disability but are rarely sensitive about lesbianism and thus do not see us as whole people. Feminist or lesbian health care services will welcome us as lesbians, but the facilities are usually inaccessible. We wind up most of the time being seen as either lesbian or disabled but not both.

The lesbian community is committed at a certain level to including all kinds of women. Lesbians usually look for wheelchair-accessible spaces in which to hold concerts and community events, and offer signing there for the deaf and hearing-impaired. Yet this risks being tokenism if a tremendous amount more is not done.

There's been both sensitivity and a lack thereof in this community. We can confront other lesbians about things that wouldn't even come up in the heterosexual world— like not just getting wheelchair access to concerts but being able to sit with our friends. Yet where were other lesbians when we picketed inaccessible movie houses? Our power and strength are used for lesbian issues at lesbian rallies, but few women rally for us.

It is time for the lesbian community to hear our voices. Don't segregate us from our other sisters. We all need each other.

Lesbian Mothers

When the rest of the world pretends we don't exist or tells us we can't exist, we as lesbian mothers need to say to each other, "Yes, come on and join us!"

Many of us were mothers before we knew we were lesbians. Some of us have become mothers since. Either way, being a mother is full of wonder and work. Although being a *lesbian* mother adds some unique satisfactions and special difficulties, the main issues we live with as our children grow are shared by most mothers in our society.

Our situations as lesbian mothers are varied. Some of us live with our children; some do not. Some of us are out to our children; others are not. Our support systems vary: many of us are single parents; some are co-parents; we receive very different amounts of support from friends, the child's father and/or blood relatives. Some of us live in neighborhoods where we can be relatively open about being lesbians, and others among us have to keep our lesbianism hidden from adult and child neighbors alike.

The heterosexual world of parent-teacher conferences, visits to pediatricians and birthday parties rarely recognizes that we are both lesbians and mothers. Even within the lesbian community we often feel like an invisible minority. While our need to come out of isolation and make ourselves known has sometimes brought us loss and pain, it has also created experiences of joy and understanding in support groups and in many friendships.

Coming Out

Should I tell my kids I'm a lesbian? When? When I have a lover? If she moves in? It is such a big part of my life that it feels crazy to hide it from them.

Being out or closeted with our children is a personal choice that ends up being based on the reality of each lesbian mother's life. All of us must weigh our concern for protecting our children from a society that validates only nuclear families against our need to be honest and open.

Being out to our children may bring problems. Children may feel they have to hide our lesbianism, and resent it.

If they [other kids] knew about my mom I'm afraid they wouldn't like me. Sometimes I feel like I'm in the closet, too, and I'm not even gay.

Our sons may feel that our choice of women implies a rejection of them. A seventeen-year-old remembers:

My mother told me she was gay when I was twelve. It made me feel very different from everyone else. I thought that if you were a lesbian then you didn't want boys around. My mother said that wasn't true, but about six months later I went to live with my father. Now that I'm older, I view it differently and I've also proved to myself that it didn't matter as much as I thought. I'm moving back home now.

For many of us, the rewards of coming out to our children outweigh the problems.

A lot of women in my lesbian mothers group have said that their kids were relieved to finally have it [our lesbianism] said instead of thinking it anyway and wondering why it couldn't be said.

I have been out to my daughter as long as I have been out to myself. I heard her at four telling a communal sister that girls could fall in love with girls and it was okay for boys to fall in love with boys. Where is the revolution? Sometimes it's right in our own backyards.

I think for those of us who are out to our kids, there are great results. Because we make ourselves open to our kids in this one area we are open to them in a lot of ways. We dare to be different, and sometimes it hurts to be different. That we share that with them creates a very special relationship. It also helps them understand prej-

udice. They begin to see that a kid who calls another kid some name about their religion or race is probably being as bigoted and narrow-minded as someone who calls their mother a dyke. They can make connections that many people are never able to make.

For all of us who are considering coming out to our children, finding support during this time can help us move toward a healthy, strong identity as a lesbian and a mother. Some of us think it is good for our kids to have a lesbian mother because they see the options; they do not grow up believing the world to be heterosexual; and they have, right in the family, someone who is willing to be different. The better we can feel about ourselves and our choices, the more we have to share with our kids and each other.

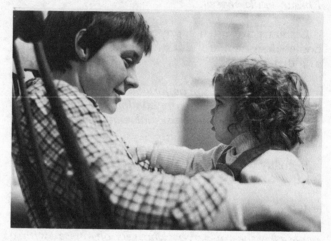

Susan Butler

Custody

Some of us have not been able to choose whether or not we will live with our children.

Having come out as a lesbian has been real difficult for me because my child was taken away by his father. I was granted visitation rights and because I didn't know to make it specific, I've gone for six months without seeing him. It takes that long sometimes for legal proceedings to work themselves out. It's amazing how the men—the fathers—get such special treatment. I mean, a battering husband is not treated the way a lesbian mother is. At the same time, though, it was being a lesbian and stepping out as a strong woman that made me able to withstand what followed.

Some of us live with the constant fear of losing our kids, and we shape our lives—coming out, jobs, lovers and living arrangements—with this in mind. Our basic right to raise our children may be challenged in the courts at any time by the father, the grandparents, relatives, neighbors or social service agencies.

However, during the past few years an increasing number of lesbians have been winning their custody battles in court. Some of us are now able to live with our children freely. Sometimes a father will win custody but sooner or later send the children back because he doesn't want the work of raising them. In addition, children who voluntarily leave may return home when they are older and clearer in identity.

It is important to recognize that *not* living with our children may be what we need or want, though in this society it can be hard to admit. Some lesbians have left their children with their fathers, which is a courageous choice since so many people believe mothers "should" keep their kids. We need to be free to make the arrangements that are the most sensible and loving all the way around.

Sometimes I feel real guilty, like a lousy mother. You know: I should be able to handle it all. I should be able to raise two kids and not be overwhelmed all the time by being a mother. On the other side of that is that I feel real good that I could be clear about the decision that my younger son would live with his father. It has worked out for all of us.

Resisting Guilt

All mothers are made to feel guilty about not being "good enough," and we may feel extra guilty if we think that our lesbianism makes our chidren's lives harder. If we are divorcing, our children express the anger and feelings of dislocation that nearly all children experience after their parents separate. We have to remember that they would be sad and angry at this time even if we weren't lesbians. All children, especially as teenagers, will have problems, because that is the nature of growing up. It is difficult to let go of the guilt because society's disapproving view of lesbians supports and reinforces it. It helps to look at our heterosexual friends: their children have nightmares, stay home "sick" from school, keep their rooms a mess, fight with their friends, get depressed, get furious at their parents, think they have the worst luck a kid has ever had—just like our kids do.

Support

So much of what we need as lesbian mothers, whether we stay with our kids or not, is the same as if we weren't lesbians.

I'm a single mother, and that's the most important factor in what makes it hard for me to be doing all that I'm trying to do.

For all of us, help from friends is one thing that makes it easier to get through a day. Co-parenting arrangements are one way some of us have worked out that support. Co-parenting can mean that women who share a living space or live near each other take some responsibility for each others' kids. It can also mean that lesbians who live together as lovers both parent the children with whom they live.

In my communal lesbian house, the other women were co-mothers to my daughter. Everyone did one night of childcare a week. Everyone also took on part of the child's rent so I didn't have to pay double.

In other cases, women haven't taken on the responsibility of co-parenting but have built stable, regular relationships with our kids and cared for them on a regular basis, such as one afternoon a week or one weekend a month. In this way we have a break we can count on, a chance to relax a little, pull ourselves together, go out with our friends or just be alone. Still another kind of support comes when groups or gatherings of women make plans for childcare so mothers aren't the only ones with responsibility for arrangements. For us, the importance of adequate childcare and reasonable locations and hours at lesbian events cannot be overestimated.

Susan D. Fleischmann

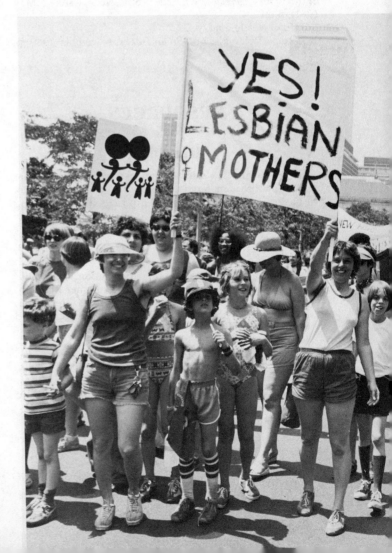

Some of us have also been part of ongoing groups where we tell about our feelings and experiences as mothers. It has helped to know that other lesbian mothers live with problems similar to ours, to realize the problems aren't "our fault," to strategize new approaches and share the daily surprises and delights we get from our kids. Here are a few things that the mothers in one group had to say about it:*

What I've always wanted for my children is a wider network of caring adults, and we're making one in this group. It's not enough just to come in and talk about being lesbian mothers; we include our kids, having parties for us all, going to the beach together....The kids must at some point look around the room and say to themselves, "All these kids have lesbian mothers," and feel less isolated....It is wonderful finding out how many lesbian mothers there are. I used to think there must be two or three in the whole city....The group is a place where neither we nor our kids have to hide any part of our lives.

NOTES

1. Joan Nestle. "Butch-Fem Relationships: Sexual Courage in the 1950s," *Heresies*, Sex Issue, Vol. 3, No. 4, Issue 12 (May 1981), p. 21.
2. Joan Nestle, *ibid*, p. 22.
3. Tacie Dejanikis, in *Off Our Backs*, November 1980, p. 25.
4. *Ibid*, p. 25.

RESOURCES

Readings

The following is a selective guide to some of the more recently published material written by and for lesbian women. We have found these books to be the most useful in discussing the many facets of our lives.

Bibliographies

Gay Task Force, American Library Association. *A Gay Bibliography*. Sixth ed., March 1980, with a summer 1981 supplement, $2.00. Write to Barbara Gittings, Box 2383, Philadelphia, PA 19103. An extensively researched and thorough compilation of books, periodicals, bibliographies, directories and films.

Grier, Barbara. *The Lesbian in Literature*. Third ed. Tallahassee, FL: Naiad Press, Inc., 1981. The most complete listing of just about everything written up to 1979. Includes over 7,000 entries and close to 100 photographs of authors.

*Women interested in forming an ongoing mothers' support group can contact the Cambridge Lesbian Mothers' Support Group, 46 Pleasant Street, Cambridge, MA 02139.

Roberts, J. R. *Black Lesbians: An Annotated Bibliography*. First ed. Tallahassee, FL: Naiad Press, Inc., 1981. A generously annotated and carefully researched guide to over 300 references to writings by and about black lesbian women.

An Overview

Allen, Paula Gunn. "Beloved Women: Lesbians in American Indian Cultures," *Conditions: Seven* (1981), pp. 67–87.

Beck, Evelyn Torton, ed. *Nice Jewish Girls: A Lesbian Anthology*. Watertown, MA: Persephone Press, 1982.

Berzon, Betty, and Robert Leighton, eds. *Positively Gay: New Approaches to Gay Life*. Millbrae, CA: Celestial Arts, 1979. A collection of topical articles dealing with coming out, relationships, lesbian mothers, older lesbians, parents of lesbians and more.

Bethel, Lorraine, and Barbara Smith, eds. *Conditions: Five, The Black Women's Issue* (Autumn 1979).

Hidalgo, Hilda, and Elia Hidalgo Christenson. "The Puerto Rican Lesbian and the Puerto Rican Community," *Journal of Homosexuality* (Winter 1976/1977).

JEB. *Eye to Eye: Portraits of Lesbians*. Washington, DC: Glad Hag Books, 1979. A lesbian photographer's portrayal of the diversity of lesbian women in the U.S.

Lewis, Sasha Gregory. *Sunday's Women: A Report on Lesbian Life Today*. Boston: Beacon Press, 1979.

Love, Barbara, and Sidney Abbot. *Sappho Was a Right On Woman: A Liberated View of Lesbianism*. New York, NY: Stein and Day, Inc., 1972. A classic. One of the first positive books written about lesbianism.

Martin, Del, and Phyllis Lyon. *Lesbian/Woman*. New York, NY: Bantam Books, 1972. One of the first affirmations of the lives of lesbian women written by the founders of the Daughters of Bilitis (DOB).

Moraga, Cherríe, and Gloria Anzaldúa, eds. *This Bridge Called My Back: Writings by Radical Women of Color*. Watertown, MA: Persephone Press, 1981. A highly recommended anthology of essays, poetry and conversations by Asian, Afro-American, Latin and American Indian women, many of whom are lesbians.

Noda, Barbara, Kitty Tsui and Z. Wong. "Coming Out: We Are Here in the Asian Community: A Dialogue with Three Asian Women," *Bridge: An Asian American Perspective*, 7 (Spring 1979).

Ramos, Juanita, and Mirtha N. Quintanales, eds. *Compañeras: Antología Lesbiana Latina/Latina Lesbian Anthology*. A collection of short stories, essays, poems, oral histories and art by Latina lesbians in both the U.S. and Latin America. Brooklyn, NY: Kitchen Table/Women of Color Press (due soon).

Rich, Adrienne. "Compulsory Heterosexuality and Lesbian Existence," *SIGNS: Journal of Women in Culture and Society*, Vol. 5, No. 4 (1980). A now classic and often cited article.

Vida, Ginny, ed. *Our Right to Love: A Lesbian Resource Book*. Englewood Cliffs, NJ: Prentice-Hall, Inc., 1978. An inclusive survey of lesbian life, including personal testimonies. A major resource produced by the National Gay Task Force.

Personal Stories

Baetz, Ruth. *Lesbian Crossroads: Personal Stories of Lesbian Struggles and Triumphs*. New York, NY: William Morrow and Co., Inc., 1980. Thematically arranged interviews with twenty-six women.

Cruikshank, Margaret, ed. *The Lesbian Path*: *Women Loving Women*. Second ed. Monterey, CA: Angel Press, 1981. Distributed by Naiad Press, Inc. Writings by thirty-seven women about their evolution as lesbians.

Stanley, Julia Penelope, and Susan J. Wolfe, eds. *The Coming Out Stories*. Watertown, MA: Persephone Press, 1980. Autobiographical accounts of the coming-out process of thirty-nine women.

Lesbian History

Cruikshank, Margaret, ed. *Lesbian Studies*: *Present and Future*. New York, NY: Feminist Press, 1982. A wonderful collection of articles about lesbians in academia, and aspects of research about our lives. An excellent resource section.

Faderman, Lillian. *Surpassing the Love of Men*: *Romantic Friendship and Love Between Women from the Renaissance to the Present*. New York, NY: William Morrow and Co., Inc., 1981. Well documented.

Katz, Jonathan. *Gay American History*: *Lesbians and Gay Men in the U.S.A.* New York, NY: Avon Books, 1976. A chronicle of lesbian and gay history in the U.S. from 1566–1976.

Schwarz, Judith. *Close Friends and Devoted Companions*: *A History of Lesbian Relationships in America*. New York, NY: William Morrow and Co., Inc. (Forthcoming as of this writing.)

Older Lesbians

Baracks, Barbara, and Kent Jarratt, eds. *Sage Writings*. (Senior Action in a Gay Environment.) New York, NY: Teachers and Writers Collaborative Publications, 1980. A collection of writings by members of the writers workshop of SAGE.

Star, Susan Leigh, guest ed. "On Being Old and Age," *Sinister Wisdom*, Issue 10 (Summer 1979).

Lesbian Youth

Wernette, Tim. "Exploring Sex with Someone of Your Own Sex," *Changing Bodies, Changing Lives*: *A Book for Teens on Sex and Relationships*. New York, NY: Random House, Inc., 1980. The voices of many lesbian and gay youths are heard in this informative chapter.

Young, Gay and Proud! U.S. edition prepared by Sasha Alyson. Boston, MA: Alyson Publications, 1980. (Order from Carrier Pigeon, 75 Kneeland Street, Room 309, Boston, MA 02111.) A supportive guide covering many concerns of lesbian and gay youths. Includes a straightforward chapter on special health concerns.

Health-Related Material

O'Donnell, Mary, et al. *Lesbian Health Matters*!: *A Resource Book about Lesbian Health*. Santa Cruz, CA: Santa Cruz Women's Health Collective, 1979. (Order from Santa Cruz Women's Health Center, 250 Locust Street, Santa Cruz, CA 95060.) An indispensible handbook. Discussions include problems of the current health care system in relation to lesbians, gynecological exams, alternative

fertilization, menopause, alcoholism and feminist therapy.

Radicalesbians Health Collective. "Lesbians and the Health Care System," *Out of the Closets*: *Voices of Gay Liberation*. Karla Jay and Allen Young, eds. New York, NY: Jove Publications, Inc./Harcourt Brace Jovanovich, Inc., 1977.

Sexuality (See also "Sexuality" chapter bibliography.)

Califia, Pat. *Sapphistry*: *The Book of Lesbian Sexuality*. Tallahassee, FL: Naiad Press, Inc., 1980. Excellent.

Corinne, Tee, Jacqueline Lapidus and Margaret Sloan-Hunter. *Yantras of Womanlove*. Tallahassee, FL: Naiad Press, Inc., 1982. Erotic photographs and text.

Karen, Jeanine, and Sue Scope. *Sapphic Touch*: *A Journal of Lesbian Erotica*, Volume 1, 1981. Pamir Productions, Box 40218, San Francisco, CA 94140. $7.00 includes postage and handling; California residents add 36¢ sales tax.

Nomadic Sisters. *Loving Women*. Sonora, CA: Nomadic Sisters, 1976.

Yarborough, Susan L. "Lesbian Celibacy," *Sinister Wisdom*, Issue 11 (fall 1979). Celibacy considered as a self-affirming choice.

Legal Guides

Boggan, E. Carrington, et al. *The Rights of Gay People*. New York, NY: American Civil Liberties Union, 1983. (Order from ACLU, 132 W. 43rd Street, New York, NY 10036.)

Curry, F. Hayden, and Denis Clifford. *A Legal Guide for Lesbian and Gay Couples*. Reading, MA: Addison-Wesley, 1981. Living-together contracts, buying real estate together, divorce and child custody, immigration, welfare and more.

Hitchens, Donna J. *Lesbian Rights Handbook*: *A Legal Guide for Lesbians*. San Francisco, CA: Lesbian Rights Project, 1982.

National Lesbian and Gay Attorney's Referral Directory. Richard Burns, ed. (Order from GLAD, 100 Boylston Street, Suite 900, Boston, MA 02116.)

Child Custody

Anti-Sexism Committee of the San Francisco Bay Area National Lawyers' Guild. *A Gay Parent's Legal Guide to Child Custody*. Second ed., 1980. (Order from San Francisco Bay Area National Lawyers' Guild, 558 Capp Street, San Francisco, CA 94110.) Includes a revised list of regional parent-support groups.

Hitchens, Donna J., and Ann G. Thomas, eds. *Lesbian Mothers and Their Children*: *An Annotated Bibliography of Legal and Psychological Materials*. San Francisco, CA: Lesbian Rights Project, 1980. An outstanding resource.

Woman-Controlled Conception

Feminist Self Insemination Group. *Self Insemination*. 1982. (Order from Full Time Distribution, Albion Yard, Building K, 17a Balfe St., London N1 9ED, England.)

Hitchens, Donna J. *Lesbians Choosing Motherhood*: *Legal Issues in Donor Insemination*. ($1.50. Lesbian Rights Project, 1370 Mission Street, San Francisco, CA 94103.) A thorough treatment of the legal implications of donor insemination. Lesbian Health Information Project, San Francisco Women's Centers. *Artificial Insemination: An Alternative Conception for the Lesbian and Gay Community*. ($2.00. SF Women's Centers, 3548 18th Street, San Francisco, CA 94110.)

Lesbian Mothers

Hanscombe, Gillian E., and Jackie Forster. *Rocking the Cradle: Lesbian Mothers—A Challenge in Family Living*. Boston: Alyson Publications, 1982.

Lorde, Audre. "Man Child: A Black Lesbian Feminist's Response," *Conditions: Four* (1979). A sensitive article about raising a son within the lesbian community; important reading for nonmothers as well.

For Family and Friends

Diamond, Liz. *The Lesbian Primer*. Second ed. Salem, MA: Women's Educational Media, 1979. (Distributed by Naiad Press, Inc.) Primarily written to dispel some classic myths about lesbian women.

Fairchild, Betty, and Nancy Hayward. *Now That You Know: What Every Parent Should Know About Homosexuality*. New York: Harvest, 1981.

Parents and Friends of Gays. *About Our Children*. (Available for 25¢ from the National Gay Task Force, 80 Fifth Avenue, New York, NY 10011.)

Media Action

Lesbian and Gay Media Advocates. *Talk Back! The Gay Person's Guide to Media Action*. Boston: Alyson Publications, 1982. (See address below.)

Recent Fiction

Please refer to Barbara Grier's bibliography, *The Lesbian in Literature*, cited at the beginning of this section, for the most comprehensive coverage. Also write to publishers, presses and bookstores for current book lists. Our list is only a taste of what is available now.

Bulkin, Elly, ed. *Lesbian Fiction: An Anthology*. Watertown, MA: Persephone Press, 1980.

Gearhart, Sally Miller. *The Wanderground: Stories of the Hill Women*. Watertown, MA: Persephone Press, 1980.

Guy, Rosa. *Ruby*. New York, NY: The Viking Press, 1976.

Hanscombe, Gillian E. *Beween Friends*. Boston, MA: Alyson Publications, 1982.

Harris, Bertha. *Lover*. Plainfield, VT: Daughters, Inc., 1976.

Ortiz Taylor, Sheila. *Faultline*. Tallahassee, FL: Naiad Press, Inc., 1980.

Rule, Jane. *Outlander*. Tallahassee, FL: Naiad Press, Inc., 1981.

Russ, Joanna. *On Strike Against God*. New York, NY: Out and Out Books, 1980.

Sarton, Mae. *Mrs. Stevens Hears the Mermaids Singing*. New York, NY: W. W. Norton and Co., Inc., 1975.

Scoppettone, Sandra. *Happy Endings Are All Alike*. New York, NY: Dell Publishing Co., Inc., 1978. (young adult novel).

Shockley, Ann. *The Black and White of It*. Tallahassee, FL: Naiad Press, 1981.

———. *Loving Her*. New York, NY: Avon Books, 1978.

Taylor, Valerie. *Prism*. Tallahassee, FL: Naiad Press, Inc., 1981.

Walker, Alice. *The Color Purple*. New York, NY: Harcourt Brace Jovanovich, Inc., 1982.

Also look for the reissues of the 1950s novels by Ann Bannon and Paula Christian. Other writers to look for: Sarah Aldrige, June Arnold, Maureen Brady, Rita Mae Brown, Jane Chambers, Rosamund Lehmann, Gail Pass and Monique Wittig.

Poetry

Bulkin, Elly, and Joan Larkin, eds. *Lesbian Poetry: An Anthology*. Watertown, MA: Persephone Press, 1981.

Because there are so many fine poets currently in print, we will list only names: Paula Gunn Allen, Gloria Anzaldúa, Robin Becker, Olga Broumas, Stephanie Byrd, Jan Clausen, Michelle Cliff, Sandra Maria Esteves, Elsa Gidlow, Judy Grahn, June Jordan, Willyce Kim, Irena Klepfisz, Joan Larkin, Audre Lord, Cherríe Moraga, Barbara Noda, Pat Parker, Adrienne Rich, Martha Shelley, Chocolate Waters, Fran Winant.

Periodicals

This list is just a representative sample of the many periodicals which are currently in print. See Clare Potter's article in Margaret Cruickshank's *Lesbian Studies: Present and Future* for a complete, up-to-date list.

Azalea. A magazine by and for Third World lesbians. Box 200, Cooper Station, New York, NY 10276.

Common Lives/Lesbian Lives. Box 1553, Iowa City, IA 52244.

Conditions. A magazine of writing by women, with an emphasis on writing by lesbians. P.O. Box 56, Van Brunt Station, Brooklyn, NY 11215.

Feminary. Lesbian feminist journal for the South. P.O. Box 954, Chapel Hill, NC 27514.

Gay Community News (GCN). The weekly for lesbians and gay males. 167 Tremont Street, Boston, MA 02111.

Lesbian Connection. c/o Helen Diner Memorial Women's Center/Ambitious Amazons, P.O. Box 811, East Lansing, MI 48823. Free to lesbians.

The Lesbian Insider/Insighter/Inciter. Box 7038, Poderhorn Station, Minneapolis, MN 55407.

Lesbian Voices. Jonnik Enterprises, P.O. Box 2066, San Jose, CA 95109.

Mom's Apple Pie. Newsletter of the Lesbian Mothers' National Defense Fund. P.O. Box 21567, Seattle, WA 98111.

SAGE Newsletter. By and for older lesbians and gay men. 487-A Hudson Street, New York, NY 10014.

Sinister Wisdom. P.O. Box 660, Amherst, MA 01004.

Publishers/Presses

Send a self-addressed stamped envelope for catalogs of publications. These publishers will also do mail-order.

Alyson Publications, P.O. Box 2783, Dept. F-12, Boston, MA 02208.

Cleis Press, 3141 Pleasant Avenue S., Minneapolis, MN 55408.

Hecuba's Daughters, Inc. "Publishers and distributors of works concerned with lesbian healing and spirituality." P.O. Box 488, Bearsville, NY 12409.

Kitchen Table/Women of Color Press, Box 592, Van Brunt Station, Brooklyn, NY 11215.

Naiad Press, Inc., P.O. Box 10543, Tallahassee, FL 32302.

Out and Out Books, 476 Second Street, Brooklyn, NY 11215.

Spinsters, Ink, R.D.1, Argyle, NY 12809.

Womyn's Braille Press, Box 8475, Minneapolis, MN 55408. Feminist and lesbian material is made available to sight-impaired women via cassette tapes, large-print formats and braille.

Bookstores

Write for current book lists. These businesses will do mail-order.

Glad Day Book Shop, 43 Winter Street, Boston, MA 02108.

Old Wives' Tales, 1009 Valencia Street, San Francisco, CA 94110.

Oscar Wilde Memorial Bookshop, 15 Christopher Street, New York, NY 10014.

Sister Moon Feminist Bookstore, 2128 E. Locust Street, Milwaukee, WI 53211.

Womanbooks, 201 W. 92 Street, New York, NY 10025.

A Woman's Place, 4015 Broadway, Oakland, CA 94611.

Archives/Special Collections/Information Clearinghouses

This list is a sampling, as more regional archives are being established.

Lesbian-Feminist Study Clearinghouse, Women's Studies Program, 1012 Cathedral of Learning, University of Pittsburgh, Pittsburgh, PA 15260. This is an important resource which exists to support research. They make unpublished manuscripts, out-of-print journal articles, etc., available to individuals and groups. Write for their informative brochure.

Lesbian Herstory Archives, P.O. Box 1258, New York, NY 10001. This is an extensive collection of material about lesbian lives. Write for information about the archives and subscribe to the newsletter, which is an invaluable source of information about their holdings.

West Coast Lesbian Collections, Box 23753, Oakland, CA 94623. The West Coast counterpart to the LHA cited above.

Women's Collection—Special Collections Dept., Northwestern University Library, Evanston, IL 60201. Extensive holdings of lesbian periodicals, posters and records.

Guides to Meeting Places/Businesses/Resorts

Gaia's Guide. Sandy Horne, ed., Eighth ed. 115 New Montgomery Street, San Francisco, CA 94105.

Gayellow Pages. Frances Green, ed. (National edition and five regional editions.) Renaissance House, Box 292 Village Station, New York, NY 10014.

Places of Interest to Women: The Women's Guide: USA & Canada. Ferrari Publications, P.O. Box 16054, Phoenix, AZ 85011.

National Organization

National Gay Task Force (NGTF), 80 Fifth Avenue, New York, NY 10011, (212)741–5800. Write for referrals and publication lists.

Specialized Organizations

Support for Physically Challenged Women

Disabled Lesbian Alliance (DLA), Room 229, 5 University Place, New York, NY 10003.

Lesbian Illness Support Group. For information write Nancy Johnson, P.O. Box 1258, New York, NY 10001.

Rainbow Alliance of the Deaf, 3007 Park Way, Cheverly, MD 20785.

Support for Parents and Friends

Federation of Parents and Friends of Lesbians and Gays, Box 24565, Los Angeles, CA 90024. Inquire for regional groups' whereabouts.

Legal Aid

ACLU-Gay Rights Project, 633 S. Shatto Place, Los Angeles, CA 90005, (213) 466-6739.

Custody Action for Lesbian Mothers, 225 Haverford Avenue, Narbeth, PA 19072.

Lambda Legal Defense and Education Fund (LLDEF), 132 W. 43rd Street, New York, NY 10036, (212) 944-9488.

Lesbian Mothers' National Defense Fund, P.O. Box 21567, Seattle, WA 98112.

Lesbian Rights Project, 1370 Mission St., San Francisco, CA 94103.

Alcoholism

Alcoholics Anonymous (Gay AA groups). Write for a referral to a local group to General Services Office, Alcoholics Anonymous, P.O. Box 459, Grand Central Station, New York, NY 10007.

National Association of Gay Alcoholism Professionals (NA-GAP), P.O. Box 376, Oakland, NJ 07436. Will provide a list of programs specializing in the treatment of gay and lesbian alcoholics.

Older Lesbians

SAGE (Senior Action in a Gay Environment), 487A Hudson Street, New York, NY 10014.

Audiovisual Materials

In the Best Interests of the Children. A 16mm film. Iris Films, Box 5353, Berkeley, CA 94705. A sensitively presented film about eight lesbian mothers and their children.

Straight Talk About Lesbians. A slide/tape presentation. Produced by Liz Diamond. Contact Women's Educational Media, 36 Colwell Avenue, Brighton, MA 02135.

Pink Triangles. Cambridge Documentary Films, P.O. Box 385, Cambridge, MA 02139. Excellent film about lesbian and gay oppression; good consciousness raiser for schools and community groups.

Woman-loving Women. A slide/tape presentation. Produced by Patricia A. Gozemba and Marilyn Humphries. Contact Lavender Horizons P.O. Box 806, Marblehead, MA 01945.

11

SEXUALITY

By Wendy Sanford, with Nancy P. Hawley and Elizabeth McGee

With special thanks to Paula Brown Doress, Jane Pincus, Janice Irvine, Bonnie Engelhardt, Shere Hite, and the women of Boston Self-Help, including Frances Deloatch, Mary Fitzgerald, Jean Gillespie, Oce, Rosemarie Ouilette, Marsha Saxton, Janna Zwerner and Joan Lastovica

This chapter in previous editions was written by Jenny Mansbridge, Ginger Goldman, Nancy London, Nancy Hawley, Elizabeth McGee and Wendy Sanford.

Our powers to express ourselves sexually last a lifetime—from birth to death. Whether or not we are in a sexual relationship with another person, we can explore our fantasies, feel good in our bodies, appreciate sensual pleasures, learn what turns us on, give ourselves sexual pleasure through masturbation. Taught to be embarrassed or ashamed of our sexual feelings, we have spent a lot of energy denying them or feeling guilty. We are learning to experience our sexuality without judging it and to accept it as part of ourselves.

We are all sexual—young, old, married, single, with or without physical disability, sexually active or not, heterosexual or lesbian. As we change, our sexuality changes. Learning about sex is a lifelong process.

When we have relationships with other people, sexuality is pleasure we want to give and get, communication that is fun and playful, serious and passionate. It can be a tender reaching out or an intense and compelling force which takes us over. It can get us into situations that delight us and ones we wish we could get out of. Sex can open us to new levels of loving and knowing with someone we love and trust. It can be a source of vital energy. Misused, it can hurt us tremendously.

At times, sexual awareness and desires are quiet and other parts of our lives take center stage. Then, after a month or a year or ten years, the sexual tide may come flowing in.

While the majority of women currently explore sexuality in relationships with men, many (at least 10 percent) do so with women. We are glad to begin to do justice to the range of possibilities of women's sexuality by including the experiences of lesbian and bisexual women in this chapter. In doing this we know we may make some readers uncomfortable, because many people still misunderstand and fear woman-to-woman sexual intimacy. Our aim here is to affirm and support *all* women's choices of whom to love, and to invite you to understand and enjoy your own sexuality more fully.

Social Influences

Society shapes and limits our experiences of sexuality. We learn, for instance, that if our looks don't conform to the ideal—if we are fat, old or disabled—then we have no "right" to be sexual. If we are women of color, stereotypes often picture us as being more sexually available and active than we are or want to be.

The so-called "sexual revolution" has had mixed results. While it did encourage people to be less restricted about sex, it has also made many women feel we *ought* to be available to men at all times. And the double standard still prevails. Women are not really "free," sexually or otherwise, as long as we remain socially and economically unequal to men. (A dramatic example of this is the way men continue to use sexual violence as a weapon against women.)

Finally, nowhere in the world have women had full access to services crucial to our enjoyment of sex— sex education, protection from unwanted pregnancy and sexually transmitted disease, abortion when we need it. Current efforts by conservative political groups threaten to limit our access even further, in an attempt to squeeze *all* our sexuality back into the confines of marriage and motherhood.

Breaking the Silence

When the women's movement surfaced again in the late sixties, women began speaking in small groups about sexual experiences and feelings. Talking more openly about sex with our friends or in small groups is not always easy at first, and shyness comes and goes, but we have much to learn from each other. Such discussions can be funny, painful and healing. We can affirm each other's feelings, help each other challenge society's distortions of our sexuality, encourage each other in our sexual adventures and learn together to be more assertive about our own sexual needs and desires.

Over the past fifteen years, we have begun to redefine women's sexuality according to our own experiences and not what male "experts" have imagined. Wanting to do more than merely react to sexist patterns that we don't like, we ask: what do *we* want? What images, fantasies, practices unlock the powerful erotic forces within us? We are delving deep into our own sexual imaginations and our satisfying sexual experiences with men and/or women for a fuller vision of what sex can be. We are working for a society free of male/female inequalities, sexual violence, homophobia and media misuse of sex, so that our sexuality can be a source of refreshment, play, passion, connection and energy.

GROWING UP

I watch my daughter. From morning to night her body is her home. She lives in it and with it. When she runs around the kitchen she uses all of herself. Every muscle in her body moves when she laughs, when she cries. When she rubs her vulva, there is no awkwardness, no feeling that what she is doing is wrong. She feels pleasure and expresses it without hesitation. She knows when she wants to be touched and when she wants to be left alone. It's so hard to get back that sense of body as home.

Ann Popkin

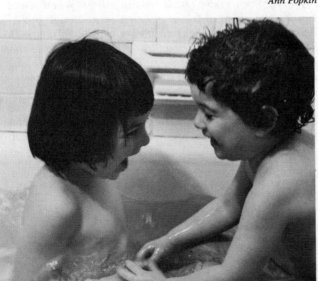

Childhood experiences and memories shape our sexuality. It is most helpful, but rare, for our families to talk comfortably about sex. From the embarrassment, what *isn't* said, the "don'ts" that come as our fingers start to explore vulva, vagina and clitoris, we learn to think of sex as forbidden, dirty and shameful.

When we become teenagers our developing bodies are usually a mystery to us.* We discover that what the media, and most people, consider beautiful falls into a narrow range. We lose respect for our uniqueness, our own smells and shapes. We judge ourselves in relation to others. We come to feel isolated ("Could anyone else be as ugly, dull, miserable as I?"). An ad for sanitary napkins reinforces our aloneness and shame: "When you have your period, you should be the only one who knows."

It takes time—sometimes years and years—and positive experiences to get rid of these shameful, negative feelings. Many of us with young children want to help them grow up feeling good about their bodies and their sexuality, though sometimes it is hard to move beyond our own upbringing.

The other day I was taking a bath with my almost-three-year-old daughter. I was lying down and she was sitting between my legs, which were spread apart. She said, "Mommy, you don't have a penis." I said, "That's right, men have penises and women have clitorises." All calm and fine—then, "Mommy, where is your clitoris?" Okay, now what was I going to do? I took a deep breath (for courage or something), tried not to blush, spread my vulva apart and showed her my clitoris. It didn't feel so bad. "Do you want to see yours?" I asked. "Yes." That was quite a trick to get her to look over her fat stomach and see hers, especially when she started laughing as I first put my finger and then hers on her clitoris.

Thanks in part to the women's movement, many of us with grown children and grandchildren talk with them more freely about sex now than we once would have. "Growing up" sexually never ends.

FANTASIES

Sometimes when I'm making love with myself or someone else, I think about the ocean roar and feel the waves swirling about me. Perhaps this means that I'd rather be floating in the sea than be in my bed. But it's also a way of heightening the experience for me. The fantasy makes me feel loose, easy, fluid. It makes me more relaxed. I usually have the fantasy just before orgasm, and it helps me let go.

*See Resources: *Changing Bodies, Changing Lives: A Book for Teens on Sex and Relationships,* for lots more on teenagers' experiences.

Today as I stretched out before my run, I closed my eyes and imagined my lover's naked body floating a few inches above me. I could feel her breasts on my face and in my mouth, our bodies reaching out, drawing close and then wrapped together. The images and feelings sailed me through an hour of strong running.

A fantasy before I made love to a plumber I know: I was entertaining myself one night by imagining I was dancing with a stillson wrench (the most enormous wrench I ever saw, very businesslike!), and it turned into the plumber. He said, "Well, men are still good for something!" We were fixing the pipe while we were dancing, and the scene changed. We were swimming in a sea of rubber doughnuts (the connector between the tank and the bottom parts of the toilet), and the doughnuts got stuck over our arms and legs. The scene changed again, to the beach, where we fell asleep.

I used to have a fantasy that I was a gym teacher and I had a classful of girls standing in front of me, nude. I went up and down the rows feeling all their breasts and getting a lot of pleasure out of it. When I first had this fantasy at thirteen I was ashamed. I thought something was wrong with me. Now I can enjoy it, because I feel it's okay to enjoy other women's bodies.

I had the fantasy of making love with two men at once. I pictured myself sandwiched between them. I acted on this one, with an old friend and a casual friend who both liked the idea. It was fun.

Nearly everyone has fantasies, in the form of fleeting images or detailed stories. They express depths within us to learn about and explore. In fantasy we can be whatever we imagine. Yet it can be difficult to accept sexual fantasies.

I was scared they would take me by surprise, tell me things about myself that I didn't know, especially bad things.

I imagined I was sitting in a room. The walls were all white. There was nothing in it, and I was naked. There was a large window at one end, and anyone who wanted to could look in and see me. There was no place to hide. There was something arousing about being so exposed. I masturbated while having this fantasy, and afterward I felt very sad. I thought I must be so sick, so distorted inside, if this image of myself could give me such intense sexual pleasure.

We have been brought up to think that sex should be "one way." We often decide we are bad or sick for imagining something different, or feel disloyal when we fantasize about someone other than the man or woman we are with. Yet our fantasies treat us to *all kinds* of erotic experiences. It takes a while to learn that this is okay, and that we can enjoy these stories and images without having to act on them.

What about rape fantasies? Some people say that if we fantasize about having sex forced on us, that means we "want" to be raped. This is untrue: totally unlike actual rape, fantasizing about rape is voluntary, and does not bring us physical pain or violation. For those of us who grew up learning that "good girls" don't want sex, a fantasy of being forced to have sex frees us of responsibility and can be highly erotic. It can allow us the feeling of being desired uncontrollably.

In one of my juiciest fantasies a woman and a man tie me up and make love to me and to each other. There is something extremely erotic in imagining being that powerless. In real life my lover and I do at times feel totally vulnerable to what the other does or wants. This fantasy lets me play around with the power dynamics that are sometimes so intense between us.

We may distrust fantasies which seem to play into male pornographic images of women as submissive or masochistic, and imagine that in a less sexist future fantasies of dominance would come to us less often. Yet this is difficult to predict. For now it seems important to accept that all kinds of fantasies may be erotic for us and free up our vital sexual energies.*

SEX WITH OURSELVES: MASTURBATION

Masturbation is a special way of enjoying ourselves.

As infants, touching and playing with our bodies, sometimes our genitals, felt good. Then many of us learned from our parents, and later from our schools and churches, that we were not to touch ourselves sexually. Some of us heeded their messages and some did not. But by the time we were teenagers most of us thought masturbation was bad, whether we did it or not. We felt guilty if we did masturbate, or we "forgot" it, or never discovered masturbation at all.

I never even knew about masturbation. When I was twenty-one, a man-friend touched me "down there," bringing me to orgasm (I didn't know that word either). Then I had a brilliant thought—if he could do it to me, I could do it to me, too. So I did, though it was a long time before I could feel a lot of pleasure and orgasm.

Masturbation allows us the time and space to explore and experiment with our own bodies. We can learn what fantasies turn us on, the kinds of touch

*If you repeatedly have fantasies which disturb or scare you, they may be a sign that you need help. Talk about them with a friend whom you trust to be wise and emphathetic, or a trained counselor or therapist.

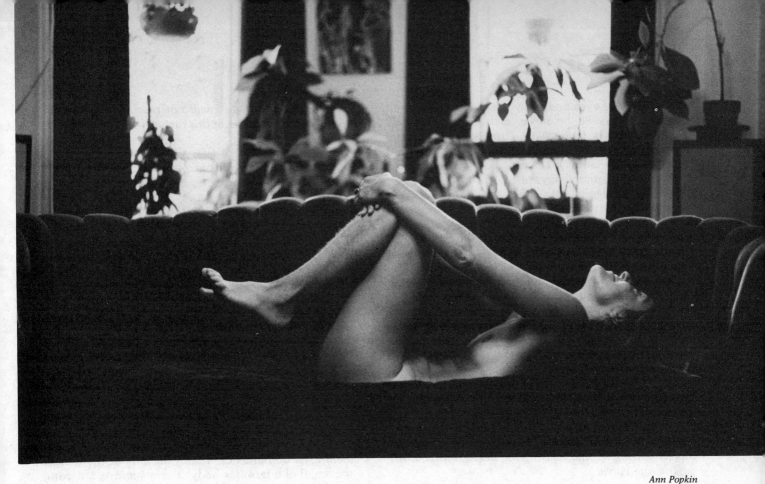

Ann Popkin

which arouse and please us, what tempo and where. We can learn our own patterns of sexual response without having to think about a partner's needs and opinions. Then, if and when we choose, we can tell our partners what we've learned or show them by guiding their hands to the places we want touched. As women, who have for so long been taught to "wait for a man to turn us on," knowing how to give ourselves sexual pleasure brings us freedom.

I used to think masturbating was okay only if I didn't have a lover, and only for a quick release. Now I see it's part of my relationship with myself, giving myself pleasure. My rhythms change. Sometimes I masturbate more when I have a lover. Sometimes I'll go for weeks without doing it.

For me at seventy-three, masturbation is better than a sexual relationship, as most of the time I'm more interested in non-sexual pursuits. Sustaining a relationship with all the time and thought involved would be a nuisance.

We can enter a sexual relationship knowing more about what we want. We aren't totally dependent on our partners to satisfy us, which can be a freedom for them, too. After menopause, masturbating also helps us avoid the drying up of vaginal tissues which can come with age.

Not everyone enjoys masturbating.

I have tried masturbating because I learned about it, not out of natural desire. Sometimes it seems like a chore. I feel like I should take the time to explore my body but I quit after a few minutes because, quite frankly, I'm bored. It just doesn't seem to have the effect another person would.

If masturbating doesn't bring you pleasure, trust your own preferences and don't do it.

Learning to Masturbate*

If you have never masturbated and want to, we invite you to try. You may feel awkward, self-conscious, even a bit scared at first. You may have to contend with voices within you that repeat, "Nice girls don't..." or "A happily married woman wouldn't want to..." You may fear losing control of yourself or you may feel shy or guilty about giving yourself sexual pleasure. Many of us have these feelings, but they change in time.

Some suggestions: find a quiet time when you can be by yourself without interruption. Make yourself as comfortable as possible: you are expecting a lover, and that lover is you! Take a relaxing bath or shower. Rub your body all over with cream, lotion, oil or anything else that feels good. Slowly explore the shape of your

*See *The Hite Report* for many examples of how women masturbate; see also *For Yourself: The Fulfillment of Female Sexuality* and *Liberating Masturbation: A Meditation on Self-Love* (listed in Resources).

167

body with your eyes and your hands. Touch yourself in different ways. Put on music you like, keep the lights soft, light a candle if you want. Think about the people or situations you find sexually arousing. Let your mind flow freely into fantasy. Let your body relax.*

Women have many ways of masturbating. We can moisten our fingers (with either saliva or fluid from the vagina) and rub them around and over the clitoris. We can gently rub or pull the clitoris itself; we can rub the hood or a larger area around the clitoris. We can use one finger or several. We can rub up and down and around and around, and try different kinds of pressure and timing. Some of us masturbate by crossing our legs and exerting steady and rhythmic pressure on the whole genital area. We may insert something into the vagina—a finger, peeled cucumber, dildo. We may rub our breasts or other parts of our bodies. Some of us have learned to develop muscular tension throughout our bodies.

At sixteen I gave up masturbation for Lent. Since I defined masturbation only as touching my genitals in a sexual way, in those six weeks I learned that I could have wonderful orgasms through a mixture of fantasy and quietly tensing up and relaxing the muscles around my vagina and vulva.

Still other ways of masturbating include using a pillow instead of our hands, a stream of water, an electric vibrator.†

I can direct our shower nozzle so the water hits my clitoris in a steady stream. I have a real relationship with that shower! I wouldn't give it up for anything! It's nice when I get up for work and don't have time for sex with my lover but do have a little time for the shower. Those few minutes are real important for me.

As you get sexually aroused, your vagina will become moist. Experiment with what you can do to feel even more. Open your mouth, breathe faster, make noise if you want or move your pelvis rhythmically to your breathing and voice.

As you are getting more aroused you may feel your muscles tighten. Your pelvic area will feel warm and full.

For me the most pleasurable part is just before orgasm. I feel I am no longer consciously controlling my body. I

know there is no way I will not *reach orgasm now. I stop trying. I like to savor this rare moment of true letting go!*

It's this letting go of control that enables us to have orgasms. If you do not reach orgasm when you first try masturbating, don't worry. Simply enjoy the sensations you have. Try again some other time.

Masturbating opens me to what is happening in my body and makes me feel good about myself. I like following the impulse of the moment. Sometimes I have many orgasms, sometimes I don't have any. The greatest source of pleasure is to be able to do whatever feels good to me at that particular time. I rarely have such complete freedom in other aspects of my life.

PHYSICAL ASPECTS OF OUR SEXUALITY

Sounds, sights, smells and touch can arouse our sexual feeling, as do fantasies, a baby sucking at the breast, the smell of a familiar body, a sexy picture, a dream, touching our own bodies, a lover's breathing in our ear, brushing against someone or hearing the person we love say, "I love you."

When I'm feeling turned on, either alone or with someone I'm attracted to, my heart beats faster, my face gets red, my eyes are bright. My whole vulva feels wet and full. My breasts hum. When I'm standing up I feel a rush of weakness in my thighs. When I'm lying down I may feel like doing a big stretch, arching my back, feeling the sensations go out to my fingers and toes.

No matter what arouses our sexual feelings or how we express them, if we continue to receive sexual stimulation our bodies go through a series of physical changes, sometimes called "sexual response." While these changes may feel different each time, they follow certain basic patterns which are helpful to know about.*

Early on in sexual excitement, veins in the pelvis, vulva and clitoris begin to dilate (open) and fill with blood, gradually making the whole area feel full. (This is called *vasocongestion*.) In the vagina this swelling creates a "sweating" reaction, producing the fluid

---

*Such a relaxed and special atmosphere isn't always possible—or necessary! Desire can overtake us at the most unexpected moments. We can find ourselves sexually aroused and masturbate while cooking a meal, traveling on a bus, working at a desk, riding a horse or bicycle, climbing a tree.

†Vibrators are sold at many drug and department stores, often as body or neck massagers. For mail-order catalogs, see Eve's Garden or *Good Vibrations Catalog* in Resources.

*The following description comes primarily from the groundbreaking laboratory research of William Masters and Virginia Johnson in the 1960s, with a number of modifications in response to more recent findings and especially to women's criticisms and additions to the Masters and Johnson model. For more details, see "Sexual Arousal and Orgasm" in the appendix to this chapter.

which makes the vaginal lips get wet—often an early sign that we are sexually excited. At the same time, sexual tension rises throughout the body as muscles begin to tense up or contract (*myotonia*). We may breathe more quickly, nipples may become erect and hard, the whole body feels alive to touch.

Orgasm

Enough stimulation of or around the clitoris and (for some women) pressure on the cervix or other sensitive areas cause pelvic fullness and body tension to build up to a peak. Orgasm is the point at which all the tension is suddenly released in a series of involuntary and pleasurable muscular contractions which expel blood from the pelvic tissues. We may feel contractions in the vagina, uterus and rectum. Some women describe orgasms without contractions.

Orgasm can be mild like a hiccup, a sneeze, a ripple or a peaceful sigh; it can be a sensuous experience, as the body glows with warmth; it can be intense or ecstatic, as we lose awareness of ourselves for a time.

Orgasm may feel different with a finger, penis, dildo or vibrator in your vagina, and different when you masturbate from when you make love with another person. It may feel totally different at different times even with the same person.

Often we become aroused at times when we can't get additional stimulation and reach orgasm. Although sexual tension subsides eventually without orgasm, it takes longer. When we get sufficiently aroused and don't have an orgasm, our genitals and/or uterus may ache for a while.

Quite a number of women have never had an orgasm. With all the publicity about orgasms in the past ten years, many of us who don't orgasm* believe we're missing something pleasurable. We can try to orgasm by masturbating, reading books about it,† asking a partner to help, joining what is sometimes called a "preorgasmic women's group." A fifty-three-year-old woman wrote to our collective that after reading an earlier edition of this book she had masturbated and reached orgasm for the first time in her life. Yet it's important that orgasm doesn't become one more "performance" pressure.

When I try too hard to have an orgasm it usually doesn't work and I end up frustrated and bored. For me it's best if I relax and let it happen if it's going to.

---

*Writer/researcher Shere Hite suggests we use orgasm as a verb, to highlight the fact that it is something women *do* and not just something which happens *to* us. We have decided to use it occasionally, along with other more familiar forms.

†See Dodson, Barbach and Hite books in Resources.

Some women can orgasm twice or more in quick succession (which men cannot do). Knowing that "multiple orgasms" are possible has made some of us feel we "ought" to have them, that we are sexually inadequate if we don't. Men may expect it, too; one woman wrote that a man she knew was considering a divorce because the woman he was married to didn't have multiple orgasms. Yet one orgasm can be plenty, and sometimes sex without orgasm is pleasurable. Seek whatever feels best to *you*.

The Role of the Clitoris

It may be arousing to stroke any part of our bodies, exciting to have our thighs caressed or our necks nibbled or our breasts sucked. However, the clitoris—the organ that is the most sensitive to stimulation—has a central role in elevating feelings of sexual tension.

Until the mid-1960s, most women didn't know how crucial the clitoris was. Even if we knew it for ourselves, nobody talked about it. Medical texts and marriage manuals (written by men) followed Freud's famous pronouncement that the "mature" woman has orgasms only when her vagina, not her clitoris, is stimulated. This theory made the penis very important to a woman's sexual satisfaction (what brought a *man* sexual release supposedly satisfied women, too). Following Freud, psychoanalytic theories belittled women's enjoyment of masturbation as "immature," and labeled lesbian sex as a pale imitation of the "real thing." In the sixties, sex researchers found that for women *all* orgasms depend at least in part on clitoral stimulation, although some women respond to internal pressure as well.

Learning about the clitoris increased sexual enjoyment for countless women and freed many of us from years of thinking we were "frigid." Our ability to give ourselves orgasms and to show our lovers how to please us has been one of the cornerstones of a new self-respect and autonomy, and has therefore been politically as well as personally important for women.

The clitoris is sometimes called the "joy button," which implies that it is one small spot. In fact, the clitoris has several parts to it. The glans (or tip, the part you can see) attaches to the shaft, which runs along internally from the glans toward the vaginal opening. The clitoris connects to a branching interior system of erectile tissue that runs through your genital area. (Erectile tissue responds to sexual arousal by filling with blood, becoming erect and hard. A penis also contains erectile tissue.) During sexual excitement, the clitoris swells and changes position. (See Chapter 12, "Anatomy and Physiology of Sexuality and Reproduction," for a fuller description of the clitoris.)

You or your lover can stimulate your clitoris in many different ways—by rubbing, sucking, body pressure, using a vibrator. Any rubbing or pressure in the pubic hair-covered mons area or the lips (even on the lower abdomen and inner thighs) can move the clitoris, and may also press it up against the pubic bone. Although some women touch the glans to become aroused, it is often so sensitive that direct touching hurts, even with lubrication. Also, focusing directly on the clitoris for a long time may cause the pleasurable sensations to disappear. As women grow older the hood of skin cov-

ering the clitoris may pull back permanently, so that if you are past menopause you may need lots of extra lubrication in order to tolerate having your clitoris rubbed.

Vagina-to-penis intercourse gives only indirect clitoral stimulation. As the penis moves in and out of the vagina it moves the inner lips which are connected to the clitoral hood, and therefore may move the hood

SEXUALITY

MAJOR AREAS OF CHANGE DURING SEXUAL AROUSAL AND ORGASM
(The dotted lines indicate most of the changes that take place. See the illustration below.)
●The blood vessels through the whole pelvic area swell, causing "engorgement" and creating a feeling of fullness and sexual sensitivity. (The blood vessels in this drawing actually represent only a fraction of what's there.)
●The clitoris (glans, shaft and crura) swells and becomes erect.
●The inner lips swell and change shape.
●The urethral sponge and the bulbs of the vestibule enlarge.
●The vagina balloons upward.
●The uterus shifts position.
Please see the diagrams in the Anatomy chapter for other views.

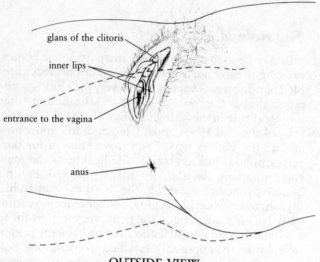

- glans of the clitoris
- inner lips
- entrance to the vagina
- anus

OUTSIDE VIEW

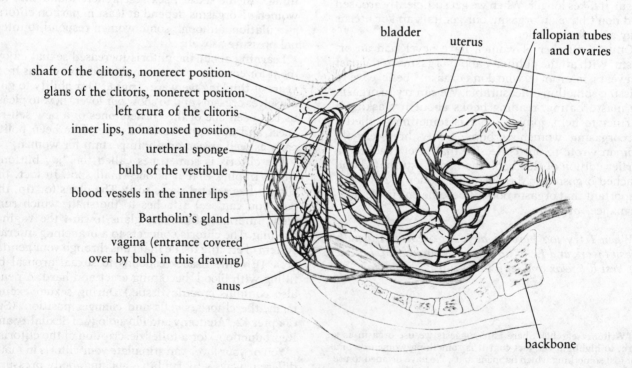

- shaft of the clitoris, nonerect position
- glans of the clitoris, nonerect position
- left crura of the clitoris
- inner lips, nonaroused position
- urethral sponge
- bulb of the vestibule
- blood vessels in the inner lips
- Bartholin's gland
- vagina (entrance covered over by bulb in this drawing)
- anus

- bladder
- uterus
- fallopian tubes and ovaries
- backbone

INSIDE VIEW

Christine Bondante

back and forth over the glans. When the inner lips become swollen and firm they can act as an extension of the vagina, hugging the penis as it moves back and forth and further increasing clitoral friction.* To reach orgasm during vagina-to-penis intercourse, many of us need *direct* and sometimes prolonged clitoral stimulation both before and during intercourse.

Many women making love to other women focus less exclusively on vaginal penetration and give more (and longer) stimulation to the clitoris. Many women who make love with men in their sixties and older (when erections happen less frequently) find that sexual pleasure increases, partly because penetration by the penis is no longer the focus of lovemaking. As more women begin to explore lovemaking beyond vagina-to-penis intercourse, it's likely that more of us will orgasm more often with our partners.

The Role of the Vagina, Uterus and Cervix

Women have the potential to respond to sexual arousal throughout the entire pelvic region. When we are aroused, the erectile tissue around the outer third of the vagina becomes full, and nerves in that area become more sensitive to stimulation and pressure. When the muscles around this part of the vagina (pubococcygeus muscles) are strong and well exercised, many women find they orgasm more easily. (See Kegel Exercises, p. 333.) Childbearing increases the venous system in the pelvis, often making arousal quicker and stronger.

Two researchers have recently identified what they call the "Grafenberg spot" ("G-spot"), a sensitive area just behind the front wall of the vagina between the back of the pubic bone and the cervix. They say that when this spot is stimulated during sex through vaginal penetration of some kind, some women orgasm with a gush of fluid from the urethra which is not urine. This is at present a controversial theory among sex researchers. It's a relief for those women who feel a urethral gushing of liquid during orgasm to find an explanation for this apparent "ejaculation," and for some others to find what may be another source of pleasure. However, if a G-spot orgasm becomes a new "ideal" for the sexually liberated woman, or is used to reinstate so-called "vaginal" orgasms as superior, it will become a new source of pressure, making us feel inadequate or unaccepting of our own sexual experiences.

Further up in the vagina, the cervix and uterus are crucial to orgasm for a number of women. While the inner two-thirds of the vagina and the cervix itself have little sensitivity, a penis, finger or dildo pressing repeatedly on the cervix "jostles" the uterus and indeed the whole lining of the abdominal cavity (peritoneum). This can create a different kind of feeling internally before and during orgasm. If you have had a hysterectomy you may have to learn to focus on different kinds of sexual stimulation and feelings, because the cervix and uterus are no longer there.*

Who Defines Orgasm? The Politics of the Great Orgasm Debate

Although Masters and Johnson asserted that all orgasms are physiologically the same (clitorally induced, with contractions occurring primarily in the outer third of the vagina), women today are speaking up about orgasms which don't "fit" the Masters and Johnson model. For example, one such orgasm is brought on by penetration of the vagina, and feels "deep," or "uterine." The build-up sometimes involves a prolonged involuntary holding in of the breath, which is released explosively at orgasm. No contractions seem to be involved.

It's not surprising that women experience a range of orgasms. But a new debate is stirring among sexologists, researchers and feminists as to how many "types" of orgasm there are and which kind is better or stronger or more satisfying. The danger is that people will once again set up one kind of orgasm as the norm, just as the "vaginal" orgasm was for so many decades.

The debate on women's sexuality has become increasingly professionalized: a number of researchers, many of them women, have claimed this as their field of "expertise," wielding studies, scientific language and statistics to make their points. We are wary of these new "experts." Are they trying to tame our sexuality by making it respectable? To make themselves a professional reputation? Might male or male-oriented researchers, threatened by women's new sexual autonomy and assertiveness, have a bias toward reasserting women's dependence on men for sexual satisfaction? In modern society professionals have enormous power to shape our understanding of ourselves. Much so-called scientific debate ends up defining women for society's purposes rather than enabling us to arrive at our own chosen development. Women doing sex research must constantly ask what people are going to do with the results, and whether their efforts may be used against women in a society where women do not have adequate social or political power.

It is crucial that women have accurate information about our sexuality, and some form of research is nec-

---

*Some feminists criticize this Masters and Johnson theory as an attempt to justify penis-in-vagina intercourse as the norm for lovemaking. See, for example, *The Hite Report*, p. 247.

*See "Sexual Response after Hysterectomy-oophorectomy: Recent Studies and Reconsideration of Psychogenesis," by L. Zussman, S. Zussman, R. Sunley and E. Bjornson, *American Journal of Obstetrics and Gynecology*, Vol. 140, No. 7 (August 1, 1981).

essary. We believe that the information we need comes most usefully and powerfully from women talking about our experiences in settings of our own making.

There is no one "right" pattern of sexual response. What works, what feels good, what makes us feel more alive in ourselves and connected with our partners is what counts.* Our sexual patterns, too, will change at different points in our life. If the "models" proposed by sexologists and researchers (*or* feminists) don't fit our experiences of orgasm, then we must trust ourselves and learn more from each other.

VIRGINITY

A virgin is someone who hasn't had sexual intercourse. Although men are virgins in this sense before they have had sex, the main pressure to *be* a virgin is on women. Today we experience conflicting pressures about virginity.

My mother told me it's a gift I can give only once, so I'd better hold on to it.

The day I left the Church was the day I had an argument in the confessional with the priest about whether having intercourse with my fiancé was a sin. I maintained it wasn't; he said I would never be a faithful wife if I had intercourse before marriage. He refused me absolution and I never went back.

I've done everything else I can do—even oral sex, which personally seems to me as close as you can get to someone. But I feel like I'll be "dirty" if I lose my virginity. Why does that one act make such a difference?

Among my girlfriends during senior year of high school, I was the only virgin. This caused me embarrassment and teasing from my friends. I was branded as a nice girl, chicken, weird, etc., even though I did all the same things they did except have sex.

The idea of virginity is an old one. People in early Greece and Rome used it to refer to a woman (or a goddess) who was autonomous, on her own, not "owned" by any man. Later it came to mean only sexual virginity and, ironically, to reflect the prevailing view of women as man's property. Remaining a virgin until she married guaranteed that a woman would uphold the family "honor" by passing from father to husband like unspoiled goods. Since there was no dependable birth control, it guaranteed also that babies would be born only to married couples.

Many parents today are less concerned about preserving their daughters' actual virginity than about how soon or with whom they have intercourse. Some parents respect and encourage a daughter's decisions about sex. But in many other families, the message is still "Stay a virgin!"* We may "do everything but" have intercourse and feel confused—though "technically" virgin, we may have become as emotionally and

---

*Many women with spinal cord injuries have no feeling in the pelvic area yet report experiencing orgasm and its sensations elsewhere in their bodies. Clearly we all have lots more to learn about sexual responses.

*This is especially true for young Latina women. In Puerto Rico, for instance, many families have a physician verify a daughter's virginity before she entertains proposals for marriage.

Jean Raisler

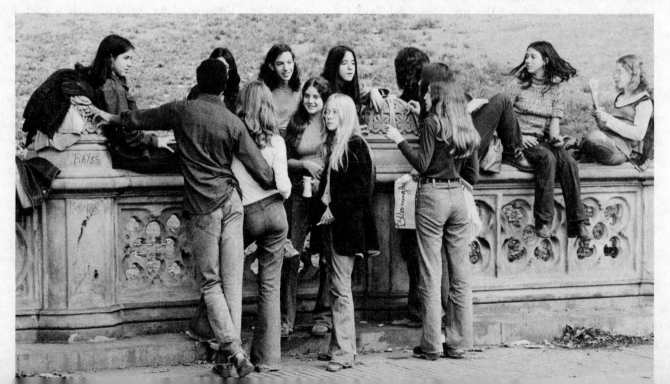

physically involved as we would have with intercourse. If we start having intercourse, we may feel troubled, guilty or ashamed about having "lost" our virginity. This may keep us from enjoying sex then or later, from asking for what we want or from feeling free to say no later on if we want to. It may keep us from finding out about birth control and using it.

Meanwhile, schoolmates and the media may pressure us to be sexually available, a pressure as strong these days as the more traditional pressure to remain a virgin.

We must be free to have sex *or not*, as we think best. Having sex usually brings many changes in the relationship and in our life. Since it is often a big decision, it makes sense to think about it, talk it over with friends and the person we're involved with, choose a method of birth control if necessary. We may well want to say no to someone who is pushing us to have sex when we don't want to.*

It might be helpful to think of "virginity" differently. Instead of virginity being something we "lose" or have to "save" for someone, it could mean our physical, spiritual and emotional wholeness, our self-respect and bodily integrity, our freedom to make a choice. When we make choices about sex out of this feeling of self-respect and "virginity," we will more likely put ourselves into situations we can be glad about. We are virgins with each new lover, sometimes even with the same lover, and in each new phase of our lives.

A NEW UNDERSTANDING OF CELIBACY

Traditionally, "celibacy" meant choosing not to marry. Today many people use it to mean not having sex for a certain period of time.† It can mean no sex with someone else, or no masturbation as well. Sometimes we choose celibacy in response to our culture's overemphasis on sex, as a break from feeling we must relate to others sexually all the time: "I was tired of having to say yes or no."

Or it's a personal adventure.

I'm exploring myself as a sexual person but in a different way. My sensitivity to my body is heightened. I am more aware of what arouses my sensual interests. I am free to be myself. I have more energy for work and friends. My spirituality feels more intense and clear.

As part of a religious commitment (for nuns, priests, and others) celibacy offers a freedom to use one's energy for other people, not so much because lovemaking

*For more on virginity and first intercourse, see Resources: *Changing Bodies, Changing Lives*.
†See *The New Celibacy* for a fuller discussion of this expanded view of celibacy.

drains energy but because sexual relationships necessitate commitments, time and attention. Yet religious celibacy has often been misunderstood or ridiculed. A nun wrote to the collective as follows:

For many religious women sex means so much that we use it as a gift of our life in the service of all people. Not to engage in an active sex life or to marry is for the purpose of being free to be of service. It is painful and depressing when others speak of this gift as though to have made this decision is necessarily to have a warped personality.

When we choose celibacy, we can experiment with any form that offers what we want.

I spend part of each day in yoga and meditation. Sometimes I go for days without thinking about my sexual identity at all. I masturbate only when inspired, which is seldom these days. Yet in meditation last week I found myself having an orgasm. It was ecstasy!

In couple relationships, we may choose celibacy when we want some distance or solitude, or when we just don't want to have sex for a while. This can be awkward and requires careful communication if a partner isn't feeling the same way.

I say to my woman lover, "I don't feel like making love this month, and I may not next month." Now, who does that? Is it okay? Am I allowed? The last thing we were ever taught was that it was okay to try what we want.

Some couples choose celibacy together, which allows both people to explore other dimensions of loving. It can help us get out of old sexual patterns, expand our sensual/sexual focus beyond genital sex if we want to and make us feel more self-sufficient and independent, which can strengthen the relationship.

Sometimes we are faced with celibacy when we *don't* choose it—after a breakup or divorce, or when a partner or lover dies. Sometimes being a parent to a new baby enforces a time of virtual celibacy. Painful if we don't want it, celibacy sometimes surprises us with its own satisfactions.

BISEXUALITY

Today many women are entering or at least thinking about sexual, intimate relationships with both men and women.

I ask myself: is it possible to be bisexual, or is it some kind of new-age fantasy that I can have a man lover and a woman lover?

I've been in lesbian relationships for ages. Then suddenly last year I fell in love with a man. A total surprise!

When I first started getting involved with women as well as men, I wanted to be more intimate with them as an extension of being friends.

Sometimes thinking of ourselves as bisexual is a safe stopping place in a transition from one identity to another.

For years I said to myself and my friends, "I think maybe I'm bisexual," meaning, "I'm probably a lesbian but I'm scared to death to admit it."

Yet for many of us bisexuality is not transitional at all.

I've tried to define myself using labels of lesbian, straight, bisexual, and I didn't feel that any of them were mine. I think of it in terms of people I could love, not sexes I could love.

Being lovers with people of both sexes opens our eyes to social and political realities which may be new to us. If we were sexually intimate only with men before, a relationship with a woman may introduce us to the world of lesbian experience, with its particular satisfactions and oppressions. We soon find that we have to be more careful in public than we ever dreamed of being; we may become aware of homophobia for the first time. Our friendships may take on new dimensions.

Sleeping with a woman for the first time allowed me to feel much more with my close women friends. Many times I'll have sexual feelings and not say anything, but they make me feel closer and more caring. I'll hug and kiss a friend and she'll have no idea what's going on inside me—the feeling of arousal is wonderful—like an opening, a blossoming.

If we have been exclusively lesbian, being lovers with a man puts us temporarily into the dominant heterosexual culture: we have the privilege of "fitting in," of being able to show our love freely in public. There also may be more struggles with sex-role stereotypes than we are used to and, before menopause, the unfamiliar need for birth control.

Invisibility is a problem. Few people know we exist, because we don't "fit" into either the heterosexual or the lesbian world. When we are open, both worlds judge us.

I'm cautious about talking about it, fear being judged, being told, "Your sexuality is wrong!"

Heterosexual friends may be shocked and scared when we have a woman lover. (See "Coming Out," p. 142.) Lesbian friends may be mistrusting, too, afraid that we may in the future slip back into the "safer" heterosexual role and hurt lesbians who have fallen in love with us. If we as lesbians become lovers with men as well, other lesbians often see us as disloyal. ("My lesbian friends have an incredible scorn for bisexuals.")

When I'm having troubles with a man and tell a lesbian friend, she usually gets a look in her eye which means, "What did you expect, being with a man?"

All these judgments isolate us. And we may feel pressured to choose: "I've had people press me to say I'm 'more' one than the other." As more women feel comfortable and safe in being open about bisexuality, we will create more of a community for ourselves, and we will further challenge both heterosexual and lesbian assumptions about who and how women can love.

SEX IN A RELATIONSHIP

Currents of sexual attraction and passion crisscross our lives and pull us into new relationships, deepen the ones we're in, teach us about ourselves. We may act on them with a look, smile, touch, kiss, or we may not want to. When we make love with someone familiar or new, woman or man, we are often at our most open, most vulnerable and also our most powerful. Sex can be dramatic, dull, comforting, scary, friendly, funny, passionate, frustrating, satisfying.

Sex doesn't take place in a vacuum. We take struggles about other things—power, money, mutuality, competition—into bed with us.

Sex in relationships can vary in meaning and intensity.

Sometimes I make love to get care and cuddling. Sometimes I am so absorbed in the sensations of touch and taste and smell and sight and sound that I feel I've returned to that childhood time when feeling good was all that mattered. Sometimes we tumble and tease. Sometimes sex is spiritual—High Mass could not be more sacred. Sometimes I make love to get away from the tightness and seriousness in myself. Sometimes I want to come and feel the ripples of orgasm through my body. Sometimes tears mix with juices mix with sweat, and I am one with another. Sometimes through sex I unite with the stream of love that flows among us all. Sex can be most anything and everything for me. How good that feels!

I enjoy sex with Mike more than I have with anyone. When we get aroused, we make the most beautiful music together! Still, sex often feels difficult for me. When I feel good about myself and close to him, when the pressures of our children and my work and friends are not demanding a lot of my energy, our sex is very fluid and strong. When I feel angry, sad, depressed or very child-like and needy, or any combination, or busy with other people in my life, I have a hard time being sexually open with Mike. We've talked about this, and he experiences a lot of the same ups and downs and distractions as I do.

Deborah's and my lovemaking has been strong, deep and varied since the first night we slept together. I've felt so sure of my sexuality with her, and increasingly trust-ing of the rhythms of our desire. Yet last year when I went to live with her in her city away from my friends, work, women's group, my own turf, I suddenly became frighteningly dependent on whether she wanted to make love with me or not. When she did, it was wonderful because I was in touch with such deep places of need and sexual vulnerability in myself that our lovemaking was profoundly moving. But when she didn't—when she wanted to go to sleep or to get up and do some work or go for a run or make some calls—I felt awful. I'd lie there feeling that I wanted sex "too much," afraid to tell her, angry, hurt, worried that she'd feel guilty. I finally dared to say something to her, only because our trust was deep enough for me to risk it. I cried as though a dam had broken. I began to see that when I'm away from my own world, the power in our relationship gets out of balance. Feeling out of touch with my own sources of strength and identity, I needed her to want me, as though her desire for me would actually make me exist. Sex and orgasm weren't the issue; identity was. We pulled out of this difficult time with a new respect for the power dy-namics in our sexual loving.

Owen Franken/Stock Boston

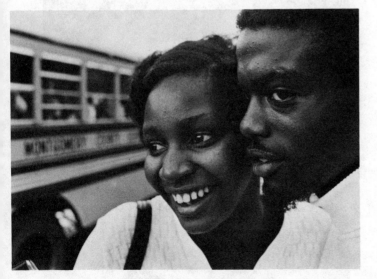

COMMUNICATING ABOUT SEX

Sexual Language

The true language of sex is primarily nonverbal. Our words and images are poor expressions of the deep feelings within and between us.

Few words in the English language feel appropriate for sex because they convey attitudes and values very unlike how we actually feel. Clinical, "proper" terms—vagina, penis and intercourse—seem cold, distant, tight; slang terms—cunt, cock, fuck, ass—seem de-grading or coarse; euphemisms like "making love" are vague. We use different words with lovers, children, friends and doctors. Though sex is a natural way of expressing ourselves, we have no natural way of talk-ing about it. Many of us are trying to put together a sexual language with which we are comfortable.

How to Say What We Really Want

There are certain issues we all face in a sexual situa-tion, whether it's with a date, longtime lover or spouse: How do I feel at the moment? Do I want to be sexually close with this person now? In what ways? What if I don't know—can I say I'm confused? Then can I com-municate clearly what I want, what I don't want? Do I feel comfortable saying it in words or letting him/her know some other way? What are the unspoken rules? Is there enough trust and caring between us for this person to listen to my feelings and respect them if I feel differently from him/her?

Often the question is whether to make love or not. When we want to ask someone to make love with us, we may have to overcome certain inhibitions, for we have been brought up to think that men, not women, should initiate sex. We have to get used to the possi-bility of being turned down. When we *don't* want to make love, we often face (in men primarily) the as-sumption that "women don't really mean it when they say no." Or someone interprets our not wanting sex as a sign of rejection or "frigidity." The more complex truth lies somewhere between the extremes of "good girls don't initiate sex" and "liberated women always want it": often we do, often we don't. Sometimes we love being coaxed into it, sometimes we hate feeling pressured. All we can do is try to be as fully aware as possible of our feelings at the moment, to be honest with ourselves about them, and to practice saying them, with clarity and no apologies, to the men or women we are with.

Communication about our sexual needs is a contin-uous process. One woman who had gotten up the cour-age to talk with her man about their sexual relationship said in angry frustration, "I told him what I like once, so why doesn't he know now? Did he forget? Doesn't he care?"

Even in the most loving relationships, asking for what we want is hard.

- We are afraid that being honest about what we want will threaten the other.
- Our partner seems defensive and might interpret our suggestion as a criticism or a demand.
- We are embarrassed by the words themselves.
- We feel sex is supposed to come naturally and having to talk about it must mean there's a problem.
- We have been making love with the same person for years (sometimes several decades) and it feels risky to bring up new insights.
- We and our partner aren't communicating well in other areas of our relationship.
- Even with a willing partner, we may as women feel a deep inhibition about asserting our sexuality openly and proudly, which is what we'd be doing if we proclaimed our erotic needs and wishes.
- We don't know what we want at a particular time, or we need to react to something our partner does. The barriers can be inside us, not just between us and our partners.

How do we work on better communications in sex? Making love is one of the special times when we have more than words to use to reach each other. Taking a partner's hand and putting it in a new place, making the sounds that let him/her know we are feeling good, speeding up or slowing down our hip movements, a firm hand on the shoulder meaning "let's go slow"—there are many ways we have of communicating, if we will use them.

I've liked just saying, "Watch," and showing.

We were both really excited. My lover began rubbing my clitoris hard and it hurt. It took me a second to figure out what to do. I was afraid that if I said something about it, I would spoil the excitement for both of us. Then I realized I could just take my lover's hand and very gently move it up a little higher to my pubic hair.

We can practice saying what feels good while exchanging massages, for example, when the atmosphere is less intense. But communicating about sex doesn't happen overnight, and it doesn't always work no matter how hard we might try.

EXPLORING LOVEMAKING

We have many ways of getting and giving pleasure—touching, caressing, looking, teasing, kissing, massaging, licking, sucking, penetrating.

My lover and I can spend hours—when we're on vacation or the kids are away on a weekend morning—looking at each other, stroking and cuddling each other, pulling and pushing and feeling our bodies stretch together. If we go past a certain point we'll both know we want to "make love," but actually we have been making love the whole time.

What we do in sex is a matter of personal preference and ingenuity, whom we are with, how much love and understanding we feel, how comfortable we both are with our bodies, how each of us feels that day. At its best, lovemaking takes its shape as we and our partners move together by mutual (often unspoken) agreement. Sexual equality is as important in bed as it is everywhere else.

Touching and Sensuality

Massages, back rubs, foot rubs, head rubs—these are wonderful anytime. As part of lovemaking, they can make sex slower and more sensual.

Joy Schneider Kendra

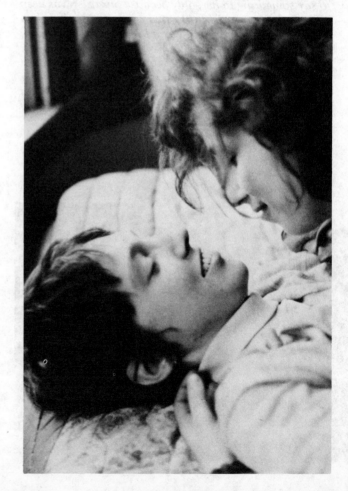

Sometimes it's a thrill to make love fast, whenever and wherever the desire hits. Other times I like to take time to emphasize every little sensual detail. We'll eat something delicious together (not too much or I'll get full and sleepy). We'll put on music, light a candle, take turns rubbing each other with oil or lotion, roll around a lot, caress each other everywhere, let our excitement build up slowly, let orgasm happen if it does. It's like a long sexual dance.

Eric likes me to rub his feet and suck his toes. I think that gives him as much pleasure or more than anything else we do in sex.

Tender touching can be a way of making love.

We always sleep right up next to each other naked. There's always a lot of touching and feeling, so even though we don't have intercourse that often, I consider us having sex all the time.

When a couple has problems in sex, it may turn out that they have been focusing entirely on each other's genitals, and not taking time or learning how to touch and stroke each other lovingly all over. Many men are more focused on genitals than women are, and need to learn the pleasures of touching.

One lover told me with great puzzlement at first that I made love slower than any woman he knew, and he didn't just mean it took me a long time to come. Later he got used to my "style" and said he liked it.

Oral Sex

We can suck or lick our partner's genitals, which when done to a woman is called *cunnilingus* (slang: going down, eating, eating out) and when done to a man is called *fellatio* (slang: going down, blow job). Sometimes oral sex is more intimate than any other kind of lovemaking. For some of us, it brings orgasm more surely than other ways of making love.

We're really into oral sex and he's always ready and willing. He'll say, "Do you want to have an orgasm?" And he'll go down on me. It's terrific.

To enjoy oral sex it helps to like our partner's genitals and feel good about our own. Yet we are often ashamed of our "private parts."

For ages I thought my lover was doing me a favor when he did oral sex on me. I couldn't imagine that I tasted good. Finally he convinced me that he loves doing it. Also, I tasted my juices and they're not bad!

At first I was repulsed by the idea of going down on a woman. I thought we smelled bad, that vaginas were nasty. It was a little pungent and intimidating in the beginning (though less so than a penis had been!). I soon learned to lose myself in the wonderful textures, tastes and formations of a woman's genitalia. I realized that lesbian sex is about loving myself, overcoming my hatred of my own body.

One of the pluses of oral sex with men is that we won't get pregnant (though with men or women we may risk a sexually transmitted disease). But like everything in sex, it's good only if we want to be doing it.

Often a guy I'm dating will say, "If you won't have intercourse, just give me a blow job." But if I don't want him in my vagina, I probably don't want him in my mouth. Oral sex can feel like rape to me if I'm not in the mood to be doing it.

My husband likes me to do oral sex on him. Sometimes it's incredibly erotic for me to have his penis moving in my mouth. Since I don't enjoy swallowing his semen, I usually spit it out or let it flow out on the sheets, and that's fine. Sometimes, however, blowing him makes me gag—I don't want his penis filling up my mouth at all. Then we do something else. Or we get in a position where I have more control, like being on top of him with the base of his penis in my hand.

What feels good in oral sex differs from time to time.

I like tongue, lips, moisture, not too much sucking and pulling, and time for exploring—my lover's got to be willing to stay with it for a while.

It can be done rather crummily! I hate it when I feel like he's eating me up with his teeth or when the pressure's too hard and it hurts or when he moves around from place to place and doesn't keep the stimulation steady.

For me there's no right or wrong place, just the places I want concentrated on on a particular day. I'm getting better at telling my lover where it feels best.

Anal Stimulation

The anus can be stimulated with fingers, tongue, penis or any slender object. For many of us, it is a highly sexually sensitive area.

I like having something small in my anus during lovemaking—no pressure or movement, just there.

177

Having the area around my anus licked during oral sex is a real turn-on. And anal intercourse when I'm in the mood is incredibly sexy. I love the sensations deep inside me, and the thrill of doing something so unusual.

The anus is not as elastic as the vagina, so be gentle. If you have anal intercourse (penis in anus),* go slowly, wait until you're relaxed and use a lubricant—saliva, secretions from the vagina or penis or a water-soluble jelly such as K-Y Jelly. Unfortunately, anal bacteria can cause serious vaginal infections and cystitis, so if you want your partner's finger(s) or penis in your vagina after being in your anus, be sure they have been washed well first, or have a male lover use a condom. Also be careful using your tongue (sometimes called rimming), as you may get a stomach infection or a sexually transmitted disease.

Anal intercourse isn't for everyone.

My husband wants to have anal sex a lot because he likes the tight fit and the exoticness of it. Once it happened and I almost didn't know it was happening. There was lubrication and everything was right and it felt fine. At other times I've really not wanted it and a few times it's been almost painful and I've stopped it. I wish I liked it better because I'd love to give him that pleasure, but I have to be honest—I just don't enjoy it.

In our one great try at anal intercourse I ended up jumping three feet in the air and squealing like a stuck pig. This so terrified him that he completely lost his erection, and we laughed and laughed. I don't think it ever really got in or anything—somehow we hadn't quite worked out the logistics of it.

Masturbating in Lovemaking

When my fiancé asked if he could help me masturbate I thought it was kinky at first. Then I showed him how I do it and he showed me how he does. We watch each other to see what feels good. He has trouble sometimes having orgasms inside me, and I know it's a relief to him that he can openly bring himself to orgasm after intercourse.

My lover rubbed her breasts and clitoris while I made love to her yesterday. After I got over feeling a little inadequate (I should be able to do it all!), I found it was like having another pair of hands to make love to her with. It was a turn-on to both of us.

When one person in a relationship wants sex or orgasm more than the other, masturbation is a possibility. Here are some different views.

It's typical for my husband to want to make love at night, but I'm too tired. Then by morning I'm very horny and he wants to get up. I always tease him in the morning, ask whether he jerked off or not. Sometimes he did. Sometimes I'll be going off to sleep and feel the bed shaking.

I guess I'm old-fashioned enough to say that no husband of mine is going to have to masturbate because I wouldn't satisfy him.

I've been sick for the past week, and how can you get really turned on when your throat's sore and your nose is running? So I said to my lover, "I don't have much energy for sex, but if you want to masturbate, please do."

Masturbation is such a private thing, and I want to keep it for when I'm alone with myself. Also, doing it with someone else would be the ultimate in showing that I'm a sexual person, and maybe I'm shy about that.

It's a relief to me to know that either of us can give ourselves an orgasm if that's what we want. It helps make coming less the center of sex for us, and frees both of us from feeling we have to "do it right" or the other person will be frustrated.

Intercourse

When you make love with a man you will probably want to have intercourse—to feel his penis in your vagina. Think of intercourse as reciprocal—you open up to enclose him warmly, you surround him powerfully and he penetrates you. It can be infinitely slow and gentle, hard and thrusting, or both—at its best, an exceptional part of lovemaking.

Your bodies and minds, your most private parts, have tremendous contact, and you connect intimately, profoundly.

I can so clearly remember moving in and around him and him in me, till it seemed in the whole world there was only us dancing together as we moved together, as we loved together, as we came together. Sometimes at these times I laugh or cry and they are the same strong emotions coming from a deep protected part of me that is freer now for loving him.

When I was trying to get pregnant I found intercourse especially exciting because of the possibility that this might be the time his sperm met my egg. It was as if my vagina was beckoning his penis to come in for an intimate hug. I felt expansive and open in my whole body.

---

*Also called *sodomy*, often by those who disapprove of it.

For intercourse to give you pleasure you must feel aroused, sexually excited, your vagina wet and open. Often it takes women longer—sometimes much longer—than men to become aroused. If you are sexually inexperienced or angry with your partner, or have a partner who practices only the "in and out" of intercourse and not the lovemaking which surrounds it, then penetration (especially when your vagina is dry) can be boring, unpleasant, even painful. Do whatever gives *you* the most pleasure. Sometimes you will feel open and ready for intercourse immediately; more often you will want your partner first to touch, rub, kiss or lick your vulva and clitoris, using his hands, mouth or penis.

Certain positions will feel more exciting to you than others (and may differ each time you make love). The "man on top" is not a "naturally" better position at all. You can sit, or lie upon him, or lie side by side. Sit up with your legs over his and his penis in you; or he can enter you from behind and reach around to caress your clitoris. If you want deep penetration and pressure on your cervix, choose positions which make these more possible. We are all different shapes and need to find positions which suit us.

Intercourse is about pleasure and connection for *both* of you, and not necessarily orgasm. Many women don't orgasm during intercourse. Sometimes trying to have an orgasm makes you self-conscious and tightens you up. On the other hand:

Sometimes it's exciting to strive for orgasms—if I don't strive I won't get them, and they feel so good!

If you are not ready for orgasm and your man is highly aroused when you begin intercourse, he might reach orgasm too soon for you if he moves back and forth inside you and you move your pelvis against his quickly. Both of you can slow your movements until you become more excited yourself. Experiment with holding your bodies still for a time when he enters you, then begin to move together slowly. Moving slowly can help men learn to delay ejaculation, which can make intercourse more pleasurable for both of you.

Pressure of the penis on the cervix can be the key to orgasm for some women, as are clitoral and vulval stimulation.

I love rubbing his penis against my clitoris and vulva. It gives both of us great pleasure and always brings me to the verge of orgasm.

It is best if you can communicate with words or movements what feels best to you. Yet sometimes talking about it is neither easy nor possible.

He would come almost instantly when we began to make love after marvelous kissing. A little while later we'd make love again, when I'd be more aroused—aching for him, in fact. I never knew how to alter this pattern, never dared talk about it, and later on found out that he had resented "having" to make love twice.

Over time you and your partner can learn your mutual rhythms of desire and arousal and explore what gives each of you the most pleasure.

After Lovemaking

The hour or so after active lovemaking can be a special time.

After sex we talk tenderly, laugh deeply, whisper, cry, sleep like babies in each other's arms. Some of the most important conversations in our relationship have come in those satisfied and intimate moments.

Some Possible Variations

● Changing roles. The one who usually initiates sex can be more receptive, the quieter one more vigorous or noisy. It can take a while to get comfortable with these changes.

I have real difficulty taking the initiative in sex, even though I know my husband would like it. Growing up I was taught that sexually aggressive women are less civilized, and I can't seem to shake my inhibition. Also, what if I initiate and he says no? What a risk; yet he takes it all the time.

Suzanne Arms

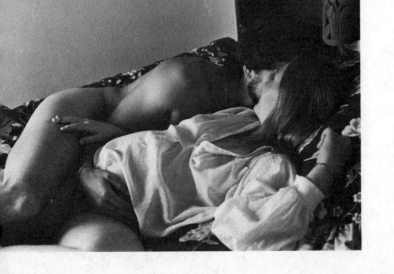

- Making love in different places or positions. (Many of us find, however, that toward the end of love-making one or two positions are best for orgasm.)
- Enjoying sexual fantasies while making love.

We've just started to talk about the fantasies we have during sex. At first it felt somehow "disloyal" that we needed fantasies when the other person was such a good lover. Now we figure, the more pleasure the better.

- Using sexually explicit materials like books, magazines or photographs, welcoming the images or words that arouse us and free up our sexual energy.

There are times when Gwen and I want a little extra turn-on. Maybe we're tired, or preoccupied with work or kids, yet we'd also like to make love. Our own fantasies are usually plenty juicy enough, but when they're not, we'll read something sexy together and have a great time.

Unfortunately, most of the erotic material that's available today is based on men's fantasies, not ours. Most of it is pornography, which depicts women's bodies as depersonalized objects and instruments of men's sexual pleasure. The exotic positions usually shown do little for a woman's clitoral stimulation. All this can aggravate the differences between what women and men want in sex.

My husband has read porn magazines since he was fourteen. He gets lots of ideas from them and keeps wanting to try things in sex which don't arouse me and I don't like much. We are both pretty disappointed in our sex life at this point.

It can be important to distinguish between "erotica"—sexually explicit materials showing sex which doesn't degrade anyone, and "pornography"—the materials which show someone (usually a woman) being forced or degraded. Women need to create more erotica of our own!*

- Playing games in sex. We can playact situations and fantasies which excite us, like being kids about to be caught or making love in a public place. We can dress up. We can be our child selves as well as our adult selves, our lusty, vigorous as well as our needy selves.

Sometimes when I'm feeling good I'll create a strip scene for my husband—and for me, since our mirror is strategically placed—and we both get very excited. Now he does it, too, standing in front of the bed, moving his body rhythmically, slowly taking off and throwing down

his clothes. I love it. His strength and vulnerability come through at the same time.

In sadomasochistic (S/M) sex play the playacting is based on fantasy situations of dominance and submission. Partners act out roles like teacher-student, police-citizen, monarch-subject. One will "enforce" her or his will on the other, often experimenting with activities involving physical pain, until the other gives the signal to stop. S/M is highly controversial among feminists, and has caused debate and even division among lesbians. Women who support S/M point out that between partners who both *fully* want to be doing it, S/M play can increase sexual pleasure and open up hidden issues of power which are present in most human intimacy. Others argue that dominance and pain infliction have no part in "healthy" sexuality. A major concern is that the many *real* inequalities in our society create a risk that S/M won't be just play, and that one partner will actually *be* dominant, while the other feels forced to acquiesce. S/M can camouflage truly oppressive behavior.

I was a battered wife. My husband, a professional with a good job, said he was into bondage. I bought into it at first. Toward the end he said that he could relate to me sexually only if he tied me up. At the end he was threatening to kill me. For him, bondage had to do with low self-esteem and wasn't a healthy expression of sexuality.

It's important to say *no* to anything you don't want to do. If you are confused or upset by pressure from a sex partner, discuss the situation with a friend who can help you decide how to respond.

A LIFETIME OF SEX

Over our lifetime we can have many changing feelings about our sexuality—how we want to explore it, with whom, and so on. Here is what several women have to say about changes in their sexual lives.

Just in the last two years—after fourteen years of marriage—we've been able to talk to each other about sex. We experience a deep kind of uncrazy passion. When you are in love it's crazy passion—you want to swallow each other up and be swallowed. This, in contrast, is a relaxed openness. Anything goes, no hurry, free of guilt. We are more sexually connected than we've ever been in our lives and able just to be with each other.

I have trouble talking about sex right now because there isn't much. I feel closeness and deep connection with my mate, and still I'm disturbed. We used to always count on being able to make love, no matter what else was wrong. And that just isn't true anymore. I feel uneasy.

*The Dodson and Friday books (see Resources) are erotic for many. For lesbian erotica, see Resources in Chapter 10.

After twenty years of being married I find myself thinking a lot about a sexual relationship with a woman.

My divorce (at forty-five) has me feeling like a teenager all over again. I go on dates; get crushes; wonder whether to sleep with someone for the first time; wait passionately for the phone to ring, hoping it's my current lover.

I want companionship from time to time. Yet I don't want an intense, continuous relationship. That means I have sporadic and spontaneous encounters with men (some sexual, some not)—momentary intimacies. This is a new experience for me, and the newness of it sometimes makes me feel shaky.

Having a baby to take care of makes us both too tired to have sex much. Yet nursing my daughter, touching her soft skin, feeling her sleeping body on mine—these are very sexual for me. My sexuality hasn't gone, but it has changed for now.

We've been married thirty-two years. I have no doubt that we'll be together until one of us dies. Yet for the past ten years our libidos have been much lower than they used to be. It's possibly the effect of medications we are taking, my husband for a heart condition and I for high blood pressure. The ten years before that were my peak sexual years, and I don't think you suddenly go from a peak to a low. I don't mean we don't have sex; it just comes in spurts.

I've gotten so angry at him in fights we've had—little fights, big ones—that I could easier kill him than sleep with him. At first these feelings scared me. Now I know they pass and change and I feel loving again.

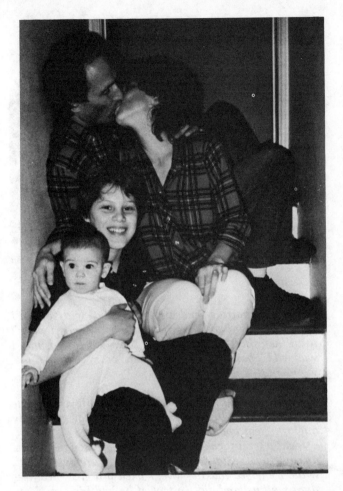

Louis Alexander

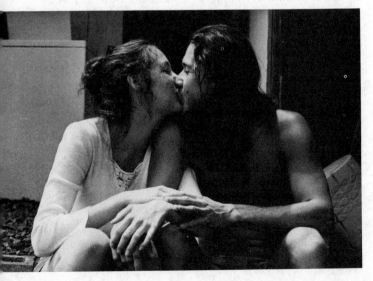

Peter Simon

When Cindy and I moved in together I went through a period of having no erotic energy whatsoever. I panicked and thought I'd never feel that passion for her again. Surprise! It came back.

We have been married for fifteen years. For several years we were passionate lovers. There was a lot of romance in our lives. Now there is less romance and very deep love and friendship. Sex is no longer the most important thing in our lives. We have sex less frequently and yet our lovemaking feels good in different ways than in those early years. We feel very warm, intimate and deeply trusting of each other.

Sally and I have been together seventeen years. Originally we had a sexual relationship. Then we broke up for five years and when we got back together it never became sexual again. I'm really glad because I can't conceive of a happier relationship. We cuddle and kiss; we hold hands on the bus; we are affectionate all the time. But we don't have sex, and I don't miss it.

181

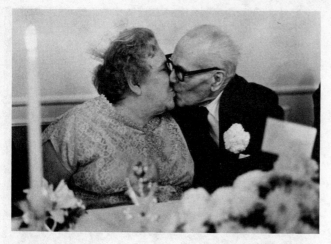

Jerry Berndt/Stock Boston

After my marriage ended I got involved with a man I felt good about and I knew felt good about me. It wasn't until then that I discovered not only was I orgasmic, I was wild, abandoned, spontaneous, crazy, witty, funny, wonderful!

We're forty-eight and fifty, and we're both very private people, but ours is such a success story that somebody ought to hear about it.

I was a virgin when I married and, as such, had quite an undefined sexuality. It quickly became apparent that, while I enjoyed making love, I liked it a great deal less than my husband did. In fact, if he had his way, I am sure he would like to make love at least once a day, now as well as then.

We immediately exploded the myth of the vaginal orgasm and learned to use manual stimulation of the clitoris, which increased my pleasure. But I was terribly afraid of making my own wishes about frequency known; above all I was afraid that, like so many other men, he would "need" to have his sexual life supplemented by extramarital sex. I never called it "rape" when he wore down my resistance over and over again or misused his superior physical strength. I now know that I did sometimes look upon it as rape.

But it doesn't happen anymore. When I was forty, for many reasons not related to marriage and sex (and maybe a few that were), I went into a depression. Sexual activity virtually ceased for us. And when I began to come out of the depression about a year later, I continued to call the shots; that is, we made love when I wanted it, and only when I wanted it. My husband had been tender and forbearing all during the worst times, and he continued to be so.

The result is that he waits to make love until I'm ready, and our sex life has never been so good. I think even he has become willing to accept the tradeoff: less frequency, more intensity. We try more daring things. But the most

interesting development is that I have begun to ask to make love more often. It may have something to do with age—I understand that we women just continue to get better and better—but I think it has more to do with the fact that I was given—no, took—more space for myself. Now I make my wishes known, he respects them and I no longer fear losing him to a more highly sexual woman. Because I'm great in bed, and so is he.

We look forward to a lifetime of ups and downs and growth and change in how we live our sexuality. We will be fascinated to see how our daughters revise this chapter!

SEX AND PHYSICAL DISABILITIES*

Some of the women speaking about sexuality throughout this chapter have a physical disability, either invisible, like epilepsy, or evident, like cerebral palsy, spina bifida or paraplegia. Those of us with physical disabilities are feeling increasingly open and proud about being sexual people.†

Whether we get a physical disability during our life or grow up with it from birth, we too often find other people assuming that we are not sexual at all.

I never get comments from guys. To them I'm an a-sexual object. It's a side of me that men don't see.

When I went out with my first ever, very good-looking boyfriend, school friends were openly amazed that I had been able to capture such a creature. I was not seen to be a woman, so I did not really see myself as a woman.

Those of us with physical disabilities discover early and more painfully something that all women face: that our identity as women and as sexual beings is measured according to our looks and our desirability to men.‡

---

*See also the table on Sex and Disability at the end of this chapter, pp. 191–94.

†Please see Chapter 1, "Body Image," for our reasons for speaking as "we" even though no one in the Collective has a physical disability, and for more on popular stereotypes of women with physical disabilities. Our special thanks to the women of Boston Self-Help for their contributions to this section on sexuality and physical disabilities.

‡It is ironic that with most physical disabilities we are considered asexual, yet if we have a condition which makes us appear unintelligent—mental retardation, emotional or speech disability—we are often thought of as *overly* sexual. For instance, one argument against sex education for mentally retarded or deaf people has been that others didn't want to encourage their "natural promiscuity." This reveals an odd warp in our society's assumptions about sexuality.

One day the gas man came to read the meter. As he was leaving the flat he asked if I was married. I told him I was, and then a funny look came into his eyes and he asked if I had sex. I was shocked. Then I was angry and said the first thing that came into my head. "Yes, do you?" He looked embarrassed and hurried away.

Growing up with certain physical disabilities keeps us from getting in touch with many of the dimensions of our sexuality.

Friends have said to me that getting their period for the first time was an important moment in their growing sense of themselves as womanly and sexual. Because my disability required my mother to catheterize me several times a day, she was the one who discovered my period. I understand now why it was so important to me a few years later to learn to change the pads myself.

I spent several months in a body cast when I was eleven and twelve years old, just when my breasts were developing. They kept having to alter the cast around my chest to make room. When my father finally came to take me home from the hospital, he brought a little sunsuit I'd worn months before. There was no way I could get my breasts in there! It was a riot. The nurses helped me fix up a hospital johnny to go under the sunsuit. That was my introduction to puberty!

Yet we may develop some dimensions of our sensuality more than others do.

A nice thing about my disability as a child was that my parents and others held me a lot, touched me all the time when they were helping me dress, kept me on their laps. Touching is still a very sensual thing for me.

Certain disabilities like multiple sclerosis and some spinal cord injuries can be so painful that there are times when we may want sex but can't stand to be touched. For the many times when the medical world can't ease the pain, some of us are turning to nonmedical alternatives like visualization, biofeedback or acupuncture. (See Chapter 5, "Health and Healing: Alternatives to Medical Care.")

Reclaiming our bodies for our own experiences of sexuality takes time and patience.

In my lesbian illness-support group we have to push past our own censored voices to discover what to do when the vulnerability of the body to pain and to medical manipulation numbs it to the touch of a lover.

I persist in feeling that my body is ugly when I'm naked. Yet my husband clearly loves making love with me. I asked him one day if I made love with a limp. "Yes," he said, "you make love with a rhythm like your walking rhythm. It's nice."

My lover, who is a paraplegic, has been subjected to enormous amounts of insensitive medical attention all her life. Health care professionals have handled her body again and again without allowing her control over the process. So obviously it is difficult for her to let go of control over her own body, and to entrust a lover with this control. I need to honor her experience, to know that it is not my fault or my inadequacy as a lover—or hers—that is the reason for sexuality being an issue in our relationship. We have discovered that honest and loving communication, with no blame or criticism, leads us to finding several ways to experience sexual pleasure with each other.

With all the obstacles, many of us choose to be sexually active.

My ex-husband and I had four children and spent twelve years raising them. The sexual side of marriage was the most satisfying part of the relationship for me and, I think, for my husband, too. If we could have spent our lives in bed I think the marriage would have been a great success!

I prefer to relate sexually to women because they are far less judgmental of my "odd" body and are really far more into sensual expression than men.

I finally lost my virginity at twenty-eight, just before going to college. Even so, it took the guy in question six months of sensitive and gentle persuasion, and then the occasion was for me a joyful and enjoyable one, coupled with a sense of relief.

The logistics of lovemaking are often a challenge, especially with a severe disability. But the "problems" are often distorted or exaggerated because of the discriminative attitudes and factors we have to face, from others' fears or unrealistic expectations to physical spaces which are poorly designed for our needs. The cultural pressure for sex to be "spontaneous" is hurtful to those of us who need some accommodation to our disability.

There is that first moment when the mechanics of your bladder management are revealed. This is the major test. How will he react to a mature woman who wears plastic knickers and pads and requires help when going to the bathroom? Reflection on this count is painful and inhibiting. Time is an important factor, because a considerable amount of physical preparation is required for intercourse. Unexpected disturbances or visitors are impossible to cope with, as I am unable to get up quickly, dress and wash. Even when sexually aroused the spontaneity can soon disappear when your partner has to help empty your bladder and carefully clean and position you.... My sexual fantasies relate to spontaneous sexual behavior—sex in an elevator, in any room of the house *and in numerous positions—on the floor, up against the wall, and so on.**

Some advanced sexual planning and open discussion may be necessary, and we need to use our imaginations and be open to whatever makes us feel good. This can be a model for all lovers whether or not they are disabled.

Whether one or both partners are disabled, often we depend on a personal care attendant (PCA) to help us prepare for sex. Having a PCA who affirms our sexuality and wants to help us is *crucial*. Then our lover has a choice about how much of the preparation to be involved in, and we can feel more independent in the sexual relationship.

Existing literature and counseling on sexuality and disability is often unsatisfactory for women.† Its terminology, for instance, can undermine our sexuality. If we experience sexual response and orgasm despite a lack of sensation in our pelvic region, for instance, we are said in medical literature to have "phantom orgasms," as though they're not quite real. The emphasis on "achievement" of orgasm and on "performance" and "sexual adequacy" make us more conscious of what we may not have rather than delighted by what we experience. The literature also focuses on sexual techniques and positions, when sexuality for *all* human beings involves above all affection, touching, communication, caring, sensuality and love.

We don't do much "hard-core sex," but find our greatest fulfillment in slow, deep touching and holding. We can't seem to get enough cuddling.

I have no sensation below my waist now, but for some reason my neck, ears and armpits are much more sensitive than they used to be, and stimulation there is really quite exciting to me.

I really like going down on my partner because I can totally control what's going on and I experience so much sensation in my mouth, whereas I can't control my vagina or feel anything there.

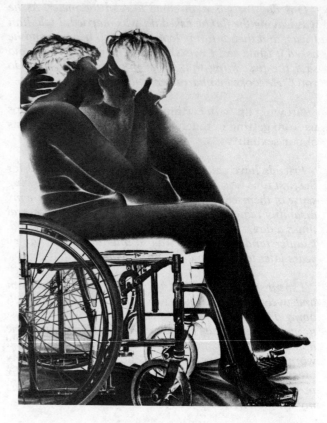

Tee Corinne

I have erratic, vague sensation in my vagina and clitoris. When I have an orgasm, I feel most of the pleasure in my knees—it's a nerve transfer thing, I guess. I'm probably the only woman in the world whose knees come....

THE POLITICS OF SEX

It can be difficult, even painful, to be sexual in a sexist, violent society. We have blamed ourselves and been blamed if sex didn't go well. We have accepted cruel labels like "frigid" or "cold" or "dysfunctional" or "cockteaser" or "insatiable." Yet when we talk with other women, we learn that many others have had the same problems we suffer over in the privacy of our bedrooms.*

---

*"Julie," in *Images of Ourselves: Women with Disabilities Talking*, p. 17. See Resources in Chapter 1, "Body Image."

†Most current literature and counseling about sex and physical disability focuses on men, penis-in-vagina intercourse and male concerns about performance and potency. Most books assume that sexual readjustment is easier for a woman, and stress how to be attractive to men rather than how to get sexual satisfaction. They deal almost exclusively with spinal cord injuries, and give little helpful information for women with other disabilities. Those of us who are blind or deaf find even less information. See Resources for a few suggestions.

---

*Most of the following factors affect heterosexual couples mainly but are often in lesbian relationships in some form.

Sexism and Power

Men as a group have more power in our society than women do. Even if you feel equal to your husband, male lover, friends, colleagues or co-workers, our culture values men more. This supposed "superiority" (even though your sex partner may not *feel* superior at all) gets played out in sex in the following ways:

- You should make love when he wants to, whether you're in the mood or not.
- You should take care of birth control because condoms interfere with his pleasure.
- You should make yourself attractive for him when he gets home from work (this despite the fact that you have been working, too, inside or outside the home or both).
- You should make sure the kids don't interrupt while you are making love.
- You should have orgasms to show him what a good lover he is.
- If you don't have intercourse, you should at least relieve him of his sexual tension by oral sex or masturbating him. (It's no more painful for a man to go without orgasm than for a woman.)

I always used to see myself as there for a man's pleasure. I would do anything to please him. Just recently, at twenty-three, I've realized that I have needs in sex and started to say something about it.

It's hard to say no to having sex with a guy when he's taken me out to dinner several times and given me so much.

I have a physical disability which makes me slow to feel sexual sensations in my genitals. With my husband I am finally going slow enough to get past my terror that I won't feel anything. But for five years I faked orgasms so men would think they were great lovers. I am angry now that I subjected myself to that kind of sexual pretense.

There are so many times I say yes when I don't really want to, just to avoid a long discussion about why not.

When I finally learned to have orgasms and wanted to make love more, my husband seemed to have less of a desire for sex. He wasn't used to my being so turned on and assertive. I think he missed the power he used to have in determining how our lovemaking would go.

Underlying all my sexual relationships with men was the assumption that my body somehow belonged to him, not me. I thought I owed my partner my sexuality, and should muster it up for him when he wanted or needed it. It was not even as crude and simple as giving over my body to be fucked. I had somehow to give him my

ardor as well, let him turn me on. In fairness to the men who were my lovers, I want to say that these were not superdemanding or overly macho men. Whether or not they thought I owed them my sexuality was irrelevant, because the assumption that I did was deep in the culture and deep in my own sense of myself. Only as I finally began to feel my authentic sexual passion as a lesbian take root and grow within me do I begin to understand the sexual need my partners used to bring to our lovemaking. I see it now less as a demand and more as a mix of excitement and desire and a powerful connecting instinct. I believe it is sexual politics, not male personality, which makes an erect penis seem to be a demand rather than a human expression of yearning and vulnerability.

We will have more satisfying sex and begin to know our full sexual potential only when we are in relationships (and eventually in a society) where sexual, racial and class prejudice and dominance are absent.

Sex-Role Stereotypes

Men are "supposed" to know more about sex, to initiate it, to have a stronger sex drive. Women are "supposed" to be passive recipients or willing students. Supposedly *they* want sex and *we* want love. Such rigid classifying of people by gender is false, silly and damaging.

Many men, for instance, seem to want sex more often than women do, and there is a myth that men have a stronger sex drive. Yet perhaps what's at issue is not "male sex drive" at all, but the fact that men are raised with few ways of expressing their emotions. Sex (i.e., intercourse and/or orgasm) is one of the few permissible ways for a man to be close to someone, the only acceptable place for men's tender, loving feelings. It may be this limitation, rather than an innate, irrepressible "sex drive," which prompts men to initiate sex so often, and leads to the false notion that women are less sexual than men. The stereotype must also arise from a deep cultural fear of women's sexual passion and power.

Conventional Definitions of Lovemaking

Most people define sex mainly in terms of intercourse, a form of lovemaking which is often well suited to men's orgasm and pleasure but is not necessarily well suited to ours.

I have orgasms easily during intercourse. Sometimes I love his thrusting deep inside me. Sometimes I don't want the penetration, I want something else. But he feels if we haven't had intercourse we haven't actually made love.

I feel shy to ask for more foreplay when I know what he's really waiting for is the fucking.

In high school we had long making-out periods and I had orgasms all the time. When we "graduated" to intercourse I stopped having them so easily because we stopped doing all the other things.

Standard (male) definitions call all the touching, licking, sucking and caressing which turns us on "foreplay" to the big act—intercourse. Most texts even call us "dysfunctional" or "frigid" if we don't reach orgasm *during* intercourse. This is not a *female* definition of female sexuality.

In one survey, 70 percent of women did not orgasm during intercourse, while most did during other kinds of sex play or masturbation.* Many of us have learned ways of increasing our satisfaction in intercourse. But the more basic answer seems to be to change our definitions of lovemaking.

Around the time when I learned I could have orgasms through oral sex but not intercourse, I was angry because so much emphasis had been placed on how to achieve them in intercourse. Why did I consume so much energy worrying about that when it seemed like you could just have a different concept of what sex is?

It took making love with women for me to see that all the other things—oral sex, having my breasts sucked, rolling around or just lying still and feeling the sensations, touching my lover and turning her on—all these are lovemaking for me. Now when I make love with men I do it more like making love with a woman—slower, more sensually and tenderly, sometimes without penetration at all.

Getting rid of the notion of foreplay and calling it *all* lovemaking may be difficult for some men to get used to. But it may be a relief to the many men who worry about keeping an erection long enough to satisfy a woman during intercourse.

Emphasis on Performance and Goals

Sex books focus on techniques and say little about feelings. We worry about being sexy enough, about "doing it" well enough to please our partners. Orgasms, too, can become a goal: some partners "work at it" for hours, wanting to please us or to show they are good lovers.

Because my previous relationships with men involved orgasm-centered sex (his orgasm, that is), I have brought

to my first woman lover lots of expectations about coming. If one of us doesn't come, I feel we haven't made love "well." I think I miss a lot of pleasure that way.

Perhaps it takes someone my age, sixty, who has lived through other times, to point out that this society's glorification of sexual orgasm borders on the excessive. It's almost enough to make a person flaunt her chastity!

The first few years we had a great sex life. We were very attracted to each other and I loved sex with Ralph. I didn't have orgasms and I didn't even know what an orgasm was. Then I learned about orgasms, partly by reading some of the new books and articles and partly by having one while masturbating. It felt so good that I wanted to have it with Ralph. The next two years were awful in bed. We had this goal—my orgasm—and it was like we'd look at our watches and say, "One, two, three, go," and work at it until we succeeded. Now, finally, we're back on an even keel. Usually I come, sometimes I don't. I let Ralph know which way I'm feeling. We can forget that goal and just do what feels good. But I wish I'd known everything I know now back when our feelings were so intense.

We may judge ourselves by new "liberated" norms.

I feel vaguely guilty if sex isn't great all the time, as though if I'm a real liberated woman I should have an incredible orgasm every time, instead of accepting that sometimes there will be little ones and sometimes big ones.

With sex coming at us from every direction in the media, we may worry whether we are doing it enough. If we're single, we "should" be finding more sex partners. If in a relationship, we "should" be making love a certain number of times per week.

Many couples these days report the "problem" of lack of interest in sex. This may reflect problems in the relationship or in ways of lovemaking. But what experts are calling insufficient interest in sex may actually be our own desires measured against today's escalated sexual standards. It may even be a reaction against the general hype about sex in the media, or simple skin hunger—the need to be touched by another human being without sex.

Objectification of Our Bodies in the Media

We bring negative feelings about our bodies into sex in a particular way. The media's "ideal" woman often robs us of sexual confidence.

For years I wouldn't make love in a position that exposed my backside to scrutiny, for I had been told it was

---

*See Resources: *The Hite Report.*

"too jiggly." Needless to say, this prevented me from being sexually assertive and creative and limited my responses.

We have a good sex life with lots of variety, fantasies, games. The fact that my disability prevents me from bending my leg limits us in some positions, but we just try different ones. Yet I don't have orgasms with my husband, only in masturbation. I am still struggling with my body. When I am unclothed I still feel like parts of me are really ugly. I think that when I can finish mourning, cry out my anguish over the disability, then sex will get better for me.

If we like the way we look and feel good about our bodies, we feel better about making love.

One of the difficult things about being large is that more often than not other people are the problem, not me. Many times I have felt that people I know wonder at my friendship with my lover. They wonder how a thin person can make love to a large one. The idea, I suppose, is that large women aren't attractive. Nonsense, of course. I enjoy my body immensely when I make love, either to myself or my boyfriend. I never think about my largeness. I simply am it and positively luxuriate in it. I love my body when I make love. It is beautiful to me and to my boyfriend. For six years we have both exulted in good lovemaking.

Violence Against Women

It is a cruel fact of our lives that many men abuse women, often using sex as a weapon. Rape, an early experience of incest, sexual harassment by a boss or co-worker or teacher, battering in the home by the man we share a bed with: any of these can devastate what sex could be for us. If we don't experience violence directly, the possibility leers at us from pornography, from news stories, movies, crude jokes.

Sometimes when I hear about a rape that's happened, I can't make love with my husband, even though I love him and usually enjoy sex. I know he is a gentle person, but for a moment I don't see him, I see all the men who use their penises as weapons to dominate and hurt women.

Making love with Rachel I am sometimes swept over by a feeling of fierce protectiveness. Her body is so precious to me. I want women and nonviolent men to become stronger and stronger and to change the things in our world which make sexual violence possible.

All of us as women face the troubling paradox of seeking to open ourselves to the deep vulnerabilities of sexual loving in a society in which we are often *not* safe.

We must work for a more equal, less violent society in which sex is used not to make money or as an instrument of dominance but in service of love—love of ourselves, love and friendship for others.

APPENDIX
Sexual-Health Care

Sexual health is a physical and emotional state of well-being that allows us to enjoy and act on our sexual feelings. We all need to follow certain procedures of routine care to stay sexually healthy.

- *A Gynecological Exam.* (See p. 476)
- *Care of Infections.* (See p. 507 and pp. 517–21) If you get an infection of the vagina or urinary tract, you need to do something about it immediately.
- *Douching.* Unless you are instructed by a doctor for a particular reason, you never need to douche (wash out the vagina). The vagina has a natural cleansing process. Frequent douching and the use of vaginal deodorants can change the acidic and alkaline balance in the vagina, leading to infections. Scents used in vaginal deodorants can also cause allergic reactions.
- *Genital Cleansing.* Rather than douche or use vaginal deodorants, you simply can wash your genital area daily with warm water. Separate the outer lips and pull back the hood of the clitoris to clean away the secretions that collect around the glans. Our body secretions and smells are a natural part of us, and if you are in good health and wash regularly, you smell and taste good. However, some of us like to wash our genitals before lovemaking. Do what makes you comfortable.
- *Birth Control.* (See Chapter 13.) If you do not want to be pregnant and you are having intercourse, you'll need to discuss with the man involved the use of birth control and who will use the selected method. If you cannot discuss it with him or he won't discuss it with you, perhaps the relationship is not ready for sex. Even if you are not having intercourse, if sperm is deposited anywhere near the vagina (even in the mons area), the sperm can swim into the vagina on vaginal secretions and up through the cervix to the uterus and fallopian tubes and join with an egg.
- *Prevention Against STDs.* (See Chapter 14.)
- *Menstruation.* It's fine to have sex during your menstrual periods if it feels comfortable to you. Some of us have found that orgasm relieves menstrual cramps. A diaphragm usually will hold back menstrual blood.
- *Pregnancy.* (See Chapter 18.)

Sexual Arousal and Orgasm

Here are some details left out of the text.

Excitement

The vagina becomes moist (lubricated). (See p. 189.) It begins to expand and balloon and eventually the inner two-thirds double in diameter.

The inner lips swell and deepen in color.

The clitoris swells, becomes erect and is highly sensitive to touch.

The breasts enlarge and become more sensitive. The nipples become erect.

The uterus enlarges and elevates within the pelvic cavity.

The heart rate increases; breathing becomes heavier and faster.

A flush or rash may appear on the skin.

The muscles begin to tighten, especially in the genital area.

If stimulation continues, the inner two-thirds of the vagina continue to balloon. The outer third narrows by one-third to one-half of its diameter, and is quite sensitive to pressure.

The entire genital area continues to swell, as do the breasts. (You may become increasingly aware of these areas of your body.)

The uterus elevates fully.

We breathe very rapidly; we may pant.

The muscles continue to contract.

With full arousal the clitoris retracts under its hood. Stimulation of the inner lips from manipulation or intercourse moves the hood of the clitoris back and forth over the glans.

Orgasm: The Release of Sexual Tension

For women, if sexual stimulation is interrupted, excitement may decline. This is especially true just before and during orgasm, when we need continuous stimulation. Direct or indirect stimulation of the clitoris (and/or, for some women, pressure on the uterus) leads to orgasm.

During orgasm, muscles around the vagina, uterus and rectum contract (the contractions cause the release of the blood trapped in the pelvic veins). For a half-hour or more after orgasm, if lovemaking doesn't continue, swelling decreases, the muscles relax and the clitoris, vagina and uterus return to their usual positions.

The Role of Testosterone in Sexuality*

Certain hormones play a role in sexual feelings, sexual activity and intensity of orgasm. The most influential is *testosterone*, sometimes called the "libido hormone" and also, erroneously, the "male hormone." Testosterone, like estrogen, is present in both men and women, though the proportions differ between the sexes. In women it is produced through the operation of both the *adrenals* (two small glands near the kidneys) and the *ovaries*, with the ovary probably the more important source.[1]

The role of testosterone in sexuality is illustrated in several ways. (1) When one adrenal is removed, women report a dramatic decrease in sexual interest, sensation and frequency of orgasm. (2) When ovaries are removed, many women report a similar loss.[2] Testosterone levels are lower in women after menopause or after ovary removal (oophorectomy) than in healthy young women with ovaries in place, showing that less testosterone is produced as ovarian function slows or stops. (3) When women who have once known libido and lost it receive moderate doses of testosterone, libido increases.[3] Pellet implants of estrogen and testosterone increase the frequency and intensity of the sexual climax, although pellets of estrogen alone or placebos have no such effect.†[4] (4) A recent study of sexually active women showed a significant correlation between blood testosterone levels and sexual responsiveness and satisfaction.[5] Knowing the importance of testosterone, ovaries and adrenals can alert us to protecting our sexuality from unnecessary removal of the ovaries or adrenals.

Problems with Sex

At one time or another all of us have problems with sex. Read about the causes and treatment for the problem you are having, particularly if it is a severe one. (See Resources.)

Sexual problems in a relationship are relationship problems. Sexual ignorance is the most frequent cause of sexual problems; poor communication patterns, male and female role expectations, a lack of trust or commitment, or unresolved conflicts between us can also lead to sexual difficulties.

How we think and feel about ourselves and sex powerfully affects how our bodies respond. Guilt, shyness, fear, conflict, ignorance, all can block or inhibit sexual responsiveness. If any of the following is a problem, we owe it to ourselves to explore further. We need not

---

*Prepared by Edith Bjornson Sunley.

†Since the long-term risks of the pellet are not known, and since taking in hormones has proved in many cases to be a health risk (estrogen, for example), the Collective does not encourage women to seek the pellet at this time. It is, in fact, not widely available, and used primarily on an experimental basis.

be in total agony or the worst on the block to look for help. Sexual problems are common.

Problems with Orgasm *

Many of us experience difficulties reaching orgasm, either by ourselves or with a lover. Shame about exploring and touching ourselves keeps us from learning to bring ourselves to orgasm through masturbation. A variety of problems keeps us from having orgasms with another. Here are some of the reasons why:

- We don't notice or else we misunderstand what's happening in our bodies as we get aroused. We're too busy thinking about abstractions—how to do it right, why it doesn't go well for us, what our lover thinks of us, whether our lover is impatient, whether our lover can last—when we might better be concentrating on sensations, not thoughts.
- We feel ourselves becoming aroused, but we are afraid we won't have an orgasm, and we don't want to get into the hassle of trying, so we just repress sexual response.
- We are afraid of asking too much and seeming too demanding.
- We are afraid that if our lover concentrates on our pleasure we will feel such pressure to come that we won't be able to—and then we don't.
- We are trying to have a simultaneous orgasm, which seldom occurs for most of us. It can be just as pleasurable if we come separately.
- We are deeply conflicted about, or angry at, the person we are sleeping with. Unconsciously we withhold orgasm as a way of withholding ourselves.
- We feel guilty about having sex and so cannot let ourselves really enjoy it.
- We rush into sex—swept off our feet just like in the movies and swept under the rug when it comes to climaxes.

Lack of Interest in Sex: Sexual Aversion

For a few of us the conflicts about ourselves and sex are so deep we never have any interest in sex. We may even feel an extreme, unpleasant sensitivity to touch, or may feel so ticklish that we can't relax. Our bodies are reacting this way for a reason, and protecting us from sexual experiences we can't handle at this point. This may well be a time to look for help.

Painful Intercourse: Dispareunia

You may experience discomfort, even pain, with intercourse for the following physical rather than emotional reasons:

*See especially *For Yourself*, by Lonnie Barbach, listed in Resources.

Local Infection

Some vaginal infections—monilia or trichomoniasis, for example—can be present in a nonacute, visually unnoticeable form. The friction of a penis or finger moving on your vulva or in your vagina might cause the infection to flare up, making you sting and itch. (See p. 517.) A herpes sore on your external genitals can make friction painful. (See page 273.)

Local Irritation

The vagina might be irritated by the birth control foam, cream or jelly you are using. If so, try a different brand. Some of us react to the rubber in a condom or diaphragm. Vaginal deodorant sprays and scented tampons can irritate the vagina or vulva.

Insufficient Lubrication

The wall of the vagina responds to sexy feelings by "sweating," giving off a liquid that wets the vagina and the entrance to it, which makes the entry of the penis easier. Sometimes there isn't enough of this liquid. Some reasons: you may be trying to let the penis in (or the man might be putting/forcing it in) too soon, before there has been enough stimulation to excite you and set the sweating action going; you may be nervous or tense about making love (e.g., it's the first time, or you're worried about getting pregnant); if the man is using a rubber (condom) you may need to add lubrication. Be sure to give the vagina time to get wet. If you still feel dry you can use saliva, lubricating jelly (e.g., K-Y) or a birth control foam, cream or jelly. (Never use Vaseline to lubricate a condom or diaphragm. It will deteriorate the rubber.) Occasionally, insufficient lubrication is caused by a hormone deficiency. After childbirth (particularly if you are nursing your baby or if your stitches hurt) and after menopause are two times when a lack of estrogen can affect the vaginal walls in such a way that less liquid is produced. Try the lubricants suggested above.

Tightness in the Vaginal Entrance

The first few times you have intercourse, an unstretched hymen (if you have one) can cause pain. And whenever you are tense and preoccupied the vaginal entrance is not likely to loosen up enough, and getting the penis in might hurt. Even if you feel relaxed and sexy, timing is important. If you try to get the penis in before you are fully aroused, you might still be too tight, though you are wet enough. So don't rush, and don't let yourself be rushed.

Pain Deep in the Pelvis

Sometimes the thrust of a finger or penis hurts way inside. This pain can be caused by tears in the ligaments that support the uterus (caused by obstetrical mismanagement during childbirth, a botched-up abortion, gang rape); infections of the cervix, uterus

189

and tubes (such as pelvic inflammatory disease—the end result of untreated sexually transmitted disease in many women); endometriosis; cysts or tumors on the ovaries. All these may be treatable.

Clitoral Pain

The clitoris is exquisitely sensitive, and for most of us direct touching or rubbing of the clitoris (especially the glans, or tip) is painful (many men don't know this until we tell them). Also, genital secretions can collect under the hood, so when washing pull back the hood of the clitoris and clean it gently.

Painful Penetration: Vaginismus

If you have vaginismus you experience a strong, involuntary tightening of your vaginal muscles, a spasm of the outer third of your vagina, which makes entrance by the penis acutely painful.

Vaginismus can be your body's defense against a sexual situation you can't handle or don't want to be in. It can also be the result of bad experiences, such as rape. If you think you are suffering from vaginismus, read about it in *The New Sex Therapy*. (See Resources.) There is a physical treatment for vaginismus which you can learn to do. Good psychotherapy may also help.

Whatever the cause, if intercourse is at all painful, don't put up with the pain! Find out what is causing it and do something about it. Until the problem is solved, figure out other ways to make love. The power that each of us has and the power that we have together to make our lives more satisfying is enormous.

Helping Ourselves

If you are feeling pain in your pelvic, genital or vaginal area, get a good gynecological exam to find out if there is a physical cause. Remember, however, that most doctors have not been trained to discuss sexual problems. Enlist the help of friends or a local women's group to find a sympathetic and competent nurse-midwife or physician.

Despite our knowledge about sex, despite the support of friends and partners, sometimes we cannot work through our difficulties. If you need someone to talk with, call your local women's health center, free clinic or the American Association of Sex Educators, Counselors and Therapists (AASECT, 11 Dupont Circle N.W., Suite 220, Washington, DC 20036, [202] 462-1171) for the name of a recommended counselor or therapist in your area. Since there are men and women without adequate training who call themselves sex therapists, we believe that contacting AASECT is better than consulting your yellow pages or, often, your health practitioner.

When there are sexual problems in a couple relationship it is often the woman who seeks help first. This may be because culturally it is easier for us to admit to our sexual concerns. It may also be because we too often assume that if sex is a problem, it's we who are in need of help. Sexual problems usually reflect or express relationship problems.

You may have a difficult time finding a good doctor or therapist. Those of us who are single or in lesbian relationships have even fewer resources than heterosexual couples. You may need to concentrate on working with friends or your partner or both, after reading the available books.

A Word About Men

Male Sexual Response

Sexual arousal in men, as in women, leads to vasocongestion (blood-engorged veins) and myotonia (muscle contraction). A woman's first reaction to arousal is vaginal lubrication, and a man's is penile erection. For both sexes the peak of sexual excitement is orgasm, which for a man includes ejaculation (when a fluid called semen, which includes sperm, spurts out of the penis). After orgasm a man has a period of a few minutes or even hours (longer as he gets older) when he cannot have another erection.

Male Sexual Problems

If we are having sex with a man who is having sexual difficulties, it is hard to have the kind of pleasure both partners would like. Further, his difficulties may complicate our own problems—even create some for us.

Men can suffer problems similar to ours, and for many of the same reasons. The common male sexual problems are: *premature ejaculation*—the inability to control the ejaculatory reflex; *impotence*—the inability to maintain, or even be aroused to, an erection; *dispareunia*—pain with intercourse; and *sexual aversion*—lack of interest in sex altogether.

Some sexual problems can be worked through with the help of good books and a caring partner, while others might call for professional help.

Sex Discussion Group for Women: Learning Together About Sex

In a women's sex discussion group, we can discuss factual information; explore our feelings; talk out problems; practice communicating (verbally and nonverbally); get help deciding how, when and with whom to share sexual feelings; and learn alternative ways to get what we want sexually.

(text cont. on p. 194)

Chronic Disease or Disability	Effects on Our Sexuality	Helpful Hints and Special Implications
Cerebral Palsy (CP)	Muscle spasticity, rigidity, and/or weakness may make certain sex acts and self-pleasuring difficult to impossible for us. Contractures of our knees and hips may cause us pain under the pressure of a partner, and spasms may increase with arousal. Our genital sensations remain intact but some of us experience a lack of lubrication. Menstruation, fertility and pregnancy are not affected. During delivery, those of us with severe CP might need a C-section.*†	Nongenital lovemaking, different positions and propping our legs up on pillows may help ease spasms. We can use a vibrator to make love alone or with another person if our arms and hands are involved. A water-soluble lubricant can often help if our vagina lacks lubrication. Inserting spermicidal foam or a diaphragm may be complicated by spasms or poor hand control. Because of an increased risk of clotting, the birth control pill is not advisable for those of us taking seizure medication (anticonvulsants) or if our mobility is greatly restricted by severe CP.§
Cerebral Vascular Accident (Stroke)	We may have difficulties in sexual positioning and sensitivity because of impaired motor strength, coordination, or paralysis. How much this affects our sexual functions will depend upon the severity of our CVA. Our sex drive may decrease, more commonly when our CVA occurs in the dominant side of the brain (for right-handers usually the left hemisphere with right-side paralysis). Menstruation and fertility are not affected, but there may be complications with pregnancy and delivery.*	If spasms or paralysis persist we can use other lovemaking positions that do not require strenuous activity. Most persons who were sexually active before CVA remain active; thus one cannot generalize about sex drive and functioning. An understanding friend or partner will often be the best help during the long recovery process. The birth control pill is never good to use, especially if our CVA resulted from diabetes or circulatory disorders.‡§‖
Diabetes	Most of the medical literature is about male sexual functioning and the few reports about women with diabetes show conflicting results. About a third of diabetic women in one study reported that their orgasms gradually got to be rarer and less intense. One possible explanation was that the threshold for orgasm increased because of damage to the nerve fibers in the pelvic region. A lack of vaginal lubrication and recurrent infections may make some lovemaking unpleasant.*	Some women say that using a vibrator allows them to reach orgasm because the stimulation is more intense. Poorly controlled diabetes may stop menstruation and cause fertility problems. Depending upon how stable our blood glucose levels are, pregnancy may be complicated and should be closely monitored. Birth control pills often aggravate other symptoms of our diabetes and should not be used because of possible cerebrovascular and cardiovascular complications.‡§‖
Renal Failure	In chronic renal insufficiency, menstruation may stop or become extremely irregular. Many women become infertile and rarely carry pregnancies to term.	Maintenance hemodialysis often brings on excessive and sometimes painful menstruations, but may improve our sex drive, though not necessarily sexual functioning. Kidney transplants usually improve both

(For footnotes see p. 194.)

Chronic Disease or Disability	Effects on Our Sexuality	Helpful Hints and Special Implications
Renal Failure (cont.)	We may have difficulties in becoming sexually excited and as in diabetes, our orgasms may become rarer and less intense. Sometimes we have a decrease in vaginal lubrication and breast tissue mass.*	our sex drive and function, and fertility improves dramatically. If our vagina is too dry, a water-soluble lubricant can help. Many of the drugs used to lower hypertension are likely to dampen our sex drive. The birth control pill is usually not advised.‡
Rheumatoid Arthritis (RA)	Swollen, painful joints, muscular atrophy and joint contractures may make it difficult for us to masturbate or make love in some positions. Pain, fatigue and medications may decrease our sex drive, but genital sensations remain intact. Menstruation, fertility and pregnancy are not affected, but birthing may be complicated if our hips and spine are involved. However, symptoms may improve during pregnancy due to changes in our immune system.	To avoid pain and pressure on affected joints, we can be creative in sexual positioning. If our symptoms respond to heat, we can plan sex after a compress, or a hot bath with our partner. Choose the best time, when you have the least pain and stiffness, for lovemaking. Try sex instead of corticosteroids—it is said to stimulate the adrenal glands and so increases output of natural cortisone which alleviates painful symptoms. The birth control pill may not be good for us if we have circulatory problems or greatly restricted mobility.‡§
Systemic Lupus Erythematosus	Many difficulties are the same as in RA (above). However, because different people have quite different symptoms, often connected to other disorders, one cannot generalize. Research on the female sexual effects of lupus is scarce, despite the fact that nine out of ten people with lupus are women. Sometimes we also have sores in and around the mouth and vagina, and a decrease in vaginal lubrication, so we may have pain during vaginal penetration.*	For helpful hints, see above as in RA. Also, we can use a water-soluble lubricant if our vagina is too dry. Choose birth control methods with extreme caution, especially if symptoms or complications other than RA exist. Birth control pills may not be advisable if we have circulatory or kidney problems, or if our mobility is greatly restricted.‡§
Myocardial Infarction (MI)	For those of us with very serious conditions, chest pain, palpitations and shortness of breath may limit our sexual activities. However, many of us can resume regular lovemaking once we can climb two flights of stairs at a brisk pace without causing symptoms. (The cardiac responses during step-climbing and lovemaking are similar, the average being 125 beats per minute.)†	We should consult our physician to see when and if we can safely begin an exercise regime. We can use lovemaking positions that require little or no exertion, especially with our arms (for example, on our side or back). Go slow in the beginning to minimize stress and fear of stress, because the majority of sexual problems arise from anxiety and misinformation about this ailment. Birth control pills should not be used.‡

(For footnotes see p. 194.)

Chronic Disease or Disability	Effects on Our Sexuality	Helpful Hints and Special Implications
Multiple Sclerosis (MS)	Depending upon the stage and severity of MS, our symptoms will vary and may come and go. Some of us experience difficulty in having an orgasm, decreased genital sensitivity, dryness of the vagina, muscle weakness, pain and bladder and bowel incontinence. There is no change in our menstrual and fertility patterns. Pregnancy and postpregnancy stress may increase MS symptoms, but the reports about this are conflicting.*†	Because sexual difficulties may come and go with other MS symptoms, it helps to be creative. Medication for spasms and topical anesthetics for pain may be helpful. If our balance is not good and we tire easily, we can use lovemaking positions that require little exertion. A water-soluble lubricant can help with a dry vagina. Some women say that intercourse is painful but having their clitoris stimulated feels good. The birth control pill is not good to use if you have paralysis or restricted mobility, but a recent study showed that it may help symptoms in the early stages of MS.*‡§‖
Ostomy	Although much more is known about sexual functioning of men with ostomies, it appears that women are better off. Surgery should not impair our genital functioning or fertility and often makes it safe to become pregnant, because a disease process, such as cancer or ulcerative colitis, has been wiped out. However, a few women report pain during intercourse or a lack of vaginal sensations after ileostomy and colostomy surgery.	An ostomy is a "hidden disability" until our clothes are off; therefore, it may help to find a comfortable way to tell potential partners before sexual relations begin. The opening or appliance may be covered or secured before lovemaking, both for aesthetic reasons and for support so it does not get in the way. We can use lovemaking positions where we feel most secure that the bag will not get pulled out. If odors are a problem we can bathe and empty the bag before making love. Consider alternatives and consult a physician if taking the birth control pill because sometimes it is not absorbed properly.‡
Spinal Cord Injury (SCI)	Our sexual functioning will depend on the location and severity of the injury, and there is great variation even for women with injuries at the same spinal level. Basically, if our injury is above the sacral area there will be reflex sexual responses, and at or below this level (conus medullaris), our reflex responses will be disrupted. SCI may result in paralysis, spasticity, loss of sensation, incontinence, skin ulcers, pain and a dry vagina, sometimes complicating making love with yourself or another. We may continue to have orgasmic sensations or they may be diffused, either in general or to specific body parts, such as our breasts or lips. Our neck, ears and the area above the injury may become more sexually exciting. Arousal, self-pleasuring	It can help to make love in ways other than vaginal penetration, which may be painful due to increased bladder infections, spasms, vaginal irritation and tearing and autonomic dysreflexia. Routine bowel and bladder programs can decrease the risk of "accidents" during sex, and a towel will help if there is any leakage. We can also tape our catheter down or move it out of the way so it does not get pulled out. Spasm medications and a water-soluble vaginal lubricant may be of some assistance. Pregnancy increases the risk of thrombophlebitis and bladder infections, but many women have relatively healthy and painless births. Be on guard for signs of autonomic dysreflexia during labor and delivery, and of uterine prolapse afterwards. Take birth control pills only with extreme caution, if at all, and never if taking antihypertensive medication or if you have circulatory problems.‡§‖

(For footnotes see p. 194.)

193

Chronic Disease or Disability	Effects on Our Sexuality	Helpful Hints and Special Implications
Spinal Cord Injury (cont.)	and lovemaking may increase spasms and the risk of incontinence. Although we may stop menstruating for several months after the injury, fertility is not permanently disrupted.†	

* The research literature is severely limited. Information presented here is only meant to be a guide, since it is based on only one or two studies or clinical observations.

† Most of the literature concerning sexuality and this disability is male-oriented, and many studies generalize their findings from men's to women's sexuality. Adequate research on sexual functioning (as opposed to reproductive functioning) has yet to be carried out with women.

‡ Many medications are directly responsible for the negative effects on sexual functioning— often much more so than the disability itself! Examples of such drugs are antihypertensives, phenothiazines, etc. Consult your physician/pharmacologist for alternative medications if you think you may have this problem. Be sure to inform your sexual health-care provider about the medications and dosage you are taking when seeking contraceptive services.

§ The diaphragm may not be a good method of birth control if you have poor hand control, recurrent bladder or vaginal infections or very weak pelvic muscles. If the use of your hands is limited ask your partner or attendant to help insert the diaphragm. There are also devices available that can make it easier to insert the coil-spring diaphragm, but some hand control is required.

‖ The intrauterine device (IUD) is not good to use for women with a loss of sensation in the pelvic area because of the risk that puncture or pelvic inflammatory disease may go unnoticed. Also, good hand coordination is needed to check the strings every month to make sure the IUD is still in place.

Table prepared by Janna Zwerner.

Here are some suggestions for organizing such a group:

Meet together and explore what you want to discuss with each other. Draw up a list of topics and a flexible plan for discussions. Select some members of the group to find out more about local resources you might want to use—films you could see or persons who might want to meet with you and offer their specialized knowledge. Choose other members to consider what materials besides this chapter you might like to read together.

Topics you may want to discuss include childhood and adolescent memories of sexuality, your feelings about your body, differences in female and male socialization, masturbation, fantasies, the nature of female sexual response, virginity, homosexuality, lovemaking, intercourse, orgasm, feelings about touching and looking at your genitals, sexual-health care, birth control, abortion, sexual problems, relationship with yourself, relationships with other women, relationships with men, the sexuality of your children.

The following "journey" through one's own sexuality is a stimulating way to begin your discussion. Before your second or third meeting, two of you get together and draw up a list of questions beginning with first memories of sensual pleasure and affection (e.g., "What kind of touching did you get as a child from your parents?" "How did you feel?"). You will want to include questions about sexual language, your parents' relationship to each other and to you, sex play with siblings and friends (e.g., playing doctor), your first menstrual period, dating, petting, intercourse, orgasm, crushes on girlfriends, marriage, sexuality as an adult, and so forth. When you all meet together again, the two of you take the rest of the group on the journey. Ask each woman to find a comfortable spot and close her eyes. The two of you alternate reading your questions very slowly, giving women time to remember. Leave a minute or two between questions. When the questions are finished, leave some more space before joining together to discuss your memories and reactions to them.

Consider activities you think would enrich your talking together. You might keep personal journals throughout the weeks you meet and share from them at a final meeting, make a collage of sex cartoons at the beginning of one week's meeting, see a porno flick or visit a bookstore that sells pornography, make a group list of all the street and slang terms you know for sex, include your lovers for a meeting or two.

NOTES

1. Christopher Longcope. "Steroid Production in Pre- and Postmenopausal Women," Chapter 2 in *The Menopausal Syndrome*, ed. by R. B. Greenblatt, V. Mahesh and R. McDonough. New York: Medcom Press, 1974.

2. L. Zussman, S. Zussman, R. Sunley and E. Bjornson. "Sexual Response after Hysterectomy–Oophorectomy: Recent Studies and Reconsideration of Psychogenesis," *American Journal of Obstetrics and Gynecology*, Vol. 140, No. 7 (Aug. 1, 1981), pp. 725–731.

3. U. J. Salman and S. H. Geist. "Effects of Androgens upon Libido in Women," *Journal of Clinical Endocrinology*, Vol. 3 (1943), pp. 253–258. Also J. W. W. Studd and M. H. Thom, "Ovarian Failure and Ageing," *Clinics in Endocrinology and Metabolism*, Vol. 10, No. 1 (1981), pp. 89–113.

4. J. W. W. Studd. "The Climacteric Syndrome," *Female and Male Climacteric*, ed. by P. A. Van Keep, D. M. Serr and R. B. Greenblatt. Lancaster, England: MPT Press Ltd., 1979, pp. 23–24.

5. Harold Persky, et al. "The Relation of Plasma Androgen Levels to Sexual Behaviors and Attitudes of Women." Reported at March 25, 1982, meeting of the American Psychosomatic Society. *Journal of Psychosomatic Medicine*, 1983.

RESOURCES

Readings

To add to this brief list, you can get extensive bibliographies on all aspects of sexuality from SIECUS, the Multi-Media Resource Center and the Kinsey Institute for Sex Research (addresses in Organizations, below). Good sources of feminist books on women's sexuality are Down There Press (P.O. Box 2086, Burlingame, CA 94010) and Naiad Press, Inc., (P.O. Box 10543, Tallahassee, FL 32302).

For books specifically on lesbian sexuality, see Resources following Chapter 10, "Loving Women: Lesbian Life and Relationships."

General

Barbach, L. G. *For Yourself: The Fulfillment of Female Sexuality*. New York: Doubleday/Anchor Books, 1976. Written for the "preorgasmic" woman, this guide to female sexuality is excellent reading for us all.

———and Linda Levine. *Shared Intimacies: Women's Sexual Experiences*. New York: Bantam Books, 1980. This fine book includes lengthy, informative and explicit quotes from women in many kinds of sexual relationships.

Bell, Ruth, et al. *Changing Bodies, Changing Lives: A Book for Teens on Sex and Relationships*. New York: Random House, Inc., 1980. Filled with quotes from teenagers and young adults, this book covers exploring sex by yourself or with another, being homosexual, family and friends, drugs and sex, emotional and reproductive health care. Emphasizes making your own decisions about sex, and enjoying sex once you've chosen.

Blank, Joani, and Honey Lee Cottrell. *I Am My Lover*. Burlingame, CA: Down There Press, 1978. About masturbation. See publisher's address above.

Brown, Gabrielle, Ph.D. *The New Celibacy: Why More Men and Women Are Abstaining from Sex and Enjoying It*. New York: McGraw–Hill, 1980.

Calderone, Mary S., and Eric W. Johnson. *The Family Book About Sexuality*. New York: Bantam Books, 1983. Friendly, clear, informative book for adults and children to consult alone or together. Liberal in approach, it does neglect certain political issues about sex, and is tolerant rather than affirming of homosexuality.

Corinne, Tee. *Labiaflowers: A Coloring Book*. Tallahassee: Naiad Press, Inc. Women's erotica.

Country Women magazine, Sexuality Issue. Box 51, Albion, CA 95410. A fine collection of erotic writing.

Demeter, Kass (formerly Teeters). *Reclaiming Women's Sexual Power*. To be published soon. For this and the book below, write to KAT, Inc., P.O. Box 21, Aptos, CA 95003.

———. *Women's Sexuality: Myth and Reality*. Palo Alto, CA: UP Press, 1977. To order, see entry above. Excellent short book for women and lovers of women. Direct, perceptive, informative, lovingly written, it emphasizes communication, touch, alternatives to intercourse.

Dodson, Betty. *Liberating Masturbation: A Meditation on Self-Love*. Bodysex Designs, P.O. Box 1933, N.Y., NY 10001, 1974. ($4.00) A classic celebration of masturbation and how to do it.

Friday, Nancy. *Forbidden Flowers*. New York: Pocket Books, 1975.

———. *My Secret Garden: Women's Sexual Fantasies*. New York: Pocket Books, 1974. Full of women's sexual fantasies, these two books are a kind of natural erotica for some.

Heresies: A Feminist Publication on Art and Politics, Sex Issue, Vol. 3, No. 4, Issue 12. Provocative articles, poems, artwork on the theme that in women's sexuality, variety is the spice of life. Thoughtful treatment of many lesser-discussed issues, such as lust, casual sex, celibacy, prostitution, sadomasochism, butch-femme.

Hite, Shere. *The Hite Report*. New York: Dell Publishing Co., Inc., 1976. Highly recommended. More than 3,000 women are surveyed about what they really like and don't like, do and don't do in sex. The results challenge many stereotypes.

———. *The Hite Report on Male Sexuality*. New York: Alfred A. Knopf, Inc., 1981.

Kerr, Carmen. *Sex For Women—Who Want to Have Fun and Loving Relationships with Equals*. New York: Grove Press, Inc., 1977. Especially helpful in identifying power dynamics in sexual loving between women and men. It includes a sensitive step-by-step program toward having orgasms with a lover (of either sex).

Kirkpatrick, Martha, ed. *Women's Sexual Experience: Explorations of the Dark Continent*. New York: Plenum Publishing Corp., 1982. ($25.00) Essays by diverse writers on women's sexual responses, teen mothers, American Indian women, Afro-American women, ageism in sexual counseling, woman abuse, incest and more.

Kitzinger, Sheila. *Woman's Experience of Sex*. New York: G. P. Putnam's Sons, 1983.

Ladas, Alice Kahn, Beverly Whipple and John D. Perry. *The G Spot and Other Recent Discoveries About Human Sexuality*. New York: Holt, Rinehart and Winston, 1982. This popular but controversial book has met criticism in much of the scientific community for proclaiming a "theory" based on skimpy data. Many feminists criticize its authors' reinstatement of the old dichotomy between "clitoral" and "vaginal" orgasms, and their apparent (though perhaps unintentional) advocacy of the latter. Other readers are more positive about the book as a useful inquiry into women's varied experiences of orgasms. See text for more on the G-spot.

Laws, Judith, and Pepper Schwartz. *Sexual Scripts*. Lanham, MD: University Press of America, 1982.

Nelson, James B. *Embodiment: An Approach to Sexuality and Christian Theology*. Minneapolis: Augsburg, 1978. Nelson's feminist perspective on sex and sexual relationships makes this an unusual and helpful book for women who are thinking through the relationship between sexuality and religion.

Off Our Backs. A monthly women's news journal. 1724 20th Street NW, Washington, DC 20009. Often runs excellent articles on sexuality.

Pond, Lily, ed. *Yellow Silk: Journal of Erotic Arts*. Verygraphics, P.O. Box 6374, Albany, CA 94706. Erotic poems, stories, essays, graphics, for women and men. The motto: "All persuasions; no brutality."

Rush, Anne Kent. *Getting Clear: Body Work for Women*. New York: Random House, Inc., and Berkeley Publishing Corp.: Bookworks, 1973. This is a workbook to help us get in better touch with our bodies and ourselves. Fun to use—highly recommended.

Shanor, Karen. *The Fantasy Files: A Study of the Sexual Fantasies of Contemporary Women*. New York: Dell Publishing Co., Inc., 1977. Includes guidance on how to interpret your own fantasies.

Silverstein, Judith. *Sexual Enhancement for Women*. Black and White Publishing, 18 Cogswell Avenue, Cambridge, MA 02140. Second printing 1982. ($16.45 includes postage.) Techniques and sensitively done explicit illustrations on self-pleasuring, pleasure with a partner, becoming orgasmic during intercourse and more.

Smith, Carolyn, Toni Ayres and Maggie Rubenstein. *Getting in Touch: Self-Sexuality for Women*. San Francisco: Multi-Media Resource Center, 1972. See address in Organizations.

Stimpson, Catharine, and Ethel Person, eds. *Women, Sex and Sexuality*. Chicago: University of Chicago Press, 1980. Important essays from a feminist/academic perspective. All first appeared in *Signs: A Journal of Women in Culture and Society*.

Vitale, Sylvia Witts. "A Herstorical Look at Some Aspects of Black Sexuality," *Heresies: A Feminist Publication on Art and Politics*, Sex Issue, Vol. 3, No. 4, Issue 12.

Walker, Alice. *The Color Purple*. New York: Harcourt Brace Jovanovich, Inc., 1982. A powerful novel which touches on many aspects of a black woman's sexuality.

Sex Research

Masters, William H. and Virginia E. Johnson. *Human Sexual Inadequacy*. Boston: Little, Brown and Co., 1970. Major research on the nature and treatment of sexual problems. The major drawback is a medicalized and performance-oriented approach to sex and sexual problems, examples being the use of such terms as "primary orgasmic dysfunction" and "ejaculatory incompetence."

————. *Human Sexual Response*. Boston: Little, Brown and Co., 1966. Masters and Johnson's revolutionary research helped open the way to more helpful understandings of women's orgasms, particularly the central role of the clitoris. Tough reading; see Brecher below.

Sherfey, Mary Jane. *The Nature and Evolution of Female Sexuality*. New York: Vintage Books, 1972. First printed in 1966, this history-making study explores the nature and origins of female sexuality. Critiquing Freudian notions, Sherfey highlights the role of the clitoris in orgasm and the potential intensity of women's sexual drives and satisfactions. A feminist classic.

Sex Therapy

Belleveau, Fred, and Lin Richter. *Understanding Human Sexual Inadequacy*. New York: Bantam Books, 1970. Shortened and more readable version of the second Masters and Johnson study, without all the clinical details.

Brecher, Ruth, and Edward Brecher, eds. *An Analysis of Human Sexual Response*. New York: Signet Books, 1966. This is a very readable analysis of the first Masters and Johnson study. Contains sections on other sex research, practical applications of sex research, and sex research and our culture.

Kaplan, Helen S. *The Illustrated Manual of Sex Therapy*. New York: Quadrangle/ New York Times Book Co., 1975.

————. *The New Sex Therapy*. New York: Brunner-Mazel (Quadrangle/ New York Times Book Co.), 1973. Male and female sexual "dysfunctions" and their treatment, primarily according to Masters and Johnson technique. Pictures are particularly fine.

Texts

Katchadourian, Heront, and Donald Lunde. *Fundamentals of Human Sexuality*. New York: Holt, Rinehart and Winston, 1980. Fine general textbook on human sexuality as a biological, behavioral and cultural phenomenon.

McCary, James L., and Stephen P. McCary. *McCary's Human Sexuality*. Fourth ed. Belmont, CA: Wadsworth Publishing Co., 1981. Highly readable general discussion of human sexuality.

Sex and Physical Disability*

Becker, Elle F. *Female Sexuality Following Spinal Cord Injury*. Bloomington, IL: Cheevar Publishers, 1978. Shows the struggle of a woman with paraplegia or quadriplegia in a world that represses and defines her sexual expression and identity, and how others can help.

Bregman, Sue. *Sexuality and the S.C.I. Woman*. Abbott-Northwestern Hospital Research and Education Department, Office of Continuing Education, 2727 Chicago Avenue, Minneapolis, MN 55407. One of the first booklets of its kind, and very helpful.

Bullard, D., and S. Knight, eds. *Sexuality and Disability: Personal Perspectives*. St. Louis: C. V. Mosby Co., 1981. Excellent book giving many different kinds of experiences.

Duffy, Yvonne. *...All Things Are Possible*. A. J. Garvin and

*Our thanks to Janna Zwerner and Barbara Waxman for assistance in compiling this section.

Associates, P.O. Box 7525, Ann Arbor, MI 48107, 1981. ($10.10) More than seventy-five differently-abled women speak candidly about their lives. Chapters on parental attitudes, masturbation, relationships, sexual intercourse, lesbianism, birth control, childbirth and childrearing contain explicit descriptions and concrete suggestions for overcoming difficulties.

Ferreyra, Susan, and Katrine Hughes. *Table Manners: Guide to the Pelvic Examination for Disabled Women and Health Care Providers*. Sex Education for Disabled People, 477 Fifteenth Street, Oakland, CA 94612, 1982. ($3.50) Written by two differently-abled women; advocates a cooperative approach.

Intimacy and Disability. Institute for Information Studies, 200 Little Falls Street, Suite 104, Falls Church, VA 22046. 1982. A "guide for people with disabilities who want to develop and maintain intimate relationships." Clear and concise, this booklet touches many issues, including ways to avoid sexual assault and exploitation. Has a chart showing sexual and contraceptive implications of fifteen disabilities. The main drawback is its exclusive heterosexual focus.

Kolodny, Robert, William Masters and Virginia Johson. *Textbook of Sexual Medicine*. Boston: Little, Brown and Co., 1979. Although not exactly feminist, the authors' attitudes toward sex and disability are excellent. Highly informative book.

Organizations

American Association of Sex Educators, Counselors and Therapists (AASECT). 11 Dupont Circle NW, Suite 220, Washington, DC 20036, [202]462–1171. Can help you find resources for sex therapy in your area.

Information Service of the Kinsey Institute for Sex Research, 416 Morrison Hall, Indiana University, Bloomington, IN 47401. Send for their list of bibliographies on many aspects of sexuality.

Institute for Family Research and Education, 760 Ostrom Avenue, Syracuse, NY 13210. Sol Gordon and his co-workers create varied and engaging materials for sex education use. Send for literature list, and for *Impact*, the journal of National Family Sex Education Week.

The Multi-Media Resource Center, 1525 Franklin Street, San Francisco, CA 94108. Distributes excellent and explicit books and films on all aspects of sexuality. Send for their long annotated bibliography and their film list.

SIECUS (Sex Information and Education Council of the U.S.), 84 Fifth Avenue, New York, NY 10011. SIECUS has sixty-five bibliographies on sex-related topics, including sexuality and illness, disability or aging, and informing children about sex. Write for an order form, also for film resources guide. SIECUS also publishes an informative monthly report.

Unitarian-Universalist Association, Department of Education, Social Concerns, 25 Beacon Street, Boston MA 02108. The UUA puts out two programs on sexuality: 1) *About Your Sexuality*, for junior high and up; includes records, filmstrips, books, etc. 2) *The Invisible Minority: The Homosexuals in Our Society*, also with a variety of materials.

Mail-order

Eve's Garden, Inc., 119 West 57th Street, New York, NY 10019. This retail and mail-order store sells vibrators, books, lotions and other means of enhancing women's sexual pleasure and power.

Good Vibrations Catalog. Order from Joani Blank, Down There Press, P.O. Box 2086, Burlingame, CA 94010. Sex aids for women's pleasure.

III
CONTROLLING
OUR FERTILITY

INTRODUCTION

Based on the work of Joan Ditzion and Janet Golden

Controlling our fertility is central to controlling our lives. The chapters in this unit present tools for understanding our fertility and making choices about whether and when to have children. We realize more every day that safe, affordable birth control and abortion, though absolutely crucial, are only part of our full reproductive freedom. All women must be free not only to prevent or end unwanted pregnancy but also to have children when and how we choose. This means, for example, that no woman should be forced into abortion or sterilization because she can't afford to raise a child (as many poor women and women of color are today). It means that no woman should become infertile due to dangerous birth control methods or misdiagnosed or untreated sexually transmitted disease.*

The following "Principles of Unity" from the Reproductive Rights National Network (R2N2) express the many facets of complete reproductive freedom:

We believe that women have a right to control our own bodies and that we must organize to secure that right in the face of attacks by church, state and the organized right wing. Therefore:

1. We support the right and access of all women, regardless of age or income, to abortion. We oppose the Hyde Amendment and any other attempt to cut off or restrict Medicaid funds for abortion, any legislation requiring parental or spousal notification, slanted "informed consent" ordinances and all other forms of restricting access to abortion.

2. We oppose all forms of sterilization abuse, including lack of informed consent, abuse of the handicapped, abuse in prisons and mental hospitals, industrial abuse and abuse resulting from the denial of abortion rights and the lack of safe, accessible forms of birth control. We support the HEW regulations on sterilization abuse.

3. We stand for reproductive freedom, including not only abortion rights and freedom from sterilization abuse but also good, safe birth control, sex education

*See also *Ourselves and Our Children,* by the Boston Women's Health Book Collective.

in the schools, the right to conduct one's sex life as one chooses and an end to nuclear, chemical and occupational hazards to our reproductive systems.

4. We support each person's right to determine his or her own personal and sexual relationships regardless of the sex of the people involved. We oppose the breaking up of families by the state in order to punish a parent for his or her sexual or political beliefs. We support the struggle for legislation guaranteeing civil rights to homosexuals.

5. Reproductive freedom depends on economics: equal wages for women, sufficient to support a family alone; a decent public health system; adequate welfare benefits; good housing; quality childcare; and a public school system that meets children's needs.

6. We see our struggle for reproductive freedom as a worldwide one. We do not believe that overpopulation is the source of the world's problems. We oppose the racist population control policies of the U.S. government and agencies aimed at Third World peoples that limit their populations through forced sterilization and the distribution of dangerous drugs, such as DES and Depo-Provera.

7. We are an activist network seeking to organize and educate women and men in health care facilities, workplaces, unions, schools and communities in support of these principles.

8. We will work in a variety of ways with other groups to achieve these ends locally, nationally and internationally.

Right to Life

A woman is not a pear tree
thrusting her fruit in mindless fecundity
into the world. Even pear trees bear
heavily in one year and rest and grow the
  next.
An orchard gone wild drops few warm
  rotting
fruit in the grass but the trees stretch
high and wiry gifting the birds forty
feet up among inch long thorns
broken atavistically from the smooth wood.

CONTROLLING OUR FERTILITY

A woman is not a basket you place
your buns in to keep them warm. Not a
   brood
hen you can slip duck eggs under.
Not the purse holding the coins of your
descendants till you spend them in wars.
Not a bank where your genes gather interest
and interesting mutations in the tainted
rain, any more than you are.

You plant corn and you harvest
it to eat or sell. You put the lamb
in the pasture to fatten and haul it in
to butcher for chops. You slice
the mountain in two for a road and gouge
the high plains for coal and the waters
run muddy for miles and years.
Fish die but you do not call them yours
unless you wished to eat them.

Now you legislate mineral rights in a
   woman.
You lay claim to her pastures for grazing,
fields for growing babies like iceberg
lettuce. You value children so dearly
that none ever go hungry, none weep
with no one to tend them when mothers
work, none lack fresh fruit,
none chew lead or cough to death and your
orphanages are empty. Every noon the best
restaurants serve poor children steaks.

At this moment at nine o'clock a *partera*
is performing a table top abortion on an

unwed mother in Texas who can't get
   Medicaid
any longer. In five days she will die
of tetanus and her little daughter will cry
and be taken away. Next door a husband
and wife are sticking pins in the son
they did not want. They will explain
for hours how wicked he is,
how he wants discipline.

We are all born of woman, in the rose
of the womb we suckled our mother's blood
and every baby born has a right to love
like a seedling to sun. Every baby born
unloved, unwanted, is a bill that will come
due in twenty years with interest, an anger
that must find a target, a pain that will
beget pain. A decade downstream a child
screams, a woman falls, a synagogue is
   torched,
a firing squad is summoned, a button
is pushed and the world burns.

I will choose what enters me, what becomes
flesh of my flesh. Without choice, no politics,
no ethics lives. I am not your cornfield,
not your uranium mine, not your calf
for fattening, not your cow for milking.
You may not use me as your factory.
Priests and legislators do not hold
shares in my womb or my mind.
This is my body. If I give it to you
I want it back. My life
is a non-negotiable demand.*

*Copyright Marge Piercy, *The Moon Is Always Female*, Alfred
A. Knopf, Inc., New York, 1980.

12

ANATOMY AND PHYSIOLOGY OF SEXUALITY AND REPRODUCTION*

By Esther Rome

With special thanks to Nancy Reame

This chapter in previous editions was written by Abby Schwarz, Esther Rome, Nancy Hawley, Barbara Perkins and Toni Randall.

FINDING OUT ABOUT OURSELVES

In talking with other women about our bodies and learning the biological facts, we arrive at a new respect for the beings we are. We equip ourselves with information of use to us in our daily lives and become active participants in our own health and medical care.

It's important to become as familiar with the appearance of our sexual organs as we are with other parts of our bodies. We have found that with just a mirror we can see how we look on the outside. The women's self-help movement encourages us to look inside at our vaginal walls and cervix (lower part of the uterus). To examine ourselves, we use a mirror, flashlight and a clean plastic speculum, an instrument which we insert into the vagina and gently open up. We can do self-exams alone or with others, once or often. With practice we can see how the cervix and vaginal walls change with the menstrual cycle, with pregnancy or with menopause, and learn to recognize various vaginal infections.†

It has taken a while for some of us to get over our inhibitions about seeing or touching our genitals.

When someone first said to me two years ago, "You can feel the end of your own cervix with your finger," I

---

*Anatomy is the physical shape and placement of our organs; physiology is how our organs work.

†This chapter touches on topics discussed throughout the book but not repeated in detail here. Please check the index if you wish to find out more about any of these subjects.

was interested but flustered. I had hardly ever put my finger in my vagina at all and felt squeamish about touching myself there, in that place "reserved" for lovers and doctors. It took me two months to get up my nerve to try it, and then one afternoon, pretty nervously, I squatted down in the bathroom and put my finger in deep, back into my vagina. There it was, feeling slippery and rounded, with an indentation at the center through which, I realized, my menstrual flow came. It was both very exciting and beautifully ordinary at the same time. Last week I bought a plastic speculum so I could look at my cervix. Will it take as long this time?

DESCRIPTION OF SEXUAL AND REPRODUCTIVE ORGANS: ANATOMY (STRUCTURE) AND PHYSIOLOGY (FUNCTION)

Pelvic Organs

The following description will be much clearer if you look at yourself with a mirror while you read the text and look at the diagrams. It is written as if you were squatting and looking into a hand mirror. If you are uncomfortable in that position, sit as far forward on the edge of a chair as you comfortably can. Make sure you have plenty of light and enough time and privacy to feel relaxed. You may want to see more with a speculum.

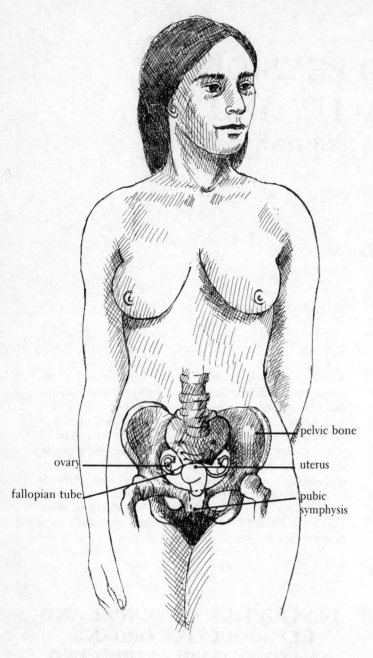

ovary

fallopian tube

pelvic bone

uterus

pubic
symphysis

Nina Reimer

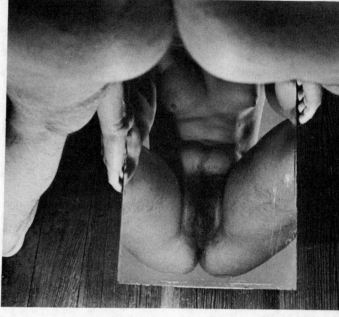

Ann Popkin

First you will see your *vulva*, or outer genitals.* This includes all the sexual and reproductive organs you can see in your crotch. Too often we confuse the vagina, only one part, with the whole area. The most obvious feature on an adult woman is the *pubic hair*,

the first wisps of which are one of the early signs of puberty. After menopause, the hair thins out. It grows from the soft fatty tissue called the *mons* (also *mons veneris*, mountain of Venus, or *mons pubis*).* The mons area lies over the *pubic symphysis*. This is the joint of the pubic bones, which are part of the *pelvic bones*, or hip girdle. You cannot feel the actual joint, though you can feel the bones under the soft outer skin.

As you spread your legs apart you can see in the mirror that the hair continues between your legs and probably on around your *anus*. The anus is the opening of the rectum, or large intestine, to the outside. You can feel that the hair-covered area between your legs is also fatty, like the mons. This fatty area forms flaps, called the *outer lips* (labia majora), which are more or less pronounced for different women. For some, the skin of the outer lips is darker. The outer lips surround some soft flaps of skin which are hairless. These are the *inner lips* (labia minora). They are sensitive to touch. With sexual stimulation they swell and turn darker. The area between the inner lips and the anus is the *perineum*.

As you gently spread the inner lips apart, you can see that they protect a delicate area between them. This is the *vestibule*. Look more closely at it. Starting from the front, right below the mons area you will see

*See Betty Dodson's *Liberating Masturbation*: *A Meditation on Self Love* (New York: Bodysex Designs, 1974) for fifteen beautiful drawings of vulvas, showing how much variety there can be in the proportions of the different parts; Suzanne Gage's drawings in *A New View of a Woman's Body*; and Tee Corinne's *Labiaflowers* (both listed in Resources).

*The formal medical term is included in parentheses if it is different from the English term. We are not including slang terms in the text. They often represent a male view of a woman's body and have been used to put women down. We can make up new words of our own, or find old words with a gentler sound, like "yoni," or use the common words, like "pussy" or "cunt," in a more positive and loving way.

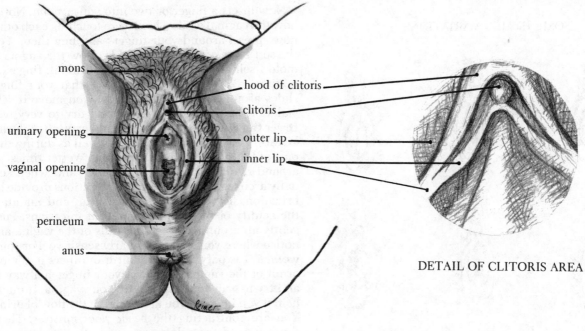

mons

hood of clitoris

clitoris

urinary opening

outer lip

inner lip

vaginal opening

perineum

anus

DETAIL OF CLITORIS AREA

Nina Reimer

VULVA

the inner lips joining to form a soft fold of skin, or *hood*, over and connecting to the *glans*, or tip of the *clitoris* (*klit*-or-iss).* Gently pull the hood up to see the glans. This is the most sensitive spot in the entire genital area. It is made up of erectile tissue which swells during sexual arousal. Let the hood slide back over the glans. Extending from the hood up to the pubic symphysis, you can now feel a hardish, rubbery, movable cord right under the skin. It is sometimes sexually arousing if touched. This is the *shaft* of the clitoris. It is connected to the bone by a *suspensory ligament*. You cannot feel this ligament or the next few organs described, but they are all important in sexual arousal and orgasm. At this point where you no longer feel the shaft of the clitoris it divides into two parts, spreading out wishbone fashion but at a much wider angle, to form the *crura* (singular: *crus*), the two anchoring wingtips of erectile tissue which attach to the pelvic bones. The crura of the clitoris are about three inches long. Starting from where the shaft and crura meet, and continuing down along the sides of the vestibule, are two bundles of erectile tissue called the *bulbs of the vestibule*. These, along with the whole clitoris and

*The glans of the clitoris is commonly referred to as "the clitoris." We will follow that convention, but please remember that the clitoris referred to here as "the whole clitoris" is really a much more extensive organ, consisting of the glans, shaft and crura, all described in the text.

For a discussion of the history of society's attitude toward the clitoris we refer you to Ruth and Edward Brecher's excellent summary of the Masters and Johnson findings, *An Analysis of Human Sexual Response* (New York: New American Library, 1966). Also see Mary J. Sherfey's *The Nature and Evolution of Female Sexuality* (New York: Random House, Inc., 1972).

an extensive system of connecting veins and muscles throughout the pelvis, become firm and filled with blood (pelvic congestion) during sexual arousal. Some pelvic congestion, giving a feeling of fullness or heaviness in the pelvic region, can occur during the menstrual cycle right before your period comes. Both the crura of the clitoris and the bulbs of the vestibule are wrapped in muscle tissue. This muscle helps to create tension and fullness during arousal and contracts during orgasm, playing an important role in the involuntary spasms felt at that time. The whole clitoris and vestibular bulbs are the only organs in the body solely for sexual sensation and arousal.

Vestibular or *Bartholin's glands* are two small rounded bodies on either side of the vaginal opening and to the rear of the vestibular bulbs. They sometimes get infected and swell. You can feel them then. Once these glands were thought to provide vaginal lubrication for intercourse, though it is now known that they produce only a few drops of fluid.

Let's return to what you can see with the mirror. Keeping the inner lips spread and pulling the hood back again, you will notice that the inner lips attach to the underside of the clitoris. Right below this attachment you will see a small dot or slit. This is the *urinary opening*, the outer opening of the *urethra*, a short (about an inch and a half) thin tube leading to your *bladder*. Below that is a larger opening, the *vaginal opening* (*introitus*). Because the urinary opening is so close to the vaginal opening, it can become irritated from prolonged or vigorous intercourse, and you may then feel some discomfort while urinating. Around the vaginal opening you may be able to see

SOME HYMEN VARIATIONS

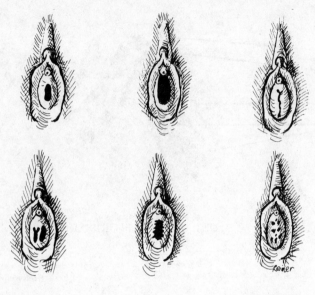

Nina Reimer

the *hymen*. When you were born it was a thin membrane surrounding the vaginal opening, partially blocking it but almost never covering the opening completely. Hymens come in widely varying sizes and shapes. For most women the hymen stretches easily. Even after being stretched, little folds of hymen tissue remain.

Now insert a finger or two into your *vagina*. Notice how the vaginal walls which were touching each other now spread around your fingers and hug them. Feel the soft folds of skin. These folds allow the vagina to mold itself around what might be inside it: fingers, a tampon, a penis or a baby. Notice that your finger slides around inside the vagina as you move it. The walls of the vagina may be almost dry to very wet. Dryer times usually occur before puberty, often during lactation and after menopause, as well as during that part of the cycle right after the flow. Wetter times are around ovulation, during pregnancy and when sexually aroused. These continuous secretions provide lubrication, help keep the vagina clean and maintain the acidity of the vagina to prevent infections. Push gently all around against the walls of the vagina and notice where you feel particularly sensitive. For some women it is only the outer third; in others it is most or all of the vagina. Now put your finger halfway in and try to grip your finger with your vagina. It might help if you imagine you are stopping the flow of urine. You are contracting the *pelvic floor muscles*. These muscles hold the pelvic organs in place and provide support for your other organs all the way up to your diaphragm, which is stretched across the bottom of your rib cage. If these muscles are weak you may have trouble having an orgasm, controlling your urine flow (urinary incontinence) or have prolapse of your pelvic organs. See p. 333 for ways to strengthen these muscles.

There is only a thin wall of skin separating the vagina from the rectum, so you may be able to feel a

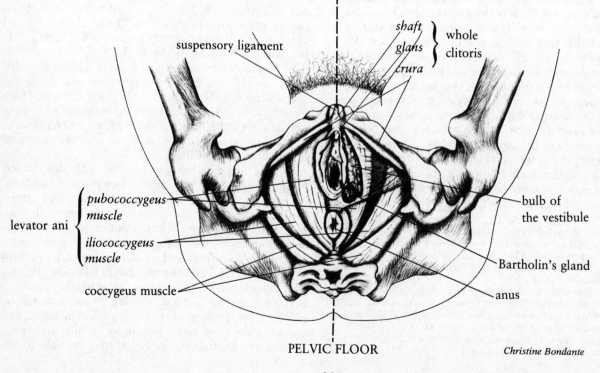

suspensory ligament

shaft
glans } whole
crura } clitoris

levator ani {
pubococcygeus muscle
iliococcygeus muscle
}

coccygeus muscle

bulb of the vestibule

Bartholin's gland

anus

PELVIC FLOOR

Christine Bondante

206

bump on one side of your vagina if you have some stool in the rectum, a small hemorrhoid or perhaps a prolapsed organ pushing on your vagina.

Now slide your middle finger as far back into your vagina as you can. Notice that your finger goes in toward the small of your back at an angle, not straight up the middle of your body. If you were standing instead of squatting, your vagina would be at about a forty-five-degree angle to the floor. With your finger you may be able to just feel the end of your vagina. This part of the vagina is called the *fornix*. (If you are having trouble reaching it, bring your knees and chest closer together so your finger can slide in farther. However, some women still may not be able to do this.) A little before the end of the vagina you can feel your *cervix*. The cervix feels like a nose with a small dimple in its center. (If you've had a baby, the cervix may feel more like a chin.) The cervix is the base of the *uterus*, or womb. It is sensitive to pressure but has no nerve endings on its surface. The uterus changes position, color and shape during the menstrual cycle and during sexual excitement as well as during puberty and menopause, so the place where you feel the cervix one day may be slightly different from where you feel it the next. Some days you can barely reach it. The dimple you felt is the *os*, or opening into the uterus. The entrance into the uterus through the cervix is very small, about the diameter of a very thin straw, and closed with a mucus plug. No tampon, finger or penis can go up through it, although it is capable of expanding enormously for a baby during labor and delivery. Most of us can see our cervixes easily during self-examination and can watch for changes if we examine ourselves fairly regularly.*

You probably will not be able to feel the rest of the organs. The nonpregnant uterus is about the size of a fist. Its thick walls have some of the most powerful muscles in the body. It is located behind the bladder, which is beneath the abdominal wall, and the rectum, which is near the backbone. The walls of the uterus touch each other unless pushed apart by a growing fetus or an abnormal growth. The top of the uterus is called the *fundus*.

Extending outward and back from the sides of the upper end of the uterus are the two *fallopian tubes* (or *oviducts*; literally, "egg tubes"). They are approximately four inches long and look like ram's horns facing backward. The connecting opening from the inside of the uterus to the fallopian tube is as small as a fine needle. The other end of the tube is fringed (fimbriated) and funnel-shaped. The wide end of the funnel wraps part way around the *ovary* but does not actually attach to it. It is held in place by connecting tissues.

The ovaries are organs about the size and shape of unshelled almonds, located on either side and some-

*See Suzanne Gage's photos of cervical changes during the cycle in *A New View of a Woman's Body*.

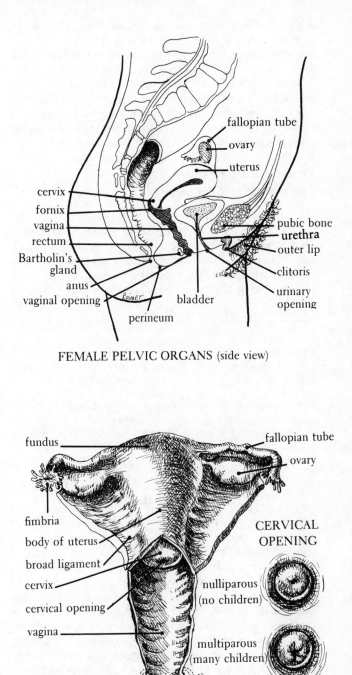

FEMALE PELVIC ORGANS (side view)

CERVICAL OPENING

nulliparous (no children)

multiparous (many children)

FEMALE PELVIC ORGANS   *Nina Reimer*

what below the uterus. They are about four or five inches below your waist. They are held in place by connective tissue and are protected by a surrounding mass of fat. They have a twofold function: to produce germ cells (eggs) and to produce female sex hormones (estrogen, progesterone and many other hormones, only some of whose functions we understand). The small gap between the ovary and the end of the corresponding tube allows the egg to float freely after it is released from the ovary. The fingerlike ends (*fimbria*) of the fallopian tube sweep across the surface of the ovary and set up currents which wave the egg into the tube. In rare cases when the egg is not "caught" by the tube, it can be fertilized outside the tube, resulting in an abdominal pregnancy.

Parallels in Female and Male Pelvic Organs

All female and male organs, including sexual and reproductive organs, are similar in origin, homologous (developed from the same embryonic tissue) and analogous (similar in function). Female and male fetuses appear identical during the first six weeks in the uterus. The following are examples of corresponding organs:

Female	Male
outer lips	scrotum
inner lips	bottom side of penis
glans of clitoris	glans of penis
shaft of clitoris	corpus cavernosum
ovaries	testes
bulb of vestibule	bulb of penis and corpus spongiosum
Bartholin's glands	Cowper's glands (bulbourethral glands)

Breasts

When we look at our breasts in the mirror we will most likely notice that they are not the same size and shape.* Often the right one is smaller than the left. If we observe our breast shape over time we will also notice that they usually become droopier over the years as our skin becomes less elastic. This happens even faster after menopause. For some of us there are pronounced changes during the menstrual cycle, with the most fullness right before our periods. Also, during pregnancy and nursing our breasts can enlarge considerably. Examining our breasts regularly can help us learn our usual patterns as well as detect anything out of the ordinary.

In the middle of the breast we notice a circle of darker skin. The color can be light pink to almost black. During pregnancy it may become larger and, in light-skinned women, darker. Sometimes the changes are permanent. This darker skin is made up of the *areola* and *nipple*. The areola may have small bumps on it. These are *sebaceous* or *oil glands* which secrete a lu-

*For stories of how women feel about their breasts and many pictures of breasts see Resources: Ayalah and Weinstock, *Breasts: Women Speak About Their Breasts and Their Lives*.

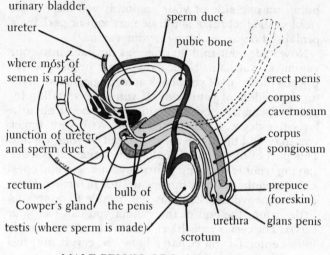

MALE PELVIC ORGANS (side view)

Nina Reimer

bricant that protects the nipple during nursing. Hairs often grow around our areolas and may increase over time or with the use of the birth control pill. Our nipples may stick out, lie flat or be inverted (go inward). Each may be different and all are normal. The only muscles in our breasts are directly under the nipple and areola. In response to cold or touch or sexual arousal, the areola may pucker and the nipples become more erect.

The inside of the breast consists of *fat*, *connective tissue* and a *milk-producing (mammary) gland*. The gland is made up of *milk-producing areas* and *ducts* which during lactation carry the milk from these areas to the nipple. During the reproductive years, even when we are not nursing, these glands periodically produce small amounts of fluid which flow from the nipples.

With the great increase of sex hormones during adolescence, the glandular tissue in the breasts starts to develop and increase in size to about the amount of a spoonful. All women have approximately the same amount of glandular tissue at the same points in their reproductive life cycles. Most of the breast consists of fat over and between sections of the gland and connective tissue. The amount of fat collected in the breasts is partly determined by heredity. This fat makes breast size vary and explains why breast size is not related to the sexual responsiveness of the breast area or to the amount of milk produced after giving birth. Because sex hormone levels change during the menstrual cycle, when starting and stopping birth control pills, during pregnancy, during lactation and after menopause, there can be variations in a particular woman's breast size and shape.

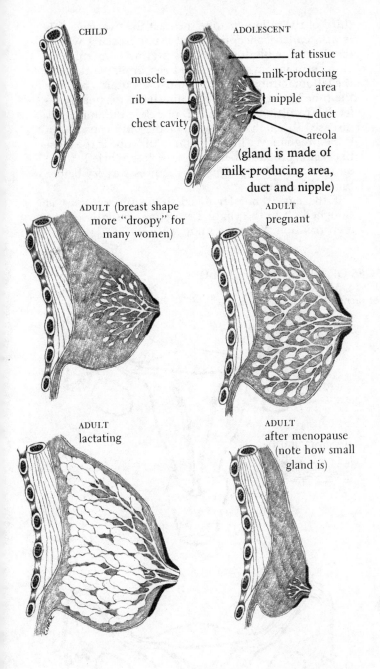

CHILD

ADOLESCENT

fat tissue

muscle

milk-producing area

rib

nipple

chest cavity

duct

areola

(gland is made of milk-producing area, duct and nipple)

ADULT (breast shape more "droopy" for many women)

ADULT pregnant

ADULT lactating

ADULT after menopause (note how small gland is)

Peggy Clark

STAGES IN THE REPRODUCTIVE CYCLE

In childhood our bodies are immature. During puberty we make the transition from childhood to maturity. In women, puberty is characterized by decreased bone growth; by growth of breasts, pubic and armpit (axillary) hair. Ovulation and menstruation (menarche) start near the end of puberty, generally when we are about twelve and a half, though any time from nine to eighteen years is normal. To menstruate, a girl must generally reach about 105 pounds, at which point about a quarter of her body weight is fat. In order to sustain menstrual cycles, a woman must maintain a slightly higher weight than when she first menstruated. Menstruation and ovulation continue until the average age of forty-eight or forty-nine, with a range of between forty and fifty-five as normal. When they stop, menopause has occurred. The transition between the reproductive and postreproductive stages, called menopause or the climacteric, often takes place over as many as fifteen years.

This entire reproductive cycle is regulated by hormones, chemical messengers and initiators in the body. The levels of sex hormones are low during childhood, increase tremendously during the reproductive years and then become somewhat lower and in a different balance after menopause. The signs and symptoms of the transitional periods are thought to be caused by the changing levels of hormones.

During the reproductive years there are monthly fluctuations of hormones which determine the timing of ovulation and menstruation. This cycle, the menstrual cycle, prepares a woman's body for the possibility of pregnancy every month.

THE OVARIAN CYCLE: OVULATION

The ovaries at birth contain about 400,000 follicles, which are balls of cells with an immature egg in the center. Only about 300 to 500 of these will develop into mature eggs.

Each month during our reproductive years, several (ten to twenty) follicles begin maturing under the influence of hormones. (See Appendix.) Usually only one develops fully and becomes a mature ovum ready for fertilization. The others degenerate before completing their development. One of the cell layers in the follicle secretes estrogen. The follicle, with the maturing egg inside, moves toward the surface of the ovary. During ovulation the follicle and the ovarian surface disintegrate at a particular point, allowing the egg to float out. If women feel this, it usually is as a twinge or cramp in the lower abdomen or back, sometimes with vaginal discharge, perhaps bloody. This is *Mittelschmerz* ("middle pain"). A few women have headaches, gastric pains or sluggishness. The symptoms can be severe enough to be confused with appendicitis or ectopic pregnancy. They may be related to infertility. Cervical mucus changes at this time, too.

Just before ovulation the same cell layer in the follicle starts secreting progesterone as well as estrogen.

After ovulation the empty follicle is called a *corpus luteum* ("yellow body," referring to the yellow fat in it). If the woman becomes pregnant, the hormones produced by the corpus luteum help to maintain the pregnancy. If no pregnancy occurs, the follicle degenerates. After several months only a whitish scar remains near the surface of the ovary. It is then called the *corpus albicans* ("white body") and eventually disappears entirely.

After ovulation the released egg is trapped by the funnel-shaped end of one of the fallopian tubes (oviducts) and begins its several-day journey to the uterus, moved along by wavelike (peristaltic) contractions of the tube. Fertilization, the union of an egg from a woman and sperm from a man, takes place in the outer

third of the fallopian tube (nearest the ovaries). This is also called conception, and usually occurs within one day of ovulation. There is a growing number of women in whom the fertilized egg implants itself in the fallopian tube while en route to the uterus because the tube has been scarred or unusually twisted by infection resulting from an IUD or pelvic inflammatory disease, although these are not the only causes of a tubal pregnancy. The midpoint of the tube is the most likely site, probably because the egg stops briefly there on its way. Tubal pregnancy requires surgery before the tube ruptures.

If the egg is not fertilized, it disintegrates or is sloughed off in the vaginal secretions, usually before menstruation. You won't notice it.

ENDOMETRIUM AT FOUR STAGES OF MENSTRUAL CYCLE:
day 5, day 14 (ovulation), day 19, day 1 of new cycle
(day 1 is first day of menstrual period)

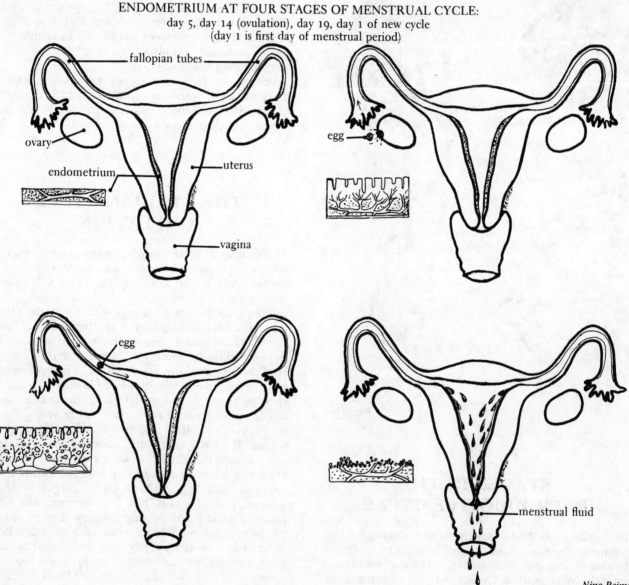

Nina Reimer

210

THE UTERINE CYCLE

Cervical Changes

The kind of mucus produced by your cervix changes through the cycle in response to hormones. Although there are general patterns, you can follow your own cycle to find out what yours is by feeling the entrance to the vagina with your finger, looking at the secretions, being aware of sensations of vaginal wetness or dryness and recording these characteristics every day for several cycles. You may also wish to taste your secretions. They can be sour, salty or sweet, changing during the cycle in a pattern typical for you. If you looked at it under a microscope, the mucus would usually look like a maze of tangled fibers. It is extremely difficult for sperm and many other organisms to get through it. At ovulation, under the influence of estrogen, it changes to form longer strands, more or less aligned, to help channel the sperm into the uterus. The mucus is a kind of gatekeeper for the uterus. It also is profuse enough at this time to coat the vagina and help protect the sperm from the acid secretions produced there. After ovulation, as estrogen drops off and progesterone rises with the approach of menstruation, your vagina gradually becomes drier. Menopausal women may find that following the changes in their cervical mucus is a simple way of monitoring their estrogen levels.

If you look at your cervix with a speculum, you may or may not be able to see the mucus change. You will probably notice that around ovulation the cervix is pulled up high into the vagina. It may also enlarge and soften and the os may open a little.

Endometrial Changes and Menstruation

Estrogen, made by the maturing follicle, causes the uterine lining (*endometrium*) to proliferate (grow, thicken, and form glands) and increases the uterine blood supply (proliferating phase). Progesterone, made by the ruptured follicle after the egg is released, causes the glands in the endometrium to begin secreting embryo-nourishing substances (secretory phase). A fertilized egg can implant only in a secretory lining, not in a proliferative one. If all goes well, the egg, after its approximately six-and-a-half-day journey, should find a well-developed secretory lining.

If conception has not occurred, the ruptured follicle, or corpus luteum, will produce estrogen and progesterone for only about twelve days, with the amount dwindling in the last few days. As the estrogen and progesterone levels drop, the tiny arteries and veins in the uterus pinch themselves off. The lining is no longer nourished and is shed. This is menstruation, the menstrual period or flow. During menstruation, most of the lining is shed; the bottom third remains to form a new lining. Then a new follicle starts growing and secreting estrogen, a new uterine lining grows and the cycle begins again.*

Any cycle that is more or less regular is normal. The length of the cycle usually ranges from twenty to thirty-six days, the average being twenty-eight days. (Menstruation is from the Latin *mensis*, for "month.") Some women have alternating long and short cycles. There are spontaneous small changes, and there can be major ones when a woman is under a great deal of stress. As you get older or after you have a baby, you may notice marked changes. An average period lasts two to eight days, with four to six days being the average. The flow stops and starts, though this may not always be evident. A usual discharge for a menstrual period is about four to six tablespoons, or two to three ounces.

The Menstrual Fluid

The menstrual fluid contains cervical mucus, vaginal secretions, mucus and cells and degenerated endometrial particles as well as blood (sometimes clotted), but this mixed content is not obvious since the blood stains everything red or brown. This regular loss of blood, even though small, can cause anemia. The fluid usually does not smell until it makes contact with the bacteria in the air and starts to decompose. Toward the end of the flow, some of the discharge may have an unpleasant odor.

Women in different cultures have handled their menstrual flow in many ways. Sometimes they don't use anything. Since earliest times, women have made tampons and pads from available materials, often washing and reusing special cloths or rags. Today, some women make them from gauze or cotton balls. Most women use commercial sanitary napkins and tampons. Directions come with the products. (Toxic shock syndrome, TSS, has been linked to the use of tampons, and rarely to sponges and diaphragms.) Do not use tampons between your periods or ones that are more absorbent than you need during your period. Unfortunately, absorbency labeling is not uniform; one brand's regular can be more absorbent than another's super. It is too absorbent if it is hard to pull out or shreds when you remove it or if your vagina becomes dry. Tampons can cause sores you probably are not able to notice on the vaginal walls when used under those circumstances. Some women experience vaginal irritation, itching, soreness, unusual odor or bleeding while using tampons. If you do, stop using them or change brands or absorbencies to see if that helps. There is no premarket safety testing of tampons. Most research is done by the manufacturers who keep it

---

*It is possible to menstruate without ovulating (anovulatory period) even after cycles have been established. In young women, anovulatory cycles average once a year, increasing to eight to ten a year as menopause approaches.

secret. Although the law requires the U.S. FDA to set uniform standards for the safety and performance on medical devices including tampons, the agency has no plans to do so.*

Recently, women have rediscovered natural sponges (not cellulose) which are reusable and economical. Because the U.S. Food and Drug Administration (U.S. FDA) does not approve sponges for this use, it will not allow them to be labeled as such.† A sponge is soft and comfortable and when damp takes the shape of your vagina, eliminating the dryness and irritation so common with commercial tampons. Unfortunately, because sponges grow in the oceans where so many pollutants are dumped, we don't know what the sponge has been exposed to, how much pollutant it has absorbed or whether residual pollutants may cause us problems. Almost no testing has been done.‡

Dampen the sponge before insertion. When you think the sponge is full, pull it out with your finger. Wash it well in cool water. Before reinserting, squeeze it to remove excess water. Some women tie a string onto the sponge, but as with tampons, the string may act as a wick for bacteria from outside the vagina. To make things simpler in public restrooms, carry an extra sponge in a plastic bag. If the sponge develops an odor, rinse it in a mild solution of vinegar and water. The sponge does not have to be made sterile. (Tampons and napkins are not sterile.) However, if you have an infection, do not reuse your sponge. Discard the sponge when it begins to fall apart.

Some women are also using a diaphragm as a cup to collect the menstrual fluid. Use a little lubricating jelly on the rim if it is hard to put in. A diaphragm holds more than a sponge or tampon. You will learn from experience when it is full. Then remove, wash and reinsert it. If it is left in too long it will overflow. Other women use a cervical cap, which has been approved by the U.S. FDA for this purpose but not for birth control! A method developed and used by women in advanced self-help groups is menstrual extraction. (See p. 295; also see Resources: *A New View of a Woman's Body*.)

Those of us who have limited sensation in the lower part of our bodies or are confined to wheelchairs often

---

*Report any tampon-related problems you have to the U.S. FDA. (See p. 579.) Write to the U.S. FDA to support uniform absorbency labeling and thorough safety testing for tampons. Even a few letters make a difference here. Please send a copy to Boston Women's Health Book Collective, 465 Mt. Auburn Street, Watertown, MA 02172.

†Although the U.S. FDA was acting according to its rules and regulations, it concentrated on menstrual sponge distributors, all very small businesses, because of the political pressure on it to take some kind of action while the issue of TSS was prominent in the media.

‡Different researchers, using only a few sponge samples each, have gotten contradictory results. Try to get Caribbean or Florida sponges, since these grow in *generally* less polluted waters than Mediterranean sponges.

---

find all of these methods either irritating or difficult to use. There is no satisfactory solution to this yet.

> Sanitary product companies are always introducing "new, improved" products. Avoid *deodorized* or *scented* tampons, napkins and feminine deodorant sprays. Many women have allergic reactions to the chemicals in them. If any of them cause problems, stop using them immediately.

> **Learning More About Your Cycle**
>
> A good way to start learning more about your own cycle and what is usual and normal for you is to keep a simple chart. Note the start of your flow on a calendar. Add whatever else you are interested in or make a separate chart or journal. Some things you might consider looking at more carefully are color, texture, taste, clots, cervical changes, breast changes, fluctuations in your general physical, emotional or sexual state. You may find no pattern where you thought there was one, or you may find that some changes occur at particular times in your cycle.

Attitudes About Menstruation

Cultural, religious and personal attitudes about menstruation are a part of our menstrual experience and often reflect negative attitudes toward women. Consider for a moment the ways you have been influenced by attitudes and customs about menstruation. How did you first hear about it? How else have you found out about it: family, friends, advertising, lovers, books, films, teachers, nurses, doctors, taboos, slang, names, jokes? What particular experiences stand out in your mind? How did they make you feel? Are your current experiences different? How is menstruation a part of your life now?

Certain cultures have isolated women entirely, or put them only in the company of other women, during their periods, because people thought menstrual blood was "unclean" and gave menstruating women supernatural powers, sometimes good but more often destructive. Women themselves may have started these practices to give themselves a time for meditation or to give older women a chance to pass on special women's secrets to younger ones.

Current taboos include refraining from exercise, showers and sexual intercourse, or hiding the fact of menstruation entirely. Notice the wording in ads for menstrual products to see how this is reinforced in our country.

In the belief that the whole menstrual cycle makes women unstable or less capable, some people deny jobs to women and treat us as inferior. The idea that women lose a lot of time from work is largely unsupported. One study of nurses shows that they lost very little time because of menstrual problems.[1] Most women do not have any measurable difference in their thinking capacity throughout their cycles[2] or in their ability to perform tasks.[3] We still work where we are "needed"—at home, in factories, in offices—with no concessions in schedules or routines to take account of individual differences in our cycles. Men, however, who are much more prone to seriously incapacitating and unpredictable diseases, such as heart problems, continue in highly responsible positions (the Presidency of the country, for example).

Feelings About Menstruation

Many of us were scared or even embarrassed when we first started to menstruate. We grew up with little or no knowledge about where the blood and tissue were coming from and why it came and why it sometimes hurt. Some of us thought we were dying when we first saw our menstrual blood. Some of us were desperately afraid that a teacher or boy would notice when we had our period. On the other hand, some of us felt inadequate if we didn't menstruate.

I used to worry about having my period. It seemed that all my friends had gotten it already, or were just having it. I felt left out. I began to think of it as a symbol: when I got my period, I would become a woman.

Beginning and ending menstruation will always be different for each person—welcome to some, not to others. We do know that as we feel better about our bodies and learn more about ourselves, our experiences of our cycles can change. During times when we feel especially good about ourselves, we may experience our periods as self-affirming, creative and pleasurable.

I really love getting my period. It's like the changing seasons. I feel a bond with other women. I feel fertile and womanly and empowered because of my potential to make a life. I even like the little aches I get because it's a reminder of having my period.

Some of us will pay less attention to menstruation and others will explore it further through art, songs, writings and new rituals. We want to be sure to tell both our daughters and sons about the many changes of the life cycle so that they can be comfortable and open about them in a way that we were not.

Menstrual Problems

Menstruation is a normal, healthy occurrence for many years of a woman's life. Yet many women, in very different cultures, experience menstrual problems which range from mild discomfort to acute pain. For those of us who have these problems either occasionally or regularly, it is important to recognize that they exist and to deal with them—arranging schedules so we can get more rest if we need it at that time, planning critical meetings for a time when we are not premenstrual, and so on.

Menstrual problems may well not be inevitable. We simply do not know enough about the interactions of our physical and emotional health and of our external environment (physical and social) and our internal environment (including cyclically changing body chemicals and heredity) to know why some have problems and others don't. We also don't know enough to understand why certain remedies work for some and not for others.

Standard medical views have not been helpful for women. In the past, doctors have attributed cramps and other problems to a variety of physical and psychological causes. Medical remedies sometimes still include general pain-killers (when other medication works better), hormones (sometimes in the form of birth control pills), tranquilizers, a "pat on the head," a hysterectomy or a recommendation to see a psychiatrist. Many doctors claim that a woman's cycle is complicated and mysterious and do not respect our self-knowledge. Researchers are finally working to understand the reasons for menstrual problems, but there is still much more to learn.

Women's menstrual problems started to get more serious attention after 1969 when a British doctor, Katharina Dalton, wrote a popular book theorizing about their causes. It was the first book which took women's complaints seriously, a big step forward. However, she still describes women stereotypically as not particularly competent, out of control and ruled by hormonal fluctuations. Unfortunately, much of the women's health movement and some of the medical profession accepted her book before reading it critically. As a result, some unsubstantiated information has been given wider credence than it should have.

Dalton divided women's menstrual problems into two sharply defined categories: *spasmodic*, which roughly corresponds to dysmenorrhea (see below), and *congestive*, which includes bloating, irritability, depression and various aches. Further research has revealed that many women don't fit neatly into one or the other of the categories.[4] Though women *do* report different types of cramping and specific constellations of symptoms, their experiences vary widely. Yet how doctors categorize a woman often determines what medical treatment she receives and whether the doctor treats her respectfully.

Premenstrual Syndrome (PMS)

Despite many shortcomings in her work, Dalton has helpfully identified and popularized PMS, the recurrence of particular symptoms around the menstrual period.* PMS symptoms often are similar to congestive problems but actually can include anything. They most commonly start when a woman is in her twenties or early thirties.[5] The latest medical trend for treating PMS is natural progesterone, sometimes used for years. However, the theoretical basis of this treatment is unproven. (See Resources: "The Premenstrual Syndrome," by Mary Brown Parlee, for one analysis of this.) There have been few controlled studies to test whether progesterone actually works better than a placebo or another remedy. Some studies show that placebos or other treatments dramatically eliminate symptoms for some women.[6] Effects of long-term progesterone use is not known; the few animal studies done indicate problems. Some women find great relief from dietary changes, vitamin supplements, daily exercise or evening primrose oil. (Human milk contains the same active ingredient.) For more on PMS, including specific recommendations for dietary and other lifestyle changes, see Michelle Harrison, M.D., *Self-Help for Premenstrual Syndrome* (listed in Resources).

Depression

Those of us who get depressed premenstrually find, when we think about it, that we are concerned with problems that have usually been there all the time. We just can't handle them as well during our premenstrual period. It is important to remember the problems that bother you, even if it means writing them down, so that when you are feeling better you don't forget to try to work toward solving them.

A week before my period comes I go through a few days of feeling more helpless, stuck or down about things in my life that have been there all along. Sometimes I appreciate being more in touch with the underside of my feelings. Other times it really gets to me. The voices inside my head which are overly critical of what I do get much more insistent when I'm premenstrual. Recently I've identified them more quickly. I'll start to get down on myself for not being a good enough mother, friend, worker, daughter, and so forth, and I'll say, "Those are your critical voices—go easy on yourself!" It helps.

You might plan to get support for yourself for the times when you feel worst. Ask close friends to drop

by, involve the rest of the family more in running the household or get a babysitter for the kids. You might start a self-help group by advertising in the paper. If fatigue is a problem, try to schedule time for extra sleeping or for energizing exercise. PMS depression may well be related to diet. (See p. 215: "Food.")

Dysmenorrhea

You can do something about dysmenorrhea, the sometimes incapacitating cramping during your period. A particular constellation of symptoms, including cramping and often nausea and diarrhea, may be caused by an excess of a certain type of prostaglandin found in the uterus and perhaps "leaking" into the intestines. (Prostaglandins are substances found throughout the body, one of which causes contractions of the uterine and intestinal muscles.) With too much prostaglandin, the usually painless rhythmic contractions of the uterus during menstruation become longer and tighter at the tightening phase, keeping oxygen from the muscles. It is this lack of oxygen which we perceive as pain. But we don't know why some women have more prostaglandins in their uterus than others. Since the uterus is a muscle, relaxation exercises help, as does massage and sometimes biofeedback techniques. Anticipation often worsens the pain by making us tense up. Antiprostaglandins, a class of drugs developed for arthritis, constitute a medical solution which helps some women. In severe cases, you must take the drug before cramping begins; still, it may only lessen the pain. Some women find some of these drugs easier to tolerate than others. The most frequent complaint is upset stomach, which is often avoided by taking the drug with milk or other food. A few women have found that one drug ceases to be effective, and they must try another.[7] Antiprostaglandins also reduce the amount of flow and shorten the period. We don't yet know how safe these drugs are for long-term, intermittent use, although they seem *relatively* safe so far.*

Endometriosis and PID also cause menstrual problems, especially cramping. Today, as doctors are beginning to find some physical basis for menstrual distresses, they are prescribing drugs that treat the particular problems. We must understand that the doctors, diagnosing on the basis of symptoms, are *only treating symptoms* and do not know the underlying causes. Although various drugs, especially antiprostaglandins, show great promise, we are cautious because we don't want their use to turn out to be another DES or thalidomide story. We don't yet know the risks

---

*Different researchers define PMS differently, often making it hard to compare studies. Some, including Dalton, insist there be a symptom-free time during the cycle; others include a premenstrual intensification of symptoms experienced to a lesser degree all through the cycle.

*These include ibuprofen (Motrin), mefanamic acid (Ponstel), naproxen (Naprosyn), indomethacin (Indocin). Drug companies are continuing to develop new antiprostaglandins. Naprosyn has been linked to pituitary tumors and swollen lymph nodes. (Dowie, et. al. "The Illusion of Safety," Part I, *Mother Jones*, Vol. 7, No. 5 [June 1982], pp. 42–43.)

of taking these drugs over a lifetime. It is best to start with the least invasive treatments, often home remedies. Acupuncture has also helped women with all types of menstrual problems.

Home Remedies for All Menstrual Problems

Women have been sharing menstrual remedies for centuries. Some of us have gained new respect for our own knowledge after trying traditional remedies and exploring new ones. Listed here are only those most frequently reported to work. Try one or more of the following suggestions and, *since each woman is unique and has different reactions, pay attention to how the remedy you choose affects you.*

Food

Make sure the food you eat is varied, sufficient and balanced. You can be malnourished and not be underweight. Pay attention to the positive and negative effects of what you eat. Many women find it helps to eat *more* whole grains and whole flours, beans, vegetables, fruits and brewer's yeast and *less* or *no* salt, sugar, alcohol and caffeine (in coffee, tea, chocolate and soft drinks). Some of us avoid salt, white flour and caffeine for at least the week before our periods and find that it helps. (See Chapter 2, "Food.") Also, you may need to eat small, frequent meals or snacks rather than two or three bigger meals.

Sleep

Get the right amount for *you*. Your rhythms may change during your cycle. Allow time for extra sleep if you need it.

Exercise

See Chapter 4, "Women in Motion," and Maddux, *Menstruation* (listed in Resources), for specific menstrual exercises. Some yoga exercises, especially the cobra position, are particularly helpful. Experiment with different positions to find out what helps you, even if it only works temporarily.

Home Remedies for Specific Menstrual Problems

Cramps and Backache

Herb teas* can help. Raspberry leaf tea is one most consistently recommended. Brew one tablespoon for

*See Resources: *Hygieia*, by Jeannine Parvati, for more on herbs.

each cup. Some women take calcium and magnesium supplements in a two-to-one ratio for several days before the flow or all through the cycle. Start with 250 milligrams of calcium and half that of magnesium. (Take the tablets separately. Dolomite, calcium containing magnesium, may be contaminated with lead or arsenic. Taking these supplements for a long time in large doses may cause problems.) Heat on your stomach or lower back may help. Orgasm, with or without a partner, may work. Some women use nonprescription drugs such as aspirin, acetaminophen (e.g., Tylenol) or alcohol. Marijuana can be effective but may cause other menstrual problems. We encourage moderation in the use of all these drugs. All kinds of massage may work. See "Menstrual Massage for Two People" on p. 216 and look for others specifically for menstrual problems in yoga, Shiatsu, acupressure and polarity therapy books.

Depression, Tension, Moodiness, Bloated Feeling

Many women find Vitamin B_6 a great help. Start with twenty-five to fifty milligrams a day and try up to 200 milligrams a day or more. Use with a general B-complex for better absorption. A lot of B_6 is found in whole grains, yeast, peanuts, fresh fish, and meats, especially liver. Try to decrease sodium by eating less salt and increase potassium. (See Chapter 2, "Food.") Some women use diuretics (plain water, water-reducing teas, foods—consult a book on using herbs—or drugs). Use them with caution; most diuretics except water deplete the body of potassium.

Tiredness or Paleness

Check your iron level for anemia.

Heavy Periods and/or Irregular Bleeding

Try eating foods or take supplements with Vitamin C *and* bioflavinoids (also called Vitamin P). Most foods with Vitamin C also contain bioflavinoids. If this problem starts after stopping the Pill,* try Vitamin A. Be cautious when taking more than 10,000 IUs of Vitamin A a day. If you start to feel nausea or other changes, discontinue using it; excessive Vitamin A is toxic.

*See also Chapter 13, "Birth Control." Irregular bleeding may come after sterilization and heavy bleeding with IUD use. Psychotropic drugs, either prescribed, such as Valium and Librium, or "street" drugs, can cause menstrual irregularities. Amphetamines and probably over-the-counter diet aids can increase menstrual flow and cramping.

Menstrual Massage For Two People

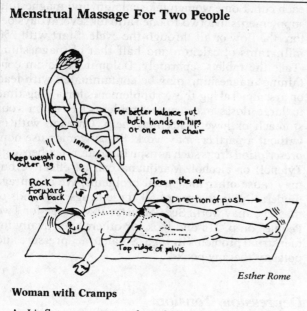

For better balance put both hands on hips or one on a chair

Keep weight on outer leg

inner leg

Rock forward and back

Toes in the air

Direction of push →

Top ridge of pelvis

Esther Rome

Woman with Cramps

A. Lie flat on your stomach, with or without clothes. Place a blanket or pad under you for extra comfort.

B. Have your arms straight out or slightly bent at the elbows. Point your toes inward if possible.

C. Tell the other person what feels good and what doesn't. It should feel good.

Person Giving the Massage

A. Basic movement:
1. Remove your shoes (or kneel and use the heel of your hand).
2. Check to see if the woman is comfortable. You might gently shake her feet or legs to help her relax and to establish physical contact.

3. Stand, placing your outer leg next to the head and *above* the shoulder of the woman on the floor.

4. Put the *heel* of your inner foot against the edge of the top ridge of her pelvis, on the same side where you are standing. (See diagram.)

5. "Hook" your heel as much under the bone as you can. If you are not sure where the pelvic ridge is, feel for it first with your fingers. It may be higher up on her back than you think.

6. Keep both of your legs slightly bent.

7. Gently push away from you, toward her feet, at regular intervals of once or twice a second.
   a. When doing this, rock with your whole body by bending *only* at the *knee* and *ankle* of the leg you are standing on.
   b. Move forward and back. Avoid a circular motion.
   c. When you are pushing firmly enough the whole body of the woman getting the massage will rock, too.
   d. Try not to push toward the floor with your inner foot. Keep your toes pointing upward to prevent this.
   e. Keep your heel in contact with her pelvic bone so the woman getting the massage won't feel bruised.

8. Increase the frequency and length of the push as long as the woman with the cramps says it is comfortable. You will probably need to work more vigorously than you first imagined.

B. When you feel comfortable with the basic movement:
1. Move your heel from side to side to different spots along the ridge of her pelvis on the side you are standing next to. Avoid her spine.
2. Stand on your other leg and repeat A and B-1.
3. Change sides as often as you want. Continue with the massage until the woman's cramps diminish or go away.

Amenorrhea

Another menstrual problem is amenorrhea (absence of menstrual periods). Primary amenorrhea is the condition of never having had a period by the time menstruation usually starts (age eighteen); secondary amenorrhea is the cessation of menstruation after at least one period. Some causes are pregnancy; menopause; breastfeeding; too little body fat; dieting; starvation; heavy athletic training, especially during early adolescence; previous use of birth control pills; use of some drugs; a congenital defect of the genital tract; hormone imbalance; cysts or tumors; disease; chromosomal abnormalities; stress or emotional factors. Since it is a frequent symptom of infertility,* medical textbooks and practitioners pay considerably more at-

tention to amenorrhea than to PMS or painful periods, although these are far more common. Doctors once again focus more on a less common but more dramatic problem and pay little attention to the kinds of emotional adjustments we may go through and the kinds of support we need.

As a home remedy for lack of periods or unusually light periods, you might want to try pennyroyal leaf tea (don't use the oil; it can be toxic). Brew one teaspoon per cup. Also, weight loss of 10 to 15 percent below a healthy minimum can stop your periods; a return to *your* minimum weight will correct this. If you've taken the birth control pill, try supplements of B_6, folic acid and Vitamin E, and decrease the amount of protein you eat. Severe anemia can stop menstruation temporarily. For menopausal symptoms, see Chapter 22, "Women Growing Older," and Reitz, *Menopause: A Positive Approach*, listed in Resources at the end of that chapter.

*For a good description of medical treatments, see Resources: *Womancare*, by Madaras and Patterson, pp. 581–601.

APPENDIX: Hormones of the Menstrual Cycle Simplified

During the reproductive part of a woman's life, baseline levels of all the sex hormones are being continuously produced. In addition to those levels, there are fluctuations which establish the menstrual cycle. The main organs involved in the cycle are the *hypothalamus* (a part of the brain) and the *pituitary* and the *ovaries* (both glands). The hypothalamus signals the pituitary, which then signals the ovaries, which in turn signal the hypothalamus. The signaling is done by hormones secreted by the different organs and carried from one part of the body to another through the blood.

The hypothalamus is sensitive to the fluctuating levels of hormones produced by the ovaries. When the level of estrogens, primarily estradiol beta 17, drop below a certain level, the hypothalamus releases GnRH, gonadatropin-releasing hormone. This stimulates the pituitary to release FSH, follicle-stimulating hormone. This triggers the growth of ten to twenty of the ovarian follicles. Only one of these will mature fully; the others will start to degenerate sometime before ovulation. The ones that degenerate are called "atretic."

As the follicles grow they secrete estrogens in increasing amounts. The estrogens affect the lining of the uterus, signaling it to grow, or proliferate (proliferatory phase). When the egg approaches maturity inside the follicle that will develop fully, the follicle secretes a burst of progesterone in addition to the estrogens. The estrogens probably trigger the hypothalamus to secrete GnRH. This releasing factor signals the pituitary to secrete simultaneously large amounts of FSH and LH, luteinizing hormone. The FSH-LH peak probably signals the follicle to release the egg (ovulation). Under the influence of LH, the follicle changes its function. Now called a corpus luteum, the follicle secretes decreasing amounts of estrogens and increasing amounts of progesterone. The progesterone influences the estrogen-primed uterine lining to secrete fluids nourishing to the egg if it is fertilized (secretory or luteal phase). Immediately after the peak that triggers ovulation, FSH returns to a baseline level. LH declines as the progesterone increases. If the egg is fertilized, the corpus luteum continues to secrete estrogens and progesterone to maintain the pregnancy. However, the corpus luteum is stimulated to do this by HCG, human chorionic gonadotropin, a hormone which is secreted by the developing placenta. HCG so far appears to be chemically identical to LH, so it's not surprising it has the same function.

If the egg is not fertilized, the corpus luteum degenerates until it becomes nonfunctioning; it is then called a corpus albicans. As the degeneration occurs, the levels of hormones from the corpus luteum decline. The declining levels fail to maintain the uterine lining, which leads to menstruation. When the level of estrogens reaches a low enough point, the hypothalamus releases GnRH and the cycle starts again.

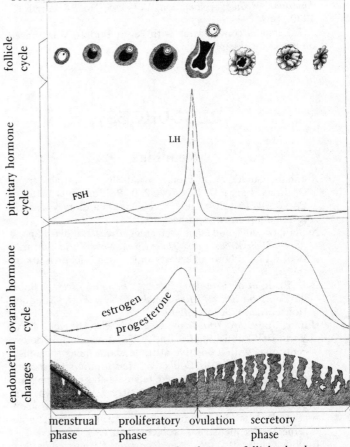

THE MENSTRUAL CYCLE—relationship between follicle development, hormone cycles, and endometrial (uterine lining) buildup and disintegration. The cervical mucus gets progressively wetter from the menstrual phase to ovulation, then becomes drier during the secretory phase.

Peggy Clark

NOTES

1. Jean Garling and Susan Jo Roberts. "An Investigation of Cyclic Distress among Staff Nurses," in Dan, et al., *The Menstrual Cycle: Volume 1*, pp. 305–11.

2. Sharon Golub. "Premenstrual Changes in Mood, Personality and Cognitive Function," in Dan, et. al., *The Menstrual Cycle: Volume 1*, pp. 237–46.

3. Effie A. Graham. "Cognition as Related to Menstrual Cycle Phase and Estrogen Level," in Dan, et al., *The Menstrual Cycle: Volume 1*, pp. 190–208.

4. Sandra K. Webster. "Problems for Diagnosis of Spasmodic and Congestive Dysmenorrhea," in Dan, et al., *The Menstrual Cycle: Volume 1*, pp. 292–304.

5. Sharon Golub. "The Effect of Premenstrual Anxiety and Depression on Cognitive Function," *Journal of Personality and Social Psychology*, Vol. 34, No. 1 (1976), pp. 99–104; Sharon Golub and Denise Murphy Huntington. "Premenstrual and Menstrual Mood Changes in Adolescent Women," *Journal of Personality and Social Psychology*, Vol. 14, No. 5 (1981), pp. 961–65.

6. Elizabeth R. González. "Premenstrual Syndrome: An Ancient Woe Deserving of Modern Scrutiny," *Journal of the American Medical Association*, Vol. 245, No. 14 (April 10, 1980), pp. 1393–96.

7. Personal conversation with Penny Budoff, M.D., based on her clinical experience.

RESOURCES

Readings

Abraham, Guy E., M.D. "Premenstrual Blues." Available from Optimax, Inc., P.O. Box 7000-280, Rolling Hills Estates, CA 90274. This 20-page 1982 booklet is a dietary and vitamin-supplement approach to PMS.

Ayalah, Daphna, and Isaac Weinstock. *Breasts: Women Speak About Their Breasts and Their Lives*. New York: Summit Books, 1979. Photos of breasts and women's feelings about their own.

Bell, Ruth, et al. *Changing Bodies, Changing Lives: A Book for Teens on Sex and Relationships*. New York: Random House, Inc., 1980. Excellent.

Blume, Judy. *Are You There, God? It's Me, Margaret*. New York: Dell Publishing Co., Inc., 1970. A wonderful adolescent novel with a positive attitude about menstruation.

Boston Women's Health Collective. *Menstruation*. For a copy send stamped, self-addressed, business-size envelope plus 50¢ to BWHBC, 465 Mt. Auburn Street, Watertown, MA 02172. A ten-page 1981 brochure including information on attitudes, examining your cycle, menstrual sponges, home remedies for menstrual problems and TSS.

Budoff, Penny, M.D. *No More Menstrual Cramps and Other Good News*. New York: G.P. Putnam's Sons, 1980. A medical approach to cramps and several other gynecological problems.

Corinne, Tee. *Labiaflowers: A Coloring Book*. Tallahassee, FL: Naiad Press, Inc. (P.O. Box 10543, Tallahassee, FL 32302). $3.95 plus postage. Nice drawings of varied labia.

Dalton, Katharina. *The Menstrual Cycle*. New York: Pantheon Books, 1969. The first book to take a woman's complaints seriously. Now much is outdated.

Dalton, Katharina. *Once a Month*. Pomona, CA: Hunter House, 1979. About PMS and progesterone treatment. Although PMS clinics usually recommend this book, Dalton has a dreadful attitude toward women and no interest in changing women's roles.

Dan, Alice, et al. *The Menstrual Cycle: Volume 1: A Synthesis of Interdisciplinary Research*. New York: Springer Publishing Co., Inc., 1980. Good research papers covering a variety of topics.

Delany, Janice, Mary Jane Lupton and Emily Toth. *The Curse: A Cultural History of Menstruation*. New York: Dutton Publishing Co., Inc., 1976. A wide-ranging exploration of attitudes.

Deutsch, Ronald M. *The Key to Feminine Response in Marriage*. New York: Random House, Inc., 1968.

Federation of Feminist Women's Health Centers. *A New View of a Woman's Body*. New York: Simon and Schuster, 1981. Excellent drawings and photos. Text sometimes confusing.

Friedman, Nancy. *Everything You Must Know About Tampons*. New York: Berkley Publishing Corp., 1981. Just what it says.

Frisch, Rose. "Nutrition, Fatness and Fertility: The Effect of Food Intake on Reproductive Ability," in W. Henry Mosley, ed., *Nutrition and Human Reproduction*. New York: Plenum Publishing Corp., 1978. A good introduction to Frisch's work. She continues to do research and publish on the trigger mechanisms for menstruation.

Gardner-Loulan, J., B. Lopez and M. Quackenbush. *Period*. Burlingame, CA: My Mama's Press, 1979 (Box 2086, Burlingame, CA 94100). A good book for girls. Shows all kinds of body types.

Golub, Sharon, ed. "Lifting the Curse of Menstruation: A Feminist Appraisal of the Influence of Menstruation on Women's Lives," *Women and Health* (special issue), Vol. 8, Nos. 2 and 3 (summer/fall 1983). The Haworth Press, 28 E. 22 Street, New York, NY 10010.

Harrison, Michelle, M.D. *Self-Help for Premenstrual Syndrome*. Matrix Press, Box 740, Cambridge, MA 02238, 1982. $6.00, including postage and handling.

Hubbard, Ruth, et al., ed. *Women Look at Biology Looking at Women: A Collection of Feminist Critiques*. Cambridge, MA: Schenkman, 1979. Selections on menstruation and menopause.

Komnenich, Pauline, et al., eds. *The Menstrual Cycle: Volume 2: Research and Implication For Women's Health*. New York: Springer Publishing Co., Inc., 1980. Another good group of research papers.

Lever, Judy, with Michael G. Brush. *Pre-Menstrual Tension*. New York: McGraw-Hill, Inc., 1981. Some parts simplistic. Gives home remedies, including B₆, but puts too much trust in medical solutions.

Madaras, Lynda, and Jane Patterson. *Womancare: A Gynecological Guide to Your Body*. New York: Avon Books, 1981. What a readable popular version of a gynecological text would be.

Maddux, Hilary C. *Menstruation*. New Canaan, CT: Tobey Publishing Co., 1975. The section on exercise is good, the rest of the book fair, the underlying attitude about menstruation negative.

Paige, Karen. "Women Learn to Sing the Menstrual Blues," *Psychology Today*, Vol. 7, No. 4 (September 1973), pp. 41–46. Investigates cultural context for menstrual problems.

Parlee, Mary Brown. "The Premenstrual Syndrome," *Psychological Bulletin* 83, 6 (1973), pp. 454–65. One of the earliest and best critiques of Dalton's work.

Parvati, Jeannine. *Hygieia: A Woman's Herbal*. Berkeley, CA: Bookpeople, 1978. The only herbal specifically for women.

Rome, Esther R. *Premenstrual Syndrome (PMS) Examined Through a Feminist Lens*. 1983. For a copy send stamped (37¢), self-addressed, business-size envelope plus $1.00 to BWHBC, 465 Mt. Auburn Street, Watertown, MA 02172.

Sampson, Gwyneth. "Premenstrual Syndrome: A Double-Blind Controlled Trial of Progesterone and Placebo," *British Journal of Psychiatry* 135 (1979), pp. 209–15. The most recent test of progesterone treatment (as of press time) showing it no more effective than placebo.

Shuttle, Penelope, and Peter Redgrove. *The Wise Wound: Eve's Curse and Everywoman*. New York: Richard Marek Publishers, 1978. A psychoanalytic but provocative approach to menstruation and menstrual problems.

Sloane, Ethel. *Biology of Women*. New York: John Wiley and Sons, Inc., 1980. One of the few (only?) anatomy and physiology texts with a feminist perspective.

Weideger, Paula. *Menstruation and Menopause: The Physiology, the Myth and the Reality*, Rev. Ed. New York: Dell Publishing Co., Inc., 1977.

Woman Spirit Magazine (Box 263, Wolf Creek, OR 97497). Often has articles on menstruation.

See Chapter 11, "Sexuality," Resources for:
 Brecher, Ruth, and Edward Brecher, eds. *An Analysis of Human Sexual Response.*
 Dodson, Betty. *Liberating Masturbation: A Meditation on Self Love.*
 Sherfey, Mary Jane. *The Nature and Evolution of Female Sexuality.*
See Chapter 22, "Women Growing Older," Resources for:
 Reitz, Rosetta. *Menopause: A Positive Approach.*
 Voda, Ann. *Changing Perspectives on Menopause.*
 Weideger, Paula. *Menstruation and Menopause.*

Audiovisual Materials

Culpepper, Emily. *Period Piece*, a 10-minute 16 mm. color film. Available from E.E. Culpepper, 64 R Sacramento Street, Cambridge, MA 02138. About attitudes, experiences and images of menstruation.

Feferman, Linda. *Linda's Film—Menstruation*, a 1974 18-minute color film. Available from Phoenix Films, 470 Park Avenue South, New York, NY 10016. A lively film for teens and preteens.

Records

Lempke, Debbie. "The Bloods—A Self-Help Song," in *Berkeley Women's Music Collective*, an LP record. Available from Olivia Records, Box 70237, Los Angeles, CA 90070. A positive attitude!

13

Birth Control

By Susan Bell

With special thanks to Judy Norsigian, Pamela Morgan, Ruth Bell and Susan Reverby

This chapter in previous editions was written by Abby Schwarz, Nancy Hawley, Pamela Berger, Wendy Sanford, Barbara Perkins and Ruth Bell.

Birth control is fundamental to our effort to understand our bodies, control our health care and have autonomy in our lives. In the U.S., women raised the issue of birth control in the early twentieth century primarily as an effort to increase our reproductive freedom through greater access to contraceptives. Today we have numerous contraceptive methods, yet many of us are dissatisfied with the choices facing us, and we still get pregnant when we don't plan to. Worrying about pregnancy can prevent us from enjoying sexual intercourse with fertile men. We may dream of a contraceptive which is perfectly safe, 100 percent effective, easy to use, instantly reversible and free. Yet controlling birth involves more than having the "right" methods and techniques. Even with them, our decision to use birth control involves our feelings about ourselves, our sexuality and our relationships. Real reproductive freedom depends on having the personal, social and political power to choose freely whether or not to have children. (See introduction to "Controlling Our Fertility.")

Since the 1950s, the population control establishment* has dominated the development and distribution of contraceptives. These organizations are more interested in limiting the size of certain groups (especially poor and minority populations) than in helping individual women control our fertility. Joining the population control establishment's efforts are a scientific community which wants to understand and control our fertility and menstrual cycles, a medical profession which views us as ignorant and incapable of taking an active role in controlling our fertility, and

*The "population control establishment" includes the U.S. government, through the Agency for International Development, for example; and private groups, such as the International Planned Parenthood Federation and the Association for Voluntary Sterilization. See Chapter 26, "Developing an International Awareness," for further discussion.

the pharmaceutical industry seeking profits from new and improved products. Together, these groups control much of our reproductive health. A noted figure in population research writes, "Basically, current research goals in contraception are often set to meet corporate goals and the perceived needs of society rather than the expressed needs of individuals."[1] This perspective has resulted in racist practices, such as forced sterilization and the toleration (even espousal) of contraceptive methods with substantial risks: "The dangers of overpopulation are so great that we may have to use certain techniques of contraception that may entail considerable risk to the individual woman."[2] To protect women everywhere, we need to recognize this kind of mentality and protest against it.

SOME OBSTACLES TO BIRTH CONTROL OR USING IT WELL

Birth Control and Sex Information

Deeply felt antisex attitudes and shame about sex prevent many of us from seeking information. On a wider scale, these same attitudes serve to keep sex information from being distributed freely in schools and community organizations. Laws, medical practices and public school policies prevent us from getting the information and services we need, especially when we are young. Many recent studies have exploded the myth that giving teenagers birth control information makes them promiscuous.

In the 1960s and 1970s some legislatures and school boards reversed restrictive laws, and parents, teachers and community people started a few good sex education programs in several U.S. school systems. More recently, groups such as the Moral Majority, sup-

220

ported by the policies of conservative federal and state governments, have sought to reinstate the old restrictive laws or pass new ones and to stop existing sex education programs.

Birth Control: Who Protects Our Interests?

We would like to think that because a method is available through a doctor's office, a medical clinic or a drugstore, its safety and efficacy have been proven. The Food and Drug Administration (FDA) regulates the methods of contraception, deciding which ones are still experimental and which are legal to prescribe and sell, so we assume that they have been carefully tested before we use them.

All birth control methods must be tested first on animals and then on women before the FDA approves them for marketing. Often, drug companies test new methods on women in Third World countries or poor women and women of color in this country. (See section on Depo-Provera, p. 247.) When the effectiveness and safety of the method satisfy federal requirements, the FDA approves it for general distribution and marketing. However, the recent history of women's contraceptives has shown that the long-term complications and negative effects are rarely thoroughly understood when methods are approved. FDA requirements take up to ten years of work before a drug is marketed, but it takes twenty years or more for some complications to become apparent. As a result, all women using the Pill or the IUD, for instance, become subjects in prolonged experiments.

When we make careful choices about birth control and seek trustworthy advice, we find conflicting information and false reassurances. Much available evidence has been researched and published by the drug companies themselves and is biased accordingly. Advice from physicians is problematic, since many physicians depend on drug company literature and sales personnel for information. Even when physicians are aware of the complications and risks associated with a particular method, some of them hesitate to tell us about them because, as one Boston gynecologist explained in testimony before Congress, "...well, if you tell them they might get headaches, they will get headaches."* This paternalistic and condescending attitude keeps us from receiving the information we need to make a responsible choice about which birth control method best suits us. Furthermore, physicians often recommend their own favorite method, which may not be the best one for us. And it is alarming that many physicians' recommendations depend on the methods they have available at the time of our visit. Thus, many of us find ourselves with inadequate or downright dangerous methods, and some of us, unwilling to go through the hassle, end up using nothing at all.

Men and Birth Control

Most women and men in this society assume that the responsibility for birth control should fall on women. One reason for this is that women have a more personal interest in preventing pregnancy than men do, for we bear the children and, in this culture, are in large measure responsible for raising them.

Placing *total* responsibility for birth control on women is unfair. It means that we must make arrangements to see a practitioner for an exam and a prescription, go to the drugstore, usually pay for supplies and make sure they don't run out. With the Pill or IUD, we feel the effects and, more seriously, take whatever risks are involved. If we don't have some kind of birth control and a man presses us to have intercourse, we must say no. If we become pregnant, it means that it's *our* fault. Total responsibility often creates anger and resentment that can't help but get in the way of our sexual feelings.

Many of us do not talk much about birth control with our partners. Yet a man can share the responsibility of birth control in several ways. When no good method is available at the moment, a supportive partner will join us in exploring ways of lovemaking without intercourse.* He can use condoms, and not just when we remind him to; help pay the doctor and drugstore bills; share in putting in the diaphragm or inserting the foam; check to see if supplies are running low. He can, if it is a long-term relationship where no children or no more are wanted, have a vasectomy. A man who truly shares responsibility for preventing

*There are many ways to have sex with a man, but this chapter is about how to prevent pregnancy when sex includes vagina-to-penis contact and intercourse.

*Dr. Frederick Robbins, quoted in Barbara Seaman, *The Doctor's Case Against The Pill* (see Resources).

Page Bond

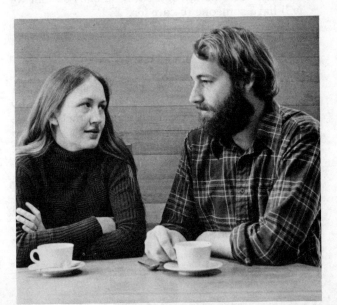

pregnancy may gain our respect. We feel better about our relationship, and use birth control better, too.

Women and Birth Control

The increased availability and effectiveness of birth control methods can encourage friends, husbands, lovers to pressure us to have intercourse whenever they want. We need to be assertive about *our* desires: being protected does not always mean we want intercourse. Many of us have found that we ourselves resist using birth control. What may appear to be personal reasons are actually due to social and political factors as well, such as poor sex education, a double standard of sex, inequalities between women and men. For instance:

- We are embarrassed by, ashamed of or confused about our own sexuality.
- We cannot admit we might have or are having intercourse, because we feel (or someone told us) it is wrong.
- We are unrealistically romantic about sex: sex has to be passionate and spontaneous, and birth control seems too premeditated, too clinical and often too messy.
- We hesitate to "inconvenience" our partner. This fear of displeasing him is a measure of the inequality in our relationship.
- We feel, "It can't happen to me. I won't get pregnant."
- We hesitate to find a practitioner and face the hurried, impersonal care or, if we are young or unmarried, the moralizing and disapproval that we feel likely to receive. We are afraid the practitioner will tell our parents.
- We don't recognize our deep dissatisfactions with the method we are using and begin to use it haphazardly.
- We feel tempted to become pregnant just to prove to ourselves that we are fertile or to try to improve a shaky relationship, or we want a baby so that we will have someone to care for.

WHAT CAN WE DO?

We can learn for ourselves and teach one another about the available methods. By speaking openly and by carefully comparing experiences and knowledge, we can guide each other to workable methods and good practitioners. We can recognize when a practitioner is not thorough enough in examinations or explanations, and encourage each other to ask for the attention we need. By talking together we can also get a better handle on our more subtle resistances to using birth control. We can begin the long but worthwhile process of talking with our male partners about birth control,

encouraging them to share the responsibility with us. We can join together to insist that legislatures, courts, high schools, churches, parents, doctors, research projects, clinics and drug companies change their practices and attitudes so that we can enjoy our sexuality without becoming pregnant. We can create self-help clinics and other alternative health-care institutions where our needs for information, discussion and personal support in the difficult choice of birth control will be better met. We can use the good clinics that do exist. We can push for decent housing, jobs and childcare so that we can choose birth control freely instead of being forced to use it by our circumstances. Whatever we choose to do, we can act together.

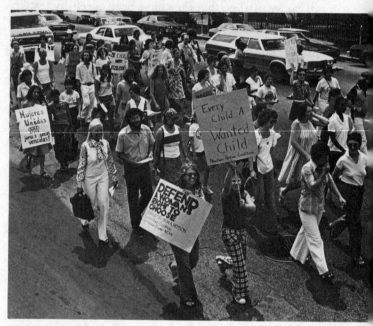

Ellen Shub

HOW PREGNANCY HAPPENS*

During sexual intercourse, sperm are ejaculated through the man's penis into the woman's vagina. If not blocked, some of the sperm swim through the cervical opening (os), through the woman's uterus and into the fallopian tubes. If the sperm encounter an egg in the outer third of the fallopian tube, one may join with the egg. The process of an egg and a sperm uniting is called *conception*. The fertilized egg takes several days to travel down the fallopian tube to the uterus, where after one-and-a-half to two days it implants in the uterine lining and develops over the course of the next nine months.

*See Chapter 12, "Anatomy and Physiology of Sexuality and Reproduction," for more details.

It is also possible for sperm to be deposited in or near the lips around the vagina during sex play. They can swim into the vagina and follow the same route to fertilize the egg. (This is even possible if the woman has an intact hymen or has never had intercourse!)

The egg leaves the ovary (*ovulation*) *approximately two weeks before the beginning of the next menstrual period.** It can be fertilized for only about twelve to twenty-four hours. Although it is unusual, *a woman can get pregnant from having intercourse during her period*, especially if she has an occasional short cycle (less than twenty-seven days). (See "Fertility Observation," p. 235.)

The Sperm

Sperm are made in the man's testicles ("balls"). Sexual stimulation makes blood flow into erectile tissue inside the penis, causing the penis to become stiff, hard and erect. The drops of liquid (semen) which come from the penis soon after erection occurs contain many sperm. If stimulation is continued, the man usually has an orgasm. As orgasm begins, sperm travel up the sperm ducts, over the bladder and through the prostate gland into the urethra and then are propelled out of the urethra by rhythmic contractions which are very pleasurable to a man. This is called *ejaculation*.

About 300 million to 500 million sperm come out in one ejaculation. This large number is needed to insure conception, since many sperm die on the trip to the egg.

Sperm come out fast and swim fast, too—an inch in eight minutes; a sperm may reach an egg in as little as thirty minutes. The acid environment of the vagina

*A common misunderstanding is that the egg leaves the ovary at midcycle, halfway between menstrual periods. This is only true when the cycle is twenty-eight days long (something which cannot be known for sure until that particular cycle is over and menstruation begins).

is inhospitable to sperm, so without favorable cervical mucus to nourish and protect them, sperm die in about half an hour. Around ovulation, cervical mucus is present which enables sperm to swim up into the cervix and uterus, where they can live four to five days.

For birth control to work, the process of conception must be stopped at some point along the way (see illustration below).

CHOOSING A BIRTH CONTROL METHOD

Since there is no one perfect method, our choice of contraceptive will be something of a compromise. Safety and effectiveness are probably the most important factors. Most of us are healthy and fertile when we begin using birth control, and we want to stay that way. We need a method that will protect us from pregnancy effectively and will not make us sick or infertile.

The following table compares the risk of death associated with different birth control methods, pregnancy and abortion. Be aware that this table does not take into account factors such as social class, race, age and pregnancy history. These factors can determine whether, for example, the Pill or pregnancy poses a greater risk for a particular woman.

When looking at *effectiveness* statistics in books and magazines, keep in mind that there is a difference between the *theoretical failure rate*, which is based on hypothetical perfect use of the method, and the higher *actual failure rate*, based on records of actual use of the method over time. Actual failure rates include accidents such as forgetting a pill, failing to put on the condom early enough, removing the diaphragm within six hours after intercourse or leaving it in the drawer instead of using it. The actual failure rate will give you a more realistic idea of how effective the method

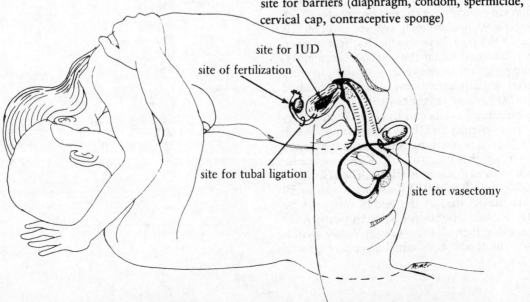

site for barriers (diaphragm, condom, spermicide, cervical cap, contraceptive sponge)

site for IUD

site of fertilization

site for tubal ligation

site for vasectomy

Nina Reimer

	Chance of Death in a Year
Birth control pills (nonsmoker)	1 in 63,000
Birth control pills (smoker) (See Chapter 3 for other dangers of smoking.)	1 in 16,000
IUDs	1 in 100,000
Barrier methods	none
Natural methods	none
Sterilization:	
laparoscopic tubal ligation	1 in 10,000
hysterectomy	1 in 1,600
vasectomy	none
Pregnancy:	
continuing pregnancy	1 in 10,000
terminating pregnancy:	
illegal abortion	1 in 3,000
legal abortion:	
before 9 weeks	1 in 400,000
between 9–12 weeks	1 in 100,000
between 13–16 weeks	1 in 25,000
after 16 weeks	1 in 10,000

This table was adapted from *Contraceptive Technology, 1982–1983*, which lists the following references: W. Cates, "Putting the Risks in Perspective," *Contraceptive Technology Update 1980* 1 (November), p. 111; B.D. Dinman, "The Reality and Acceptance of Risk," *Journal of the American Medical Association* 244 (1980), pp. 1226–28; C. Tietze, "New Estimates of Mortality Associated With Fertility Control," *Family Planning Perspectives* 9 (1977), pp. 74–76; National Center for Health Statistics, Final Mortality Statistics, United States, 1976–78; Center for Disease Control, Abortion-Related Mortality, United States, 1976–78.

is, and will invite you to consider the crucial question of how effectively *you and your partner* will use it.

> If you think your method of birth control is making you sick, go to a clinic or health practitioner. If the clinic/practitioner doesn't give you an adequate answer, get a second opinion. Stop using that method, and be sure to use another one to avoid pregnancy.

The table at right gives both actual and theoretical rates. A 5 percent pregnancy rate, or failure rate, which is the same as a 95 percent effectiveness rate, means that studies in the past have shown that five women out of every hundred using that particular method have become pregnant in one year. Note that, in comparison, heterosexually active women using no method at all have a 90 percent pregnancy rate.

Some researchers have begun to argue that the actual failure rates of pills and IUDs are probably much higher than 5 to 10 percent, because so many women discontinue using them as a result of their troublesome and sometimes dangerous effects. The *discontinuation rate* for the Pill and IUD may be as high as 50 percent. This means that at the end of one year 50 percent of the women who started using these methods are no longer using them. If these women do not switch to alternative methods, they can become pregnant.

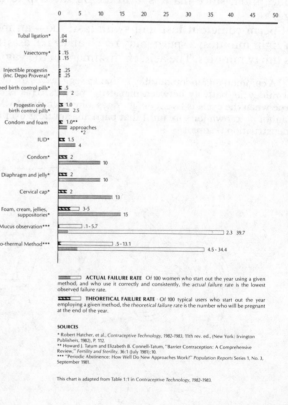

THEORETICAL AND ACTUAL FAILURE RATES OF STERILIZATION AND REVERSIBLE BIRTH CONTROL METHODS

ACTUAL FAILURE RATE Of 100 women who start out the year using a given method, and who use it correctly and consistently, the actual failure rate is the lowest observed failure rate.

THEORETICAL FAILURE RATE Of 100 typical users who start out the year employing a given method, the theoretical failure rate is the number who will be pregnant at the end of the year.

SOURCES
* Robert Hatcher, et al., *Contraceptive Technology, 1982–1983*, 11th rev. ed., (New York: Irvington Publishers, 1982), P. 112.
** Howard J. Tatum and Elizabeth B. Connell-Tatum, "Barrier Contraception: A Comprehensive Review," *Fertility and Sterility*, 36:1 (July 1981): 10.
*** "Periodic Abstinence: How Well Do New Approaches Work?" *Population Reports* Series 1, No. 3, September 1981.

This chart is adapted from Table 1:1 in *Contraceptive Technology, 1982–1983*.

Susan Bell

Barrier methods like the diaphragm, condom, foam, cervical cap and contraceptive sponge may have lower discontinuation rates than the Pill and IUD, making them more effective in the long run.[3]

The Collective favors certain methods of contraception over others and has chosen to place them first. Most of us who use birth control choose a diaphragm, cervical cap, or foam and condom, because they are both effective and safe. We have become increasingly discouraged about the Pill and IUD after receiving hundreds of letters from women who have been harmed by these methods. Research also documents Pill and IUD risks. We believe that the Pill and IUD are dangerous enough to warrant their use as methods of "second choice" rather than "first choice," and so we describe them toward the end of the chapter.

As you read, you will, of course, form your own opinions and make your choices. No one method is likely to satisfy us through all our fertile years.

THE DIAPHRAGM AND SPERMICIDAL CREAM OR JELLY

Before the diaphragm* was invented in the nineteenth century, women had to depend on men (using condoms and withdrawal) to prevent pregnancy, and on crude abortion and infanticide for backup. The diaphragm was a major breakthrough, giving women responsibility over birth control and freeing us from unwanted pregnancies. It was popular until the 1960s—at one time, a third of all U.S. couples practicing birth control used it. By 1971, however, Planned Parenthood reported that only 4 percent of its clients were choosing diaphragms. What had happened?

In the late 1950s and 1960s, the drug industry, the medical profession, private foundations and the U.S. government began to pour money into researching, developing and distributing the Pill and the IUD, virtually excluding any research on the diaphragm and other barrier methods. Usually, these interests were more concerned with developing new technologies and/or making profits than with the health and well-being of women. Many of us believed the drug industry's and physicians' proclamations about Pill and IUD safety and hoped that the Pill and IUD would allow us more sexual spontaneity and protection against pregnancy than diaphragms.

Recently, many women have begun using the dia-

phragm again. Our more positive feelings about our sexuality and our increasing ability to communicate openly with the men we sleep with allow us to use the diaphragm more easily. Also, we have learned that diaphragms, correctly fitted and worn, are more reliable than IUDs and safer than the Pill or IUD.

Yet there are still obstacles to diaphragm use. Only a practitioner can legally prescribe it. Some practitioners, especially physicians, do not include time for fittings in their schedules and often charge high fees for their services. A practitioner's attitudes about sexuality *can* affect his/her attitudes about certain methods of birth control and affect ours in turn. Many practitioners don't trust our ability to use a barrier method well; they frequently assume that IUDs or pills are "better" and that we wouldn't want to "mess" with the diaphragm. Research on barrier methods continues to be inadequate: out of a total of 30.2 *million* dollars spent in 1976 on contraceptive research, the U.S. spent only fifty *thousand* dollars on barrier method research.[5]

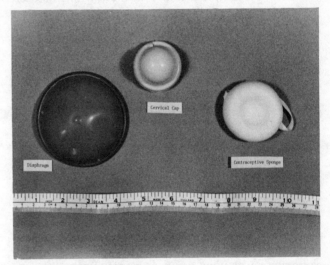

Diaphragm/cap/sponge   *Phyllis Ewen*

Description

A diaphragm, *which must always be used with spermicidal cream or jelly*, is made of soft rubber in the shape of a shallow cup (see illustration above). It has a flexible metal spring rim (arcing, coiled or flat). When properly fitted and inserted, it fits snugly over your cervix, sitting in place behind the pubic bone and reaching back behind your cervix. It comes in a variety of sizes measured in millimeters (mm), ranging from fifty to 105 millimeters, or two to four inches, depending on the size of your upper vagina.

Diaphragm Alert! The 86,000 Koro-Flex diaphragms bearing the serial numbers F6, C6, H6 or I6 were *recalled* in May 1977 because 1 percent of them are defective. They have pinprick-size holes along the rim. If your diaphragm is Koro-Flex (note: Koro-Mex devices are not included in the recall) and has one of these four serial numbers on the rim, return it to the place you got it or to a Planned Parenthood clinic for replacement or refund.

How It Works

When the diaphragm is in place, holding spermicidal jelly or cream up to your cervix, the sperm cannot go into your cervical canal. Sperm swim up around the rim of the diaphragm and run into the cream or jelly, which kills them. Some women also smear jelly on the outside of the diaphragm to help kill sperm remaining in the vagina. Always use a diaphragm with cream or jelly: *they* are the important contraceptives; the diaphragm exists only to hold them in the proper place.

Effectiveness

The diaphragm can have a failure rate as low as 2 percent if fit properly, its use carefully taught and used perfectly.[6] Most likely, the 2 percent failure rate exists because the diaphragm moves around a bit with frequent insertion of the penis, positions in which the woman is on top and expansion of the upper vagina during intercourse. The actual failure rate is higher, about 10 percent, if it is not used *every time* or used without cream or jelly.

You can combine use of the diaphragm with fertility observation (see p. 235). You can increase the effectiveness of the diaphragm substantially when your partner also uses a condom on your fertile days.

Reversibility

The diaphragm doesn't affect your fertility at all. Simply don't use it if you want to become pregnant.

Safety and Possible Problems

The diaphragm is almost completely safe. It cannot slide up inside us and disappear (as some of us may fear) because the vagina stops about an inch beyond the cervix. A particular cream or jelly may irritate your vagina or your partner's penis. Try a different brand if this happens. The diaphragm itself might push forward and cause cramps in your uterus, bladder or urethra. For some women, this can lead to urethritis or recurrent cystitis. The diaphragm could also push backward on your rectum, which can be uncomfortable, too. If this happens to you, it may mean that the diaphragm is the wrong size. Try out different types of diaphragms as well to see if one is less uncomfortable than another. Some women get recurrent yeast infections when using the diaphragm, which you can avoid by making sure that you wash and dry your diaphragm thoroughly between uses. (For possible negative effects of creams and jellies, see p. 233.)

Who Shouldn't Use the Diaphragm

If you have a severely displaced uterus (severe prolapse, for instance), you cannot use a diaphragm. If you have a protrusion of the bladder through the vaginal wall (cystocele) or other openings in the vagina (fistulas), you cannot use this method.

If you don't feel comfortable touching your genitals and do not think you can get used to it, you would most likely have trouble using a diaphragm effectively. You may feel very squeamish and embarrassed the first time you put your finger into your vagina, but as you get used to it and realize that your body is yours to touch, you should get over any uneasiness about inserting the diaphragm. Starting or joining a self-help group may help you to discuss negative feelings about touching yourself.

Since there is about a 2 percent failure rate associated with the diaphragm, women who must not or who do not wish to become pregnant and who would not choose abortion as a backup might prefer using a more effective barrier method of contraception, such as the foam and condom or diaphragm and condom combination, or might choose to avoid all vagina-to-penis contact during fertile times. (See "Fertility Observation," p. 235.)

How to Get the Diaphragm

The size of diaphragm you should use depends on the size and contour of your vagina and the muscle strength of the surrounding vaginal walls. In this country it is usually a doctor, nurse-practitioner or other women's health care provider who measures (or "fits") you for a diaphragm. If your uterus is tipped forward or backward slightly, the person fitting the diaphragm can choose one of the three kinds of metal spring rim (arcing, coiled or flat) to fit your particular anatomy. If one kind doesn't fit, try another kind.

Very important: When you have been measured and fitted, practice putting the diaphragm in and taking it out before you leave the practitioner's office, so s/he can tell you if you are doing it right. (Or go home, practice and come back in a few days with the diaphragm in place.) Reach in and see what it feels like when it is in correctly and get help immediately if you have problems, so that when you actually use it you won't be "experimenting." Many practitioners neglect this important step.

The practitioner will have the diaphragm available right there or will give you a prescription for the proper size.

How to Use the Diaphragm

Somebody once said that if someone handed you a toothbrush with no instructions and you had never seen one before, you might not use it very well for a

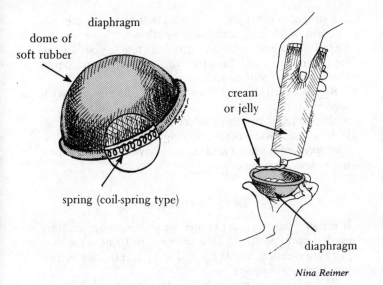

dome of soft rubber

diaphragm

spring (coil-spring type)

cream or jelly

diaphragm

Nina Reimer

while. Like any tool, the diaphragm is simple to use once you've practiced with it. Putting it in and taking it out might feel awkward at first, but it will become easier and quicker every time. You must put the diaphragm in *within six hours** before intercourse or vagina-to-penis contact, since the creams and jellies may start to lose their spermicidal potency in the body after that time. The most conservative estimates say to put it in as close to intercourse as possible, but if you tend to get carried away with sexual intensity, it's probably best to insert the diaphragm in advance.

Preparation and Insertion

Put one teaspoonful to one tablespoonful of cream or jelly (three-quarters of an inch from the tube) into the

*This is a change from the previously recommended time, two hours. See *Contraceptive Technology, 1982–1983*; see also Seaman and Seaman, *Women and the Crisis in Sex Hormones* (both listed in Resources).

shallow cup (see illustration at left). Spread the cream around. (Some books say to put the cream on the rim also; others say that cream on the rim makes the diaphragm slip. An effective compromise might be to put cream around the inside of the rim and not on top of the rim.) Then squeeze the cup together by pressing the rim firmly between your thumb and third finger. If you have trouble, you can buy a plastic inserter (good only with a flat-spring diaphragm). You can squat, sit on the toilet bowl, stand with one foot raised or lie down with your legs bent. With your free hand, spread apart the lips of your vagina and push the diaphragm up to the upper third of your vagina with the cream or jelly facing up. If you have not used tampons or reached into your vagina before, remember that it angles toward your back (see illustration below). Now push the lower rim with your finger until you feel the diaphragm lock into place. You should then reach in to make sure you can feel the outline of your cervix through the soft rubber cup. (For more protection, some women insert a little extra cream or jelly with an applicator when the diaphragm is in place, but this is *not* necessary.) When it's in right and fits properly, you should not be able to feel the diaphragm at all. Your partner probably won't either, although some men notice that the tip of their penis is touching soft rubber instead of cervical and vaginal tissue. (This is not painful.) *Never use petroleum jelly (like Vaseline) with a diaphragm, as it destroys the rubber.*

Leave the diaphragm in for at least six hours after intercourse, because it takes the spermicide that long to kill all the sperm. You can leave it in up to twenty-four hours, but not longer. Douching is unnecessary, but if you want to douche, you must wait six hours.

Subsequent Intercourse

If you have intercourse again, you *must* add more cream or jelly with an applicator. Put it into your vagina, leaving the diaphragm in place.

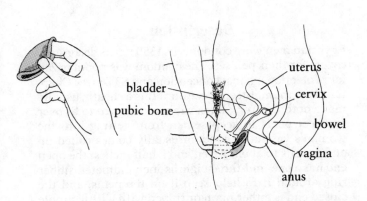

bladder

pubic bone

uterus

cervix

bowel

vagina

anus

INSERTION OF DIAPHRAGM

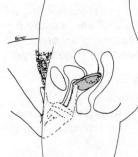

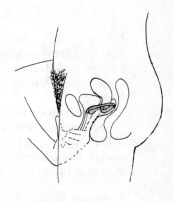

CHECKING OF DIAPHRAGM

Nina Reimer

Removal

Remove the diaphragm by choosing a comfortable position, perhaps the same way you chose to insert it. If you have trouble reaching the diaphragm, try another position or bear down as if you were going to have a bowel movement. Slide a finger into your vagina and hook it under the lower rim of the diaphragm, either between the diaphragm and your vaginal wall or over the rubber dome. Pull the diaphragm forward and down. If you have long nails, take care not to rip the diaphragm.

Care

Wash the diaphragm with mild soap and warm water, rinse and dry carefully, dust it with cornstarch if you wish (but never talcum powder) and put it into a container (away from light). Don't boil it. *Check it for holes* every so often by holding it up to the light or filling it with water and looking for leaks, especially around the rim.

Life of Product

Get your diaphragm size rechecked every year or two. You may need a new size if you gain or lose a lot of weight or have vaginal surgery, and after pregnancy, abortion or miscarriage. The diaphragm will last at least a couple of years with proper care.

Cost

A diaphragm costs about twelve dollars.* The medical examination for the diaphragm can cost from fifty to a hundred dollars depending on whether you go to a clinic or a private physician and on how extensive the examination is.

Spermicidal jellies and creams vary in price from about eight dollars, depending on the size of the tube. A 4.4-ounce tube contains approximately twenty-four applications.

Advantages

It is a good method if you have intercourse with a partner who is cooperative and helpful about using it, and/or if you have intercourse relatively infrequently, since it only has to be used around the time of lovemaking.

It is very effective if used well and every time.

There are almost no side effects or dangers.

The diaphragm is helpful if you want to have intercourse during your period and don't want a heavy menstrual flow to interfere.

*In some federally funded clinics, diaphragm kits (including diaphragm and jelly) can be had for eight dollars or even less.

Using a diaphragm can be a good kind of body education. If you are unfamiliar with what your vagina feels like, using a diaphragm will teach you. In the long run, the more familiar you are with your body, the more you will enjoy sex.

Repeated studies indicate that the diaphragm with cream or jelly reduces your chances of getting gonorrhea or trichomoniasis infections in the vaginal canal. It increases your protection against PID (pelvic inflammatory disease) and cervical dysplasia, and may help clear up adenosis.

Disadvantages

If either you or your partner want sex to be uninterrupted and absolutely spontaneous, putting in the diaphragm can be a hassle if you don't put it in long before you start having sex.

You must remember to use it every time, be sure not to run out of cream or jelly and have it with you when you need it.

The discharge of cream or jelly can be a nuisance, although it does not stain. Try different brands and, if necessary, use a pad or a tissue for leaking after intercourse.

Some people who enjoy oral sex find the taste of the jellies and creams unpleasant. One way around this is to wash carefully after putting in the diaphragm. Another is to put the diaphragm in after oral sex play and before intercourse. This is a definite interruption, however, and that increases the possibility that you won't put it in at all.

Responsibility

The woman goes to be fitted. After that, you and your partner can share the responsibility of insertion, although a lot of women do the whole thing themselves.

THE CONDOM (RUBBER, PROPHYLACTIC, "SAFE")

Description

Egyptian men wore condoms in 1350 B.C. as decorative covers for their penises. The condom was popularized for protection against conception and STDs (see Chapter 14) in the eighteenth century. It is a sheath, usually made of thin, strong latex rubber, designed to fit over an erect penis to keep semen from getting into the woman's vagina. A condom usually comes rolled up and unrolls to about seven and a half inches; the open end has a one-and-three-eighths-inch-diameter rubber ring around it to help keep it on the penis, and the closed end is either plain or tipped with a little nipple that catches the semen and helps to keep the condom

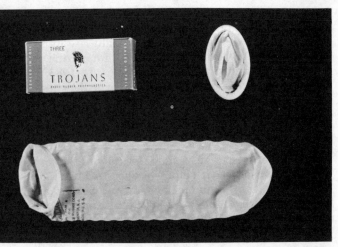

Condoms   *Elizabeth Cole*

How to Use the Condom

The man or woman unrolls the condom onto the erect penis before *any* vagina-to-penis contact or intercourse—*not* just before ejaculation, since long before ejaculation the male may discharge a few drops with enough sperm to cause pregnancy.

Cautions

Leave space at the end of the plain-ended condom for the semen: a half-inch of air-free space between the end of the penis and the condom will keep the ejaculate, which comes out fast, from bursting the condom. Catching air in the end may also cause bursting.

If you do not use a lubricated condom, use a lubricant to prevent tearing—spermicidal foam, cream or jelly or K-Y Jelly, but *never* Vaseline (petroleum jelly), which can corrode the rubber. Saliva is always available but may increase your chances of developing a monilia (yeast) infection. Apply the lubricant after the condom is on the penis.

One of you must hold the rim when you move away from him or he withdraws his no-longer-erect penis after ejaculation; otherwise the condom might slip off, and sperm could get into the vagina.

In case of accident, insert cream or jelly or foam into your vagina as quickly as possible. Do not douche.

from bursting. "Skin" condoms (made of lamb membrane) are more expensive but much thinner. Lubricated rubber condoms minimize the risk of tearing but tend to slip off the penis more easily and have to be used extra carefully. A new type of condom uses a spermicidal lubricant which kills most sperm on contact and is probably more effective than other types of condom. (Ramses Extra is the only product like this so far.)

The condom is the only temporary means of birth control a man can use. Since it can be purchased over the counter or found on a drugstore shelf, or even purchased by mail, men don't need to visit a medical facility to obtain a prescription. Furthermore, women can also easily buy and carry condoms. It should not be surprising, therefore, to find that the condom is the most frequently used barrier method in the U.S.

Once even more widely used, the condom, like all other methods, fell into disfavor when the Pill and IUD appeared. Men could share in the spontaneity and relative sexual freedom brought about by the Pill and IUD without having to experience their negative effects. Furthermore, manufacturers and researchers have conducted almost no studies to try to improve the condom's effectiveness or to develop a tough yet thinner substance which would eliminate the reduction in sensation that some men find objectionable.

Responsibility

The man uses the condom. It is much more enjoyable to use it if both partners join in putting it on. For a couple who have intercourse more than a few times, condoms are a good way for the man to share in birth control. In a shorter-term relationship, when you may not know whether you'll be having intercourse or not, condoms can be very convenient. But don't expect the man to have a condom in his pocket—you may be disappointed. If you don't know him well enough to be sure he'll have a condom, it makes sense for you to have some with you. But it is hard for many of us to pull out a rubber and suggest that the man use it.

Effectiveness

A good-quality condom has a failure rate of about 2 percent when used as directed, but in actual use its failure rate is about 10 percent. We suggest combining condoms with a spermicidal foam, cream or jelly for close to 100 percent protection. Used with an IUD or diaphragm, condoms provide extra protection at ovulation.

Advantages

It is fairly cheap, readily available and easy to use.

It is a method of birth control that gives some protection against gonorrhea and syphilis when used in *every instance* of vagina-to-penis contact. It also prevents partners from infecting and reinfecting each other with an infection such as trichomoniasis or herpes.

If the man tends to ejaculate too quickly, a condom may decrease the stimulation of his penis enough to help him delay ejaculation and prolong intercourse.

A condom catches the semen, so if the woman wants

Reversibility

Perfectly reversible. To get pregnant, just don't use condoms.

to go somewhere right after intercourse, she won't feel drippy.

You don't need a doctor's prescription to buy a condom.

Disadvantages

You have to use the condom right at the time of intercourse, which ruins the spontaneity of sex for some couples unless the woman puts it on the man and makes it a part of sex play.

It may lessen the man's sensation, as his penis doesn't touch the vaginal walls directly. Many men resist using condoms for this reason, forgetting the effects that women's birth control methods can have on a woman's enjoyment of sex. Some men say they do not feel such a great reduction in sensation.

The condom eliminates one source of lubrication for intercourse (the drops of fluid that come out when the man gets an erection), and the resultant friction can irritate a woman, especially during the entrance of the penis into her vagina. You can use the lubricants mentioned above.

How to Get Condoms

You can find condoms in drugstores, at family planning agencies or in vending machines. Many men say they were embarrassed the first time they bought condoms, particularly if the druggist asked, "What size?" and the man didn't know s/he was referring to the size of the package. Condoms are made in a standard size, they come in packages of three or twelve, and they cost about one and a half to two dollars for a package of three and four to six dollars for a package of twelve, depending upon the brand. Some high-quality condoms are Ramses Rubber Prophylactics, Trojans Rubber Prophylactics, Trojan-Enz Rubber Prophylactics. Some condoms are colored, but both men and women have reported that the dyes stain and cause burning and irritation. Some manufacturers are making ribbed condoms, which they claim make intercourse more enjoyable for women, though some of us who have experienced them could not feel any difference.

Life of Product

Condoms have a shelf life of five years if kept away from heat. Since heat causes them to deteriorate, do not store them for very long in a wallet or pocket. If you carry them around, use the kind sealed in foil.

THE CONTRACEPTIVE SPONGE

Investigation to develop a contraceptive sponge began a few years ago, prompted by a number of factors: women moving away from using the Pill and IUD, a growing recognition by the medical establishment that women are seeking alternatives, a slight rise in publicly and privately funded research for improving barrier methods and producing new ones. In 1983, the FDA approved the sponge for general over-the-counter marketing.*

Description

The disposable sponge is made of polyurethane, an artificial substance. It comes in one size, two and a quarter inches in diameter and three-quarters of an inch thick, with an indentation (dimple) in the center and a loop of tape attached (see photograph on p. 225).

How It Works

The sponge covers the opening of the cervix (os), where it traps sperm. It is held in place by the walls of a woman's vagina and the "dimple" covering the cervix. It also contains a spermicide (nonoxynol-9), which it releases slowly to kill sperm.

How to Use the Sponge

Wet the sponge with water and compress it. Then insert it into your vagina by hand or with an applicator. Once the sponge is inside your vagina, it expands in the space around the cervix, blocking the opening (os). It does not require an exact fit as the diaphragm and cervical cap do. You should *not* use the contraceptive sponge during menstruation. To reduce the risk of toxic shock syndrome during your period, use another method of birth control.

Once the sponge is in place, you can have intercourse as often as you like, without having to add any more spermicide. After intercourse, you *must* leave it in place for at least six hours; you *can* leave it in your vagina for up to twenty-four hours (one day). Take it out by pulling on the tape which is attached to it, and throw it away.

Effectiveness

Preliminary reports show the sponge has an actual failure rate of about 16.8 percent.

Reversibility

There is no indication that the sponge will interfere with a woman's fertility when it is not being used. If you want to become pregnant, just stop using the sponge.

*As of early 1984, 400,000 women in the U.S. had used the new contraceptive sponge. Nine hundred thousand sponges had been sold by that time. In one recent study comparing the sponge and diaphragm, the sponge had a 16.8 percent *actual failure rate* versus 13.2 percent for the diaphragm.

Safety

No long-term studies have been conducted on the safety of the material used in the contraceptive sponge. It is unclear whether the high concentration of non-oxynol-9, which is considerably more than used with other barrier methods, poses any increased risks. Also unknown is the effect of polyurethane. The possible association between the sponge and toxic shock syndrome has not been adequately tested yet. About 2 percent of women using the sponge have reported allergic reactions. Some sponges have shredded while they are in place.

Advantages

The contraceptive sponge has most of the advantages of the diaphragm: safety and effectiveness, easy reversibility, encouragement for learning about your body, possible prevention of sexually transmitted diseases.

It remains effective for up to twenty-four hours, allowing vagina-to-penis contact and sexual intercourse to be spontaneous.

It comes in one size, so it doesn't need to be fitted.

You can buy it over the counter.

It doesn't leak, so it's less messy than most other barriers and doesn't interfere with oral sex.

Disadvantages

Some women notice an unpleasant odor after intercourse.

About 2 to 3 percent of women in clinical trials report expelling the sponge, usually during a bowel movement.

If you don't feel comfortable about touching your genitals, you will have trouble using the sponge.

Some women, such as those with a prolapsed uterus, cannot wear it.

THE CERVICAL CAP

The cervical cap is a barrier contraceptive which may soon be more widely available in the United States. It is a thimble-shaped rubber or plastic cap that fits snugly over the cervix. Like the diaphragm, it blocks sperm from entering the cervical opening. Usually, a small amount of spermicide is used on the inside of the cap to kill any sperm that might break through the suction seal. Used in some European countries, the cap was also used during the early twentieth century in the U.S.* With the rise in use of the Pill and IUD,

*The idea of the cervical cap is thousands of years old. In ancient Sumatra, women molded opium into cuplike devices to cover their cervices. See Seaman and Seaman, *Women and the Crisis in Sex Hormones*, p. 190 (listed in Resources).

the cervical cap, like the diaphragm, declined in popularity. By the mid-1960s, U.S. companies had completely stopped producing it for contraceptive purposes.

Although the cap is an "investigational" device not yet approved by the FDA for general contraceptive use, it is, however, available in the United States in major metropolitan areas as of late 1982. Some practitioners participating in FDA-approved studies* currently import the cap from England. Although we clearly need more data on the effectiveness and long-term safety of the cap, it is ironic that a device which is probably very safe should be so much harder to get than the more dangerous Pill and IUD.

Description

By far the most commonly used cervical cap is called the Prentif cavity rim, made of flexible rubber. It looks somewhat like a thimble with a rim and fits over the cervix the same way a thimble fits over your finger. It is about one and a half inches long and covers almost the entire cervix (see illustration, p. 225). Since cervices are different sizes, this rubber cap comes in four different sizes, from twenty-two millimeters to thirty-one millimeters in diameter (less than one inch to about one and a quarter inches). Other kinds of caps are the vault (or Dumas) cap and the Vimule cap.† These variations are used mainly when a woman cannot get a good fit with the Prentif cervical cap. (The information below is about the Prentif cervical cap, unless another type is specifically mentioned.)

How It Works

Like other barrier methods, the cervical cap keeps sperm out of the uterus. The cap is designed to create an almost airtight seal around the cervical opening (os). Suction, or "surface tension," hugs it close to the cervix, and sperm can't swim past the edge of the cap the way they can with the diaphragm. The spermicide both inactivates sperm and strengthens the suction seal between the cap and the cervix.

Effectiveness

Only a few studies have been done on the cervical cap. The newest edition of *Contraceptive Technology* lists a *theoretical* failure rate of 2 percent and an *actual* fail-

*Since January 19, 1981, only practitioners granted an official Investigational Device Exemption (IDE) have been allowed to continue fitting caps.

†Some practitioners have noticed that the Vimule cap, with its flanged rim, has caused small lacerations or abrasions around the cervix. This alarming news may be a good reason not to use the Vimule cap at all. In February 1983, the FDA requested that any woman fitted with a Vimule be notified of this possible adverse effect and be reexamined by her practitioner.

ure rate of 13 percent. A certain percentage of failures may be due to the cap being dislodged during intercourse by the penis thrusting against the cervix.

How to Get the Cap

You can get a list of practitioners and clinics which fit cervical caps from New Hampshire Feminist Health Center, 38 South Main Street, Concord, NH 03301, (603) 428-2253.

The cervical cap must be fitted to your cervix by a trained practitioner. One of the different models will usually fit a particular woman, but the practitioner may not have all of them in stock. Whenever you are fitted for a cap, be sure that the practitioner gives you time to try inserting and removing it. A cervical cap is somewhat more difficult to use than a diaphragm, since you have to be able to reach your cervix with your fingers to put the cap into place. With practice it becomes easy for most women.

How to Use the Cap

Most health workers advise using a small amount of spermicidal jelly or cream. Practitioners debate the amount. Some think the cap should be filled one-third full; others, two-thirds full. If you use too much, it may break the suction. The spermicide should be spread around the inside of the cap up to the rim. You may insert the cap hours or even a day or two before intercourse or vagina-to-penis contact. There is no reliable data to indicate how long a cap remains effective. Some women prefer replacing spermicide each day, just in case.

You *must* keep the cap in place for eight to twelve hours after intercourse. Douching is unnecessary, but in any case, never douche while the cap is in place, since this could dilute the spermicidal jelly or cream. For backup, some women insert cream or jelly into their vagina one-half to one hour before removing the cap.

Practitioners debate how often to remove the cap. They generally advise removing it after no more than three days, partly because strong odors tend to develop after that. Many women remove the cap once a day or every other day to allow cervical secretions to flow freely. This may help prevent infections and toxic shock syndrome.* During your period, remove the cap often or don't use it at all, since the menstrual flow may break the suction seal. A diaphragm may be better contraception at this time.

Some women help prevent odors by soaking the cap for twelve hours in rubbing alcohol, water and vinegar, or lemon juice. After soaking, rinse and dry the cap before using.

For a month or two after you start using the cap,

*Some researchers have found high concentrations of *Staphylococcus aureus*, the bacteria involved in toxic shock syndrome, in women who have left the cap in for three days or more.

and whenever you have intercourse with a new partner, use extra spermicide in your vagina or have your partner use a condom for extra protection. Especially if the cap doesn't fit exactly right, and depending on the angle of penetration and your particular anatomy, the cap can become dislodged when a man's penis thrusts against your cervix. Since you might not feel this, check the cap with your finger after intercourse; if it is out of place, put in extra cream or jelly. You may have to see if a different-size cap fits better, or switch to a diaphragm.

Who Shouldn't Use the Cervical Cap

Many women, even those who can't wear the diaphragm, can use the cervical cap, but the existing sizes may not fit all women.* If you have a cervical erosion or laceration, you shouldn't use the cap, since it doesn't allow the free flow of cervical secretions, which may be a cause of irritation.

If your cervix is very long or of an irregular shape, you may not be able to use the rubber cap, but will probably be able to wear the vault or Vimule caps. Also, it is possible for a woman's vagina to be so long that she can't reach deep enough inside to place or remove the cap easily. A cap inserter would solve this problem and may be developed in the near future.

Other reasons for not using the cervical cap are the same as for not using the diaphragm (see p. 226).

Advantages

When used properly, the cap is very effective and you can insert it long before intercourse, which means it need not interfere with lovemaking.

The cap itself is relatively inexpensive, costing between seven and ten dollars, but the fee for the initial fitting can be high in order to pay costs of research required by the FDA. Since it requires so little spermicide, it's less messy than the diaphragm, and one tube will go a long way.

Like the diaphragm, the cap helps us get to know our bodies better.

Disadvantages

The cap is not widely available, so depending on where you live, it may be difficult to obtain.

*A doctor and dentist in Chicago are working on a technique to mold individual caps for each woman according to the size of her cervix. (See The University of Chicago Division of Biological Sciences and the Pritzker School of Medicine, *Reports* 27 [Spring 1979], p. 2.) Since the size and position of the cervix changes throughout the cycle for many women, a *single* custom-fitted cap size may not make sense at all. The Contracap is designed to stay in place throughout a woman's menstrual cycle, a fact which alarms us somewhat. Even though this cap has a valve which can be opened to permit menstrual fluid to pass through, we wonder about the effects of leaving a cervical cap in place for a long time. Will this be irritating, cause cervical or vaginal lacerations or be otherwise unhealthy?

The cap may cause an unpleasant odor if you don't remove it fairly often.

Some women dislike the idea of trapping cervical secretions for as long as the cap is worn, because this may lead to infections. A few health workers wonder if the constant cervical contact with rubber might be harmful, causing cervical erosions or irritations. Recent studies have demonstrated no such changes as measured by repeated Pap smears.

Occasionally a partner feels discomfort if his penis hits the rim of the cap during intercourse.

You have to keep checking the cap carefully to feel whether it has become dislodged. If the airtight seal is broken, the cap's effectiveness is reduced.

(See the section below on possible negative effects of creams and jellies.)

JELLIES AND CREAMS

Spermicidal cream or jelly is really designed for use with a diaphragm or cervical cap (and can be used for

HOW TO INSERT SPERM-KILLING FOAM, CREAM OR JELLY

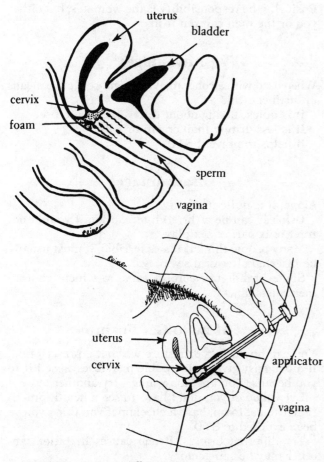

Nina Reimer   jelly, cream, or foam

extra protection with a condom). Alone, creams and jellies have a high failure rate, so *please don't depend on them.*

Cream or jelly comes in a tube with a plastic applicator. Jellies are clear, creams are white. They are available without prescription at all drugstores. (See "How to Get Foam," p. 234, for purchase hints.)

Deposited just outside the entrance to your cervix at the top of your vagina, cream or jelly keeps sperm from entering the cervix and kills them as well.

How to Use Jellies and Creams

For use with a diaphragm or cap, see above. For use with a condom: as short a time as possible (under fifteen minutes) *before* vagina-to-penis contact or intercourse, you or your partner should fill the applicator, insert it into your vagina and push the plunger. Use an additional full plunger for each additional act of intercourse. Leave the jelly or cream in for six to eight hours; if you want to douche, you must wait.

Possible Negative Effects

In 1981 a *much criticized* study linked spermicide use with birth defects.[7] Since then, better studies have found no such link.[8] Some brands sold in the U.S. at one time contained mercury. As a result of Japanese studies showing that mercury could cause kidney damage, it was removed. It may still be found in some jellies and creams sold outside the U.S.

Advantages

Like condoms, you can get cream or jelly on short notice; also, they increase your protection against gonorrhea and trichomoniasis.

Disadvantages

There can be problems of leakage, allergy or reaction to the smell or taste. Jelly may be less irritating but tends to be more gooey than cream.

FOAM: AEROSOL VAGINAL SPERMICIDE

Description

Foam is a white aerated cream which has the consistency of shaving cream and contains an effective sperm-killing chemical. It comes in a can with a plunger-type plastic applicator.

How It Works

Deposited just outside the entrance to your cervix at the top of your vagina, foam keeps the sperm from entering the cervix and kills them as well.

Effectiveness

Recent studies indicate that foam used alone has a theoretical failure rate of 3 to 5 percent but an actual failure rate of at least 15 percent. We strongly recommend using foam in combination with a condom. When used together, their effectiveness approaches 100 percent. Foam is also very effective when used as a supplement during the first months of Pill use or as an extra precaution with an IUD.

Problems with effectiveness arise from using too little foam, not realizing that the container is almost empty, failing to shake the container enough, not inserting the foam correctly or inserting it after vagina-to-penis contact has begun.

Encare Oval, a vaginal suppository containing a foaming spermicide, has been heavily advertised by its manufacturers as being 99 percent effective. The May–July 1978 issue of the FDA *Drug Bulletin* states that the FDA considers this claim to be unsupported. Many physicians, unaware of the FDA announcement, continue to recommend the Encare Oval. *We strongly recommend that vaginal suppositories (Encare Oval, S'positive, Semicid, Intercept) be used only in combination with a condom.* Insert a suppository into your vagina ten to thirty minutes before vagina-to-penis contact.

How to Use Foam

Insert no longer than thirty minutes before vagina-to-penis contact. If the foam is in a can, *shake the can very well*, about twenty times. The more bubbles the foam has, the better it blocks sperm, and the spermicide tends to settle in the bottom of the container, so it must be mixed. Put the applicator on top. When the applicator is tilted (Delfen) or pushed down (Emko and Koromex), the pressure triggers the release valve and the foam is forced into the applicator, pushing the plunger up. Some brands of foam come in preloaded applicators.

Lie down, use your free hand to spread the lips of your vagina, insert the applicator about three to four inches and push the plunger. Then remove the applicator *without pulling on the plunger*, or you may suck some of the foam back into the applicator. Insert one full applicator of Emko, Emko Pre-fil, Because or Dalkon, or two applicators full of Delfen or Koromex. If you have never used tampons, you may want to practice inserting the applicator. You'll find that your vagina angles up toward your back, not straight up in your body. Your aim is to deposit the foam at the entrance of your cervix.

Wash the applicator with mild soap and warm but not boiling water before putting it away. You don't have to wash it immediately.

Cautions

Put in more foam every time you have intercourse or vagina-to-penis contact, no matter how recent the last time was. Leave the foam in for six to eight hours. If you want to douche, you must wait. If the foam is dripping and bothers you, use a minipad or tissue in your underpants.

Keep an extra can on hand. Some brands indicate when they're running out; others just come out of the can more slowly.

Use foam with a condom for maximum effectiveness of both.

Negative Effects

Foam (especially the suppositories) irritates some vaginas and some penises, leading to pain, itching or the sensation of heat.

Responsibility

Basically the responsibility is the woman's, but either you or the man can put it in.

Advantages

When used with a condom, it is a highly effective means of birth control.

It is quick, taking about thirty seconds to use.

It is less drippy than cream or jelly.

It helps to prevent STD.

Disadvantages

Alone, it is quite ineffective.

Using it can be a (brief) interruption if you do not treat it as part of sex play.

Many people think it tastes terrible; it must usually be inserted after oral sex play.

Some brands use aerosol cans, to which environmentalists object.

How to Get Foam

You can buy it in a drugstore without a prescription. If a druggist gives you trouble or refuses to sell it to you because you are "too young," try another store.

Even though you don't have to see a health practitioner to get foam, have a checkup if you think you've been exposed to STD.

Try different brands. If one causes irritation, another may be satisfactory.

Cost

Foam costs about seven dollars for a medium-size can (with applicator) which contains enough for about twenty uses.

FERTILITY OBSERVATION (sometimes called NATURAL BIRTH CONTROL)

We can learn to observe and understand the hormonal changes in our bodies which are linked to fertility by observing the amount and quality of vaginal discharge, noting changes in the texture and position of the cervix and monitoring body temperature. In this way, we can accurately decide whether we are fertile (able to become pregnant) or infertile on a day-to-day basis. It takes only a few minutes each day to make and record our observations.

Most of us have heard of the rhythm method, notorious for its high failure rate. It tries to predict a woman's cycle based on information from past cycles. However, since no one has absolutely regular cycles all the time, it *fails* frequently. Bad experiences with rhythm have led many women to discount so-called "natural" methods of birth control; yet natural methods that work *have* been developed, and their scientific basis is well documented. *They should not be confused with the rhythm method.*

Using fertility awareness we learn that we are fertile only during part of our menstrual cycle and that we can recognize this time. Fertility observation has far-reaching implications: we can use it to learn basic body information even if we aren't interested in birth control, and to prevent or achieve pregnancy or to predict menstruation. Lesbians can also use it to achieve pregnancy using self-help methods (see Chapter 17, "New Reproductive Technologies").

Avoiding Pregnancy Through Fertility Observation

Fertility depends on three factors: a healthy egg, healthy sperm and favorable cervical mucus. The relationship between cervical mucus and fertility was well known before modern times. For example, among the Bantu people in East Africa, grandmothers taught granddaughters to wipe the outer lips of their vaginas with a smooth stone to collect mucus.

Cervical mucus nourishes and guides sperm which would otherwise die in about a half-hour or swim in circles and probably never reach an egg. A woman ovulates once each cycle. (If there is a second ovulation, it occurs within forty-eight hours of the first ovulation.) The egg lives twelve to twenty-four hours and then disintegrates if not fertilized. Under favorable cervical mucus conditions, sperm can survive as long as five days within the body. Therefore, it is possible to become pregnant from vagina-to-penis contact or intercourse as long as five days before ovulation.

Once a woman can recognize when she is in a fertile phase of her menstrual cycle (see p. 236), she avoids all contact between vagina and penis during that time, and therefore avoids pregnancy. Some women use barrier methods during their fertile time, but jelly or foam in the vagina can mask indications of fertility and make it impossible to tell whether you are still fertile. Some women report no problems in combining a barrier method with fertility observation, especially if using a condom.

It is crucial for women to learn fertility observation methods directly from other women and to chart their observations daily.* It is *not* advisable to learn a method just by reading a book. Although a number of books in Resources can be very helpful and are recommended, books (including this one) cannot give you the personal feedback, support and experience-sharing you need. Check your local women's center or write to the Ovulation Method Teacher's Association (OMTA), Box 14511, Portland, OR 97214, for information about groups. If you are willing or want to hear Catholic morality mixed in with the information, most Catholic hospitals or churches can help you find a teacher.

Here are some issues to consider in choosing a group:†

1. Is the teacher a woman with experience herself? A male-female couple? A medical person? A nun or priest?

2. Does the format include participatory classes or groups and more than one meeting?

3. Is there an option to learn in an all-woman group? If all classes are open to men, is the orientation toward monogamous heterosexual couples? What efforts are made to insure support for other sexual lifestyles?

4. Can you get help from the teacher in the months or years after the training process is over?

5. Where does the registration fee go? (Are you unwittingly supporting a cause you would find offensive?)

6. What is the sponsoring organization's or teacher's position on birth control and abortion? Will they refer you to a facility that provides a full range of birth control options and/or abortion services? If you do not get straightforward answers to questions 5 and 6, be suspicious. If you hear the term "prolife" used, remember that this indicates an antiwoman, antiabortion philosophy.

---

*Depending on which method you use, write down the day of your cycle; whether you "feel" wet or dry; describe the color and consistency of any external mucus, your temperature and changes in your cervix.

†Adapted from S. Bell, et al., "Reclaiming Reproductive Control: A Feminist Approach to Fertility Consciousness," *Science for the People* 12:1 (1980), pp. 6–9, 30–35.

THE OVULATION METHOD (AWARENESS OF MUCUS)

Twenty-five years ago, an Australian couple, Evelyn and John Billings, sought a method of child spacing that would be effective in preventing pregnancy and also acceptable to the Catholic Church—one that would reinforce the Catholic philosophy about sexuality, marriage and women. They developed the ovulation method, a way of interpreting the vaginal sensations of wetness or dryness and the consistency of the mucus discharge so as to determine whether you are fertile or infertile.

You may already be aware that you normally have a discharge from your vagina which varies throughout your menstrual cycle. You may notice nothing for several days and then suddenly experience a discharge—a bubbling sensation, a stickiness or a feeling of your vaginal lips being "wet." This is caused by mucus, made in the cells of the cervical canal in response to your hormonal changes. Here is a brief outline of the relationship of mucus to fertility. (See the chart on p. 217.)

1. Menstruation. A cycle begins on the first day of your period. Since menstrual discharge may mask mucus discharge, the menstrual period is not necessarily safe for unprotected intercourse or vagina-to-penis contact.

2. In some cycles, as menstruation stops you may feel "dry"; that is, you may have no sensation of discharge, no mucus present at the vaginal opening, no discharge noticeable on your underwear. Since there is no mucus present, sperm will not be able to survive in the acid environment of the vagina. These days are considered infertile and therefore safe for unprotected intercourse or vagina-to-penis contact. (*Note*: you will almost always find something resembling mucus if you look *inside* your vagina. The mucus which promotes sperm survival is fluid enough to flow to the *outside* and should be checked outside only.)

3. As you begin to approach ovulation, your cervix produces enough mucus to flow down and "coat" the vagina with a protective covering which promotes sperm survival. It is fluid enough to flow out of your vagina. When you begin to feel a *sensation* of discharge from the vagina, *see* it on your underwear or *wipe* it off with toilet paper, your fertile time has begun. The mucus may start off as whitish or yellow, tacky, crumbly or creamy. It usually becomes more fluid, clearer or thinner as ovulation approaches. It also has a very characteristic slippery or lubricative feel when ovulation is near. Some women can take a sample and stretch it between two fingers. The last day of mucus with any of these characteristics is called the peak day. Ovulation usually occurs on the day *following* the peak day. The peak day is always identified by looking back over the cycle. You are *fertile* from the time the mucus first appears until the fourth day after the end of the peak symptom. The number of fertile days varies from cycle to cycle and from woman to woman.

4. At ovulation, your mucus will undergo a distinct change from the peak symptom: you may become dry again, or develop a thicker discharge. In either case, a change is evident. Your period will start eleven to sixteen days after the peak day. (This is one way to know that you have correctly identified ovulation.) From the fourth day past the peak day until your period begins, you are infertile. Every woman's mucus pattern is slightly different from this "classic" description we have given—*but every woman can learn to recognize her own pattern.*

If you have a vaginal infection, you probably won't be able to tell the difference between cervical mucus and the discharge from your infection or with any medication you are using to treat it. During this time, you should not rely on mucus observation for contraception. You must also be careful not to confuse mucus with semen or secretions during sexual arousal. While spermicidal foams, creams and jellies are in your vagina, you probably won't be able to observe cervical mucus.

THE SYMPTO-THERMAL METHOD (STM)

This method usually combines mucus observations with predictions based on past cycle history (using a calendar calculation) before ovulation, and uses changes in basal body temperature combined with cervical mucus to confirm ovulation. Sometimes it also includes recognizing and interpreting other changes in your menstrual cycle, such as breast tenderness or fullness after ovulation, pain and/or spotting around the time of ovulation and cervical variation (see p. 211). If you are using the STM, you must consider yourself fertile when calendar calculations indicate or when mucus starts, whichever comes earlier. Women have used the postovulation change in temperature as an indication that ovulation is past. By taking your temperature on a basal body thermometer (about five dollars at a drugstore) each morning at the same time and recording it on a chart, you will see that your temperature rises slightly following ovulation and stays high until menstruation begins. (It falls as your period starts and stays low until the next ovulation.) Your fertile time ends *either* on the fourth day after the mucus peak *or* on the evening of the third day in a row of elevated temperatures, whichever is later. (Elevated temperature means one-tenth of a degree [Fahrenheit] above the highest of at least six preovulation readings after the first four days of menstruation.) The temperature method by itself is of no use in determining which days *before* ovulation are fertile or infertile.

Effectiveness

Many health professionals rate all natural methods of birth control as poor. In most cases, they have confused the word "natural" with the word "rhythm." Key factors in effectiveness of the natural methods are personal motivation, correct information and a commitment to observe and chart physical signs faithfully. Recent studies (based on women avoiding all vagina-to-penis contact on fertile days) indicate that the Ovulation Method or Sympto-Thermal Method can be extremely effective when taught carefully, understood thoroughly and used correctly (called "theoretical effectiveness"). The Ovulation Method has a theoretical failure rate of 0.1 percent to 5.7 percent and an actual failure rate ranging from 2.3 percent to 39.7 percent. The STM has a theoretical failure rate of 0.5 percent to 13.1 percent and an actual failure rate of 4.5 percent to 34.4 percent. When women use barrier methods or withdrawal on fertile days with either the STM or the Ovulation Method, the actual failure rate is from 6.8 percent to 23.9 percent. The upper figure in the actual failure rate is due to women not using or understanding the method properly. You can reduce this by making sure you find good teachers, group support and partners who are as committed to it as you are.

You can use fertility observation to *increase* the effectiveness of the IUD and barrier methods by avoiding any vagina-to-penis contact on fertile days.

Reversibility

Excellent reversibility. Just have intercourse on fertile days.

Responsibility

Basically the responsibility is the woman's. It requires cooperation from the man.

Advantages

It has no negative effects.

Many of us enjoy being more aware of our body's cycles.

It can lead, during fertile days, to exploration of other ways to give and receive pleasure, such as mutual masturbation and oral sex. (Be sure to avoid *all* vagina-to-penis contact.)

The cooperation necessary for this method can bring understanding and closeness between partners.

Disadvantages

The major disadvantage is the risk of pregnancy if you are not diligent.

It takes at least two to three cycles to learn and use confidently.

It may be impractical if you are not in a committed, cooperative relationship with your sex partner.

If you choose not to use a barrier method and to abstain from intercourse and vagina-to-penis contact when you are fertile, it can be sexually frustrating unless you enjoy other forms of sex.

Mechanization of Fertility Observation

Numerous machines and devices are being developed to measure hormonal changes and to pinpoint fertility. They are based on the same principles as the Ovulation Method and the STM, but they're more expensive and more profitable for the manufacturers without necessarily being more accurate.

ABSTINENCE

There is nothing wrong with abstinence. In fact, sometimes it is just what we want. Abstinence means making love without having intercourse. It is the most effective form of birth control, has been used for centuries and is still very common. It has no physical side effects as long as prolonged sexual arousal is followed by orgasm to relieve pelvic congestion. Take care not to have any vagina-to-penis contact, as sperm can swim inside your vagina and go on to fertilize the ovum.

BIRTH CONTROL PILLS

The Food and Drug Administration approved the Pill for marketing in 1960 without adequate testing or study. A synthetic pill almost 100 percent effective in preventing pregnancy when taken daily, it created tremendous excitement among the medical, scientific, pharmaceutical and population-control communities. Very few professionals cautioned against using it too widely or too quickly; to do so meant fighting against the prevailing ideology which supported rapid development and distribution of new drugs generally and risking the charge of holding back progress. To women, it seemed like a wonderful alternative to the methods then available.

The Pill became a gigantic experiment: within two years about 1.2 million American women used it, and by 1973 the number rose to an estimated 10 million. Though the increase in its use has ended, the Pill is still the most widely used reversible contraceptive both in the U.S. and worldwide.

Many women first heard about its dangers not from physicians but when they read Barbara Seaman's book, *The Doctor's Case Against the Pill*, published in 1969 and again, updated, in 1979 (see Resources), and elected to stop taking the Pill or to find another alternative. Although medical literature confirmed the dangers of the Pill as early as 1962, it was not until 1970 that the FDA issued package warnings, which one FDA official now admits "didn't say much of anything important." Since 1978 the FDA has required physicians and pharmacists to hand out comprehensive information sheets on its possible negative effects and complications.

In late 1980, the drug company G.D. Searle financed a publicity campaign to falsely reassure women about the Pill's safety. Searle misrepresented the findings of a ten-year government-funded project carried out in Walnut Creek, California, one of three major studies begun in 1968. (The other two were done in England.) New information about the Pill is emerging all the time—in fact, it is now the most widely researched drug on the market. We need to evaluate carefully both the methods and purposes of this research.

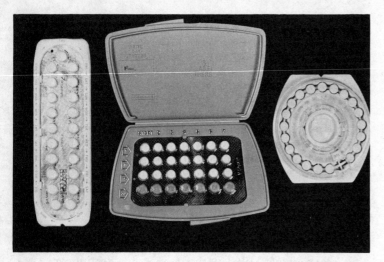

Pill packets   *Elizabeth Cole*

How They Work

To understand how birth control pills work, you need to know how menstruation works. Chapter 12, "Anatomy and Physiology of Sexuality and Reproduction," and its appendix describe what hormones are and how the female hormones, estrogen and progesterone, guide a woman's menstrual cycle.

The way the most widely used pills ("combination pills") work to prevent pregnancy is outlined in the chart on p. 239, which puts an average menstrual cycle and the Pill cycle side by side. It shows how the Pill interrupts your menstrual cycle by introducing synthetic versions of the female hormones.

Combination birth control pills prevent pregnancy primarily by inhibiting the development of the egg in the ovary. During your period, the low estrogen level normally indirectly triggers your pituitary gland to send out FSH, a hormone that starts an egg developing

to maturity in one of your ovaries. The Pill gives you just enough synthetic estrogen to raise your estrogen level high enough to keep FSH from being released. So during a month on the Pill, your ovaries remain relatively inactive and there is no egg to be fertilized by sperm. This is the same principle by which a woman's body checks ovulation when she is pregnant: the corpus luteum and placenta put estrogen into her blood, thereby inhibiting FSH. So in a way, using much lower levels of hormones, the Pill simulates pregnancy, and some of the Pill's negative effects are like those of early pregnancy. If ovulation occurs, it is because your body needed a higher dose of estrogen than your Pill gave you to inhibit FSH, or because you have missed one or more pills.

Synthetic progesterone, called progestin, is used differently in different varieties of the Pill. The *combination pill* combines estrogen and progestin for the entire twenty or twenty-one days. Progestin provides two important extra contraceptive effects: increased thickness of cervical mucus and incomplete development of the uterine lining (see chart below). The *progestin-only pills* depend on these two effects and do not inhibit ovulation. They are therefore not quite as effective in preventing pregnancy. The *sequential pill* uses estrogen alone for several days and then a combination of estrogen and progestin. Less effective than combination pills, and with more dangerous effects than the other two, sequentials were taken off the market by the FDA in 1976.*

COMBINATION PILLS

Effectiveness

The combination pills have the very low theoretical pregnancy rate of 0.5 percent, but in actual use, they show a failure rate of 2 percent. Pregnancy can occur if you forget to take your pill for two or more days, if you don't use a backup method of birth control for your first packet of pills or while taking antibiotics for an acute infection, and occasionally when you change from one brand of pill to another. (In this case, use an extra method for two weeks to be safe.)

---

*Some pharmacies still have them in stock and physicians may be prescribing them. If you are using Oracon, NorQuen, Ortho-Novum SQ or other sequentials, get your prescription changed to a combination or progestin-only pill or use another form of birth control.

WOMAN'S MENSTRUAL CYCLE AND THE WAY THE COMBINATION
BIRTH CONTROL PILL AFFECTS THAT CYCLE TO PREVENT PREGNANCY

Normal Menstrual Cycle*	With the Pill
Day 1. Menstrual period begins.	Day 1. Menstrual period begins.

Day 5. An egg in a follicle (pocket, sac) in one of your ovaries has begun to ripen to maturity. The egg starts developing in response to a hormonal message (FSH) from your pituitary gland, which in turn has been triggered indirectly by the low level of *estrogen* (an ovarian hormone) at the time of your period.
 	
Days 5–14. The follicle in which the egg is developing makes first a little, then more and more *estrogen*:
1. *Estrogen* stimulates the lining of your uterus to get thicker and the cells of your cervix to produce mucus that is receptive to sperm.
2. As *estrogen* increases, it slows down and then cuts off FSH.
 	
Day 14. Ovulation: *estrogen* peak and a spurt of progesterone occurring during days 12–13 indirectly trigger ovulation. Ripe egg is released from ovary, starts 4-day trip down fallopian tube to uterus. Fertilization by sperm from the man must occur in first 24 hours.
	Day 5. Take your first pill. In the pill, you take two synthetic hormones every day: *estrogen* and *progestin* (synthetic progesterone).
	  Estrogen: The pill contains more *estrogen* than there usually is in your body on Day 5—enough to stop the usual message from your pituitary gland (FSH) for an egg to develop. By taking this amount of *estrogen* every day for 21 days, you prevent an egg from developing at all that month. Therefore there is no egg to be fertilized by the sperm.
	  Progestin: A little *progestin* every day provides two vital backup effects:
	1. keeps the plug of mucus in your cervix thick and dry, so sperm have a hard time getting through;
	2. keeps the lining of your uterus from developing properly so that if an egg does ripen (if *estrogen* level of pill is too low for you, or if you forget a pill) and sperm do make it through the cervical mucus and fertilize the egg, the fertilized egg will not be able to implant.

Days 14–26. The ruptured follicle, now called *corpus luteum* ("yellow body"), makes two hormones for about 12 days: *Estrogen* continues. *Progesterone* increases and peaks about day 22: 1. makes your cervical mucus (plug of mucus in cervix) thick and dry, a barrier to sperm; 2. stimulates the glands in lining of your uterus to secrete a sugary substance and further thickens the lining.	Days 6–25. Continue taking one pill a day.
Days 26–27–28. If pregnancy did not occur, *corpus luteum's* manufacture of *estrogen* and *progesterone* slows down to a very low level. The lining of your uterus, which needs the stimulation and support of these hormones, starts to disintegrate.	Day 26. Take your last pill.† Days 27–28. Sudden drop in *estrogen* and *progestin* makes the lining of your uterus start to disintegrate.
Day 29–Day 1. Menstrual period begins. Low level of *estrogen* (see Day 26) will begin indirectly to stimulate pituitary's egg-development hormone (FSH) to start a new cycle.	Day 29–Day 1. Menstrual period begins. Your period is lighter than normal, because of effect #2 of progestin in the pill.

*This is a simplified version of the menstrual cycle. See the appendix to Chapter 12 for a more thorough description.
†With the 28-day combination pill, you take pills without hormones in them from day 27 to day 5.

Reversibility

If you want to become pregnant, stop taking pills at the end of a packet. It may be several months before your ovaries are functioning regularly, and your first non-Pill periods may be a week or two late or missed completely. It is a good idea to use another method of birth control for three to six months after you go off the Pill to allow your body to return to normal before you try to get pregnant.

It is unclear at present whether women who have taken the Pill have a higher rate of temporary or permanent infertility or a higher number of miscarriages. Most women do have successful pregnancies after they go off the Pill. However, some women, especially those who menstruated irregularly before taking the Pill, have difficulty conceiving after they stop taking it. If you have not started to ovulate within one year after going off the Pill, you can request treatment with clomiphene citrate (Clomid; see Chapter 21, "Infertility and Pregnancy Loss").

Safety

Many of us are uneasy about taking a medication which affects almost every organ in our bodies each day for months and years, since its effects have not been conclusively tested and it has been in wide use for only twenty years. Yet some of us choose to take whatever risks are involved because we falsely believe we are getting 100 percent effectiveness and absolutely don't want to become pregnant. What price do we pay for this alleged perfect protection?

A great deal of information exists on the adverse effects of the Pill, as the following pages demonstrate. In most cases of Pill-related injury or death, women had not been examined carefully enough by the doctor who prescribed the Pill for them, had not had checkups while taking the Pill, or had not been told that there was some risk involved in taking it. Some women ignored pains that were, in fact, warning signals, and sought help too late. Some of the Pill-related deaths were unpredictable and unpreventable.

How Long to Take the Pill

If you are not now experiencing problems, you may want to enjoy the freedom of the Pill indefinitely. Yet if you take the Pill for many years at a time, you are in a sense part of a huge experiment on the long-term effects of daily hormone ingestion in healthy women. Researchers disagree on how long a woman should stay on the Pill. Some suggest two- or three-year intervals with three-month breaks in between; others say in some cases it is safe to take it for ten years without stopping. If you want to have a baby at some point later on, you may choose not to stay on the Pill

for more than two to four years at a time. Once you pass forty, you are at higher risk of Pill-related death. Some researchers believe that complications and problems increase the longer you take the Pill, and you may continue to have problems for years after you stop taking it.

Going Off the Pill

It is a sad fact that many women get pregnant in the first few months after going off the Pill because they feel awkward using another method of birth control, especially one of the safer barrier methods. We need discussion, information and support in making the switch to another method. It helps to have a partner or partners who understand and appreciate our desire to change to a safer form of contraception.

Warning Signals

Any problem lasting more than two or three cycles should be reported to a physician or medical facility. The following are symptoms of serious problems: severe pain or swelling in the legs (thigh or calf), bad headache, blurred vision (or loss of sight), chest pain or shortness of breath, abdominal pain. *Report these immediately*, for they are signs of heart attack, stroke or liver tumors and mean you should stop taking the Pill. (*Note on leg pain*: Some leg cramps may be caused by fluid retention induced by the estrogen in the Pill. Don't confuse this with severe leg pain, but also don't hesitate to call a medical practitioner if your leg cramps become painful.)

Who Should Absolutely Not Use the Pill

The Pill is dangerous for certain women. The FDA requires drug companies to publish a list of contraindications and conditions that prohibit the use of the Pill and include the list with your package of pills. Do not use the Pill if you have:

Any disease or condition associated with poor blood circulation or excess blood clotting: Bad varicose veins, thrombophlebitis (clots in veins, frequently in the leg), pulmonary embolism (blood clot which has traveled to the lung, usually from the leg), stroke, heart disease or defect, coronary artery disease.

Hepatitis or other liver diseases. As it is the liver which metabolizes sex steroids (progesterone and estrogen), no one with liver disease should take the Pill until the disease is cleared up. Use a good alternative method of contraception, because pregnancy can be a great strain on the liver. A woman who tends to get jaundice during pregnancy should not use the Pill.

Liver tumors; undiagnosed abnormal genital bleeding; cancer of the breast or of the reproductive organs; pregnancy.

Who Is Strongly Advised Not to Use the Pill

Women with the following conditions are strongly advised not to use the Pill:

Migraine headaches.*

Hypertension. A woman with high blood pressure (hypertension) or mild varicose veins must take the Pill with caution.*

Diabetes,* prediabetes or a strong family history of diabetes. Sugar metabolism is extensively altered in women on the Pill. The progestin tends to bind the body's insulin and keep it out of circulation, which increases a diabetic woman's insulin requirement. If you are a diabetic, or if close relatives are diabetic, you should have regular periodic blood tests if you go on the Pill. Many doctors do put diabetic women on the Pill because pregnancy is especially hazardous to a diabetic.

Gallbladder disease.*

Cholecystitis during previous pregnancy, congenital hyperbilirubinemia (Gilbert's Disease).

Mononucleosis in the acute phase.

Sickle cell anemia or trait. Black women planning to go on the Pill should have a sickle cell test. If it is positive, you should discuss the hazards of going on the Pill, which include an increased risk of intravascular blood clotting.*

Elective surgery planned in the next four weeks.

Major surgery requiring immobilization.*

Long leg casts or major injury to the lower leg.

Impaired liver function in the past year.

Women over forty run a statistically higher risk of thromboembolism and other complications when taking the Pill. Since such risks also increase during pregnancy, women over forty should consider a barrier method or sterilization—tubal ligation for you or vasectomy for your partner.

Smokers, especially women who smoke fifteen or more cigarettes a day, run a statistically higher risk of stroke and heart attack on the Pill (see table, p. 224).

Who Should Probably Not Use the Pill

Women with the following situations or conditions should probably not use the Pill:

Lactation. The Pill may dry up the mother's supply of milk, especially if administered soon after she gives birth. Even if it does not dry it up, the Pill decreases the amounts of protein, fat and calcium in the milk. Some estrogen will also come through in the milk. At present this is a controversial subject, since no one knows the long-term effects of this substance on children.

Pregnancy ended within the past ten to fourteen days.*

Weight gain of ten pounds or more while taking the Pill.*

Women who don't have regular periods (at least ten periods a year). This includes women who are just beginning to menstruate and women whose menstrual cycles suggest that they aren't ovulating or that they might have infertility problems.*

Cardiac or renal disease or a history of these diseases.*

Conditions likely to make a woman unreliable at following Pill instructions: major psychiatric problems, alcoholism, mental retardation.

It may not be wise for women with the following conditions to take the Pill: **depression,* chloasma, or hair loss related to pregnancy or a history of such;* asthma;* epilepsy;* uterine fibromyomata;* acne; varicose veins, history of hepatitis but normal liver function tests for at least one year; a woman who is a DES daughter.**

Complications and Negative Effects

The Pill enters our bloodstream, travels through the body and affects many tissues and organs, just as natural estrogens and progesterone do. However, the hormones in the Pill are synthetic and have exaggerated effects on some women.

Even though there is an FDA-required package insert, health workers and doctors must clearly explain the risks we take in choosing the Pill. Unfortunately, they don't always know themselves. Also, they sometimes believe that effects are psychosomatic and that telling us what might happen will influence our perceptions. This attitude is insulting and dangerous. Find out what the risks are before you get a prescription for the Pill.

Many of us experience none or only a few effects from using the Pill. Some women have pregnancy-like symptoms during the first three months, but after that they don't notice anything. Also, many women choose to put up with mild effects in exchange for the Pill's convenience and effectiveness. If you want to use it, try it for a few months to see how your body responds.

The Pill and Circulatory Disease: Heart Attack and Stroke

In general, the risk of death due to circulatory disease (heart attacks, strokes, pulmonary embolism, other

---

*Starred conditions are contraindications to combination pills and may not be contraindications to progestin-only pills.

*Starred conditions are contraindications to combination pills and may not be contraindications to progestin-only pills.

clotting disorders) is much higher in women who use or have used the Pill than among women who have never used it. (This may be related to higher triglyceride [blood fat] and cholesterol levels in Pill users.)[9] This risk probably increases the longer you take the Pill, and persists even when you stop if you have taken it for at least five years.[10] Cardiovascular disease is responsible for most Pill-related deaths. If you are a smoker and use the Pill, your chance of death due to a circulatory disease is ten times that of nonsmokers who have never used it. Women between thirty-five and forty-four on the Pill have a five times' greater death rate due to circulatory disease.* See above for warning signals.

The Pill and High Blood Pressure

Between 5 and 7 percent of women on the Pill will develop hypertension (abnormally high blood pressure) and will be at greater risk for heart attack and stroke. Women who develop hypertension should go off the Pill. Women with a family history of hypertension or who already have high blood pressure are strongly advised by practitioners to choose some other form of birth control.

It is not yet clear whether the effects of hypertension created by the Pill continue even after you stop taking it. Some studies indicate that certain effects persist. Also, the incidence of high blood pressure tends to increase with increased duration of Pill use and with age. Low-dose pills cause fewer problems, but are not quite as effective in preventing pregnancy.

The Pill and Cancer

A study done in 1968 showed that cervical cancer was about three to five times more common in women who had used oral contraceptives for at least four years than among women who had never used the Pill. This study scared many of us unnecessarily, because when the statistics were examined more closely, it became apparent that the deciding factor was not Pill use but the frequency of sexual intercourse and, in particular, the number of sexual partners. The Pill is implicated here only in that it allows some of us to feel freer to have sexual experience, since it provides constant protection against pregnancy.

Recently, however, more studies are showing that there may be particular connections between the Pill and certain forms of cancer. For example, if a woman has cervical dysplasia (abnormal cells in the cervix), the Pill may cause that dysplasia to become cancerous.[11]

There may be a relationship between skin cancer

*In other words, the risk of circulatory disease is low for nonsmokers who are healthy and younger than thirty-five, even if they take the Pill. (Contraceptive Technology 1982–1983, p. 49)

and the Pill, although researchers disagree and are currently studying this.[12]

Researchers disagree about the relationship between the Pill and breast cancer. The most recent research indicates that there is no relationship between the Pill and breast cancer.[13] However, some unanswered questions still remain about the long-term effects of using the Pill, especially its use before a woman's first full-term pregnancy.

The sequential pill (which has been removed from the market) has been linked to cancer of the uterus. Several recent studies show that the combination pill may *protect* women from endometrial and ovarian cancer. However, one of these studies, in which age was considered as a factor, found no protection from ovarian cancer for women under forty years of age.[14] Theoretically, the progesterone in the combination pill balances the estrogen. It's not yet known how long after women stop taking the Pill that this possible protection lasts.

The Pill and Your Present or Future Children

Birth defects (sex malformation or cardiac defects) have been reported in increased incidence among babies of mothers who were taking the Pill while pregnant, who took hormones to prevent miscarriages, who were given progesterone as a pregnancy test or who became pregnant within three months of stopping the Pill.

There may be a higher rate of jaundice among infants whose mothers took the Pill before pregnancy.

Don't use the Pill while breastfeeding (see p. 241).

Children who find pills and eat them may become nauseated. We do not know what harm this may cause. You should go to or call a medical facility if your child swallows more than a few pills.

Other Effects

Headaches

Around 5 percent of women on the Pill develop bad migraines or other frequent headaches.

Migraines are throbbing headaches which result from a problem in the circulation of blood to the brain. Migraines are painful. Further, *migraines can be a warning signal for impending stroke* and should cause a woman to switch to a lower-dose estrogen pill or to stop taking pills altogether.

Diabetes

In some women, the Pill, like pregnancy, can precipitate diabetes. (See also "Who Is Strongly Advised Not to Use the Pill," p. 241.)

Depression

Possibly one in four women are more irritable, anxious or depressed on the Pill. These symptoms often continue instead of improving with succeeding cycles. Switching to a pill with a *less* potent progestin may help. Vitamin B₆ supplementation can also help (see p. 244).

Change in Intensity of Sexual Desire and Response

Many women feel and act sexier as soon as their fear of pregnancy is removed. But increasing numbers of women on progestin-dominant, low-dosage estrogen pills don't feel like making love, orgasm less easily and complain about dry vaginas and less sensation in the vulva.

Nausea

This is a common early negative effect of the Pill. The estrogen in the Pill may irritate your stomach lining or make you feel sick to your stomach, just like a pregnant woman whose body is getting used to the high levels of estrogen that the placenta puts into her blood. Nausea usually goes away after three months; antacid tablets or taking the Pill with a meal or just before bedtime usually give relief.

Fatigue

Another common symptom of pregnancy—tiredness and lethargy.

Vaginitis and Vaginal Discharge

Vaginitis is a vaginal inflammation that may be caused by infection with a fungus, trichomoniasis, bacteria or a virus. The Pill changes the normal vaginal environment and provides excellent conditions for rapid growth of microorganisms. It does not always occur, but any of the pills could make the vagina more susceptible, particularly to the yeast monilia (*Candida albicans*). Vaginitis is treatable, but if it persists you may have to go off the Pill. Increased vaginal discharge is fairly common, can be due to estrogen and does not necessarily indicate infection—though if it is bothering you, you should have it checked.

Urinary Tract Infection

Some reports indicate that women on the Pill tend to have more infections of the bladder and urethra, the tube which leads urine out of your body.[15]

Changes in Menstrual Flow

Your periods will be lighter with most pills (estrogenic pills cause more normal flow). Occasionally your flow will be very slight or you will miss a period. Missing a period when you haven't missed a pill does not necessarily mean you are pregnant; sometimes it is due to taking pills for a long time or taking pills high in progestin. If you miss two periods in a row, consult a practitioner.

Breakthrough Bleeding

This is vaginal bleeding or staining between periods. If there isn't enough estrogen or progestin in the pills you are taking to support the lining of your uterus at a given point in your cycle, a little of the lining will slough off. (This may also occur if you miss a pill.) With combination pills, it usually happens in your first or second pill-cycle and often clears up after that, as your uterus gets used to the new levels of hormones. If breakthrough bleeding doesn't stop after a few months, see a practitioner to find out whether you need to try a different brand or whether you may have another problem. With progestin-only pills, this is very common. Breakthrough bleeding does not mean that the Pill isn't working as a contraceptive.

Breast Changes

Increased breast tenderness or fullness may occur, but it usually lasts for only the first three cycles.

Skin Problems

The Pill may be associated with eczema, urticaria (hives or rashes) and, more rarely, chloasma, changes in skin pigmentation, sometimes described as "giant freckles."

The progestin-dominant pill can cause or increase skin oiliness in some women. An estrogenic pill can decrease acne.

Gum Inflammation

The Pill, like pregnancy, can cause gum inflammation. Women on the Pill should brush their teeth extra carefully, use dental floss regularly and see a dentist every six months to a year.

Liver and Gallbladder Disease

The Pill is associated with an increased incidence of gallbladder disease and of liver tumors (both benign and malignant). Jaundice may be an early symptom of liver complications, so at the first sign of jaundice you should stop taking the Pill. Benign liver tumors are rare, but they can increase rapidly in size and may rupture spontaneously.

Epilepsy and Asthma

The Pill can cause epilepsy and aggravate existing epilepsy and asthma. Low-estrogen pills should be used, and the woman should stay under close medical supervision.

Virus Infections

An increased incidence of chicken pox and other viral infections among Pill users suggests that the Pill may affect your body's immunity.

Cervical Dysplasia

This problem, growth of abnormal cells on the cervix, is more common in women using oral contraceptives than women not using the Pill.[16]

The Pill also has been linked to pleurisy; suppression of bone growth in young women; arthritic symptoms (swelling of joints); visual disturbances; ulcers in the mouth; bruising; antagonism with Rifampin, a drug for tuberculosis, so that neither works as it should; lupus erythematosus, a disease of unknown origin which may be caused by an allergic reaction; abdominal cramping during the first three months; changes in thyroid function; photodermatitis (sunlight sensitivity with hypopigmentation); one form of hair loss, called alopecia; excessive hair growth (hirsutism); benign growths consisting of muscular tissue; and autophonia, an ear or nasal disorder which causes increased resonance of your voice, breath sounds, etc. There is no conclusive proof that the Pill causes these effects; nevertheless, if you should encounter one of these problems, consider that it might be connected with taking the Pill.

Beneficial Effects

Besides greater freedom from pregnancy, the Pill has a number of beneficial effects. Women taking it have shorter menstrual periods with less bleeding and cramping. Premenstrual tension tends to decrease. Iron deficiency anemia is less likely, probably because of decreased menstrual flow. Benign breast growths are less frequent. The Pill also protects against pelvic inflammatory disease (PID), and may protect against ovarian and endometrial cancer, functional ovarian cysts and rheumatoid arthritis.

Nutrition and the Pill

The Pill alters the nutritional requirements of women who take it, which may contribute to some of the complications and negative effects. Pill use has been linked to increased requirements for Vitamins C, B_2 (riboflavin), B_{12} and especially B_6 (pyridoxine) and folic acid* (folate or folacin). Women who face the greatest nutritional risks are teenagers, poor women, women recovering from a recent illness or surgery or who have just given birth, women who have taken the Pill for two years or more who take brands with moderate to high estrogen levels. Since metabolic changes occur within the first few months after beginning the Pill, it is a good idea to have a physical exam and blood tests after you have used the Pill for six months to see if you are suffering from any particular deficiencies.

Studies show that women on the Pill have impaired glucose tolerance tests. This means that their carbohydrate metabolism is adversely affected, resulting in weight gain and/or elevated glucose and insulin levels (ranging from mild to diabetic). These alterations are most often seen when women take combination pills, especially those containing seventy-five micrograms or more of estrogen. Trying a different brand and eating wholesome foods may help to decrease glucose and insulin levels.[17]

While on the Pill, try to maintain a healthy nutritional balance: 1. by eating wholesome foods—especially those containing complex carbohydrates; 2. by reducing sugar intake; and 3. by taking vitamins, especially B-complex, C supplements and folic acid. Doing the same thing for a few months after you stop taking the Pill is also a good idea, especially if you plan to become pregnant. A higher than average number of women who conceived within four months after discontinuing the Pill developed folic acid and B_6 deficiencies during pregnancy.[18]

Water Metabolism and Weight Gain

The Pill alters water metabolism. Estrogenic pills (Enovid, Ovulen) can cause fluid retention because of increased sodium, a temporary and usually cyclic effect. You may experience swollen ankles, breast tenderness, discomfort with contact lenses or a weight gain of up to five pounds. Changing your brand of Pill, reducing your salt intake moderately or taking a diuretic drug are all ways of controlling water retention. (Diuretics have their own risks, such as robbing your body of potassium, so use them sparingly if at all and only with a health practitioner's advice.)

*Up to 20 percent of women taking the Pill show abnormal Pap smears, which may be caused by folic acid deficiencies.[19] The Pill seems to impair our ability to absorb the type of folic acid found in food, but does not do so when the folic acid is already broken down in a vitamin pill. Some nonprescription vitamins contain 400 micrograms of folic acid, the Recommended Daily Allowance (RDA).

Progestin-dominant pills (Ortho-Novum, Norlestrin, Ovral) can cause appetite increase and permanent weight gain because of the buildup of protein in muscular tissue. If you want to gain weight, this is helpful. Pill-related depression may also lead to increased appetite and weight gain.

How to Get Pills

As we have seen, certain physical conditions make taking birth control pills very dangerous, so *it is in your vital interest to have a careful exam before taking pills.* Don't borrow them from a friend. Be sure a health practitioner gives you an internal pelvic exam, breast exam, eye exam, Pap smear and blood-pressure, blood and urine tests. The interview should include questions about you and your family's medical history of breast cancer, blood clots, diabetes, migraines and so on. If you were born between 1945 and 1970, find out if your mother took DES while she was pregnant. If so, you should have a colposcopy test, as you might have adenosis, a condition that the Pill can aggravate. (See the section on DES in Chapter 23.) *Too many people prescribe and use birth control pills hurriedly; make sure you are carefully checked for each one of the contraindications.* When you are on the Pill, you should have an exam every six months to a year.

How to Use Pills

Combination pills come in packets of twenty-one or twenty-eight pills. With twenty-one-day pills, you take one pill a day for twenty-one days and then stop for seven days, during which time you will menstruate. With twenty-eight-day pills, which give you twenty-one hormone pills followed by seven different-colored placebos (without drugs), you take one pill a day with no pause between packets. You will have your period during the time that you are taking the seven different-colored pills. The twenty-eight-day pill is good if you feel you would have trouble remembering the on-and-off schedule of the twenty-one-day pill. There is no medical difference between them.

Most pill regimens start the first pill on the fifth day after your period starts, counting the day you start your period as day one. (Some pills start on the first Sunday after your period comes or on the first day your period begins.) Take one pill at approximately the same time each day. If you feel nausea, take the pill with a meal or after a snack at bedtime. Here is an almost foolproof schedule: take a pill at bedtime, check the packet each morning to make sure you've taken a pill the night before, and carry a spare packet of pills with you in case you get caught away from home or lose pills. *Read the directions carefully.*

If You Forget a Pill

Take the forgotten pill as soon as you remember it, and take the next pill at its appointed time, even if this means taking two pills in one day. If you forget two pills, take two pills as soon as you remember, then take two pills the next day to catch up and use an additional method of contraception (foam, condoms) for the rest of that cycle. You may have some spotting. If you forget three pills or more, withdrawal bleeding will probably begin, so act as though you are at the end of a cycle. Don't make up the missed pills; stop taking your pills and start using a second method of birth control immediately. Start a new package of pills the Sunday after you realized you missed three or more pills, even if you are bleeding. Use an extra method of birth control from the day you realize you forgot the pills through two weeks of the next cycle. If you miss a pill or two and skip a period, start using another method of birth control and get a pregnancy test. If you've been taking your pills correctly and you skip a period, it is unlikely that you are pregnant, but you may need a different brand of pill.

Protection

Your first packet of pills may not protect you completely, as an egg may have started to develop before you take the first pill. To be safe, use another method of birth control for the first month. After this, you will be protected against pregnancy all month long, even during the days between packets. Recent evidence suggests that if you are taking antibiotics for an acute infection, or if you get sick and have several days of vomiting or diarrhea, you should use another method of birth control for the rest of the cycle to be safe.

Responsibility

Birth control pills are primarily the woman's responsibility. You see the doctor, get examined, remember to take the pill, feel the effects and run the risks.

Advantages

Almost complete protection against unwanted pregnancy.

Regularity of menstrual cycles—a period every twenty-eight days.

Lighter flow during periods. This effect pleases most women, bothers some.

Relief of premenstrual tension.

Fewer menstrual cramps or none at all.

An estrogenic pill will clear up acne for some women.

You may enjoy sex more because the fear of pregnancy is gone.

Taking the Pill has no immediate physical relationship to lovemaking, which is especially relaxing if you are just starting to have intercourse and have a lot to learn about your body and a man's. Later on, when you are more comfortable with sex and more able to communicate openly with your partner(s), the interruptions involved in using a diaphragm or foam and condoms may not seem so prohibitive.

Disadvantages

Most of the disadvantages have been described under the section on effects. The only one to add is that you do have to remember to take a pill every day. Some women are forgetful, or live lives that are too chaotic for them to remember to do so. Younger women who live at home and feel a need to hide their pills from their parents sometimes leave them behind or are unable to take them on time.

Differences Among the Several Brands of Pills

How do you and your medical practitioner determine which pill you should take? Be aware that different pills have different kinds, strengths, and quantities of synthetic estrogen and progesterone in them. The first and firmest guideline has been suggested by the British Committee on Safety of Drugs, which warns that high-estrogen pills are more likely to cause blood clots. The Committee advises that only products containing fifty micrograms or less of estrogen be used; that products containing seventy-five micrograms or more of estrogen are associated with a higher incidence of thromboembolic disorder. Pills with fifty micrograms of estrogen are: Ortho-Novum 1/50, Norinyl 1/50 (same as Ortho-Novum 1/50), Demulen, Norlestrin and Ovral. Pills with more than this recommended dose of estrogen are Ortho-Novum, Ortho-Novum 1/80, Norinyl 1/80, Ovulen, Enovid 10, Enovid-E, Enovid 5, Norinyl and all sequential pills.

Recently several pills with doses of synthetic estrogen lower than fifty micrograms ("low-dose" pills) have come on the market. These are Loestrin 1.5/30, Loestrin 1/20, Norinyl 1/35, Ortho-Novum 1/35, Ovcon 35, Lo-Ovral, Modicon and Brevicon. You may wish to try these, especially if you are having trouble with estrogenic side effects. These pills may produce more spotting between periods, and the pregnancy rate, especially of the lower doses, may be a bit higher.

Many practitioners are still prescribing high-dosage estrogen pills, either because they don't know about the British report or because they disagree with it. Others prescribe higher-dosage estrogen pills if a woman has had bad side effects from a higher-dosage progestin pill or if there is an indication that she will have them (see below). In these cases, the practitioner must be sure to inform the woman of the higher risk of blood clots.

The effects of a particular pill are related to the amount and potency of the progestin relative to the estrogen in that pill. There are several kinds of synthetic progesterone (progestins). Some, such as norgestrel (used in Ovral and Lo-Ovral), norethindrone acetate (Norlestrin) and norethindrone (Norinyl and Ortho-Novum), tend to produce *androgenic* ("male") effects—for example, hairiness, scanty periods, acne, permanent weight gain. With pills in which the estrogen dominates (Enovid, Demulen, Ovulen), either because of a lower progestin-to-estrogen ratio or because of the use of a less potent progestin, the effects tend to be *estrogenic* ("female"), such as heavier periods, fluid retention, breast swelling and tenderness.

It is not always possible to predict the estrogen or progestin potency by the dose, because the synthetic compounds vary in potency and effect. Also, each woman's body has its own normal estrogen and progesterone levels. You and your medical practitioner may want to experiment with different brands to minimize undesirable effects.

PROGESTIN-ONLY PILLS

Progestin-only pills are sometimes called "mini-pills," but this term will not be used here in order to avoid confusion with the "low-dose" estrogen combination pill and with a pill that was taken off the market several years ago.

Description

These pills contain small doses of the same progestins available in combination pills. Micronor and Nor-Q-D. each provide 0.35 milligrams of norethindrone, and Ovrette provides 0.075 milligrams of norgestrel. They contain no estrogen. You take one a day continuously, starting on day one of your period, at the same time each day (particularly important), without stopping during your period, which may come irregularly.

Exactly how they work is not known, but progesterone may change cervical mucus so that it is hard for sperm to get through, inhibit the egg's travel through the tubes, partially inhibit the sperm's ability to penetrate the egg, and partially inhibit implantation. You may feel safer taking them knowing they have no estrogen and a very small dose of progestin, and that they may have about the same rate of effectiveness as an IUD. On the other hand, the irregular cycles may get you down, or you may not wish to be one of the testers of a very new pill.

Effectiveness

The theoretical pregnancy rate is 1 to 1.25 percent, higher than the combination pill. The actual failure rate is 2.5 percent. The pregnancy rate may be lower for women who switch from the combination pill to the progestin-only pill than it is for women have never taken the combination pill. Pregnancy rates are highest in the first six months, so using an alternative method of contraception during this period is recommended.

Contraindications

Women who absolutely should not take combination pills (see p. 240) should absolutely not take progestin-only pills. Women with the following conditions are strongly advised not to take progestin-only pills: diabetes (or suspected diabetes), acute mononucleosis, irregular periods, past history of ectopic pregnancy.

Possible Effects

The progestin-only pills were developed in part to avoid estrogen-associated complications. Some women who had estrogen-related problems while taking combination pills are now using progestin-only pills. However, some of the negative effects seen with the combination pill are being reported for the progestin-only pill: headaches, change in weight, cervical erosion and change in cervical secretion, jaundice, allergic skin rash, chloasma, depression, gastrointestinal disturbances and breast changes. There may also be an increased risk of ectopic pregnancy. A common complaint is that menstrual bleeding is very irregular in amount and duration of flow and length of cycle.

RESEARCH AND DEVELOPMENT OF SYNTHETIC HORMONES

Most money for contraceptive research goes into projects to develop variations on the Pill which introduce synthetic hormones into a woman's body. We should view all of them *extremely cautiously* and judge them in light of lessons that we've learned from the Pill. Most likely, once the FDA approves a new product for marketing, it will be advertised widely as both safe and effective. But since all of these products are new, their short-term risks and long-term effects are *unknown*. Some of these new products are described below:

The biphasic pill (Ortho-Novum 10/11) is a low-dosage combination pill designed to reduce breakthrough bleeding and spotting associated with other low-dosage pills. It has a *constant* low dose of estrogen (thirty-five micrograms); it provides less progestin during the first ten days of the cycle (half a milligram) and more in the next ten days (one milligram). So far, it appears to have the same effectiveness rates as combination pills. It comes in twenty-one-day packs and twenty-eight-day packs and has been marketed in the U.S. since April 1982.

The triphasic contraceptive pill (Trinordiol) is a low-dosage combination pill in which the amount of estrogen and progesterone varies during each third of the menstrual cycle. Estrogen increases at midcycle and progesterone slowly increases throughout the cycle. It has a lower dosage of estrogen than other combination pills and a lower dosage of progesterone than the progestin-only pills. In clinical trials there have been no pregnancies so far, and the breakthrough bleeding associated with it ranges from 1 to 6 percent. Currently, it is being sold in Britain and West Germany by its sole manufacturer, Wyeth International.

Other products being developed are subdermal (under the skin) implants lasting up to ten years; a once-a-month pill; progestin-coated vaginal rings and cervical devices; postcoital (after intercourse) pills.

Research is also being conducted on ways to synthesize a brain hormone, LHRH (luteinizing hormone-releasing hormone) and using it to inhibit ovulation. Unlike synthetic estrogen and progesterone, LHRH has a direct effect on the pituitary gland. Like other new hormone products, its long-term and short-term risks are unknown.

DEPO-PROVERA AND OTHER INJECTABLE CONTRACEPTIVES

Depo-medroxy progesterone acetate (DMPA), better known as Depo-Provera or "the shot," is a long-acting synthetic hormone (progesterone) used as an injectable contraceptive in over eighty countries. It is manufactured and distributed by the Upjohn Company. No one understands exactly how it works. It probably suppresses ovulation, makes cervical mucus inhospitable to sperm and makes the lining of the uterus unsuitable for implantation. It is usually given as an injection every three months and is about as effective as the combination pill.

Although the FDA has refused for many years to approve DMPA for contraceptive use in the U.S., the drug has been on the market for several other approved uses (for example, the treatment of uterine cancer). Since DMPA is available, some physicians have chosen to use it as a contraceptive. However, they often do not follow informed consent procedures, so women may not understand fully what they are getting.*

---

*The practice of prescribing drugs for *nonapproved* uses is legal, but physicians who do this are supposed to obtain signed consent forms demonstrating that the drug's unapproved status, as well as potential risks, are known to the woman.

Safety

According to current evidence, DMPA causes fewer major health problems than the Pill. However, women can experience serious problems with DMPA, including extreme weight gain, hair loss, severe depression, acne and very heavy periods, irregular periods or no periods at all.

In one ten-year study of fifty-two rhesus monkeys, two monkeys developed uterine cancer. Without fifteen- and twenty-year studies which monitor thousands of women given DMPA, we will not know the real nature of the cancer risks for women.

Immediately after a DMPA injection, a woman has very high levels of the drug in her bloodstream and, if lactating, in her breast milk. Although we have no long-term studies establishing the safety of DMPA for breastfeeding infants, Upjohn continues to market DMPA in some Third World countries as the "ideal contraceptive for lactating women."

Reversibility

Although most studies indicate that ovulation resumes within one year after discontinuing DMPA injections, there have not been enough studies to prove conclusively that DMPA did not contribute to long-term infertility in some cases.

The Controversy

Many women's health activists have opposed the widespread use of DMPA in the absence of more long-term studies. The National Women's Health Network played an active role in opposing the approval of DMPA in the U.S. as a contraceptive at a special Board of Inquiry hearing convened by the FDA in 1983.* At the same time, some family-planning providers believe that many women would choose DMPA over other contraceptives *even with full information about possible risks*. Although this is true, important concerns still remain to be addressed. The example of the Pill (also marketed prematurely) should warn us to be very careful with new hormonal contraceptives. Also, DMPA is different from other reversible contraceptives, since a woman can't change her mind after receiving a shot. Whereas we can stop using other methods immediately when we have problems, DMPA must remain in our system for at least several months until it is fully metabolized.

Quickly and easily administered, injections may be attractive to both providers and users. However, for those of us who are not informed about DMPA and who are considered by providers as "ideal acceptors" for DMPA (this usually means we are poor white, black or Latin women or mentally retarded women who "cannot use other methods responsibly"), it may *not*

*As of mid-1984, a decision from this board is still forthcoming.

be in our best interests to have DMPA widely available. Until we can be sure that true informed consent for *all* women will be the rule rather than the exception, the approval of DMPA represents a serious threat to those women already most vulnerable to abuse.

PILLS FOR MEN

A pill for men could inhibit the production of sperm or prevent sperm from maturing and surviving. Compared with efforts directed at women, very little research is being done on contraceptive methods for men.[20] Many women have been talking about lobbying for more research on male methods. We suspect that male scientists and doctors would be unwilling to offer men a contraceptive which exposed them to as many effects and potential risks as the Pill or IUD do to women. So far, there has not been any birth control pill developed for Western men, and there probably won't be for at least the next decade.

Researchers in the People's Republic of China have shown that gossypol (extracted from cottonseed) stops sperm production and changes sperm motility. No clinical trials are underway in the U.S. with pills made from gossypol.

What if there were a pill or shot for men? Not all of us can absolutely trust our sex partners. As part of the active-passive, pursuer-pursued, predator-prey, male-female stereotypes that we act out in sex, men say many persuasive things to women to get us into bed. If the man lied about taking birth control pills, the woman would still be the one to get pregnant. Getting men to share the responsibility for birth control involves a lot more than finding methods for them to use. (See "Men and Birth Control," p. 221.) For now, many of us prefer to keep the control in our own hands.

AFTER UNPROTECTED INTERCOURSE: THE "MORNING-AFTER PILL"

The morning-after pill is a series of very high doses of synthetic estrogens (DES), progesterones, or combination pills (Ovral) which must be started *within three days* of unprotected intercourse.

Because the long-range effects of even one-time use of DES on the user have not been adequately studied, you should consider DES *only in an emergency, if at all*. Because DES has been used widely as a morning-after pill for ten years, many doctors and clinics (especially university health services) prescribe it. The FDA *has never approved* using DES or Ovral as morning-after pills.

The negative effects of morning-after pills containing estrogen are the same as those for combination birth control pills—nausea and vomiting, headache and breast tenderness. (Ovral seems to cause fewer of these effects, perhaps because of its lower dose of estrogen.) With DES, the nausea and vomiting may be severe.

The most common treatment is 250 milligrams of diethylstilbestrol (DES) taken for five days (two twenty-five-milligram pills each day). Its failure rate ranges from 0 to 2.4 percent, partly because of the relatively low rate of pregnancy involved: about four out of a hundred women who have a single act of unprotected intercourse during a cycle get pregnant. There has been a high incidence of ectopic pregnancies (outside the uterus) when DES fails, perhaps because it prevents implantation in the uterus but not in the fallopian tubes.[21] (See p. 427.) Another treatment is Ovral, a combination birth control pill. Ovral's failure rate ranges from .16 to 1.6 percent. *You should be examined* before taking a morning-after pill. If you should not take combination birth control pills, you should not take a morning-after pill. (See p. 238.) If warning signals of heart attack and stroke occur (see p. 240), *stop taking the pills immediately and see a health practitioner*.

Pills containing progestin alone have also been used twenty-four hours after each time a woman has intercourse, with a failure rate ranging from zero to 45.2 percent. Progestins may prevent fertilization by immobilizing sperm or prevent implantation by making the uterus inhospitable. Especially when used regularly, progestins can cause irregular bleeding. (For contraindications to taking progesterone, see p. 247.) For signs of heart attack and stroke see p. 240.

If you have had unprotected intercourse, you may prefer not to take a morning-after pill, wait to see if you are pregnant and, if so, have an abortion. Although abortion is more expensive and more difficult emotionally, it may be safer in the long run. The estrogens and progestins in the morning-after pills can cause birth defects, and DES can cause vaginal or cervical cancer in daughters. (See section on DES in Chapter 23.) If you take morning-after pills and get pregnant anyway, *you should seriously consider having an abortion because of the potential danger to offspring*.

THE INTRAUTERINE DEVICE (IUD)

Centuries ago, when camel drivers in the Middle East started out on a long journey across the desert, they would insert pebbles into the uterus of a female camel to keep her from becoming pregnant on the trip. A foreign body in the uterus seems to prevent pregnancy most of the time. IUDs became popular contraceptives for women in the 1960s, and today about sixty million women worldwide use more than a hundred types.

In the mid-1960s, the IUD seemed to be the perfect alternative to the Pill. It was almost as effective and didn't introduce synthetic hormones into women's bodies. Once the IUD was inserted, women couldn't forget to use it. It was an inconspicuous method: it couldn't be discovered by the wrong person. Since it requires minimal involvement on our part, it seemed especially "appropriate" for young or poor women (especially women of color) in the U.S. and Third World countries, whom population control advocates view as uncooperative and irresponsible.

Like the Pill, IUDs were marketed before sufficient research had been done to demonstrate their effectiveness and safety over a long period of time. In some cases, these problems have been so drastic that several IUDs have been removed from the market. In other cases, the device is still marketed, but the list of contraindications continues to grow.

An extreme example is the Dalkon Shield, an IUD marketed from 1971 to 1974 and manufactured by the A.H. Robins Company. It was soon implicated in a high number of cases of pelvic inflammatory disease (PID) and spontaneous septic abortions (miscarriages). At least seventeen young women have died as a result of Dalkon Shield–related septic abortions. In 1974, the Shield was taken off the market (although devices already sold were not recalled). It was still distributed abroad, however. Today, more than 1,570 women in the U.S. have lawsuits pending against A.H. Robins, claiming the Shield caused them illness and sterility in some cases.

In 1981, the National Women's Health Network filed a class-action lawsuit against A.H. Robins, seeking a worldwide recall of the Shield, still inside an estimated 50,000 women in the U.S. and 500,000 women in other countries. In addition to providing a major educational campaign about the Dalkon Shield directed at both women and physicians, the suit seeks reimbursement for medical expenses for those who have it removed. If successful, the suit will represent a major step forward in establishing the public's right to hold corporations accountable for their defective products, not just in the U.S. but internationally.

If you have a Dalkon Shield in place, we urge you to have it removed by a knowledgeable health practitioner. Removal is less difficult during menstruation. It can be painful, so you should consider asking for a painkiller and bringing a friend along.

Description

IUDs are small devices which fit inside the uterus. Some are made of white plastic alone; others contain copper or synthetic progesterone. One or more strings are attached to IUDs. When the IUD is in place, these strings extend into the upper vagina. IUDs come in different sizes and shapes (see p. 250).

How It Works

No one is absolutely sure how the IUD works. The most widely accepted theory is that the IUD causes an inflammation or chronic low-grade infection in the uterus. This causes the body's defense system to produce higher numbers of white cells in the uterus. These cells destroy sperm and the fertilized egg, should it arrive in the uterus, and may also hinder the normal buildup of the uterine lining which must occur before implantation of the fertilized egg. (This does not preclude conception, however, and it allows the possibility of ectopic pregnancy [see p. 427], one problem associated with IUD use.) IUDs may also work by speeding up movement in the fallopian tube, causing the egg to arrive at the uterus too soon; or by increasing the production of prostaglandins, which inhibit implantation; or by causing an implanted egg/sperm unit (blastocyst) to dislodge.[22]

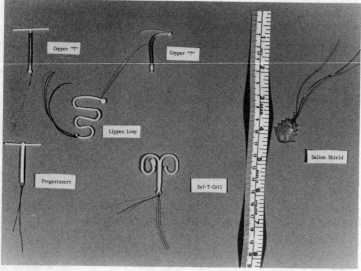

IUDs   *Phyllis Ewen*

Different Types of IUD

The Lippes Loop and the Saf-T-Coil are the most commonly used IUDs. They are made of white plastic. The Loop is available in four sizes; the Coil comes in three. A variation of the Lippes Loop contains copper.

IUDs covered with thin copper wire are the Copper-7 (also called the Cu-7 or Gravigard) and the Copper-T (also called the TCu-200, Gyne T or TCu-200B). Available in one size, they are recommended for women who have never been pregnant because these women tolerate them better. Copper IUDs seem to cause less cramping during insertion and menstrual periods. Be aware that the long-term effects of even the small amounts of copper used in these devices are as yet unknown.

The Progestasert or Progesterone-T is a plastic IUD containing synthetic progesterone. (See p. 246 for contraceptive effects of progesterone.) This IUD has a higher rate of ectopic pregnancies than other IUDs.

All plastic IUDs are coated with barium so that they will be visible under X-ray. (See "Perforation," p. 252.)

The Majzlin Spring, the Birnberg Bow and the Dalkon Shield have been removed from the market and should *not* be used because they are linked with the most serious IUD-related complications: perforation and infection.

Effectiveness

The IUD is considered a very effective form of birth control. In theory it has a failure rate of 1.5 percent; its actual failure rate is 4 percent.

Pregnancy rates for IUDs are lower among women over thirty and (except for the Saf-T-Coil) those who have previously given birth.

For almost 100 percent effectiveness, use contraceptive cream, jelly or foam, or have your partner use a condom along with the IUD—all the time or when you know you are fertile. (See "Fertility Observation," p. 235.) *It is a good idea to use a supplemental birth control method for at least the first three months after IUD insertion*, as that is the time when the IUD is most likely to be expelled and conception most likely to take place.

Medications and IUD Effectiveness

Since some practitioners suspect that aspirin or antibiotics may interfere with the IUD's effectiveness, it might be a good idea to use an additional method of birth control when you take aspirin or antibiotics.

Expulsion

A major drawback of the IUD is its high expulsion rate. Our bodies have a natural tendency to expel foreign objects. After one year of use, between 5 and 20 percent of women with IUDs will have expelled them, sometimes without knowing it has happened. These women are vulnerable to pregnancy without being aware of it. The Progestasert-T and Copper-7 seem to be expelled less frequently than the other IUDs.

If your body is not going to tolerate the IUD, it will usually expel the device during the first three months after insertion. This happens most frequently during menstruation. Since you might not feel it coming out, check for it in the toilet and on your tampon or sanitary napkin. Be sure to feel the length of the string a few times each month, especially right after your period.

Signs of IUD expulsion include an unusual vaginal discharge, cramping or pain, spotting, a longer string or an ability to feel the IUD in your vagina or cervical

IUD EFFECTIVENESS

Device	Size	Pregnancy Rate*	Color of String†
Lippes Loop	A (small)	8.0	Blue
	B	5.8	Black
	C	4.1	Yellow
	D (large)	3.6	White
Saf-T-Coil	For women who have never given birth	0.1	Green
	Previously given birth	1.3	Green
Copper-T	One size	1.5	Light blue (variable)
Copper-7	One size	1.5	Black
Progestasert-T	One size	2.5 (never given birth)	Translucent
		1.9 (previously given birth)	

This table is adapted from *Contraceptive Technology 1982–1983*, Tables 6.1 and 6.2, pp. 76–77.
*Per 100 woman-years.
†You can see the IUD string(s) if you use a speculum and a mirror to look at your cervix. (See Chapter 12, "Anatomy and Physiology of Sexuality and Reproduction.")

os. When an IUD is being expelled, your male partner may feel pain or irritation during intercourse.

The longer your body retains the IUD, the better your chance of not expelling it.

Reversibility

The IUD can harm our fertility through pelvic inflammatory disease, perforation, embedding or ectopic pregnancy. These serious complications can cause impaired fertility or sterility and may lead to hysterectomy. Health practitioners should tell this to every woman who chooses an IUD as her form of birth control, especially to those of us who hope someday to have children.

If you don't have any of these problems during the time you use an IUD, your chance of becoming pregnant after it is removed is probably the same as it was before using the IUD (although there is some controversy on this).

Safety

More and more studies are documenting serious negative effects suffered by IUD users. Some women have died from IUD complications; others have had serious injury (see below).

How Long to Keep Your IUD

A growing number of practitioners are recommending that you get the plastic types of IUDs replaced every three to five years to prevent pelvic infections. However, each time you have a new IUD inserted there is the possibility of perforation. For this reason, some practitioners recommend *not* replacing them routinely.

Copper devices must be replaced every three years. They probably lose some of their contraceptive quality after that, either because a corroded crust has formed over the device, prohibiting the copper from being released, or, as some research suggests, because the copper has dissolved, presumably having been absorbed by the body. IUDs containing progesterone should be changed every year because the supply of progesterone in the device is used up after twelve months.

Warning Signals

The following are signs of serious problems: late period or missed period; abdominal pain; increased temperature, fever, chills; noticeable or foul discharge; spotting, bleeding, heavy periods, clots. *Report these immediately*, for they are signs of infection, perforation or pregnancy. Report *any* problem lasting more than a few cycles to a health practitioner or clinic.

Who Should Absolutely Not Use the IUD

IUDs should *absolutely not* be used by women who are pregnant and women with active pelvic infection, including known or suspected gonorrhea. (Remember that more than 70 percent of gonorrhea in women is *asymptomatic*.)

Who Is Strongly Advised Not to Use the IUD

Women with the following situations or conditions are *strongly advised not* to use IUDs: abnormal Pap smears, abnormal pelvic bleeding, acute cervicitis, difficult ac-

251

cess to emergency treatment, disorders of blood or impaired coagulation, endometritis, exposure to DES *in utero* (DES daughter), gynecological malignancy, history of ectopic pregnancy, impaired response to infection (in diabetics or women taking steroids), multiple sexual partners (because of risk of infection), recent or recurrent pelvic infection (or single pelvic infection if you want to become pregnant someday), sickle cell anemia.

Who Should Probably Not Use an IUD

Women with the following situations or conditions *should probably not* use the IUD: anemia, bicornate uterus, cervical stenosis, a desire to get pregnant in the future, endometrial polyps, endometriosis, inability to check IUD string or to check for warning signals, leiomyomata, past history of fainting or severe vasovaginal reaction, severe menstrual cramps or bleeding, small uterus, valvular heart disease. Women who have a copper allergy or Wilson's disease (a rare inherited disorder of copper excretion) should probably not use *copper* IUDs.

Complications and Negative Effects

Infections

Infections of the uterus or pelvic areas (pelvic inflammatory disease, PID; see p. 502) are between three and nine times more likely to occur in women with IUDs than in women without IUDs.[23] *Infections can spread more rapidly* with an IUD in place than they ordinarily would. The string dangling from the IUD into the vagina often acts as a well-placed ladder for germs to climb and enter the uterus. PID will not go away by itself. It can lead to tremendous pain, future ectopic pregnancy, sterility and even death. See "PID" for symptoms and treatment.

Another form of infection that may occur is an infected miscarriage, called a septic abortion. Women who become pregnant with an IUD in place are more susceptible to septic abortion, especially during the second trimester. In extreme cases, this can cause death to the woman as well as the fetus, and in most cases leads to hospitalization. That is why most doctors recommend having the IUD removed if you become pregnant.

Excessive Bleeding and Cramping

A common problem for women with IUDs is increased menstrual bleeding, sometimes excessive, and painful cramping and/or backache. Some women experience longer periods and bleeding or spotting and/or cramping between periods, too.

Usually these symptoms are more intense during the first three to six months after the IUD is inserted. Between 5 and 15 percent of IUD users have the IUD removed within one year because of bleeding and cramping.

The Lippes Loop and Saf-T-Coil increase blood loss by about 75 to 100 percent each cycle, and the Copper-7 increases it by roughly 50 percent. Heavier menstrual flow may make you anemic. Because many menstruating women are marginally anemic anyway, it is a good idea to have a blood test before you get an IUD and at each follow-up appointment. Eat plenty of iron-rich foods.

Embedding

This is a common problem in which the lining of the uterus begins to grow around the IUD. If an IUD becomes partially embedded in the uterine wall, the device will usually still be effective. But embedded IUDs can cause more pain during removal. In some cases, you may need a D and C to get it out (see p. 478). In several cases we know of, women had hysterectomies because of embedded IUDs, a devastating blow for anyone who wants to have a child.

Check the string carefully at least once a month. A shorter string may indicate an embedded IUD, and you should have it checked by a health worker, who may remove it to avoid further complications, such as perforation. You can have the IUD replaced, or you may want to choose another method of contraception.

Perforation

One of the most serious complications of IUD use is perforation of the uterine wall. This can happen partially, with part of the IUD pushing through the wall and part staying in the uterus; or it can happen completely, with the entire IUD pushing out of the uterus into the abdominal cavity. In the latter case, the IUD can migrate to other organs and become embedded in them, sometimes causing medical emergencies. Perforation occurs or begins to occur most frequently during insertion, due primarily to a practitioner's poor technique. It happens less often when a uterine sound has been taken, so always insist on this procedure. (See p. 356.)

Unfortunately, there are usually no symptoms accompanying perforation. The first sign may be a shorter string or no string at all during your monthly check (a good reason to check the string more than once a month). If this happens, be sure to see a health worker immediately. You should also use another form of birth control, because if the IUD has left the uterus, you are no longer being protected against pregnancy. In fact, some women only become aware of perforation after finding out they are pregnant.

Missing String

Since a missing string can mean either expulsion or perforation, there is no way of knowing what has happened unless you see the IUD come out. Otherwise there are several procedures available for trying to locate it. A medical practitioner can probe your uterus with a uterine sound or a biopsy instrument. If sounding fails to locate the IUD, an X-ray or ultrasound (see p. 356) may work. If the IUD is still in the uterus s/he can then try to pull the string down to remove the IUD. This may involve dilating the cervix, which can be painful.

If no IUD can be located, this probably means it was expelled. If you are pregnant and elect not to have an abortion, you should not have an X-ray. Ultrasound may be used instead, although this procedure can be expensive, and as yet no one knows the long-range effects, if any, of ultrasound on developing fetuses.

If the IUD is located outside the uterus, it should be removed, as it increases your chances of developing an internal infection. Copper and progestin are particularly damaging. Also, the IUD may prevent other organs from performing their functions properly or may puncture or strangle organs in the abdominal cavity, such as the bowel.

Recovery of an IUD which is not in the uterus and not expelled requires surgery. This can often be done in the outpatient services of your hospital or clinic. A laparoscopy operation is performed in this case (see p. 481). If the IUD is not accessible by laparoscopy, more extensive surgery may be required.

Pregnancy

If your period is late and you have an IUD, have a pregnancy test. If you know you are pregnant and you have an IUD in place you should have the IUD removed *whether or not* you wish to continue the pregnancy. If you do *not* have it removed, your chances of miscarriage are about 50 percent, and during the second trimester your chances are ten times greater than normal. The miscarriage could become infected. If you *do* have the IUD removed, your chances of miscarrying are about 25 percent.

If you carry a pregnancy close to term with an IUD in place, there may be a higher likelihood of premature birth.[24] There have been some cases of stillbirth associated with the IUD.

Ectopic Pregnancy

If you get pregnant with an IUD in place, there is a 5 percent chance of ectopic pregnancy. *An ectopic pregnancy is a serious problem* which can cause hemorrhage and lead to infection, sterility and sometimes death. Frequently it is misdiagnosed, so IUD users should be aware of possible symptoms of ectopic pregnancy. (See p. 427 for more information.)

Other Possible Effects

The copper in the Copper-T and the Copper-7 may produce an allergic skin reaction, and there is some question as to how it might affect a developing fetus. One investigator has suggested that the copper may have an inhibitory effect on gonorrhea, but don't count on it.

There is no evidence that the IUD can cause cancer, but it has not been studied long enough to know the long-term effects of either the material it's made of (polyethylene) or the material some IUDs contain (progestin and barium).

How to Get an IUD

Because of the risk of perforation, a well-trained person must insert the IUD. Choose a practitioner who has experience with IUDs and find out in advance which device s/he uses. If s/he doesn't insert IUDs or the kind of IUD you want, go to someone else.

You must have a full medical, pelvic and breast examination, including a Pap smear, pregnancy test and blood test, and tests for STD before being given the IUD. This is very important, since if you have an STD or if you are pregnant, you should not use the IUD. That means at least two visits, since it takes a few days to receive results from the Pap smear and the STD cultures. You should, by law, be given an informed consent form to sign at this time. (See "Our Rights as Patients," p. 584.)

The practitioner should do a sounding of the uterus to measure its depth and position. If your uterus is small, as it is if you have never been pregnant, you'll get a small IUD (unless your uterus is too small and you can't be fitted with an IUD at all). An IUD can be put into a tipped uterus.

Insertion takes place through the os (the opening in the cervix) which is in diameter about the size of a thin straw. Just before insertion, the IUD is straightened out in a plastic tube like a straw. The practitioner gently puts the tube into the vagina and up into the uterus through the cervix (see illustration). Then s/he pushes the IUD through the tube and it springs back into shape within the uterus. The practitioner removes the tube and the IUD stays in the uterus, with its string dangling into the vagina. Make sure that you understand how to check the string.

The process can hurt, sometimes a lot, because the inserter stretches the os open and the device irritates the uterus. You may have cramps during the insertion and for the rest of the day. Bring a friend with you if you can, someone who can accompany you home after the appointment. You might choose to have a local

IUD INSERTION

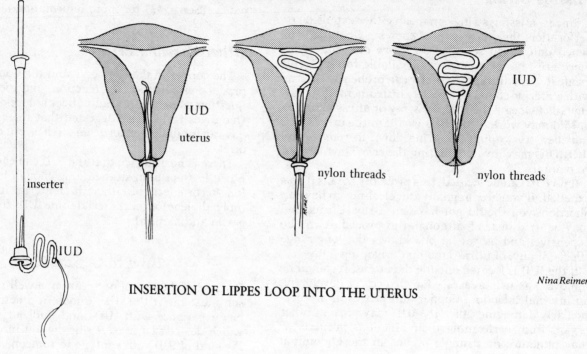

INSERTION OF LIPPES LOOP INTO THE UTERUS

Nina Reimer

anesthetic (rare) or take a mild painkiller, or you can pant quickly or relax and take deep breaths.

When to Get an IUD

This is controversial. Many advise inserting the IUD during or just after your period; the os is slightly opened at that time, so insertion may be less painful. Also, the fact that you are having your period probably means you aren't pregnant (although sometimes women have one or even two scant periods during pregnancy). Some suspect there may be a greater chance of incurring infection during menstruation, however, and avoid inserting IUDs at that time. Similarly, practitioners used to think that IUDs should be inserted right after childbirth or abortion. However, now many practitioners are afraid of infection at that time and believe that, because the uterus is soft then, there is a greater chance of perforation and a higher rate of expulsion.

Consequently, the best time for insertion may be between periods and at least six weeks after childbirth or abortion.

Checking Your IUD

At first you'll want to check your IUD string before intercourse (you may want to ask your partner to do it) and after each period. After three months or so, once or twice a month is enough.

You can try to feel the string with your finger or look for it during a cervical self-exam using a specu-lum (see p. 478). To check with your finger, squat, bringing your bottom down near your heels to shorten the length of your vagina, and reach into your vagina with your longest (clean) finger. The bathtub or shower is a good place, or bear down while you are sitting on the toilet. You may be confused by the folds in your vagina, but when you reach your cervix you will know it, as it is harder and firmer than anything else you'll touch. Find the dimple in your cervix; this is the entrance to your uterus, and the strings of the IUD should be sticking out a little way. Some days your uterus may be tipped in such a way that you can't reach the cervix or find the hole; try again the next day. If you cannot find the strings for a few days or if they are much longer or shorter, or if you feel a bit of plastic protruding, call your health practitioner or clinic.

Advantages

You don't have to worry about forgetting to take a pill, check your signs of fertility or use a barrier method at the time of intercourse.

Checking the string a few times each month encourages you to get to know your vagina and cervix and to feel comfortable about touching your genitals.

Disadvantages

Most of the disadvantages in terms of pain and risk have been described above. Note particularly the likelihood of long-term infertility due to PID. Women without access to abortion sources or who would elect not to have an abortion risk having a baby, a miscarriage or a septic abortion.

Responsibility

The woman sees a practitioner for insertion and at least once a year afterward. She experiences the insertion and any negative effects. The woman or her partner must check the string periodically.

Cost

Private doctors can cost anywhere from thirty-five to a hundred dollars. Family-planning clinics may charge as little as ten dollars. In some places there may be no charge at all. After the initial visits for testing and insertion, there's no cost except for your yearly checkup.

New IUD Design

Researchers are always designing new products to improve the effectiveness and reduce the problems of IUDs. View *all* new IUDs cautiously, since experience has shown that many of their long-term negative effects will show up only after they're put on the market. Some new designs we've heard about include IUDs that can be inserted immediately after childbirth, IUDs containing synthetic estrogens and IUDs made out of a copper/zinc combination.

The IUD as Postcoital (Morning-After) Birth Control

Since the IUD may inhibit the implantation of a fertilized egg, it has been used as a postcoital contraceptive. So far only the copper IUDs have been used in this way on a few women, but they have proven successful at preventing pregnancy within one to five days after conception occurs.

Of course, using the IUD postcoitally involves the risks discussed above. However, some people think that this method is safer overall than the morning-after pill, and it continues to provide birth control protection for as long as the IUD is left in the uterus.

It is not wise to use the postcoital IUD if there is a chance you may have contracted STD.

WITHDRAWAL (COITUS INTERRUPTUS, OR "TAKING CARE" OR "PULLING OUT")

Worldwide, this is the most universally used of all methods, a folk method passed on from one generation to the next. Withdrawal involves removing the penis from the vagina just before ejaculation so that the sperm is deposited outside the vagina and away from the lips of the vagina as well.

Withdrawal is not very effective because the drops of fluid that come out of the penis right after it becomes erect can contain enough sperm to cause pregnancy. Also, the man cannot always get out in time to avoid contact with the vagina *and* vaginal lips (sperm can swim all the way from the vaginal lips up into the fallopian tubes). Multiple acts of intercourse in a short period of time increase the likelihood of failure, since more sperm are mixed in with the lubricating fluid. Withdrawal has a theoretical failure rate of 16 percent but an actual failure rate of 23 percent.

Withdrawal has a number of drawbacks in addition to its high failure rate. The man must keep in control and therefore cannot relax. When used over a long period, it may lead to premature ejaculation by the male. Withdrawal can also be uncomfortable for the woman: the man may have to withdraw before she reaches orgasm, interrupting the flow of her sexual response; also, a part of her is wondering whether he's going to withdraw in time, so that she, too, cannot entirely relax. Some couples who have used withdrawal for a long time have been able to work out these problems.

NON-METHODS

Douching

Some women douche with water or other special solutions immediately after intercourse, in an attempt to remove semen from the vagina before sperm enter the uterus.

Douching does not work. Sperm swim fast, and some will reach your uterus before you've reached the bathroom; and the douche, which is liquid squirted into your vagina under pressure, will push some sperm up into your uterus even as it is washing others away.

Douching is the least effective of all methods, and it puts the burden exclusively on the woman, who must hop up to the bathroom immediately. Don't use it!

Avoidance of Orgasm by the Woman

Some people think that in order to conceive, a woman must have an orgasm. This is false. One of the major differences between men and women in reproduction is that a man must have an erection and ejaculation to cause a pregnancy, whereas a woman can conceive without any sexual arousal.

Breastfeeding

Although occasionally breastfeeding on demand with no supplementary food for the baby may prevent ovulation for some women, you should not count on this.

Astrological Birth Control

The previous edition of *Our Bodies, Ourselves* included a brief section on astrological birth control, which just doesn't work.

STERILIZATION

Since 1973, the use of sterilization as a permanent* method of contraception has increased rapidly. Today it is the most frequently used method of birth control among married couples in the U.S. Sterilization is a *virtually 100 percent* effective form of birth control, available for both women and men. In women, the fallopian tubes are cut and/or blocked so the egg and sperm cannot meet. This is called *tubal ligation*. In men, the vas deferens is cut and/or blocked so sperm cannot mix with seminal fluid. This is called *vasectomy*. Currently physicians and the population control establishment are promoting sterilization as the best form of birth control. As one advocate put it: "Sterilization is the most cost-effective method of birth control, considering the number of years of protection it provides."[25] However, many women are choosing this procedure without adequate information about the possible risks and consequences involved, or under coercive circumstances.†

Choosing to be sterilized is a major step. Recent studies have shown that nearly one-third of the women who were sterilized at one point in their lives regretted this decision later on, particularly if they were under thirty years old when sterilized. Some women turn to sterilization in desperation because there is no suitable form of contraception for them. (Nothing else points out so clearly our need for better temporary methods of birth control.) Many feel they have no other choice: "The lack of employment opportunities, education, day care, decent housing, adequate medical care; safe, effective contraception and access to abortion all create an atmosphere of subtle coercion."[26]

*Although there have been some successful attempts at reversing both vasectomies and tubal ligations, *the operation should be considered permanent and not reversible.*

†Most (but not all) documented cases of coerced sterilization in the U.S. involve women. Here we focus on the experiences of women.

For some women, however, the choice to be sterilized is a positive wish to avoid pregnancy forever. Some have already had children; others decide they never want children.

Under whatever circumstances sterilization is chosen, the decision usually brings up deep feelings, as this thirty-six-year-old mother of two described to us:

The week before my sterilization I was very nervous, irritable and jumpy. I'd yell at my husband. I tried to pull out of myself all my fears about having an operation: I would die, there'd be a mistake, I'd be out of control, I'd get the wrong anesthetic; and fears about this particular operation: my husband would think that I wasn't a real woman anymore, he'd leave me for a fertile woman, I'd get all dried up and wrinkled. I felt angry at my husband for not wanting to deal with his feelings of loss of manhood by having a vasectomy (though that was a little irrational on my part, for his vasectomy couldn't give me my sexual freedom if I wanted to make love with another man).

Now, almost two years later, I am glad I made the choice I did. I feel much freer when I make love....

Since 1974, women have revealed and studies have documented a terrible pattern of sterilization abuse. Victims of sterilization abuse are usually poor or black, Puerto Rican, Chicana or Native American, often with little or no understanding of English.* Sometimes physicians consider women mentally unfit.† Physicians pressure women into giving consent during labor or childbirth; welfare officials threaten the loss of benefits if women refuse; no one informs women that the operation is permanent. Black women in the South

*Sterilization abuse is not a new development. Beginning in the nineteenth century, people known as "eugenicists" tried to popularize the idea that social problems such as crime and poverty could be eliminated by preventing certain "unfit" people from having children. The eugenics movement, which has proponents even today, argued that criminals, "imbeciles," blacks and immigrants would produce more "inferior" people like themselves if allowed to reproduce. Eugenicists urged the passage of laws empowering the state to sterilize such individuals against their will. These eugenics laws were passed in thirty-seven states and as of 1979 were still on the books in about twenty.

†A major investigation and report, produced only after great pressure from people such as Connie Uri, a Native American physician, found that large numbers of women living on Indian reservations had been sterilized without consent by government-sponsored programs. (See the U.S. General Accounting Office Report to Hon. James G. Abourezk, B164031 [5], November 1976.) At a major teaching hospital in Los Angeles, a resident went to the local newspapers to expose cases of sterilization abuse involving many poor Chicana women. (See "A Health Research Group Study on Surgical Sterilization: Present Abuses and Proposed Regulations," Health Research Group, 1973.)

GAO reports (single copy) are free. Write to U.S. GAO, Distribution Section, Room 1518, 401 G Street NW, Washington, DC 20548. Indicate the report number and date. Health Research Group reports are available from HRG, 2000 P Street NW, Washington, DC 20036.

are all too familiar with the "Mississippi Appendectomy," in which the fallopian tubes are tied or the uterus is removed without them knowing it. Sometimes sterilizations are done primarily for the purpose of training residents or interns. Of the million hysterectomies done each year, perhaps one out of five is done for sterilization only, with no legitimate medical reason. Hysterectomy, a major surgical procedure, is unnecessary for sterilization purposes. The risk of death or complication from a hysterectomy is ten to a hundred times greater than from a tubal ligation. (See "Hysterectomy and Oophorectomy," p. 511.) Especially if women are poor, public and private programs make it easier to get sterilization services than abortions or prenatal care and financial assistance so that we can have healthy children; or they refuse to perform abortions until women agree to be sterilized. In recent years legislators in at least ten states have proposed compulsory sterilization for all women on welfare. (No such measure has yet passed.) Occasionally physicians refuse to sterilize fully informed white middle-class women with no children who request this procedure. Sterilization and its abuses are experienced differently by different groups of women.

Sterilization abuse also occurs internationally. See Chapter 26, "Developing an International Awareness," for U.S. government participation.

Feminists, health activists and others joined together to expose sterilization abuse and to organize against it in hospitals, communities, courts and legislatures. In 1975, responding to this pressure, New York City became the first city in this country to produce guidelines. On March 9, 1979, federal sterilization regulations went into effect. The most important requirements of the federal regulations include:

- obtaining voluntary informed consent using a mandatory, standardized consent form in a person's preferred language;
- prohibiting overt or implicit threat of loss of welfare or Medicaid benefits if someone doesn't consent;
- explaining alternative methods of birth control and the risks, side effects and irreversibility of sterilization, orally and in writing, also in a person's language;
- waiting at least thirty days after a person signs the consent form before sterilization (except for premature delivery and emergency abdominal surgery);
- prohibiting obtaining consent while someone is in labor, before or after an abortion or while the person is under the influence of alcohol or other drugs;
- prohibiting hysterectomies for sterilization in federally funded programs;
- imposing a moratorium on federally funded sterilizations of people under twenty-one who have been declared legally incompetent or are involuntarily institutionalized;

- auditing sterilization programs in the ten states where most federally funded sterilizations are performed.[27]

The government does not monitor or enforce these regulations, and often doctors and hospitals ignore them. If you are considering sterilization, make sure that the clinic or hospital performing it complies with these regulations. If you suspect that it doesn't, contact your local women's health group or one of the following organizations:

- American Civil Liberties Union
  Reproductive Freedom Project
  132 West 43rd Street
  New York, NY 10036

- Committee for Abortion Rights and Against Sterilization Abuse (CARASA)
  17 Murray Street
  New York, NY 10007

- Indian Women United for Social Justice
  P.O. Box 38743
  Los Angeles, CA 90038

- Mexican American Women's National Association (MANA)
  L'Enfant Plaza Station SW
  P.O. Box 23656
  Washington, DC 20024

- National Women's Health Network
  224 Seventh Street SE
  Washington, DC 20003

TUBAL LIGATION

Female sterilization is effective immediately. It can be done under general, spinal or local anesthesia, and women usually go home the same day.

Laparoscopy, or "Band-Aid" surgery, is the most common surgical technique for sterilization in the U.S. General anesthesia is usually administered, although a laparoscopy can be done under local or spinal anesthesia. The actual procedure takes about thirty minutes and involves making a small incision in a woman's belly button and inflating her belly with gas (carbon dioxide or nitrous oxide) so the fallopian tubes can be more easily seen. The woman is tilted back, head down, allowing her intestines to move away from her fallopian tubes. The tubes are moved into view by inserting a clamp (tenaculum) onto the cervix and an instrument (sound or intrauterine cannula) through the vagina, and then manipulating the uterus and tubes. Next,

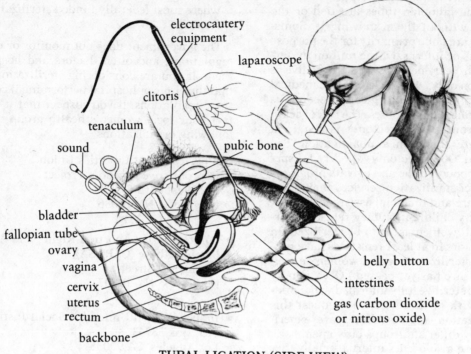

electrocautery equipment

laparoscope

clitoris

tenaculum

sound

pubic bone

bladder

fallopian tube

ovary

vagina

cervix

uterus

rectum

backbone

belly button

intestines

gas (carbon dioxide or nitrous oxide)

Christine Bondante

TUBAL LIGATION (SIDE VIEW)

her belly is inflated with gas to make the tubes visible. A laparoscope (a thin tube containing a viewing instrument and a light) is inserted through the incision to view the tubes. An instrument to block the tubes is introduced through the laparoscope or through a second tiny incision below the belly button. The tubes can be blocked by burning (electrocoagulation or cautery) or cutting them, clipping them shut or applying rings to them. The incisions are sewn closed (see illustration).

The *mini-laparotomy,* or "mini-lap," involves making a small incision just above a woman's pubic bone, moving the tubes into view with a tenaculum and sound (see above), pulling the fallopian tubes up through the incision and blocking them (usually by tying and cutting them). The incision is sewn shut. Women seem to have more cramping and pain afterwards than with a laparoscopy, sometimes lasting a few days.[28]

Laparoscopy and mini-laparotomy have a failure rate of about 0.025 percent.

Tubal ligations can also be performed through a woman's vagina (*colpotomy* or *culdoscopy*) or cervix (*hysteroscopy,* an experimental procedure). Sterilization by *laparotomy* involves major surgery. (See Chapter 23, surgery section.)

Sterilization probably does not affect a woman's hormone secretions, ovaries, uterus or vagina. Her menstrual cycle continues but may become irregular. An egg ripens and bursts out of an ovary every month, but stops partway down the tube, disintegrates and is absorbed by her body.

Complications and Negative Effects

Whenever surgery involving anesthetic is performed, certain complications are possible. Major complications happen relatively rarely and depend a great deal on the skill and experience of the practitioner performing the sterilization. Cardiac irregularity, cardiac arrest, infection, internal bleeding and perforation of a major blood vessel are a few of the potential hazards. Laparoscopic techniques may involve specific problems such as internal burn injuries or punctures to other organs or tissue, skin burns, puncturing of the intestine, perforation of the uterus and carbon dioxide embolism (which may cause immediate death). Some women experience a postlaparoscopic syndrome including heavy irregular bleeding and increased menstrual pain, which may create the need for repeated D and Cs or, in some cases, complete hysterectomies.

Reversibility

No woman should undergo sterilization with the hope that the procedure can be reversed. If you think there is any chance you may want to have children someday, use a reversible form of birth control.

Nonetheless, recent advances in microsurgery have increased the possibility of tubal reconstruction, called *reanastomosis.* It is major surgery, requiring extreme skill on the part of the surgeon, highly specialized and expensive equipment and a woman in good health. The operation can cost ten thousand dollars or more.

258

This means that only women with substantial resources will be able to reverse sterilization.*

Before undergoing this operation, a woman and her partner should be tested for fertility potential. Also, the woman should have a laparoscopic examination to determine if her tubes are too damaged to be repaired. Cauterization tends to destroy a significant amount of the tube. Clips and rings seem to destroy much less of the tube.

NEW TECHNIQUES IN FEMALE STERILIZATION

Possible new techniques involve injecting substances into the fallopian tubes, inserting pellets or plugs, modifying surgical procedures and using new types of clips or rings. We have heard of experiments using methylcyanoacrylate (MCA), also known as Crazy Glue or Superglue; and silicone plugs. The negative and long-term effects of these substances are unknown. Although female sterilization is far more complex than male sterilization and has more potential risks, much larger sums of federal money are spent researching the negative effects and complications of male sterilization.[29]

MALE STERILIZATION: VASECTOMY

Male sterilization is a much simpler process than female sterilization. Usually done in a doctor's office or in a clinic, the operation takes about half an hour. The practitioner applies a local anesthetic (such as Novocaine), makes one or two small incisions in the scrotum, locates the two vasa deferentia (singular: vas deferens; tubes that carry sperm from the testes to the penis), removes a piece of each and ties off the ends. Men are not sterile immediately, since sperm are already in the vasa deferentia. For this reason, use another method of birth control for two months or until the man has had two negative sperm counts.

Vasectomy leaves the man's genital system basically unchanged. His sexual hormones remain operative, and there is no noticeable difference in his ejaculate because sperm make up only a small part of the semen.

*A possible form of sterilization abuse may develop along these lines: technology for sterilization reversal will improve greatly, due to a combination of physicians' recognition that many women do want reversal, scientific fascination with new surgical techniques and population establishment preference for sterilization as the most cost-effective form of birth control (see p. 256). The improved reversal techniques will lead to a popular misunderstanding that *all* women can count on reversal when and if they want it. Yet due to economic inequalities and racism, reversal will *not* be available to poor women and women of color in this country and around the world.

Some men, even though they know these facts, are still anxious about what a vasectomy will do to their sexual performance. Talking with someone who has had a vasectomy can help allay such anxieties.

In some men, antibodies to their own sperm can be found after a vasectomy. Some research suggests that these antibodies may lead to certain diseases of the immune system, yet many fully fertile men also have such antibodies, and so far this suggestion is without support.

A report in 1980 by Clarkson and Alexander[30] indicated that vasectomy may induce atherosclerosis (hardening of the arteries) which can lead to heart attack or stroke. More recent experiments were unable to substantiate that finding, however.[31]

Experimental operations have placed a piece of plastic into the tube to plug it up temporarily so that if the man later wants to have a child he can have the plug taken out. Several valves have also been tried which can be implanted in the tube and turned back on if the man wishes to regain fertility. These techniques have not yet been successful.

Vasectomy should be considered irreversible.

NOTES

Note: Space limits mean that we can print only some of the documentation for points made in this chapter. Additional documentation is on file at the Boston Women's Health Book Collective office.

1. Malcolm Potts. "Why the World Is Not Getting the Contraception It Needs," *People* 8:4 (1981), p. 28. Published by the International Planned Parenthood Foundation. Available from WHR, Inc., 105 Madison Avenue, New York, NY 10016 ($15 each year).

2. Dr. Frederick Robbins, quoted in Barbara Seaman. *The Doctor's Case Against the Pill*, rev. ed. New York: Dell Publishing Co., Inc., 1979, p. 11.

3. Malcolm Potts and Robert Wheeler. "The Quest for a Magic Bullet," *Family Planning Perspectives* 13:6 (November/December 1981), pp. 269–71; Robert Hatcher, et al., *Contraceptive Technology 1982–1983*, 11th rev. ed. New York: Irvington Publishers, 1982, p. 36.

4. One recent analysis has argued that "The low priority given to research on barrier methods reflects a bias of reproductive scientists and health professionals in favor of high technology, sophistication and a belief that 'science' will solve our health problems." Judith Bruce and S. Bruce Schearer. "Contraceptives and Common Sense: Conventional Methods Reconsidered," a public issues paper of the Population Council, PI-03 (1979), p. 2. Available from the Population Council, 1 Dag Hammarskjold Plaza, New York, NY 10017.

5. *Ibid.*, p. 65.

6. Mary E. Lane, et al. "Successful Use of the Diaphragm and Jelly by a Young Population: Report of a Clinical Study," *Family Planning Perspectives* 8:2 (March/April 1976), pp. 81–86.

7. H. Jick, et al. "Vaginal Spermicides and Congenital Dis-

orders," *Journal of the American Medical Association* 245 (1981), pp. 1329–32.

8. S. Shapiro, et al. "Birth Defects in Relation to Vaginal Spermicides," *Journal of the American Medical Association* 247:17 (1982), pp. 2381–84. J.L. Mils, et al., "Are Spermicides Teratogenic?" *Journal of the American Medical Association* 248:17 (November 5, 1982), p. 2148.

9. J. Schwartz, et al. *Connections: Nutrition, Contraception, Women, Eating*. Boston, MA: Boston Family Planning Project, 1982.

10. D. Slone, et al. "Risk of Myocardial Infarction in Relation to Current and Discontinued Use of Oral Contraceptives," *New England Journal of Medicine* 305:8 (1981), pp. 420–24.

11. E. Stern, et al. "Steroid Contraceptive Use and Cervical Dysplasia: Increase in the Risk of Progression," *Science* 196 (1977), p. 1460.

12. C. Bain, et al. "Oral Contraceptive Use and Malignant Melanoma," *Journal of the National Cancer Institute* 68 (1982), pp. 537–39; E.A. Holly, et al., "Cutaneous Melanoma in Relation to Exogenous Hormones and Reproductive Factors," *Journal of the National Cancer Institute* 70 (1983).

13. The Centers for Disease Control. "Long-Term Oral Contraceptive Use and the Risk of Breast Cancer; The Centers for Disease Control Cancer and Steroid Hormone Study," *Journal of the American Medical Association* 249 (1983), pp. 1591–95.

14. D. Kaufman, et al. "Decreased Risk of Endometrial Cancer Among Oral Contraceptive Users," *New England Journal of Medicine* 303:18 (1980), pp. 1045–47; L. Rosenberg, et al., "Epithelial Ovarian Cancer and Combination Oral Contraceptives," *Journal of the American Medical Association* 247:23 (1982), pp. 3210–12; D.W. Cramer, et al., "Factors Affecting the Association of Oral Contraceptives and Ovarian Cancer," *New England Journal of Medicine* 307:17 (October 21, 1982), pp. 1047–51.

15. World Health Organization. *Oral Contraceptives: Technical and Safety Aspects*, p. 20. Available from United Nations Bookshop, United Nations Building, First Avenue between 42nd and 43rd Streets, New York, NY 10017.

16. N.H. Wright, et al. "Neoplasia and Dysplasia of the Cervix Uteri and Contraception: A Possible Protective Effect of the Diaphragm." *British Journal of Cancer* 38 (1978), p. 273; Meisel, et al., "Dysplasia of Uterine Cervix," *Cancer* 40 (1977), p. 3076.

17. J. Schwartz, et al. *Connections: Nutrition, Contraception, Women, Eating*. Boston, MA: Boston Family Planning Project, 1982; Kay Behall, "Oral Contraceptives and Nutrition: A Report on Research in Progress," U.S. Department of Agriculture (undated).

18. Kay Behall. "Oral Contraceptives and Nutrition: A Report on Research in Progress," U.S. Department of Agriculture (undated), p. 2.

19. *Contraceptive Technology Update* 3:4 (April 1982), p. 54.

20. Belita Cowan. "Ethical Problems in Government-Funded Contraceptive Research," in H.B. Holmes, B.B. Hoskins and M. Gross, eds. *Birth Control and Controlling Birth. Women-Centered Perspectives*. Clifton, NJ: Humana Press, 1980, p. 39.

21. Shan Ratnam and R.N.V. Prasad. "Finding an Alternative to Post-Coital Sneezing," *People* 8:4 (1981), p. 22.

22. "IUDs—Update on Safety, Effectiveness and Research," *Population Reports*, Series B, No. 3 (May 1979). Available from Population Information Program, the Johns Hopkins University, 624 N. Broadway, Baltimore, MD 21205. (Multiple copies are 50¢ each; free to developing countries.)

23. D.W. Kaufman, et al. "Intrauterine Contraceptive Device Use and Pelvic Inflammatory Disease," *American Journal of Obstetrics and Gynecology* 136 (1980), pp. 159–62.

24. H. Foreman, et al. "Intrauterine Device Usage and Fetal Loss," *Obstetrics and Gynecology* 58:6 (1981), pp. 669–77.

25. Pourbe Bhiwandiwala. "New Approaches to Female Sterilization," *People* 8:4 (1981), p. 14.

26. Rahemah Amur, et al. "Sterilization Rights Abuses and Remedies," *Sourcebook for the 11th National Women and the Law Conference*, Spring 1980.

27. R.P. Petchesky. "Reproduction, Ethics and Public Policy: The Federal Sterilization Regulations," *Hastings Center Report* 9:5 (October 1979), pp. 29–41. Copies of the regulation may be obtained from Marilyn L. Martin, Hubert Humphrey Building, Room 722-H, 200 Independence Avenue SW, Washington, DC 20201.

28. M.H. Saidi and C.M. Zainie. *Female Sterilization: A Handbook for Women*. New York: Garland STPM Press, 1980, p. 52.

29. B. Cowan. "Ethical Problems in Government-Funded Contraceptive Research," in H.B. Holmes, B.B. Hoskins and M. Gross, eds. *Birth Control and Controlling Birth*. Clifton, NJ: Humana Press, 1980, pp. 37–46.

30. T.B. Clarkson and N. Alexander. "Long-Term Vasectomy: Effects on the Occurrence and Extent of Atherosclerosis in Rhesus Monkeys," *Journal of Clinical Investigations* 65 (1980), pp. 15–25.

31. "No Atherosclerosis Risk in Vasectomized Men, Preliminary Studies Find," *Family Planning Perspectives* 13:6 (1981), p. 276.

RESOURCES

General

Bell, Ruth. *Changing Bodies, Changing Lives*. New York: Random House, Inc., 1980. A handbook on health, sexuality and birth control especially for teens.

Committee for Abortion Rights and Against Sterilization Abuse (CARASA), 17 Murray Street, New York, NY 10007. An activist group working for abortion rights and against sterilization abuse. Publishes *CARASA News*.

Davis, Angela. "Racism, Birth Control and Reproductive Rights," in A. Davis, *Women, Race and Class*. New York: Random House, Inc., 1983.

Ed-U-Press, 760 Ostrom Avenue, Syracuse, NY 13210. Send for literature list, including birth control material for teens.

Foster, Henry W., Jr. "Contraceptives in Sickle Cell Disease." *Southern Medical Journal* 74:5 (May 1981), pp. 543–45.

Gordon, Linda. *Woman's Body, Woman's Right: A Social History of Birth Control in America*. New York: Penguin Books, 1977.

Hatcher, Robert, et al. *Contraceptive Technology, 1982–1983*, 11th rev. ed. New York: Irvington Publishers, 1982. A comprehensive handbook on birth control methods.

Holmes, Helen B., et al. *Birth Control and Controlling Birth. Women-Centered Perspectives*. Clifton, NJ: Humana Press, 1980.

Impact, the journal of National Family Sex Education Week. Available from the Institute for Family Research and Education, 760 Ostrom Avenue, Syracuse, NY 13210. Send $1.00 for postage and handling. A periodical that always includes articles on teenage pregnancy, Margaret Sanger, the current backlash against homosexuality, high school censorship and more.

Luker, Kristin. *Taking Chances: Abortion and the Decision Not to Contracept.* Berkeley, CA: University of California Press, 1975. A study of the complicated reasons why some women have sexual intercourse without using birth control, even when contraceptives are available.

Mass, Bonnie. *Population Target: The Political Economy of Population Control in Latin America.* Ontario: Charters Publishing Co., 1976.

Norsigian, Judy. "Redirecting Contraceptive Research," *Science for the People* (January/February 1979), pp. 27–30.

Reproductive Rights National Network (R2N2), 17 Murray Street, New York, NY 10007. A feminist health activist network with newsletter, slide show tour and other resources.

Seaman, Barbara, and Gideon Seaman. *Women and the Crisis in Sex Hormones.* New York: Bantam Books, 1978 (paper). An excellent resource on the Pill, IUD, barrier methods, etc.

Barrier Methods

Belsky, R. "Vaginal Contraceptives: A Time for Reappraisal," *Population Reports*, Series H, No. 3 (January 1975), pp. 14–40.

Bruce, Judith, and S. Bruce Schearer. "Contraceptives and developing countries: The role of barrier methods." A public-issues paper of the Population Council, 1983. 1 Dag Hammarskjold Plaza, New York, NY 10017.

"Cervical Cap," *Population Reports*, Series H, No. 4 (January 1976). Available from Population Information Programs, Johns Hopkins University, 624 N. Broadway, Baltimore, MD 21205.

Eagen, Andrea Borgoff. "The Contraceptive Sponge: Easy—But Is It Safe?" *Ms.* 12:7 (1984), pp. 94–95.

Fairbanks, Betsy, and Beth Scharfman. "The Cervical Cap: Past and Current Experiences," *Women and Health* 5:3 (1980), pp. 61–80.

"FDA Approves Vaginal Sponge as a Contraceptive Device," *Contraceptive Technology Update* 4:5 (May 1983).

Jick, H., et al. "Vaginal Spermicides and Congenital Disorders," *Journal of the American Medical Association* 245 (1981), pp. 1329–32.

Lane, M.E., et al. "Successful Use of the Diaphragm and Jelly by a Young Population: Report of a Clinical Study," *Family Planning Perspectives* 8 (1976), pp. 81–86.

New Hampshire Feminist Health Center. Information packet on the cervical cap. Send $7.50 to the Center, 38 S. Main Street, Concord, NH 03301.

Redford, M.H., et al. *The Condom: Increasing Utilization in the United States.* San Francisco: San Francisco Press, 1974.

Shapiro, S., et al. "Birth Defects in Relation to Vaginal Spermicides," *Journal of the American Medical Association* 247:17 (May 7, 1982), pp. 2381–84.

"Spermicides—Simplicity and Safety are Major Assets," *Population Reports*, Series H, No. 5 (September 1979). Available from Population Information Programs, Johns Hopkins University (address above).

Tatum, Howard J., and Elizabeth B. Connell-Tatum. "Barrier Contraception: A Comprehensive Review," *Fertility and Sterility* 36:1 (July 1981), pp. 1–12.

"Update on Condoms—Products, Protection, Promotion," *Population Reports*, Series H, No. 6 (September–October 1982). Available from Population Information Programs, Johns Hopkins University (address above).

Vessey, M., and P. Wiggins. "Use-effectiveness of the Diaphragm in a Selected Family Planning Clinic in the United Kingdom," *Contraception* 9 (1974), pp. 15–21.

Wortman, J. "The Diaphragm and Other Intravaginal Barriers—A Review," *Population Reports*, Series H, No. 4 (January 1976). Available from Population Information Programs, Johns Hopkins University (address above).

Natural Birth Control

Note: These are some of the publications or resources currently available. Please understand that they are *not* meant to take the place of a group in which these skills are shared on a woman-to-woman basis. We do not recommend that you use the information for contraception until you have participated in such a group.

Bell, S., et al. "Reclaiming Reproductive Control: A Feminist Approach to Fertility Consciousness," *Science for the People* 12:1 (1980), pp. 6–9, 30–35. Available from Science for the People, 897 Main Street, Cambridge, MA 02139.

Billings, Evelyn, and Ann Westmore. *The Billings Method.* New York: Random House, Inc., 1980. A popularized introduction to the ovulation method.

Billings, John, Evelyn Billings and Maurice Catarinich. *The Atlas of the Ovulation Method.* Published in Australia. Available from WOOMB–USA, Room 119, 1750 Brentwood, St. Louis, MO 63144, for $10. This teaching manual can be very helpful to women who want to learn the method.

Department of Health and Hospitals, 1400 W. 9th Street, Los Angeles, CA 90015. A large resource center for the ovulation method. Slides and cassettes in English and Spanish, a newsletter and a teacher's guide.

Garfink, Christine, and Hank Pizer. *The New Birth Control Program.* New edition. New York: Bolder Books, 1977. A good account of the sympto-thermal method. The information about mucus is not very good; the emphasis is on temperature.

Gillette, Nealy, ed. *The Ovulation Method Newsletter.* Published quarterly. Available for $3 per year from the Ovulation Method Teachers Association, Box 14511, Portland, OR 97214.

Guren, Denise S., and Nealy Gillette. *The Ovulation Method Cycles of Fertility.* Published by the Ovulation Method Teachers Association, 4760 Aldrich Road, Bellingham, WA 98225. Send $2.95 plus 60¢ postage and handling; discounts available for bulk orders. Clear, concise and without moral or religious overtones. The best book we've seen yet about the ovulation method.

Kippley, John, and Sheila Kippley. *The Art of Natural Family Planning,* 2nd ed., 1979. Couple to Couple League, Box 11084, Cincinnati, OH 45211. Send $6.95 plus $1.25 for shipping.

"Periodic Abstinence: How Well Do the New Approaches Work?" *Population Reports*, Series I, No. 3 (September 1981). Available from Population Information Programs, Johns Hopkins University (address above).

The Pill and Other Hormones

American Academy of Pediatrics, Committee on Drugs. "Breast Feeding and Contraception," *Pediatrics* 68:1 (July 1981), pp. 138–40.

Boston Collaborative Drug Surveillance Program. "Oral Contraceptives and Venous Thrombo-embolic Disease, Surgically Confirmed Gall Bladder Disease, and Breast Tumors," *Lancet* 1 (1973), pp. 1399–1404.

"Breast Cancer and the Pill—A Muted Reassurance," an editorial in *British Medical Journal* 282 (1981), pp. 2075–76.

Cowan, Belita. Testimony on the morning-after pill before the U.S. House of Representatives, December 15, 1975.

Evrard, J.R., et al. "Amenorrhea Following Oral Contraception," *American Journal of Obstetrics and Gynecology* 124 (1976), p. 88.

Gold, R., and P.D. Wilson. "Depo-Provera: New Developments in a Decade-Old Controversy," *International Family Planning Perspectives* 6:4 (December 1980), pp. 156–60.

Heinonen, O.P., et al. "Cardiovascular Birth Defects and Antenatal Exposure to Female Sex Hormones," *New England Journal of Medicine* 296:2 (January 13, 1977), pp. 67–70.

Janerich, D.T., et al. "Fertility Patterns After Discontinuation of Use of Oral Contraceptives," *Lancet* 1 (1976), pp. 1051–53.

Kaufman, D., et al. "Decreased Risk of Endometrial Cancer Among Oral-Contraceptive Users," *New England Journal of Medicine* 303:18 (1980), pp. 1045–47.

"Liver Tumours and the Pill," an editorial in *British Medical Journal* 2:6803 (August 6, 1977), pp. 345–46.

Minkin, S. "Nine Thai Women Had Cancer....None of Them Took Depo-Provera: Therefore, Depo-Provera Is Safe. This Is Science?" *Mother Jones* (November 1981), pp. 34ff.

Mintz, M. "Annals of Commerce: Selling the Pill," *Washington Post*, February 8, 1976.

O'Malley, Becky. "Who Says Oral Contraceptives Are Safe?" *The Nation*, February 14, 1981.

"Oral Contraceptives and Endometrial Cancer," an editorial in *New England Journal of Medicine* 302:10 (1980), pp. 575–76.

"Patient Skin Changes May Be Indication for Discontinuing OC," *OB/GYN News* (April 15, 1976).

Royal College of General Practitioners' Oral Contraception Study. "Further Analysis of Mortality in Oral Contraceptive Users," *Lancet* 1 (March 7, 1981), pp. 541–46.

Schwartz, J., et al. *Connections: Nutrition, Contraception, Women, Eating*, 1982 Boston Family Planning Project, Department of Health and Hospitals, 818 Harrison Avenue, Boston, MA 02118.

Seaman, Barbara. *The Doctor's Case Against the Pill*. New York: Peter Wyden, 1969; rev. ed, New York: Dell Publishing Co., Inc., 1979.

"Searle Concedes Bribe Payments," *The New York Times*, January 6, 1976.

"Serious Adverse Effects of Oral Contraceptives and Estrogens," *Medical Letter* (February 27, 1976).

Slone, D., et al. "Risk of Myocardial Infarction in Relation to Current and Discontinued Use of Oral Contraceptives," *New England Journal of Medicine* 305:8 (1981), pp. 420–24.

Vessey, M.P., et al. "Breast Cancer and Oral Contraceptives: Findings in Oxford Family-Planning Association Contraceptive Study," *British Medical Journal* 282 (June 1981), pp. 2093–94.

Zachran, M. "Effects of Contraceptive Pills and Intrauterine Devices on Urinary Bladder," *Urology* 8 (1976), p. 567.

IUD

Bevia, Maria, and Gordon Myron. "Common Complications from IUDs," *Resident and Staff Physician* (June 1976).

Cates, W., et al. "The Intrauterine Device and Deaths from Spontaneous Abortion," *New England Journal of Medicine* 295 (1976), p. 1155.

Dowie, Mark, and Tracy Johnson. "A Case of Corporate Malpractice," in C. Dreifus, ed., *Seizing Our Bodies: The Politics of Women's Health*. New York: Random House, Inc., 1977. Story of the Dalkon Shield.

Foreman, Harry, et al. "Intrauterine Device Usage and Fetal Loss," *Obstetrics and Gynecology* 58:6 (1981), pp. 669–77.

"IUDs: An Appropriate Contraceptive for Many Women," *Population Reports*, Series B, No. 4 (July 1982). Population Information Programs, Johns Hopkins University (address above).

Kaufman, D.W., et al. "Intrauterine Contraceptive Device Use and Pelvic Inflammatory Disease," *American Journal of Obstetrics and Gynecology* 136 (1980), pp. 159–62.

"Progestasert—A New Intrauterine Device," *Medical Letter* (July 30, 1976).

Roberts, Katherine. "The Intrauterine Device as a Health Risk," *Women and Health* 2:1 (July/August 1977), pp. 21–30.

Sterilization

Ad Hoc Women's Studies Committee Against Sterilization Abuse. *Workbook on Sterilization and Sterilization Abuse*, 1978. Available for $1.75 from Women's Studies, Sarah Lawrence College, Bronxville, NY 10708.

CARASA. *Sterilization: It's Not as Simple as "Tying Your Tubes."* Myths and facts about sterilization. Available for $1.00 from CARASA. (See p. 260 for address.)

CARASA. *Women Under Attack: Abortion, Sterilization Abuse and Reproductive Freedom*. In-depth information about the history and politics of these issues. Available for $2.50 from CARASA.

National Women's Health Network. *Resource Guide 9: Sterilization*, 1978. Available for $3.00 from NWHN, 224 7th Street SE, Washington, DC 20003.

"No Atherosclerosis Risk in Vasectomized Men, Preliminary Studies Find," *Family Planning Perspectives* 13:6 (1981), p. 276.

Petchesky, Rosalind P. "Reproduction, Ethics and Public Policy: The Federal Sterilization Regulations," *Hastings Center Report* 9:5 (October 1979), pp. 29–41.

Winston, R.M.L. "Why 103 Women Asked for Reversal of Sterilization," *British Medical Journal* 2 (July 30, 1977), pp. 305–07.

14

SEXUALLY TRANSMITTED DISEASES

By Mary Crowe, with Judy Norsigian

With special thanks to Hilde Armour, William McCormick, Esther Rome, Pam White and Paul Wiesner

This chapter in previous editions was called "Venereal Disease" and was written by Esther Rome and Fran Ansley.

Many people are surprised to learn that sexually transmitted disease (STD) is one of the most common kinds of infection going around today. Every year more than 10 million Americans get STD, which is passed from person to person primarily through sexual contact. Until recently these infections were called venereal disease, or VD, a term many people associate with gonorrhea and syphilis. Actually, there have been more than twenty STDs identified; many are at epidemic levels in this country. In addition to the diseases themselves, which can range from mild to life-threatening, there is the possibility of complications for women which can impair their fertility.

Many of us still believe that "nice" girls don't get STD. When we do, we are labeled "promiscuous" if we are single, or "unfaithful" if we are in a monogamous relationship. Worst of all, we may not get help when we are sick and need it most. As long as our society continues to look upon STDs as "punishment" for people who have casual sex, the problem will be hard to talk about, much less eradicate.*

No woman should be ashamed of having sexual feelings or choosing to be (or not to be) sexually active. But it is important to keep our sexual relationships healthy. That means learning how to prevent STDs, which are infections, before they happen, as well as how to get cured after the fact. Nearly all STDs can be cured with drugs. We can help prevent the spread of infection without giving up our sex lives.

Since STD is hard to talk about, it can be difficult

*In Western culture this goes back a long way. Even before sexual nature was understood, syphilis and gonorrhea were considered just punishment for blasphemy. (See Theodore Rosebury, *Microbes and Morals: The Strange Story of Venereal Disease*, listed in Resources.)

to find the information we need. Sometimes it seems easier to avoid the issue and forget about prevention.

One day, while I was getting my car fixed by my regular mechanic, I realized I was feeling horny. I hadn't slept with anyone for a long time. I got up my courage and propositioned him. When we got into bed I noticed his penis looked a little funny, but I couldn't really tell because the light wasn't very good. The thought of VD flickered through my mind, but it was just casual and I didn't want to be bothered. I wanted some sex, not a lot of hassle.

STD has so many dirty, sleazy overtones. Even when we feel comfortable talking about sex we may not want anyone to know that we might have an STD.

I've been so upset these last few days. My husband told me he'd slept with someone else and might have gotten VD. I didn't know what to do. How could I call up my regular doctor and expose myself? If I asked any of my friends what to do, they would be mortified. I saw an ad yesterday for a VD hotline, and after a lot of hesitation I called. It was a relief to get information without anyone knowing who I was.

Having an STD can affect the way we feel about ourselves, our sexuality and our relationships. We may feel victimized, angry or depressed, and even blame ourselves unfairly.

If one person in a supposedly monogamous couple gets an STD, it often serves as a dramatic focus for any problems the couple might have.

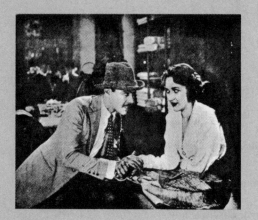

Beware of Chance Acquaintances

"Pick-up" acquaintances often take girls autoriding, to cafès, and to theatres with the intention of leading them into sex relations.   Disease or child-birth may follow

Avoid the man who tries to take liberties with you
He is selfishly thoughtless and inconsiderate of you

Believe no one who says it is necessary to indulge sex desire

Know the men you associate with
AMERICAN SOCIETY FOR SOCIAL HYGIENE 1926

Unknown

My husband and I, our toddler and sixteen-year-old babysitter went to the country at the end of the summer. When we returned home I started having a vaginal itch. Then I noticed my husband was itching, too. I asked him if he had slept with anyone else recently. He admitted to me he had slept with the babysitter. Otherwise he would never have told me.

Even when we feel comfortable about facing these issues, getting an STD usually means trouble. We will have to spend time and money for medical care; we will need to tell our sex partners so they can be treated too; and we will have our own feelings to deal with. Friends, counselors from a women's health center or a self-help group can all help when we have an STD.

WHAT ARE STDS?

STD is a term used to describe any disease acquired primarily through sexual contact. Most are caused by bacteria, a few by viruses and a few by tiny insects.

Brief Summary

1. STDs are very common. If you are sexually active in anything but a totally monogamous relationship, you have a good chance of getting an STD. Also, you can get some of these diseases (such as genital warts or herpes) without sexual contact at all.

2. The best way to deal with an STD is to avoid getting it in the first place. Use preventive methods wherever possible.

3. If you think there is the slightest possibility you have an STD, get medical attention as soon as you can. In the meantime, try to figure out if the person you had sex with thinks s/he has been exposed to an STD. That can help to indicate how likely you are to get it.

4. Don't have sex until you have been tested or are sure you are cured (usually indicated by two negative follow-up tests).

5. If you do have an STD, inform all your recent partners personally or through a case finder.

6. Before accepting treatment, make sure you understand what you are taking and for how long, the side effects and any follow-up tests or treatment required. Don't be embarrassed about asking questions. It's your life, not theirs.

7. Remember, if you are cured you can get the same STD again. Also, having one STD doesn't protect you from getting any others.

To find out where you can get more information on symptoms, testing and treatment, see the Resources section at the end of this chapter; call the hotlines listed in Resources.

THE MOST COMMON STDS

Mucopurulent Cervicitis (MPC)/Nongonococcal Urethritis (NGU)*	Syphilis
	Pediculosis Pedis (Crabs)
	Scabies
Gonorrhea	Chancroid
Genital Herpes	Lymphgranuloma
Genital Warts	Venereum
Trichomoniasis	Granuloma Inguinale
Gardnerella Vaginalis (also called Hemophilus)	Hepatitis B

*Mucopurulent Cervicitis (MPC)/nongonococcal urethritis (NGU) refers to a range of diseases, including chlamydia, which affects men and women, and ureaplasma, which causes disease in men and may cause infertility in women. Technically, NGU is a disease of men only and MPC is the female equivalent, but in most medical literature, all these infections are lumped together under NGU.

264

HOW STDS ARE SPREAD

The organisms (bugs, germs) that cause these diseases (except for crabs and scabies) generally enter the body through the mucous membranes—the warm, moist surfaces of the vagina, urethra, anus and mouth. Thus you can catch an STD through intimate contact with someone who already has the infection, especially during oral, anal or genital sex. When your partner has more than one STD you can become infected with all you are exposed to; gonorrhea and chlamydia are often transmitted together. Some STDs can also be transmitted nonsexually. (See individual descriptions for more information.)

The stories about how you can get STDs from toilet seats, doorknobs or other objects are not true except under certain extremely rare conditions.* Nor can you catch STDs from heavy lifting, straining or being dirty. Animals don't transmit STDs to humans. Organisms which cause most STDs live best in a warm, moist environment like the linings of the genitals or throat. Outside the body they usually die in less than a minute.

HOW LIKELY AM I TO GET STD?

Statistically, if you are young (between fifteen and twenty-four), are sexually active with more than one partner and live in an urban setting you are at highest risk for STD. Your chances of getting an individual infection will also depend on your access to information and screening. Basically, however, if you are heterosexual and have sexual contact with a man who has an STD your chances of catching the infection are good. For example, after just one exposure to gonorrhea you have a 40 to 50 percent chance of catching the disease.

If you are lesbian, you are much less likely to get an STD because most STDs are not easily spread between women. It is possible to transmit herpes during oral genital sex or through skin contact between an open sore and broken skin. It is also theoretically possible, though almost unheard of, to transmit gonorrhea to the throat during oral sex, or syphilis through skin contact. For more information see "Lesbian Health Matters," listed in Resources under Booklets, Pamphlets and Reprints. If you have sex with both men and women, your chances of getting STD are the same as for heterosexuals.

*The inanimate object would need to have on it fresh, wet contaminated body fluid. See individual diseases for an explanation of when this could occur.

BIRTH CONTROL AND STDS

While the Pill does not seem to promote gonorrhea, one recent study suggests that women using the Pill may be more susceptible to chlamydial infections.[1]

The IUD, on the other hand, does help spread gonorrhea and chlamydia into the fallopian tubes, possibly by dislodging the protective mucus plug that covers the opening of the cervix and acting as a wick for bacteria. The IUD also irritates the uterus, sometimes causing small ulcerations which can make the uterus more vulnerable to STD infection.

Unlike barrier methods of contraception (condoms or diaphragms with spermicide), neither the Pill nor the IUD provides any protection against STD.

HOW BIG IS THE PROBLEM?

Statistics show that the incidence of nearly every STD is on the rise. Of the ones we will be discussing in detail in this chapter, only gonorrhea has remained relatively stable at an epidemic level, thanks to massive federal programs for screening and control. Syphilis, considered under control in the late seventies, is now increasing rapidly, especially among women, while the more newly recognized STDs, chlamydia and herpes, are growing so fast that they are called the "new epidemics." The incidence of genital warts is thought to have doubled in the past few years, particularly among women.

One of the reasons that some STDs are continuing to grow at such a rapid rate is that women often don't have symptoms or, if they do, the symptoms may suggest other diseases. For each of the STDs detailed in this chapter, there is on the average a 40 to 60 percent chance that you will have no discernible symptoms or will mistake them for something else.

WHY PREVENTION?

1. Most literature on STDs stresses treatment and cure, which is not at all an effective way of controlling and reducing these diseases in this country. Because so many women (and quite a few men) have no symptoms, we can unknowingly start a chain of infection which affects many people. We can stop this chain if each of us uses protection in addition to seeking a cure when we know we're infected.

2. By using prevention, we can protect ourselves from the serious STD complications such as pelvic inflammatory disease and infertility, and our children from diseases of the newborn.

3. It takes a lot out of our bodies to be sick. It is also stressful to take the large doses of antibiotics required to cure some of the STDs. (For this reason, the so-

The following methods are medically effective against STD in laboratory or clinical tests.*[2] No method is 100 percent effective, but using any of them should greatly reduce your chances of catching STD.† A recent study reports that women who use vaginal spermicides catch gonorrhea only one-eighth to one-fourth as much as those who use other contraceptive methods.[3]

1. Use vaginal spermicides (contraceptive foams, creams and jellies), especially those containing Nonoxynol 9.‡ You can purchase the following products in a drugstore without a prescription and use them with or without a diaphragm: Conceptrol, Delfen Cream, Emko Cream, Koromex II Jelly, Ortho Cream, Ortho Gynol Jelly, Preceptin Gel. For maximum protection, use them with a diaphragm. If you take the Pill or have an IUD, it is wise to use them, too. Before sex, put one of these inside the vagina for vaginal intercourse or in the anus for anal intercourse.

2. Use other products good for STD prevention but not birth control: Lorophyn Vaginal Suppositories, Progonasyl (by prescription only—see number 4 below).

3. Use barrier methods: condoms (rubbers) used during vaginal and anal intercourse are an effective barrier to STD organisms. The man must put on the condom before his penis touches your vulva or anus. A diaphragm (preferably with spermicide) can protect you against STD, which primarily affects the cervix (as with gonorrhea and chlamydia). Some researchers have found that women who use diaphragms have a lower incidence of chlamydial infection than those who use other forms of birth control.[6]

4. Progonasyl,[7] an iodine preparation which becomes a gel on contact with moisture, may block and destroy STD organisms when used in the vagina. Available by prescription only, it is not useful for birth control.

5. Washing genitals before and right after sex,[8] also urinating right after sex. These methods are of questionable use for women, but it is important for men to wash their testicles and penis, particularly after anal sex and before going on to vaginal or oral sex. Douching in most cases does not prevent STD, as it washes away normal vaginal secretions which help our bodies fight off infection.

6. Penigen, a foaming vaginal tablet containing antibiotics, has been used for years in Japan to prevent STD but is not approved for use in this country.

7. We do not recommend the "morning after" pill for gonorrhea and syphilis (different from the "morning after" pill for birth control). Taken just before or within nine hours after exposure to an infected person, the pill contains enough penicillin or one of the tetracyclines *to prevent* these diseases, but *not enough to cure* an established infection. This method has serious drawbacks. Each time we use an antibiotic, we increase our chances of becoming allergic to that particular family of antibiotic, and then we cannot use that antibiotic for another illness for which it may be the most effective treatment. Also, if you take antibiotics frequently or in less than the optimal dosage, you may encourage the development of resistant strains of gonorrhea, and you may also become a chronic or asymptomatic carrier of these diseases. *We do not recommend this method except possibly in cases of emergency such as rape.*

---

*Most traditional STD clinics emphasize treatment rather than prevention techniques. Show your practitioner this list and supporting footnotes. Pass the word along that prevention works.

†Edward Brecher has compiled a summary of methods tested plus an extensive bibliography on prophylaxis. See *Journal of Sex Research*[4] for more documentation than we list. Also see Cutler, et al., "Vaginal Contraceptives as Prophylaxis Against Gonorrhea and Other STDs"[5] and Cutler, "Venereal Disease Prevention," previously cited in Note 2.

‡The creams, foams and jellies listed here have been proven effective against organisms which cause gonorrhea, syphilis, trichomoniasis, candidiasis and chlamydia, and perhaps against the herpes virus. We do not know how effective they are against other STDs. These products have not been tested for use in anal sex, but they probably won't do you any harm. Be gentle when inserting anything into your anus. Some people may be allergic to one of the products. If you or your lover gets an itching or burning after using one, switch to another brand. If you can't find one of these brands, look for one that contains Nonoxynol 9.

called "morning after" shot of antibiotics to prevent STD should not be used except perhaps in emergencies like rape.)

4. Herpes has no known cure at this time, but using contraceptive creams, jellies, foams and condoms *may* stop its spread.

HOW TO PREVENT STD

We can protect ourselves from catching STD in a number of ways. Some involve common sense. Talk to your lover about STD before having sex. Ask if s/he has been exposed to an STD. This is especially important if you are pregnant! Look carefully at your body and your lover's, checking for bad smell, unusual discharge, sores, bumps, itching or redness. If you think you or your partner may have an infection, don't touch the sores or have sex.

It's one thing to talk about "being responsible about STD" and a much harder thing to do it at the moment. It's just plain hard to say to someone I am feeling very erotic with, "Oh, yes, before we go any further, can we have a conversation about STD?" It is hard to imagine murmuring into someone's ear at a time of passion, "Would you mind slipping on this condom or using this cream just in case one of us has an STD?" Yet it seems awkward to bring it up any sooner if it's not clear between us that we want to make love. So I use a birth control cream the first time and then bring up the subject afterward for us to consider together.

For some ideas on how to talk about sex more comfortably with a lover, see Chapter 11, "Sexuality."

TREATMENT: CONVENTIONAL VS. ALTERNATIVE AND "SELF-HELP"

In most cases, high doses of antibiotics cure STDs caused by bacteria by helping the body fight off bacteria or by actually killing them. Antibiotics are not effective against viral infections like herpes. Some people are allergic to penicillin or related drugs, while others suffer unwanted side effects from other antibiotics. Sometimes antibiotics just don't work. (For information on antibiotics, see p. 270.) Most herbalists do not recommend treating serious infections like gonorrhea, chlamydia or syphilis with natural remedies— at least without first trying antibiotics.

No matter what treatment you use, remember, *curing STD does not provide immunity against future infection.*

SOCIAL PROBLEMS

Medical Care and the Morality Issue

The social stigma attached to STD often affects the quality of medical care more than we would like to think.

1. Until recently, medical schools virtually ignored STDs. As a result, physicians who received training prior to the past few years may not know much about diagnosing and treating STDs, especially when there are no symptoms, or symptoms characteristic of other infections. Though physicians and medical care workers in clinics which regularly treat STD probably have the most up-to-date information, they are rarely informed about preventive methods (such as condoms or vaginal contraceptives).

2. Many medical care providers consider STD an appropriate punishment for "immoral sex." This is particularly true when they are dealing with women, since we are more readily labeled "promiscuous" than men. It is even more true for poor women and women of color than for white middle-class women. Too often, this attitude affects the quality of medical care provided.

3. Instead of blaming patients for the spread of STD, the medical profession must examine the reasons for their own poor record of adequate screening, diagnosis, treatment, reporting and follow-up of patients with STD. Some studies show that only a small percentage of doctors diagnose and treat STD patients according to the recommendations of the Centers for Disease Control (CDC).[9] Since untreated STDs can have such serious consequences, our crisis-oriented medical care system must change and make prevention a priority.

People at all levels of responsibility, too moralistic or too ashamed about sex, have blocked research into improved methods of prevention and curtailed the spread of information about available methods of prevention and cure.

With the advent of widespread birth control, which reduced the fear of pregnancy, fear of STD became the last deterrent to sex outside of marriage. Yet information and access to contraceptive devices which also help prevent STD may soon be harder to get, especially for teenagers.

Money and Politics

During 1981, only 40,600,000 dollars was federally appropriated in grants to the states for STD. In 1982, budget cuts reduced grants 23 percent to 31,600,000 dollars, drastically affecting research, clinical training, screening, control and educational programs. Many experts suggest that a bare minimum of 100 million dollars yearly is needed, though adequate prevention programs might reduce this amount. When you consider that it costs 500 million dollars a year, now paid out by individuals, to treat gonococcal PID (just *one* complication of *one* STD), it becomes clear just how inadequate the current level of funding is.

Clearly, we need to spend more money on better, easier and cheaper screening methods, and on finding out how existing products which are available and cheap (such as vaginal contraceptives) prevent the spread of STD. The federal budget allocates no money for research in this area. Instead, it has concentrated its money on the development of new antibiotics, antiviral drugs and STD vaccines (all very expensive, long-term projects).

Changes We Can Make Now

Although some medical professionals maintain that the only solution for our current STD epidemic is to develop a preventive vaccine, others believe that we can and should attempt to contain the diseases now.

It is possible to reverse the trend toward an increased incidence of gonorrhea. Several European countries and China have done so by educating the people about prevention, symptoms, testing and treatment. Sweden, by promoting the condom, has reduced the incidence of STDs without restricting sexual activity.

In order to use the tools we have now, we need to change the attitude that STD is a punishment for "immoral" sex. We must demand and initiate public education programs without moral overtones in our schools and communities. There are some nonjudgmental films, pamphlets and brochures (see Resources), though few deal with preventive measures women can use. We can distribute them in public places such as libraries, schools, movie houses, social centers and health facilities; we can talk with friends, parents and children to make sure they have as much accurate information as possible. We can support women's centers as they work for more complete sex and health education. When our society accepts sexuality it will be more likely to encourage STD prevention.

Practitioners must learn more about STDs. Self-testing kits have been developed and should be made available. More paramedics and lay health workers should be involved in running community screening programs to make tests, screening and treatment available to all economic and social groups. We can ask for routine screening tests for STD when we go for medical care; medical workers will be more apt to include tests automatically if a large number of clients request them.

SEXUALLY TRANSMITTED DISEASES: SYMPTOMS AND TREATMENT*

Gonorrhea

Gonorrhea is caused by the gonococcus, a bacterium shaped like a coffee bean, which works its way gradually along the warm, moist passageways of the genital and urinary organs and affects the cervix, urethra, anus and throat. You can transmit this disease to another person through genital, genital-oral and genital-

*For more information about tests, drugs and how STDs affect men than we can include in this chapter, see "A Book About Sexually Transmitted Diseases," listed in Resources under Booklets, Pamphlets and Reprints.

rectal sex. You can get a gonorrhea infection in your eye when you touch it with a hand that is moist with infected discharge. A mother can pass it to her baby during birth. Occasionally very young children can contract gonorrhea by using towels contaminated with fresh discharge. More frequently, children with gonorrhea are found to have been sexually abused. Evidence of gonorrhea has also been found in donor semen used for artificial insemination.[10]

The disease is more likely to persist and spread in women than in men. Untreated gonorrhea can lead to serious and painful infection of the pelvic area called pelvic inflammatory disease (PID). Seventeen percent of the women known to have gonorrhea develop PID; of these, 15 to 40 percent become sterile after just one episode.

A less common complication is proctitis, inflammation of the rectum. If the eyes become infected by gonococcal discharge (gonococcal conjunctivitis), blindness can result. Disseminated gonococcal infection, rare but serious, occurs when bacteria travel through the bloodstream, causing infection of the heart valves or arthritic meningitis. Gonorrhea can be treated at any stage to prevent further damage, but damage already done usually cannot be repaired.

Remember, it is important to use preventive measures, since a woman often does not have early symptoms. By the time pain prompts her to see a doctor, the infection has usually spread considerably. A woman who has had a hysterectomy can be infected in the cervix (if it is left), the anus, urethra or throat.

Symptoms

Although women often have gonorrhea without any symptoms, as many as 40 to 60 percent don't notice symptoms because of their mildness, or confuse them with other conditions. Symptoms usually appear anywhere from two days to three weeks after exposure. The cervix is the most common site of infection. In cervical gonorrhea, a discharge develops which is caused by an irritant released by the gonococci when they die. If you examine yourself with a speculum you may see a thick discharge, redness and small bumps or signs of erosion on the cervix. You may at first attribute symptoms to other routine gynecological problems or to the use of birth control methods like the Pill. The urethra may also become infected, possibly causing painful urination and burning. As the infection spreads, it can affect the Skene's (on each side of the urinary opening) and Bartholin's glands. Vaginal discharge and anal intercourse can infect the rectum. Symptoms include anal irritation, discharge and painful bowel movements. If the disease spreads to the uterus and fallopian tubes, you may have pain on one or both sides of your lower abdomen, vomiting, fever and/or irregular menstrual periods. The more severe the infection, the more severe the pain and other

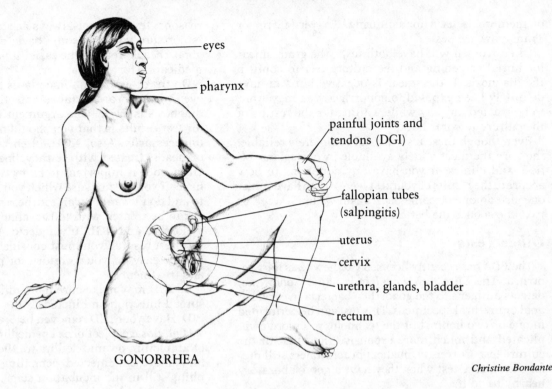

eyes

pharynx

painful joints and
tendons (DGI)

fallopian tubes
(salpingitis)

uterus

cervix

urethra, glands, bladder

rectum

GONORRHEA

Christine Bondante

symptoms are likely to be. These symptoms may indicate PID.

Gonorrhea can also be spread from a man's penis to a woman's throat (pharyngeal gonorrhea). You may have no symptoms, or your throat may be sore or your glands swollen.

One to 3 percent of women with gonorrhea develop disseminated gonococcal infection (DGI). Symptoms of DGI include a rash, chills, fever, pain in the joints and tendons of wrists and fingers. As the disease progresses, you may have sores on the hands, fingers, feet and toes.

Men's Symptoms

A man will usually have a thick milky discharge from his penis and feel pain or burning when he urinates. Some men have no symptoms. Gonorrhea in a man is often confused with nongonococcal urethritis (NGU), which also produces a discharge and requires a different drug for cure. If you have had sex with a man who has a discharge from his penis, get him to go for a test right away. His discharge can be tested and diagnosed the same day. If he does not have gonorrhea or NGU, then you will not have to take unnecessary medication.

Testing and Diagnosis

It is important to be tested before taking medication, because a test done while treatment is being given is not accurate.

Don't douche right before a test, because you can wash away the accessible bacteria, giving a false negative test result. The gram stain and the culture are two standard tests for gonorrhea in current use. A woman can have them done during a pelvic examination or a throat exam. The widely used gram stain is very accurate for symptomatic men but only 50 percent accurate for women and asymptomatic men. In this test a smear of the discharge is placed on a slide, stained with a dye and examined for gonorrhea bacteria under a microscope. If your regular male partner's test is positive, you may want to be treated at the same time regardless of the test results.

The culture test (more reliable, but it takes longer) involves taking a swab of the discharge, rolling it onto a special culture plate and incubating it under special laboratory conditions for sixteen to forty-eight hours to let the gonorrhea bacteria multiply. Even the culture test can be inaccurate, primarily because it is difficult to maintain specimens in good condition during transportation to the lab. Test accuracy also depends greatly on which sites are chosen for testing. If you have the most commonly affected sites (cervix and anal canal) cultured, there is about a 90 percent chance of finding any existing infection. (Many women with gonorrhea also have trichomoniasis and/or chlamydia.) The swab from the cervix is the best single test, about 88 to 93 percent accurate. About 50 percent of women with infected cervices also have infection in the anal canal. If you have had a hysterectomy, ask for a urethral culture, too. If you have had oral-genital sex, ask for a gonococcal throat culture. Ask what kind of medium is used for culturing. Thayer-Martin or Transgrow are best.

Often women will have both tests, the gram smear for initial screening and the culture test to confirm the diagnosis. If the smear is negative but you have definitely been exposed to gonorrhea, you may want to be treated anyway while waiting for the results of the culture to come back.

Even though these tests are not completely reliable, they are the most widely available in physicians' offices and clinics. If you have any doubts as to how accurate the results of your test were, try to have someone else do one or come back again within a week or two, the sooner the better.

Other Tests

The FDA has recently licensed two new tests for gonorrhea. The *Eliza technique* (trade name Gonozyme) detects antigens to the gonorrhea bacteria in cervical, anal or urethral specimens. This test can be performed in one or two hours, but the technology is more complicated and much more expensive than that of the culture test. Currently, medical practitioners still prefer the culture test when they have a good laboratory nearby to do it.

The second test, the *Gonosticon Dri-Dot test*, is cheap enough (about one dollar) for office use, but it is not yet widely available. The test involves examining a patient's blood for antibodies to gonorrhea. According to the Center for Disease Control, which does *not* recommend the test, there are two problems with this procedure: one is that a blood test cannot detect a recent infection because antibodies take time to build up in your system; another is that if antibodies from a previous infection are present, the test may give false results. Some doctors, however, recommend the test on the basis that it may be useful for diagnosing women who have abdominal PID or arthritis as a result of gonorrhea.

Another test, not yet approved, is the *Transformation test* (also called the C Test). It detects infection in a cervical specimen by isolating DNA from gonorrhea bacteria. Research is being done to see if this method could be adapted for use in a self-test kit, perhaps using a tampon to collect specimens. No field trials have been conducted to date. So far, it is cheaper and simpler but not quite as accurate as the culture test.

A *monoclonal antibody* test, also not yet approved, shows great promise for diagnosing gonorrhea in one to two hours. For this, a smear of the infected area is exposed to mouse antibodies and is examined under a fluorescent microscope for evidence of the bacteria."[11]

Treatment

Many physicians prescribe medication before the culture test is back or diagnosis is certain for three reasons: tests are not always accurate; the physician is not sure you will come back; and the sooner the gonorrhea is treated, the easier it is to cure. Ask about medication for your partner.

On the other hand, some places refuse to treat you, even when you are certain of infection, until a positive diagnosis is made. One argument in favor of waiting for test results is that you should not take antibiotics unnecessarily. Also, NGU, often confused with gonorrhea, is treated with tetracycline rather than penicillin, so it is important to know which infection you have. If you are not sure which you have been exposed to and don't want to wait for the results of the culture, ask to be treated with tetracycline, effective for both gonorrhea and NGU. If you decide to wait for the culture test results, you must consider whether or not it will be easy for you to return for possible later tests and treatment.

An IUD may make cure more difficult since it helps spread infection and increases the chances of getting PID. Have your IUD removed before treatment.

High-dosage injections of penicillin or high oral doses of ampicillin or amoxicillin are the usual treatments for gonorrhea. Injected penicillin can also cure syphilis still in the incubation stage. You may also receive oral probenecid, a drug which slows down the urinary excretion of antibiotics and allows them to remain in the bloodstream in high enough concentrations to do the job.

Some doctors recommend tetracycline as a treatment of choice because it avoids the risk of serious side effects of allergy to penicillin. Its disadvantage is that you must take it regularly for two weeks or so for it to be effective. Tetracycline also has a high failure rate in cases of anal and rectal gonorrhea. For more information on these drugs and possible undesirable effects (such as yeast infections), see "Drugs Women Should Know About" and "A Book About Sexually Transmitted Diseases," listed in Resources.*

Over the past twenty-five years, gonorrhea has required increasing doses of penicillin to cure, and new strains of gonorrhea have emerged which are resistant to the drug. In 1972, 22 percent of the strains of gonorrhea were resistant to penicillin. That number has now dropped to 4 percent. One strain, penicillinase-producing N. gonorrhea (PPNG), remains highly difficult to treat. Soldiers stationed in the Far East brought it back with them to the U.S.† In this case, the gonococcal organism produces an enzyme (penicillinase) that destroys penicillin, making the drug

---

*Those of African and Mediterranean ancestry should check for sensitivity to sulfa drugs and probenecid. Pregnant women should not take tetracycline.

†Outbreaks of STD have always been clearly related to war zones, where normal life is disrupted, where women are raped or forced to earn a living through prostitution and where medicine is available only through a black market.

useless for treatment. Tetracycline is also ineffective. If a culture indicates PPNG, other medications such as spectinomycin, cefoxitin and cephalosporin will be prescribed.

Test for Cure

Every woman treated for gonorrhea should have *two* negative culture tests, including a rectal culture, a week or two apart before considering herself cured. If cultures remain positive, get retreatment with another antibiotic such as spectinomycin and a culture for PPNG. Pockets of infection in reproductive organs may be difficult to cure. If your partner has gonorrhea, you can become reinfected very soon after a cure, so it's crucial that he be tested and treated as well.

Gonorrhea and Pregnancy

Pregnant women should receive at least one routine gonorrhea culture during pregnancy. A pregnant woman with untreated gonorrhea can infect her baby as it passes through her birth canal. In the past, many babies went blind due to gonococcal conjunctivitis. All states now require the eyes of newborns to be treated with silver nitrate or other antibiotic drops in order to prevent this disease, even when the mother is sure she does not have gonorrhea and knows the treatment is unnecessary.

Chlamydia

Until recently, the bacterium *Chlamydia trachomatis* was thought to affect only men, causing half of the cases of male nongonococcal urethritis (NGU), while women were silent "carriers." Now we know that chlamydia can cause very serious problems for women, including urethral infection, cervicitis (inflammation of the cervix), PID and infertility as well as dangerous complications during pregnancy and birth. (See below.) It has been linked to some cases of Reiter's syndrome (an arthritic condition) and cervical dysplasia (precancerous changes in cervical cells). If you practice anal sex, this organism can cause proctitis (inflammation of the rectum).

Chlamydia is transmitted during vaginal or anal sex with someone who has the infection. It can also be passed by a hand moistened with infected secretions to the eye, and from mother to baby during delivery.

Ureaplasma

If your partner has NGU, you can also become infected by *Ureaplasma urealyticum* (also called *T-Mycoplasma*), transmitted separately from or together with chlamydia. It has been found in the genital tracts of many apparently healthy people who have no symp-

toms of infection. While ureaplasma causes up to one-quarter of the cases of NGU in men,* it is not generally thought to cause cervicitis or PID in women.† However, some researchers believe it can cause other genital tract infections and pregnancy complications (see below).‡[12]

Symptoms

Women often don't know they have these infections. The cervix may or may not appear inflamed upon examination. If you have no symptoms, you must rely on your partner to tell you if he has symptoms or has been diagnosed for NGU. Women who do have symptoms may experience dysuria (painful urination), cystitis, a thin vaginal discharge and/or lower abdominal pain ten to twenty days after exposure.

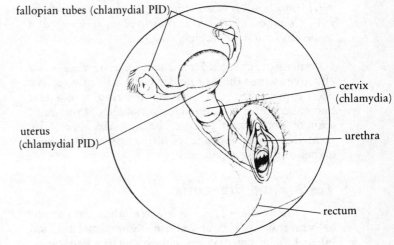

fallopian tubes (chlamydial PID)

cervix (chlamydia)

urethra

uterus (chlamydial PID)

rectum

CHLAMYDIA AND UREAPLASMA

Chlamydia can also be transmitted to the eyes via the hands.

Christine Bondante

Men's Symptoms

Men will usually have a burning sensation upon urination and a urethral discharge that appears one to three weeks after exposure. Symptoms may be similar to those of gonorrhea, but are usually milder. The incubation period is also generally longer—at least seven days. About ten percent of men have no symptoms, even though they can still transmit the disease. Fre-

*Fifty percent of cases of NGU are caused by chlamydia, 25 percent by ureaplasma and 25 percent by as yet unidentified organisms.

†Some researchers dispute this assumption.

‡A less common but related organism, *Mycolasma hominis*, may cause infections leading to PID and, according to some researchers, infertility and/or premature birth.

quently only one member of a couple will have symptoms, while the other carries the infection. Both partners must be treated to prevent passing the disease back and forth.

Many practitioners are not yet aware of the dangers of chlamydia. In addition, because chlamydial infection is so easy to confuse with gonorrhea and other diseases, they often misdiagnose it. They also overlook women's symptoms or attribute them to other causes.

It started out as cystitis. A few months later I started having fever, chills and a lot of pain in my lower abdomen. The doctor never said anything about the possibility of chlamydia or PID. Instead they did tests for gonorrhea, which were negative. After six months of being really sick, they gave me ampicillin, which didn't help. They kept saying, "There's nothing wrong with you. You must be having emotional problems." After nine months I had a good case of PID, which they called "a little pelvic infection." It wasn't until my husband came down with symptoms of NGU that they took me seriously and treated us both with the right drugs.

Remember, the usual treatment for gonorrhea is *not* effective against these organisms. If you think you have been exposed to NGU, wait for the results of a test before accepting treatment for gonorrhea. If you can't wait or don't want to come back, make sure to be treated with tetracycline, effective against both gonorrhea and these organisms.

Testing and Diagnosis

At present there is no *widely* available test specifically for chlamydia or ureaplasma. Sometimes a skilled lab technician can diagnose chlamydia by a Pap smear. In most cases, if you or your partner has a discharge, you will be tested for gonorrhea, and if that is negative, the practitioner will diagnose NGU/MPC by elimination. Incubation of the disease is also a clue. NGU takes longer to show up than gonorrhea, although the time period can vary, depending on whether chlamydia, mycoplasma, a combination of the two, or other bacteria are causing the infection. Some experts think that when a man suspects he may have NGU, he should have his seminal fluid (obtained by masturbation) checked.[13] The CDC, however, maintains that a urethral smear is the only accurate test. Tests for chlamydia and ureaplasma involve taking a swab from the cervix and culturing the specimen, and are performed only at large medical centers and some public health laboratories. For information on where to get tested, call your public health department. Unfortunately, these cultures are expensive (thirty-five to forty dollars). For these reasons, many physicians are reluctant to recommend them. Some prefer to wait until a woman's partner develops symptoms of NGU. This trend may be slowly changing, particularly when women

are pregnant. The blood tests presently available for chlamydia are currently considered too impractical for widespread use.

New Tests

The FDA recently approved a *monoclonal antibody* test for chlamydia that the manufacturer reports is 92 to 98 percent effective and gives results in less than an hour. The test uses a cervical smear. It should become widely available in 1984 and be much less expensive than the culture test. If the test performs as expected it is likely to replace the culture test in a few years (see p. 274).

Treatment

Tetracycline is the standard treatment for chlamydia and ureaplasma infections. Doxycycline and minocycline, also prescribed, are much more expensive and can cause serious negative side effects. Erythromycin is often prescribed when tetracycline cannot be given. Sulfa drugs such as sulfamethoxazole-trimethoprim (Septram, Bactrim) are effective against chlamydia but not ureaplasma. Many of the other antibiotics commonly used for STD infections, including penicillin, are not effective. People with chlamydial eye infections are treated with local antibacterial agents such as chlortetracycline.

Take all the medication prescribed, or the infection may come back at a later date, cause more trouble and be harder to get rid of. Usually it clears up within three weeks. If not, go back to the practitioner, who will prescribe a different antibiotic or a longer treatment time. Regular sexual partners should take tetracycline whether or not they have symptoms. Because 10 percent of ureaplasma is resistant to tetracycline, some practitioners recommend a follow-up culture one to four weeks after treatment.

Before taking any antibiotics, check with your doctor about possible undesirable effects.* Pregnant women should not take tetracycline. Avoid alcohol until the infection is cured, as it may irritate the urethra. Use condoms until you and your partner are cured. If you seem to keep having recurrent episodes of chlamydia or MPC and antibiotics have not cleared up the infection, you may have another bacterial infection or possibly a stubborn case of PID.

Chlamydia, Ureaplasma and Pregnancy

Recent studies indicate that 8 to 10 percent of all pregnant women may be infected with chlamydia[14] which, if untreated, can then be transmitted to the baby during birth. Infected babies may develop conjunctiv-

*See note, p. 270, regarding sensitivity to some of these drugs.

itis or pneumonia. Chlamydia has also been linked to miscarriage, ectopic pregnancy, premature delivery and postpartum infections. Because of these risks, testing for chlamydia may soon be recommended for all pregnant women.

Because ureaplasma has also been strongly implicated as a cause of infertility, miscarriage and premature birth, some researchers feel that any woman with a history of infertility or ectopic pregnancies should be tested for ureaplasma as well.[15]

Herpes

Herpes (from the Greek word "to creep") is caused by the herpes simplex virus, a tiny primitive organism whose nature is still more or less a mystery. The virus enters the body through the skin and mucous membranes of the mouth and genitals, and travels along the nerve endings to the base of the spine, where it sets up permanent residence, feeding off nutrients produced by the body cells. There are two types of herpes simplex (HSV) viruses. Type I (HSV I) usually is characterized by cold sores or fever blisters on the lips, face and mouth, while Type II (HSV II) most often involves sores in the genital area. While HSV I is usually found above the waist and HSV II below, there is some crossover, primarily due to the increase in oral-genital sex. In this chapter we will be concerned with genital herpes.

You can get herpes during vaginal, anal or oral sex with someone who has an active infection. You can spread it from mouth to genitals (or eyes) via the fin-

gers. It can also be spread through linens and towels, although this happens rarely. Although the disease is normally contagious only from the time the skin reddens until the sores crust over, herpes can possibly be transmitted when no symptoms are present, but the chances of this happening are minuscule.

Symptoms

Symptoms usually occur two to twenty days after a primary exposure, although some people may not have symptoms or may not be aware of them until much later. An outbreak of herpes usually begins with a tingling or itching sensation of the skin in the genital area. This is called the "prodromal" period and may occur several hours to several days before the sores erupt, or it may not occur at all. You may also experience burning sensations, pains in your legs, buttocks or genitals and/or a feeling of pressure in the area. Sores then appear, starting as one or more red bumps and changing to watery blisters within a day or two. Blisters are most likely to occur on the labia majora and minora, clitoris, vaginal opening, perineum and occasionally on the vaginal wall, buttocks, thighs, anus and navel. Women can also have sores on their cervix, which usually cause no discernable symptoms. Ninety percent of women have sores on both vagina and cervix during a first infection. Within a few days, the blisters rupture, leaving shallow ulcers which may ooze, weep or bleed. Usually after three or four days a scab forms and the sores heal themselves without treatment.

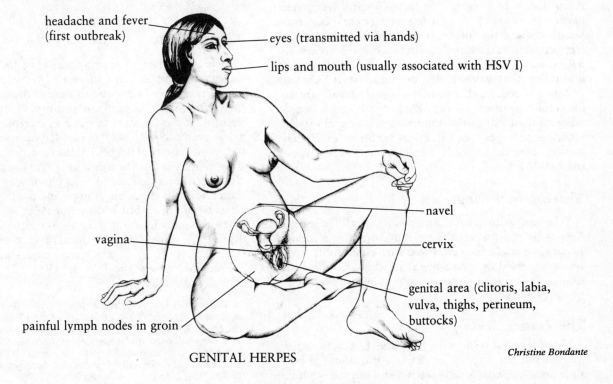

headache and fever (first outbreak)

eyes (transmitted via hands)

lips and mouth (usually associated with HSV I)

navel

vagina

cervix

genital area (clitoris, labia, vulva, thighs, perineum, buttocks)

painful lymph nodes in groin

GENITAL HERPES

Christine Bondante

273

While the sores are active, you may find it painful to urinate, and you may have a dull ache or a sharp burning pain in your entire genital area. Sometimes the pain radiates into the legs. You may also have an urge to urinate frequently and/or a vaginal discharge. You may also have vulvitis (a painful inflammation of the vulva). During the first outbreak, you may also experience fever, headache and swelling of the lymph nodes in the groin. The initial outbreak is usually the most painful and takes the longest time to heal (two to six weeks).

Men's Symptoms

Men may experience pain in the testicles during the prodromal period, followed by sores which usually appear on the head and shaft of the penis but can also appear on the scrotum, perineum, buttocks, anus and thighs. Men can also have sores without knowing it, usually because they are hidden inside the urethra. There may also be a watery discharge from the urethra.

Recurrences

Some people never experience a second outbreak of herpes, but most people (75 percent) do, usually within three to twelve months of the initial episode and usually in the same area of the body. Recurrent episodes are usually milder, last from three days to two weeks and usually do not involve the cervix. They often seem to be triggered by stress, illness, menstruation or pregnancy. Most people find that the number of yearly recurrences decreases with time. Because recurrent herpes is associated with lowered resistance, some people believe the infection can lead to secondary infections such as trichomoniasis, bladder infections, venereal warts, yeast infections and vaginitis. Poor diet and drugs that weaken the immune system (such as caffeine, speed, birth control pills and diet pills) may also make you more susceptible to recurrences. People who are deficient in B-vitamins or who are unusually tense seem to get more frequent recurrences. Recent studies show that HSV II is much more likely to recur than HSV I.[16]

Testing and Diagnosis

You and your practitioner can usually diagnose herpes by sight when the sores are present, although herpes is occasionally confused with chancroid, syphilis or venereal warts. Several lab tests confirm the diagnosis or indicate the presence of herpes even when no sores are active.

The Tzanck Test

This test is similar to a Pap smear. A scraping is taken from the edge of an active sore, smeared on a slide sprayed with a cell fixative and sent to a lab for evaluation. A fairly accurate method of diagnosis, it can be used for both men and women, and is inexpensive (three to fifteen dollars). It cannot differentiate between HSV I and HSV II.

Viral Culture

A viral tissue culture can be taken using living cells to grow the virus. This test has an advantage in that it can distinguish between Herpes I and Herpes II, but it is expensive (about forty-five dollars) and few laboratories or doctors are equipped to perform it. The test is more accurate than the smear and should be done when the sores *first* appear.

Other Tests

You can get a blood test to measure the level of herpes antibodies in the blood. (Once you have been exposed to the virus, your body manufactures antibodies to fight off the infection.) For this test, two ampules of blood are drawn, one during the initial attack and the second two to four weeks later. If you have herpes, the second sample will show a much higher antibody level. (It takes about two weeks to build antibodies.) This test is only effective when performed during the initial attack of herpes. Later, the test results are difficult to interpret. This test costs thirty-five to fifty dollars and may not be covered by all federal or state medical assistance programs. Some public health departments in metropolitan areas, however, provide the test free of charge.

A *monoclonal antibody* test is being investigated now to determine how accurate it is. It still cannot detect latent cases (see p. 272).

Treatment

At present there is no medical cure for herpes, although researchers are investigating vaccines, antiviral therapy and immune-system stimulants.* In the meantime, keep sores clean and dry. If they are very painful, you may want to get a prescription for xylocaine cream or ethyl chloride. If you are having an outbreak of genital herpes for the first time, your practitioner may prescribe a new antiviral drug called acyclovir (trade name Zovirax). Acyclovir seems to reduce pain and viral shedding (the period during which the virus is infective) but it does not delay or prevent recurrences and it won't help if you already have the disease. Acyclovir in oral form *may* prevent recurrences, according to one study, and should be approved for use by the FDA in 1984.[17] It is still not considered a cure, however.

*In the past few years more than thirty experimental treatments for herpes have been tested and found ineffective in clinical trials. For a list of these experimental treatments, some of which are still used, and other information, send for "Questions and Answers on Genital Herpes," Technical Information Services, Division of Sexually Transmitted Diseases, CDC, Atlanta, GA 30333. It is free.

Another promising experimental treatment involves the use of laser beams which, when applied to sores within forty-eight hours of a first outbreak, may help prevent recurrences. This method also seems ineffective for women who already have recurrent herpes.[18]

Self-Help and Alternative Treatment

When sores first appear, take warm sitz baths with baking soda three to five times a day. In between, keep sores clean and dry. A hair dryer helps to dry sores. Sores heal faster when exposed to air, so wear cotton underpants or none at all. If it hurts to urinate, do it in the shower or bathtub or spray water over genitals while urinating (using any plastic squeeze bottle). When sores break, apply drying agents such as hydrogen peroxide or Dom Burrows, which is available in drugstores. For pain relief, take acetaminophen (e.g., Tylenol) or aspirin.

Many women have found the following alternative treatments very helpful for herpes.* They may or may not work for you. Because some of the products mentioned below must be purchased at a health food store, they may be expensive. We suggest that you pick one or two. Remember, all are most effective when combined with good nutrition and rest. (If you are pregnant, don't take medicinal teas or high doses of Vitamin C without consulting your practitioner.)

1. Echinacea is a blood-purifying plant. Capsules made from it are available at health food stores. Take two capsules every three hours, make a tincture and apply (one teaspoon every two hours for three to four days) or make a soothing tea (four cups a day).

2. Take 2,000 milligrams of Vitamin C or two capsules of kelp followed by sarsaparilla tea (four to five cups during the day).

3. Chlorophyll (in powder form) and wheatgrass are good antiviral herbs. Drink them with warm water. Also, eating blue-green algae (3,000 milligrams daily) may be helpful.

4. Lysine is an amino acid that many women find very effective in suppressing early symptoms. If you stop using it, symptoms may reappear. Take 750 to 1,000 milligrams a day until sores have disappeared. Thereafter take 500 milligrams a day. Lysine seems to work by counteracting the effects of argenine (a substance found in foods such as nuts—especially peanuts—chocolate and cola) which stimulates herpes. During any herpes episode it is wise to avoid argenine-rich foods.

5. Zinc: take five to sixty milligrams daily.

6. Grape skins may be antiviral. Some women recommend eating red grapes.

*Information adapted from "Herpes," Santa Cruz Women's Health Center; "Her Pease," Women's Health Services, Santa Fe, NM; and "Herpes, Something Can Be Done About It," by N. Sampsidis. To order copies of these booklets, see Resources.

7. Acupuncture treatments administered at the first signs of an attack sometimes prevent recurrences. Fingertip stimulation of acupressure points in the feet may also prevent outbreaks (three thumbs forward of the ankle bulge, along the line between the ankle bulge and little toe).

For Symptomatic Relief

1. Make compresses out of tea made with cloves, use black tea bags soaked in water (tannic acid is an anesthetic) or take sitz baths with uva-ursi (also known as kinnikinnick or bearberry).

2. Apply peppermint or clove oil, Vitamin E oil, A and D Ointment, baking soda, cornstarch or witch hazel to the sores. (Some people believe that keeping the sores moist may make them feel better but last longer.) Before applying any salve, some people suggest you rub the area with mouthwash containing thymol.

3. Make poultices using pulverized calcium tablets, powdered slippery elm, goldenseal, myrrh, comfrey root or cold milk. Make a paste using any of these and apply to the sores. After applying, keep the paste moistened with warm water.

4. Aloe vera gel soothes and helps to dry out sores and promote healing.

Herpes and Pregnancy

Studies show that women with herpes have an increased risk of miscarriage and premature delivery. Equally important, when a mother has active sores at the time of delivery, herpes can be transmitted to the baby during passage through the birth canal, causing brain damage, blindness and death in 60 to 70 percent of cases. Scary as this sounds, it is important to know that this is rare, occurring only in one out of every 7,000 normal births. The risk is much higher when mothers have a primary outbreak at the time of delivery; when they have open sores, their babies have a 50 percent chance of contracting herpes during a vaginal birth. For a mother with recurrent sores, the risk goes down to about 4 percent because she has passed antibodies on to the baby through the amniotic fluid and the baby's blood.[19]

Pregnant women who don't have herpes should avoid unprotected sex during the last six weeks with partners who have herpes. If you are pregnant and have recurrent herpes, get a Pap smear or viral culture done regularly from thirty-two weeks of pregnancy to delivery. If you have prodromal symptoms or active sores at the time of delivery, you will usually have a Cesarean section within four to six hours of the time the waters break. Some studies suggest that women who have negative cultures within three days of birth can and should deliver vaginally. After birth, take care not to infect the infant. After about three weeks, babies usually do not develop serious infections.

Cytomegalovirus (CMV), another virus related to herpes which may be an STD, seldom causes symptoms in the mother but is also thought to be a major cause of birth defects.

Herpes and Cancer

Studies show that women with genital herpes have a five times' greater risk than others of getting cervical cancer. This does not mean that just because you have herpes you will get cancer, but it is advisable to get a Pap smear every six months. It is possible that the factors that make us susceptible to herpes are similar to those which make us susceptible to cancer.

Prevention

A herpes vaccine is being tested on people now, but it will be at least 1986 and probably later before we know how effective it will be. Only then will the FDA approve it for general use. Because there is no cure for herpes, it seems especially worthwhile to protect yourself from getting it. That does *not* mean that you should never have sex with someone who has the virus in a latent stage; it simply means using your common sense in evaluating the risk and taking simple precautions when possible. The following suggestions (along with the general methods outlined on p. 266) may also reduce your chances of getting herpes.

1. You will be less susceptible to herpes when you are in good health, eating well and have ways of dealing with stress in your life (such as yoga, deep breathing, meditation—whatever works for you).

2. Avoid sex with someone who has active sores. If you decide to go ahead anyway and your partner is male, use condoms and/or a diaphragm with spermicide containing Nonoxynol 9, which may possibly be effective against the herpes virus.

3. Because herpes can be spread by skin contact from one part of the body to another, try to avoid touching an open sore. Wash your hands after examining yourself or touching the genital area. Always wash your hands before inserting contact lenses.

Protecting Others (If You Have Herpes)

1. If you have active sores, you might try to keep towels separate and wear cotton underpants in bed at night, since herpes may be transmitted through shared towels or linen.

2. Do not donate blood during an initial outbreak.

3. Some people recommend avoiding swimming pools, hot tubs and saunas during an initial outbreak.

Preventing Recurrences

1. Herpes attacks seem to be triggered by stress. If possible, figure out what precipitated your attacks and try to eliminate or reduce tension in your life.

2. Limit the use of stimulants such as coffee, tea, colas and chocolate.

3. Increase your intake of Vitamins A, B, C and pantothenic acid as well as zinc, iron and calcium to help prevent recurrences.[20]

4. Avoid foods which have a lot of argenine (such as nuts, chocolate, cola, rice and cottonseed meal).[21] Instead, eat foods high in lysine: potatoes, meats, milk, brewers' yeast, fish, liver and eggs.

Living with Herpes

Accepting herpes as a permanent part of your life may be difficult. You may feel shocked when you discover you have herpes, and then frantically search for a cure. You may feel isolated, lonely and angry, especially toward the person who gave you the infection. You may become anxious about staying in long-term relationships, having children or getting cervical cancer. Not everybody experiences herpes in these ways, nor do these responses necessarily last forever.

After the first big episode of herpes, I felt distant from my body. When we began lovemaking again, I had a hard time having orgasms or trusting the rhythm of my responses. I shed some tears over that. I felt my body had been invaded. My body feels riddled with it; I'm somehow contaminated. And there is always that lingering anxiety: is my baby okay? It's unjust that the birth of my child may be affected.

If you are in a close relationship with someone who doesn't have herpes, it can affect you both in subtle ways.

Sometimes it bullies both of us. When my lover feels she has to protect me from stress because I'm about to get herpes, she doesn't always ask for attention, time or comfort when she needs them.

How much herpes affects your relationships can depend a lot on how much you trust each other and how comfortable you feel about sharing your concerns.

My lover really trusts me when I say the episode has passed and it's okay to have oral sex. She doesn't second-guess me and say, "Let's wait a few days so I won't get it." What a blessing.

The way we experience herpes may have a lot to do with our attitude about disease. For example, people who see herpes as a symptom of stress, illness or other problems rather than as a medical disaster seem to have a much easier time finding their own ways of coping with it.

Herpes is an inconvenience and a pain, but it's something you learn to live with. I think of it as an imbalance.

Since I know it's related to stress, I keep myself in as good physical condition as possible and try not to get too upset about it.

The one good thing I can say about herpes is that it keeps me honest in taking care of myself. When I feel my vulva start to tingle and ache, it's immediately a reminder to me to slow down. I take long, hot baths. I try to think relaxing, releasing thoughts and send healing, calming energy to that area. Sometimes I meditate.

Humor is the best way of coping with herpes. There is so much serious, scary stuff about it. You've got to recognize that it's just one of the bad tricks people have to live with.

Herpes may be easier to cope with if you feel comfortable enough to talk about it openly. Some people manage to talk themselves out of recurrences.

What turns out to be really useful is when my family and I talk about the viruses. We say things like, "They don't want to come down now. It's much cozier up by the spinal cord where they are. The weather is pretty bad out here and everyone's too busy to pay them much attention." I think what it probably does is calm me and ease whatever is bothering me. Who knows? Maybe they hear! All I know is that sometimes after I get the warning aches we sit at dinner having those discussions about how my little herpes viruses should stay where they are, and they don't come!

The Herpes Resource Center (HRC), an organization with local chapters throughout the country, provides support, information and self-help groups for people with herpes. It also publishes an informative newsletter called *HELPER*. You can join by sending five dollars and a stamped, self-addressed envelope to HRC (see Resources).

Syphilis

Syphilis is caused by a small spiral-shaped bacterium called a spirochete. You can get syphilis through sexual or skin contact with someone who is in an infectious (primary or secondary and possibly the beginning of the latent) stage. A pregnant woman with syphilis can also pass the disease to her unborn child.

Syphilis spreads via open sores or rashes containing bacteria which can penetrate the mucous membranes of the genitals, mouth and anus as well as broken skin on other parts of the body.

Symptoms

Once the bacteria have entered the body, the disease goes through four stages.

Primary

The first sign is usually a painless sore called a chancre (pronounced "shanker") which may look like a pimple, a blister or an open sore, and shows up from nine to ninety days after the bacteria enter the body. The

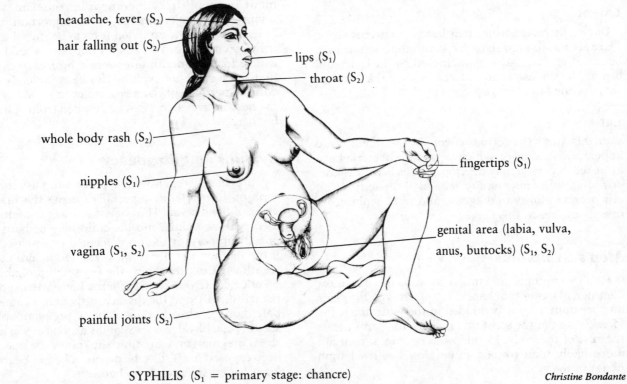

headache, fever (S_2)

hair falling out (S_2)

lips (S_1)

throat (S_2)

whole body rash (S_2)

fingertips (S_1)

nipples (S_1)

genital area (labia, vulva, anus, buttocks) (S_1, S_2)

vagina (S_1, S_2)

painful joints (S_2)

SYPHILIS (S_1 = primary stage: chancre)
(S_2 = secondary stage: red, sore area; rash)

Christine Bondante

sore usually appears on the genitals at or near the place where the bacteria entered the body. However, it may appear on the fingertips, lips, breast, anus or mouth. Sometimes the chancre never develops or is hidden inside the vagina or folds of the labia, giving no evidence of the disease. Only about 10 percent of women who get these chancres notice them. If you examine yourself regularly with a speculum, you are more likely to see one if it develops. At the primary stage, the chancre is very infectious. The preventive methods outlined on p. 266 work only if the chemical or physical barrier covers the infectious sore. With or without treatment, the sore will disappear, usually in one to five weeks, but the bacteria, still in the body, increase and spread.

Secondary

The next stage occurs anywhere from a week to six months later. By this time the bacteria have spread all through the body. This stage usually lasts weeks or months, but symptoms can come and go for several years. They may include a rash (over the entire body or just on the palms of the hands and soles of the feet); a sore in the mouth; swollen, painful joints or aching bones; a sore throat; a mild fever or headache (all flu symptoms). You may lose some hair or discover a raised area around the genitals and anus. During the secondary stage the disease can be spread by simple physical contact, including kissing, because bacteria are present in the open syphilitic sores which may appear on any part of the body.

Latent

During this stage, which may last ten to twenty years, there are no outward signs. However, the bacteria may be invading the inner organs, including the heart and brain. The disease is not infectious after the first few years of the latent stage.

Late

In this stage the serious effects of the latent stage appear. Depending on which organs the bacteria have attacked, a person may develop serious heart disease, crippling, blindness and/or mental incapacity. With our present ability to diagnose and treat syphilis, no one should reach this stage.

Men's Symptoms

Men's symptoms are similar to women's. The most common place for the chancre to appear is on the penis and scrotum. It may be hidden in the folds under the foreskin, under the scrotum or where the penis meets the rest of the body. In the primary stages, men are more likely than women to develop swollen lymph nodes in the groin.

Diagnosis and Treatment

Syphilis can be diagnosed and treated at any time. However, because syphilis is less common now than in the past, medical care workers may confuse early symptoms with several other STDs, including chancroid, herpes and LGV (lymphogranuloma venereum).

Early in the primary stages a practitioner can look for subtle symptoms like swollen lymph glands around the groin, and examine some of the discharge from the chancre, if one has developed, under a microscope (a dark-field test). Do not put any kind of medication, cream or ointment on the sore until a doctor examines it. (The syphilis bacteria on the surface are likely to be killed, making the test less accurate.) Spirochetes will be in the bloodstream a week or two after the chancre has formed. They will then show up in a blood test, which from then on, through all the stages, will reveal the infection. If you suspect that you have been exposed to syphilis and have been recently treated for gonorrhea with medication other than penicillin, you should have four tests one month apart to cover the possible incubation period. (Some drugs used to treat gonorrhea do not cure syphilis.) Remember, incubation can be as long as ninety days. A good description of the different blood tests used can be found in "A Book About Sexually Transmitted Diseases" (see Resources). If you are sexually active with more than one partner or if your sexual partner is, request a syphilis blood test during regular health checkups.

Penicillin by injection or a substitute such as tetracycline pills for those allergic to penicillin is the treatment for syphilis. Since people sometimes have relapses or mistakes are made, it is important to have at least two follow-up blood tests to be sure the treatment is complete. You should not have sexual intercourse for one month after receiving treatment. The first three stages of syphilis can be completely cured with no permanent damage, and even in late syphilis the destructive effects can be stopped from going any further.

Syphilis and Pregnancy

A pregnant woman with syphilis can pass the bacteria on to her fetus, especially during the first few years of the disease. The bacteria attack the fetus just as they do an adult, and the child may be born dead or with important tissues deformed or diseased. But if the mother gets her syphilis treated before the sixteenth week of pregnancy, the fetus will probably not be affected. (Even after the fetus has gotten syphilis, penicillin will stop the disease, although it cannot repair damage already done.) Every pregnant woman should get a blood test for syphilis as soon as she knows she is pregnant and any time she thinks she may have been exposed. If she has the disease, she can be treated for it before she gives it to her fetus.

Genital Warts and Human Papillomavirus Infections*

Genital warts are caused by the human papillomavirus, or HPV, similar to the type which causes common skin warts. The same virus causes invisible warts or flat lesions on the cervix. HPV usually spreads during sexual intercourse with an infected partner. While HPV-caused infections have not been associated with serious complications in the past, studies now show that women with HPV-caused lesions on the cervix probably have a higher-than-normal risk for developing cervical cancer. Unfortunately, these invisible cervical lesions are not easily detected by either the health care practitioner or the woman with the infection.

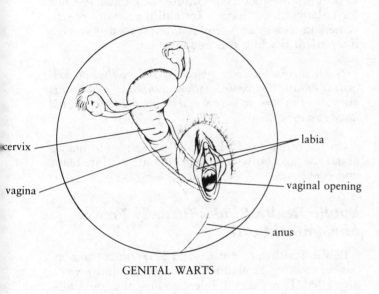

GENITAL WARTS

Christine Bondante

Symptoms of genital warts usually appear from three weeks to three months after exposure. During the pre-symptomatic period (as well as while they are present), warts can be very contagious, so it is advisable for your male partners to use condoms if any of you have been exposed to the virus. The visible genital warts look like regular warts, starting as small, painless, hard spots which usually appear on the bottom of the vaginal opening. Warts also occur on the vaginal lips, inside the vagina, on the cervix or around the anus, where they can be mistaken for hemorrhoids. Warmth and moisture encourage the growth of warts, which often develop a cauliflowerlike appearance as they grow larger. Cervical lesions, though more prevalent than the visible warts, cannot be seen by the naked eye and have no symptoms.

*See "Who Is at Risk of CIN or Cervical Cancer," p. 487.

Men's symptoms

Warts usually occur toward the tip of the penis, sometimes under the foreskin and occasionally on the shaft of the penis or scrotum. Using a condom can help prevent the spread of warts.

Diagnosis and Treatment

Diagnosis of warts is usually made by direct eye exam. An abnormal Pap smear may indicate the presence of cervical lesions, but a colposcopy is usually necessary to confirm this. Occasionally you will need a biopsy to check for unusual cell growth, especially if there are ulcerations (open sores) or a discharge, but these are rare. If you have cervical warts or lesions, get a Pap smear every six months for early detection of unusual cell changes.

There are several treatments for warts:

1. Practitioners most often prescribe podophyllin solution (some say ointment is better). Apply it to the warts and wash it off two to four hours later to avoid chemical burns. Protect the surrounding skin with petroleum jelly (eg., Vaseline). Sometimes several treatments are necessary, and they are not always successful.

2. Trichloracetic acid (TCA) is currently used by only a small percentage of practitioners but appears to be better than podophyllin in several respects. It is usually equally effective and yet causes fewer problems than podophyllin. The strength of TCA is more easily controlled; it works on first contact with the skin and then stops in about five minutes, reducing the danger of scarring. It does not seem to provoke severe reactions as podophyllin occasionally does. Some doctors use TCA during pregnancy, although no studies have been done to verify its safety at that time.

3. Cryotherapy (dry ice treatment) or acid can freeze or burn off small warts. This hurts briefly and sometimes causes scarring. You may want a local anesthetic.

4. You can apply 5-fluorouracil cream. It may cause irritation and discomfort.

5. Surgery or electrodesiccation (using an electric current to destroy tissue) becomes necessary for very large warts which fail to respond to other treatments. This procedure requires an anesthetic. If you have a cardiac pacemaker, the electric current may disturb it, so be sure to tell your practitioner.

6. Recent studies suggest that laser beams applied to warts is an effective treatment that does not affect normal tissue or cause scarring. Some practitioners recommend it particularly for HPV infections of the cervix (warts and lesions). Local or general anesthesia may be necessary, depending on the number and size of the warts. Only physicians specially trained to do laser therapy should perform this treatment.

No matter what treatment you get, it is important

279

to remove all warts, even those inside the vagina and on the cervix, to keep the virus from spreading. Sexual partners also should be treated.

Genital Warts and Pregnancy

Warts tend to grow larger during pregnancy, probably due to the increasing levels of progesterone. If the warts are located on the vaginal wall and become very large or numerous, the vagina may become less elastic, making delivery difficult. Do *not* use podophyllin to remove warts, as it is absorbed by the skin and can cause birth defects or fetal death.

Other Sexually Transmitted Diseases

There are many more STDs than we can cover in this chapter. See Chapter 23, which deals with common medical and health problems, for information on common infections which can be transmitted nonsexually as well as sexually. Other STDs which are rare or tend to affect men more than women (such as chancroid, lymphogranuloma venereum [LGV], granuloma inguinale, intestinal STDs and hepatitis B) are discussed in the newly revised "A Book About Sexually Transmitted Diseases" (see Resources).

Acquired immune deficiency syndrome (AIDS) is another recently identified STD. It is primarily a disease of homosexual men; however, some women and a few very young children have gotten it (probably while in the uterus or from breastfeeding). The total number of cases is a very tiny percentage of the general population, but a very high percentage of those who have gotten it have died. A person loses her or his ability to fight off common organisms that cause disease when a person is run down, and sometimes the victim develops a rare cancer called Kaposi's sarcoma. Researchers are working on a vaccine for AIDS, but developing this will take years.

Women who have gotten AIDS generally have had sex with bisexual men and/or use intravenous drugs. A few people have gotten it from blood transfusions.* There is no evidence that AIDS can spread in any way other than in the transfer of body fluids. This normally requires close, intimate contact between people. The warning signs of AIDS are not very distinctive; if you have any of the following problems you could have any of several illnesses other than AIDS. Symptoms include a serious form of pneumonia; rapid weight loss; persistent fatigue; fevers; drenching night sweats; diarrhea; dry cough not otherwise explainable; enlarged, painful lymph nodes in the neck and/or armpits; and/or purplish nodules on or under the skin.

---

*The recent discovery of a virus that is probably the cause of AIDS makes it possible to develop a test to screen blood collected for transfusions.

What to Do If You Think You Have an STD

Get a diagnosis as early as possible. Most STDs are easy to cure, though it can be difficult to wade through the medical system to get care. Women who think they may have an STD have several choices when it comes to medical treatment. Some of the advantages and disadvantages of each are listed below.

Private Physicians, Gynecology Clinics and Hospital Emergency Rooms (Varying Fees)

Many private doctors' offices, gyn clinics and hospital emergency rooms lack the equipment necessary to do a routine gonorrhea culture (GC), much less test for chlamydia or herpes. In addition, many practitioners in these places tend not to test readily enough if a patient is white and middle-class.

The first time I asked a gynecologist for a routine gonorrhea culture, he smiled with a comradely look in his eye. "But I'm sure no man you'd be involved with would have gonorrhea."

On the other hand, they may be overly suspicious about the possibility of STD in patients who are black and poor.

Public Health Clinics (Usually Free or of Nominal Cost)

Public health departments run STD clinics throughout the country (sometimes located in hospitals) which are called "L" or "skin" clinics. Because they deal with STD on a daily basis, most clinics have personnel experienced in diagnosing STDs and good diagnostic equipment for major diseases. They also offer the services of a public health adviser who answers questions about STD. Most of the clinics do not test for hepatitis or the intestinal STDs, and some of the smaller ones may only be equipped to deal with gonorrhea, syphilis and common complications like PID.

Women who use public health clinics on a regular basis sometimes say they feel a definite stigma attached to them (as opposed to the experiences of patients at a hospital or neighborhood or private clinic).

Everyone looks at you when you're sitting in the Health Department clinic as if you're dirty or something. Then there are so many people reading your file: secretary, nurse, doctor. It's like they all know about you. It's very embarrassing.

Because clinics tend to be overcrowded, you may have a long wait before being seen by a hurried doctor or health care worker who may not take the time to answer your questions. The quality of service varies, of course, from clinic to clinic. To find the public health facility nearest to you, call the Clinic Locator: (1-800) 227-8922.

Feminist Health Centers

Women's health centers undoubtedly offer the most sympathetic care for women with STD. If they lack the necessary diagnostic equipment for your STD, they will refer you to a sympathetic doctor or clinic. For a list of feminist health clinics, write to us (the Boston Women's Health Book Collective) at 465 Mt. Auburn Street, Watertown, MA 02172, or write to the National Women's Health Network, 224 Seventh Street SE, Washington, DC 20003.

Going for Treatment

Before going to a physician or clinic, it's a good idea to call ahead to get an idea of services offered and charges. Tests are often free, but there may be a fee for the visit. If you are a minor and don't want your parents notified or sent the bill, ask about the policy on this.

If you are a minor, you can receive examination and treatment without your parents' permission in every state. The law, however, does not *prevent* the physician from telling your parents.

Wherever you decide to go for care, you have a right to courteous and thorough treatment. Expect to have a medical history taken and a pelvic exam. The practitioner should explain any test, treatment and negative side effects. Before leaving, know what your follow-up care will be. If your doctor or medical care worker is too busy to answer your questions, ask to speak to someone else. It's always a good idea to take someone with you. Don't leave before your questions are answered. Even then, however, you may still feel uncertain about your treatment. Sometimes tests are not accurate; sometimes treatments don't work. That can mean more medical visits, time and money. Treatment can be painful—two big shots in the buttocks for gonorrhea, for example. But the alternative—not getting treatment—is worse.

STDs and the Law

State law requires that physicians and clinics report all cases of gonorrhea and syphilis to the state or local health officer. Chancroid, granuloma inguinale and lymphogranuloma venereum (LGV) are also reportable in most states.

If you do not want to be identified, use a false name when you go for treatment; pay with cash (to avoid identifying yourself by your check, which may show your home address). Another reason for using an as-sumed name is that state boards of health can demand medical records from physicians or clinics, and courts can subpoena them. If you have gonorrhea or syphilis, a social worker may interview you and ask for names of your "contacts" (people you may have caught the disease from or given it to). Usually contacts are notified anonymously—your name is not mentioned. If you do not wish to give names of contacts, say you will contact them yourself. Then it is your responsibility to contact each person you've had sex with and ask them to seek treatment.* Remember, you may be saving their fertility or even their lives.

NOTES

1. British Journal of Venereal Disease, June 1981.
2. John C. Cutler. "Venereal Disease Prevention," Cutis, Vol. 27 (March 1981), pp. 321–27.
3. Hershel Jick et al. Journal of the American Medical Association, Vol. 248 (1982), pp. 1619–21.
4. Edward Brecher. Journal of Sex Research, Vol. 11, No. 4 (November 1975), pp. 318–28.
5. John C. Cutler et al. "Vaginal Contraceptives as Prophylaxis Against Gonorrhea and Other Sexually Transmissible Diseases," Advances in Planned Parenthood, Vol. 12, No. 1, Excerpta Medica (1977), pp. 45–56.
6. William McCormack. "STD, Women as Victims," Journal of the American Medical Association, Vol. 248, No. 2 (July 7, 1982), pp. 177–78.
7. Sexually Transmitted Disease Newsletter, Vol. 2, No. 8 (September 1979), pp. 1–3.
8. M. A. Reasoner. "The Effect of Soap on Treponema Pallidum," Journal of the American Medical Association, Vol. 68, 973 (1917).
9. William Darrow. "Social and Psychologic Aspects of Sexually Transmitted Diseases: A Different View," Cutis, Vol. 27 (March 1981), pp. 311–19.
10. Modern Medicine, April 1977.
11. For more information on monoclonal antibody tests for gonorrhea, chlamydia and herpes, see Robert Nowinski et al. "Monoclonal Antibodies for Diagnosis of Infectious Diseases in Humans," Science, Vol. 219, No. 4585 (February 1983), pp. 637–44.
12. "Mycoplasma Infection Linked to Prematurity Risk," Ob-Gyn News (August 1, 1981); Ruth Kundsin, "Mycoplasmas in Humans: Significance of Ureaplasma Urealyticum," H. L. S., Vol. 13, No. 2 (1976), p. 144; Jan Freiburg, "Mycoplasmas and Ureaplasmas, Infertility and Abortion," Fertility and Sterility, Vol. 33, No. 4 (April 1980), pp. 351–52.
13. Atila Toth and Martin Lesser. "Asymptomatic Bacteriospermia in Fertile and Infertile Men," Fertility and Sterility, Vol. 36, No. 1 (July 1981), pp. 88–91.
14. H. Hunter Hansfield. "Nongonococcal Urethritis," Cutis, Vol. 27 (March 1981), p. 270.
15. "Mycoplasma Infection Linked to Prematurity Risk," Ob-Gyn News (August 1, 1981); Ruth Kundsin, "Mycoplasmas in Humans: Significance of Ureaplasma Urealyticum,"

*Some lesbian organizations suggest that gay women not give out information to health authorities. For more information on lesbians and legal issues surrounding STDs, write Ain't I a Woman, P.O. Box 1169, Iowa City, IA 52240.

H. L. S., Vol. 13, No. 2 (1976), p. 144; Jan Freiburg, "Mycoplasmas and Ureaplasmas, Infertility and Abortion," *Fertility and Sterility*, Vol. 33, No. 4 (April 1980), pp. 351–52.

16. William Reeves et al. "Risk of Recurrence after First Episodes of Genital Herpes," *New England Journal of Medicine*, Vol. 305, No. 6 (August 1981), p. 159.

17. A. E. Nilson. "Efficacy of Oral Acyclovir in Treatment of Initial and Recurrent Herpes," *The Lancet* (September 11, 1982), p. 571.

18. "Laser Beam: A New Treatment for Viral Venereal Diseases," *Contraceptive Technology Update* (December 1981), p. 159.

19. John Grossman et al. "Management of Genital Herpes Simplex Virus Infection During Pregnancy," *Obstetrics and Gynecology* (July 1981), p. 159.

20. Santa Cruz Women's Health Center. "Herpes" (1977), p. 9.

21. Nicholas Sampsidis. "Herpes, Something Can Be Done About It." New York: Sunflower Books, 1980, pp. 4–14.

RESOURCES

Organizations to Contact for Bibliographies and Information

American Foundation for the Prevention of Venereal Disease, Inc., 335 Broadway, New York, NY 10013.

American Social Health Association (ASHA), 260 Sheridan Avenue, Palo Alto, CA 94306.

American Venereal Disease Association, P.O. Box 200, San Diego, CA 92134.

Centers for Disease Control, Bureau of State Services, Venereal Disease Control Division, Atlanta, GA 30333.

Ed-U-Press, Box 583, Fayetteville, NY 13066.

Herpes Resource Center (HRC), P.O. Box 100, Palo Alto, CA 94302.

Institute for Family Research and Education, Syracuse University, 760 Ostrum Avenue, Syracuse, NY 13210, (315) 423-4584. (Subdivision: Family Planning and Population Information Center.)

National Clearinghouse for Family Planning Information, P.O. Box 225, Rockville, MD 20852.

Planned Parenthood: your local office is listed in the white and yellow pages of your phone book.

Public Health Department, Venereal Disease Division (state level): listed in the white pages of your phone book.

Books

Bell, Ruth, et al. *Changing Bodies, Changing Lives: A Book For Teens On Sex And Relationships*. New York: Random House, Inc, 1980. $7.95, paperback. An *Our Bodies, Ourselves* for teens.*

Corsaro, Maria, and Carole Korzeniowsky. *STD, A Commonsense Guide*. New York: St. Martin's Press, Inc., 1980. $9.95, hardcover. A comprehensive, practical and down-to-earth approach. Includes appendices on self-examination, prevention and where to find health care for STD.*

Gardner, Joy. *Healing Yourself*. Seattle: Snohomish Publish-

ing Co., 1980. $4.00, paperback. A good chapter on natural remedies for some STDs, including herpes, trichomoniasis and vaginitis.*

Hamilton, Richard. *The Herpes Book*. Los Angeles: J.P. Tarcher, Inc., 1980. Paperback. A comprehensive treatment of causes, symptoms, treatment and prospect for cure of herpes.

Lumiere, Richard, and Stephanie Cook. *Healthy Sex...And Keeping It That Way: A Complete Guide to Sexual Infections*. New York: Simon and Schuster, 1983. Clear and to the point.

Mayer, Ken, and Hank Pizer. *The AIDS Fact Book*. New York: Bantam Books, 1983.

Rosebury, Theodore. *Microbes and Morals: The Strange Story of Venereal Disease*. New York: The Viking Press, 1971; Ballantine Books, Inc., 1973, paperback. An excellent historical look at STD, including examination of origin and spread.

Stein, Mari. *VD: The Love Epidemic*. Palo Alto, CA: Page Flicklin Publications, 1973, 1977. Paperback. Wonderful cartoons accompanied by simple, nonjudgmental and informational text on eight STDs.

Wear, Jennifer, and King Homes. *How to Have Intercourse Without Getting Screwed*. Seattle: Madrona Publishers, 1976. Paperback. Address: 113 Madrona Place, Seattle, WA 98112. Good chapter on STD.

Booklets, Pamphlets and Reprints

American Foundation for the Prevention of Venereal Disease, Inc. "The New Venereal Disease Prevention for Everyone." Free. Address listed under Organizations. Excellent pamphlet on prevention.

American Social Health Association (address under Organizations). "Some Questions and Answers About VD" gives general information on STD, little on prevention; "Women and VD" gives concise information on seven STDs, little on prevention; "The Sexually Active and VD" discusses symptoms, prevention (condom only), risks and ways of informing partners; "How to Cope with Herpes" describes precautions, symptoms, treatment, complications during pregnancy and childbirth; "CMV" describes transmission and complications of the little-known STD virus that is a major cause of birth defects; voice of the establishment. All are free.

Boston Women's Health Book Collective, 465 Mt. Auburn Street, Watertown, MA 02172. "Sexually Transmitted Diseases and How To Avoid Them." Concise information and chart on five STDs. Emphasizes prevention. Send fifty cents plus a stamped, self-addressed, business-size envelope.*

Cherniak, Donna. "A Book About Sexually Transmitted Diseases." Montreal Health Press, P.O. Box 1000, Station LaCité, Montreal, Quebec, Canada H2W 2N1, 1983. $2.00. Also available in French: "Les Maladies Transmises Sexuellement." Best single publication on STD, some on prevention.*

Chico Feminist Women's Health Center, 330 Flume Street, Chico, CA 95926. Packet of information on STD. $1.50. One of the few pamphlets for lesbians.

Commonwealth of Massachusetts. "The Facts About VD" and "Los Datos Sobre EV." For a copy in English or Spanish,

*Highly recommended.

*Highly recommended.

write to the Department of Public Health, Division of Communicable Disease, 600 Washington Street, Boston, MA 02111. Prevention, including condoms and diaphragm.

Ed-U-Press (address under Organizations). "Facts About VD for Today's Youth." Up-to-date information on symptoms and treatment of some STDs. $3.50. Also "VD Claptrap," a comic book, 30¢.

Feminist Health Works, 487 A Hudson Street, New York, NY 10014, (212) 929-7886. "Herbal Remedies for Women." Includes discussion of alternative treatments for vaginitis and PID. Also fact sheets on "What You Should Know About Antibiotics."*

National Institute of Allergy and Infectious Diseases, Information Office, Bethesda, MD 20014. "Sexually Transmitted Diseases." Symptoms, diagnosis, complications and treatment (no prevention) of several STDs. Free.

New York State Health Department, Office of Communications and Education, Tower Building, Empire State Plaza, Albany, NY 12237. "Worried About VD" explains a visit to a public health clinic, 1978; "It's a Fact of Life—VD Gets Around" discusses syphilis and gonorrhea; "Other Types of STD" describes seven other STDs. Free to New York residents, single copies free to nonresidents.

Pennsylvania Department of Health, P.O. Box 90, Harrisburg, PA 17120. "Common Sexually Transmitted Diseases." A concise chart of thirteen STDs with pertinent information. Nothing on prevention. Free.

Planned Parenthood of Minnesota, 1965 Ford Parkway, St. Paul, MN 55116. "What Is Herpes?" Transmission and care of herpes, plus chart of other STDs. 25¢.

Sampsidis, Nicholas. "Herpes, Something Can Be Done About It." New York: Sunflower Books, 1980. Nutritional approach to herpes prevention and treatment.*

Santa Cruz Women's Health Center, 250 Locust Street, Santa Cruz, CA 95060. "Herpes," a comprehensive 1978 eighteen-page booklet on prevention, symptoms, traditional and nontraditional treatment of herpes, $2.00; "Lesbian Health Matters," a comprehensive 106-page book on health care for lesbians, including a discussion of STD, $4.00; "Pelvic Inflammatory Disease," a description of symptoms, causes and treatment of PID, $2.00.*

U.S. Department of Health and Human Services, Public Health Service, Centers for Disease Control, Venereal Disease Control Division, Atlanta, GA 30333. "Sexually Transmitted Diseases Treatment Guidelines 1982," HHS Publication #(CDC)82–8017, Morbidity and Mortality Weekly Report Supplement, Vol. 31, No. 25 (August 20, 1982). There probably will be updates to this.

Women's Health Services, 316 E. March Street, Santa Fe, NM 07501. "Her Pease," from spring 1981 edition of Hot Flash. Best single article on herpes, including prevention, symptoms, traditional and nontraditional treatments.*

Women's Place Resource Center, 460 S. Division, Portland, OR 97202. "Natural Treatments for Vaginitis," available from the Women's Health Clinic at the above address; "Herpes Rising," an excellent article on herpes.*

Periodicals

The HELPER. Quarterly newsletter of HRC, focusing on all aspects, medical and psychological, of dealing with herpes.

*Highly recommended.

Includes updates on latest research. Very comprehensive. Free to HRC members. Single issues available at $1.50 per copy. Send to The HELPER, P.O. Box 100, Palo Alto, CA 94302.*

Sexually Transmitted Diseases. Quarterly publication of the American Venereal Disease Association, P.O. Box 200, San Diego, CA 92134.

Sexually Transmitted Diseases, Abstracts and Biography. Center for Disease Control, Technical Information Services, Bureau of State Services, Atlanta, GA 30333. Free.

STD Newsletter. Monthly newsletter of the City of New York, Bureau of Venereal Disease Control, New York City Health Department, 93 Worth Street, Room 806, New York, NY 10013.

Hotlines

The following offer confidential counseling and referral related to STD: HELPLINE (for herpes), (415) 388-7710 (8 A.M. to 4:30 P.M., Pacific time). VD National Hotline, (800) 227-8922 except in California which is (800) 982-5883 (8 A.M. to 8 P.M., Pacific time).

Audiovisual Materials

Facts About Sexually Transmitted Disease, a 25-minute 16-mm color-and-sound 1980 film. Purchase and rental. Available from Benchmark Films, 145 Scarborough Road, Briarcliff Manor, N.Y. 10510. Describes eight STDs and their complications.

Management of Recurrent Herpes, an audiocassette tape. $5.00 for HELP members, $10.00 for nonmembers. Available from ASHA (address under Organizations). Focuses on the effects of emotions on the immune system, and herpes in particular. Discusses wholistic approach to herpes.

VD and Women, 8 mm, 6 mm or videocassette, 17 minutes, 1978. Purchase and rental. Available from Perennial Education, Inc., 477 Roger Williams, P.O. Box 855, Ravinia, Highland Park, IL 60035. Focuses primarily on gonorrhea and herpes. Excellent on prevention.*

VD: A Newer Focus, a 16-mm 1977 film. Purchase and rental. Available in English and Spanish from American Educational Films, 132 Lake Drive, Beverly Hills, CA 90212. Includes information and exposes myths surrounding STD.

VD: Prevent It, purchase only. Available from Alfred Higgins Productions, Inc., 9100 Sunset Boulevard, Los Angeles, CA 90069. Demonstrates various preventive measures.

VD Quiz: Getting the Right Answers, a 25-minute 1977 film. Purchase and rental. Available in English and Spanish from American Educational Films (see above). Facts about several STDs, options for treatment and solutions to the STD epidemic.

When Love Needs Care, a 17-minute 8-mm or 16-mm color-and-sound film, or videocassette. Purchase and rental. Available from Perennial Education, Inc. (see above). Experience of two teenagers being examined and treated for STD. Not much on prevention.

*Highly recommended.

15

IF YOU THINK YOU ARE PREGNANT: FINDING OUT AND DECIDING WHAT TO DO

By Jane Pincus and Jill Wolhandler

Some of us want to have a child and, within a matter of months or years, become pregnant.

Some of us become pregnant unexpectedly or when we don't want or can't have a child.

There are several ways of finding out whether you are pregnant. It is best to find out early. If you want to have a baby, you can take extra good care of yourself. If you decide not to continue the pregnancy, you can get an early abortion, the easiest and safest kind. *If you suspect pregnancy but haven't yet had a test, don't assume you definitely are pregnant. Use birth control if you have intercourse and don't want to be pregnant.*

Usual signs of early pregnancy (one to two weeks after conception) are 1. missing a period; 2. a period with less bleeding or fewer days than usual; 3. swelling, tenderness or tingling in your breasts; (about two weeks after conception) 4. frequent urination; 5. fatigue; 6. nausea or vomiting (morning sickness); 7. feeling bloated or crampy; 8. increased or decreased appetite; 9. changes in digestion (constipation or heartburn); 10. mood changes. Keep in mind that some women become pregnant and are not aware of it for the first few months. Signs of pregnancy vary from woman to woman and pregnancy to pregnancy.

WHERE TO GET A PREGNANCY TEST

Pregnancy tests are available through many clinics and medical practitioners (doctors, midwives, nurse-practitioners, physicians' assistants). In many places family-planning organizations (Planned Parenthood, for example), women's health centers and abortion clinics offer the most frequently used pregnancy testing services. The yellow pages may also list labs that do pregnancy testing. You can buy a kit in a drugstore and do a test yourself at home (see below). In some places you may have to call a doctor or hospital to get a test.

You may be able to get a free test, but be aware that free services may be offered as a way to promote some-

thing else. For example, groups like Birthright advertise free pregnancy testing and counseling and offer help with problem pregnancies. These groups give out antiabortion propaganda, hoping to frighten you and convince you not to consider abortion even if you do not want to have a baby.

Wherever you go, the person who tells you the result of your test may make assumptions which do not apply to you: s/he may tell you about abortion but not about prenatal care and having a baby; tell your husband, boyfriend, or parents without your permission; act as if you are in a crisis situation and feeling terrible; or congratulate you on the "happy news." Remember that it's your body and your choice. You may feel not at all the way anyone else expects you to feel.

KINDS OF PREGNANCY TESTS

All urine and blood tests react with a hormone called HCG (human chorionic gonadotropin), which is secreted into a pregnant woman's blood by the developing placenta. HCG shows up in the urine, through which it is excreted. *Urine slide tests* are the fastest, easiest and least expensive pregnancy tests. A drop of urine is mixed with the test serum on a slide; after two minutes the presence or absence of little clumps in the mixture indicates whether there is HCG in the urine. These tests are accurate for most women at about twenty-seven days after conception (when a period is about thirteen days late). In a *urine tube test* the urine is mixed with purified human HCG in a test tube. After one to two hours the cells sink to the bottom of the tube in a doughnut pattern if there is enough HCG for a positive test. These tests are generally accurate a few days earlier in pregnancy than the slide tests. Recently, new and more expensive urine tests have been developed which may be accurate as early as fourteen days after conception.

To collect a good urine sample use a *very clean, dry jar.* Do not use an old medicine container or shampoo bottle, because traces of chemicals or soap can contaminate the sample. Especially if it is early in the pregnancy, take the sample when you first wake up in the morning, because your urine is more concentrated then. A small amount (several tablespoons) is sufficient for the test. Cover the urine and keep it refrigerated. It is best not to use aspirin or marijuana the day before you take the sample, because they can interfere with the test.

Pregnancy test results can be positive, negative or inconclusive. A positive result almost always means pregnancy. A false positive—that is, a positive result when a woman is not actually pregnant—is rare. False positives can be caused by an error in reading the test, drugs (marijuana, methadone, Aldomet, large amounts of aspirin, synthetic hormones like birth control pills, some tranquilizers and other drugs that affect the nervous system), protein or blood in the urine, soap or other substances in the container, hormone changes of menopause* or certain tumors or other rare medical conditions.

A negative test may mean that you are not pregnant, but false negatives are fairly common. Often, it is too early in your pregnancy for the test to measure the small amount of HCG in your urine. Later, the amount of HCG starts to decrease after a couple of months; by four to five months the HCG level may be so low that a test may give a false negative. Other reasons for false negatives are 1. the urine became too warm; 2. the urine was not concentrated enough; 3. there was contamination from the jar or from certain medications; 4. it is an unhealthy pregnancy that may miscarry; 5. it is an ectopic pregnancy (pregnancy outside the uterus); 6. there has been a mistake in doing the test. A health worker can help you evaluate your chances of a false negative and discuss why your period may be late if you are not pregnant. If you suspect that you are pregnant even though a test is negative, have a pelvic exam and/or repeat the urine test. Don't just keep waiting for your period.

In two weeks I had three pregnancy tests; all of them were inconclusive, according to the lab reports I got. By the time I was given a blood test which established my pregnancy as real rather than imagined, I felt angry at the medical establishment for disbelieving me.

Home Pregnancy Tests

Some women appreciate the option of a home pregnancy test because it gives privacy, convenience and control over the experience. However, other women feel isolated doing a home test. The test itself is not hard to do, but home tests may give false results more often than lab tests. The instructions do not include enough information to evaluate whether the result is accurate, so you may need additional information.

Blood Tests

Two kinds of blood tests—radioimmunoassays (RIAs), which test for the beta subunit of HCG, and radioreceptorassays (RRAs)—are more sensitive than slide or tube tests. They can detect low levels of HCG in the blood even before the first missed period. (HCG appears earlier in the blood than in urine.) Blood tests may be needed to detect an ectopic pregnancy or missed abortion. They are expensive and require sophisticated equipment and personnel, although cheaper versions are being developed. The RIA test is accurate seven to twelve days after conception, while the RRA test, called Biocept-G, is accurate fourteen to seventeen days after conception. Like all tests, they sometimes give false results.

Pills and Injections

If the doctor suggests injections or pills to see whether they will bring on your period, *do not agree*. This procedure, sometimes called a hormone withdrawal test, is *not* an accurate test for pregnancy, and it is dangerous. The drugs used are synthetic hormones (usually progestin) which can cause negative effects in a woman who takes them, and birth defects if she is pregnant and decides to have the baby. Though the FDA issued warnings against this procedure in 1973 and withdrew approval in 1975, a 1976 survey showed that doctors were still using it.*

Pelvic Exam

To check on the results of a pregnancy test or to find out how far along your pregnancy is, have a pelvic exam at around six weeks after your last menstrual period (six weeks LMP). If you are pregnant, 1. you, your doctor, midwife or other practitioner will feel that the tip of your cervix (neck of the uterus) has become softened; 2. your cervix may change from a pale pink to a bluish color because of increased blood circulation (you can see it yourself if you have a speculum and mirror); 3. your uterus feels softer to the person examining you; and 4. the size and shape of the uterus change.

Some women just know they are pregnant. Some of us feel we know the *moment* we become pregnant. Perhaps one sign—a missed period, tender breasts—tunes us in to the fact that our bodies feel different.

With my first child I missed a period and my breasts hurt. With Jesse, I knew the moment I conceived him.

---

*All the tests except the beta subunit tests cross-react with LH (see p. 424). For this reason, premature menopause and actual menopause can give false positives. Also, it is possible, though very rare, that a test at the LH surge at ovulation could give a false positive.

*See *Biology of Women*, by Ethel Sloane, New York: John Wiley & Sons, Inc., 1980, p. 264.

There's no way of pinning that down, no way of explaining how I felt. I just knew.

Now you know you are pregnant. If you are going to have the baby, see Unit IV, "Childbearing." If you plan to have an abortion, turn to Chapter 16, "Abortion." In either case, you may want to consider the information below.

IF YOU'RE NOT SURE WHAT YOU'RE GOING TO DO

Think through the various possibilities and what they would mean to you. You may be able to decide what to do very quickly; you may think you know what you are going to do, but after more thought and talking about it, you may change your mind; you may be torn for a long time and find it incredibly difficult to make a decision. You are not required to talk to anyone in order to decide, but talking with people you think will be supportive can be immensely helpful. You may or may not want to include family members or the man involved. Talking may make you closer than before, or you may not get support when you most want or expect it. Often others have such strong feelings about your pregnancy that they are not helpful and may even upset you. Sometimes it is wisest to talk to others *after* you have made your decision.

Whatever choice you make, it should be *yours* and no one else's. Other people (family, friends, lover, counselors) can help you figure out what you want, but you should not have to justify your decision to anyone. *If you don't make any decision, you are in fact deciding to have a baby, without acknowledging it.*

HAVING AND REARING CHILDREN

Get some idea about what it's like to raise children; observe and talk to mothers, fathers, children you know. Offer to take care of friends' children. If you are married or living with someone, think about how having a baby will change your life together. If you are single, think about how you would support and care for a child; where you would live; who, if anyone, you would live with. If you already have children, what will a new child mean to you and to them? Always keep in mind that we all need help at different times to bring up our children.

ABORTION

For many women abortion is a positive choice. Having an abortion can be much less traumatic physically and emotionally than having an unwanted child. The safest and easiest time to have an abortion is within the first three months (first trimester) of the pregnancy.

This is the first time I really told people because it was such a big thing for me. There are so many women who've had abortions. These women have made these choices, too—so nothing's wrong with me....When you are willing to talk about it, it makes another feel she can talk to you.

I was the mother of three little boys. Being a mother and having children has always been very important to me, and this made the decision that much more difficult. Loving children as I do, I also knew that having the baby and then giving it up for adoption would not be an option for me.

Before I made the decision to have the abortion, I cried a lot. I would wake up around four-thirty in the morning and think about what to do, and cry. I'm sure experiencing the loss of a potential child was part of it.

My lover was opposed to having the child (as a team) and I didn't want another child without his help, so I decided on abortion. I was not happy with this because I wanted the child and was in love with the father.

I knew that abortions were legal, but that's all. I was afraid to mention it to my doctor. I thought he'd accuse me of being evil. (He didn't.) I also thought I'd be in terrible pain. The hospital had a program explaining the procedure the day before to the whole group of us. It was very helpful.

I get so bitter hearing people piously stating how those poor babies have a right to live and there are lots of people who want babies and can't have them. A baby isn't just produced and given away and that's that. You're talking about a part of the woman's body. That baby is part of her, and to expect her to give it up after going through a pregnancy is really ridiculous. I know many women could, but many couldn't. I couldn't have. I know that without my abortion I would have gone through nine months of hell, dealing with my boyfriend, my parents, my friends, my job, my financial situation, my health, my whole future and then thinking about the baby, its future, would I keep it or not, how to support it, and so on—one headache after another. At that time in my life, I don't think I could have handled it all. I couldn't even handle it now, and I'm better off now than I was a year ago.

ADOPTION AND FOSTER CARE

(Be sure to see p. 429 for more about adoption.)
Explore the adoption alternatives and services avail-

Adoption Abuse

by Carole Anderson and Lee Campbell, with Mary Anne Cohen. Reprinted from *Womenwise*, Vol. 5, No. 3, Fall 1983.

You may never have heard the term birthmothers before, but we are the mothers who have surrendered children to adoption. We have joined together to form a national, non-profit group called Concerned United Birthparents, Inc. (CUB). We are the living proof of why all feminists must oppose legislation that now threatens to destroy the gains made for women in the past few years.

Most people assume that mothers who surrender their babies to adoption do so because they don't want their children. Or they assume that mothers choose adoption as a means of providing more for their children than they could offer. In our view, these assumptions are dangerously simplistic.

In a male-dominated society, a woman's expression of sexuality is permitted only within strict bounds. Traditionally, only when she is married is sexual activity considered legitimate; indeed, it is expected at a husband's whim as his right.

For thousands of years men have sought to control women's sexuality and fertility. Out-of-wedlock pregnancies have historically merited harsh punishment. In some cultures, that punishment is even death. An unmarried pregnant woman is still considered, in some Moslem countries, to be such a stain on the family's honor that it can be cleansed only through the woman's death, and the murderer is rarely prosecuted.

America's preferred punishment appears more civilized. We favor removal of the evidence: before birth, in maternity homes, segregated educational programs, or away at Aunt Sally's; after birth, by adoption. When these preferences are ignored, we mount subtle but effective campaigns to condemn the perpetrators. We sympathize with infertility among married couples in the same breath that we bemoan the so-called "unwed teenage pregnancy epidemic," as though the issues are related. We proclaim that "adoption builds families" without reference to the female-headed families adoption has separated, as though they never existed. We begrudge the subsidies that help economically deficient single-parent families to remain together, while we uncomplainingly subsidize foster care and adoption.

Most younger single mothers have little knowledge of rights. They are accustomed to following the advice of parents, teachers, and other authority figures. Frightened, vulnerable, and economically dependent, mothers whose parents are not supportive are easy prey to the social workers, attorneys, and doctors who arrange adoptions and collect placement fees of as much as $30,000 for healthy white infants.

Most CUB members surrendered children at a time when they were unaware of financial help that would have enabled them to keep their children, or when such help did not exist. Most encountered social workers who failed to give information about alternatives that could have aided mothers to keep their families together. Children of single parents, it was said, would be ridiculed at school as bastards, or grow up to be homosexual because they lacked a father image, or would live in poverty forever because no decent man would marry their mother. Through the 1960's most schools expelled pregnant students, thus denying them a chance to graduate. And day care opportunities were rare even if a mother could find a job that would support her and her child. Denied education, denied jobs and denied any knowledge of financial assistance, few had any option but to surrender their children.

The loss of a child to adoption is a unique and unnatural one. Unlike death, which is final, adoption creates a loss that is renewed daily, as each day is a new day of trying to live without the surrendered child whose life continues separately. It is a limbo loss, in which there are constant questions but no answers. Is my child well or ill? Happy or miserable? Alive or dead?

For ten years I tied up all my emotional energy in trying to pretend it never happened, and I almost believed it. I had to stay emotionally detached to survive. I was afraid to face all this pain, but I was numbing myself to everything else in life too.

Part of me died. I feel empty inside, I'm afraid to make decisions about anything, and I can't trust anyone. I was told so many lies. I can't let anyone get close to me, especially men, and I cringe if a man touches me.

When I was eighteen I believed what the social worker said about adoptive couples. That they were screened so they were totally perfect parents who had everything my child needed, and I had nothing. Now I know adoptive parents are the same as everyone else. They're not perfect. I feel cheated. Why did I have to compete with other people for the right to raise my own child?

Forcing me to surrender my child was an ultimate act of rape. I wish that when they were through with me, they had put a bullet in my head so I wouldn't have to live in such anguish.

When a mother surrenders her child, she is allowed no options in the terms of that surrender. She has no right to participate in selecting who will raise her child, to know anything about her child's adoptive parents, to know anything about her child's health or welfare. She has no right to choose whether or not she wishes to be anonymous to the adoptive parents or to her child, even after her child is an adult. She has no right to legal counsel, no right to be informed of alternatives, no right to copies of information about her. She has no right to her child's original birth certificate, nor to the falsified version that will later be substituted to state that the adoptive parents gave birth. She has no right to know the legal process involved in adoption. She even has no right to receive a copy of the surrender document that separates her child from her.

Social workers defend this process by claiming that adoption is a positive choice for a young woman with an unplanned pregnancy since it permits the mother to correct her mistake. They insist that the mother's pain is temporary, and that she will be able to begin a new life. That same child who was described as a burden to the mother is transformed into a blessing for a married couple able to pay a placement fee.

Many adoptive mothers, too, have sought to keep birthmothers in the role of brood mares. While some adoptive mothers have joined in CUB's efforts, others loudly proclaim that they alone are really mothers, that birthmothers do not deserve to know of their children's welfare, that God gave the child to adoptive parents, or that birthmothers should be grateful to adoptive parents for having saved their children from the stigma of illegitimacy. These adoptive parents demand that birthmothers respect adoptive parents' efforts, while they ignore birthmothers' sacrifices.

These women, too, are victims. Many have reported feelings of inadequacy and insecurity as a result of their inability to bear children of their own. Made by our society to feel their value as women depended on their ability to bear children, some feel they have to adopt babies and act as if they had borne them. The final proof of motherhood—the child's birth certificate—is permanently sealed, and a false one issued to reinforce the idea that birth alone confers motherhood.

Feminists have been slow to recognize adoption's exploitation of their sisters. Perhaps one reason is that women have been not only the victims of adoption abuse but also its chief perpetrators and beneficiaries. Just as it is women like Phyllis Schlafly who have led efforts to defeat the Equal Rights Amendment and advances for women's rights, it is women who have fought to continue adoption abuse.

Reflecting the changes brought about by the women's movement, in the recent past single mothers have succumbed less frequently to adoption abuse. But know these things: Although only 3 percent of mothers under twenty now choose adoption, 43 percent of 125 cities with a population of 100,000 or more offer adoption services. The clientele being served today are infertile couples who, unwilling to adopt the many older or special-needs children who are available, wait in frustration on ever-lengthening lists for healthy, white infants. Joining agency workers' and infertile couples' demand for adoptable babies are anti-choice proponents who blithely tout adoption as the answer to abortion.

In response to this burgeoning undercurrent are Right-Wing-sponsored legislation and programs that are dangerous to single-parent families. One is the Adolescent Family Life bill which asserts that "adoption is a positive option for unmarried pregnant adolescents," and seeks an allocation of $30 million for three years for demonstration projects. Under the act's provisions, teens are to be advised not to be sexually active, but if they must, to get parental consent for contraceptive use. If these provisions are ignored, then the mothers are to be "encouraged" to separate forever from their children by adoption.

The Family Protection Act is evidence of further bias. It would permit a $1,000 tax exemption for the year in which a child is born or adopted, but only if the parents are married. The tax exemption is increased to $3,000 for the adoption of a bi-racial or handicapped child. Thus a single mother raising her child could not receive the tax consideration to which her married counterparts are entitled.

The potential abuse of a Human Life Amendment is obvious to feminists everywhere. Supporters of HLA are often eloquent in their defense of the fertilized egg but are seldom willing to aid the woman whose body nourishes it.

The Family Protection Act, Adolescent Family Life bill, and Human Life Amendment attempt to impose an official governmental view of morality on women, especially those who are most impressionable and least powerful because of their youth. They attempt to punish the "immoral" by forcing them to give birth and then depriving them of their children.

Unless we exert the same effort in this area of reproductive rights as we do in others, single-parent families will be unnecessarily separated by adoption in the same manner they have always been. Adoption is especially susceptible to exploitation because there are no laws granting rights to birthmothers, no system of accountability for agency workers, and no recognition among lay people of the conflict of interest that inevitably arises when counselling centers and maternity homes double as adoption agencies.

Despite claims by the New Right to the contrary, adoption as it is traditionally practiced is not the panacea for all of society's ills. The unnecessary separation of mothers and children is a cruel, but regrettably usual, punishment that can last a lifetime.

A lifetime of suffering is too much to demand for any woman's expression of her sexuality. Even if contraception is obtainable, no fertile woman is ever safe from the possibility of unintended pregnancy, since there is no method that is 100% reliable. Even abstinence has its failures since rape exists.

We birthmothers are openly fighting for the rights of the young women of the future who may be threatened with our fate. Our lives are testimony to the devastating effects of the oppression of women that is our mutual foe. Help us, and let us help you, in our common cause. We are your mothers, your daughters, your sisters, perhaps even yourselves.

Lee Campbell is a founder and President of CUB. Carole Anderson is Vice President for Public Education for CUB and the editor of *The Communicator*, CUB's monthly newsletter. Mary Anne Cohen is a poet, feminist and an original member of CUB.

Concerned United Birthparents, Inc., is a national organization with forty branches throughout the U.S. For more information about this organization or to arrange for presentations, write CUB National Headquarters, 595 Central Ave., Dover, NH 03820.

able to you. Find out about your legal rights from your *own* lawyer, a legal aid office, or an informed women's group, but not from anyone who will benefit or profit from your decision, such as a lawyer or social worker suggested by an adoption agency. Adoption agencies are geared primarily to performing adoptions rather than serving the needs of a woman with an unwanted child, although some claim to do both. All rights and laws vary from state to state. Some states allow only agencies to arrange adoptions while others allow private placement arranged by a lawyer, physician or the woman who is pregnant or has had the child. Never sign any papers until you are *absolutely sure* of your decision. In some states there is a grace period even after you sign during which you can change your mind. (New York State, for example, has a thirty-day grace period.)

Many women have joined together recently to talk about what it meant to them to give their children up for adoption many years ago. Whether or not they felt they had done so of their own free will, whether or not they felt that it had been the right decision for them at the time, they all agree that giving your child up for adoption doesn't mean that you aren't a mother anymore; you will always be the child's birthparent.

They use yourself against you—your fears, insecurity, guilt! You give all your power away. You don't see it happening overtly, so you're never at the point where you'll run out the door with the baby. I can't believe I signed that paper. I thought I was doing the best thing; I didn't want her to be taunted and marked for life. For years afterward I couldn't remember anything about how I gave her up. I heard about one woman who forgot she even had had a baby.

When I hear people say that adoption is the option women should choose instead of abortion, I get a knot in my stomach and all my memories come back. Adoption may be an option for some people, but it wasn't a good answer for me.

Foster Care is a way of having someone else raise your child temporarily. If your relatives take care of your child you avoid the necessity of going through an agency. When you go through an agency, you are giving up control of your baby, and your future wishes may not be respected.

RESOURCES

Berends, Polly B. *Whole Parent, Whole Child*, rev. ed. New York: Harper and Row Publishers, Inc., 1983.

Bernard, Jessie. *The Future of Motherhood*. New York: Dial Press, 1974.

Boston Women's Health Book Collective. *Ourselves and Our Children*. New York: Random House, Inc., 1978.

Burgess, Linda Cannon. *The Art of Adoption*. New York: Acropolis, 1977. A social worker reviews 900 adoptions and their effects on families years later.

Callahan, Sidney C. *Parenting: Principles and Politics of Parenthood*. New York: Penguin Books, 1974.

Childbearing Rights Information Project. *For Ourselves, Our Families, and Our Future: The Struggle for Childbearing Rights*. Boston: Red Sun Press, 1981.

Chodorow, Nancy. *The Reproduction of Mothering*. Berkeley, CA: University of California Press, 1978.

Concerned United Birthparents. *Choices, Chances, Changes*. CUB, Inc., 595 Central Avenue, Dover, NH 03820, 1981. A useful effort to present *all* the options possible for deciding how to resolve unwanted pregnancies.

Daniels, Pamela, and Kathy Weingarten. *Sooner or Later: The Timing of Parenthood in Adult Lives*. New York: W. W. Norton and Co., Inc., 1982.

Deykin, Eva, Lee Campbell and Patti Trish. "The Post-Adoption Experience of Surrendering Parents," *The American Journal of Orthopsychiatry* (January 1984). A new study of birthparents' survival and coping strengths.

Dowrick, Stephanie, and Sibyl Grundberg, eds. *Why Children?* New York: Harcourt Brace Jovanovich, Inc., 1980.

Dusky, Lorraine. *Birthmark*. New York: McEvans Co., 1979. One birthmother's story, recalled as she searches for her daughter years later.

Fabe, Marilyn, and Norma Wikler. *Up Against The Clock: Career Women Speak on the Choice to Have Children*. New York: Random House, Inc., 1979.

Fisher, Florence. *The Search for Anna Fisher*. Greenwich, CT: Fawcett Publications, 1974. A twenty-year search story told by an adoptee who founded ALMA, the adoptees' rights and search group, after finding her original parents.

Friedland, Ronnie, and Carol Kort, eds. *The Mothers' Book— Shared Experiences*. Boston: Houghton Mifflin Co., 1981.

Gilligan, Carol. *In a Different Voice*. Cambridge, MA: Harvard University Press, 1982. A detailed study of decision-making and moral development of women, using the example of abortion.

Hope, Karol and Nancy Young. *Momma: The Sourcebook for Single Mothers*. New York: New American Library, 1976.

Kelly, Marguerite, and Ella Parsons. *The Mother's Almanac.*. New York: Doubleday and Co., Inc., 1975.

Kirk, H. David. *Adoptive Kinship: A Modern Institution in Need of Reform*. Toronto, Canada: Butterworth, 1981. (Soon to be distributed in the U.S.) A sociologist and adoptive father uses surveys and interviews with adoptive parents and other social science resources to raise crucial issues.

———. *Shared Fate*. New York: The Free Press, 1964. A new theory of adoption as an institution based on ten years of sociological research.

Klein, Carole. *The Single Parent Experience*. New York: Avon Books, 1976.

Klerman, Lorraine V. "Adoption: A Public Health Perspective" (editorial), *American Journal of Public Health*, Vol. 73,

No. 10 (1983), pp. 1158–60. An urgent call for research in the wake of federal programs promoting adoption.

Krementz, Jill. *How It Feels to Be Adopted*. New York: Alfred A. Knopf, Inc., 1982. Through interviews, nineteen adopted children, ages eight to sixteen, of various races and cultures (some in mixed racial adoptive families), describe their thoughts and feelings about adoption, adoptive parents, birthparents and searching. Beautiful photos.

Lazarre, Jane. *The Mother Knot*. New York: Dell Publishing Co., Inc., 1967.

Lifton, Betty Jean. *Lost and Found: The Adoption Experience*. New York: Dial Press, 1979. The best single overview of adoption issues today, by an adoptee who has done extensive research.

Lindsay, Karen. *Friends as Family*. Boston: Beacon Press, 1981.

McBride, Angela. *The Growth and Development of Mothers*. New York: Harper and Row Publishers, Inc., 1973.

Miller, Shelby Hayden. *Children as Parents: A Final Report on a Study of Childbearing and Child Rearing Among 12- to 15-Year-Olds*. New York: Child Welfare League of America, 1983.

Pogrebin, Letty Cotton. *Family Politics*. New York: McGraw-Hill, Inc., 1983.

———. *Growing Up Free*. New York: McGraw Hill, Inc., 1980.

Putnam-Scholes, Jo Ann S. "An Epidemic of Publicity (The Rate of Births to Girls 15–19 Has Fallen)," *The Atlantic Monthly*, July 1983, pp. 18–19. A careful statistical and political analysis showing how the need for white adoptive infants lies behind teen pregnancy publicity.

Robie, Diane, and January Roberts. *Open Adoption, Open Placement*. Brooklyn Park, MN: Adoption Press, 1981. A new and more humane approach to adoption.

Silverman, Phyllis R. *Helping Women Cope with Grief*. Sage Human Services #25. Beverly Hills, CA: Sage Publications, 1981. Covers birthparenthood as a process of grieving.

Sorosky, Arthur, et al. *The Adoption Triangle: The Effect of Sealed Records on Adoptees, Birthparents, and Adoptive Parents*. New York: Doubleday/Anchor Books, 1978. The best single compilation of research from a psychosocial perspective by professionals.

Triseliotis, J. *In Search of Origins: The Experiences of Adopted People*. London/Boston: Routledge and Kegan Paul, 1973.

Willis, Ellen. "The Politics of Abortion," *In These Times*, June 1983, pp. 15–28.

16

ABORTION

Physical and emotional aspects of abortion by Jill Wolhandler, with Ruth Weber
Abortion history and politics by Trude Bennett, with Jill Wolhandler and Dana Gallagher

With special thanks to Vickie Alexander, Diane Balser, Terry Courtney, Margie Fine, Linda Gordon, Debra Krassner, Jane Pincus, Meredith Tax, and members of the Reproductive Rights Action Group at Brooklyn College

This chapter in previous editions was written by Carol Driscoll, Nancy P. Hawley, Elizabeth McGee, Pamela Berger and Wendy Sanford.

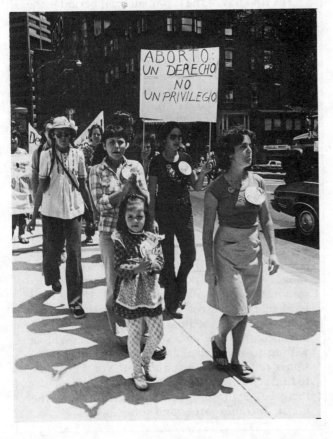

Ellen Shub

Women have always used abortion as a means of fertility control. Unless we ourselves can decide whether and when to have children, it is difficult for us to control our lives or participate fully in society. Legal, safe and affordable abortions help to give us that control.

Women of various ages, races, religions, economic and marital status and sexual preference choose to have abortions for many reasons. We may become pregnant because of inadequate birth control methods, information and access. Since no birth control method is 100 percent effective, abortion is a necessary backup when birth control fails. We may be pregnant, want a child and not be able to afford it, or decide that even a planned pregnancy is a mistake after our economic or personal circumstances change. We may find out through amniocentesis that our fetus has a serious genetic defect. We may become pregnant against our will because of rape, incest or other kinds of sexual coercion so common in our society. Little or nonexistent sex education leaves young women particularly vulnerable to sexual pressures.

Deciding whether to have a baby or an abortion is always a serious choice. You have to decide what you believe is responsible, moral and best for yourself and the important people in your life, depending on your needs, resources, commitments and hopes. We believe that compulsory pregnancy and forced motherhood are morally wrong.

I have never regretted my abortion. I am just determined that my daughters and my granddaughter can have safe and legal abortion available should they need it. The freedom from unwanted pregnancies that today's woman enjoys is something I wish my mother could have lived to see, as it is something she never dreamed would ever happen. Her struggle to limit her reproduction has left its imprint on me, as we were very close. My father was a tyrant. Birth control was her problem. But it was her wifely duty to satisfy his sexual desires. She used self-

291

induced abortion as a means of limiting her family. She was determined not to have a houseful of cold and hungry kids as her own mother had—eight children and she finally died in childbirth.

My mother suffered a great deal of guilt because of society's attitude about abortion—miscarriage, it was called. She reasoned it a greater sin to bring into the world children to suffer cold and hunger than to abort.

Even though the abortion was long and uncomfortable, it was incredible and wonderful to have so much support around me from other women. I felt that I was sharing in the process of creating a new/rediscovered female experience that I don't even think we have words for yet. We think of "pregnancy" as a state which leads to birthing a child, which is beautiful when that is what the woman wants. But that's not always what happens, and it's not the only way to understand what being pregnant is about.

The fact that I was able, for so many reasons, to choose to have an abortion has made an enormous difference in my life since then. Other decisions that I've made (where to live, to go back to school, to come out as a lesbian, what kinds of work to do) might all have been different if abortion hadn't been available to me in the past. As a woman-identified woman, I feel so strongly that those options should be open to other women. Of course, this means not just abortion but childcare, decent incomes and housing and education, struggling with racism and more. But I know from my own direct experience what is involved, on so many levels, for a woman to decide on an abortion and follow it through. Knowing that afterwards my feelings weren't as simple as I'd expected just makes it clearer for me that no one else has any right to interfere with a woman doing what she needs to do, according to her own wisdom and judgment.

When I found out I was pregnant, I was frightened and angry that my body was out of my control. I was furious that my IUD had failed me, and I felt my sexual parts were alien and my enemy.

I had strong feelings against abortions and knew that I myself could never have one. Pregnancy to me meant that a little soul had chosen to come into my body, and how could I say no to that? But when I found myself pregnant and with two teenage children, a year-old baby and myself and my husband working night and day with barely any time for each other, I knew that I had to have an abortion. It wasn't too hard a thing to do.

I was extremely anxious and upset. Although a health professional (nursing degree and master's in public health), I panicked. I felt hopeless—depressed, guilty and angry.

I've never wanted to have children. Deciding to have an abortion was the easy part. The hard part was living

How Pregnant Are You?

The length of a pregnancy is usually counted from the first day of the last normal menstrual period (LMP) and not from the day of conception (fertilization). LMP dating is inaccurate and misleading. It can make you think that you are two weeks further along in the pregnancy than you really are. It assumes that every woman not only has a twenty-eight-day cycle but ovulates exactly two weeks after her period began. (Nobody has a regular cycle *all* the time.) The *first trimester* is the first thirteen weeks; the *second trimester* is the fourteenth through twenty-fourth weeks LMP; twenty-five weeks LMP and later is the *third trimester.* Abortion is safer, easier and less expensive in the first trimester. It may be difficult to find a facility that provides second-trimester abortions, and impossible to get a third-trimester abortion unless your life is endangered by your pregnancy.

The first day of the last menstrual period is the most common way to date a pregnancy, but you must consider whether that period was normal for you. If it came at an unexpected time or was lighter than usual, conception may have happened *before* that bleeding.

If you chart your body changes with a fertility awareness method (see p. 235) you will have a written record of ovulation and will be able to recognize pregnancy quite early on. If you do cervical self-examination, you may notice that your cervix has changed color and become bluish-purple, which happens early in pregnancy.

Signs of pregnancy can help confirm the date of conception (see p. 284).

An experienced health worker or medical practitioner can estimate the length of a pregnancy by feeling the size of the uterus during a pelvic exam. This is usually accurate within a two-week range. Ultrasound, another method for determining the length of a pregnancy, also has a two-week margin of error. The practitioner doing the abortion makes the final decision about how far advanced the pregnancy is and whether s/he is willing to perform the abortion. If the practitioner refuses to do the abortion, you may have to find someone else. Statistically, abortion risks increase as the pregnancy progresses and the uterus becomes larger and softer.

through the physical aspects of pregnancy and mentally dealing with fears and anger that popped up. Life was hell before the abortion. I had morning, afternoon and evening sickness; I didn't eat for days.

To this day I have conflicted feelings about the murder issue, but the decision was fairly simple....And since I couldn't deal with another delivery/adoption, I said a prayer that the spirit of the child would pass to someone who could be receptive.

It was so hard for me to get an abortion, since I had been so excited about the pregnancy and very much wanted to be a mother. But when the amniocentesis showed that I would have a Down's syndrome baby, I knew I wasn't prepared either emotionally or financially to raise a child who is likely to have serious physical and mental problems.

It seemed like a punishment. I used birth control and got pregnant anyway. I no longer trusted my diaphragm, my lover, my body. My guilt about being pregnant turned into anger when I learned that no method of birth control is 100 percent effective! I took all the precautions and still needed an abortion. At the clinic, so many women had similar experiences.

Deciding to have an abortion wasn't a difficult decision or a big deal. From the way everyone I told reacted, though, I started wondering if something was wrong with me for not being upset.

MEDICAL TECHNIQUES FOR ABORTION

When you are considering an abortion or choosing where to have an abortion, you have a right and a need to know the procedures used at each stage of

Procedure	Techniques	Weeks LMP	Where Performed	Common Anesthesia (see p. 297)
1. Preemptive Abortion Endometrial Aspiration Menstrual Regulation (See section on Menstrual Extraction)	suction	4–6	clinic MD office	none (local)*
2. Early Uterine Evacuation (EUE)	suction	6–8	clinic MD office	none local
3. Vacuum Aspiration	dilation, suction, sometimes curettage	6–14	clinic MD office (hospital)*	none local (general)*
4. Dilation and Curettage (D and C)	dilation, curettage	6–16	(clinic) (MD office)* hospital	(local) general
5. Dilation and Evacuation (D and E)	dilation, suction, curettage, use of forceps	12—upper limit varies from 16–24	clinic MD office hospital	local general
6. Induction Abortion (Instillation Procedure) (Saline Abortion) (Prostaglandin Abortion)	injection of liquid through the abdomen into amniotic sac; uterine contractions (labor) expel the fetus and placenta	16–24	hospital	local for the injection and pain-killers for the labor and delivery
7. Prostaglandin Suppositories (rarely used)	drug inserted into the vagina to cause labor and miscarriage	13–?	hospital	pain-killers for labor and delivery
8. Hysterotomy	uterus is cut open	16–24 or later if woman's life in danger	hospital	general

*Parentheses mean "less common."

LMP: last normal menstrual period.
Dilation: enlarging the cervical opening by stretching it with tapered instruments called dilators, or with laminaria (see p. 479). Many medical technicians use the word "dilatation" to mean the same thing.
Suction: drawing out the contents of the uterus through a narrow tube attached to a gentle vacuum source.

Curettage: scraping the inside of the uterus with a metal loop, called a curette, to loosen and remove tissue.
Forceps: grasping instruments used to remove tissue.
Amniotic Sac: sac of fluid surrounding the fetus.
Prostaglandin: hormonelike substance that causes uterine contractions.
Saline: salt water.

Procedure	Complications	Possible Costs
1. Preemptive Abortion Endometrial Aspiration Menstrual Regulation	infection retained tissue (incomplete abortion) perforation hemorrhage continuing pregnancy (missed abortion) cervical tear reaction to anesthesia or other drugs postabortal syndrome (blood in uterus)	$125–$150
2. Early Uterine Evacuation (EUE)		$175–$300
3. Vacuum Aspiration		$175–$300
4. Dilation and Curettage		varies greatly
5. Dilation and Evacuation		$185–$800
6. Induction Abortion	infection, retained tissue, hemorrhage, cervical tear, drug reaction, others (see p. 296)	$450–$800
7. Prostaglandin Suppositories	often unsuccessful, severe gastrointestinal side effects	NA
8. Hysterotomy	risks of major surgery (see p. 297)	$2,000 or more

pregnancy, the risks and possible complications and the cost.

In pregnancy, a tiny ball of cells attaches itself to the lining of the uterus about one week after conception. A mass of tissue called the *placenta* develops in the uterine lining to nourish the *embryo*. By the end of the second month, the embryo, now called a *fetus*, is surrounded by a protective fluid-filled sac, the *amniotic sac*. At about twenty weeks the woman begins to feel the fetus move. Sometime between the twenty-fourth and twenty-eighth weeks the fetus reaches the point where it may live outside the mother for at least a short while under intensive hospital care.

In an abortion, the contents of the uterus (embryo or fetus, placenta and built-up lining of the uterus) are removed. Different methods are used, depending on how large the pregnancy tissue has grown, the training of the person performing the abortion, the approaches favored by the local medical community and the equipment available. The following chart summarizes medical abortion procedures. The numbers in this section refer back to the chart. These procedures may not all be available in your area, or different names may be used for some of them. Ask for explanations of words and terms that you don't understand.

During an aspiration abortion (1, 2 and 3 on the chart) the contents of the uterus are removed through a strawlike tube that is passed through the cervix into the uterus. The tube, called a cannula, is attached to a source of gentle suction—an electric or mechanical pump or a syringe—which draws out the tissue.

Aspiration is now the most common abortion technique. Of all the methods it carries the least chance of complications and considerably less risk than pregnancy, labor and delivery. In fact, it is now the safest of all operations, safer than tonsillectomies or circumcisions. It only takes a short time (five to fifteen minutes).* Aspiration abortions are now available throughout the U.S., though some women still have to travel many hours to get to an abortion facility. *THIS KIND OF ABORTION IS THE SAFEST AND LEAST DISRUPTIVE FOR A WOMAN, BOTH PHYSICALLY AND EMOTIONALLY. IT CAN ONLY BE DONE DURING THE FIRST THREE MONTHS OF PREGNANCY.*

1. An aspiration procedure before five to six weeks LMP, when pregnancy cannot yet be verified by a pelvic exam, is called *preemptive abortion*, *endometrial aspiration* or *menstrual regulation*. (Some people also call it *menstrual extraction*, but that term describes a different procedure and should not be used for this one. See p. 295.) A syringe is attached to the cannula to suction out the lining of the uterus, including the small amount of fetal and placental tissue if there is a pregnancy. Since a syringe rather than a motorized pump is used to create a vacuum, electricity is not needed.

No dilation (stretching of the cervical opening) is needed to insert a small (four to five millimeters) flexible plastic cannula into the uterus. Local anesthetic

*First-trimester aspiration abortions can be done by trained paraprofessionals as easily and safely as by doctors. Unfortunately this is illegal in most states. In Vermont, women trained as physicians' assistants have performed one-third of the abortions for years, with an excellent safety record. However, anti-abortion politicians have been trying to change Vermont laws to restrict the performance of abortions to MDs only. This would make abortions harder and more expensive to obtain, prevent women from turning to other skilled women for abortions and reinforce the power of doctors.

294

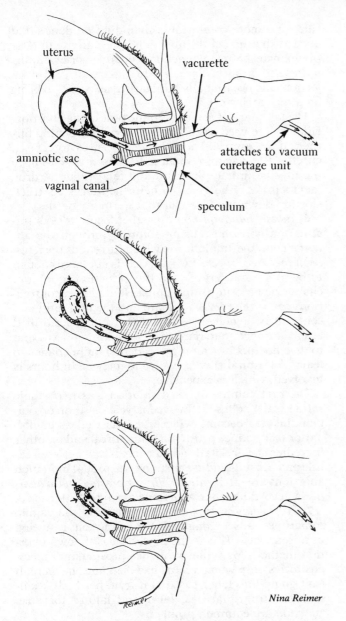

uterus

vacurette

amniotic sac

attaches to vacuum
curettage unit

vaginal canal

speculum

Nina Reimer

VACUUM SUCTION ABORTION

is rarely used, because there is no dilation and the procedure only takes a few minutes. The same complications can occur as with an aspiration abortion performed a few weeks later, after pregnancy is confirmed. However, because only flexible instruments are used, there is less risk of perforating the uterus, and problems that might result from dilating the cervix are avoided. But there is slightly more chance that the practitioner may miss aborting the pregnancy, if there is one, since the fetal tissue is so tiny.

Some women want to remove a pregnancy as soon as possible or prefer not to know whether they actually are pregnant. However, having an abortion before you know for sure that you are pregnant does not neces-

---

Menstrual Extraction

In the early 1970s self-help groups at the Feminist Women's Health Center in Los Angeles and elsewhere developed a technique using a small flexible plastic cannula to remove the lining of the uterus at about the time that the menstrual period is due. Women practiced on each other in order to develop safe instruments and techniques. Menstrual extraction is done on an experimental research basis by women in advanced self-help groups; it cannot be obtained at a medical facility. Menstrual extraction helps women avoid the discomfort of a menstrual period, provides information about menstruation and enables women to learn basic health care skills. A very early pregnancy, if present, would probably be removed along with the lining of the uterus. We need to do more research before we can know whether frequent extraction of the uterine lining creates any long-term or delayed health problems, although there is no evidence of any so far. Several aspects of the techniques developed for menstrual extraction have been incorporated into medical practice for early abortion with flexible cannulas. Menstrual extraction is a powerful example of medical research done by women on and for ourselves.

---

sarily mean that you won't have any feelings about pregnancy and abortion to deal with. One drawback is that you may indeed not be pregnant; there are many reasons for a period to be late, including anxiety about being pregnant! (If blood tests for very early pregnancy are available in your area, you can avoid an unnecessary procedure by confirming your pregnancy in this way.) Also, tests for the Rh blood type are not usually part of preemptive abortions and Rh-negative women are not usually offered Rhogam (see p. 354).

2. Abortions by *early uterine evacuation (EUE)*, done when a pelvic exam confirms pregnancy, use a tech-

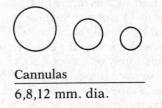

Cannulas

6,8,12 mm. dia.

Robbie Pfeufer

nique similar to number 1, except that a five- to six-millimeter flexible cannula is used. Population control projects have exported this technique to many Third World countries because it is easy to train laypersons to do it and it does not require a motorized suction pump or much equipment.

3. During a *vacuum aspiration abortion*, the cervical opening is stretched (dilated) so that a larger cannula can be used. An electrically powered aspirator is the source of suction.

There are several variations of this method. For over a decade women have been working to create the safest, least physically traumatic vacuum aspiration techniques. A number of woman-owned and -controlled feminist health centers have trained practitioners to use minimal dilation and small flexible cannulas, which reduce the chance of tearing or perforating the uterus or cervix. (An eight-millimeter cannula can be used for abortions through eleven to twelve weeks LMP.) Curettage, or scraping the inside of the uterus with a metal loop called a curette, is not routinely necessary. Experiences at these clinics and others show that this approach is more comfortable for women than that of most conventionally trained abortionists, who use larger, rigid plastic or metal cannulas (which require more dilation) and a curette after the suction.*

4. *Dilation (dilatation) and curettage (D and C)* is a standard gynecological procedure used to treat conditions such as excessively heavy bleeding and to diagnose various uterine problems. It is usually done in a hospital under general anesthesia. Because medical students routinely learn D and C, this used to be the most common method for first-trimester abortions. Now it has been virtually replaced by the quicker, easier and safer aspiration techniques, which are usually done in clinics with local or no anesthesia. Some doctors will do a D and C for abortions from twelve to sixteen weeks.

5. *Dilation (dilatation) and evacuation (D and E)* is a newer method that combines D and C and vacuum aspiration techniques for abortions later than twelve weeks LMP. Because the fetal tissue is larger and the uterus is softer and easier to injure than in the first trimester, a D and E is more complicated and requires a high level of skill on the part of the person performing the abortion. An ultrasound examination (sonogram) may be required beforehand.

The cervix needs to be dilated more than with an earlier abortion so that larger instruments can be put into the uterus to remove the pregnancy. Often dilation is begun by placing one or more laminaria sticks into the cervical opening the day before the D and E. (This extra visit may be inconvenient for some women and difficult or even impossible for others.) Laminaria is a sterilized seaweed that absorbs moisture and expands, gradually stretching the cervix. Dilation taking place this way over a number of hours is probably

safer and more comfortable than dilation done all at once at the time of the abortion, especially with later pregnancies. Some women feel pressure or cramping with laminaria in place. There is a small risk of infection, and occasionally laminaria itself starts to bring on a miscarriage.

The laminaria is removed at the time of the abortion. Dilators are used to enlarge the cervical opening further, if necessary. Then the doctor uses forceps, a curette and vacuum suction to loosen and remove the uterine lining, placental and fetal tissue. A drug (oxytocin) may be given to help the uterus contract, slowing down the bleeding that normally occurs.

6. In an *induction abortion*, the doctor injects (instills) an abortion-causing solution through the abdomen into the amniotic sac which surrounds the fetus. (Before sixteen weeks LMP this sac is not large enough to be located accurately, so the induction procedure cannot be used until this time.) Hours later, contractions cause the cervix to dilate and the fetus and placenta to be expelled. A D and C is often performed after the abortion to remove any remaining tissue and to give doctors in training (residents) more chance to learn. A hospital stay of twelve to forty-eight hours is involved, which is expensive.

The first commonly used solution was hypertonic saline (salt) solution. In recent years use of prostaglandins has become widespread, as well as combinations of saline, prostaglandins, urea and/or other ingredients. For details and a comparison between saline and prostaglandin abortions, see p. 304. Induction abortions are often called *saline* or *prostaglandin abortions*, according to the abortion-causing solution used.

7. *Prostaglandin suppositories* placed in the vagina sometimes cause strong uterine contractions resulting in miscarriage. This is the newest, least known abortion method. Many hospitals use prostaglandin suppositories only when a fetus has died and the woman isn't going into labor to expel it from her body. Nausea, vomiting, diarrhea, fever and failure to cause abortion are common problems.

8. In a *hysterotomy* the surgeon removes the fetus and placenta through an incision into the abdomen and uterus, like a small Cesarean section. The incidence of serious complications for this kind of major surgery is considerably higher than for other methods of abortion. You may need a hysterotomy when induction methods have been repeatedly unsuccessful or can't be used for medical reasons.

RISKS AND COMPLICATIONS

As with any medical procedure, there are possible risks and complications. The chance of a complication for a first-trimester abortion is about 1 percent. The later the abortion, the more chance of complications. Signs of a complication will generally appear within a few

---

*Doctors are trained to consider new information about medical procedures only if it comes from so-called medical authorities. They are not trained in give and take, or in learning from health workers "below" them in the medical hierarchy, or from women on whom they do the procedures (patients).

days after the abortion. Listed below are possible risks and complications of aspiration abortions, their symptoms and treatments. (See p. 304 for additional risks and complications of induction abortions.)

Infection

Infection is one of the more common complications. Even though sterile instruments and antiseptic are used, bacteria sometimes travel into the uterus. Signs of an infection are fever of 100.5 degrees Fahrenheit or higher, bad cramping and/or vaginal discharge with a foul odor. Treatment consists of antibiotics, usually tetracycline or ampicillin. It is important to have an exam after finishing the medication to make sure the infection is gone and there is no sign of retained tissue. Left untreated, an infection can cause serious illness, sterility or even death.

Retained Tissue

Since the practitioner can't actually see inside the uterus during the abortion, occasionally s/he leaves some tissue behind. Signs of retained tissue include very heavy bleeding, passage of large blood clots, strong cramps, bleeding for longer than three weeks or signs of pregnancy (for instance, sore breasts, nausea, tiredness) lasting longer than a week. Tissue remaining inside the uterus is likely to become infected. Sometimes drugs (Methergine or Ergotrate) are given to stimulate the uterus to contract and push out the retained tissue. The other treatment is removing the tissue by an aspiration procedure similar to an aspiration abortion but shorter, or occasionally a D and C.

Perforation

Perforation of the uterus occurs if an instrument goes through its wall. There is more risk of perforation in a D and E than in a first-trimester abortion. If a woman is awake, she is likely to feel a sharp pain or cramp. If perforation occurs, the medical staff will monitor pulse, blood pressure, cramping and bleeding very closely. The uterus is a very strong muscle and often heals quickly on its own. However, if there are any indications that a large blood vessel or another organ may have been injured, you will need hospitalization and possibly surgery. If the abortion has not been completed when the perforation occurs, it is usually finished in a hospital.

Hemorrhage

Uterine hemorrhage (excessive bleeding) during or after an abortion is more likely to occur in second-trimester abortions. Excessive bleeding can sometimes be a sign of retained tissue, perforation or failure of the uterus to contract. Drugs may be given to stimulate the contractions of the uterus, or an aspiration procedure may be done to slow down the bleeding. Check before you leave the clinic and inform the recovery room staff of the amount of bleeding.

Cervical Laceration (Tear)

There is more chance of the cervix being injured during a second-trimester abortion than an earlier abortion. A woman may not feel a tear when it happens, but the practitioner should inform her and record it in her medical record. A small tear heals without treatment. A more serious tear may require stitches, and there may be some bleeding from the tear.

Missed Abortion—Continued Pregnancy

In very rare instances, some tissue is removed and yet the woman remains pregnant. This is more likely early in pregnancy (less than four weeks after conception, six weeks LMP). All clinics should inspect the tissue removed from the uterus right after the abortion to be sure that all the pregnancy tissue has been removed. Sometimes one pregnancy is removed but another remains. If this happens, signs of pregnancy are likely to continue. The abortion will have to be repeated in a week or so.

Postabortal Syndrome (Blood in the Uterus)

If the uterus doesn't contract properly or if a blood clot blocks the cervical opening and prevents blood from leaving the uterus, blood collects within it. As blood accumulates, pain, cramping and sometimes nausea increase. Sometimes you can push the clots out by deep massage directly over the uterus (pressing hard with your fingers just above the pubic bone). If this doesn't work, the clots need to be removed by reaspirating the uterus.

Possible Effect On Future Pregnancies

Having an abortion does not decrease the chances of having a healthy baby in the future. There is some indication that having several abortions may slightly increase chances of miscarriage or premature birth, but enough good research on this issue has not been done. (Dilating the cervix should be done as little and as gently as possible in order to minimize the chances of weakening it.)

ANESTHESIA

If you are going to have an abortion by a suction method, you may have the choice of using anesthesia (pain-reducing drugs). If you understand what your options are and how they may affect you, you can decide which type of anesthesia you prefer, or decide not to have any at all.

There are two basic types of anesthesia: *local*, which affects only the cervix, and *general*, which makes you unconscious ("asleep"). There is also a newer method that combines a local anesthetic with drugs that cause partial loss of consciousness. This is called *augment*.

Local anesthesia is injected into the cervix (neck of the uterus). It relaxes the cervical muscle, easing cramps that may occur when instruments such as dilators are passed through the cervix. Cramps caused by contractions of the uterus as it is emptied are not lessened by this method, however.

General anesthesia is usually given intravenously (injected into a vein in the arm). It causes unconsciousness; you won't see what's happening or feel pain but you may well hear what is being said. Augment anesthesia, such as narcotics or tranquilizers, is also given intravenously.

Any anesthetic drug has risks and complications, in addition to the risks of the abortion. With a local you may briefly experience ringing in your ears, tingling in your hands or feet or light-headedness. Seizures or serious allergic reactions are rare. If you have general anesthesia you may feel groggy, nauseated and disoriented after you wake up; some people do not feel well even a couple of days later. You may wake up with cramps.* Rarely, a serious reaction may damage the liver or other organs. In addition, general anesthesia increases some of the risks of the abortion itself. For example, there is more bleeding because the uterine muscle is more relaxed. There is also a greater chance of a serious perforation because doctors, unfortunately, have been known to be less gentle with the instruments if the woman is asleep and cannot complain about unusual pain. The risks, negative effects and recovery from augment vary with the particular drugs used, but generally last several hours or less.

For a first-trimester abortion, general or augment anesthesia is not medically necessary. For a second-trimester D and E, which takes longer and may be more uncomfortable, these strong drugs are more commonly used. Some women, for their own reasons, choose not to be awake. Most women find the cramps quite bearable with a local or no anesthetic.

I felt real good about my decision not to be put to sleep for my abortion. I found out that I have the strength to face my fear of pain. My cramps were bad for a few minutes, but I concentrated on deep breathing and held my counselor's hand. Ten minutes later I felt fine and ready to go home.

*These cramps may not be different from cramping after an abortion with local or no anesthesia, but it can be much harder to deal with them when you are waking up mentally affected by the anesthetic drugs.

With general or augment anesthesia you have little control over the abortion experience because you will most likely not be aware of what occurs during the procedure. Sometimes doctors or nurses will express hostility during those emotionally vulnerable minutes just before the drugs take effect and as they are wearing off.

During my last abortion...I was put to sleep....I couldn't deal with being awake....Before I went under, the doctor said to me, "This is your third abortion, isn't it? What birth control are you using?"

Unfortunately, it is hard to get evidence of how frequently this kind of emotional abuse occurs. Women are often either unconscious or partially conscious when it occurs, and any witnesses are medical personnel who find this kind of behavior acceptable or who will not risk their jobs and professional status by telling on other professionals.

Each woman's abortion experience is a unique one, within a known range of possibilities. No one can predict whether you will find the cramping painful or mild, or what the effects of anesthesia will be for you. Try to find out what drugs are used in the facility you go to. Information about drug effects and risks should be a part of your preparation for an abortion and will help you make the best choices if decisions are left up to you. Some facilities have a set way of doing things, and they may or may not respond to your requests.

Sometimes abortion facilities have their own reasons for using general or augment anesthesia for first-trimester abortions. A nurse-counselor at one abortion facility said:

Black and Hispanic women are all screamers. We try to give them general anesthesia so that they don't upset the other patients or the staff. Teenagers and Medicaid patients also should have a general.

There can also be financial motives for encouraging women to accept general anesthesia. With the woman unconscious there is no need to be reassuring or gentle during the procedure, and the doctor can work faster, performing more abortions and making more money.

ABORTION FACILITIES

This section refers to legal abortions, although with the current political situation our right to legal abor-

*This is an example of racist stereotyping as well as a value judgment by a woman whose culture approves of quiet and forbids loud noises to express emotions. Why should all women of a certain race, culture, economic status or age automatically be subjected to the health risks of general anesthesia, while middle-class white women are given the choice of a local anesthetic?

tions is in serious danger. How much choice you have about where your abortion takes place may depend on where you live, how much money you have or what your insurance will cover, how old you are, how far along you are in your pregnancy and which referral sources are available to you. Other people can be invaluable in helping you find an abortion service that fits your needs or, if only one facility is available, in helping you get your needs met as fully as possible.

Agencies That Can Help You Get an Abortion

There are a variety of responsible sources of information about where to get an abortion, but there are also profit-making referral agencies that get financial benefits from doctors or clinics for referrals. And some antiabortion groups masquerade as referral agencies, and then try to convince women not to have abortions. Feel free to leave or to hang up the phone if you're not getting the information you want. Whenever possible, take someone you trust with you.

Women's centers and feminist health centers often make referrals for abortion. They are listed in phone books, local newspapers and college campus directories. You can also get information from National Women's Health Network, 224 Seventh Street S.E., Washington, DC 20003, (202) 543-9222; National Abortion Federation Hotline, (800) 772-9100; Planned Parenthood; the yellow pages under Family Planning, Abortion, Birth Control or Pregnancy Testing; the gynecology clinic at a local non-Catholic hospital or neighborhood health center. Planned Parenthood has offices in almost every state, providing referrals and, in some areas, operating abortion clinics. (Quality of care at Planned Parenthood clinics may vary, but in some areas Planned Parenthood is the only resource.) If you are having difficulty finding facilities that perform second-trimester abortions, the NAF Hotline or Planned Parenthood in New York or San Francisco, cities where abortion is available up to twenty-four weeks at a fairly low cost, may be good places to call.

If abortion is made illegal again, many of these resources will not be available and counselors will not be able to offer information as easily or directly.

What to Look for in Choosing a Facility

There are different kinds of abortion facilities with a variety of medical procedures, prices, atmospheres and attitudes toward women. Most first-trimester abortions are done in free-standing clinics which are not part of hospitals. Their focus on abortion usually means lower prices, specifically trained counselors and medical practitioners with a lot of experience with abortions and a less intimidating atmosphere than a hospital. Abortions are also done in doctors' offices,

What You Need to Know

Whether you have to search to find one abortion service or you can choose among several facilities, ask questions beforehand. Not only must you get an idea of what to expect, but you can also prepare yourself to negotiate for options that may not be part of the standard procedures.

1. Cost? Must the fee be paid all at once? Will Medicaid or health insurance cover any of it? Is everything included or may there be additional charges (for example, for a Pap smear or for Rhogam)?

2. Are there age requirements or special consent requirements? Do I have to tell my parents or husband, get their consent and/or bring proof of age?

3. How long should I expect to be at the facility? Will everything be done in one visit?

4. Will childcare be provided for my child(ren)?

5. What do I need to bring with me?

6. Is there anything in my medical history that would interfere with my getting an abortion at that facility?

7. Can I bring someone with me? Can s/he stay with me throughout the counseling and the abortion procedure if that's what I want?

8. Will there be a counselor or nurse with me to provide information and support before, during and after the abortion?

9. Will there be staff people who speak my native language? If not, will the facility provide an interpreter?

10. Can the facility accommodate any special needs I have (for example, wheelchair accessibility)?

11. What type of abortion procedure will be done?

12. What anesthesia and other medications are available? What choices do I have?

13. Will the facility be responsible for routine follow-up? For treating complications? What type of backup services are available in case of emergency?

14. Will a breast exam, Pap smear and gonorrhea culture be done?

15. Will birth control be available if I want it?

Ask about *anything* that concerns you. Often the way the staff answers questions indicates their attitude toward women coming for abortions. Trust your feelings about the way you are treated on the phone as well as in person.

hospital outpatient clinics, and in hospitals, sometimes with an overnight stay. *A hospital setting is not necessary for first-trimester abortions except when certain serious health conditions require hospital emer-*

gency facilities to be immediately available. Second-trimester D and E abortions can also be performed safely in a properly equipped clinic or doctor's office. If you need a second-trimester abortion, try to locate a facility that has plenty of experience with these abortions. Because of price variations, local delays and differences in quality of service, it may be worthwhile to travel for a second-trimester abortion, especially if you can have a D and E by an experienced doctor rather than an induction abortion.

Women-owned and -controlled health centers offer pregnancy testing, counseling and, often, abortion services (see p. 609 for a list). Feminist clinics are owned and run by the women working there. As consumers themselves, they are aware of our need for good, supportive and affordable health care. They usually include health education as an essential part of quality health care. Unfortunately, there are not enough of these health centers, and their numbers are dwindling as economic pressure and political harassment intensify.

Clinics run by doctors or corporations, usually for profit, may have names similar to women-controlled clinics. The motivations of the people who own a facility affect the type of abortion procedure, information and counseling provided. You can ask who owns the business, their reasons for providing abortions and whether they support population control research, or political action on women's health issues.

The attitudes of counselors and medical staff toward women can greatly influence how we feel after the experience. Many clinic staff assume that women coming for abortions are irresponsible about birth control, ambivalent about abortion, heterosexual, and have only one male partner. Often clinic personnel are trained to believe that abortion is an emotionally traumatic experience for every woman. In fact, these assumptions are not true for most of us. Birth control methods do fail sometimes. Some of us thought that our fertility had ended early in menopause and were shocked to find ourselves pregnant. Lesbians, heterosexual women with more than one sex partner, women who have been raped—any woman may at some time need an abortion. Although abortion is not always an easy choice, it is often a very positive one. However, unsupportive, insensitive treatment by clinic staff can make an abortion unpleasant or worse.

Just because they give you a white woman to talk to don't mean you got counseled. She was nice; she gave me good information. I'm explaining to her how I feel about this whole thing. She tells me that she thinks that I'm not ready to have an abortion and she's going to send me home. Well, I hit the roof! "You're going to send me home? Do you know how hard it is to get here?" She didn't understand what I was saying to her. I was saying, "Yeah, if I had a baby I could deal with it. I have to deal with anything that comes up. This is how my life has been, *how my mother's life, all the people I knows life has been. You deal with whatever shit happens. But if I had a choice, I would prefer not to have this baby. And since I do have this choice, this is what I want to do."*

She interpreted that as being not sure and feeling maybe I do want to have a baby. "Yeah, I want to have a baby, but not now, not now! I love kids." And she didn't understand. They sent me home. It was a really big mess. I was furious....

I honestly believe that she thought she was being sensitive. She thinks she's doing a great job. I just don't think she understood. And then, when I was trying to tell her that she wasn't hearing what I was saying to her, she didn't hear that, because she was in the position where I was the person that was "in need of help" and she was the "counselor," so of course what she thought was right, period. And I think she did throw some of her judgments on me. I think that a lot of the problem was she was white and I was black. She didn't understand what it meant to me, a black woman, and I guess to black women, period, to have a baby.

A staff member at a feminist health clinic says:

At our clinic counselors are trained to help each woman sort out her feelings. We do not invade anyone's privacy if she tells us that her decision is clear, not coerced, and that she does not want to discuss her reasons or feelings. Women talk with each other, not just with the counselor. We provide very detailed and accurate information about the abortion procedure, including risks and complications. Local anesthetic, a mild tranquilizer and mild painkillers are offered as options, with discussion of possible benefits and disadvantages of each drug. If a woman wants, she can have a friend stay with her during the abortion, although we have found that some friends are a distraction rather than a help. Counselors learn many specific ways to help a woman cope with nervousness or pain. Our practitioners are required to respond to requests to slow down, except when this would endanger the woman's physical safety. When there is a decision to be made, the woman herself is an active participant.

We have made changes in our procedures because of input from clients and from nonmedical staff. Our goal is to treat each woman with the same kind of respect that we ourselves want shown to us, and I think we do a pretty good job! I wish women could walk into any medical facility feeling that we deserve to be treated with respect and demanding it when it isn't there. We should stop feeling grateful every time we are not overtly abused.

HAVING A VACUUM ASPIRATION ABORTION

The large majority of abortions currently done in the U.S. are first-trimester vacuum aspiration proce-

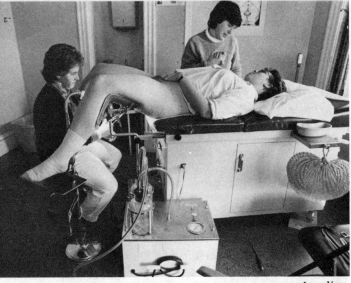

Lynn Vera

dures in an outpatient clinic. Clinics vary a great deal, and your experience may be very different from another woman's, even at the same clinic.

Medical Preliminaries

After arriving at the clinic, you will fill out a medical history form. A health worker will draw blood to check for the Rh factor* and for anemia, do another pregnancy test and check your pulse, blood pressure and temperature (vital signs).

Counseling

Most clinics provide individual and/or group counseling. The counselor explains the abortion procedure and what to expect afterward. She may also talk about birth control options. The counseling session is a time for you to ask questions and express any fears or concerns, especially about the pregnancy or the abortion. Being in a group provides an opportunity to talk with other women who are having abortions. Discussing your experiences together can help you feel clearer, stronger and less alone.

*Blood is either Rh positive or Rh negative. When an Rh-negative woman carries an Rh-positive fetus, antibodies against the Rh factor can build up in her blood. The most likely time for this to happen is at the end of the pregnancy, whether by abortion, miscarriage or birth. In a later pregnancy these antibodies can react against an Rh-positive fetus, causing serious harm and even endangering its survival. An injection of a blood derivative (one brand name is Rhogam) within seventy-two hours after the end of every pregnancy usually prevents antibody formation. If you need Rhogam, it should be given before you leave the clinic.

The two rooms where the abortions were done opened onto the porch where the six of us were waiting. One girl from the group, who had said she never had a pelvic examination in her life, was just coming out of the abortion room. She had just had her abortion and looked okay. That was comforting. A seventeen-year-old girl came in. She was very scared. I held her hand and comforted her. I hadn't had my abortion yet and was scared, too (although I'd had one operation, two children and a D and C with a spinal). Something amazing happened when I held her hand. Any fear I'd had disappeared as if it were drawn out of me. We were all such different women who for varying reasons were having the identical physical thing done to us.

The Abortion

The counselor will take you to the exam room after you go to the bathroom. Before the abortion itself, the practitioner performs a bimanual exam to feel the size and position of your uterus, confirming the stage of pregnancy. S/he needs this information to decide how large a cannula to use and the angle at which to insert instruments safely. If you've never had a pelvic exam, tell your counselor. Whether this is your first exam or you have had others, make sure that the practitioner goes slowly, is gentle, explains what is happening and allows you to have some control over the procedure.

Next, the practitioner inserts a speculum into your vagina, separating the vaginal walls to see the cervix. You may feel pressure but this should not hurt. Have the practitioner readjust the speculum if it pinches. A gonorrhea culture should be taken, and a Pap smear if you haven't had one recently.

The practitioner thoroughly wipes your vagina with antiseptic solution to help prevent infection. If you are having a local anesthetic, it is injected into the cervix. Since the cervix has very few nerve endings, you may not feel this at all, or it may feel like a pinch or pressure. Next, a tenaculum is attached to the cervix to keep the cervix steady. You may feel a pinch, cramp or nothing at all. Some practitioners then measure the inside of the uterus with a thin rod called a sound; others believe that this is not necessary. Sounding may cause a short cramp. The cervical opening is gradually stretched by inserting and removing dilators of increasingly large sizes. You will probably feel some kind of cramping, perhaps similar to mild or stronger menstrual cramps. Two to eight dilators may be used. Dilating usually takes less than two minutes.

A sterile strawlike tube is inserted through the cervix into the uterus. Cannulas are made in different diameters, from the size of a small drinking straw to the size of a large pen (five to twelve millimeters). The later the pregnancy, the larger the cannula needed to remove it. Tubing connects the cannula to a bottle. The aspirator, a motorized suction machine, creates a vacuum in the bottle. As the cannula is moved along

301

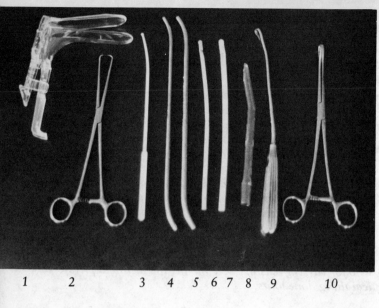

1   2   3 4 5 6 7 8 9   10

Lynn Vera

1: speculum
2: tenaculum
3: sound
4 and 5: dilators
6 and 7: flexible plastic cannulas
8: rigid plastic cannula
9: curette
10: forceps

the uterine walls, gentle suction draws pregnancy tissue out through the cannula and tubing into the bottle. The aspiration usually takes no more than a few minutes, depending on how many weeks pregnant you are.

Forceps may also be used to remove tissue. Some practitioners insert a curette and scrape the inside of the uterus to check that it is completely empty. Others think that this additional step is unnecessary. It causes extra bleeding, increases the risk of perforation, lengthens the abortion and causes discomfort or pain.

As the uterus is emptied, it starts to contract to its nonpregnant size. These contractions can range from hardly noticeable to painful cramps—each woman is different. Breathing deeply and in a regular pattern, especially with the help of a counselor or friend, can help you to relax your body, "riding through" the cramps. It is also important to keep your stomach muscles as relaxed as possible and not to move around. Cramps should lessen immediately after the cannula is removed or within the next ten minutes or so.

After the Abortion

After wiping out your vagina and checking for bleeding, the practitioner will remove the speculum. Then you can move into a more comfortable room to sit or lie down for a while. You may feel weak, tired, crampy or nauseous for a while, or you may be ready to get up immediately. Before you leave, a counselor should explain aftercare instructions (what to expect and watch for). Your vital signs, cramping and bleeding should be checked before you leave.

The abortion itself was very uncomfortable, like having an IUD put in but more intense. It didn't last long and the doctor was good.

I received no counseling of any kind from the doctor. There was, however, a beautiful, middle-aged nurse there who explained the whole procedure carefully and stayed with me. I especially appreciated her because while I was not particularly frightened of the abortion itself, I was, and still am, terrified of doctors and hospitals.

The abortion itself was amazingly quick and painless (considering the propaganda to the contrary). I spent an hour lying down to recover. I remember being elated—it was over and it had been so simple!

It hurt so much. It was incredible. The people at the clinic were really sweet and helpful but they should have told me how much it was going to hurt. What hurt the most was that I could feel when they were scraping around inside. I've talked to a lot of girls who said the same thing happened to them when they were really far along. That's why it pays to have an abortion as early as possible.

I experienced some pain with the procedure but mostly it was just a series of new sensations. I had never been so aware of my uterus.

When I found out I was pregnant I was numb, unfeeling. This scared and confused me. I had never blocked my feelings so totally or unconsciously before. I wonder now if that's why the abortion itself was so physically painful.

SECOND-TRIMESTER ABORTIONS

Very often, women choose second-trimester abortions because they were unable to get the money together in time to have first-trimester abortions. Ironically, a later abortion is an additional financial drain: it costs more, requires more time off from work and may involve extra expenses for travel to an appropriate facility. Other reasons for second-trimester abortions may include errors in pregnancy detection: false-negative pregnancy tests or inaccurate uterine sizing by medical practitioners. Women who were pregnant when they started taking birth control pills or who were not told that it is possible to get pregnant with an IUD in place sometimes do not even suspect pregnancy for several months. Some states now require women under eighteen to get parental consent or a court order, which can result in delays of weeks or even months. Occasionally a woman (especially a teenager) may not admit the possibility of pregnancy. Because she lacks support, money or information, she may feel afraid, overwhelmed and unprepared to deal with pregnancy, so she denies it, hoping it will somehow go away on its own. Given these all-too-common situations, a woman may come to the experience of a later abortion already emotionally exhausted.

A large percentage of women who are forced to seek second-trimester abortions are young, poor or women of color. They bear the brunt of attitudes that "blame the victim." A woman may be treated as though she is stupid and/or irresponsible and deserves to be "punished" by an unsupportive atmosphere and a painful experience.

Most doctors and hospitals choose not to perform second-trimester abortions. Someone from Planned Parenthood told us, "Many doctors wish the problem would go away." In February 1975, a Boston jury convicted Dr. Kenneth Edelin of manslaughter for performing a routine hysterotomy on a woman whose pregnancy was between twenty and twenty-eight weeks LMP. Though the Boston jury's decision was reversed in a higher court and Dr. Edelin was acquitted of the charges, hospitals around the country (never enthusiastic about late abortions in the first place) have reacted by closing down their second-trimester abortion services, or by bringing in costly equipment to try to keep alive fetuses which show signs of life when expelled (costs to be passed on to the woman).

Abortion, Amniocentesis and Disability

We believe that the availability of amniocentesis (see p. 356) with the option for abortion if serious genetic defects are found should not conflict with our commitment to build a better world for people with disabilities. The disability rights movement has pointed out the danger in equating the presence of a genetic defect with the notion of a life not worth living. A woman should have the right to bear a child with a disability and not be punished by lack of support for that choice. All of us can reach out and create networks of information so that a woman confronting the diagnosis of Down's syndrome or any other serious disability in her fetus can meet other parents and children living with these conditions, and learn realistically about the quality, cost and availability of the services that make such lives better.

The Advantages of the D and E Procedure

The D and E has several advantages over the induced-miscarriage procedures more commonly used for abortions in the second three months of pregnancy. Not only is the D and E safer, but it is physically and emotionally easier for a woman than an induction

TABLE 17:5* EFFECTIVENESS AND COMPLICATIONS OF ABORTIONS PERFORMED AT THIRTEEN WEEKS GESTATION BY D AND E, SALINE AND PROSTAGLANDIN F2A†

Outcomes	Intraamniotic Instillation		
	D and E‡		PGF$_2$a‡
Effectiveness			
Success rate	99.90	97.60	92.50
Induction–abortion time (hours)	0.50	29.20	24.80
Specific complication§			
Incomplete abortion	0.90	28.27	36.10
Hemorrhage	0.71	1.86	5.80
Transfusion	0.19	0.96	1.53
Cervical laceration or fistula	1.16	0.55	0.64
Convulsions	0.02	0.08	0.32
Uterine perforation	0.32	0.05	0.16
Any complication	5.83	37.45	53.26

*This table appears in Robert A. Hatcher, et al., *Contraceptive Technology*, New York: Irvington Publications, Inc., 1982, p. 178.

†Source: W. Cates, D. A. Grimes, K. Schulz, H. W. Ory and C.W. Tyler. "World Health Organization Studies of prostaglandins versus saline as abortifacients," *Obstet Gynecol* 52.493, October 1978.

‡Data derived from the Joint Program for the Study of Abortion under the auspices of the Centers for Disease Control.

§Complications per 100 procedures.

abortion, where she goes through labor and delivery of a fetus, often while in a hospital room by herself. D and E is much quicker (ten to forty-five minutes, compared to many hours with an overnight stay in a hospital for induction abortion), and complications are less likely, although more studies are needed. D and E can be done in a properly equipped doctor's office or clinic with local anesthetic and perhaps also a tranquilizer, although most are still done in hospitals using general anesthesia. A few doctors are doing the D and E procedures through twenty-four weeks LMP with good results, although a limit of sixteen, eighteen or twenty weeks is more common.

The biggest problem with D and E, however, is that it is not widely available. There are not enough people yet trained to do D and E procedures, especially in the eighteen- to twenty-four-week LMP range. Many doctors dislike the idea of removing a second-trimester fetus by performing a D and E. They would rather provide induction abortions, which do not require their presence after the injection. (The woman and the nursing staff are left to deal with the aborted fetus.) Unfortunately, not enough doctors are willing to accept the personal strain of doing D and E's. We need more doctors who place greater priority on the fact that *a D and E is both safer and less upsetting for women.*

In some places a D and E costs more than an induction abortion. Or a D and E may be available to women who can afford private gynecologists or to women who can afford to travel to another state but not to women who must get their medical care from local government-funded clinics and teaching hospitals. This kind of unconscionable discrimination means that women who have less money are forced to accept an induction procedure, which involves more pain, more time and more chance of health complications.

HAVING A SECOND-TRIMESTER INSTILLATION ABORTION

Choosing a Facility

Having an induction abortion from sixteen to twenty-four weeks of pregnancy is a more difficult experience than a first-trimester abortion or a second-trimester D and E abortion. There may be hours of uncomfortable labor as the uterus contracts to open the cervix and expel the fetus. The complication and mortality rates, though no higher than for full-term pregnancy and delivery, are higher than for earlier abortions or D and E by a skilled doctor. Emotionally, too, it can be a hard experience, even when you are very sure you do not want to have a baby. The pain and/or discomfort, the length of time, the similarity of the experience to delivery of a baby, an intimidating or unsupportive hospital atmosphere and the influence of a very vocal part of society that says that later abortions are "bad"—these factors can make induction abortion upsetting.

Pay attention to both emotional and physical needs when choosing a facility. (Unfortunately, it may be difficult to find *any* medical facility near you where second-trimester abortions are performed). Doctors usually do induction abortions in general hospitals where the quality of care and degree of personal attention vary greatly. A few small hospitals and clinics specializing in abortion try to make late abortion as comfortable as possible. Some hospitals have a separate second-trimester abortion unit with counseling and special staff. They avoid insensitive treatment such as placing abortion patients in rooms with women who are having babies. In any hospital you may be left alone a lot, not told clearly what is being done to you, not offered enough pain medication (if you want it). Unfortunately, if you do not have the time and money to travel for an abortion, you may have to accept whatever kind of care you can find. Talk with the doctor beforehand, as well as the hospital, about the type of care you want to receive. Try to bring a friend who can give you support and help see that your needs are respected and responded to.

A COMPARISON OF SALINE AND PROSTAGLANDIN ABORTIONS

In an induction abortion the practitioner injects a miscarriage-causing solution through the abdomen into the amniotic sac and uterine contractions expel the fetus. The two most commonly used solutions are a saline (salt) solution, which usually causes fetal death followed by uterine contractions, or the prostaglandin F_2a, which causes labor contractions. Sometimes urea or saline is added to a prostaglandin solution. In some hospitals you will have a choice of methods if you are firm about requesting it. Also, refer back to the table of complications on p. 303.

Saline solution has a lower complication rate, a lower rate of incomplete abortion and consequent D and C, and a lower chance of having to repeat the injection. The disadvantages of saline include a longer wait before labor begins and a slight risk of serious emergency, such as shock, and possibly death if careless instillation allows salt to enter a blood vessel. Liver or kidney problems, heart failure, high blood pressure and sickle cell anemia are medical reasons not to have a saline abortion.

The prostaglandin F_2a works more quickly and does not have the same risk of serious emergency carried by saline. However, it has more negative effects, including nausea, vomiting and diarrhea; a higher rate of failure of the first instillation; a higher rate of excessive bleeding and retained placenta (requiring immediate D and C). The labor contractions are usually faster, sharper and more painful, and there is a risk of the cervix tearing. (Use of laminaria to stretch the cervix before contractions begin may reduce this risk.) In very rare cases the fetus is expelled with signs of life and does not expire until shortly afterward. Medical reasons to avoid prostaglandin are a history of convulsions, epilepsy and asthma.

Preliminaries

Read the box (p. 299) for suggestions of questions to ask when you set up an appointment. Plan to be at the hospital overnight. If you are having an out-of-town abortion, make sure before you go that you have the name and phone number of a doctor or clinic at home to call in case of questions or complications after the abortion.

The same tests and examinations are necessary as for suction abortion. In taking your medical history, the medical staff should check for conditions which would contraindicate use of saline or prostaglandin methods. If you are going to have a prostaglandin abortion, the hospital may ask you to come in the day before for insertion of laminaria.

The Procedure

Instillation

The doctor cleans your abdomen, numbs a small area below your navel with a local anesthetic and then inserts a needle through the skin into your uterus. This may sound scary, but you will probably feel only a slight cramp when the needle enters your uterus. For saline, some amniotic fluid is removed. The miscarriage-inducing solution is slowly injected into the amniotic sac. You may experience pressure or a bloated feeling. If you are having saline and feel waves of heat, dizziness, backache, extreme dryness or thirst, tell the doctor right away; this may indicate that the salt is entering a blood vessel, which is dangerous.

Waiting

It will take hours before the labor contractions begin; from eight to twenty-four or more with saline and less with prostaglandin. Medication can relieve nausea and diarrhea caused by prostaglandin. If labor contractions don't begin within the expected time, oxytocin may be given to stimulate contractions. This carries a risk of rupture of the uterus if contractions are too strong. Sometimes the instillation is done a second time.

Contractions

At first contractions will probably feel like mild cramps. Later you may feel a lot of pressure in the rectal area and then a gushing of liquid from the vagina—this is the breaking of the amniotic sac (bag of waters). Each woman's labor is different in terms of how long it takes and how it feels. When prostaglandin or oxytocin is used, contractions are quicker and sharper than with saline.

As a rule the contractions are not as strong as those of full-term labor and delivery, but they can be painful. Relaxation, deep breathing or panting can help make the later contractions easier to tolerate. Sitting or squatting may be the most comfortable, though hospital staff may want you to lie down. Support and comfort from a friend can help, too. No general anesthesia is given, but tranquilizers and pain medication should be offered if they won't slow down the labor.

Expulsion

Eventually the contractions will expel the fetus and, within an hour, the placenta.

Recovery

You will probably stay in the hospital for some hours after the abortion. If all of the placenta was not expelled, you may need an aspiration procedure or a D and C to remove the retained tissue. Aftercare is the same as for a suction abortion.

AFTER AN ABORTION

Aftercare

Women have a variety of experiences after an abortion. Most of us feel fine and do not have any problems, but some feel tired or have cramps for several days. Bleeding ranges from none at all to two to three weeks of light to moderate flow, which may stop and then start again. Signs of pregnancy may last up to a week. Some women experience a variety of changes four to seven days after an abortion because of the drop in hormone levels that happens at this time. Because of the drop in hormone levels at this time, bleeding, cramping, breast soreness and/or feelings of depression may increase or appear if they have not been present.

Here is a list of ways to take care of yourself after an abortion:

1. Try to follow what your body needs—rest for a day or so if you feel tired. (If you can't rest because you have no one to help take care of your children or you have to go to work to keep from losing your job, you may recover more slowly.) Avoid heavy lifting or strenuous exercise in the next few days, as it may increase your bleeding. Drinking alcohol may also have this effect. Sometimes Ergotrate or Methergine (drugs that stimulate the uterus to contract) is prescribed on the theory that it may keep bleeding to a minimum and help expel any tissue retained in the uterus.

2. To help prevent infection, don't put anything into your vagina. This will avoid introducing germs that may travel up into your uterus before it has had a chance to heal completely. Don't use tampons, take tub baths, swim, douche or have intercourse for two to three weeks.*

3. Watch for signs of complications. If you have fever of 100.5 degrees Fahrenheit or higher, severe cramping or pain, foul-smelling vaginal discharge, vomiting, fainting, excessive bleeding (soaking an entire pad in an hour or less or passing quarter-sized clots) or signs of pregnancy that last longer than a week, report this to the clinic or doctor immediately. If you often get high on alcohol or drugs during this time, you may

---

*You may have been given antibiotics (usually tetracycline or ampicillin). Some people think that this cuts down the chance of developing infection; others think you should never take unnecessary antibiotics. They may also mask signs of infection. If you do decide to take antibiotics, be sure to take them according to directions.

not be alert enough to pay attention to these warning signals. Remember that complications are rare, but they do happen to some of us. It is not your fault if you have a complication. If a complication is not taken care of as soon as possible, it might turn into a serious situation, so don't ignore possible warning signs. Often a call to the clinic will reassure you that what is happening to you is not a complication after all, but within a range of normal experience.

After the abortion, I had retained tissue. I needed a reaspiration [basically, a second abortion] to prevent an infection and remove the remaining tissue. Although the national rate of complications is very low, I was enraged to be a statistic. I had decided to terminate my pregnancy, but I didn't expect another abortion one week later. I didn't have any choice but to see it through and get my body back to normal.

4. Often the place where you had the abortion is the best source of information and medical advice or care in case of a possible complication. Call them if anything is bothering you, even if you cannot go back there for care. If you need follow-up medical attention, try to consult people who are experienced in treating women who have had legal abortions. Stay away from hospitals, clinics and practitioners who believe in forced motherhood and are against abortion. They may try to make you feel that you "deserve" the complication as "punishment" for having had an abortion, and they may not be well informed about proper treatment for postabortion problems.

5. It is important to get a checkup in two to three weeks. A pelvic exam gives information about the small possibility of retained tissue or infection that may not be causing any symptoms yet. Also, you can get any routine gynecological care which was not done at the time of the abortion. This is often a good time to discuss birth control, which may have been difficult to talk about at the time of the abortion. A feminist health center should offer you a chance to learn more about your body, including breast and cervical self-examination techniques. You may also be asked to talk about what's been happening since your abortion—both body changes and feelings. It can be especially helpful to talk with other women who have had abortions recently. Most of us are reassured by having questions discussed and learning that our experiences have happened to other women, too. If you are one of the few women who has a continuing problem or complication, you need good information and medical help until the problem is over.

6. Your next period will probably start four to eight weeks after your abortion. *You can get pregnant immediately after an abortion, even before your next period, so you need to use reliable birth control if you have intercourse and don't want another pregnancy.* You may say and believe, "I'll never have intercourse again, so I don't need birth control." And although there are many wonderful ways of making love without intercourse (see Chapter 11, "Sexuality,"), you may later change your mind. *One thing that you have in common with all women having abortions is that you know you can get pregnant.* If you weren't sure before, you know beyond any doubt that you need to use birth control if you have intercourse again and do not want to become pregnant.

Choosing a birth control method is a very individual matter (see Chapter 13, "Birth Control"). Some facilities will encourage you to use certain methods, especially pills, which you can start taking the day of a first-trimester abortion. If you do this, you will be protected after the first cycle of pills, four weeks later. However, the hormonelike drugs of the pills affect your whole body and can cause changes that are similar to signs of pregnancy, which could be confusing right after an abortion. It is probably not a good idea to have an IUD inserted at the time of an abortion, because of greater risks of infection and perforation. Also, the IUD effects of cramping and bleeding may mask the symptoms of an abortion-related infection. A diaphragm or cervical cap can be fitted or refitted at the postabortion checkup. You can start a natural birth control class after an abortion or obtain foam and condoms from a drugstore without a prescription. If the clinic or practitioner encourages you to use "the Shot" (Depo-Provera) or be sterilized, be sure to find out about the risks and the other methods that are more likely to allow you to become pregnant later if you want to. (See Chapter 13 for discussion of the reversibility of various methods of birth control.)

Feelings After an Abortion

Positive, negative or mixed feelings are all natural after an abortion. For most of us the end of an unwanted pregnancy brings relief. Many women experience sadness as well as a sense of loss. We may feel new strength in having made and carried out an important, often difficult decision.

I left the clinic with my friend, feeling two ways about the whole experience: one, that I'd had as good and supportive an abortion experience as a woman could have; and two, I never want to put myself in the position of having to go through it again.

The ambivalence I felt throughout this experience will probably never be resolved. This abortion occurred at a difficult time for me. I had just lost my mother and was entering the end of my reproductive years....The experience has left me with a sense of loss. I do not consciously regret the decision I made, but I often think of the child I might have had.

It was best for my peace of mind. It meant my two children would have a life of quality rather than a mother with too many responsibilities. In the six years that have passed I have never regretted it.

There aren't too many people who know that I've had an abortion. No matter how legal it is, I was raised with the notion that abortion is a bad thing to do.

I was so relieved not to be pregnant anymore that I didn't think I had any sad feelings at all. Then, a few days later, on my way to a friend's house, I saw a young couple walking a new baby and I burst out crying there on the street.

The major mistake was in not handling my grief (which was real, even though there was no question about the rightness of the decision) at the time. It's only come up in the past two years.

Severe depression after an abortion is extremely rare. In fact, it is much less likely than severe depression after childbirth. A few women experience feelings of sadness or depression years later at around the time of year when they had the abortion or when they would have given birth.

Women sometimes feel guilty, which is understandable in a society that doesn't particularly accept the choice of abortion. So much emphasis is put on motherhood that many people act as though a fetus is more important than a woman. Some women feel guilty about ending the potential for life.

Guilt can sometimes give rise to fears of "punishment." Some of us become afraid that we will not be able to have a baby if we want to in the future. The antiabortion movement plays on these fears. Some women are so affected that they become pregnant again soon after an abortion to reassure themselves that they have not lost their fertility.

If you were not able to work through your feelings before the abortion, you may feel troubled afterwards. Being able to talk about your feelings with a sympathetic and objective friend, relative, counselor or group is the most important thing you can do to help you feel better, resolve difficulties and move on.

Fortunately, all my conflicts about the abortion were resolved about a year and a half later, when I found the courage to speak of it in a women's group I was in. Because of the calmness and caring the other women shared with me, as well as some of their own experiences with abortion, I came away from that meeting feeling that this thing that had haunted me for so long was finally resolved. I no longer felt bitter about the only choice I could possibly have made in order not to totally wreck my own life and that of others.

If you would like help from someone with special training, the facility where you had the abortion or any of the groups mentioned earlier in this chapter can refer you to someone to talk with—social worker, counselor, clergy person—or to a postabortion support group.

Unfortunately, many of us do not have an opportunity to be part of a support group or to talk about our feelings. Some of us grew up in families or cultures where feelings were never talked about at all, and it may be hard for us to say anything about our feelings, even if we do have a supportive place to talk. We may have other ways besides talking to resolve difficult feelings: yelling, crying, prayer, music, meditation, art, athletics or physical activity. Some of us block our feelings rather than feel them, joke about them rather than talk seriously, put them away and deal with them later or take pride in getting through something on our own without expressing our feelings. We must respect the different ways women deal with feelings.

Sometimes the abortion provokes other changes. Relationships may end. The whole experience may strengthen a relationship or give us strength to make other positive changes in our lives.

My boyfriend's attitude afterward was depressingly callous. His idea was, Well, it's over now; why bother thinking about it? That's when I started to have to pull away from him emotionally.

By learning to share my experiences with other women, I've been able to develop more intimate relationships and resolve my emotional dilemma. I've also found a women's clinic where the nurse-practitioners don't treat you like an object and are genuinely concerned about their patients' welfare and will answer any questions patiently and thoroughly.

I feel good in recalling the support I received from my husband, friends and family. And just for the record— all my doctors are now women.

Some of us have negative feelings about sex, or intercourse in particular, for a while after the abortion.

For a good month or two I felt like sex was repulsive. We'd start to make love and I'd feel, I hope I don't have to pay for this. Also, I was using a diaphragm for the first time, and I didn't really trust it yet.

On the other hand, some of us had a chance to choose a reliable method of birth control for the first time after the abortion, and we are more relaxed about sex. We may be angry and bitter if we had to have an abortion because we did not have the resources—decent jobs, daycare, education, food—to raise a child. We may be angry about the reactions of friends, family or the man with whom we became pregnant, and about disrespectful treatment or bad medical care from the abortion facility.

The service they gave me and the follow-up they gave me, plus the method of birth control they gave me—all that stuff was not adequate....They told me I had an infection but yet still they gave me an IUD.

If your birth control method failed, if you didn't use birth control, if you were pressured into having intercourse when you didn't really want to or if you were raped, you may feel angry about the abortion. And you may be angry if you did not get needed support.

Even though my husband was very supportive, I felt angry—not so much because he put the sperm into me as because he in no way could understand what I had experienced.

Some of us choose to translate our feelings into action: do political work to keep abortion legal, work for improvements in abortion services, demand daycare and jobs, fight against restrictions that prevent Medicaid or insurance from paying for abortions, educate our daughters about sex, help a friend who is dealing with an unwanted pregnancy.

I started doing counseling a short while after my first illegal abortion. Someone would call me to find out where to get an abortion. I would automatically ask them to come to my home and would spend time talking about it....I would spend anywhere from an hour or two to a whole day doing the "counseling." I would, of course, ask for a report back as to the conditions they found and how they felt. I very seldom got this feedback but found it very helpful when I did get it, sometimes to the detriment of the doctor....If a woman had a bad experience, I would not refer to that doctor again until I had been able to check him out some other way.

HISTORY AND POLITICS OF ABORTION

Anthropological studies show abortion to be widespread in ancient and preindustrial societies throughout the world, throughout history. In the Western world, before Christianity, Greeks and Romans considered abortion acceptable during the early stages of pregnancy.

Over several centuries and in different cultures there is a rich history of women helping each other to abort. Until the late 1800s women healers in Western Europe and the United States provided abortions and trained other women to do so, without legal prohibitions.

In other parts of the world today skilled women abortionists still practice, despite the expansion of institutionalized medicine. In Thailand, Malaysia and the Philippines, for example, village abortionists continue their traditional technique of abortion by massage.

From its beginnings Christianity was ambivalent about abortion, though for many centuries the Catholic Church permitted abortion until the fetus became "animated" by the "rational soul."* American and English common law dating back to the thirteenth century tolerated abortion up until "quickening," the moment at about twenty weeks when a pregnant woman first feels the fetus move.

Neither Church nor State prohibited abortion until the nineteenth century, nor did the Catholic Church lead in this new repression. Britain first passed anti-abortion laws in 1803, which then became stricter throughout the century. The United States followed, as individual states began to outlaw abortion at any stage of pregnancy. By 1880 most abortions were illegal in the U.S., except those "necessary to save the life of the woman." But the tradition of women's right to early abortion was rooted in American society by then; abortionists continued to practice openly with public support, and juries refused to convict them.

When, in 1869, Pope Pius IV declared all abortion to be murder and removed the concept of animation from Church law, the Catholic Church assumed its crusading role against abortion.

Abortion suddenly became a crime and a sin for a number of reasons. A trend of humanitarian reform in the mid-nineteenth century broadened liberal support for criminalization of abortion, because it was at that time a dangerous procedure done with crude methods, few antiseptics and high mortality rates. But this alone cannot explain the attack on abortion. For instance, other risky surgical techniques were considered necessary for people's health and welfare and were not prohibited. "Protecting" women from the dangers of abortion was actually meant to control them and restrict them to their traditional childbearing role. Antiabortion legislation was part of an antifeminist backlash to the growing movements for suffrage, voluntary motherhood and other women's rights in the nineteenth century. The prevailing public prudery and antisexual moralism condemned feminism and considered sex for pleasure evil, with pregnancy as punishment.† At the same time male doctors were

---

*Abortion was considered murder and severely punished only after "animation," thought to occur forty days after conception for a male fetus and eighty or ninety days after conception for a female. (Once again the Church thinks that males must come first! But no one knows how they determined the sex of the fetus.)

†Anthony Comstock, fanatical secretary of the New York Society for the Prevention of Vice, was responsible for legislation in 1873 which banned "obscene" materials from the U.S. mail—including anything to do with contraception or abortion. Also see Linda Gordon's *Woman's Body, Woman's Right*, New York: Penguin Books, 1977.

tightening their control over the medical profession. Doctors considered midwives, who attended births and performed abortions as part of their regular practice, a threat to their own economic and social power. The medical establishment actively took up the antiabortion cause in the second half of the nineteenth century as part of its effort to eliminate midwives.

Finally, many countries were concerned about declining populations in the nineteenth century. In the interest of increasing its own numbers, the Catholic Church justified its ban on abortion with the biological rationale that life begins at conception. Developing industries and expanding territories in the U.S. needed workers and farmers. With the declining birth rate among whites in the late 1800s, the U.S. government and the eugenics movement urged white, native-born women to reproduce, and warned against the danger of "race suicide."* Budding industrial capitalism relied on women to be unpaid household workers, low-paid menial workers, reproducers and socializers of the next generation of workers. Without legal abortion, women found it more difficult to resist the limitations of these roles.

Then, as now, making abortion illegal neither eliminated the need for abortion nor prevented its practice. In the 1890s, doctors estimated that there were two million abortions a year in the United States. A recent study in New York City showed that over 45 percent of women who had legal abortions would have tried to get them even if they had been illegal.

Women who are determined not to carry an unwanted pregnancy have always found some way to try to abort. Lacking better alternatives, all too often they have resorted to dangerous, sometimes deadly methods, such as inserting knitting needles or coat hangers into the vagina and uterus, douching with dangerous solutions like lye and swallowing strong drugs or chemicals. The coat hanger has become a symbol of the desperation of millions of women who have risked death to end a pregnancy. When these attempts harmed them, it was hard for them to obtain medical treatment; when these methods failed, women still had to find an abortionist.

Illegal Abortion

Many of us do not know what it was like to need an abortion before legalization. Women who could afford to pay skilled doctors or go to another country had the safest and easiest abortions. Most women found it difficult if not impossible to arrange and pay for medical abortions.

*"Race purity must be maintained, we must have more native white births." (Teddy Roosevelt, 1905, quoted in Angela Davis, *Race, Sex and Class*, Chapter 12, footnote 13, in Melvin Steinfeld, *Our Racist Presidents*. San Ramon, CA: Consensus Publishers, 1972, p. 212.)

With one exception the doctors whom I asked for an abortion treated me with contempt, their attitudes ranging from hostile to insulting. One said to me, "You tramps like to break the rules, but when you get caught you all come crawling for help in the same way."

The secret world of illegal abortion was frightening and expensive. Many of the laywomen and some of the doctors who performed abortions were both skilled and dedicated. But most doctors (and those who claimed to be doctors) cared only about being well rewarded for their trouble. In the 1960s abortionists often turned women away if they could not pay 1,000 dollars or more in cash. Some male abortionists insisted on having sexual relations before the abortion.

Abortionists emphasized speed and their own protection. They often didn't use anesthesia because it took too long for women to recover, and they wanted women out of the office as quickly as possible. Some abortionists were rough and sadistic. Almost no one explained what was happening, discussed birth control techniques or took adequate precautions against hemorrhage or infection.

Typically, the abortionist would forbid the woman to contact him or her again. Often she wouldn't know his or her real name. If a complication occurred, harassment by the law was a frightening possibility. The need for secrecy created isolation for women having abortions and those providing them.

The woman who did my abortion did not charge very much. No one in our neighborhood had much money, and finding a "doctor" to do an abortion was impossible. After I got home, I developed a high fever. I was so sick I was delirious with the pain and fever. My mother took me to the emergenccy ward. The doctors asked her who had done the abortion. When she didn't tell them, they refused to treat me. They said that they would let me die if she didn't tell them the name and address of the abortionist. Frightened, she gave them a false name and address and then they started treatment for me. When the police went to arrest the abortionist and found out that my mother had given false information, they went to my house and arrested my husband. They kept him in jail for several days until he agreed to give the information they wanted. The police took him with them to the woman's house to be sure he had told the truth. He called out to her in Spanish to warn her that the police were there, but they made him be quiet. Even though I almost died, I felt that the woman had done the best she could and had been trying to help me when I was desperate and had nowhere else to turn. It would have been impossible for me to have another child then. I hope other women will never have to go through what I experienced—to be treated like a criminal even when you need immediate medical care.

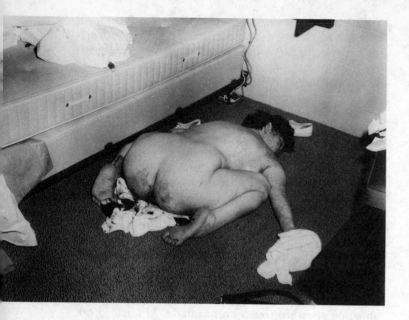

Woman dead on motel room floor. Her death was due to an air embolism suffered during an illegal abortion.

Files of Dr. Milton Halpern, Former Medical Examiner, New York City

In the 1950s about a million illegal abortions a year were performed in the U.S., and over a thousand women died each year as a result. Women came into emergency wards only to die of widespread abdominal infections, victims of botched or unsanitary abortions. Many women who recovered from such infections found themselves sterile or chronically and painfully ill. The enormous emotional stress often lasted a long time.

Poor women and women of color ran the greatest risks with illegal abortions. In 1969, 75 percent of the women who died from abortions (most of them illegal) were women of color. Ninety percent of all legal abortions in that year were performed on white private patients.

Attempts to Make Illegal Abortion Less Dangerous

Many communities had informal networks of people who knew where women could obtain an abortion. In the 1960s, clergy groups and feminist groups set up their own referral services to help women find safer illegal abortions. Some groups found that they needed to learn more about women's bodies and about abortion techniques in order to evaluate abortionists and help women avoid dangerous procedures. As they learned, they began to seek and create better, safer alternatives. In Chicago a group of women formed the Jane Collective, which provided safe, effective and supportive illegal abortions. When they discovered that one of the skilled abortionists they used was not a doctor, Jane women realized that they could learn to perform the abortions with adequate training, and they did. Over a four-year period the Jane Collective was able to help over 11,000 women get illegal first- and second-trimester abortions with a safety record comparable to legal abortions done in medical facilities. They also reduced the cost to fifty dollars and never turned any women away because of inability to pay the fee. In this way, they put many of Chicago's expensive and unsafe illegal abortionists out of business.

Groups like the Jane Collective and other less well-known women's groups demonstrated that determined and dedicated laywomen with no formal medical training can, with careful instruction and practice, perform abortions competently and humanely. Because what they were doing was illegal, they had to set up security measures to protect the identities and safety of those involved. They could not discuss their role in providing abortions over the phone or in writing. Nor could they speak publicly about what they were doing, to encourage other women and help them in similar work. A common rule was not to tell any person, *no matter how close a friend*, any information about abortion activities that she did not need to know, because this could make her an accessory to the "crime" as well as a potential source of danger to the safety of the group. Complicated arrangements protected the anonymity of women providing the abortions and the locations where they were performed. Instruments and supplies had to be obtained, stored and transported in secrecy. If a woman had a complication during or after her abortion, or when she wanted a routine postabortion follow-up, she needed to know where to go for help and what information to give to the medical personnel to get care while protecting security. And, most impressive of all, these groups of women insisted that all these arrangements include emotional support, reassurance and kindness.

Despite the existence of groups like the Jane Collective most women having to seek an illegal abortion endured substantial risk and trauma. It is crucial that we keep abortion safe, legal, and accessible, so that abortion will never have to go underground again.

Some women have written about learning how to do nonmedical abortions and claim to have had good results with alternatives, especially one to four weeks after conception. Yet information about many nonmedical abortion techniques, especially herbal ones, is incomplete, vague or even inaccurate. While attempting to induce an early abortion with acupuncture, acupressure or Vitamin C may not be successful, it is not likely to involve serious risks. Taking herbal preparations, however, may be dangerous, sometimes even deadly, when women do not have extensive knowledge of herbs and cannot recognize signs of complications. In 1978 the Center for Disease Control reported three cases of pennyroyal oil poisoning from unsuccessful attempts to induce abortions. One of the women died. Pennyroyal is a potent herb listed in many books and articles as an abortion-causing substance (abortifacient) without clear instructions about safe dosages, dangers of overdose and differences between the oil and a tea brewed from the leaves.

My personal opinion is that most of the plants abortion-seeking women are using today are either unsafe or unreliable. The lack of safety has to do with the drastic side effects of some of the plants, the lack of specific dosage guidelines and the lack of experienced herbal practitioners in this area. The unreliability stems from the fact that the same plant can't be counted upon to always produce an abortion, that this seems to be an area of vastly differing biochemical individuality and that not achieving the desired effect seems to encourage women on to more drastic herbs and more drastic doses.*

The Push for Legal Abortion

In the 1960s, inspired by the civil rights and antiwar movements, we began to fight more actively for our rights as women. The fast-growing Women's Movement took the taboo subject of abortion to the public. Rage, pain and fear burst out in demonstrations and speakouts, as women burdened by years of secrecy got up in front of strangers to talk about their illegal abortions. We condemned the abortionists who had exploited and mutilated us, the laws which had forced us to resort to back-alley abortions and the system which placed so little value on our lives. We marched and rallied and lobbied for abortion on demand. Civil-liberties groups and liberal clergy supported us.

Reform came gradually. A few states liberalized abortion laws, allowing women abortions under certain circumstances (e.g., pregnancy resulting from rape or incest, being under fifteen years of age) but leaving the decision up to doctors and hospitals. Costs were still high and few women actually benefited.

In 1970 New York State went further with a law which allowed abortion on demand through the twenty-fourth week from the last menstrual period if it was done in a medical facility by a doctor. A few other states passed similar laws. Women who could afford it flocked to the few places where abortions were legal. In 1972, 223,000 abortions were reported in New York City alone; 61.8 percent were obtained by women from out of state. Safety and efficacy of legal abortion services improved each year. Feminist networks offered support, loans and referrals, and fought to keep prices down. But for every woman who managed to get to New York, many others lived in isolated communities and had limited financial resources. Without money or mobility, these women could not be helped as easily. Illegal abortion was still common. The fight continued; a number of cases be-

*Billie Potts, *Witches' Heal: Lesbian Herbal Self-Sufficiency*, Hecuba's Daughters, Inc., P.O. Box 488, Bearsville, NY 12409, p. 95.

fore the Supreme Court urged repeal of all restrictive state laws.

As the tide began to turn, medical organizations (like the American Medical Association and the American College of Obstetricians and Gynecologists) joined the campaign for legalization. Although some physicians were truly concerned about women's need for safe abortions, others saw financial incentives for planned, legal and state-funded abortions and wanted to make sure doctors were in control of the procedures. Population-planning groups also threw their weight behind legalization, seeing abortion as a tool for better population control.

On January 22, 1973, the U.S. Supreme Court, in the famous Roe vs. Wade decision, stated that the "right of privacy...founded in the Fourteenth Amendment's concept of personal liberty...is broad enough to encompass a woman's decision whether or not to terminate her pregnancy." The Court held that through the end of the first trimester of pregnancy, it is only a pregnant woman and her doctor who have the legal right to make the decision about an abortion. States can restrict second-trimester abortions only in the interest of the woman's safety. Protection of a "viable fetus" (able to survive outside the womb) is allowed only during the third trimester. If a pregnant woman's life or health is endangered, she cannot be forced to continue the pregnancy.

Though Roe vs. Wade left a lot of power in doctors' hands, it was an important victory for us. While the decision did not guarantee the right to abortion, it decriminalized it and paved the way for federal Medicaid funding. With legalization and the growing consciousness of women's needs came better, safer abortion services. Severe infections, fever and hemorrhaging from illegal or self-induced abortions became a thing of the past. Women health workers improved abortion techniques. Some commercial clinics hired feminist abortion activists to do counseling. Local women's groups set up public referral services and women in some areas organized women-controlled nonprofit abortion facilities. These efforts have turned out to be just the beginning of a longer struggle.

After Legalization

Although legalization has greatly lowered the cost of abortion, millions of women in the United States today—especially women of color, young, rural and/or poor women, do not have access to safe, affordable abortions. Difficulties and delays stall many women beyond the first twelve weeks. Southern and rural states and counties have often ignored the Supreme Court decision. State regulations and funding vary widely. It is still hard to get second-trimester abortions. By 1977, when federal funds did pay for abortions, fewer than 20 percent of U.S. (public) county and city hospitals actually provided them. In other words, some 40 percent of American women—perhaps 93 percent of women living in rural areas—never benefited from liberalized abortion laws. Adequate counseling is rare, and few people respect the rights of teenagers to make their own choices.

Many clinics emphasize making money at the expense of quality care. Feminists on staff have protested these trends and often been fired. At the Preterm Clinic in Boston, a 1976 strike united demands about working conditions and patient care, as both clinic workers and clients protested that management was cutting back counseling to increase the volume of abortions.

We have learned that legalization, though essential, is not enough. Laws and their enforcement vary, depending on who is in power. A strong movement needs to maintain constant public pressure.

In 1978, Italy passed a law giving women the right to free first-trimester abortions. The law requires a doctor's approval, a waiting period and parental consent for women under eighteen. Abortions can only be performed in public hospitals where anyone involved, from administrators to surgeons to anesthesiologists, can claim "conscientious objector" status and refuse to participate. In this Catholic country where the Church exerts a lot of pressure, 72 percent of Italian doctors became objectors within a year and refused to perform legal abortions. Some of these same doctors, however, continued to perform illegal abortions outside of hospitals, collecting high fees from women who could not obtain legal abortions.

Passage of the law was just the beginning of the fight for Italian feminists. They had to keep demanding abortions from clinics and hospitals. In 1978 they occupied and operated the abortion clinic in the Policlinico, Rome's largest hospital, whose director had promised to provide abortions and then changed his mind. After three months (and three police attacks), the women were finally ousted.

The hospital occupation helped consolidate the Italian prochoice movement. When a measure came up to repeal legal abortion in May 1981, it was defeated two to one. This was an impressive victory in a Catholic country with wealthy and powerful antiabortion forces.

Race, Class and Population Control

One tactic the government and medical establishment have used to limit the numbers of people they consider to be "undesirable" has been to pressure certain women to have abortions. Yet abortion is still a valuable tool

when freely chosen. In the words of a black woman activist:

Many black people on hearing the word "abortion" immediately think of genocide—the killing of a people. With a racist history and the continuing virulence of racism in the U.S., there is little question as to why blacks link abortion to genocide. While such precaution is warranted, at the same time many black women are choosing to have abortions. In the struggle to become full participants in the labor force and to overcome tremendously adverse social conditions, the availability and accessibility of adequate and supportive abortion services is essential for black women. A black woman's decision to have an abortion is integrally bound up with her continuing struggle to improve the quality of life for herself as well as her family. It is for these reasons that black women and all women of color join in the fight to maintain abortions—safe, legal and on demand.

Today, sterilization is a favored method among population planners. Its relationship to abortion availability is revealing. While the federal government stopped reimbursing states for Medicaid abortions in 1977, it has continued to pay for sterilizations, which, unlike abortion, permanently end women's ability to bear children.

Knowing it will be difficult or impossible to get an abortion if you need one creates tremendous pressure to go ahead and do something permanent. There are many reports, too, of physicians or social workers pressuring women on welfare to be sterilized at the time of an abortion; some have even implied falsely that welfare benefits would be cut if they didn't. It seems no coincidence that when the Illinois government cut funding for Medicaid abortions in 1980, the number of government-funded sterilizations doubled in the state. Lack of abortion availability to poor women and women of color compounds sterilization abuse.

The Current Antiabortion Crusade

When the Supreme Court legalized abortion in 1973, the antiabortion forces led by the Catholic Church hierarchy and the right-wing so-called "National Right-to-Life Committee" began a serious mobilization. The first major setback to abortion rights came in July 1976 when Congress passed the Hyde Amendment, banning Medicaid funding for abortion unless a woman's life was in danger. Henry Hyde stated at that time:

I certainly would prevent, if I could, legally anybody having an abortion, a rich woman, a middle-class woman, or a poor woman. Unfortunately, the only vehicle available is the DHEW Medicaid bill...and so we proceed.

The Department of Health, Education and Welfare, now the Department of Health and Human Services (DHHS), predicted that without Medicaid abortions 250 women might die and 25,000 suffer complications each year from illegal and self-induced abortions.

A temporary injunction stalled the Hyde Amendment for a year. Meanwhile, in June 1977 the Supreme Court ruled that states did not have to fund what they considered "medically unnecessary" (varies from state to state) abortions, which paved the way for more discrimination against poor women. The first reported death as a result came in November 1977. Rosie Jimenez, a twenty-seven-year-old Chicana from Texas, died following an illegal abortion in Mexico after Texas stopped funding Medicaid abortions.

It is impossible to count the number of women harmed by the Hyde Amendment, but 260,000 women a year used to receive Medicaid abortion funds. In December 1977 a "compromise" version of the amendment added exceptions for promptly reported rape and incest and cases in which two doctors testify that the woman's health would be seriously impaired. A broad spectrum of groups fought against the Hyde Amendment but the final ruling of the Supreme Court upheld it in the 1980 Harris vs. McRae decision.

Legislation recently passed by states and cities includes parental consent bills for abortion and contraception. Some laws required waiting periods during which parents or husband are informed of a woman's intention to have an abortion. The woman had to be shown pictures of fetuses, warned that the procedure is "dangerous" to herself and her future fertility and "informed" that the fetus is considered a person. Other laws required that second-trimester abortions be performed in hospitals rather than clinics. The constitutionality of these bills was contested in the Supreme Court, which ruled once again, in June 1983, that the government cannot interfere with the fundamental right to abortion, striking down these forms of restrictive legislation, and reaffirming the Roe vs. Wade decision.*

As of 1983, antiabortion legislation pending in Congress included the *Human Life Statute* (HLS). This bill would make the fetus a legal "person." Abortion, even to save the life of the pregnant woman, would be manslaughter or murder. Some birth control pills, the IUD or any form of birth control that interrupted growth of the fertilized egg would also be outlawed. The *Human Life Amendment* (HLA) would amend the Constitution itself in a similar fashion. The *Human Life Federalism Amendment* (the Hatch amendment) would allow states to have abortion laws equal to or more restrictive than federal law. This was also defeated in late June 1983, by an all-too-narrow margin.

Lobbying for legislation is only one tactic of the antiabortion forces. A network of New Right groups has been raising large sums of money for electoral campaigns in the 1980s. At every level of public office they target prochoice abortion candidates, using expensive and powerful techniques, such as eleventh-hour media blitzes, to smear liberal candidates.

The Catholic Church still plays a major role in antiabortion activities. The National Conference of Catholic Bishops' "Pastoral Plan for Pro-Life Activities" maps out an organizing plan to eliminate legal abortion including political lobbying and campaigning, picketing abortion clinics and collecting money. Church dioceses raise large amounts of money from church collections. The Church hierarchy does not truly represent the views of American Catholics on this issue. Catholic women have abortions just about as frequently as do other women.*

Other religious groups like the Mormons and some representatives of Jewish orthodoxy have traditionally opposed abortion. Rapidly growing fundamentalist Christian groups, which overlap with the New Right and "right-to-life" organizations, are the most recent and visible boosters of the antiabortion movement.

Antiabortion groups talk as if all truly religious and moral people disapprove of abortion. This is not true now and never has been.

The National Right-to-Life Committee, which includes most antichoice groups, claims a membership of 11 million and has a three-million-dollar annual budget. The Committee has affiliates in all fifty states; Minnesota alone has some 200 chapters of Citizens Concerned for Life. "Right-to-lifers" also routinely harass staff and patients at abortion clinics. They try to prevent women from entering and disrupt abortions in progress. After struggling with her complex feelings and then deciding to have an abortion, a woman approaching a clinic may be faced with cries of "murderer." Since 1977 hundreds of clinics have been bombed, burned and vandalized. Prochoice supporters have responded with physical defense of clinics and escorts for patients.

Taking Action

To the New Right, abortion symbolizes women's independence and sexual freedom, the breakdown of the male-dominated family and women's bolder demands as workers and mothers. Their attacks on women's freedom to choose abortion are in part a reaction to the strength of the women's movement. Antiabortion forces have created an atmosphere which is moralistic, volatile, irrational and sometimes violent, so that being vocally prochoice can be risky.

Yet activist women are constantly forming new

*For an analysis of this decision, see *Off Our Backs*, August/September 1983, 1841 Columbia Road NW, Rm. 212, Washington, DC 20009, pp. 18–19.

*Catholics for a Free Choice (see p. 315) has several studies on this subject.

Thousands March in Support of Women's Lives

We are people demonstrating IN SUPPORT OF WOMEN'S LIVES against the National Right to Life Committee outside of their convention hall. We support every woman's right to safe, legal, affordable abortion. We reaffirm that commitment today. *We are the majority.* A recent Associated Press and NBC News poll showed that 80% of people in the U.S. support legal abortion.

Women fought hard to make abortion legal. Now that right is in jeopardy. Poor women have already lost the right to federally funded abortion under Medicaid, teenagers are losing their right to decide without parental consent.

The National Right to Life Committee is launching a major campaign to pressure the Senate to pass the Hatch Amendment. This constitutional amendment would allow both the states and Congress to ban abortion. They are also backing legislation to make the ban on Medicaid abortion permanent. At their convention, the Right to Life Committee is teaching its members to disrupt abortion clinics, interfere with abortions in progress and harass women seeking abortion services. Their goal is to make all abortions illegal, to prosecute women seeking abortions as criminals, to bring back the days of back-alley abortions. *Their goal is compulsory pregnancy.*

They call themselves pro-life, but the anti-abortion movement's concern for life ends at birth. Their money and support elects politicians who vote against everything women and children need: equal rights, quality child care, prenatal care, social security, food stamps, education and Aid to Families with Dependent Children.

Eliminating abortion is only one part of their plan to put women in "their place." They want to deny teenagers access to contraceptives and sex education. They are working to legalize discrimination against lesbians and gay men. They want to end funding for battered women and child abuse shelters.

WE ARE HERE:

- because we remember the days when women died from back-alley abortions;
- to support poor women's right to full health care coverage, including abortions, under Medicaid;
- because we believe that every woman has the right to decide if and when to have children.

We've come to Cherry Hill so that our voices will be heard.

Together we will continue the fight for full reproductive freedom for all women!*

---

*From the Cherry Hill Demonstration Leaflet handed out on July 1, 1982, where prochoice supporters demonstrated at the annual Right to Life Convention.

groups—community, student, worker, religious and rural—each with its particular needs and tactics, as more and more of us combine our rage and share our vision for the future. These groups circulate petitions, organize letter-writing campaigns to legislators and visit their offices, combine legislative work with educational and grass-roots organizing, write letters to local papers, leaflet on streetcorners, bombard radio talk shows with phone calls, organize speakouts on campuses and neighborhood house meetings which give women a chance to talk for the first time about their abortion experiences, create hotlines, referral services and more clinics.

Right wing attacks challenge us to mobilize our strength, expand our numbers, regain and extend our rights. While we work for abortion rights, we also make the connections with issues like sterilization abuse, welfare rights, disability rights, gay rights and daycare. These coalitions give us a chance to make alliances with a broad range of groups.

An exciting aspect of the last ten years is the international nature of our growing prochoice movement. We have participated in international days of protest and gatherings that build solidarity and communication among women all over the world. All of us who believe that safe abortions contribute to the preservation of human life must be active in the political battle for accessible legal abortions.

Since 1979 the *Reproductive Rights National Network* (R2N2) has linked together reproductive rights groups from all over the country. Over seventy active groups in the R2N2 now work on a local, regional and national level. They distribute a national newsletter, pamphlets, buttons and bumper stickers. If you are interested in finding a reproductive rights group in your area or want to start one, you can contact R2N2 at 17 Murray Street, New York, NY 10007, (212) 267-8891.

Abortion Rights Mobilization (ARM) is an organization formed to implement and guarantee a woman's right to legal abortion as decreed by the U.S. Supreme Court. Their focus is on lawsuits and lobbying. Contact ARM, 175 Fifth Avenue, Suite 712, New York, NY 10010, (212) 677-0412.

The *American Civil Liberties Union's* (ACLU's) Foundation Reproductive Freedom Project is involved in litigation relevant to abortion rights and publishes a number of pamphlets. Twice a year they publish a docket that describes every active court case on reproductive rights in the U.S., indexed by geographical area and by topic. Contact the ACLU, 132 West 43rd Street, New York, NY 10036, (212) 944-9800.

Catholics for a Free Choice helps train counselors who deal with Catholic women seeking abortions and actively seeks to educate and inform people about the prochoice views of 79 percent of American Catholics. Contact Catholics for a Free Choice, 2008 17th Street NW, Washington, DC 20009, (202) 638-1706.

The *Committee to Defend Reproductive Rights* (CDRR) does grass-roots organizing around reproductive rights issues. They provide information on how to organize, and publish *The Media Book: Making the Media Work for Your Grass-Roots Group.* Contact CDRR, 2845 24th Street, San Francisco, CA 94110, (415) 826-4401.

The *National Abortion Federation* (NAF). Although activities are geared toward members (clinics, doctors, Planned Parenthood), the newsletter, training seminars on medical issues and public action seminars on political and legal issues are open to the public. Contact NAF, 900 Pennsylvania Avenue SE, Washington, DC 20003, (800) 772-9100.

The *National Abortion Rights Action League* (NARAL) focuses on single-issue political lobbying and fund-raising to support prochoice candidates. They publish a regular legislative update, a newsletter and pamphlets. Contact NARAL, 1424 K Street NW, Washington, DC 20005 (202) 347-7774.

The *National Organization for Women* (NOW). One of NOW's hottest priorities is keeping abortion and birth control safe and legal. NOW works on obtaining grass-roots support and lobbying on state and national levels. A Reproductive Rights Resource Kit and pamphlets are available. Contact National NOW Action Center, 425 13th Street NW, Suite 723, Washington, DC 20004, (202) 347-2279.

The *National Women's Health Network* (NWHN) works for abortion rights as one of many women's health issues. They try to maintain national communications about antiabortion legislation and aid groups doing local organizing. The Network is currently updating its Abortion Rights Organizers Kit, and publishes a newsletter. Contact NWHN Abortion Rights Project, 224 7th Street SE, Washington, DC 20003, (202) 543-9222.

The *Religious Coalition for Abortion Rights* (RCAR) is an ecumenical coalition of thirty-one religious denominations and organizations supporting a woman's right to choose. They publish a newsletter and many publications on positions of religious organizations in regard to abortion rights. Contact RCAR, 100 Maryland Avenue NE, Suite 307, Washington, DC 20002, (202) 543-7032.

RESOURCES

Most of the organizations listed in the "Taking Action" section of the chapter offer publications, bibliographies or other sources of information.

Readings

Ambrose, Linda. "The McRae Case: A Record of the Hyde Amendment's Impact on Religious Freedom and Health Care," *Family Planning/Population Reporter* 7, No. 2 (1978), pp. 26–30.

Bart, Pauline. "Seizing the Means of Reproduction: An Illegal Feminist Abortion Collective—How and Why It Worked." Available for $2.00 from Boston Women's Health Book Collective, 465 Mt. Auburn Street, Watertown, MA 02172. An excellent discussion of the Jane Collective.

CARASA. *Women Under Attack: Abortion, Sterilization Abuse, and Reproductive Freedom,* 1979. Available from CARASA, 17 Murray Street, 5th floor, New York, NY 10007.

David Beach

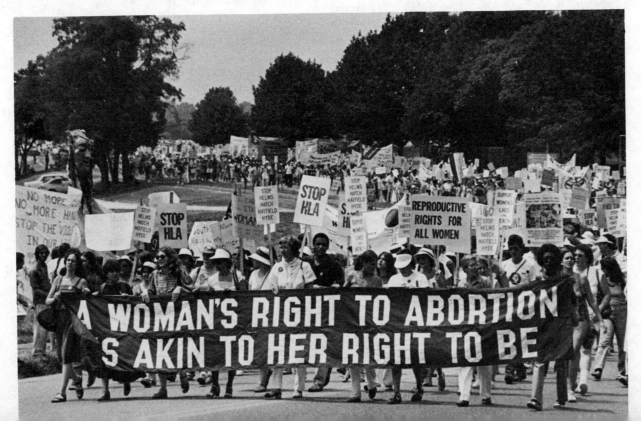

Cava-Rizzuto, Virginia, and Nancy Borman. "The Majority Report Guide to Abortifacient Herbs," *Majority Report* (August 6–19, 1977).

Centers for Disease Control: Abortion Surveillance. CDC, Public Health Service, U.S. Dept. of Health and Human Services, Bureau of Epidemiology, Family Planning Evaluation Division, Atlanta, GA 30333. Issued every year. Free.

Erlien, Marla, et al. *More Than a Choice: Women Talk About Abortion*. Abortion Action Coalition, Boston, 1979. Personal stories and politics.

Federation of Feminist Women's Health Centers. "Menstrual Extraction," in *A New View of a Woman's Body*. New York: Simon and Schuster, 1981.

Gage, Suzann. *When Birth Control Fails: How to Abort Ourselves Safely*. Hollywood, CA: Speculum Press, 1979. Available for $2.00 from Speculum Press, P.O. Box 1063, Hollywood, CA 90028. An important resource for thinking about abortion if it again becomes illegal, but dangerous if used as a do-it-yourself guide. Write to Boston Women's Health Book Collective, 465 Mt. Auburn Street, Watertown, MA 02172 for reviews of this book.

Gallagher, Janet. "Abortion Rights: Critical Issue for Women's Freedom." WIN, March 8, 1979, pp. 9–11, 24–26.

Gordon, Linda. *Woman's Body, Woman's Right: A Social History of Birth Control in America*. New York: Penguin Books, 1977.

Alan Guttmacher Institute. *Abortions and the Poor: Private Morality, Public Responsibility*. New York: Alan Guttmacher Institute, 1979. Available for $2.50 from the Institute, 515 Madison Avenue, New York, NY 10022.

National Women's Health Network. *Abortion. Resource Guide 8*, 1980. Available from National Women's Health Network, 224 7th Street SE, Washington, DC 20003.

———. *Self-Help: Resource Guide 7*, 1980. Includes reprints of two excellent articles on menstrual extraction: "Menstrual Extraction: Procedures" by Lorraine Rothman, and "Menstrual Extraction: Politics" by Laura Punnett, both reprinted from *Quest*, Vol. 4, No. 3 (summer 1978).

Sifford, Belinda. "Abortion in Italy: Humiliation, Not Liberation," *HealthRight*, Vol. 4, Issue 4 (fall 1978). Available for $1.00 from Boston Women's Health Book Collective (address above).

Women Speak Out About Abortion (first abortion testimony survey). Available for $3.00 from Rose Soma/Americans United to Save Abortion, P.O. Box A-W, Miller Place, NY 11764. A number of the experiences in this chapter were taken from this book, which includes many moving stories.

Women workers in abortion clinics. *Getting Stronger: Women Workers Organize the Abortion Clinics*. Red Sun Press, 94 Green Street, Jamaica Plain, MA 02130, 1978.

Women's Research Action Project. *The Abortion Business: A Report on Free-Standing Abortion Clinics*. Cambridge, MA: Goddard-Cambridge Graduate Program, 1975, rev. ed. 1977.

Audiovisual Materials

Abortion, a 1971 black and white film. Available from Boston Women's Film Collective, c/o BWHBC, 465 Mt. Auburn Street, Watertown, MA 02172. A women-made noncommercial film about how things used to be and still are for many women, including an excellent discussion of sterilization abuse. As timely now as when it was made, though in different ways.

Abortion Clinic, a 52-minute 1983 color videocassette from the PBS series "Frontline." Available from Fanlight Productions, 47 Halifax Street, Jamaica Plain, MA 02130. Presents perspectives of both prochoice and antiabortion advocates. Includes voices of women making the decision, women having an abortion, counselors and practitioners in a clinic, and antiabortion picketers.

It Happens to Us, a 30-minute color film. Available from New Day Films, P.O. Box 315, Franklin Lakes, NJ 07417.

Our Lives on the Line, a 45-minute videotape. Rental $25 plus shipping. Available from Boston's Women's Health Collective (address above). Four black women living in Boston openly discuss their abortion experiences, their relationships with men and their families, the effects of racism on the health care treatment they received and what having an abortion means to them. An excellent, powerfully moving videotape, from which a number of the experiences in this chapter were taken.

17

NEW REPRODUCTIVE TECHNOLOGIES

By Ruth Hubbard, with Wendy Sanford

With special thanks to Gena Corea

From *in vitro* fertilization and sex preselection to distant future possibilities of cloning or even artificial placentas, scientists and physicians are working hard on new technologies which could drastically change women's relationship to childbearing. These technologies raise a dilemma for those of us who are writing and consulting on this book. On the one hand, we know that some technologies have helped or have the potential to help women who badly want biological children and would otherwise be unable to have them. We want to support a woman's right to choose to have children and by the means she sees best. We know also that certain technologies can help parents avoid passing on hereditary diseases to their children.

Yet we have serious questions. The technologies involve a degree of invasiveness and medical manipulation of women's bodies which alarms us. Most of the money that goes into developing these technologies would be better spent on preventive measures and basic health care services for all women. What's more, white, professional, affluent men make up the overwhelming number of the scientists who research these technologies, the physicians who apply them, the legislators who approve and fund the research and the drug company directors who translate them into products to be advertised, sold and profited from. Despite claims that these technologies are to "serve" women, our experience with the use of other medical technologies has taught us to be suspicious; physicians and hospitals now virtually force birthing technologies on us, and sterilization has been outrageously misused against women of color. Most doctors offering even something as technically simple as donor insemination have so far restricted their services to married women. We can reasonably predict that those in control of the technologies of the future will show a continued resistance to sharing them with women in nontraditional relationships, particularly lesbians.

We have questions, too, about the long-range goals of this research. One source lists as the final goal of reproductive engineering "the ultimate manufacture of a human being to exact specifications."[1] Who will decide these specifications? Our guess is that without a major political revolution it won't be women, and it especially won't be women of color or women who are poor. Will these new reproductive technologies truly serve us? Or, in a society where women have less power than men, will they be a means of further controlling our freedom to make choices about our bodies?

We are also critical of the way the society measures our worth as women by our fertility. We are made to feel inadequate or unwomanly if we can't bear children "of our own." The mother of the first test-tube baby expressed the guilt she had felt:

"I'm not a normal woman," I told John.... "I wouldn't even blame you now if you went off with someone else."...It wasn't John's fault. He could have as many children as he liked with another woman. A whole football team....[2]

Wanting a baby and not being able to have one can be intensely painful. But society heaps an extra load of guilt on us. Is this one of the reasons why some of us are so willing to go through all kinds of time-consuming, painful and at times degrading tests and medical manipulations to have a child? Even the less invasive infertility techniques expose a very private corner of our lives and open us to endless questions and advice from relatives, friends and physicians, who may also recommend surgery, drugs or other risky and invasive procedures. Our male partner may share our sense of violation as he ejaculates on command, so his semen can be examined and his sperm counted.

There is no inner recess of me left unexplored, unprobed, unmolested. It occurs to me when I have sex that what used to be beautiful and very private is now degraded and terribly public. I bring my [menstrual cycle] charts to the doctor like a child bringing home a report card. Tell me, did I do well? Did I ovulate? Did I have sex at the right times as you instructed me?[3]

It would be a lot better if we felt less pressured to produce our "own" children and could express our needs to love, nurture and be loved by becoming close to children of neighbors, friends or relatives, by adopting children who need parents or by becoming foster parents. At present, adoption and foster parenting involve personal and legal problems that many of us aren't willing or able to take on. And yet the biotechnical solutions aren't easy, either.

We must judge the value of the reproductive technologies in the context of the social, political and economic setting in which they are produced and used. We must look at who owns them and who profits from them, whether they give professionals more power over us or whether they increase the power and self-sufficiency of those of us who use them. We must assess their dollar cost and judge how easily ordinary people can have access to them. We must also recognize that researchers may be seeking the fame and funding that come from achieving scientific breakthroughs and triumphs rather than working for the well-being of women.

In this chapter we have tried to help inform women considering the use of these technologies, while at the same time raising the strong doubts we hold.

DONOR INSEMINATION (DI)

This is the simplest, least invasive and most widely used of the technologies we are considering. It doesn't require professional help, and we can do it at home.

To use DI on your own, you should have no fertility problems and your menstrual cycle should be fairly regular. Then you begin by charting your basal temperature and mucus consistency for a few months (see "Fertility Observation," p. 235) so that you know when you are likely to ovulate. You must also find a fertile man who is willing to donate sperm. You can do this yourself or, if you want anonymity, through a friend. When you know from past cycles that you are about to ovulate, the sperm donor must masturbate into a condom or a clean (preferably boiled, *but cooled*) jar. Within an hour after ejaculation, you suck the semen into a needleless hypodermic syringe (some women use an eye dropper or a turkey baster), gently insert the syringe into your vagina while lying flat on your back with your rear up on a pillow, and empty the syringe into your vagina to deposit the semen as close to your cervix as possible. Then continue lying down comfortably for about half an hour, so that as little sperm as possible leaks out of your vagina.

It's a good idea to repeat this with fresh sperm samples on two or three days, during and after the time you ovulate. Most women become pregnant after trying DI during three to five cycles. If you aren't pregnant after having tried it five or six months, you may want to consult a fertility clinic to check on your and your donor's fertility.

This kind of DI is often called "artificial insemination by donor," or AID. At present, probably more than 15,000 babies a year are conceived by DI in the U.S.

by women whose husbands either have fertility problems or are at risk of passing on a serious hereditary disease, as well as by women who are single or part of a lesbian couple. Some married couples are occasionally advised to use the husband's sperm for DI. This is useful when there are structural or psychological barriers to sexual intercourse. In addition, if the husband provides normal motile sperm, but not enough, he may be advised to collect the first few drops of the ejaculate separately from the rest. Since the first portion contains most of the active sperm, that's what you use for donor insemination.

When a procedure is this simple, why do some of us take on the expense and other drawbacks of involving physicians and lawyers? For one thing, when a physician does the insemination, it is easier to provide anonymity for both donor and recipient (see below). Ideally, the donor also would be properly screened for possible health problems, although in fact most physicians ask prospective donors only a few questions about their health and family histories for various diseases.* Indeed, since donors usually receive twenty-five to forty dollars per ejaculate, some men may conceal health problems in order to be eligible. A survey of physicians' practices shows that most of them don't offer you more protection than you could provide yourself.[4]

Physicians do have access to sperm banks which store frozen sperm, so that you don't need a donor on call to produce sperm when you ovulate. Unfortunately, however, frozen sperm is less effective than fresh sperm, so that it usually takes more attempts to achieve fertilization, costing you more time and money. (At about seventy dollars per insemination, DI through a physician costs about 140 dollars a month at two inseminations per cycle.)

Mutual anonymity between you and the man who donates the sperm may be important for both of you, and can forestall legal and emotional complications. Problems have arisen when a man who gave his sperm had a change of feelings later and sued for visitation or wanted to give the child his surname. Single and lesbian women especially have to guard against this kind of harassment. The sperm donor, too, may need protection, because a court may later assert a donor's responsibility for child support.†

There are also arguments against anonymity. Many unmarried women, both heterosexual and lesbian, want the donor to be a friend who will possibly be involved in the child's life. Also, just as adopted chil-

*There is preliminary evidence that more women are contracting PID as a result of DI (see p. 502).
†The legal status of DI differs in different states and is sometimes unclear. Some states have considered children conceived by DI to be "illegitimate"; others acknowledge paternity of the social father. The legal ground is shifting as DI becomes more widespread, so it is a good idea to be aware of the situation in your state.

dren are making increasing efforts to locate their biological parents, some children conceived by DI may be disturbed and angry if they cannot find out who their biological fathers are. Also, health problems may arise that may make us or our children want to have access to the biological father's medical history.

As you think about the entire situation, as well as about other alternatives such as adoption or structuring your life without a child, you may want to talk with others who have used DI or with an infertility counseling or educational group such as Resolve, Inc. (see Resources). The procedure isn't right for everybody and raises different questions for different people.

Some married women have said that they felt as though they were committing adultery. (The Roman Catholic and Orthodox Jewish religions, as well as the laws in some states, do consider DI adultery.) A partner may not feel as involved in the pregnancy or parenthood as you had hoped, because the baby isn't his or her biological child. If you value genetic continuity and family resemblances highly, then DI is not for you. Think about what you will tell close friends and family, and—most importantly—what you will tell your child. Many parents in the past have kept DI a secret, perhaps to protect the man from the embarrassment of having people know he is infertile. (Fertility and sexual potency—particularly in the sense of the ability to achieve erection and ejaculation—are very often mistakenly linked and overvalued.) Don't assume from the start that you must be secretive or, conversely, tell all.

Some people feel more comfortable with a carefully worded consent form, signed by all parties—the woman who plans to be inseminated, her partner (if she has one), the sperm donor and preferably also his partner (if he has one). Such a contract can spell out future financial obligations and visitation rights for the donor (if he is to have any) and for partners in case of separation or divorce. However, courts don't have to honor such a contract if they decide that some other arrangement would be in the child's best interest. What's more, some lawyers think that it is a mistake for the recipient or donor of sperm to sign anything, since a signature could be construed as an admission of paternity that could be used against either of them in later litigation.*

Under proper circumstances, DI may be right. Two lesbian partners, who plan to raise children together, told about the bond it created between them for the one to help the other with her insemination. Another woman, more ambivalent, said:

*Donna J. Hitchens of the Lesbian Rights Project in San Francisco (1370 Mission Street, San Francisco, CA 94103) has written an article entitled "Lesbians Choosing Motherhood: Legal Issues in Donor Insemination," which contains good information for anyone thinking about using DI. You can get a copy by writing to the Project, enclosing $1.50 for xeroxing and postage.

Our daughter is really extraordinary—enormous energy, very strong-willed and totally different-looking from either of us. I am reminded constantly that her father was a stranger.

And one wrote:

My husband and I had more than our share of doubts right up until the moment of our daughter's birth. When we saw our baby girl, all our doubts disappeared.[5]

SURROGATE MOTHERHOOD

In this procedure as it is practiced so far in the U.S., one woman—the surrogate—bears a child which another woman raises as her own. This possibility appeals to some heterosexual couples in which the woman cannot conceive or carry a fetus to term, whereas her partner produces normal amounts of active sperm.

The service now offered requires that Mr. and Ms. Doe find a Ms. Roe, who is willing to be inseminated with Mr. Doe's sperm and to go through the pregnancy and birth. Immediately after the birth, Ms. Roe gives up the baby to the Does, who are henceforth its parents. Ms. Roe gets paid at least her expenses and usually a fee. Often an agency, physician and/or lawyer mediate the transaction.

As you may imagine, this enterprise raises a host of social, legal and financial questions. Our strongest concern is that this option puts pressure on some of us to "rent out" our bodies for most of a year as a way to earn money. Can we really contract to give up a child before we become pregnant and be sure that we'll be able to live with the decision once the baby is born? Aren't the issues currently being raised by birthmothers, who have given up children for adoption, likely to surface for surrogate mothers?

Some surrogate mothers have in fact changed their minds and decided to keep the child. Probably no contract we sign beforehand is legally binding on the biological mother, because in any litigation concerning children courts have the final say.

[Mr. and Ms. John Doe] of Rochester, N.Y., cannot have children together. [Jane Roe] agreed, by way of a lawyer who specializes in these arrangements, to bear Mr. [Doe's] child and give up all parental rights. Thanks to the kind of technological triumph to which we're now accustomed, Mr. [Doe's] sperm was frozen and flown to California, and [Ms. Roe] was impregnated.

Recently she changed her mind and wants to keep the child. [Ms. Roe] is, strictly speaking, the baby's mother. But she had promised it to [Ms. Doe]. Mr. [Doe] claims parenthood, but since California law does not treat semen donors as natural fathers, [Ms. Roe's] lawyer has asked that his suit be dismissed. And until the legal tangle is unraveled, Baby [Roe], who is still residing in a rented womb, may on delivery be moving to a foster home....[6]

It is also far from obvious what the couple's obligations are should they separate or change their minds during the pregnancy. And what if the baby they contracted for is born with an unanticipated health problem? Can they go back on the contract? And must the biological mother then care for it, or does a judge decide whose child it is?* A 1983 case widely reported in the press raises many of these complications—and others.†

The economics are also complicated. Some surrogate mothers have asked to be paid only for their expenses, saying that they want to give the child as a gift to women who cannot bear children. For others it is a way to earn money. One surrogate mother said, "It's a business endeavor that satisfies monetary needs and emotional needs." But what is a fair price? Figures quoted in the media have been from 5,000 dollars up, and though that may seem a lot, it isn't much for a year of a woman's life. (Illicit adoptions of "desirable" babies now cost up to 20,000 dollars.) Physicians' and lawyers' fees get added on and are sometimes exorbitant. One physician has said bluntly that the process costs "what the traffic will bear."[7] Since some well-to-do couples are prepared to pay a good deal for a baby that is genetically at least partly theirs, "baby brokers" stand to make money from the situation.

IN VITRO FERTILIZATION (IVF)

IVF is a biologically and technically complicated procedure which is still new and experimental.

It is available to women whose ovaries and uterus appear to function normally, but whose fallopian tubes are blocked or don't function properly so the egg cannot get to the uterus. Under present regulations in the U.S. women must also be married.

About 600,000 American women are in this situation, but at present only very few centers offer the procedure. Though IVF costs between 2,500 and 4,000 dollars, plus the medical expenses associated with pregnancy and birth, thousands of women are waiting to be screened to determine whether they meet the clinics' criteria.

*In a 1981 Inaugural Symposium on Surrogate Parenting speakers pointed out that new laws are needed to exempt surrogate motherhood from existing restrictions on buying or selling babies. To make the procedure safer and more acceptable, legal rights of all participants must be spelled out and uniform rules established.

†The couple contracting for the baby was in fact separated before the insemination; the physician had not advised the surrogate mother to avoid intercourse with her husband prior to insemination; the baby was born with serious health problems; the sperm donor refused to approve treatment for the baby, but the biological mother and her husband consented; tests revealed that the woman's husband and *not* the sperm donor was the baby's biological father; the donor filed a multimillion-dollar suit against the parents for breach of contract; and the parents are suing the physician.

In vitro is Latin for "in glass." In *in vitro* fertilization, the technical feat is to extract a ripe egg from the ovary, fertilize it with sperm in a glass dish and get the embryo back into the womb. The first successful *in vitro* fertilization and subsequent implantation was achieved in England in November 1977 and resulted in the birth of Louise Brown. Since then, babies conceived *in vitro* have been born in different parts of the world, and at this writing several hundred women are carrying fetuses conceived by IVF.

Different physicians and clinics are developing their own modifications, but the procedure involves these steps:

A woman who wants to try IVF first undergoes a battery of screening procedures, which often include surgery to make her ovaries accessible for collecting eggs. The practitioner must collect the egg just before it would normally be released. (Human eggs are so small that they are hard to find once they've left the follicle.) To pinpoint the precise time when a follicle will release an egg, the practitioner examines the ovaries with ultrasound* and measures hormone levels. To have more control of the timing of ovulation, most physicians now administer hormones called gonadotropins. Unfortunately, gonadotropins somewhat increase the chances that the eggs will have chromosomal abnormalities, such as the chromosome duplication responsible for Down's syndrome. They also induce several eggs to mature at the same time, something that ordinarily happens only rarely.

The physician then collects ripe eggs from the ovary by a surgical procedure known as *laparoscopy*, which at present is done under general anesthesia. During the laparoscopy s/he punctures the follicle(s) and draws out the egg(s) by gentle suction.† S/he places the egg in a clean, sterilized dish containing a nutrient solution and mixes it with a sample of newly ejaculated sperm. The covered dish is placed in an incubator at normal body temperature and examined from time to time under a microscope.

If all goes well, one of the 20,000 or so sperm in the sample will enter the egg, the egg and sperm nuclei (the organelles where the chromosomes are) will fuse and within a few hours the fertilized egg will divide first into two cells, then four and so on. The cells remain attached to each other and form the early em-

*Physicians now use ultrasound as though they know it is safe and assure pregnant women of its safety. But one cannot yet be sure. It took several decades before the risks of X-rays were obvious. We must worry about this especially when it's a question of irradiating our ovaries or early embryos with ultrasound, because their cells divide frequently and dividing cells tend to be especially sensitive to all forms of radiation.

†The image the surgeon sees with the laparoscope can be projected onto a screen so that the entire operating team can see it. In the "Nova" program on IVF, first screened in January 1982, the TV audience saw Ms. Carr's ovary and watched the collection of the egg that resulted nine months later in the birth of her daughter.

bryo. Some clinics transfer the embryo into the womb at the two-cell stage; others wait until it has four or six cells. If the cells look normal under the microscope, one or two embryos are introduced into the mother's womb, so that one or both can attach and develop further. At this time, no one knows how to make a human embryo survive outside the womb past these earliest stages.

In order for the physician to transfer an embryo into the womb, the woman lies on her back with her knees up, as she would for a cervical exam, on a table that sometimes is tilted about twenty degrees head down. Her vagina and cervix are swabbed with sterile salt solution, and the physician sucks the embryo and a drop of the solution in which it has been growing into a tube that is the width of a thin straw; then s/he inserts this tube into the womb through the vagina and cervix. By means of gentle positive pressure, the embryo in its drop of fluid is expelled into the womb, and the tube is slowly pulled out. This takes only a few minutes and is done without anesthesia.

At this point everyone waits to see whether the embryo will implant—the step that most often fails during the entire procedure. Even with natural fertilizations, probably only about one in four embryos implant properly and the rest are lost. At this time with IVF, chances are more like one in ten.

If the embryo doesn't implant, the entire procedure, including the laparoscopy, must be repeated.

Once we decide to try IVF, many of us are prepared to come back if we don't become pregnant the first time, though clinics usually limit the number of times a woman can try. To avoid the need for repeated anesthesia and surgery, physicians are giving women so-called "fertility drugs" which make several eggs mature simultaneously (gonadotropin hormones—see above). They can then collect several eggs during one laparoscopy and fertilize them all *in vitro*. Some physicians then transfer two (or more) embryos into the womb, hoping that at least one will implant. Of course, if both implant you can end up with twins, and multiple pregnancies sometimes involve increased health risks for mothers and babies. Others also freeze a few for storage and possible later insertion if the first implantation doesn't succeed, but so far physicians have had little or no luck getting frozen and thawed embryos to implant. At present no one knows the risks of this procedure.

The physicians who use IVF believe that the risks are negligible. They argue that if an egg or embryo is damaged, it simply won't develop. But we won't know whether that's true until thousands of babies conceived *in vitro* have had a chance to grow up. This is why some critics of IVF, as of other reproductive technologies, have said that in this procedure, women and their babies become guinea pigs.

And what of the ethical, legal and emotional issues? A procedure that requires this much technical exper-

tise is completely under professional control. We and our partners will never have much say about where or how we want it done. Because the pregnancies are so precious (emotionally, technically and economically), couples are under pressure to manage the prenatal period and birth just as the physicians order. Many women who have IVF are having Cesareans.* And when Ms. Brown was expecting Louise, she even had to agree in writing that she would have an abortion if Drs. Steptoe and Edwards thought she should!†

As thousands of women try to enroll in IVF programs, we must question why it is that many of us gladly accept painful medical interventions and unknown health risks in order to bear a child. We must look at the socialization we undergo as women which makes childbearing seem more important than our own health and well-being. We mustn't feel pressured by the fact that this technology now is available. *There is nothing wrong with us as women if we decide not to become involved with complicated, expensive and experimental procedures whose risks cannot be known with certainty for a long time.*

Clearly the procedure is sufficiently expensive, complex and of such uncertain outcome that it can serve relatively few of us. Meanwhile, many of us will risk invasive exploratory procedures and repeated attempts at IVF only to end up disappointed. IVF is yet another example of the way the medical profession develops high-technology "solutions" to preventable problems instead of stressing simple preventive measures that could serve many more of us. Most of us who end up wanting IVF would not need it if we had known earlier about possible *preventable* long-term effects of untreated or mistreated pelvic inflammatory and sexually transmitted diseases, and about risks from IUDs and other birth control methods that physicians often urge on us.

SEX PRESELECTION

Some couples try to choose the sex of their child for medical reasons, because certain inherited diseases—

*Cesareans always give doctors more control over the birth without necessarily improving birth outcomes. Many physicians prefer to do Cesareans with "precious pregnancies," regardless of how the woman wishes to give birth. Some women who require IVF also have medical complications that may make a Cesarean necessary.

†Though Steptoe and Edwards no longer require this, it is frightening that they were able to assume that much control. But they needed this control because their entire program would have been threatened had "their" first baby not been "perfect."

for example, hemophilia and a type of muscular dystrophy—are much more likely to affect boys than girls. But some people just feel strongly that they want to have a child only if they can be sure it will be the gender they "prefer." This pressure to choose the sex of one's child for reasons of sex preference is becoming more acute as more of us decide to have small families. Yet every child is an experiment! To know the sex of the child tells us nothing about what sort of person s/he will be. Surely our best chances of successful parenting will come if we can accept our children whatever their sex or personality, so that we can help them accept themselves and, hopefully, us as well.

Some population planners advocate sex selection as a way to limit population growth. One argument is that people often have more children than they really want because they keep trying for a girl (or boy) if they don't have one. The other, uglier, argument goes like this: Most people seem to prefer having boys. So let them have boys. Not only will they themselves have fewer children but, if fewer girls are born, there will be fewer women to bear children in the next generation.*

Techniques for choosing the sex of a child before conception depend on the fact that a child's sex is determined by the father. The reason is as follows. All our cells contain forty-six chromosomes which come in twenty-three pairs. We get one member of each pair from our mother, the other from our father. One of the twenty-three pairs determines sex. They are the "sex chromosomes," called X and Y. Women have two X chromosomes; men have one X and one Y. Mature eggs and sperm contain only one member of each chromosome pair, and therefore only one sex chromosome. Since a woman has only X chromosomes, all her eggs contain an X. Since a man is XY, about half his sperm cells contain an X chromosome and half a Y. If an egg (which is always X) is fertilized by a sperm that contains an X, the child will be a girl (XX); if it is fertilized by a sperm that contains a Y, the child will be a boy (XY).

Methods of sex preselection try to favor the X- or the Y-bearing sperm, but none is very effective. They rely on observations that Y-bearing sperm tend to swim faster and would be more easily damaged by the acidic environment of the vagina than X-bearing sperm, whereas X-bearing sperm appear to live longer and be more sensitive to the alkalinity in the cervix, uterus and fallopian tubes.

One recommendation is that to improve the likelihood of conceiving a girl, you should have intercourse thirty-six to forty-eight hours before ovulation and, for a boy, try delaying intercourse until two to twenty-four hours before you ovulate.[9] (See "Fertility Observation," p. 235.) Confusingly, other researchers have come up with the opposite recommendation: that intercourse a few days before ovulation weights chances in favor of boys, intercourse at the time of ovulation very slightly in favor of girls.[10]

Another recommended technique makes use mainly of the differences in the sensitivities of X and Y sperm to acid and alkali. Proponents suggest that to load the dice in favor of a girl, you use a mildly acid douche (two tablespoons of white vinegar in a quart of lukewarm water) before intercourse, allow only shallow penetration of the penis (so that the sperm must spend a longer time in the acidic environment of the vagina), be in a face-to-face position and avoid orgasm, which increases the alkalinity of the uterus. If you prefer a boy, you use an alkaline douche (two tablespoons of baking soda in a quart of water) and reverse the other conditions.[11] Neither method guarantees success but they may improve chances.

Obviously these methods deal only in probabilities. If your genetic history is such that a male child would have a fifty-fifty chance of inheriting a disease you want to avoid, you may want to be more certain. In that case, you can have a physician determine the fetus's sex after you are pregnant, so that you can have a choice of having an abortion if it is male or be more prepared for coping with the disease both emotionally and practically should you decide to continue the pregnancy. Increasing numbers of sex-linked diseases can now be diagnosed in the fetus, so that you don't need to consider abortion unless prenatal tests show that the fetus you are carrying has the disease.* (See p. 355 for a discussion of prenatal diagnosis.)

In the U.S., fetal sex usually is determined by amniocentesis, which cannot be done until about the fourteenth week of pregnancy. Since it takes another three or four weeks to complete the chromosomal analysis, if you decide to abort it means a second-trimester abortion—more painful, risky and psychologically difficult than early abortion.

Occasionally couples try to obtain amniocentesis and abortion merely because of sex preference, though some physicians won't do amniocentesis for that reason alone. Though we who are writing this book support

*In China, physicians have developed a method of diagnosing sex as early as forty-seven days after conception, by sampling fetal cells that can be scraped off the cervix early in pregnancy. They are offering first-trimester abortions (see Chapter 16, "Abortion") for purposes of sex selection "to help women who desire family planning." In a pilot study with 100 pregnant women, of forty-six found to carry girls twenty-nine elected abortions, whereas of fifty-three who were carrying boys, only one chose to abort.[8] But under what social pressures must these women be—and how must they view their own lives—to "plan" not to have girls?

*A group of women advising us on living with a physical disability expressed a concern about the pressure to have an abortion in cases of predicted disability, as each one was glad herself to be alive. If this society were less demanding of physical "perfection" and more helpful to parents and children with special needs, women might worry less about having a child with special health problems.

a woman's right to choose abortion, we believe strongly that sex selection is a poor reason to have one.

THE FUTURE: ARTIFICIAL PARTHENOGENESIS, EGG FUSION AND CLONING

If developed, these techniques would produce children from women's eggs without the use of sperm. Although they are only at the fantasy stage for people, some of us would be glad if they become available. One woman said:

I have a real longing for egg fusion because I am in a deep and long-term partnership with a woman and would love to have a child which comes truly from both of us. I know if we use DI or if we manage to adopt, I will love our child tremendously, but I do yearn to create a new being with her from the start.

However, these technologies involve serious biological and social risks to ourselves and our future children. There would also be such a high degree of technological complication and invasiveness that women choosing them would be subject to unprecedented control by professionals. Yet this fact has not prevented the experiments that scientists have done already. As women, we must insist on being involved in deliberations on these issues so that public policy addresses the social and economic problems which affect us and our children *now*, before entering into expensive experiments that are likely to create immense new ones.

With *parthenogenesis*, a woman could produce a child entirely by herself. She would have to stimulate an egg, following ovulation, to divide spontaneously, resulting in the formation of an embryo that could implant in her womb. Since all her eggs are X, all such embryos would be female.

Parthenogenesis involves serious health risks. To round out the normal human complement of forty-six chromosomes per body cell, each of the twenty-three chromosomes in the egg would have to double itself. Each woman's eggs carry any number of genes that could produce abnormalities or diseases in our children, though we ourselves are not ill. Ordinarily we do not pass them on to our children because the egg is fertilized by a sperm. And though that sperm carries its own assortment of "trouble genes," since every egg and sperm contain millions of different genes, chances are that a normal gene in the egg will cover for a "trouble gene" in the sperm, and the other way around. (Obviously this doesn't always happen, since two healthy parents sometimes have a child with an unexpected genetic disease due to the fact that both hap-

pened to have the same "trouble gene" without either of them knowing it.)

Since in parthenogenesis all the genes, including the problem ones, would be duplicated, the resulting baby would show all the egg's potential genetic problems.

Egg fusion would involve joining two eggs—either both from the same woman or one each from two of us. A physician would get the eggs by laparoscopy and fuse them *in vitro*, as with IVF. Biologically this would be safer than parthenogenesis since one egg could negate the other's "problem" genes. But it cannot be done at this time. Even with mouse eggs, scientists so far have only gotten two eggs to fuse and go through a first division into two cells before they die.

In *cloning*, the practitioners would replace the nucleus of an *in vitro* fertilized egg with the nucleus from a skin or other body cell of a chosen person (you, your lover or anyone else you choose). Since the nucleus contains the genetic material (all forty-six chromosomes), the resulting baby would be genetically identical with the chosen person, no matter who furnishes the egg or the sperm or in whose body the fetus grows.

Needless to say, this cannot yet be done with people. But toads and other animals have been cloned in this way. Of course, there also is no way to know what it would mean that the baby is genetically identical with the person of your choice. Genetically they would be like identical twins, but they would be likely to live in much more varied environments than most identical twins do. (So lots of psychologists and sociologists would want to test and study them!)

In concluding this chapter, we as authors feel impelled to say that we would not advise using any of these technologies except DI. We cannot forget that this society has an enormous economic and social investment in making us believe that women's natural, principal function is to bear children. How better to get us to accept low-paying "women's jobs" and second-class social status? We also cannot forget that while poor women—and especially poor women of color—are being sterilized against their wills, new reproductive technologies are promoted for those who can pay.

Although some of us know from personal experience the strong desire many women feel to have a biological child, these techniques involve so much social and medical manipulation of women and of our reproductive systems that we think the risks and costs are too high.

NOTES

1. "Genetic Engineering: Reprieve," *Journal of the American Medical Association*, Vol. 220, No. 10 (June 5, 1972), p. 1355; quoted in "Genetic Engineering: Evolution of a Tech-

nological Issue," U.S. House of Representatives, 92nd Congress, second session, 1972.

2. Lesley and John Brown with Sue Freeman. *Our Miracle Called Louise*. London: Magnum Books, 1979, p. 83.

3. Barbara Eck Menning. "The Emotional Needs of Infertile Couples," *Fertility and Sterility* 34, No. 4 (October 1980), pp. 313–19.

4. Martin Curie-Cohen, Lesleigh Luttrell and Sander Shapiro. "Current Practice of Artificial Insemination by Donor in the United States," *New England Journal of Medicine* 300, No. 11 (March 15, 1979), pp. 585–90.

5. Barbara Eck Menning. "Donor Insemination: The Psychosocial Issues," *Contemporary Ob/Gyn* (October 1981), p. 9.

6. "Love for Sale," *The New York Times*, April 2, 1981, reprinted in *Resolve Newsletter*, June 1981, p. 6.

7. Barbara Eck Menning. "Surrogate Motherhood: What Are the Ethical Issues?" *Resolve Newsletter*, June 1981, p. 9.

8. Department of Obstetrics and Gynecology, Tietung Hospital of Anshan Iron and Steel Company, Anshan, China. "Fetal Sex Prediction by Sex Chromatin and Chorionic Villi Cells During Early Pregnancy," *Chinese Medical Journal* 1 (1975), pp. 117–26.

9. Sophia J. Kleegman. "Can Sex Be Planned by the Physician?" *Proceedings of the Fifth World Congress on Fertility and Sterility, Excerpta Medica Foundation*, International Congress Series No. 133 (1966), pp. 1185–95.

10. Rodrigo Guerrero. "Association of the Type and Time of Insemination within the Menstrual Cycle with the Human Sex Ratio at Birth," *New England Journal of Medicine* 291, No. 20 (November 14, 1974), pp. 1056–59.

11. Landrum B. Shettles. "Conception and Birth Sex Ratios: A Review," *Obstetrics and Gynecology* 18 (1961), pp. 122–30. All these techniques of sex preselection are described and evaluated in *Boy or Girl?* by Elizabeth Whelan, (New York: Pocket Books, 1977, pp. 94–156).

RESOURCES

Arditti, Rita, Renate Duelli Klein and Shelley Minden, eds. *Test Tube Women: What Future for Motherhood?* Boston: Routledge and Kegan Paul, 1984. Contains articles by feminists and disability rights activists reflecting on the ways in which recent medical and social practices are reshaping experiences of pregnancy, birth and disability.

Holmes, Helen B., Betty B. Hoskins and Michael Gross, eds. *The Custom-Made Child? Women-Centered Perspectives*. Clifton, NJ: Humana Press, 1981. This is part of a two-volume collection that came out of a meeting in which community workers, physicians, scientists, ethicists and government planners—most of them women and feminists—spent several days discussing women's reproductive health issues. It contains discussions of sex preselection, *in vitro* fertilization, artificial parthenogenesis, cloning and other novel manipulations, real and imagined.

Menning, Barbara Eck. *Infertility: A Guide for Childless Couples*. See Resources for Chapter 21, "Infertility and Pregnancy Loss," for more information.

Milunsky, Aubrey, and George Annas, eds. *Genetics and the Law II*. New York: Plenum Publishing Corp., 1980. A collection of articles and discussions from a meeting of physicians, lawyers, ethicists and other invited speakers, dealing with donor insemination, *in vitro* fertilization and other new reproductive technologies, largely from a medical and legal perspective.

Resolve, Inc., is an infertility self-help group. See Resources for Chapter 21, "Infertility and Pregnancy Loss," for more information.

Teichler-Zallen, Doris, and Colleen D. Clements, eds. *Science and Morality: New Directions in Bioethics*. Lexington, MA: Lexington Books, 1982. Contains up-to-date discussions of the techniques and ethics of genetic manipulation and *in vitro* fertilization.

IV
CHILDBEARING

INTRODUCTION

By Jane Pincus

This introduction in previous editions was written by Jane Pincus and Robbie Pfeufer

Pregnancy, labor and birth are normal bodily processes, uncomplicated most of the time when healthy, self-confident women receive skilled and caring support for the entire childbearing year.

We have great strengths when we bear children—body knowledge about what feels best, flexibility, determination, humor and endurance. We also have great needs.

We need:

- love;
- enough money and/or community support to take care of ourselves;
- a healthy unpolluted environment;
- nourishing food in adequate amounts and to be in as good physical shape as possible and to get sufficient rest;
- a skilled, wise practitioner whom we trust and like, a place of birth which feels comfortable and safe and continuity of care throughout the whole childbearing year;
- confidence in our ability to give birth well. During labor we need people around us who respect us, who have confidence in us and patience with the natural unfolding of our labor. We need food and drink to keep up our strength. We need physical and emotional support to help us relax, to sustain and guide us. We need freedom to adopt the most comfortable labor positions. We need surgically skilled medical personnel with appropriate equipment reasonably nearby in case of emergency.
- After the baby is born we need the opportunity to be with her or him whenever we want, and a helping hand during the days and weeks which follow birth so that we can be sure our families are cared for. We continue to need plenty of good food, rest and help in caring for our babies.
- Control over our fertility so that we have pregnancies we want and plan for.

What if we were to make meeting these needs a priority? We have the necessary resources and information: physiological and psychological knowledge about the childbearing process so that none of us need

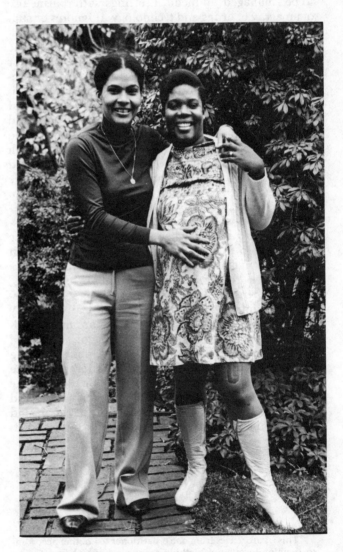

Peter Simon

be ignorant and fearful; enough food (if it were wisely distributed) to nourish every pregnant woman, every man and child. We have medicines and technologies available for crises. A large network of midwives could attend the majority of normal births (85 to 95 per-

327

cent)* and obstetricians could take care of problems requiring medical attention or surgery. Women could have their babies wherever they found it most comfortable and safe, with the assurance that, whatever their choice, they would receive skilled assistance and backup. The whole maternity system would revolve around women, babies and families.

A dream? Yes. Instead, our medical system trains its (mostly male) physicians to consider every birth a potentially life-threatening situation for the mother. The medical world thinks of labor and birth as dangerous, unbearably painful processes, if not illnesses, to be "managed" in medical settings with routine use of an array of drugs and technology. It ignores or suppresses the sexual and spiritual dimensions of childbearing. It reflects this society's social and economic inequality, so that poor women and women of color not only run greater risks during the childbearing process, but have to confront racist and classist practitioners. It presents medical solutions to obstetrical crises provoked by social ills, and looks askance and often with hostility at women and practitioners who choose and create alternatives like out-of-hospital birth centers and informed home births. It has not changed much despite clear evidence that many alternative practices can be as good or better—and safer—than routine, conventional obstetrical practices.

Since money and power underlie our medical system, it changes only when "consumers" make noise and threaten to take their business elsewhere. With childbirth, it has bent only so far by letting fathers into delivery rooms, building hospital birthing rooms, buying expensive birthing chairs, inviting some nurse-midwives into some hospitals. These are all relatively good changes, but token ones: fathers are merely "allowed" in; it is not considered their right. A hospital birthing room is offered only if a woman meets a long list of conditions, so it's not a real alternative. The presence of a commercial birthing chair requires the woman to sit in it as she would a dentist's chair and be controlled, instead of being free to move around and find the labor positions most comfortable and ef-

fective for her. And nurse-midwives must perform a delicate balancing act in hospitals so as not to encounter resistance or lose their jobs. When a laboring woman asks for what she wants, she may be called aggressive or uncooperative or told that her preferences will be "unsafe for the baby." Nurse-midwives attempting to set themselves up in private practice may be denied physician backup; if anything untoward happens when a lay midwife attends a home birth, she may be viciously attacked by the medical establishment (which monitors its own members poorly).

Doctors are our allies in a necessary sense, for we must turn to them in emergencies. But when we are pregnant or in labor, they often ally themselves instead with our fears of risk or pain, and profit from our weakening and giving in. Women used to have good reason to fear childbirth. Becoming pregnant almost every year, they knew next to nothing about pregnancy and birth; they were often less healthy than women of today; there were no antibiotics or blood banks, and many women died. But in these times we have little to fear and much to gain by believing in our health and our strengths, by working for control over our experience and for a more just social and political system in which all of us would get our childbearing needs met. What is best for us is often best and safest for our babies. It is a pity and a challenge that so many of us—parents, midwives, nurses, childbirth educators, a few doctors—have to fight a seemingly endless uphill battle with the medical establishment when, if we lived in a saner society, we could be working together.

It can be wonderful to be pregnant and to prepare for having children. The goal of the next four chapters is to enable you to take charge of your childbearing experience as fully as possible while understanding some of the obstacles which prevent you from doing so. We can help one another improve the quality of care for all mothers-to-be and mothers, and together support those practitioners and other people in our communities who have our interests at heart.

*This figure varies from one practitioner to another according to their philosophy of birthing and actual experience. The incidence of complications is low in places where women's needs are met. For instance, at The Farm, a rural community in Tennessee, there was a 1.5 percent Cesarean rate in the first 1,000 births. At Michel Odent's clinic in Pithiviers, France, there is a 6 percent Cesarean rate. Nurse-midwife-attended deliveries show fewer complications than do physican-attended deliveries, even with relatively "high-risk" women: since 1971, the Frontier Nursing Service's perinatal mortality rates have averaged only six per 1,000, half the average of the rest of the country.

18

PREGNANCY

By Jane Pincus, with Norma Swenson and Bebe Poor

With special thanks to Jenny Fleming, Linda Holmes and Becky Sarah

This chapter in previous editions was written by Ruth Bell and Jane Pincus.

PRENATAL CARE: PREPARATION FOR PREGNANCY, LABOR AND BIRTH

Prenatal care means caring for yourself. We no longer believe that it is enough just to "see the doctor regularly" or "leave it all to the doctor." When you visit your practitioner (doctor or midwife) every month and then every week, s/he is simply monitoring the care you give yourself.* When you have conditions which require watching or medical attention, you especially need to care for yourself to keep in top shape and minimize complications. Caring for yourself means that your good mothering has already begun.

Eating Well

(Also be sure to read Chapter 2, "Food.")

It is essential to eat well during pregnancy.† Think of it as eating for yourself—when you are healthy, most likely your baby will be healthy, too. Also think of it as eating for three—you, your baby and the placenta which links you together, through which your baby receives all its nourishment.

By eating well:

- You expand your blood volume to meet the increased demands pregnancy makes on your body. Blood bathes and washes over the placenta where the exchange of oxygen and nutrients takes place.

- You help make sure that your uterus—and all other tissues—grow and increase in elasticity, that your baby grows to its full genetic potential and weighs as much as it should.

- Adequate birth weight and placental "sufficiency" increase the likelihood that labor and birth will be uncomplicated. You lower the risk of complications such as infections, anemia and toxemia in the mother, and prematurity, low birth weight, stillbirth, brain damage and retardation in the baby.

- You improve the future health of your child.

- Your body stores the fats and fluids you will need when you begin to breastfeed. You will need to continue to eat and drink a lot of healthy foods and fluids after your baby is born.

Eat as well as you can even if finances are tight. Don't deprive yourself to feed other family members. You may be eligible for the WIC (Women, Infants and Children) program, a supplemental food program sponsored by the government. Designed for pregnant and lactating women, it provides milk, fruit, cereal, juice, cheese and eggs. Contact a public prenatal clinic, your local health department, or your public health nurses to find out how you can join. If you are on public assistance, a physician may request a higher food allowance from welfare for you.*

You may not be able to eat large meals, especially during early pregnancy if you are nauseous, or toward the end when your uterus takes up so much room. Instead, eat smaller amounts more often. Eat regularly. Don't go for long stretches of time without food, because your baby needs to eat *all* the time.

---

*In some places, women conduct part of their own prenatal exams (test their urine, take their own blood pressure and keep their own charts). See Maternity Center Association's self-help list (MCA address in Resources in Chapter 19, "Childbirth").

†Even when you are trying to get pregnant, you can begin to change and improve your eating habits.

---

*For more information, contact the Children's Foundation, Suite 800, 1426 New York Avenue NW, Washington, DC 20005, (202) 347-3300, and/or your public health nurse.

AS FOR WEIGHT GAIN, DON'T FIXATE ON A MAXIMUM NUMBER OF POUNDS. EVERY WOMAN'S METABOLISM IS DIFFERENT. IF YOU EAT WELL AND NUTRITIOUSLY, YOUR WEIGHT WILL TAKE CARE OF ITSELF. PREGNANCY IS NOT THE TIME TO DIET.

A Suggested Daily Diet for Pregnancy

1. Two to four protein servings of meat, fish, poultry, cheese, tofu (soybean curd), eggs or nut-grain-bean-dairy combinations. (See p. 17.) If you do not drink one quart of milk a day, add additional protein foods.
2. A quart of milk (whole, skim, buttermilk) or milk equivalents (cheese, yogurt, cottage cheese). Use dry milk powder when cooking other foods. If you are allergic to dairy products, take calcium lactate. Seaweed, sesame seeds, butter, molasses and shellfish contain calcium; some tofu is also made with calcium lactate.
3. A serving of fresh, leafy green vegetables—spinach; dark, loose-leaf lettuce; broccoli; cabbage; Swiss chard; kale; collard; mustard or beet greens; alfalfa sprouts.
4. One or two vitamin-C-rich foods—whole potato, grapefruit, orange, melon, green pepper, cabbage, strawberries, fruit, orange juice.
5. A yellow or orange vegetable or fruit.
6. Four to five slices of whole-grain bread, pancakes, tortillas, cornbread, or a serving of whole-grain cereal or pasta. Use wheat germ and brewers' yeast to fortify other foods.
7. Butter, fortified margarine, vegetable oil.
8. Salt to taste. (Avoid foods and drinks with needless sodium.)
9. Six to eight glasses of liquid—fruit and vegetable juices, water and herb teas. Avoid sugar-sweetened juices and colas.
10. For snacks, dried fruits, nuts, pumpkin and sunflower seeds, popcorn.

Special Food Needs During Pregnancy

Pregnancy increases your need for *calories* and *protein*. Almost all foods contain some protein. You'll also need to eat a wide *variety* of foods, as other nutrients are scattered around in different foods. In general, eat sixty to eighty grams of protein a day. If you are a teenager or carrying twins, you should eat closer to 100 grams a day.

Folic Acid

Found in green leafy vegetables, folic acid consists of a group of compounds in the B-complex family. It is essential for protein synthesis in early pregnancy and also for the formation of blood and new cells. Your baby needs folic acid to grow. Symptoms of folic acid deficiency are anemia and fatigue (anemias may also have other causes). Our bodies don't store folic acid, so if we are anemic, daily supplements are necessary.

If you have taken birth control pills and are now pregnant, you may have depleted your supply of Vitamins B_6 and B_{12} and folic acid and may need supplements.

Iron

Iron is obtained from prune juice, dried fruits, legumes, blackstrap molasses, lean meat, liver, egg yolk and cooking food in iron pots and pans—the longer you cook food, the more it absorbs. It is a main component of hemoglobin which, composed of complex molecules of protein and iron, carries oxygen to your baby and your cells. The baby also draws on your iron reserve to store iron in its liver to last for the duration of his/her milk diet after birth. You'll also need a lot of oxygen (supplied by hemoglobin) during labor for your uterus; the baby's brain cells need oxygen, too. Many young women are iron-deficient before pregnancy. If you eat a well-balanced iron-rich diet, your system may contain enough iron. If not, you'll require a supplement; ask for ferrous gluconate or ferrous fumarate rather than ferrous sulfate, which tends to take vitamins out of your system. Organic iron, a natural form of iron, is available in health food stores.

Calcium

Similarly, your need for calcium increases during pregnancy and lactation.

Fluids

Fluids aid the circulation of blood and body fluids and the distribution of mineral salts, and stimulate the digestion and assimilation of foods. Use care in drinking caffeine. Colas—*all* of them—have too much sodium.

Practitioners, the Medical System and Nutrition

Midwives, nurse-practitioners and family practitioners emphasize eating well much more than the vast majority of obstetricians do. Illogical and unscientific as it may seem, obstetrical training includes little or nothing about the science of applied nutrition.* Many obstetricians consider eating well barely worthy of mention beyond the admonition to "eat a balanced diet." They are taught that they can "rescue" women and babies through technology, drugs and operations when problems arise during pregnancy, labor and birth, instead of learning to prevent, from the outset, conditions that cause many of these problems. Almost totally out of touch with how poor the typical American diet is, doctors do not recognize symptoms of malnutrition and treat it appropriately; they assume that even their middle-class clientele is eating well.

We who are writing this chapter are outraged at a medical and social system which doesn't consider good nutrition to be a basic necessity and right. Women, men and children should have adequate, nutritious food for their entire lives. Physicians and hospitals spend huge amounts of money (more than in any other country) on facilities, research and monitoring equipment for "high-risk" women and low-birth-weight babies when so much of this money could be spent more directly and humanely on guaranteeing us food in the first place. The women who don't have much money, who are under seventeen years of age, who don't gain much weight during pregnancy, who don't eat well, who have infections and diseases—who have never had adequate diet or adequate health care—these are the women who have most of the low-birth-weight babies. Women of color have *twice* as many low-birth-weight babies than do white women. Premature, low-birth-weight babies of color comprise most of the infant deaths in this country. The WIC program, essential to so many women, *has* made a difference, though it is only a drop in the bucket. But stricter eligibility requirements and cuts in funding have reduced WIC's effectiveness. Our society's *first* priority must be to provide basics for ourselves and our children so that we can prevent most crises, which will certainly be cheaper and less stressful than having to cope with them.

Weight-Gain Restriction, Salt-Free Diets, Diuretics and Diet Pills

Most doctors in previous decades restricted weight gain, caloric and salt intake during pregnancy. Many gave pregnant women dangerous diet pills (amphetamines) and diuretics (which eliminate liquids from the body). Some doctors continue these practices in the belief that weight gain and salt intake cause or

*At a January 1982 meeting in which ACOG (the American College of Obstetricians and Gynecologists) members met with local Boston women to have a dialogue about meeting women's real needs, ACOG President George Ryan stated that "nutrition information has been offered in a graduate-level course, but not too many physicians or students were interested." We think that such courses should become part of every obstetrician's *basic* training so that they will have to pay attention to the importance of good nutrition.

Some Facts About the Lack of Prenatal Care for Poor Women and Women of Color*

Many women of color and poor women avoid prenatal care because of prior bad experiences with health professionals who attempted to make them feel inferior, wasted their time and did little for them. Often women who have had little or no prenatal care enter hospitals—usually public hospitals and teaching institutions—with little knowledge of their rights or ways of learning them.

The babies of women of color in this country have almost twice the neonatal mortality rate of babies of white women. In 1976, the neonatal death rate was 9.7 per 1,000 for white women and 16.3 for women of color; in the same year, the maternal mortality rate was 9.3 per 100,000 live births for white women and 15.2 for women of color.

In Washington, D.C., one of the most affluent U.S. communities, the neonatal mortality rate is the highest in the country, evidence of a two-class medical system and gross neglect of the city's mostly black population. In 1981, the white infant mortality rate was 14.1, and the black, 25.5.

In California, Native American infant mortality is higher than in any other reported ethnic groups except blacks. In December 1979, 38 percent of all pregnancies at the Pine Ridge Sioux reservation in South Dakota resulted in miscarriage before the fifth month or excessive hemorrhage, and 60 to 70 percent of the children born suffered breathing problems. A 1980 WARN (Women of All Red Nations) study indicated that the reservation water contained pollutants and radioactive materials.

---

aggravate a condition called toxemia (see p. 346). Studies by nutritionists and a few doctors over the past forty years show toxemia to be a disease caused in part by malnutrition (especially by lack of protein). It can be almost totally eliminated by eating a nutritious diet. These studies also show that calories, salt and increased body fluids are essential to pregnant

*Excerpted from Kathleen Newland, Worldwatch Paper #47: *Infant Mortality and the Health of Societies*; NIH Task Force Report on Cesareans; Barbara McCormic, "Poor, Pregnant Women Experience Powerlessness," *ICEA News*, 19:2, 1980; the California Indian Maternal and Child Health Plan, California Urban Indian Health Council, Oakland, CA; National Health Law Program, *Hard Facts: The Administration's 1984 Health Budget*, "Infant Mortality and Lack of Prenatal Care," March 1, 1983. 2639 S. La Cienega Boulevard, Los Angeles, CA 90034; Winona LaDuke, "They Always Come Back," *Sinister Wisdom* 22/23, P.O. Box 660, Amherst, MA 01004, p. 53.

women and growing babies and that some edema (swelling of the face, hands and feet) is normal during pregnancy. (This edema is different from the accumulation of fat and also from the *sudden* edema weight gain of toxemia, almost always accompanied by high blood pressure and protein in the urine.)

If toxemia, one of those diseases of an economically unequal society, can be prevented by good nutrition, then clearly one of our national priorities should be to provide good food for *all* pregnant women *at the very least*. Though a few women would still develop toxemia, a major factor in this sickness would be eliminated.

Substances and Procedures to Avoid

Drugs*

Commonplace substances such as coffee, tea and over-the-counter medications like aspirin are drugs. They contain many chemicals which have been investigated as possible agents causing birth defects. In the United States a pregnant woman ingests, on the average, seven to eight different drugs during her pregnancy.

Most of the drugs we take during pregnancy will cross the placenta. Fetuses are extremely susceptible to drugs, especially during the first three months when vital organs are forming. We can classify direct effects of substances on pregnancy and the fetus into three different types: *teratogenic* (causing birth defects), *toxic* (having a more severe pharmacological effect on the fetus) and *withdrawal* (causing dependence). Although only a handful of drugs have been shown to be teratogenic, there is much we don't know about possible subtle or long-range effects of many drugs and environmental agents. Therefore, take as few drugs as possible during pregnancy. Sometimes you have to weigh the risks of an illness versus known or unknown risks of the drug in question. For example, if you have a high fever during the first months of pregnancy, your best course of action may be to take aspirin to reduce the fever, because prolonged high fever can be teratogenic. If you have a serious condition such as diabetes or hypertension, you may need to take prescribed drugs to control the disorder, since your illness can affect the baby's development. If you are bothered by more common disorders such as headaches, nausea or constipation, first try nonmedical remedies. If they don't work, consult your practitioner before taking *any* medication, prescription or nonprescription.

Alcohol: a heavy drinker may have a normal child

after one pregnancy and a child with fetal alcohol syndrome (see p. 33) after the next, though her alcohol consumption remains the same. It is not possible to state a level of alcohol regarded as safe during pregnancy. An occasional glass of wine or beer should not cause you anxiety, but you would be wise to limit your drinking to little or nothing. *Caffeine* is a common drug found in coffee, tea, chocolate and over-the-counter drugs. Present evidence, though limited, indicates that moderate amounts of coffee (three cups a day) seem to present no special risks.* *Smoking*, on the other hand, has consistently been shown to have detrimental effects on fetuses. Heavy smokers (more than fifteen cigarettes a day) have a higher rate of miscarriage, stillbirths, premature and low-birth-weight babies. If you can't stop smoking altogether, then reduce the number of cigarettes you smoke, and eat well.

X-Rays

Consider them carefully, and avoid them or delay them until after you have given birth. Have the minimum number if you absolutely have to have them. Diagnostic X-rays are under one rad; many physicians put ten rads of radiation to the fetus as the "safe" exposure limit and offer a therapeutic abortion if amounts have exceeded this limit. Therapeutic irradiation for cancer can cause deformities and spontaneous abortions.

Physical Activity and Exercise

See also Chapter 4, "Women in Motion."

Physical activity and exercise are essential when you are pregnant. Throughout pregnancy, women do everything from swimming, running or walking briskly to dancing and yoga. Use common sense when exercising. If what you are doing makes you feel good, then continue. If you become too tired or uncomfortable, choose a less strenuous activity.

In her book *Essential Exercises for the Childbearing Year* (see Resources), Elizabeth Noble describes many exercises in detail. Chapters include "Pregnancy Creates a Special Need for Exercise, "The Pelvic Floor," "The Abdominal Muscles," "Posture and Comfort," "Relaxation and Breathing." In *New Life* (see Resources), Arthur and Janet Balaskas describe how to get used to practicing varied labor positions, and demonstrate the effectiveness of the squatting position for labor (it increases the pelvic outlet by as much as 30 percent) with excellent illustrations of the pelvis. They also discuss relaxation, massage and breathing. Also see Sheila Kitzinger's book *The Experience of Childbirth* (listed in Resources) for a lot of good ideas about breathing and relaxation.

---

*Drug research gives us conflicting results because it is difficult to do scientific studies using human beings. Drug dosage can be controlled in animal studies, but as animals metabolize drugs differently from humans, results cannot be directly applied. Also, not all fetuses will be affected by the same dosage.

*See "Nutritional Services in Prenatal Care," National Research Council, National Academy Press, Washington, D.C., 1981.

Kegel Exercises

It is simple to do *Kegel exercises*—contracting your pelvic-floor muscles. They help you prepare for childbirth.

A good way to locate these muscles [the pelvic-floor muscles] is to spread your legs apart and to start and stop the flow of urine—your ability to do this is one indication of how strong your muscles are. Another method is to try tightening around a man's erect penis during intercourse (this will feel very pleasant to him and can help to enhance your pleasure, too). Or use one or two of your fingers.

Begin exercising these muscles by contracting hard for a second and then releasing completely. Repeat this ten times in a row to make up one group of exercises (this takes about twenty seconds). In a month's time, try to work up to twenty groups during one day (about seven minutes total). You can do this at any time—while sitting in a car or bus, while talking on the telephone, or even as a wake-up exercise. Some of us have noticed improved muscle tone (and occasionally increased pleasure during sex) in only several weeks. For more detailed instruction on Kegel exercises, consult your local childbirth group.

Putting Yourself at Ease During Pregnancy

Explore your own and your partner's greatest hopes and deepest fears about pregnancy and birth, about becoming parents. Picture what you want the birth to be like. Learn about the baby growing within you, about what happens during childbirth. Learn relaxation skills, read books. Create a community around you by finding a variety of people—your partner, friends young and old—to advise and encourage you. If you don't know any other women who are pregnant, put up a sign at the market or laundromat. *Women were never meant to go through childbearing alone.*

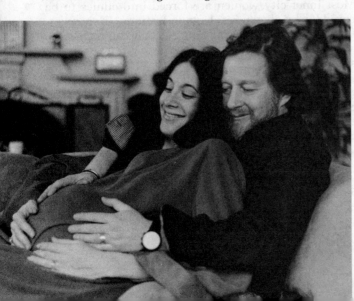

Childbirth Classes

Many women have learned about pregnancy and birth and met other pregnant women by attending childbirth classes.

You may or may not have a choice of classes where you live. In large cities there is a wide range: private classes taught by nurses, midwives or physicians; hospital-based classes; prepaid health-plan classes; and community-based classes taught by childbirth education organizations, Bradley and Lamaze method advocates, home birth groups and independent teachers. If no classes exist, *you can create your own* with the assistance of a layperson or professional who knows about childbearing and with the help of groups already active.*

Community-based classes are likely to be smaller and more personal than hospital classes and much richer in content. You may meet people going to different kinds of birthplaces as clients of a variety of midwives and physicians. You get a better idea of the possible choices. You may make friends who will enjoy trading childcare and providing mutual parenting support for years to come.

Home birth classes can often give you the most positive and complete information about normal labor and birth; people planning other kinds of birth attend them also. They touch on a wide range of concerns—the physiology of labor and birth; visualization of the process (you imagine yourself giving birth); relaxation techniques; the importance of someone (other than hospital staff) to assist you and be your advocate; the practice of supported positions during labor; discussions of fantasies and feelings; risks of routine drugs and interventions, and their occasional benefits; what it's like to breastfeed, to be parents. Couples visit with their new babies to describe their own experiences and answer questions. Films are shown; sometimes tapes of women in labor are played.

It was the first time I'd ever seen anything be born. Hearing people talk, hearing the sounds, made it real. I see that it's a lot of work; people are working hard to make the birth happen. A person can go through all that and be fine!

Those sounds she made were upsetting. I wanted her to stop. They were so intimate, sexual. I could be making those sounds.

*To find out what's available in your area, ask public health nurses, other nurses, midwives and physicians you respect. Contact your local childbirth organization. HOME (Home Oriented Maternity Experience), ICEA (International Childbirth Education Association), NAPSAC (InterNational Association of Parents and Professionals for Safe Alternatives in Childbirth), VBAC (Vaginal Birth After Cesarean), CPM (Cesarean Prevention Movement) or your local women's center. For information on starting your own class, contact Birth Day, P.O. Box 388, Cambridge, MA 02138.

Jim Harrison/Stock Boston

Childbirth preparation has become equated in the popular mind with the Lamaze method (psychoprophylaxis, "prepared" or "natural" childbirth), which teaches women how to breathe and relax in specified ways during labor and birth. In the 1960s, prepared childbirth advocates did fight for women to be awake and conscious during birth—an important advance, since during the previous forty years they had been drugged to the point of unconsciousness. Yet critics of the method point out that it fits all too well with the American way of birth, coexisting with *all* forms of intervention. We are led to believe that we are having "natural" births when in fact we are lying in bed, horizontal, motionless; our labors are accelerated by Pitocin; we are shaved, hooked to monitors, cut (episiotomy) and sometimes partially drugged. Mentally active—concentrating on breathing, panting away like machines—but physically inactive, we are not "in control" but doubly controlled by the interventions and by the breathing method itself. In the words of a labor attendant and childbirth preparation teacher:

I've seen women told to "do your breathing" as they were objecting to painful exams and procedures.

From a conversation with a midwife:

Teach women how to breathe? Why, we know *how to breathe, honey—we've been doing it all our lives!*

Every class we got to know each other better. During breaks we'd talk about our dreams, problems, questions, over apples, tea and crackers. After our babies were born we continued to meet every month for two years.

Most hospital classes tend to focus on labor and delivery and prepare you to accept hospital "management" of birth, presenting their procedures and techniques as if they were a normal and inevitable part of childbirth. Occasionally in hospitals you will find instructors strongly dedicated to your having the best possible experience.

If your hospital class doesn't suit you, change to another if you can, or take more than one kind. Here's an example of the best kind:

The hospital class was useful in preparing couples for the emotional aspects of childbearing.... There were twenty people. The teacher told us about her own experiences. She stressed taking care of yourself afterwards and gave support in being assertive with hospital personnel. In the *Lamaze class, the teacher was more distant but gave better information, role-played us through difficult situations. Classes were indispensable in getting Joel involved.*

Choice and Limitations

The alternatives or choices available in childbirth may not address parents'...concerns about maternity care adequately because the choices offered are limited, and because parents are not really free to choose. Obstetric care is organized in ways that limit choices, being a hierarchical system dominated by an engineering model of birth, in which caregivers contact parents very briefly and are themselves interchangeable, where efficiency is paramount, and where the technology that has been adopted is confining rather than freeing. Safety is a spurious issue in limiting most choices.*

In certain areas of the country where women have been working to expand birthing alternatives, you may be able to choose both practitioner and birthplace—from family practitioners and obstetricians to nurse- and lay-midwives, from freestanding birth centers to home births backed up by hospitals, to hospital birthing rooms and the usual labor and delivery rooms.

However, your town or the city nearest you may have only one clinic, one hospital and one physician (or a group of physicians who have the same ideology). Economic pressures may reduce your options—the local maternity clinic has been closed down for lack of funding, the prepaid health plan you belong to limits your choices because of its stringent rules, you can only afford to use the public hospital clinic and birthing facilities, your insurance coverage restricts you to one type of care. Also, practitioner and place are usually linked: most physicians will not attend you at home and most lay-midwives cannot or will not attend you in hospitals. Laws in most states limit nurse-midwives to attending women in hospitals or birthing centers, though some states permit them to attend home births. The greatest range of choices is available mostly in a narrow, concentrated band in suburbs and edges of cities. Women in rural areas and inner-city areas have little if any real choice of attendant or place of birth. Most inner-city women are forced into clinics to be cared for by ob/gyn residents in training. In these situations, the best you and your partner can do is to be as informed and assertive as possible, and seek out supportive nurses.

Our choices are also limited by the fact that the medical establishment is just that—a *medical* system. Some books and childbirth classes generate a liberal-type illusion that it's possible to make nonmedical choices within that system. It may be possible—up to

*M.P.M. Richards, "The Trouble with 'Choice' in Childbirth," *Birth: Issues in Perinatal Care and Education*, Vol. 9:4 (Winter 1982), p. 253.

a certain point. But once in the hospital, despite our books, classes, "best doctor in town" and even written statements sent beforehand to hospital administrators and nursing staff, we often have very limited control over the environment. Chance and luck play huge roles in what happens during labor: a wonderful, encouraging nurse may be on duty, or there may be a nurse who knows practically nothing about normal labor and doesn't respect our wishes. Our physician, whom we trust, may be busy with another birth or on vacation, and a doctor we've never seen before thinks our ideas absurd and does things his own way, at our expense. In addition, the presence of drugs and equipment nearby and personnel trained and eager to use them alters our choices if we don't have enough support when labor becomes intense.

When we understand these limits, we can work for the changes which make *real* choice possible.

If you do have real choices where you live, learn as much as you can. Ask yourself, what is most important? Where and with whom will you feel most secure? You are the only one who can decide. Each situation is unique; your priorities may be different from another woman's. Also, each region has its own history of obstetrical and midwifery practice which you will need to take into account. Your choices may not always be clear and simple. In many cases, no absolute answers exist. Once you make a decision, you can remain flexible in case you want to or have to change your mind.

Types of Practitioners

When women go to practitioners for checkups, they should walk out from every visit feeling ten feet tall! ...Every site of care and style of care, no matter who gives it, ought not only to give surveillance but should educate and empower, should enhance every woman's feeling of her ability to do what she's doing well.

Physicians

Every good-sized community has physicians.

Obstetrician/gynecologists, trained primarily as surgeons, see women for brief periodic checkups, are usually in and out during labor and often arrive just before delivery. Often they practice in groups, and may control childbirth practices in one hospital or throughout a whole region. They do not usually practice in rural areas. In most suburban and metropolitan areas only ob/gyns have delivery room privileges in hospitals; in teaching hospitals and medical centers all MDs will be ob/gyns or ob/gyn residents in training. Though most obstetricians are not trained to deal with *normal* labors (see p. 364, "Physicians' Obstetrical Training Contributes to the Climate of Doubt"), their surgical skills are invaluable in real emergencies. Their prenatal care is often lacking.

From a conversation among pregnant women:

a. I really didn't think much of the doctors at the clinic. They were very impersonal and ...it's a real mill....They want you out of there in 20 minutes.
b. So do private obstetricians. They want you out of there in *10.*
c. Mine didn't even know my *name* through the whole pregnancy.*

When I go for checkups at the health plan office, nurses check my weight, urine and blood pressure. The doctor listens to my baby's heartbeat. They never ask me how I am feeling, what I eat, if I get enough exercise and rest or if I have any questions or problems.

Family practitioners (MDs and DOs [osteopaths]) and *general practitioners* (almost extinct) are "primary-care" physicians trained in family medicine, which means that they can give basic, comprehensive care to any person of any age. They are more likely to see you as a whole person and to know other family members. Most of them have a fair amount of obstetrics experience and some specialize in obstetrics. They have delivery room privileges in most community hospitals.

There *are* family practitioners and obstetricians who have our true interests at heart, who listen to what we want, alter their practices accordingly, teach us a lot and learn from us.

A family practitioner:

In my relationship with families I get as much as I give. I see people doing marvelous jobs: during labor and birth they are autonomous, assertive, really pleased with themselves. To be part of their birth experiences is exciting for me in turn. My presence helps them to feel safe having babies at home.

A male family practitioner:

When I attend women in labor I am as much my woman-self as I can be. Sometimes I know when they are fully dilated, for my own stomach feels crampy. I've asked the midwives about this and they say it happens to them, too.

A mother:

When I was ready to give birth the nurse said, "Push with your mouth shut." But I thought to myself (it wasn't exactly thinking), "That's not the best way for the baby to get oxygen." I wanted to groan, so I groaned deep, loud primal groans and pushed my daughter out. My doctor was amazed. He'd never heard such sounds before. They worked so well he said he would suggest them to other women.

*Jo Ann Bromberg, "Having a Baby: A Story Essay," in *Childbirth: Alternatives to Medical Control*, Shelly Romalis, ed., University of Texas Press, Austin, TX, 1981, p. 40.

In a hospital birthing room:

Dr. E. checked me out during my pregnancy because I had a particular medical problem. (Otherwise the midwives he works with would have seen me.) Though he stayed with me during labor, Bonnie, my labor coach, acted as midwife, suggesting what to do, applying hot compresses. Dr. E. showed her a lot of respect, the respect she deserved to have. It tickled me to overhear him say to the medical student present, "Now, here's birth with dignity! I certainly don't need to be here."

Such physicians are rare.* Many of them are either scorned or harassed by their colleagues.

Midwives

Women have cared for childbearing women for centuries. In many communities they were recognized as "wisewomen" and consulted about issues other than childbearing—illness, abortion and child health.

In the U.S. today there are two main types of midwives—*certified nurse-midwives* and *lay (empirical) midwives*. They often share similar philosophies about childbearing, although their education and training differ.

At the heart of midwifery lies the belief that the passage through the birth canal is a healthy experience for mother and baby. The midwife believes in the ability of a woman's body to move toward health, to compensate for irregularities and to overcome pain. She sees birth as an expression of spirit in a physical act [and] believes that the baby benefits from this creative expression and actually likes being born.†

In the words of a nurse-midwife working in a hospital:

I want to be where women are. I want to be where women want to be. I am fascinated to watch them be powerful. I see them emerge from their birth experiences and make changes in their own lives.

When midwives are free to practice as they want, they offer us continuous care during pregnancy, labor and birth and after the baby is born.

Midwives, *at their best,*

- pay attention to the woman in her family context, to family dynamics. They help expectant and new parents sort out their feelings and deal with practicalities;
- bring to their work a strong combination of prac-

*See Michel Odent's *Birth Reborn*, and Sagov, et al., *Home Birth: A Practitioner's Guide to Birth Outside the Hospital*, for informed descriptions of attitudes toward childbirth and how medically trained people can change their attitudes. (Both listed in Resources in Chapter 19, "Childbirth.")
†Peggy Spindell, "Midwives and Physicians: Making Home Birth Work Together," Chapter 3 in Sagov, et al., *A Practitioner's Guide to Birth Outside the Hospital.*

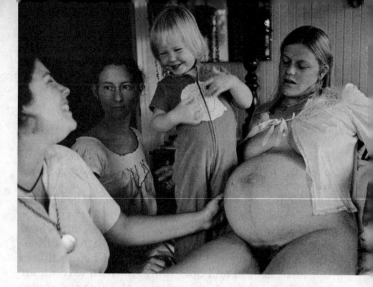

Suzanne Arms

ticality and spirituality. They are concerned with the woman's well-being and satisfaction as well as with the safety of mother and baby;
- encourage women to take charge of their care, to believe they are equal to the responsibility, to feel in control of their experience;
- are knowledgeable about normal pregnancy, labor and birth;
- respect the process of birth, trust the unique course of each labor, patiently watch it unfold, sustain and guide us, encourage us to find comfortable, efficient labor positions and help us ease the baby out;
- bring us through difficult moments, sometimes turning what looks like a complicated labor into a normal one;
- recognize complications which require a doctor's attention and call upon doctors for help when necessary.

[A midwife's] skills, besides medical techniques, include elusive abilities to intuit, evoke and channel. Her hands are among her most precious tools.*

For me, Janet, my nurse-midwife, meant the support I'd hoped for; for instance, coming to our apartment for my actually fairly short labor. When I thought I was really not holding up under the stress she'd say, "That was pretty intense," verifying that it was okay to be "falling apart" and that I was doing great. We ended up going to the hospital birthing room when I was pretty far along—unpleasant having to move, but it certainly kept my labor going. For me, even the pushing hurt, but again I felt such confidence that everything was going well....After Jackie was born, I felt only Janet understood what I'd been through and what I was going through.

Certified Nurse Midwives (CNMs)

More and more communities and hospitals have CNMs, nurses educated in graduate programs as specialists in normal pregnancy and birth and in well-woman care. They follow an organized program of

*Elizabeth Davis, *A Guide to Midwifery, Heart and Hands*, p. 4. (See Resources in Chapter 19, "Childbirth.")

study designed to meet preset standards for knowledge, skill and judgment. Graduates are evaluated and certified after passing examinations, and each state licenses nurse-midwives to practice under its own regulations.

CNMs work in their own private practices, in private physician practices, freestanding birth centers, hospitals, health departments and sometimes homes. They *always* practice in conjunction with physicians, referring women who have problem pregnancies to them and calling upon them in situations and emergencies which require medical care, advice and/or surgical attention.

CNMs in the U.S. got their start in the 1920s, when nurses associated with the Frontier Nursing Service and Maternity Center Association began attending poor women in Appalachia and New York City, later working in and out of hospitals for fifty to sixty years. The American College of Obstetricians and Gynecologists (ACOG) waited until 1971 to recognize the profession officially. Nurse-midwives have been instrumental in creating out-of-hospital birth centers and in-hospital alternative maternity care programs in response to parents' complaints about conventional hospital care. They often attend poor women when physicians will not, and fight along with clinic patients for simple changes in obstetrical routines.

It is a victory for us to enable clinic women to labor upright....Otherwise they'd be flat on their backs the whole time.

STUDIES OF NURSE-MIDWIFERY PRACTICE, PAST AND PRESENT, CONSISTENTLY SHOW OUTCOMES AS GOOD OR BETTER THAN PHYSICIAN OUTCOMES, WITH FEWER FORCEPS DELIVERIES, CESAREAN SECTIONS AND EPISIOTOMIES, FEWER STILLBIRTHS AND LOW-BIRTH-WEIGHT BABIES.* Despite this excellent record, and although nurse-midwives are in increasingly high demand (most women attended by nurse-midwives prefer them to physicians), there are simply not enough of them, for the following reasons: 1. too few training programs exist, though there is a huge backlog of applicants; 2. for a number of years many state laws restricted or prohibited nurse-midwifery practice (rarely the case now); 3. nurse-midwifery is an interdisciplinary profession and NMs may find it difficult to obtain adequate physician backup. While some physicians appreciate the quality care nurse-midwives offer, many others, especially obstetricians, consider nurse-midwifery an economic threat as well as a challenge to their competence as clinicians. As a result they may either refuse to develop the necessary cooperative relationship, attempt to prevent other physicians from doing so, or punish them when they do.

*See "Information Concerning the Quality of Nurse-Midwifery Care" (MCA), available from the Boston Women's Health Book Collective.

Insurance companies in some states are beginning to reimburse nurse-midwives. However, Blue Cross/Blue Shield companies offer a lower rate of coverage since many of the "Blues" have physicians on their boards who want to limit financial competition.*

Lay (Empirical) Midwives

Lay midwives attend the childbearing women in their communities who have babies at home and want assistance.

Though the rise of obstetricians, the outlawing of midwives and the move to hospitals eliminated most traditional midwives by the mid-1960s, they continued to practice in regions where there were no doctors nearby, where women were too poor to pay doctors' fees and where black and Chicana women could not get into segregated hospitals or were so mistreated in hospitals that they felt more comfortable delivering at home attended by women they trusted. "Granny" midwives continue to work, licensed and sometimes supervised by state departments of health, but each year there are fewer of them. In these rural areas, the lack of Medicaid reimbursement directly contributed to their demise. Clients who once used them turned to doctors and hospitals for "free" care. Yet in many cases, the care they gave was outstanding. For instance, in North Carolina between 1974 and 1976, black granny midwives were among those lay-midwives who had a neonatal mortality rate of four per thousand in planned home births, despite the high-risk profile of their clientele.†

Over the past twenty years a new group of lay-midwives has come into being to answer the needs of healthy pregnant women who want to deliver at home or who cannot afford a hospital birth. At their best, these midwives apprentice with more experienced midwives, read everything they can, learn from and work with supportive physicians, keep their skills fresh and create educational programs for themselves (Seattle and Rhode Island now have midwifery schools). They become specialists in normal pregnancy, labor and birth. (Sometimes they are the most skilled, knowledgeable and competent *normal* birth attendants in their community.) They know their limits, screen pregnant women for risks, encourage them to obtain physician backup or obtain backup for themselves. They know how to recognize labor complications, and they call upon physicians when necessary.

In somewhat the same way that nurse-midwives are

*For a listing of health insurance companies providing direct or indirect reimbursement for certified nurse-midwives, see Doris Haire, "Health Insurance Coverage for Nurse-Midwifery Services," *Journal of Nurse-Midwifery*, Vol. 27, No. 6, November/December 1982, pp. 35–36.

†See Claude A. Burnett, et al., "Home Delivery and Neonatal Mortality in North Carolina," U.S. Department of Health, Education and Welfare, Center for Disease Control, Bureau of Epidemiology, Atlanta, Georgia.

In this set-up that man has to do away with the midwives, God is yet on his throne....So don't you worry about Alabama doing away with the midwives. God is in Alabama—unhun—and in other places, too.

Miss Annie Lee James, midwife
Louisville, Alabama

Miss James and many other southern granny midwives believe in keeping the faith. In fact, many of these women can trace their faithkeeping heritage to great-grandmothers who were midwives during slave times. The granny women say God gave midwives their work and the powers of the supernatural will always be present to guide them.

As recently as 1950, the majority of all black babies born were attended by granny midwives, primarily older, self-educated black women. Today, however, granny midwives' hands provide care for less than 1 percent of childbearing mothers. White granny midwives practicing mostly in Appalachian areas and Hispanic grannies in the southeastern United States have also been legally eradicated.

Besides their profound sense of spirituality, granny midwives were particularly sensitive in understanding their clients' emotional, social and psychological needs. Grannies, for example, often waited on generations of the same family. ("Waited on" is an expression used by the granny women to describe their childbirth attendant activities.) Other aspects of their community roles as midwives included counselor for baby ills, household support person for postpartum mothers, adviser on gynecological problems, community herbologist and general healer. These granny midwives who maintained culturally based expressions around the birth event were also recognized by community members as ritual specialists.

As for actual midwifery practices, many of them were precursors to the current wave of birthing alternatives. Grannies kept their mammas stirring, as they say, during labor. These women were masters of various massage techniques which they applied during pregnancy as well as in the course of childbirth. And many grannies assisted mothers in using the traditional birthing positions taught to them by their mothers or the community's elder midwives; midwives recognized that stooping, kneeling or squatting made birthing much easier. Most of these traditions are African and are still alive in African culture today. Some midwives have also even quietly maintained their knowledge of the use of various teas as purgatives, labor stimulants and muscle relaxants. Of course, the granny midwife differs from other American birth attendants in her training. These granny midwives acquired their skills through apprenticeships with other midwives, with varying degrees of medical input from local nurses, nurse-midwives and doctors. Often, however, the primary basis of their education was the experience gained through helping friends and relatives in childbirth and in waiting on themselves—many women had no assistance at the time of birth. Yet, despite their lack of formalized training, these midwives somehow managed to attend normal childbirths successfully, as well as the birth of twins and breech deliveries when medical assistance was unavailable.

—Linda Holmes

meeting standards and offering peer support, so women in the best lay-midwifery communities keep in constant communication about their work.

Since most doctors, especially obstetricians, are hostile to lay midwifery, midwives in some areas have a difficult time finding any medical support at all. In some states lay midwifery is legal; in others its legal status is unclear. Some lay midwives work in hospitals as well as homes.* Others must work in semisecrecy.

Some Considerations About Midwives

Though midwives are often the best practitioners for childbearing women, they differ greatly in philosophy, personality and practice. You'll want to screen a midwife as carefully as you would a physician, looking for competence, flexibility and empathy.

Some CNMs have a more medicalized approach than others, especially when they work in hospitals rather than in freestanding birth centers or homes. Some lay midwives are able to keep a clearer vision of what normal childbirth can be than can midwives working in more medicalized settings. On the other hand, because their learning is often individual and unstructured, lay midwives can differ greatly in levels of experience. Occasionally a woman who decides to act as a midwife without fully realizing the importance of lengthy experience, study and training may be incompetent.

When nurse-midwives and lay midwives are too much in demand, they can overcommit themselves, get overtired and "burnt out" and end up spending less time with you than you or they expected.

*For example, in San Francisco General Hospital and Gifford Memorial in Randolph, Vermont.

Making an Active Choice

(See Appendix for questions to ask practitioners and hospitals.)

Check out the options where you live. Get names of practitioners from people you know and trust; from local childbirth groups, childbirth teachers, women's health groups, the American College of Nurse-Midwives, MCA, NAPSAC, ICEA or the BWHBC (see Resources in Chapter 19, "Childbirth.").

Once you know what choices are available, look around. Be as clear as you can about the kind of pregnancy, birth and postpartum experience you want. Ask other women who have had babies recently, *"What happened?"* Then visit practitioners or phone them, and ask them about their beliefs and practices. Some will treat you well and welcome your questions. Some physicians may be resentful, even hostile, at your efforts to evaluate them, because they aren't used to it. Persist—you have a right to make an informed choice.

As you speak with practitioners: 1. State your preferences. Ask questions clearly and tactfully; aim to communicate well from the start. Ask for equally clear and specific answers. 2. Bring someone with you, preferably the person who will share pregnancy, birth and childcare with you, for company and support, and to help you remember what you want to ask. 3. Trust your own instincts. If you think that the practitioner resists or resents your questions, it should not have to be your task at this time to educate him or her, though if you live in an area of limited choice you may have to. 4. Especially important: if, during the course of your relationship with your practitioner you feel dissatisfied with answers to your questions, or demeaned, then consider changing if possible.

It can be hard even to think of switching. Sometimes we feel unaccountably "loyal" even to a person who makes us uncomfortable, hurts us in some way, or whom we actively dislike. More emotional than usual during pregnancy, you may hesitate to make such a big change, especially if you are feeling unsure of yourself. Ask your partner and friends to help you. Once

you decide, you may find it easy and strengthening to choose someone else. It is never too late to switch.

I was in labor for two days at the hospital. My labor wasn't progressing fast enough for my doctor. He was angry at me because I refused to have it speeded up by Pitocin. I knew I was doing fine. Finally the hospital decided I wasn't in labor (at five centimeters' dilation!). My doctor sent me home. As soon as I got home my labor picked up and became so intense I knew I was about to give birth. My husband rushed me to another hospital (I was afraid to return to the first—no way!) and I had the baby then and there, attended by the very surprised nurse-midwife on duty!

HOSPITAL BIRTHS

When you choose a practitioner or a clinic, you are usually choosing a hospital, too. Most hospitals find it easier to treat all women the same way. Hospital routines may or may not coincide with those of your practitioner. Learn as much about the hospital as you can. (See Appendix for questions to ask.) Take a tour early so that the surroundings become familiar and you feel comfortable. Ask questions. Talk with the nurses, too, if you can.

Deciding

Actually, if there were a birth center nearby, I'd have my baby there. But since there isn't, and since I'm completely healthy, I don't want to go to a hospital and be made to feel unhealthy. We're having a home birth with a very fine midwife. The more I learn, the more I'm sure that's what I want.

I chose the hospital because I wanted the whole experience to be separate from the rest of my life, and I felt safest there.

CHOOSING A BIRTHPLACE

Place	Practitioner	Place of Birth
hospitals	doctors (ob/gyn, resident, GP or family practitioner [sometimes a medical student]); nurse-midwife	labor and delivery rooms; labor room; birthing room (alternative birth center, or ABC); operating room
free-standing birth center	doctor; nurse-midwife	birthing room or bedroom
home delivery service; home	nurse-midwife; doctors, lay or nurse-midwives	living room, bedroom, bathroom—anywhere

339

It would freak out our landlords if we gave birth in our apartment. I don't feel at home there anyway, and have no special attachment to it. I'm also a little nervous. So we're planning to use the hospital birthing room. Our doctor is a family practitioner.

I had my first two children in a hospital. Both were good experiences, but after having a home birth I know what a truly good experience is. I felt rested, healthy, ready to have a baby. My husband was as involved, eager and interested as he could be. I wanted to have the least intervention possible. My friends were all around me. It's incredible to think about doing the hardest, most concentrated intense work you will ever do in your life in an unfamiliar place—the most intimate experience and you are sharing it with strangers. Here I was in my own bed, my own clothes, in an atmosphere so familiar.

Another factor against home birth was having to deal with such "stuff." It was complicated-sounding getting everything set up—backups, etcetera. And I didn't really want to deal with all the people who would be appalled, the explaining we'd have to do. Everyone (like my mother) was satisfied with the idea of a nurse-midwife. I could say, "Oh, yes, the doctors are there if needed"; "It's in a medical facility"; etcetera.

I was aware of the home birth movement, but for me I couldn't do it comfortably. If anything happened I'd never forgive myself. My parents would never forgive me. But I know childbirth is a fairly normal process so I didn't want to go to the Boston crisis centers. I wanted a labor coach because I wanted to stay home as long as possible during labor. So I chose Dr. M. and the birthing room of the small hospital he worked at.

Hospital Birthing Rooms

For the past five years, many hospitals have offered birthing rooms, sometimes called "alternative birth centers" (ABCs), *not* to be confused with freestanding birth centers. The mere existence of a birthing room does not guarantee you a more autonomous labor and delivery. If someone else has gone into labor ahead of you, it may not even be available. In some places birthing-room regulations are so stringent that you must meet rigid criteria to be "eligible." Then, when you are "allowed" to use it, the moment your labor deviates from a mythical "norm" you may be transferred to a conventional labor room. You may feel you have to prove yourself, an added stress which can make you tense and slow your labor. Only when hospital staff and administration respect the noninterventionist policy behind a birthing room is it a *real* alternative.*

*See Jane Dwinell, "A Model Program for Family Centered Hospital Care," in Janet Isaacs Ashford, *Whole Birth Catalog*, p. 91. Also Diony Young, *Changing Childbirth*, pp. 141–65 (see Resources in Chapter 19, "Childbirth").

FREESTANDING BIRTH CENTERS

Freestanding birth centers provide a homelike atmosphere for women and families, where skilled practitioners treat birth as a normal, healthy process and don't practice routine intervention. There are now at least 107 birth centers in the U.S. These centers always have a system whereby women can be transferred to a hospital if they need more specialized procedures. As birth centers in the U.S. are new and vary in their practices, check out their philosophies, protocols and procedures.* Nurse-midwife-directed centers, for example, offer the best comprehensive care at the lowest rates, using physicians as consultants. Physician-directed centers tend to rely on nurses (who may or may not have midwifery skills) for care, thereby creating a "minihospital" rather than a home as the midwives do. Many physicians do not have adequate midwifery skills to attend births outside of hospitals.

HOME BIRTHS

Home births offer us the opportunity to labor in familiar surroundings, to choose our own attendants, to do things to soothe and encourage ourselves. At home we avoid the annoying and sometimes dangerous hospital routines. At home, birth is a family event with the father, grandparents, older children and friends all welcome to share the wonder of birth and greet the new baby. Once the baby is born, we can relax in our own way, eat the food we like and get to know our new baby without the need to conform to an institution's schedules.

We are also concerned with the safety of home birth.† The outcome of childbirth is determined primarily by the care we give ourselves and the training of our birth attendant rather than by the place of birth. We must be screened prenatally for contraindications to home birth (for example, toxemia, kidney disease, severe anemia, heart disease, hypertension, diabetes, drug addiction, severe infection, abnormal presentations, multiple births, Rh sensitization, placenta previa or a history of premature babies). However, this screening is not a substitute for the care we give ourselves throughout pregnancy. If genuine high-risk conditions are identified, then we should plan for the birth to take place in facilities equipped to deal with possible complications. Most birth attendants will not agree to

*Contact the National Association of Childbearing Centers (NACC), formerly the Cooperative Birth Center Network (CBCN), Box 1, Rte. 1., Perkiomenville, PA 18074, (215) 234-8068, if you are looking for a birth center in your area. Send a stamped, self-addressed envelope for information.

†See Sagov, et al., *Home Birth: A Practitioner's Guide to Birth Outside the Hospital*, for an informed discussion of this issue.

attend a woman at home if she has any of these conditions.

In this country the woman who wants to give birth at home has to take a great deal of initiative. Most physicians oppose home birth outright.* They may frighten you with horrible tales of what might happen without discussing ways of making home birth safe. They may not be able to prescreen adequately for risks or provide emergency backups. They will ignore excellent statistics from Europe and our own Kentucky Frontier Nursing Service. Behind this smoke screen lie other, sometimes unspoken, factors: home births are inconvenient for physicians; it is frightening for them to be away from all their hospital equipment; it is psychologically threatening for them to be the invited guest in your home, where you set the tone and they are not in complete control. Fear of malpractice suits and hospital backup are added issues.

Most insurance policies will pay all or part of a physician's fee—but not the midwife's—regardless of where the birth takes place.

Once you've decided to have your baby at home, preventing complications and handling unexpected problems is your next concern. The best preventive measures are to eat a sufficient quantity of high-quality food, exercise regularly, and avoid cigarettes and alcohol.

Emotional and spiritual strength and well-being are important.

Women who plan to give birth at home are often denied prenatal medical care or backup emergency care by local obstetricians, who are openly hostile and say, "We can't afford the risk; we may be sued if something goes wrong."

Most complications of childbirth are minor and can be handled without difficulty by a practitioner experienced in normal births at home. (See "Midwives," p. 336.) Even in the cases of more serious complications, however, there is almost always enough time to get more specialized help. The times when hospital care unexpectedly becomes instantaneously necessary are rare. A matched, controlled study by Mehl, comparing the outcomes of 1,046 home births to 1,046 hospital births, found no significant differences in maternal or infant mortality or morbidity.†

*In 1982 ACOG and the obstetrical establishment circulated throughout the media raw and undifferentiated statistics from several state health departments which purport to show that there is a higher risk of death when babies are born at home. These statistics represent unplanned, premature, precipitous home births. ACOG hired expensive public relations experts to mislead the public and their colleagues in other specialties. What these figures actually show is what happens when women are denied adequate medical care by physicians and welfare bureaucrats. Meanwhile, major policy decisions are being made by state and welfare officials on the basis of ACOG's report.

†See Lewis E. Mehl, "The Outcome of Home Delivery: Research in the United States," in Sheila Kitzinger and John A. Davis, *The Place of Birth*, pp. 93–117 (see Resources in Chapter 19, "Childbirth").

While hospital emergency rooms are required by law to accept anyone who appears for emergency care, both parents and birth attendants feel more comfortable knowing that they have made arrangements in advance for such an emergency transfer in case it becomes necessary.

Birth attendants have differing criteria for transferring a birth to the hospital. Their decisions may vary depending on the nature of the problem, their training, the available equipment, their agreements with supporting physicians and the nature of the emergency backup facility as well as its distance from the birth.

It was a really beautiful thing to do—not only to be freed from the atmosphere and personnel of the hospital (and who knows what it means for a newborn to see wood walls and carpeted floor, to smell real human smells, to feel wool and cotton and flannel clothes instead of starchy, white, deodorized...) but also to know that my body and her body knew what to do, and probably did it better than any doctors could. She was crying before the push that sent her into the world had faded, and was wide awake from the start.

Now that it's over I can think of the risks we took—being an hour and a half from the hospital on a cold night if we needed help—and I can get angry again at the system and the attitudes that forced me to choose the risk. But still, the pride, the job, the beauty, the wonder of it all overshadow the anger and fear. I hope lots more women do this—I feel strangely stronger (in terms of self, not physically) than ever before.

THE PREGNANCY ITSELF

I sit here on the porch as if in a deep sleep, waiting for this unknown child. I keep hearing this far flight of strange birds going on in the mysterious air about me. How can it be explained? ...Suddenly everything comes alive...like an anemone opening itself, disclosing itself, and the very stones themselves break open like bread.*

During your pregnancy, several processes are going on at once: you are going through physical changes and emotional changes and your fetus is growing within you. Though your pregnancy will have much in common with other women's, it is yours and unique (and each pregnancy you go through will differ from the others). In talking to women who have been pregnant and who are pregnant at the same time you are, you will discover that there's no one right way to be pregnant.

Many changes take place in your body as the fetus develops in you. Some of these changes are just changes but, though we are adapted to bearing children, dis-

*Meridel LeSueur, "Annunciation," *Ripening*, Feminist Press, Old Westbury, NY, 1982, p. 128.

341

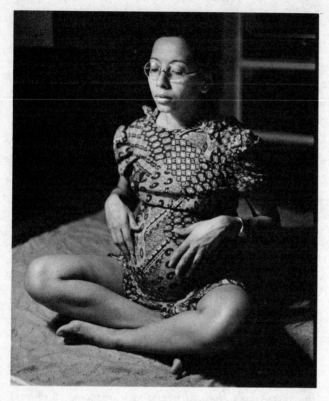

George Malave/Stock Boston

comforts can arise. You may feel many changes and discomforts, few or none at all. You'll want to know what they are, why they occur, when they are likely to occur. Eating well and exercising reduce or eliminate many discomforts. Some minor discomforts, if neglected, can lead to major complications. And you should know that in every pregnancy there's a possibility of miscarriage (though the likelihood decreases with the passing months), so that if it happens to you, you won't be totally unprepared.

As for your feelings, they will vary tremendously according to who you are; how you feel about having children; your previous pregnancies and/or abortion experiences, if any; how you feel about your own childhood, your parents or the people who reared you; whether or not you are with a partner—and if you are, how you feel about him or her.

At each stage you may feel conflicts as well as harmonies. Sometimes you'll feel positive, sometimes negative. You'll have doubts and fears. It's important to know that these doubts and fears occur during a "good" pregnancy, too, for in a very real sense your body has been taken over by a process out of your control. You can come to terms with that takeover actively and consciously by knowing what's happening to your body, by identifying your specific feelings (especially the negative ones, because they are the most difficult to deal with) and also by learning what the

fetus looks like as it grows. Its growth is dramatic and exciting. (See p. 351 for more on feelings.)

Our society tends to treat pregnancy as a solitary, clinical experience. Many nonindustrialized societies have invested it with religious significance, respect it as an altered physical and psychic state and celebrate it as significant not only for the couple but for the entire community. Making and deepening bonds with people who make you feel special can be an important source of strength.

Due Date

The length of a normal pregnancy can vary from 240 to 300 days. It's good to know approximately when your due date will be, but don't get fixated on a particular day. Only 5 percent of women give birth on their projected due date! (Some practitioners advise rounding it off to the nearest month!)* Since there are so many changes and feelings to talk about, it's more convenient to talk within the framework of trimesters.

First Trimester (First Twelve Weeks)

Physical Changes

You may have none, some or many of the following early signs of pregnancy. If you have had regular periods, you will probably notice that you have missed a period. However, some women do bleed for the first two or three months even when they are pregnant, but bleeding is usually short and there's scant blood. Also, about seven days or so after conception, the *blastocyst*, the tiny group of cells which becomes the embryo, attaches itself to the uterine wall, and you may have slight vaginal spotting, called implantation bleeding, while new blood vessels are being formed. *Be sure to get a pregnancy test* (see p. 284).

You may have to urinate more often because of increased hormonal changes; pituitary hormones affect the adrenals, glands which change the water balance in your body, so you retain more body water. Also, your enlarging uterus presses against your bladder.

*If you and your obstetrician disagree seriously about the conception date, this can affect your baby's well-being. For example, if your obstetrician thinks the baby is "postmature," s/he may advise induction. If you are right and s/he is wrong, the birth may be premature. If your doctor thinks you are *less* pregnant than you are, you may give birth before anyone is prepared for it.

We have talked with dozens of women whose doctors refused to believe that they knew when their babies were conceived and thus approximately when they were due. Some had problems as a result. *Don't let the due date tyrannize you.*

Nowadays, obstetricians tend to dismiss their judgment *and* yours, and rely on ultrasound to assess fetal maturity. Unfortunately, some doctors recommend *monthly* ultrasound pictures and depend on these rather than on physical exams. This is not sound medical practice.

Your breasts will probably swell. They may tingle, throb or hurt. Your milk glands begin to develop. Because of an increased blood supply to your breasts, veins become more prominent. Your nipples and the area around them (areola) may darken and become broader.

You may feel nauseated, mildly or enough to vomit, partly because your system is changing. One theory is that the higher level of estrogen accumulates even in the cells of the stomach and causes irritation as acids tend to accumulate. The rapid expansion of the uterus may be involved. If you feel nauseated, eat lightly throughout the day rather than taking large meals. Eat food high in protein. Munching crackers or dry toast slowly before you get up in the morning can help a lot. Avoid greasy, spiced food. Don't fast, and at least drink juice. Take Vitamin B_6 and other B-vitamins. Apricot nectar helps some women. Powdered ginger in capsules or as a tea can help too.

You may feel constantly tired.

You may have increased vaginal secretions, either clear and nonirritating or white, yellow, foamy or itchy. The chemical makeup as well as the amount of your vaginal fluids is changing. If you are very uncomfortable or if such a condition persists, see your practitioner.

The joints between your pelvic bones widen and become more movable about the tenth or eleventh week. Occasionally the separating bones come together and pinch the sciatic nerve, which runs from your buttocks down through the back of your legs; this can cause pain.

Your bowel movements may become irregular, in part because the heightened amount of progesterone relaxes smooth muscles; therefore, your bowels may not function as efficiently as they did. Also, if you are resting more often, your decreased activity may cause some constipation. Eat foods high in fiber content and/or simply add bran to other foods. Eat salads and fresh fruits frequently and drink fruit juices.

During the first ten weeks you'll feel relatively few body changes. All those above are fairly common and not too annoying, though nausea and tiredness can wipe some women out.

Early pregnancy surprised me. I was expecting to feel very different and instead was feeling things I'd felt before. It was like premenstrual tension. I was a little nauseous. But it's amazing—once I realized I was pregnant the symptoms were tolerable, because they are not signs of sickness but of a life growing.

I felt at the same time more vulnerable and more powerful than ever.

Exam Schedule

Obstetricians and clinics usually set up a fairly cursory routine examination schedule. Midwives and family practitioners will see you just about as regularly, but most likely will spend more time with you.

During your first visit the practitioner should take a complete medical, reproductive and family history, including menstrual history, previous babies, pregnancies, operations, abortions, illnesses, drugs taken, family illnesses such as heart disease (see p. 542). Bring any medical records that you have and describe as completely as possible what's happened to you physically in the past. You should have a general physical exam and then an exam for pregnancy, which includes examination of the breasts to see if there are changes in the glands, and a pelvic exam, which shows the position and consistency of the uterus, the condition of the ovaries and fallopian tubes and the consistency and color of the cervix. A blood sample will be taken to determine your blood type and the presence or absence of the Rh factor, and to provide blood for a blood count and hemoglobin analysis. You'll probably have tests for rubella* and possibly for toxoplasmosis (a disease resulting from cat feces or raw meat which causes retardation in newborns) and an AFP titre (see p. 355). You'll also get other tests and cultures for STDs. (See Chapter 14, "Sexually Transmitted Diseases," for a description of the effects of untreated STDs on newborns.) The urinalysis will check for protein and glucose in the urine and a urine culture will reveal any urinary tract infections.† Your weight and blood pressure will be checked and you will have a Pap smear. If you have a history of diabetes and a specific risk factor (large babies, family history of diabetes, previous history of stillbirths), get your urine checked two times in a row before getting a blood sugar (glucose tolerance) test. Get frequent blood and sugar tests and eat carefully.

---

*If you are not immune to German measles (rubella), try to avoid exposure. When you have it, you may have a rash, tenderness of the lymph nodes in the back of your neck and possibly mild joint pains. If you are exposed in the first trimester of pregnancy and if you get the disease, chances are high that the fetus will be deformed. At this point you will have to make a decision about whether or not to continue your pregnancy. A blood test will tell you if you have or have had rubella.

†When you are pregnant you become more susceptible to urinary tract infections because the hormone progesterone relaxes smooth (involuntary) muscle and the collecting area in the kidneys and the tube connecting the kidneys to the bladder becomes larger. Urine tends to stagnate there, aggravating any latent infection. Signs of infection are increased urination, pain and/or a burning sensation. More extreme signs are back pain, chills and fever, bloody urine.

To prevent UTIs, it helps to drink fairly large quantities of fluids throughout pregnancy, especially acidic juices. You can make your own cranberry juice by boiling cranberries in water, straining and adding honey. Or add the juice of one whole lemon or lime to a half-gallon of water, keep it cold and drink three to four glasses a day. Also empty your bladder completely and frequently. Acupuncture may help, too.

In the first trimester of pregnancy your infection should be treated with sulfa drugs if juices and frequent urination don't work.

Some practitioners help you evaluate your diet by asking you to make a chart of everything you eat over a three-day period and then discussing it with you.

Insist that you get complete information about the purposes as well as the results of all the tests.

Your next visits will be monthly. The heartbeat and position of your baby will be checked, as well as your urine, weight and blood pressure. If you or your partner has a history of herpes, you must have a culture at the thirty-fourth and thirty-sixth week, and then weekly after that.

At the beginning of your eighth month you'll see the practitioner every two weeks.

During the ninth month you'll see him or her once a week. It's best at this time to keep internal exams down to a minimum to prevent infection. Most often you will go into labor when you are ready.

At the other extreme of exam scheduling, many women from poor areas never see a nurse or doctor until it's time to deliver. Conditions in some hospitals and clinics are so bad—crowded, long waits, careless medical people, lack of respect for women and families—that women become discouraged and don't want to take the time to come for appointments.

What I hated most about City Hospital was the "cattle run." There was always a mad rush for the elevator immediately before clinic was about to begin. When we arrived every patient was assigned a number. We waited, seated in rows on long, hard benches. The bathroom stank. The rooms were dirty, drab and overheated. The medical staff were often overworked and overwhelmed; the nurses and doctors were impersonal. I rarely saw the same doctor twice. Another concern was, why didn't I ever see any women doctors or physicians of color?

Your Feelings About Yourself and Your Pregnancy

At the beginning of a first pregnancy, or of any pregnancy, there are many variations in feeling, from delirious joy to deep depression.

Some Positive Feelings

You may feel an increased sensuality, a kind of sexual opening out toward the world, heightened perceptions, a feeling of being in love. A lot of new energy. A feeling of being really special, fertile, potent, creative. Expectation. Great excitement. Impatience. Harmony. Peace.

It gave me a sense that I was actually a woman. I had never felt sexy before. I went through a lot of changes. It was a very sexual thing. I felt very voluptuous.

It meant I could get pregnant finally after a lot of trying, that I could do something I wanted to do. It meant going into a new stage of life. I felt filled up.

Some Questions

What's going to happen to me? How will being pregnant change me? Will I be able to cope well? Can I physically handle birth? Will I miscarry? How long can I keep my job? Who am I? What image can I form of who I want to be? What is my baby going to be like? What about my partner?

Some Negative Feelings

Shock. I'm losing my individuality. I'm not the same anymore. I'm a pregnant woman; I'm in this new category and I don't want to be. I don't want to be a vessel, a carrier. I won't matter to people now, only my baby will. I can't feel anything for this thing growing in me. I can't feel any love. I'm scared. I'm tired. I feel sick. I wish I weren't pregnant. I'm not ready. I don't understand motherhood.

Negative feelings are natural. When you deal with them and don't avoid or ignore them, you'll be better prepared to handle them close to the birth and afterward. Also, miraculously they usually change a lot from one trimester to the next, most often in a positive direction.

Sometimes it seemed like I had gotten pregnant on a whim—and it was a hell of a responsibility to take on a whim. Sometimes I was overwhelmed by what I'd done. A lot of that came from realizing that I had chosen to have the baby without the support of a man. I was scared up until the third trimester that I wasn't going to make it.

Some of you will be too busy to think often about your pregnancy. Others will have more leisure. Some of you will be interested in your pregnancies in different degrees, your awareness switched inward at different times.

When I first felt her move, I knew there was life inside me. But I didn't realize I was having a baby until my doctors literally pulled her out of me upside down and she sneezed, and then she lay next to me and I felt her tiny breath on my fingers.

Maybe the last three weeks I started looking at other babies.

At the beginning of pregnancy it's sometimes a relief not to think about it, and you can even forget it if you want to. At some point during pregnancy you may wish you could escape from the inevitability of what is happening to you.

Growth of the Fetus

You can't feel the changes going on inside you. Both the placental systems and the complicated systems of your fetus are developing on a miniature scale. See *A Child Is Born* for wonderful photographs (listed under Ingelman-Sundberg in Resources in Chapter 19, "Childbirth.").

Second Trimester (Thirteenth to Twenty-Sixth Week)

Testing during Pregnancy*

(See Appendix, pp. 352–60.)

Because of newly developed tests and technology, we are faced with choices we didn't have to make ten years ago. Many of these tests are too often overused, but they are sometimes necessary.

Physical Changes

At about the fourth month the fetus begins to take up much more space. Your waist becomes thicker, your clothes no longer fit you, your womb begins to swell below your waist and, around the fourth or fifth month, you can begin to feel light movements ("quickening"). The fetus has been moving for months, but it's only now that you can feel it. Often you will feel it first just before you fall asleep.

*For an excellent discussion of these tests and procedures, see Rita Arditti, Renate Duelli Klein and Shelley Minden, eds., *Test Tube Women*, Boston: Pandora Press, Routledge and Kegan Paul, 1984.

WOMAN IN 16TH WEEK OF PREGNANCY

Nina Reimer

You are probably gaining weight now. Eat as well as you can.

Your circulatory system has been changing and your total blood volume increasing, as your bone marrow produces more blood corpuscles and you drink and retain more liquid. Because of the increase in blood production, you may need more iron. Your heart is changing position and increasing slightly in size.

In some women the area around the nipple, the areola, becomes very dark due to hormonal changes. The line from the navel to the pubic region gets dark, too, and sometimes pigment in the face becomes dark, making a kind of mask. The mask goes away after pregnancy. Usually the increased color around your nipples and in the line on your abdomen will not go away, but it may fade.

Some women salivate more. You may sweat more, which is helpful in eliminating waste material from your body. Sometimes you'll get cramps in your legs and feet when you wake up, perhaps because of disturbed circulation. Calcium relieves these cramps; or drink raspberry leaf tea at bedtime. Just relax—the cramps will go away. Keep your feet elevated and warm, or pull your toes toward your knees.

Your uterus is changing, too. It's growing. Its weight increases twenty times, and the greater part of this weight is gained before the twentieth week.

As your abdomen grows larger the skin over it will stretch and lines may appear, pink or reddish streaks. Your skin may become very dry; add oil to your bath and rub your skin with oil.

By midpregnancy your breasts, stimulated by hormones, are functionally complete for nursing purposes. After about the nineteenth week a thin amber or yellow substance called *colostrum* may come out of your nipples; there's no milk yet. Your breasts are probably larger and heavier than before. If you are planning to breastfeed, it's a good idea to begin gently massaging your nipples. If your nipples are inverted (turned in), pull them out gently several times a day by putting your thumbs on each side of them, pressing down into the breasts and away from the nipple. Wash your breasts daily with mild soap or clean water. It's also a good idea to wear a supportive bra, as your breasts can begin to feel very heavy.

Your bowels and your entire digestive system may move more slowly. Indigestion and constipation can occur. You may have heartburn because of too much acid in your stomach. Again, a good diet and regular exercise ease these situations. Eat frequent small meals if possible. Avoid greasy foods and coffee. Drink a lot of fluids and increase bran and fiber. Avoid taking strong, oily laxatives or laxatives containing sodium, such as baking soda or Alka-Seltzer. Papaya pills (available at health food stores) may be helpful.

As a result of pressure of pelvic organs, veins in your rectum (hemorrhoidal veins) may become dilated and sometimes painful. To prevent hemorrhoids, practice

345

rectal Kegel exercises, which resemble the pelvic floor exercises (see p. 333) except that you contract your rectal muscles instead. When you go to the bathroom, prop your feet up on a stool. Eat a lot of roughage. When you have hemorrhoids, lie down with your rectum high and apply ice packs or heat. Tucks pads and Preparation H are okay. Or take warm baths and apply Vaseline. Vitamin-E oil may help. Eat fewer spices. Continue to exercise.

Varicose veins are veins in your legs that have become enlarged and can hurt. Because of pressure, the veins and blood vessels that carry blood from your legs to your heart aren't working as smoothly as before. A tendency to varicose veins can be hereditary. Many women find it very helpful to wear support stockings a half-size larger than their ordinary stockings. And lots of rest, with legs elevated, is good, alternated with walking or mild exercise.

Many women have nosebleeds because of the increased volume of blood and nasal congestion, or perhaps because of increased hormone levels. (It's also possible to have "sympathetic" nosebleeds during periods.) A little Vaseline in each nostril may stop the bleeding.

Edema (Water Retention)

Your feet, ankles, fingers, hands and even your face may swell somewhat. When you are eating well, including adequate protein intake, edema is normal and no cause for worry, especially during the last half of pregnancy. Pregnancy hormones manufactured by the placenta, principally estrogens, cause connective tissue throughout your body to retain extra fluid, which benefits you and your baby. It serves as backup for the expanded blood volume needed to nourish the placenta, protects you from going into shock if you lose blood and assures you an adequate milk flow during early breastfeeding. With twins, edema will increase as will your weight gain. Normal edema is associated with good infant outcome—higher birth weight and lower infant mortality.*

If you are uncomfortable, try to lie down with your feet raised several times a day. Exercise helps squeeze water from the tissue spaces in your blood vessels. Cut down on refined carbohydrates and get more rest.

Toxemia

After the twenty-fourth week of pregnancy, some women develop a combination of high blood pressure, edema and protein in the urine. While these conditions can occur separately and sometimes all together for many reasons, they may also be symptoms of toxemia (also called mild pre-eclampsia or severe pre-eclamp-

*Dr. Leon Chesley, author of the section on toxemia in *Williams Obstetrics*, the most widely used ob/gyn textbook, as quoted in Gail Brewer, *What Every Pregnant Woman Should Know*, p. 34 (see Resources in Chapter 19, "Childbirth").

sia). Be sure to check with your practitioner. S/he should observe your blood pressure on at least two occasions a minimum of six hours apart, and check the amount of albumin (a protein) in the urine. Toward the third trimester of pregnancy, if you develop very high blood pressure, a large amount of protein in your urine with a decrease in the amount of urine, a severe continuous headache or swelling of your face or fingers, you may have severe pre-eclampsia. These conditions can develop in just a few hours, and unless you have them checked immediately, eclampsia—convulsions and coma—may occur. Some mild conditions can be treated at home after medical evaluations; others and all serious pre-eclamptic conditions *must* be treated in the hospital; your life and the baby's are at stake.

All medical people agree that the incidence of toxemia in pregnancy is much lessened by constant prenatal care and supervision and good diet.

Clothing

Your clothes should be loose and comfortable, warm in winter and cool in summer. Many women modify their own pants by piecing in an elastic stretch panel in the front. Simple unbelted smocks are useful as dresses. Large men's shirts are useful, too. Maternity clothes in stores are often expensive. Ask your friends for any clothes they may have.

Get as much rest as you possibly can. If you are very busy, try to set aside segments of time for total relaxation, even if it's only fifteen minutes at a time.

Your Feelings About Yourself

How will you feel about your changing body?

I was excited and delighted. I really got into eating well, caring for myself, getting enough sleep. I liked walking through the streets and having people notice my pregnancy.

But many of us watch ourselves growing outward so quickly with mixed emotions.

I don't like being pregnant. I feel like a big toad. I'm a dancer, used to being slim, and I can't believe what I look like from the side. I avoid mirrors.

Your Feelings About Your Baby

If you are feeling really good or ambivalent or even bad, the first movements you feel your baby make can be beautiful and moving.

I was lying on my stomach and felt...something, like someone lightly touching my deep insides. Then I just sat very still and for an alive moment felt the hugeness of having something living growing in me. Then I said, "No, it's not possible, it's too early yet," and then I started to cry....That one moment was my first body awareness of another living thing inside me.

And after the first movement—in the fourth or fifth month—you may wait days for another sign of quickening.* Then the movements will become frequent and familiar. The baby begins to feel real. You can feel from the outside the hard shape of your uterus.

If you are angry or upset by pregnancy, then your baby's movements serve to focus your anger.

Last night its kicking made me dizzy and gave me a terrible feeling of solitude. I wanted to tell it, "Stop, stop, stop, let me alone." I want to lie still and whole and all single, catch my breath. But I have no control over this new part of my being, and this lack of control scares me. I feel as if I were rushing downhill at such a great speed that I'd never be able to stop.

Perhaps feeling the baby move for the first time will change you.

Sitting on a rock overlooking the domesite, trees growing right out of the rock. They cling and flourish on nothing. Images of the growing life inside me, also coming from nothing, getting nutrition from my body the way the tree does from the rock....Occasionally I give it warmth, mostly when it moves. The more it moves, the more I like it. I also resent it an awful lot; I feel big, ugly and uncomfortable, and in spite of Len's protestations, I feel alone.

Even during the most positive pregnancies there may be moments, hours and days of depression, anxiety and confusion. These depressions may be connected to all the submerged anxieties you have in relation to your own childhood, doubts that come from our society's ignorance about pregnancy and childbirth, doubts you have about your own identity, economic problems, having too many children already and problems in your relationship with your partner.

It seems that my feelings about my pregnancy, my body, the coming of the baby, were inextricably wound into my feelings, problems, hopes and fears for our relationship....It's hard to separate which feelings were a result of my unhappiness about us (a lot of the bad feelings about my body arose because Bob showed very little interest in my enlarged, changing body), which ones were my own negative feelings about having a less functional body (I wanted to keep working and active, but my body was so cumbersome that I was always worn

*Even if you aren't sure when you conceived your baby, you can be almost certain that quickening occurs between the eighteenth and twentieth weeks of your first pregnancy, earlier in subsequent pregnancies.

out and tired) and which ones were just moods caused by pregnancy.

We all have general fears, too; there is fear of the unknown, especially if it's a first pregnancy. No matter how much we do know about the physiological changes in our bodies, there's something incomprehensible about the beginnings of life. And by becoming pregnant we open ourselves to changes and complications. We become much more aware of being vulnerable.

I remember feeling overwhelmed by sad things I saw, and was overwhelmed by things that could happen to innocence. I'd wake in the night and think people were going to come in and take things, take the baby from me. I was beginning to be out of control. I was terribly afraid of chance. I've always been afraid of irrationality, of fate.

You may have vivid dreams.

For two nights now my falling asleep has given rise to that old childhood dream-image of falling down a deep, dark, square hole ever diminishing in size.

I'm in a hospital in a room all alone, a cold room. The nurse gives me a shot; I have my baby and I don't feel a thing. I look up and see my baby floating in a beaker, alive. I can't go to her; I'm sad and frustrated.

The baby starts coming out of my belly. I have to hold it in. My skin is transparent.

We fear that our babies will be deformed. Between 3 and 4 percent of babies are born with diseases and 1 percent with physical malformations. Some of us have dreams, fantasies and nightmares about deformity. These are normal and universal.

When I was about six months pregnant and Dick was starting school again, I was home alone, isolated for days at a time. My nightmares and daydreams started around then, really terrible fears of the baby being deformed. All my life I've always been the good girl. I knew I wasn't really good. I knew I had bad thoughts, but I was never allowed to express them. So I thought that my baby's deformities would be the living proof of the ugliness and badness in me.

We fear our own death, the child's death.

In fact, we do have to face the fact that some women miscarry and some babies die. While it's difficult, threatening and sad to think of, we know it happens. Though it's very hard and not usually useful to try to prepare ourselves for death, it helps to know what has happened to some of us, so that if we or our friends experience such tragedy, we can in some way be acquainted with the event. This knowledge is a kind of preparation. It's vitally important to be able to reach out to friends when tragic things happen to them, and to help ease their feelings of isolation. It also helps us to know that we can and need to ask for help if such a thing happens to us.

I went into the hospital for the birth of my first child....The child's lungs became infected and he died two days later. I never saw him. When I began to return to myself I found that despite all those times I had told myself that nothing could really happen, I had nothing but an empty belly. I don't know if we should be warned ahead of time to worry needlessly about something that happens to a very few women, but as one of those women, I definitely need to feel some sense of sharing with others in the same position—not to cry over what happened but to work out how to face other people. That's the hardest part—nobody wants to deal with death, especially when your friends are at the childbearing age themselves and can't help being afraid of you for what you stand for. I found that my friends wanted me to pretend nothing had happened—even that there had been no pregnancy. I don't think it was just my particular friends—it's natural to want to avoid those things. And so my fantastic pregnancy, in which a lot of things went on in my head and body that helped me to change and get myself together, had to be buried. Even now, after a year, I can see their pain and fear for me as I start into my eighth month of pregnancy with my second child. I have to be the one who keeps them calm, and I especially must assure everyone that this one will be okay.

We may also feel guilty about having fears. Don't they in some way suggest that as mothers we will be weak and inadequate? The myth is that we can't allow ourselves these depressions because we are supposed to be strong, mature, maternal, accepting, loving all the time.

Our feelings are legitimate. We must feel free to know them, to express them and to be strengthened by them.

Men's Feelings About You and Your Pregnancy

How will the man you are involved with respond to you? That depends on how you feel about yourself, on the relationship between you, on how he feels about himself and about fatherhood and what he sees his part to be in your pregnancy. If he wants to get involved, it's a good idea to prepare with him and learn together, especially if he will live with you after your baby is born. He may feel close and attracted to you, and fascinated by your growing body. Or for reasons having to do with his own upbringing and particular problems, he may feel repelled, confused and threatened by all your changes and by what's to come. Or he may feel positive sometimes, negative sometimes.

Sometimes I thought you were very beautiful and your belly was beautiful. And sometimes you looked like a ridiculous pregnant insect. Your navel bulging out looked strange.

If you are having problems it's certainly best if you can talk together and realize that often your and his complex feelings are changeable. Talk can also lead to some deep, good questioning about the conventional ideas of beauty we are all exposed to. It's possible that he won't be able to talk about or to cope at all with the changes and responsibilities that your pregnancy implies. He may be jealous or resentful. For many reasons, some men seek out women other than the pregnant women they are living with, whether they're married or unmarried. Some men, while not actually leaving you, may withdraw from you emotionally at this crucial time.

Being Lesbian and Pregnant

More and more lesbians are becoming pregnant through artificial insemination or intercourse with a man and are having babies together.* You will have most of the same joys and anxieties as heterosexual couples do. In some places, practitioners, clinics and birth centers will accept you as a couple when you go for prenatal care; other people may be prejudiced and punitive. Depending on the situation, you may not want to come out to your practitioner (or you may end up changing practitioners). But sometimes when you do, it can have a positive effect.

I had requested early in pregnancy to have Mary with me during labor and birth. I asked the hospital, wrote them a letter, and was told it had to go to the Board. They kept giving me the runaround. Meanwhile I was developing a good relationship with my obstetrician. At the beginning he had negative value judgments about me. As he got to know and like me, everything changed. He went to bat for me, got permission for Mary to be with me. I was also told afterward that he had spoken to the obstetrical staff to prepare them for our being there together. He told them that if any of them had negative feelings about lesbianism, they should not be there when we were. The result was that everyone at my labor and birth was extremely supportive.

Making Love During Pregnancy

You will have many different feelings about making love during pregnancy. Your moods and desires will shift.

I wanted to make love more than ever.

*See Chapter 17, "New Reproductive Technologies," for information on artificial insemination.

I remember feeling very sexy. We were trying all these different positions. Now that we were having a baby, I felt a lot looser, a lot freer. I used to feel uptight about sex for its own sake, but when I was pregnant I felt a lot freer.

I felt very ambivalent about making love. I had miscarried several times. I wanted to make love and I was scared to make love. As a single woman it was hard to find men who found me attractive with my belly so big. I had no sexual contact at all during the last two months.

You may feel more open, giving and sensuous than ever before (some women have orgasms or multiple orgasms for the first time). You may turn inward. With each month, each trimester, you may feel different. You may be afraid that making love will hurt the baby. It won't.

You can use pregnancy as a time to experiment with many different ways of loving, from touching and sensual massage to exploring a whole range of lovemaking positions. For instance, at the end of pregnancy, the man-on-top position is the most uncomfortable of all for women. Instead, try propping yourself up on pillows, you on top, both of you relaxed side by side like two spoons fitting into each other, mutual masturbation or anything you want to think up that feels sensual and satisfying.

Use pregnancy as a time to learn what your genitals look like and how to contract and release pelvic-floor muscles (see Kegel exercises, p. 333).* Having orgasms during masturbation and lovemaking may even strengthen uterine muscles; your uterus contracts during orgasm and then relaxes. Lovemaking brings you closer to your partner at a time when closeness is needed, and can prepare you for the giving, taking, opening up and deep relaxation of labor. Childbearing can be a vivid expression of your sexuality.

After making love your uterine contractions may continue. You can feel your uterus tighten, then relax. But lovemaking can bring on labor toward the end of pregnancy *only if your body is ready to go into labor.* Some researchers believe that prostaglandins concentrated in semen can cause uterine contractions, but have found no conclusive link.

What Physicians Tell Us

Physicians still advise us not to have sexual intercourse from six weeks before birth until six weeks afterward, three months altogether.† They base this

---

*Also see Sheila Kitzinger, *Experience of Childbirth*, and Elizabeth Noble, *Essential Exercises for the Childbearing Year*, for good descriptions of pelvic-floor exercises. It's a skill one has to learn.

†A widely published report appeared in the *New England Journal of Medicine* in 1979, linking sexual intercourse with infection of the amniotic fluid (the waters surrounding the fetus), the theory being that sperm or enzymes in semen may enable bac-

recommendation not upon scientific fact but upon four unproven beliefs: the thrusts of the penis against the cervix induce labor; uterine contractions of orgasm induce labor; membranes may rupture, causing infection; and intercourse between man and woman can be uncomfortable.

We find lurking behind these beliefs the attitude that there is only one way to make love, i.e., sexual intercourse (penile penetration) in the "missionary" position, and that women can't be both sexual beings and mothers at the same time.

There are some indications for not having *intercourse.* You shouldn't if you have vaginal or abdominal pain; if you have any uterine bleeding; if your membranes have ruptured (then there *is* danger of infection); if you have been warned about miscarriage or think that one may occur. If you know that your partner works in an environment where toxics may concentrate in sperm, he should wear a condom (see p. 82). When you have oral-genital contact, your partner should not blow air into your vagina, because it can cause an air embolism which can lead to death (although this is extremely rare). If either you or your partner have open herpes sores, avoid all contact with the sores.

Third Trimester (Twenty-Seventh to Thirty-Eighth Week)

Physical Changes

Your uterus is becoming very large. It feels hard when you touch it.

I remember my friends' surprise when they put their hands on my belly to feel it. They expected it to be soft and somehow jellylike and were amazed at its hardness and bulk.

It's a strong muscular container. You can feel and see the movements of your fetus from the outside now, too, as it changes position, turns somersaults, hiccups. Sometimes it puts pressure on your bladder, which makes you feel that you need to urinate even when you don't, and which can hurt a little, or sometimes a lot, for very brief periods. Sometimes toward the end of pregnancy it puts pressure on the nerves at the top of your legs, which can be painful, too.

---

teria to penetrate the cervix and reach the womb. This is another theory which confuses association with causation. Just because women with infections had sexual intercourse doesn't mean that intercourse caused the infection. We mention this study as an example of both nonscientific research and alarmist reporting. A recently published *Lancet* study shows no greater risk of infection among those having intercourse.

Your baby will be lying in a particular position, sometimes head down, back to your front, sometimes lying crossways. It moves around often. Your practitioner can help you discover which position the baby is in.

Sometimes your baby lies still. It's known that babies sleep *in utero*. If you don't feel movement for three to four days and you're anxious about it, call your practitioner if you can and ask whether s/he thinks it's a good idea to check the fetal heartbeat. Usually these are periods of "rest" for the baby and can last several days.

Postures to Turn a Breech Baby

Begin after the thirtieth week of pregnancy for up to four weeks before birth, or until version (turning, a shift in position) takes place, whichever happens first.

1. PRACTICE TWICE A DAY FOR TEN MINUTES EACH TIME.

Lie on your back on a hard surface with the pelvis raised by pillows to a level nine to twelve inches above the head. Stomach should be empty. (This posture corrected breech to head-first position of baby for 89 percent of patients in one study.) Lying head down on a collapsed ironing board with one end propped on a couch or chair is sometimes more comfortable than the pillow position.

2. PRACTICE TWICE A DAY FOR TEN MINUTES EACH TIME.

Knee-chest position: on all fours, fold your arms and place head on them, knees about eighteen inches apart, back straight. Bladder should be empty. If you do this posture so that your head is at the edge of your bed, a book can be placed on the floor below and it is possible to read comfortably.

Your uterus will tighten every now and then. These are painless contractions called Braxton-Hicks contractions. They are believed to strengthen uterine muscles, preparing them for eventual labor.

It becomes increasingly uncomfortable for you to lie on your stomach. You may experience shortness of breath. There's pressure on your lungs from your uterus, and your diaphragm may be moved up as much as an inch. Even so, because your thoracic (chest) cage widens, you breathe in more air when you are pregnant than when you are not. Sometimes when you lie down you may not be able to breathe well for a moment. Prop yourself up with pillows or turn on your side, and the pressure on your diaphragm will be lessened.

The peak load on your heart occurs in about the thirtieth week. After that the heart usually doesn't have to work so hard until delivery.

You are still gaining weight. If you have hemorrhoids or varicose veins, try to avoid standing up for long periods of time, and when you sit or lie down, be sure your feet are raised.

Your stomach is pushed up by your uterus and flattened. Indigestion becomes more common. If you have heartburn, sleep with your head and shoulders raised. Eat small amounts. Don't take mineral oil—it causes you to excrete necessary vitamins.

Vaughn Sills

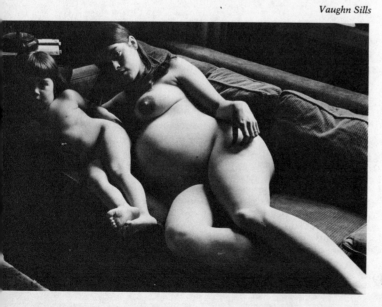

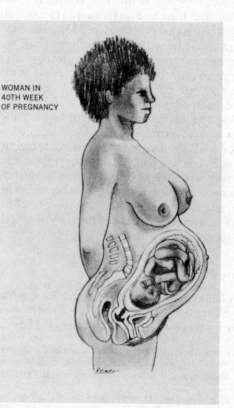

WOMAN IN 40TH WEEK OF PREGNANCY

Nina Reimer

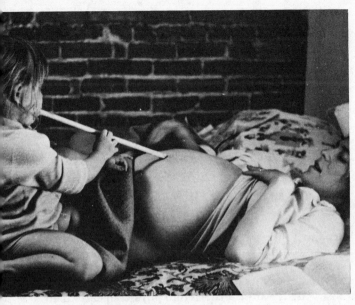

Ed Pincus

If you have insomnia or trouble sleeping because the baby's movements make you uncomfortable, take walks and hot baths. Drink warm milk or raspberry tea. Avoid sleeping pills. Brisk exercise during the day will help you sleep better.

I think there is a reason for this nonsleeping: there's work getting done. That restlessness needs to happen. Your energy builds up for the coming crisis. I remember pacing around my house at midnight, burning with energy, finally finding the tiny sandals my first child had worn as a toddler. I carefully cleaned and polished them for the new baby. Then I slept fine.

Your navel will probably be pushed out.

Since your body has become heavier, you'll tend to walk differently for balance, often leaning back to counteract a heavier front. This can cause backaches, for which there are exercises. Your pelvic joints are also much more separated.

At about four to two weeks before birth, and sometimes as early as the seventh month, the baby's head settles into your pelvis. This is called "lightening" or "dropping." It takes pressure off your stomach. Some women do feel much lighter. And if you have been having trouble breathing, pressure is now off your diaphragm. This "dropping" can cause constipation; your bowels are more obstructed than they were.

As for water retention, an average pregnant woman retains from 6.5 to 13 pints of liquid, half of this in the last ten weeks. Swollen ankles are common.

Your Feelings About Yourself and Your Pregnancy

I had a feeling of being at the end, of nothing else being terrifically important.

I thought it would never end. I was enormous. I couldn't bend over and wash my feet. And it was incredibly hot.

At the end I started to feel it was too long. Dick took pictures of me during the eighth month. I saw my face as faraway and sad.

I had insomnia. I couldn't get comfortable. I couldn't sleep, he'd kick so much.

I wonder what it looks like. How fantastic that it only has to travel one-and-a-half feet down to get born.

My kid is dancing under my heart.

The relationship of mother carrying child is most beautiful and simplest.
I pity a baby who must come out of the womb.

David Alexander

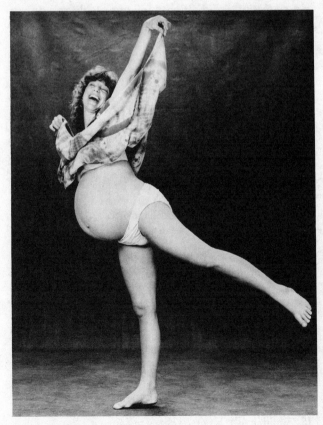

Fairly confidently and calmly awaiting the baby—quite set on a home delivery. Doctor said Thursday I was already dilated two-and-a-half centimeters, so it must be getting close. Getting a bit anxious, listening to every Braxton-Hicks contraction, awaiting with hope—and fear, too—its change into the real thing.

I feel exultant and tired and rich inside. My belly is large, and last night the baby beat around inside it like a wild tempest. I thought the time had come and was panicked and nauseated, then very excited. I woke Ed up. Then at five I fell asleep. Meanwhile I move in slow motion and wait.

APPENDIX

Questions for Practitioners Who Work in Hospitals*

(These questions are purposely broad and vague. Use them to lead into a more detailed interview once you have read these chapters and other books.)

What is your philosophy of childbirth? What kind of prenatal care do you offer? What kind of childbirth preparation do you favor? Do you consider good nutrition and exercise important and can you help me with them? Do you recommend childbirth preparation classes? What kind? What kind of tests do you do during pregnancy and just before birth? Will you be easy to reach if I need you?

How many births have you attended? Where? Where has your training been? How do you usually conduct labor and birth? Do you stay with women throughout labor or appear at the end of labor? Do you approve of labor coaches? Of family, friends, children being present? What percentage of your clients walk around during labor? Eat or drink during labor? Labor in positions of their choice? Have no drugs at all? Have no episiotomy? Hold their babies and breastfeed right away? Under what circumstances and what percentage of the time do you use drugs and interventions: IVs? Amniotomy? Electronic monitors? Pitocin to start or speed up labor? Episiotomy? Forceps? Cesareans? Who backs you up if you can't be present at prenatal visits or at labor and birth? Do they share your beliefs? Can you give me the names of some women who have used your services? What is your overall fee for prenatal care and a vaginal delivery? For a Cesarean? If

I've had a Cesarean, do you encourage trial labor and vaginal delivery?

How often will I see you after my baby is born?

Two important points: 1. Be sure to compare what the practitioner says with hospital rules and anesthesia department requirements, which may be different. 2. No matter what your physician says, the attitudes and practices of nurses attending you during labor can influence or determine what happens.

Questions for Nurse-Midwives Who Give Care in Private Offices, Clinics or Hospitals

Very much like the above questions. Add: Will I need to make contact with someone other than you? What percentage of your clients require physician care? Under what circumstances do you call in the doctor to assist you? If I am transferred to physician care in an emergency, will you still be able to be with me?

Questions for Nurse-Midwives and Physicians Who Work in Freestanding Birth Centers

Most of the same questions as above. Add: What are your requirements for birth center admission? What are your screening protocols? What percentage of your clients have been "risked out" prior to labor? Why? What are backup arrangements? What are your protocols for hospital admission? When do you advise women to go into the hospital?

Questions for Lay Midwives Who Attend at Home

What is your philosophy of birth? Of prenatal care? Do you offer comprehensive care, including laboratory work, either on your own or in connection with a facility, interpreting urine, blood, diagnostic tests? Can I do these tests myself? Do you provide nutritional counseling? How often do you visit before and after the birth? What kind of childbirth preparation do you favor? Do you recommend classes? What kind?

What has your training been? Whom have you trained with? Are you in communication with other midwives in your area? How many births have you attended? How many births have you been responsible for?

What medical/hospital backup do you have? What have your experiences been?

How do you conduct labor and delivery? When do you check the baby's heartbeat, my blood pressure and pulse, dilation, baby's position and descent?

How do you define complications? How do you han-

---

*All these questions are derived from: 1. Doris Haire, "Getting What You Want From Your Birth Experience," National Women's Health Network, 224 7th Street SE, Washington DC 20003; 2. Tracy Hotchner, *Pregnancy and Birth*, New York: Avon Books, 1979; 3. Gail Brewer, *Right from the Start* (see Resources in Chapter 19, "Childbirth"); 4. Diony Young and Charles Mahan, *Unnecessary Cesareans: Ways to Avoid Them* (see Resources in Chapter 19, "Childbirth"); 5. ourselves and our friends!

dle complications? Under what conditions would I see a physician or go to the hospital?

How do you reduce or prevent perineal tearing? What about repair? How do you define newborn distress? Handle it? Do you know how to do mouth-to-mouth resuscitation on newborns? Do you make postpartum visits? When? For how long a period of time? Who is your backup? Does s/he share your beliefs? Can I meet her/him? Can you give me the names of some women you have assisted? What do you charge?

Questions for Hospitals*

May I preregister, or will I have to fill out forms when I arrive in labor? Do you have a birthing room? What are the criteria? What percentage of women use it? What percentage of doctors use it?

Routines

What procedures are routine here? Do you remove personal belongings? Do preps (shave pubic hair)? Give enemas? Do you have a place for women in early labor—a special room or a lounge? May my partner/relatives/friends/labor coach be with me during labor and delivery? May my child(ren) be present? Do you routinely require IVs and fetal monitors? May I walk around during labor? Take showers or baths? May we take photos? May I stay in the labor room for the whole time instead of going to the delivery room?

If it's a teaching hospital, how will that affect me? (In some teaching hospitals women are approached during labor and asked if they will take part in studies; in others, they may undergo certain procedures unnecessarily for the sake of a study, without being told.)

What is the Cesarean rate at your hospital, both for primary and repeat Cesareans? Have there been nursery staph infections during the past year?

Can my partner and coach be with me in the delivery and recovery rooms if I have to have a Cesarean? Can my partner hold the baby right afterward?

May I hold my baby immediately after delivery, and nurse her/him? May we stay together in privacy after the delivery? Are mothers and babies separated after delivery? For how long? Why?

Do you have rooming-in? What kind: Complete? Modified? What hours? Can my baby feed on demand? Do you have experienced advice available for breast-feeding mothers?

What are visiting hours? May my partner and family visit whenever they want? Can I decide the length of time I want to stay? Do you have early discharge? What is your exact policy?

*If hospitals really met women's needs, we wouldn't have to ask all these questions!

You can write a letter to your practitioner, hospital administrator and head of nursing staff stating your preferences and priorities concerning labor and birth. Bring a copy with you when you go to the hospital to have your baby. (Birth Day—see Resources in Chapter 19, "Childbirth"—has a sample letter to give you some ideas.) Decide what your bottom line is—what you absolutely *won't* give up.

Testing Before or During Pregnancy

Sickle Cell Trait and Sickle Cell Anemia

One in twelve black people in the U.S. carries only a single gene for sickle cell anemia and consequently has sickle cell *trait*. This is a benign condition that rarely has any effect and that most people don't know they have. The sickle cell gene developed thousands of years ago in people who lived in Africa and in countries around the Mediterranean Ocean, apparently because having sickle cell trait helped protect them from malaria. However, if you have sickle cell trait and your partner does, too, each of your children will have one chance in four of having sickle cell anemia.

About one in 165 black people is born with the inherited disease of sickle cell *anemia*. Symptoms can include poor physical development, jaundice, weakness, abdominal pains, lowered resistance to infections, bouts of swelling and pain in muscles and joints. The red blood cells, shaped like a farmer's sickle, don't live as long as normal cells and are destroyed at a faster rate, so movement of oxygen is reduced. The clinical picture is variable. Some people who have severe anemia during childhood may find the symptoms becoming milder as they grow older. For others, the anemia is tiring at times but tolerable, or it can be extremely painful. In order to have the disease, you must inherit a *pair* of genes for sickle cell, one from each parent.

If you are black and if you are planning a pregnancy with someone of similar background, you may want to be tested for sickle cell trait. The blood test is simple and you can have the results in thirty minutes. Then, if your test is positive, your partner may want to be tested, too.

If you have the trait and your partner doesn't, then your children have a fifty-fifty chance of having the trait. If one of you has sickle cell anemia and the other has neither sickle cell anemia nor the trait, all your children will have the trait and therefore have no problems. If you both have the trait, every time you have a child, s/he will have one chance in four of having completely normal blood, one chance in two of having the trait and one chance in four of having sickle cell

353

anemia. If one of you has the trait and the other has sickle cell anemia, each child will have a fifty-fifty chance of having sickle cell anemia.

Ideally, your test for sickle cell trait or anemia should be part of a program which will do several things for you. It will inform you as soon as possible of test results and keep them absolutely confidential. If you and your partner both have the trait, it will provide counseling if you want it as you decide about having children. If you have sickle cell anemia, it will identify which form you have, as some are not as troublesome as others. It will help you learn about the problems and risks of going through a pregnancy; some of your symptoms may be intensified by pregnancy (circulatory problems may become worse; you may be more tired or depressed than usual and more prone to miscarriage). Finally, a good program will provide counseling and support services to you and your family if your children or your partner have sickle cell anemia and you need these services.

To locate a sickle cell program in your area, check with your local hospital, neighborhood health clinic or department of health.

Tay-Sachs Disease

Tay-Sachs disease is another genetic disease, rare in the general population (one in 100,000) but much more common in Jews of Eastern European origin (one in 3,600 births). It results from the deficiency of an enzyme (hexosaminidase A) involved in the metabolism of some of the fatty substances essential for the nervous system's proper functioning. Infants with Tay-Sachs disease are born seemingly normal, but early in infancy their development slows down and paralysis, blindness, severe behavioral changes and disorders of the nervous system follow. It is always fatal, usually by age three or four.

If you are a Jew of Eastern European descent and plan to have a baby, you and your partner can be tested for the trait. If you both have it, your baby has one chance in four of having Tay-Sachs disease. In 1970 a relatively simple test became available to detect carriers of the trait (the test determines the concentration of hexosaminidase A in the blood). It is also possible to detect affected fetuses *in utero* through amniocentesis (see below).

Rh Factor in Blood

The Rh factor is a substance in the blood. At least 86 percent of us have this substance coating our red blood cells; we are called Rh positive (Rh+). Those of us who don't have it are Rh negative (Rh−).

If someone with Rh− blood receives transfusions of blood containing Rh+, the Rh− blood gradually builds up antibodies which defend the blood from the hostile Rh+ factor, causing some red cells to be broken down and their products spread through the body.

This same process can occur during pregnancy, because a certain amount of blood is transferred between you and your fetus through the placenta, though each circulatory system remains fairly separate. Most of the change goes from the mother to the fetus. At birth, however, because of the separation of the placenta from the uterus, there can be a much larger spillover, and a quantity of the baby's blood can be absorbed by the mother. This mixing does not occur often. If you have Rh− blood, are pregnant for the first time and have not had a transfusion containing Rh+ blood, your first child will probably be all right. But at birth you can absorb your baby's Rh+ blood, causing your own blood to react and begin developing antibodies. These antibodies will be present in your blood during your next pregnancy. They can get into the bloodstream of your second child as it grows and attack and destroy some of its red cells. As a result, the baby may be stillborn, severely anemic or retarded.

Thus every Rh− woman should have her blood checked regularly, beginning early in pregnancy. If you are Rh−, pay careful attention to the following: 1. The father's Rh factor should be checked. If he is also Rh−, all your offspring will be Rh− and there's no need for further checking. If he's Rh+, it should be determined whether he has both Rh+ and Rh− genes, in which case the fetus will be Rh+ only 50 percent of the time. If the man has only Rh+ genes, the fetus will always be Rh+. 2. You should know whether you have had previous blood transfusions. It's possible (though rare now that people are aware of the Rh factor) for a woman with Rh− blood to have received Rh+ blood in a transfusion, and thus to have already developed antibodies. 3. You should have your own blood tested for Rh sensitization (the presence of antibodies) during your pregnancy. 4. A fetal amniotic fluid sample can be taken during amniocentesis to see whether the blood cells of the fetus are being altered. If the bilirubin level in the fluid is high, it indicates that the fetus is affected, and a blood transfusion may be given to the baby *in utero*.

Rhogam

A drug called Rhogam has been developed which prevents you from producing antibodies. *For Rhogam to be effective, you must get it within seventy-two hours after a miscarriage from the second month on, and after every abortion or pregnancy.* In some states you can get free Rhogam shots. Check with your health department.

What can be done if the blood of the fetus is being invaded by maternal antibodies? There are now techniques for exchanging invaded fetal blood for healthy blood while the fetus is still in the uterus, and for exchanging the baby's blood after it is born. Check with your practitioner about the risks and benefits of these techniques. Ask for names of other women with the Rh− factor and find out from them what their experiences were. Thanks to Rhogam and these new techniques, most Rh incompatibles are now born healthy.

Testing During Pregnancy*

Deciding

Testing during pregnancy poses a dilemma for many women. Testing is reasonable when we anticipate that a fetus may be at risk for a particular health problem. There are advantages to knowing beforehand if there are certain problems with the fetus and to have the chance to decide whether or not to continue the pregnancy. On the other hand, having a child is always a gamble, and even with the available testing, many problems cannot be detected. Often we come to believe, in our technological, medicalized culture, that the newly developed prenatal tests magically "prevent" disease and birth defects; that by having them we assuage the gods so that we won't be "punished"; and that we are irresponsible when we decide not to have them. Though tests are appropriate and even lifesaving in specific instances, it is not reasonable for them to be done routinely—they may not always be safe for us or our babies, they further medicalize the pregnancy experience and they can cause us to worry when we don't have them *and* when we do. Unfortunately, often their very existence pressures us into having them done. When we decide against them, we have to resist that pressure.

My son was born fourteen years ago. In the past three years I had an abortion and a miscarriage. Once again I became pregnant. Though I had planned to have an amniocentesis done that last pregnancy, the miscarriage changed my mind: when the medical center sent out an informational pamphlet about amniocentesis which said that there was a 1.5 chance of miscarriage or fetal damage,† and after Steven and I had done a lot of reading, I realized that if I had to go through another loss I'd be a basket case. So I decided not to have it done.

Then came the enormous pressure: here I was, thirty-eight. My doctor urged me; so did my father, my husband's parents; my sister had had one and so had all my friends, without questioning. I even knew abstractly that I'd rather have a miscarriage than a Down's syndrome baby.

*Be sure to read Ruth Hubbard's article, "Legal and Policy Implications of Recent Advances in Prenatal Diagnosis and Fetal Therapy," Women's Rights Law Reporter (Spring 1982), Vol. 7, No. 3, pp. 201–24, for another perspective on prenatal testing. Arditti, Klein and Minden's Test Tube Women (see Resources) is also an invaluable book.

†If you are at a place which presents this high a risk, go elsewhere if you can.

For three weeks I was a wreck. Then one of my friends asked me, "What would be the worst thing?" I said, "The worst thing would be if the baby were healthy and amniocentesis caused a miscarriage."

That did it: no amniocentesis. I'd really made the decision. We lived with it fine.

And Sarah is wonderful and healthy.

There is no easy answer.

Physicians want us to have ultrasound and amniocentesis after age thirty-five. (Though some of them are concerned about our babies' welfare, others may be simply protecting themselves, "doing everything possible" in case something goes wrong.) It can be overwhelming.

My doctor insisted I should have amniocentesis and downplayed any risks. "Well, when are you going to do it?" he kept asking. Finally, during one checkup, he got me when I was feeling very vulnerable. Yet even when I got up on the table to have it done, I hadn't really made up my mind about it.

It is important to think about why we have these tests, to learn about the procedures, not to feel pressured and to be comfortable with the decisions we make.

I was thirty-seven, healthy, had had two children and was pregnant again after seventeen years. I just knew I didn't want a needle poking into my womb.

I am planning a home birth and thought long and hard about amniocentesis. You have to use technology selectively. I finally decided to have it done—that if there was something wrong, I owed it to my family to find out. I wanted to have the chance to decide about continuing the pregnancy. After it was over, what a relief! We don't have the results yet, but I'm not at all wondering or worried!

At present, 3 to 4 percent of infants in the U.S. are born with a problem necessitating medical or surgical intervention. Several prenatal tests can provide specific information about the condition of the fetus: *ultrasound* or *sonography* (UTS), *amniocentesis* and *alpha-fetoprotein* (AFP) *screening* are the three most common procedures. With these tests, doctors can detect certain fetal abnormalities such as neural tube defects (NTDs) and severe brain deformities, Down's syndrome and some serious metabolic disorders.

Ultrasound and AFP screening (a blood test) are simple medical procedures (although a positive AFP test can lead to a further series of tests, including ultrasound and amniocentesis). Amniocentesis is a more difficult, time-consuming and costly procedure, and carries a small (less than 1 percent) risk of miscarriage or infection.

The main purpose of prenatal testing is to detect birth defects early enough to enable women to decide whether to terminate pregnancy if the test is positive.* Also, some women who do not plan to abort ask to be tested so as to be able to prepare for the birth of a child with health problems. Unfortunately, you can't learn the results of amniocentesis and AFP screening until approximately twenty weeks into pregnancy, so that if you decide to end the pregnancy you will have to have D and E or a saline or prostaglandin abortion (see p. 304), which is an induced miscarriage late in the second trimester. This procedure can be extremely difficult emotionally and requires support and counseling.

The tests are intended for women who have reason to be concerned about the health of their fetus, because they have already given birth to a child with a disability, because a particular disability runs in their or their partner's family or because they have some other reason to believe their children to be at risk for a particular disability. For approximately 95 percent of women who are tested, the results are negative. However, a negative result on a particular test does not guarantee that the baby does not have some other problems, though it's unlikely. Many abnormalities cannot yet be tested for.

When considering each test you must ask these questions:

- What medical facility is best for the particular test I'm considering? Which practitioner is best?
- What will I learn from the test? How accurate is it?
- What are the risks to me and my baby if I take the test?
- What are the risks if I don't have the test done?
- How long do I have to wait to learn the results?
- What procedures will be either necessary or available if the test yields positive results? And how far am I prepared to go along with the routines that now exist?

Be sure that you want and need the test in question. Talk it over with your physician, especially if s/he performs tests routinely. Ask to talk with a genetic counselor. Be sure you understand what is happening and why. If you have any doubts, get a second opinion. Try to talk with other women who have had the test.

Ultrasound

Ultrasound uses intermittent high-frequency sound waves to create pictures of the body's inner organs by recording their echoes, much as sonar measures shapes in the water. A technician or physician runs a *transducer* back and forth over your abdomen and a computer translates the resulting echoes into pictures on a video screen so that the fetus's and your inner organs are made visible. When performed by a capable technician, ultrasound is a valuable noninvasive tool which can give immediate, important information. It appears to be one of the safest procedures for the amount of information it provides, *yet we don't know enough about its long-term effects and must question many physicians' routine use of it, especially during early pregnancy.*

Amniocentesis

This procedure can be used to reveal chromosome abnormalities and certain metabolic disorders in the fetus. Physicians now offer it to women who will be thirty-five and over at the time of delivery, because older women have an increased chance of having babies with Down's syndrome (a form of mental retardation). Age thirty-five is the cutoff because at this age the likelihood of having a baby with a chromosome abnormality (such as the one responsible for Down's syndrome) is about the same as the risk that the test will injure the fetus or induce a miscarriage. (The risk to the fetus is estimated to be one loss in 400 amniocentesis procedures at large city hospitals specializing in prenatal testing. In places where the staff is not well trained and has much less experience with performing the test, the risk is higher. Down's syndrome, also called trisomy 21, is the most common chromosome abnormality found by amniocentesis, and has an incidence of approximately one in 400 births for women of thirty-five. The risk increases with age and reaches one in 100 at age forty.*

Physicians bring up amniocentesis when you are close to age thirty-five because of recent lawsuits in which parents who have had a child with Down's syndrome have sued doctors who have not warned them and told them about amniocentesis. Many doctors recommend it by age thirty-eight. Some physicians will not accept women in their forties as clients if they refuse amniocentesis. If your obstetrician has suggested amniocentesis because of your age or a genetic condition in your family, your decision to have the test or not depends on many personal considerations, such as your family situation, your feelings about medical procedures and risks, your feelings concerning abortion and the way you feel about the possibility of having a child with a disability.

Disabilities differ a lot in their severity. Getting to know children with disabilities and/or their parents

---

* "...the technique has more often been responsible for people's having children than it has been a prelude to abortion. Before the reassurance of prenatal diagnosis became widely available, people who knew they had a history of serious genetic disease in their families, or who had already given birth to a seriously diseased child, simply did not dare to initiate pregnancies." (Christopher Norwood, *At Highest Risk*, New York: Penguin Books, 1980, p. 82.)

* Recent studies have shown that the father is responsible for about one in four babies with Down's syndrome. Amniocentesis, of course, permits diagnosis in either case.

can often help you to acquaint yourself with what the situation would mean to you and your partner. Different people feel very different about this matter, and it is important that you not feel pressured into a decision you won't be comfortable with.

Do not assume you should not have amniocentesis when you are certain you would not have an abortion. No physician should refuse the test on this condition.

When I became unexpectedly pregnant at forty-three, my doctor told me about amniocentesis, but I told him that because of my religion I wouldn't consider having an abortion no matter what the results of the test. He then suggested I consider having the test just to find the condition of the baby—that probably we would be reassured that it was all right. I talked it over with my husband and he thought this idea made sense. It was very upsetting when we first learned the baby had Down's, but this didn't change our original feelings. Learning the baby's condition early made all the difference. I attended a clinic which helps parents care for children with Down's and talked with many parents. As well as preparing ourselves, my husband and I were able to help our three teenage children know what to expect. We all picked out the baby's name together and the children are waiting for him to come home so they can help take care of him.

It is also important to discuss your and your partner's family's medical history and ethnic background with your physician, since amniocentesis can also test for approximately eighty rare disorders, among them Tay-Sachs disease and sickle cell anemia, though the latter can be done only in a few specialized centers. Tests other than routine chromosome analysis and AFP screening for neural tube defects will be performed only if your physician indicates that they are necessary, because they are costly and time-consuming. Ordinarily you would not consider any of them unless you had special reasons to believe that your baby is at risk.

The procedure: a physician performs amniocentesis on an outpatient basis in a hospital or his or her office. S/he must keep taking ultrasound pictures to check the location of the fetus and the placenta. *The amniocentesis must be performed immediately after the UTS while you are on the table.* If you get up and walk to another room, or if you wait, the baby may shift around. (Some physicians use a local anesthetic to numb the skin, others don't.) The physician then inserts a long, thin needle through your abdominal wall into the womb and draws off approximately four teaspoons of fluid into a syringe. On rare occasions s/he may have to try a second time to get enough fluid. You may have some or all of the following sensations during the procedure: pricking or stinging of your skin, cramping when the needle enters the uterus and pressure when the fluid is withdrawn. These reactions are normal and don't mean that anything is amiss, but they should

diminish and disappear within a day. If they don't, call your physician.

While some women find the procedure easy, others find it an unpleasant, upsetting experience.

I was nervous. But my obstetrician met us in the waiting room and told me that discomfort is unusual. First they showed it on the ultrasound screen and then made a pen mark on my stomach where the needle was to go in. The whole procedure turned out to be completely painless. My doctor talked his way through: "Now I'm going to do…Now you'll feel…" It was reassuring. Then he told me to take it easy for a day. After, we spoke to a genetics counselor and asked a lot of questions. She told us as much as we wanted to know and showed us "pictures" of imperfect chromosomes which cause birth defects. It was abstract but it hit home. It helped that nothing had gone wrong during the procedure. We didn't worry at all about what the results would be.

I hadn't been anxious about the procedure but looking back I'm glad my husband decided to come. No one had prepared me for how important it was to have someone there holding your hand and being supportive. The doctor couldn't get the needle in the right place and kept moving it around for a long time. This really hurt and I was upset and anxious. Finally he took the needle out and tried again. The second time there was no problem but I was quite distraught by that time. The staff and doctors were wonderful but I wish I had talked beforehand to someone who had gone through the experience.

The procedure itself wasn't bad. My husband went with me. I found it kind of creepy thinking of that long needle so I didn't look. It took longer than I thought. Having my own doctor there made a difference; I would have been more nervous in a clinic in somebody else's hands. Afterwards, however, I had bad cramps and was in great pain. I found it traumatic to hear (from the counselor) about all the genetic deformities that could not be picked up and why the test might have to be done again. The cramps did go away but I stayed in bed for two days because I had lost a baby a few years before and was afraid of miscarriage. When it became clear that things were all right I felt better.

The correct use of ultrasound and proper needle size are important. When hospitals use improper techniques, risks to the fetus increase. You may want to consider traveling to a hospital other than the one near you if the facilities are better and the personnel more experienced. Find out who specializes in the procedure and the number of amniocentesis procedures they do. Talk to other women who have had amniocentesis.

The sample of amniotic fluid contains some of the baby's cells and fluids. The cells are cultured and a photograph is made of their chromosomes. You may receive a picture of the chromosomes (karyotype) if you wish. Some people choose not to see it, since you can tell the sex of the baby from the chromosomes. Others prefer to know their baby's sex before it is born.

Maternal Serum Tests (Alpha-Fetoprotein Tests) for Neural Tube Defects

Approximately two in 1,000 infants in the U.S. are born each year with a neural tube defect (NTD). In this disorder, the developing neural tube, which forms the brain, spinal cord and spinal column, does not close over completely. The defect, which usually leaves an open lesion, can occur anywhere along the neural tube. If the tube remains open at the top, the baby will be born with only a rudimentary brain and open skull. This condition, called *anencephaly*, is always fatal. If the opening is along the backbone, the severity of the defect will depend on several factors: whether the lesion is covered with skin, whether nerve tissue protrudes from the defect, and the size and location of the lesion. This condition is known as *spina bifida* or *meningeomyelocele*. Children with open lesions almost always have severe medical problems: some are mentally retarded, many have no bladder or bowel control and most have some degree of paralysis. Therefore they require extensive medical and surgical procedures. However, many forms of spina bifida are much less disabling, and people with the condition lead rich, full lives.* Unfortunately, the AFP test gives no indication of the severity of the problem, although ultrasound can help with the diagnosis in some cases.

During the last decade, researchers discovered that the amount of alpha-fetoprotein was higher for women who carried an affected fetus. The alpha-fetoprotein test can diagnose about 85 percent of fetuses with an open lesion. About 10 percent of fetuses with neural tube defects have lesions covered with skin. They are not detectable and usually less serious.

Although the blood test itself is routine and easy to do, the results are difficult to interpret for the following reasons:

1. The amount of AFP varies during pregnancy. Therefore it is important to know when you became pregnant. An ultrasound may help find out how old the fetus is.

2. The blood test may give "false positives," or detect an increased amount of AFP for reasons other than NTDs in 5 percent of the tests. Multiple births, certain rare disorders and an incorrect estimate of fetal age can result in false positives.

Because of the many false positives, further tests are done on women who have a high AFP reading. These include a second blood test, ultrasound to check the

fetus's age and finally amniocentesis. Each step increases the accuracy with which the relatively few cases are diagnosed.

Medical and laypeople have raised objections to routine AFP screening, which subjects numbers of women to several tests when so few will actually have the problem and will have to wait so long for the results. Inadequate counseling, lack of information and the procedures themselves can cause inordinate stress for the women who decide to have repeat testing.

If you decide to have an AFP blood test, remember that a series of tests may be necessary to be sure that a normal baby will not be diagnosed as having a neural tube deficiency. If you are having amniocentesis anyway, the AFP blood test is unnecessary since the AFP level in the amniotic fluid should be measured routinely.

Researchers do not know what factors can produce neural tube defects, and believe them to be brought on by a combination of genetic and other unknown factors. One study found that supplementary vitamins around the time of conception and for the first month of pregnancy may help prevent the disorder.* This should not be interpreted as meaning that megavitamins are useful to women who eat a complete diet. Most of the vitamin research has been done with women whose diets are poor and lacking in certain essentials.

Testing Before Birth (Antepartum Fetal Testing)†

Another set of tests exists, originally designed as screening and diagnostic tools for women with health problems (diabetes, heart or kidney disease or excessively high blood pressure) or for women who have had a previous problem, such as stillbirth. These tests are also performed when a woman or her practitioner thinks that a baby is overdue—usually after forty-two weeks of pregnancy—or that a fetus still in the uterus has stopped growing (IUGR—intrauterine growth retardation), for the placenta can reach a point where it no longer functions at its peak. The goal of these tests is to discover whether the baby is healthy enough to remain in the uterus. While sometimes successful

---

* Contact the Spina Bifida Association of America, 343 South Dearborn, No. 317, Chicago, IL 60604, (312) 663-1562, for more information.

* Smithells, R.W., S. Sheppard and C.J. Schorah. "Possible prevention of neural tube defects by preconceptual vitamin supplementation," *Lancet*, February 16, 1980.

†For further reading, see Judith Lumley, "Antepartum Fetal Heart Rate Tests and Induction of Labor," in *Women and Health: Obstetrical Intervention and Technology in the 1980s*, Vol. 7, Nos. 3/4, Diony Young, ed., New York: Hawthorne Books, Inc., 1983, pp. 9–28; also Adrian Grant and Patrick Mohide, "Screening and Diagnostic Tests in Antenatal Care," in *Effectiveness and Satisfaction in Antenatal Care*, Murray Enkin and Iain Chalmers, eds., Philadelphia: J.B. Lippincott, 1982, pp. 22–59; also Margot Edwards and Penny Simkin, *Tests and Technology, A Consumer's Guide*, The Pennypress, 1100 23rd Avenue E, Seattle, WA 98112, 1980.

TESTS DURING PREGNANCY

Ultrasound	Amniocentesis	AFP Screening
Indications • Profuse bleeding (possible placenta problems) • Suspected multiple birth • Suspected abnormality in fetus or placenta • Woman's size not compatible with dates	**Indications** • Previous child of either parent with a neural tube or chromosome abnormality • History of certain diseases • History of repeated spontaneous abortions (could indicate chromosome abnormality) • Woman a carrier of an x-linked disorder • Woman 35 years or older when baby is born • Need to access fetal lung maturity	
Routine Uses • Preparation for amniocentesis • To check baby's position (early for ectopic pregnancy, close to delivery for complications) • To check position of placenta • Woman with diabetes		**Routine Uses** • Women with diabetes
Time of Test • Anytime during pregnancy	**Time of Test** • Around 14–16 weeks of pregnancy for chromosome analysis • Before delivery for fetal lung assessment	**Time of Test** • 16–19 weeks into pregnancy for most accurate results
Risks Woman: none known Fetus: short-term: none long-term: unknown	**Risks** • Mild: cramping, spotting and leaking of fluid fairly common but should disappear in one day • Serious: miscarriage, maternal bleeding, injury to fetus • Need for a repeat: infrequent, caused by not enough fluid or laboratory problems • Ultrasound: long-range risks unknown	**Risks (of blood test)** • None to woman or fetus
Accuracy (assuming experienced technician) • Baby's and placenta's position: very accurate • Dating pregnancy: plus or minus 10 days	**Accuracy (assuming experienced technicians and doctor)** • Results of all tests done with amniocentesis very accurate	**Accuracy (see p. 358)** • Will detect 85% of NTDs, although some women will need several tests before a final diagnosis is made. Risk of diagnosing normal children as affected is so small it cannot be measured.
Time Required for Results • Pictures obtained immediately; other physicians may be consulted for second opinion	**Time Required for Results** • Chromosome analysis and other tests: 2–3 weeks • Fetal lung assessment: 2 hours in lab-equipped hospital	**Time Required for Results** • 3–5 days in a lab-equipped hospital
Routine Information Gained • Information as to general development of fetus—gross development of kidneys, heart, brain, spinal column, digestive tract can be checked. • Limb and some other defects can be detected via visualization after 16 weeks	**Routine Information Gained** • Analysis for chromosome disorders • Diagnosis of neural tube defects • Sex of baby	**Routine Information Gained** • Detects AFP level in maternal blood

in reassuring worried women and practitioners, and sometimes leading to a truly lifesaving Cesarean (as in the case of pre-eclampsia), these tests, like the tests previously discussed, do not *guarantee* a healthy baby. In addition, researchers have not performed enough randomized clinical trials to prove that testing and knowing the results actually do reduce perinatal death. The tests have high false-positive rates and medical people disagree as to which results constitute "normalcy" and which mean danger. Despite such cautions, many doctors have begun performing some of these tests routinely on healthy women toward the very end of their pregnancies. This practice does reassure some women, and because some tests are performed in the hospital, can serve to acquaint women with the birthplace and practitioners there, if the hospital is small enough. But tests also cost more money; further medicalize pregnancy; worry many women excessively, causing them to mistrust their bodies and their health; and sometimes lead to unnecessary medical induction of labor or to further (unnecessary) interventions.

If you do have any of these tests, first do what is simplest. As a start, some women simply check three times a day to see if the baby moves at least ten times in an hour. When they see their practitioner s/he will listen with a stethoscope or doptone to the baby's heartbeat after each of several movements to determine whether the heart tones speed up (accelerate) after each movement, an indicator of good health.

Estriol Determination Series

The placenta provides a high amount of the hormone estriol toward the end of pregnancy. Estriol is excreted in the blood and urine, and the level can be determined by tests, the blood test being the most accurate. The estriol level indirectly indicates whether the placenta is functioning properly or not. You must have several tests; just one isn't enough. A gradual or sudden drop may indicate a problem. Estriol counts by themselves are never accurate enough to provide the basis for a decision to perform a Cesarean section.

Non-Stress Test

This test may also be performed, based on the idea that when a healthy baby moves in the uterus, its heart rate will speed up with each movement. The test takes twenty to forty minutes and is usually performed in a hospital maternity ward or wherever an external fetal monitor is available. Go for the test at a time when you know your baby is "awake." The nurse determines fetal heart rate by hooking you up to the fetal monitor as you lie on your left side or sit up. The baby either moves by itself or when you or your practitioner push at it. (Drinking a glass or two of orange juice very often makes the baby move, according to one maternity nurse we know.) The test is "reactive" if fetal heart tones accelerate fifteen beats above baseline (120 to 160 beats a minute) twice or three times within twenty minutes. However, practitioners don't all have the same standards as to what a normal response should be, or they may misinterpret their findings. Negative results—a "nonreactive" baby—don't necessarily mean that the baby is in danger. This test is almost always performed before the contraction stress test.

Contraction Stress Test

This test takes two forms. The first, less interventive than the second, simply consists of *nipple stimulation*, causing you to secrete oxytocin which leads to uterine contractions. You are lying on your left side or sitting up, hooked up to an external fetal monitor. You stimulate your nipples with your fingers, a warm or dry washcloth or a breast pump. Contractions begin within twenty to forty minutes, and usually much sooner. You should have three moderate contractions within ten minutes, each lasting around forty-five seconds. The monitor records the fetal heart's response to each contraction. The aim of this test is to determine your baby's condition by seeing how the placenta responds to the stress of a contraction. If nipple stimulation doesn't succeed in bringing on contractions, then you will have the oxytocin challenge test, or OCT, in which a small amount of Pitocin (synthetic oxytocin) is introduced via an intravenous drip. Once contractions begin the fetal heart tones are checked. The OCT has a high false-positive rate with results sometimes difficult to interpret and different observers giving different readings. Its risks lie in the fact that it is an unnatural intervention. It can lead to artificial induction of an entire labor, to Cesareans and to hospital-caused (iatrogenic) prematurity—a baby simply may not be ready to be born.

Use your own judgment in relation to these tests. Their very existence and availability may mean that you will be more likely to use them, that you will be pressured into using them. It is most important that you feel as calm as possible toward the end of your pregnancy. The tests may or may not contribute to your peace of mind. You may not want to have any done at all, especially if you are feeling fine. You may choose to have some. Be sure to get good information and support from family and friends before you make your decisions.

19

CHILDBIRTH

By Jane Pincus, with Norma Swenson

With special thanks to Jenny Fleming, Judy Luce and Becky Sarah

This chapter in previous editions was called "Prepared Childbirth" and was written by Ruth Bell and Nancy P. Hawley.

CLIMATE OF CONFIDENCE

To birthing...we bring our histories, our relationships, our rituals...needs and values that relate to intimacy, sexuality, the quality and style of family life and community, and our deepest beliefs about life, birth and death....[1]

When you believe in your basic health and strength, in your ability to give birth in your own way, trusting yourself and the people around you to provide guidance and support; when your practitioners believe in you, bringing to the birth of *your* baby their cumulative experience of seeing many normal births and healthy babies, then you and they together create a climate of confidence.

I had a long, drawn out labor. Each person there got a chance to rest. They switched on and off being with me. I'd take hot showers. I could do what I wanted. I was standing most of the time and walking around. I was so pleased not to be in bed. They encouraged me to eat; I did drink some tea. Finally they convinced me to lie down and I got a little sleep.

Labor was painful. Pain isn't an adequate word. I was bowled over by the intensity of the physical experience. I remember thinking as labor got heavy, women are fantastic, they get pregnant over and over again and are strong enough; people go through this all *the time. Nobody could have prepared me for it in words.*

I could imagine myself understanding how I'd take drugs if someone urged them on me in a hospital. But here, because everyone was saying, "Everything is fine," it was easy to keep going.

Finally it was dragging on. Laura (my midwife) said, "You and Lewis run around the back yard." We did. We tromped around. Every time I had a contraction I leaned against the pear tree. Then I ran up and down the stairs a few times. Labor became more intense.

Laura called Peter (the doctor). He came over, sat in a corner and read a magazine, saying, "This could take up to two hours. Don't worry, you have plenty of time."

Then came the best time of all. Pushing wasn't at all painful. Mary was holding the mirror; each time I pushed I could see the effects. Laura: "Try breathing—blow out from really deep inside you. Let your cheeks puff out." It worked. I started squatting, then sitting up with Lewis behind me. My final delivery position was on my side, one leg up on Laura's shoulder. With every single push I could see Emma coming out, bigger and bigger. After every push Laura would massage my perineum. The little—no, the big head came out. She was cooing. It was the sweetest thing I ever heard. Laura said to Lewis and me, "Reach down and pull out your baby." It was a big surprise to us! We did! We pulled her out! I brought her to my breast. We were enthralled. The afterbirth came out with no problem. Laura showed it to us.

The whole experience changed my life. It taught me how deeply physical life is, and connected me much more with my body. I'd learned a refined kind of Catholicism where nothing was earthy, nothing was said aloud. But there's nothing subtle about being pregnant and having a baby!

Another woman and her husband created their own climate of confidence when they had their second baby in a large, busy city hospital where they were more or less left to themselves.

Labor really began at twelve-thirty A.M. on Monday. At two A.M. we went to the hospital. At two P.M. the next day I was working harder but still four centimeters dilated. The obstetrician wanted to give me morphine, saying, "This has gone on too long for a second labor. I'll put you to sleep for five hours and you'll wake up in active labor." Jack and I looked at each other and said, "This guy's really hot to trot." But we knew that when the baby's ready to be born, it will be born. We said we'd decide at three P.M. At three P.M. I was five centimeters dilated. Nurses were changing shifts. Though they were wonderful there were never many of them around. I was sitting up all the time. Jack and I used a lot of imagery. He helped me to breathe into the pain. We imagined wind and waves. I made sure the sensation would go down and through my cervix, and pictured my cervix opening, pictured myself being born. That helped a lot. Looking at Jack was best, or burying my face in his neck, or closing my eyes and going inside. If he hadn't been there, forget it. We were so concentrated on what we were doing. We knew it was our experience. He knew exactly what to do. He never left me.

At three-thirty they said they were thinking of breaking my bag of waters, but because of the change in shifts, they never got around to do it. Then my waters broke by themselves and labor got harder. I knew it was toward the end. I felt pressure against my pubic bone, which was relieved by counterpressure and singing. Singing was exactly what I wanted to do with this one. All of a sudden I needed to push. "Don't push," they said. "I can't not," I said. They took me to the delivery room. I delivered my baby quickly. It was intense. I did my share of yelling. Her head came through while the doctor was still getting dressed, so I had no episiotomy. I made the doctor show me the placenta. My baby nursed in the recovery room, just as I had dreamed about it last summer.

And a midwife states:

All efforts are made to see birth as a continuum. I tell people who have prepared for home birth, who begin labor at home and then end up at the hospital, "Who you are never changes: your planning, ideals, values, beliefs, principles never change just because you end up in the hospital, or with a Cesarean. You are stronger than you would have been because you've gone through all those decisions and made the choices you did."

CLIMATE OF DOUBT

These women giving birth with confidence in themselves, both in and out of medical settings; these practitioners—midwives, doctors, nurses—show us that childbearing can be qualitatively different from what the medical world offers us, much richer than we ever imagined and as free as possible from medical interventions. They show us mothers drawing on their own strengths, listening to their bodies and, when tired or tense, being supported by caring attendants to relax, renew themselves, and above all to have confidence in their own birthing powers. Their experiences make it vividly clear to what extent the purely medical view of childbirth focuses mainly upon fears—fears of something going wrong, fear of pain—the most negative aspects of birthing.

How did this negative focus come about? In fact, the climate of doubt has been in the making a long time. To begin with, obstetrics in the U. S. began as a surgical specialty practiced by males.

Brief History

More drugs and technologies are now used in "normal" births in America than anywhere else in the world. This reflects in part the desire to master, conquer and control nature that was present among the colonists from the beginning.[2]

The present system was born in and shaped by the competition between male and female healers.[3]

In colonial, preindustrial America, midwives and community women attended childbearing women with excellent results. Sometimes—rarely, when all else failed—they called upon barber-surgeons: "Small wonder that the men who were called by midwives to assist in births regarded births as deadly and dangerous. They lacked the midwives' experience of hundreds of routine births that required no assistance."[4] "Man-midwives," as they were called at first, used forceps and hooks, as few women would or did. A formal training period was deemed necessary, and obstetrics became the first specialty to be taught in medical schools in the U.S. in the eighteenth century.

Many of our own and our doctors' present attitudes

Suzanne Arms

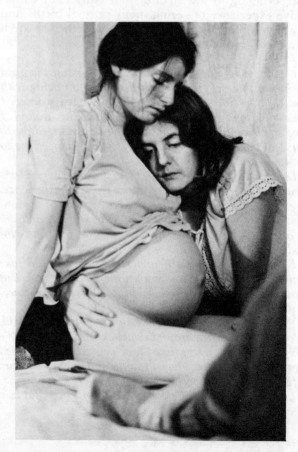

originated during the nineteenth century.* Male doctors gradually gained control of childbirth among the upper and middle classes, a control which represented political and economic triumph rather than scientific necessity. They deliberately, systematically excluded women from medical training.[5] "Doctors feared, not without reason, that if women were admitted to the profession, woman patients would prefer physicians of their own sex, especially for childbirth."[6]

Although in the 1830s and 1840s a strong grass-roots popular health movement campaigned against medical elitism and many kinds of healing sects flourished, and although the medical "regulars"—upper- and middle-class men—had nothing to recommend them over lay practitioners—"they still couldn't claim to have any uniquely effective methods or special body of knowledge"[7]—the "regulars" won out through political influence.

Around the same time, doctors performed cruel experimental surgery upon many women, especially black slaves and poor women, in the name of science[8] (an experimentation which continues in gynecology and obstetrics to this day[9]). Out of this early experimentation grew "cures" for gynecological conditions, many of which were actually created by barbarous childbirth practices (although this was not recognized at the time). These skills increased gynecologists' powers enormously, since the promise of cures and even of prevention lay with them.

The Victorian era saw gynecologists and obstetricians gain even more control over women. Middle- and upper-class women, admiring education and science and able to afford doctors' fees, changed their allegiance from midwives to scientifically-trained doctors, men of their own class, who eventually became advisers in all sorts of matters and went so far as to become judges of their moral conduct (also a role which continues to this day). These women were rarely physically active. Meanwhile working-class women continued to work day and night in factories and fields, their pregnancies and births attended by local midwives. Physicians continued to look upon midwives both as economic threats and threats to the masculine, medical order they were in the process of establishing.† They waged a virulent campaign against midwives, stereotyping them as ignorant, dirty and irresponsible. Physicians deliberately lied about midwifery outcomes to convince legislators that states should outlaw it, when in fact midwives often had safety records superior to those of physicians.[10] In addition, though most people of that time believed that birth was usually a healthy, natural process:

> Obstetricians campaigned to reverse that belief. They set out to make mothers "fear" the dangers of pregnancy and childbirth, and think of "no precaution as excessive"; and then to comfort them with the assertion of their right to the care of the only ones who could provide it, the professional obstetricians.[11]

As medical boards and state legislators systematically suppressed midwifery, women had to move out of their homes into hospitals to give birth, which did not prove to be safer or better for them and their babies.[12] In 1900, 5 percent of babies in the U.S. were born in hospitals; by 1935, 75 percent; and by the late 1960s, 95 percent.[13] By giving birth in hospitals women took the last step toward total dependence on the man-made obstetrical system, which became a de facto monopoly. Our struggle to escape this monopoly continues to this day.

Some Attitudes Which Create and Sustain a Climate of Doubt

Taking their own bodies as the norm, most doctors see women's bodies as abnormal. Influential obstetricians in this century have come up with some striking descriptions of labor and birth, among them Joseph B. DeLee who in 1920 compared labor to a crushing door and birth to falling on a pitchfork, the handle driving through the perineum:

> In both cases, the cause of the damage, the fall on the pitchfork and the crushing of the door, is pathogenic, that is disease provoking, and anything pathogenic is pathologic and abnormal.[14]

The well-known author of *Birth Without Violence*, Dr. Frederick Leboyer, says:

> One day, the baby finds itself a prisoner...the prison comes to life...begins, like some octopus, to hug and crush...stifle...assault...the prison has gone berserk...with its heart bursting, the infant sinks into this hell...the mother...she is driving the baby out. At the same time she is holding it in, preventing its passage. It is she who is the enemy. She who stands between the child and life. Only one of them can prevail. It is mortal combat...not satisfied with crushing, the monster...twists it in a refinement of cruelty.[15]

> The orthodoxy reflects an anxious view of birth...as a treacherous course mined with sudden, unexpected disasters requiring the medical equivalent of a military alert.[16]

These ideas and others less dramatic but equally negative underlie and shape many routine obstetrical practices. The practices then reinforce our fears that our bodies won't work right and something will go

---

*See G. J. Barker-Benfield, *Horrors of the Half-Known Life*, for a fascinating and informative description of the U.S. male mentality in the nineteenth century. Also read Barbara Ehrenreich and Deirdre English, *For Her Own Good*, and *Witches, Midwives and Nurses*; and Richard and Dorothy Wertz's *Lying-In: A History of Childbirth in America* (see Resources).

† "It is at present impossible to secure cases sufficient for the proper training in obstetrics, since 75% of a material otherwise available for clinic purposes is utilized in providing a livelihood for midwives." (Dr. Charles E. Zeigler, quoted in Barbara Ehrenreich and Deirdre English, *For Her Own Good*, p. 95.)

wrong, cause new doubts, disrupt the physiology of labor, distort our experiences or completely prevent them from taking place normally. Attitudes themselves—our own and our practitioners'—affect the course of labor—slowing it down, speeding it up—as much as any drug or mechanical intervention.* When we accept medical descriptions of what we should feel, do and take during labor and birth we allow our powers to be diminished and tamed.

Institutions Contribute to the Climate of Doubt

During the 1950s and 1960s, operations research techniques used to expedite the manufacture of various forms of weaponry in WW II were applied to developing more effective obstetrical suites....Priorities were formulated to facilitate the efficient processing of as many women as possible rather than to allow for an adjustable tempo for each individual birth. The factory approach was soon incorporated into textbooks on hospital design: "The conveyer belt concept has its use in analyzing our problems. It emphasizes the repeated transference of a mother (as in motor-car assembly) from place to place, and also that unequal time periods at any station can render the process uneconomical."[17]

Hospitals reduce labor and birth to a medical, debilitating event. As healthy, strong women with good energy, we enter these places for sick people and our strength is systematically depleted; often we are put into wheelchairs. Our personal effects are taken away. We are cut off from friends and the people closest to us, isolated among strangers and made dependent and anonymous. When medical personnel give us enemas and shave (prep) us, they desex and infantalize us. We are not allowed food and drink, which weakens us, slows labor down and endangers our health. We are hooked up to IVs, which immobilize us: "You don't want to get exhausted, do you?" We are given epidurals: "It will get worse before it gets better (and you won't be able to handle it)." As one nurse-midwife said, regretfully, "The most natural aspects of birth—sexuality, blood, sweat, shit, movement and sounds—have no place here." We are assaulted by assumptions about our inability to give birth without intervention (at times even by the best intentions of hospital staff wanting to "do something useful"). Each "stage" of labor *has* to take place within a given amount of time.

"Continuity of care," one of medicine's own standards for quality care, does not exist. We see many

*Ann Oakley's *Subject Women*, New York: Schocken Books, 1980, has an excellent discussion of women's attitudes about themselves and professionals' attitudes toward them. Diana Scully's *Men Who Control Women's Health* describes obstetrical residents' attitudes toward the women they see in hospitals. Gayle Peterson, in *Birthing Normally*, details some of the ways in which *our* beliefs and attitudes can affect pregnancy and labor.

people and have to cope with different personalities, which is neither easy nor particularly good for us. During pregnancy, one doctor or series of doctors checks us out, often hastily and impersonally. During labor in the hospital all kinds of strangers—anesthesiologists, nurses, nursing students, residents, medical students and lab technicians—walk in and out of the room. Some nurses do all they can, but there are not enough of them.

The nurses came and went and didn't stay. My husband did fine, but I was a crab. He couldn't relieve my backache from back labor. One nurse gave me good massages—she knew just where to press—but she was so busy that she had to leave all the time. That upset me.

We also may have no one at all with us for periods of time. *Few cultures leave laboring women so alone.* The doctor, appearing briefly or just at the end of labor, may be someone we have never seen before. When the baby is born, we often have a new set of nurses and an unfamiliar pediatrician. In large hospitals a doctor who specializes in newborns (neonatologist) may appear as well.

This terrible care distracts us, causes insecurity and confusion at a time when we should be relaxing, comfortable, concentrating on ourselves and our babies.

Isolation and immobility during labor increase pain, which increases tension and fear, which brings on more pain. In such surroundings, women end up "needing" pain relief, and obstetricians, anesthesiologists, researchers and drug companies hasten to provide it in abundant variety.

Physicians' Obstetrical Training Contributes to the Climate of Doubt

Men and women trained in medical schools, clinics and hospitals rarely, if ever, see a normal spontaneous labor and birth. To most students, childbirth means a woman lying on her back during labor, her bag of waters broken artificially, labor "accelerated" by Pitocin, often hooked up to a fetal monitor, drugged or anesthetized, feet in stirrups for delivery in the lithotomy position, given an episiotomy, with a possibility of forceps or perhaps a Cesarean section.

As a result, physicians don't know how to relate to a fully conscious, unanesthetized woman. They don't sit through labor from beginning to end to learn how or what a woman feels, to become acquainted with the rhythm of her labor, the positions she chooses and the sounds she makes, to monitor the baby's descent, encourage her and simply to do nothing at times—"mastering the art of inactivity," as one childbirth educator said.

My first home birth, in a trailer in Maryland, was also the first time I had ever been alone with a woman throughout her whole labor. It took hours. There were no nurses, no shifts, no system to shield me from how long having a baby really takes. I remember opening my obstetrics book, examining the course of labor charted on the page and feeling reassured, for the hours of labor were no longer than the hours of the curve.[18]

Nor do medical students learn "hands-on" skills so important to laboring women—massage, physical support, perineal massage. In sum, they do not learn midwifery skills. Most find it boring and undramatic to sit through a labor. Even when they want to, they don't have enough time. Instead, they learn to use mechanical interventions of all kinds routinely to speed up labor, unaware of just how invasive and even dangerous these interventions can be (see pp. 379–82). Also, since obstetrics is a surgical specialty, they must meet a quota for procedures performed, practicing their craft not because women need certain procedures done but because students need experience. Many of them learn to manipulate us into accepting and submitting to interventions "for our own good" and "for the safety of the baby," strongly suggesting that if we don't agree to undergo certain procedures we do not care about the baby. They also learn that unless they use or have close at hand every available tool and instrument, they may be sued for malpractice at some point in their future career. Drugs and intervention used routinely in the name of safety become instruments of control and debilitation.

After such training it is no wonder that physicians genuinely believe that we cannot and should not give birth without medical interventions and hospital assistance.

Women Internalize the Medical Model

Childbearing has always involved a perfectly natural fear of something going wrong, of the unknown, of pain and the risk of death. We can never be completely certain of the outcome wherever and however we have children. Medical attitudes and practices encourage, indeed thrive on these fears. One mother says:

It is as if our confidence is a large, bright piece of fabric. When little pinprick holes of fear and doubt appear, the medical mentality makes them larger and larger until the once beautiful cloth is nothing but gaping holes.

When we are isolated and have no experienced, empathetic women around us to answer questions, listen to us and help us keep feeling positive; when we put our faith only in doctors who don't believe in our ability to give birth; when we depend, as they do, only on their medical techniques; then we reinforce their belief that we can't do without them. TV, with its images of groaning women giving birth draped in white sheets, and women's magazines repeat the message:

The single factor most responsible for recent advances in helping mothers and infants through the prenatal period (defined as from conception through the first month of the infant's life) is sophisticated technology. It allows physicians to closely monitor fetal development through pregnancy and labor. If the pregnancy is developing *entirely* normally and if the delivery is *totally* uncomplicated, the *full weight* of this technology need not be brought to bear, *although it sometimes is.*[19][Emphasis ours.]

Millions of women read articles like this one, which sets up an impossible "model" of pregnancy and labor while suggesting that almost no one will have one. Such propaganda subtly demoralizes us, making us believe that technology must be inevitable. In absorbing the medical model of childbearing we allow our fears of what might go wrong to win over our knowledge that *all* living is risk, that life is to be lived fully with reasonable care rather than with unreasonable caution.

Childbearing is *your* experience—you, not anyone else, are having your child. If you want to give birth in a climate of confidence you must know it is possible, create it, seek it out, surround yourself during pregnancy with friends and practitioners who feel positive about childbirth. You must know how pervasive the climate of doubt is these days so that you can recognize it in all its forms and resist it. Many experienced lay and nurse-midwives; a few physicians, especially family practitioners; some nurses and special labor attendants can help you have the childbirth you want, either in your home, in freestanding birth centers or sometimes even in hospitals.

LABOR

Your body prepares for labor. During labor, uterine muscles gradually stretch the cervix open for the baby to come out, and the muscles also push the baby down into the vagina so it can be born.

Throughout your pregnancy you have been having contractions regularly—called Braxton-Hicks contractions—as uterine muscles tighten, then loosen, exercising the uterus and preparing it to work efficiently during labor. Toward the end of pregnancy you may feel these contractions pulling and stretching more intensely and frequently; occasionally they are uncomfortable. Your cervix is softening, ripening.

Both effacement (thinning and drawing up of the cervix) and dilation (opening of the cervix) can occur before you *feel* your labor beginning. Some women remain slightly dilated for weeks before labor begins. Others go into labor *before* dilation starts and have their babies a few hours later!

When you feel contractions stronger than Braxton-Hicks, more like menstrual cramps, you may think you

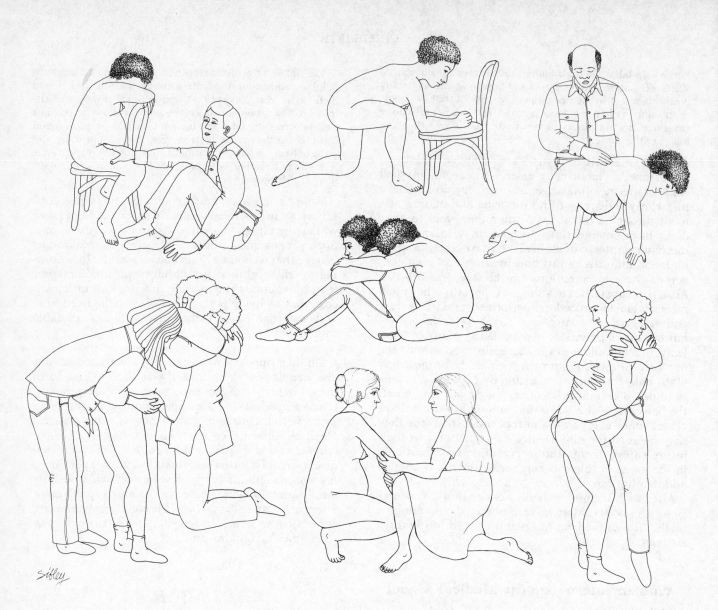

Sifley

Dana Sibley

are beginning early labor (and sometimes you are!). Called "false labor" by the medical profession, these contractions are another form of preliminary labor and play an important role in initial dilation and effacement. They make your cervix contract and relax rather than contract and pull back. These contractions usually stop after a while, though they can last for hours. When you feel them, get up and walk around, and see if they continue or if the intervals between contractions become longer or shorter.

What Causes Labor?

We know a lot about labor, but we don't know exactly what sets it off. It may be that when the fetus matures, its own glandular system sends out hormonal messages into the woman's bloodstream, altering maternal hormone levels. As a result, the woman's pituitary

gland secretes the hormone oxytocin, which causes the uterus to contract. A higher estrogen level may stimulate contractions. The uterine lining may secrete prostaglandins which cause secretion of oxytocin. And the baby's head pressing on cervical nerve endings may help initiate labor. Our emotional state as well as physical position can also affect labor, stopping or slowing it down if we feel afraid and tense, speeding it up when we relax.

Some First Signs of Labor

Some body signals let you know that you are about to go into labor. Your Braxton-Hicks contractions may become more intense and frequent. You may have diarrhea for a few days or on the day labor begins, your body's way of emptying itself so that labor is less obstructed. You may feel an extraordinary burst of

366

energy and want to cook, clean house, organize—a kind of nesting instinct. You may suddenly want to do nothing.

Bloody Show

As your cervix begins to stretch open, the small mucus plug which seals it comes out, not usually in one piece but as pink mucus, "bloody show," blood-tinged from the broken capillaries formerly attaching it to the cervix. Many women never have a "show." Others have it all through early and active labor.

Waters Breaking

As your baby's head presses down against the membranes containing amniotic fluid, they may break. (Most often they break when you have been in active labor for a while. Rarely, they remain intact until after the baby is born.) Your "waters" may rush out or, more commonly, just trickle out, usually clear and odorless, or milky. Some women think they are wetting their pants. Check color and smell. If you can't stop it by holding it back, it is probably amniotic fluid. *No matter how much fluid comes out, your body replaces it every few hours. There is no such thing as a "dry birth."* After your membranes break, labor will probably begin within a few hours, though some women trickle for a few days or even weeks. Practitioners disagree about what should be done after your waters break. Physicians are more likely to say that you should come right to the hospital to prevent infection. Some of them routinely induce labor after twenty-four hours if you haven't started on your own. Midwives and birth attendants are more likely to tell you to relax, that labor will begin soon.

Even if you are planning to give birth in the hospital, consider staying at home; there's usually *less* chance of your getting an infection at home in your customary environment. *Don't* take baths, put anything into your vagina (no internal pelvic exams) or have sexual intercourse. Stay clean. Drink a lot of fluids. Take your temperature regularly, twice a day or more. After twenty-four hours, another thing you can do is to get a white-blood-cell count every day to make sure there's no infection. Your practitioner may want to check your baby's heartbeat periodically.

If your waters broke suddenly you may want your practitioner to check externally that the baby's head fits right into your cervix so that the umbilical cord isn't swept through your cervix (which happens sometimes if the baby is in breech position or presenting "high"). Also, if you notice any brown or green staining, let your practitioner know, as it means that meconium (the tarry substance in your baby's bowels) has been squeezed out—common but occasionally an indication of fetal stress or distress.

Contractions (One of the Most Common Signs of Labor)

Your uterus will begin to contract regularly and/or strongly after a while. At first it may feel like gas pains, menstrual cramps, backache, a pulling and stretching in your pubic region. In early labor, contractions may be as regular as clockwork—perhaps ten minutes apart—or they may be irregular, inconsistent, widely spaced. (For some women they remain irregular or widely spaced all during labor.) If you begin labor during the daytime, go about your daily routine, especially if this is your first baby, when labors usually take longer. More often, labor begins at night when you are relaxed. It's a good idea to get some more sleep if you can.

At five A.M. I felt period cramps, was really excited. They weren't particularly painful. I knew something was happening! I waited for other signs. Had "bloody show." Beryl, my birth attendant, examined me. I was fully effaced and not dilated at all. Rick and I thought about what we wanted to do with the day. I baked a birthday cake, we took naps, had a quiet day together. I ate lightly all day, had spaghetti for dinner. We went to sleep; I woke up at eleven-thirty P.M. truly in labor.

An unplanned home birth:

I was probably in labor all day and didn't realize it. I went to take a shower, to wash my hair and shave my legs to be presentable. Lo and behold, my son was born then and there. The three of us went to the hospital, my head covered with shampoo.

Some women know when they are about to go into labor, and some can make it happen.

My body felt different the night before, as if I'd become lighter and the baby had shifted position.

I went into labor with my second child very consciously because I needed to. I don't believe in trying to control a process like labor, but it was wonderful to know I could invite it/allow it to start. My blood pressure had been climbing the last weeks of the pregnancy because of overwork and extreme stress. The midwife said to me firmly, "Just have the baby," so I went home to try. I thought about it, we made love, I let go of the reasons why it wasn't a good day, and in two hours my water broke with mild contractions starting up soon.

I know a midwife who covers the delivery service for only twelve hours a week at a large city hospital. She has delivered four babies for this one woman with whom she has a deep rapport. The woman has managed to time all four labors to fit into the midwife's twelve-hour segments, which shift around from week to week.

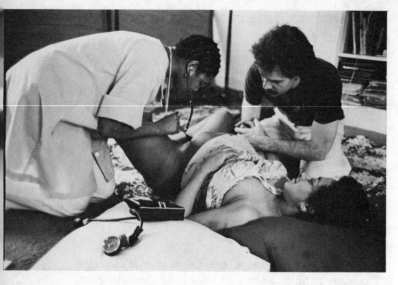

Ann McQueen/Stock Boston

Early Labor

In early labor, walking around, taking long walks, taking long baths or making love if your waters haven't broken, orgasm without intercourse if your waters have broken, showering, hugging, kissing, stroking your nipples or having them sucked all can stimulate your contractions and relax you. (Says one nurse: "Pizza, beer and orgasms—our favorite induction!")

When we went for a walk it was fun running into friends: "What are you doing up? I thought you were in labor." It was fun changing people's image of a woman in labor.

We went to the movies because our apartment was small, and it was too cold out to take a walk. I don't remember much of the film.

We made love while I was in labor. We went to bed and had a wonderful time. I was happy to be giving— to him and to myself—and not just concentrating on contractions.

When you rest or go to bed, the baby's head no longer presses on your cervix, and contractions may slow down. Alternate moving around with brief naps. Stay rested.

Some women prefer to stay at home until contractions become frequent and strong. *The longer you stay out of the hospital, the less likely you are to have your labor intervened in.* Others prefer to go and settle in before contractions become so strong that walking and riding in a car is uncomfortable. (Afterwards, some wish they had never gone to the hospital, others that they had left home sooner.)

Labor

During each contraction your upper uterine muscles pull the cervical muscles upward ("thinning," "taking up," effacement) and pull open the muscles around the cervix (dilation). Effacement is often measured by percentage (50 percent, 80 percent effaced) and dilation in centimeters or fingers (two centimeters equal one finger). When you've dilated ten centimeters, or five fingers, your baby is ready to be born, and then the uterus can push her/him through your vagina and out of your body. A while later your uterus contracts a few more times to expel both placenta and membranes (the transparent bag which contained your baby and the protective amniotic fluid).

Medical tradition divides labor into three stages: 1. the time it takes to become fully effaced and dilated, 2. pushing the baby out, and 3. expelling the placenta. Most physicians and hospital personnel set strict time limits in which they expect each of these stages to take place. These limits vary from one practitioner and place to another. Some hospitals may wait twenty-four hours before "accelerating" labor with Pitocin; others wait only twelve hours, or even less, or do a section for "failure to progress." Most physicians don't like "second-stage" labor to last more than one or two hours.*

Some midwives say there are only two stages: before the baby is born and afterwards. A practitioner skilled in normal labor knows that each labor has its own rhythm and takes its own time. S/he will not set arbitrary limits for the length of each phase but will decide whether labor needs to be helped along at a certain point. S/he also knows that these medically defined stages refer only to the relation of the baby to the woman's body, and not at all to labor as the woman experiences it. Some first stages can last up to forty hours with a one-hour second stage, or last for just two hours with a four-hour second stage. Other midwives and childbirth educators refer to the end of the first stage as "transition."

All practitioners agree that the placenta must come out within a reasonable time. (See p. 375.)

---

*Often this is because if you have received anesthesia, it has a depressant effect on the baby.

Active Labor

When labor really gets going, contractions are strong and rhythmic. You feel them building like a wave, pulling and tightening first in one place, then expanding throughout your uterus, into your back or your groin, and then lessening. In between you can rest, sleep, stay still, walk, talk. *Make sure to empty your bladder regularly.* Relaxing deeply *between* contractions gives you energy for each new one. Relaxing deeply during them helps reduce pain sensation.

Contractions when most intense felt like a belt around my lower back and abdomen. Most of the feeling was in my lower back. Contractions had a curve: strong at the beginning and then slowing down. You get to know them. What surprised me was that you're in two worlds. You have to concentrate on them when they happen, but when they stop, you're just regular. I've never felt so lucid, so clear, as in between contractions.

…Language was really important, and I didn't like the word "contraction." …I found when I was having my babies that if I thought "contraction" it meant making something tight. It's true the uterine muscles are contracting, but if everything's working right, at the same time the cervix is expanding. It's much more useful to think of the expansion….[20]

You adapt to labor. The hardest part comes early sometimes. Then you accept that it's really happening, it's a baby, it hurts—no abstractions. Later it can get easier, though contractions may be much *stronger.*

Suzanne Arms

There is a lot else going on besides the pain in the belly. I felt my nose and teeth going numb, rather as from drinking too much wine. I also saw the colors in the kitchen getting brighter and stronger. I'm not into mystical things, or thinking about auras, but yes, labor is a kind of high if you flow with it, and a room full of loving people does produce energy…gives you strength.[21]

Some Ideas for Coping with Hospital Routines

- Go in with your partner and/or birth attendant. It's better to be with someone familiar, never necessary or helpful to be separated. It helps if you can bring two support people—one to help you physically during labor and one to troubleshoot in case you have problems getting what you want.
- They may bring you a wheelchair. Ignore it if you feel comfortable standing and walking; take advantage of it if you want to. There is no medical reason for you to use it.
- They may give you a hospital "johnny" to wear. You can wear your own clothes. If you wear the johnny, take two, and use one as a robe. Be sure to bring soft, stretchy socks, preferably knee socks. Hospital rooms are often air conditioned.
- You may be asked to sign a patient consent form. If you haven't preregistered, it's standard. It states that you always have the right to informed consent, to say no and to know the risks and advantages of all drugs and procedures. It may also ask you for an "ether permit"—your agreement to be anesthetized in an emergency. You can withdraw your consent at any time.*
- A nurse or resident will ask you some questions about your pregnancy and your labor.
- A lab technician will probably take a blood sample, just in case it becomes necessary to match your blood.
- Hospital staff may listen to the fetal heartbeat with a fetoscope or doptone or see if the fetal heart remains steady during and after contractions. Since the doptone is a form of ultrasound, you may want to ask for a regular fetoscope instead. (Some nurses have never been trained to use regular fetoscopes, however.)
- During all these procedures you can stand or sit. You don't need to get into bed or lie down, though you may be urged or expected to. (You will need to lie down for a fetoscope but not for a doptone.) A mother who labored and gave birth two times lying flat on her back observed:

*Be sure you don't automatically sign a circumcision consent form. If you are a Jehovah's Witness you need to sign a specific form for yourself and baby to refuse blood products. Signing a form does *not* prevent you from taking legal action in the future should that become necessary.

I've often thought that the best thing a woman can do for herself when she gets into the hospital is to stay upright, standing, sitting, kneeling, squatting. That way she remains active, in control.

- In some hospitals the nurses may want to do a "test strip," using the external fetal monitor to check the course of the baby's heartbeats during a series of contractions. They will ask you to lie still for twenty minutes to an hour. Remember that when you lie down, your contractions change. If you are in early labor they may slow down and even stop altogether. They may become more uncomfortable, making you tense up, which affects their efficacy. Ask for a human monitor instead! If the nurses aren't around and you have a birth attendant who knows how to listen to the fetal heartbeat, she can check the fetal heart rate.
- You will probably have an internal exam to check dilation. In some hospitals nurses do them; in others, residents or doctors.

One resident must have been magic. He was a small, silent young man. I didn't feel his exams at all.

I'd brought tapes and music, was walking and dancing. We'd created a wonderful mood. Then the resident came in and blew it. He examined me internally, causing more pain than ever in my life.

- You have the right to turn away residents, to say, "I want my own doctor." But in teaching hospitals, residents are often the only doctors you get, and several of them may want a look at you. You have the right to say no.
- You can refuse to participate in teaching programs. You can always refuse any procedure from anyone, even in life-threatening situations.* Your partner and/or birth attendant can advocate for you and protect you.
- Nurses will be your most constant medical attendants if you have no midwife or labor coach. Let them know what you want. Many nurses are encouraging and helpful.

I was in labor for thirty-six hours altogether, most of them in the hospital. One nurse stayed in the room with me the whole time, sleeping in the other bed, keeping people from coming in. She'd tell them, "This is my patient; I'm in charge!" She helped me to have a beautiful vaginal delivery. Without her I could not have done it.

If you have a bad rapport with one nurse, ask for

*Sometimes the staff proceeds anyway. The hospital is usually protected against any legal action in the future, on the grounds that they acted to save your life.

another. It's not always easy to do so (or possible to get another) but it's worth a try.

- If, during any of the procedures mentioned above, you are having a contraction, let the people around you know. They may not be aware of it. Hold up your hand, tell them. Your partner can tell them. They should stop what they are doing and wait. You should not be distracted. Focus on what you want and need. This is your labor and your birth.

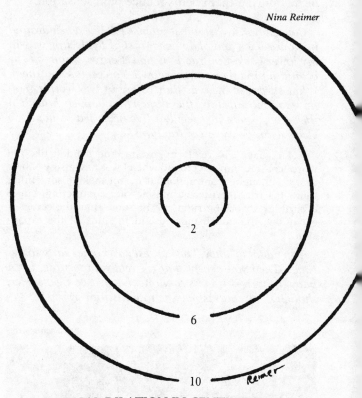

Nina Reimer

CERVICAL DILATION IN CENTIMETERS,
SHOWN ACTUAL SIZE

Achieving Full Dilation and Effacement (Sometimes Called Transition)

A range of signs indicates that your uterus is coming to the end of stretching and opening fully. You may have a powerful "opening up" feeling, contractions may come rapidly or be more intense than before. The more relaxed you are at this time, the better you'll feel. You may need others especially now to help you breathe deeply and focus your energies, to hold you, encourage you.

You may be very vocal during contractions, and doze or be very still in between. Or you may be inward and concentrated throughout. Many women choose one particular position at this time—kneeling, on hands and knees, on their side in bed. This time has been associated with nausea, shaking, trembling of thighs

What You Can Do to

- relax during labor;
- make pain bearable;
- eliminate most if not all interventions;
- help prevent a Cesarean and have a vaginal birth after a Cesarean (VBAC) (see p. 385), and what your partner and birth attendants can do for you.

Choose comfortable surroundings. When you feel comfortable and safe, with familiar people around you, you are better able to relax. Women give birth at home to be in familiar territory where they are free to be themselves. Out-of-hospital birth centers are usually like homes; you can cook your own food, use the living room, spend time with your children and friends. If you go to the hospital, bring "home" along with you—favorite clothes, photographs, pictures, beloved objects, a rug or blanket, records or tapes for music.

Choose people you feel comfortable with. It is important that the presence of others, their touch, advice and actions give you comfort and strength and make you happy and confident, and that they feel comfortable with you.

The pain was like a hurricane shaking me apart. I yelled a lot and walked around and took showers. I remember looking at Paul and thinking, What are you so happy about? This is terrible. Yet I know that the grin on his face sustained me. I needed his touch and his joy, and I needed—very differently— the midwife's words and knowledge and reassurance.

Choose support people who can understand what you want and don't want without having their feelings hurt. Too many and/or the wrong people (sometimes even your partner) can hinder labor by being too solicitous, too anxious, too noisy, too bossy.

Breathe deeply. Whether or not you've practiced breathing beforehand, deep breathing can help you to relax. Imagine your breath carrying oxygen to every part of your body. Breathe in whatever way is comfortable. Loosen your jaw. Open your mouth and throat. Smile. Laugh.

I found my own way of breathing. I knew I had to relax into the tenseness.

Some women may use the breathing they've practiced and become too controlled, too tense. Combine breathing with different positions, with sounds.

I was with a woman doing rigid strong labor breathing she had learned in a childbirth class. She was tight, exhausted. I said, "You don't have to do that." "What will I do?" "Just see what happens." She began to relax. When she let go trying to keep her control, her energy started to flow. Over the next few hours she started doing little sighs which became moans at the end. On the floor, kneeling, she breathed into her husband's lap and rocked her pelvis. He started to breathe and rock with her.

Endorphins. You may feel exhilarated during labor, mellow and peaceful between contractions, especially when your labor is progressing naturally and uninterruptedly. Some researchers now believe that when you are relaxed, your body produces its own substances for pain relief, called endorphins, which have a morphinelike effect. (High levels have been found in the placentas of animals and humans after birth.[22]) Tension and fear may inhibit the secretion of endorphins, causing you to secrete adrenalin instead, which tenses you up, slows your labor and makes it more painful. If labor is painful, don't blame yourself. Deep relaxation can be difficult, even in an ideal environment.

Change position and move around. Positions in which your spine is upright, as when you are walking or rocking, can help you relax, alleviate pain and make contractions work more effectively. Being on hands and knees also helps, especially when you have back labor. You can rock back and forth, dance slowly and rhythmically and move in ways you'd never dream you'd move! Many women find sitting on the toilet most comfortable.

Eat and drink. When you drink and eat—light foods at the beginning of labor, juices, tea with honey, juice popsicles as it becomes more intense—you keep up your strength and blood sugar level. You don't become dehydrated and you are better able to handle contractions. Drink, and remember to pee often.

Birth is a time of great energy: No one would be expected to run a marathon or swim the English channel if she had been deprived of sustenance and was unable to continue to nourish herself from time to time.[23]

Express emotion if you want. Some women don't want or need to make noise, but many find that expressing strong emotions of the moment—anger, exaltation, fear, pain—groaning, grunting, shouting, moaning, laughing, singing, chanting—can loosen them up. During second-stage labor as you breathe or push the baby out you'll probably be making sounds along with the pushing. Low sounds seem to work better than high-pitched ones—more of a *downward* feel to them, say some midwives.

Learn how terrific water is. Baths and showers can relax and soothe us during labor. Some women stay in the shower for hours. (When your bag of waters has broken, avoid baths.) When tub water is shallow, someone can pour warm water over your belly during contractions. (A midwife we know says, "It's better than Pitocin for getting contractions going!") When the water is deep, your uterus will be lifted up and away from your body, which can reduce the intensity of labor, especially back labor. Lying mostly under water, leaning against supports, you can float slightly and relax deeply.

Ask for physical support, touch, massage and holding. Ask your partner, friend, birth attendant or nurse to help you when you squat, stand or kneel; to lean against you; hold you under your arms; let you hang from his/her shoulders; hold you however you want to be held.

"Drink in" touch and massage. Human contact can make you feel at ease, sustained and loved. Your partner or attendant may know exactly what to do without being asked. Or s/he may not. If the touch doesn't feel right, ask until something feels better.

This kind of caring enables you to relax and makes pain more bearable.

I asked my two friends to massage deeply and hard, putting a lot of pressure on my lower back muscles to counter all that force. I liked feeling their hands supporting my belly at the same time.

Actively imagine opening up. In South India, birth attendants place a flower near the laboring woman; as its petals unfold, her cervix opens. Opening is a ceremony, a celebration.

Imagine being in a place you love the best, where you are most happy. Imagine you are a flower opening, light exploding. Open your mind to images. Imagine your baby hugged by your uterus, pushing down, ready to be born in its own way, opening you. Say to yourself, "I feel my baby moving down my pelvis, I feel my muscles letting go; my cervix is stretching, opening, opening MORE—open...open...OPEN."

Suggestions for people attending a birth: what they can do. Look at her. Does she look comfortable? Check her beathing. Is she relaxed? Say, "Relax." Use your hands. Run them down her back, over her muscles. Stroke or massage her in a way that helps her relax more. Move slowly, breathe slowly, stay calm. As you touch her, think of what your hands are communicating. Don't expect her to be stoic. Don't expect her to tell you politely what she wants. Sometimes she may not want you to touch her at all. If she tells you to go away, don't take it personally. It's just labor. Don't feel sorry for her. Yes, it hurts, but show your belief in her strength. Or she may say, "I can't stand this anymore." Tell her she can. She is. Change what's happening. Make it better. Maybe a walk, a shower, a bath, a change of position will make her feel better. Keep her focused on the present. If she is losing her concentration, help her focus. Hold her, sing, chant, laugh, moan, rock with her. Just before the baby is born, at the most intense time, she may need touch, eye contact. Breathe along with her. Hold hot compresses against her perineum; she can relax into the heat. Or let her lean against/on you.*

---

and legs, chills and irritability, though these things can happen at other times, too. Some women are comforted by the incredible intensity, even by their own irritability, because they know it means that they are close to the end of this part of labor.

When you reach full dilation labor often slows down, with contractions farther apart for a while, as if your body were taking a rest. Or contractions may come so close together they feel like one long one. Or you may scarcely have time to take a breath before your enormous uncontrollable "pushing" contractions begin.

The Baby Moves Down Through Your Vagina

You may suddenly feel an amazing urge to bear down. Breathe lightly or blow if your attendant says that you are not completely dilated. Many women are disappointed when this phase turns out to be more painful or longer than they expected. Others, who expect the expulsion to be the most painful part, are surprised by how exhilarating and painless it can be to push out a baby. A few women never feel that strong urge to push.

Women who attend childbirth preparation classes are often taught to practice pushing by taking huge, deep breaths, holding them and bearing down as hard as they can. Yet strenuous active pushing doesn't necessarily get the baby out faster.[24] In fact, it can lead to the baby's being deprived of oxygen.[25]

Your uterus contracts involuntarily and will push the baby out itself most of the time if not interfered with. *Feel* it pushing and bear down only when you

*Special thanks to Becky Sarah!

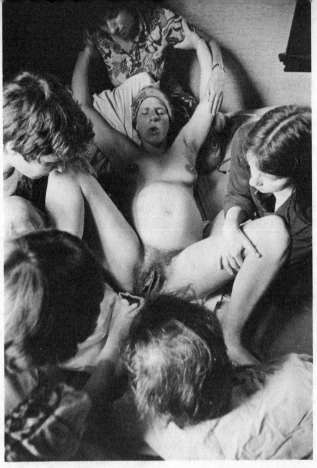

Jim Harrison/Stock Boston

fewer or no perineal tears. During contractions, let your belly bulge out; relax your whole body, especially your mouth and jaws. Consciously direct your energy downward, outward.

I was holding back. This thought raced into my mind and out the other side: If I push hard enough, I'm going to become a mother. Ann said, "Next time you have a contraction, push a little bit; think open; you'll feel better." Amazing—I could feel her coming down; it did feel better.

You can be in any position to let the baby come out, but upright ones often work best. When you are on hands and knees or squatting with knees apart, your pelvis is at its widest. You may feel most comfortable kneeling or on the toilet at first, then go to kneel on the bed or sit, or lie on your side with one leg up on an attendant's shoulder.

feel the urge. Don't close your throat unless your body wants to. (Breathe deeply or sigh between contractions.) You may want to grunt, moan, howl or simply "breathe" the baby out.*

Today many physicians emphasize having a short second stage (typically two hours or less) without evidence to prove that a longer one hurts the baby.† This phase of labor can, in fact, take a few minutes or five hours, as long as the baby's heartbeat is fine. When you relax between contractions and don't push hard, you don't get as tired as you would if you were pushing. Your perineum has more time to stretch around the baby's head as it moves down during the contraction, then back a little, down during the next, then back again. (Don't be disappointed if the process takes a long time; many women think it only takes a couple of pushes and wonder what is wrong if it takes longer.) Sometimes your attendant will ask you to breathe lightly so as not to be pushing at all as s/he gently stretches or massages with oil and hot compresses the area around the baby's head. Gentle pushing means

*See Sheila Kitzinger's books, Rahima Baldwin's *Special Delivery* and Elizabeth Davis's *A Guide to Midwifery: Heart and Hands*, for more detailed descriptions of this phase of labor.

†Roberto Caldeyro-Barcia, a well-known South American ob/gyn, says that fetal lack of oxygen (hypoxia) has been a "reason" to push the baby out quickly and thus have a short second stage, when in fact it's the sustained pushing which can cause hypoxia in the first place. Physicians often feel hysteria at the idea of the baby "trapped" in the "birth canal" and rush to pull it out. Nurses also contribute to the rushed atmosphere by calling MDs in too soon. Since they're all there they say, "Let's get her delivered," especially when they are very busy.

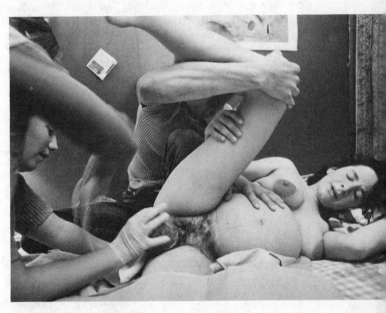

Suzanne Arms

> THE LITHOTOMY POSITION—LYING ON YOUR BACK WITH YOUR FEET UP IN STIRRUPS—IS THE WORST, MOST INEFFECTIVE AND MOST DANGEROUS POSITION FOR LABOR. IT IS USED IN MOST HOSPITALS FOR THE CONVENIENCE OF THE DOCTOR.

Pushing was the strangest and in some ways the nicest sensation I've ever had. I could actually feel the shape of the baby, feel myself sitting on the head as it moved down...the thought of moving, especially from a good, comfortable, well-supported seated position, to flat-out on a bed seemed ridiculous. So there I was on my rocking chair, with my feet up on two little kitchen chairs, with Hersch on one side and the doctor on the other...it was like moving a grand piano across a room: that hard, but that satisfying.[26]

BIRTH

Your baby's head will be born first, unless the baby is in breech position (see p. 377). You must usually wait for the baby to rotate a quarter-turn in order for the rest of it to be born—shoulders, one at a time, then body. During this time your practitioner may ask you to pant and not push as s/he checks to see if the cord is around your baby's neck and perhaps also to suction mucus from its nose and mouth.

Within a few minutes, the baby was coming. I knelt on the bed, leaning forward against Thomas. It was a wonderful position, very solid and stable, yet my hands were free to reach down and feel her head. My older daughter was ready with a blanket to wrap the baby, and I will never forget the feeling of the little body sliding out and into my hands just as the sun came up. It's a great moment—the baby is there, it doesn't hurt anymore, both in the same instant. The room was full of light.

Vaughn Sills

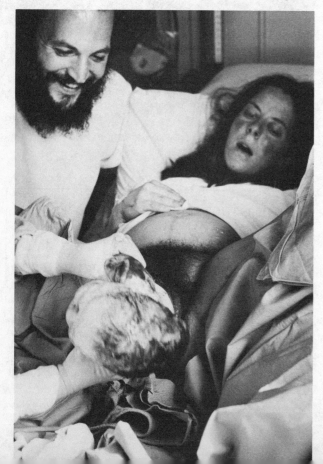

I got to shouting, "That's enough, that's enough." "My hemorrhoids hurt," I got to blubbering. Marya said, "Run some water; take a bath." It felt good to have all that water sloshing around. Nothing was happening on the bed; it seemed so much easier in the water. Everything I needed was there at the time. I said, "I feel kind of open!" Then I saw my son float out. It was great. He was so peaceful and calm. His eyes were open under the water.

I felt godlike—a miracle worker. It was the best moment of my life. I felt my baby's head, then saw his face— I got to cut his cord and put him to my breast. I felt like I did the impossible. I couldn't believe he was finally out into the light. I felt holy.

RIGHT AFTER

If your baby breathes as soon as the head is completely out, s/he may be born looking pink. Otherwise s/he will look very still and bluish until breathing becomes regular and sustained. No one knows for certain why newborns take their first breath. Not all newborns cry. Some cry for a moment, then stop. They may just breathe, blink and look around or snuffle.*

Right after birth, hold your baby close. S/he's your own; you have waited all this time and labored hard. At home, in birth centers and in some hospitals you can hold your baby right away. It can be easier to hold your baby when you are sitting up. Cover her/him with blankets for warmth and hold her/him naked against your breasts and belly in order that s/he may touch your skin, smell you, feel you, hear you, look at you and your partner. You'll want to caress, touch, talk to her/him. Enjoy this slow time. If you are exhausted, your partner can hold the baby against you or close to him/herself.

So much has been written about this moment. We want hospitals to respect how crucial it is for us, our partners and children to be close to our babies and, in this way, begin (and continue) a family together. Most babies have the capacity to form a strong attachment to another human being after birth. Yet this process, called "bonding," cannot be forced or created just by going through the motions. As Sheila Kitzinger said in one of her talks, "Some hospitals act as if it's a special glue that can be sprayed on and will take in five minutes. After that they think it's too late." One mother fighting separation from her baby was told, "You're bonded to her now, so what's the problem?"

And if for some reason the first moments after birth don't turn out the way you want, you will have many

*Gail Brewer's *Right from the Start* has a detailed description of the changes which take place in the baby's body and a critical discussion of routine medical practices during the first hours after birth.

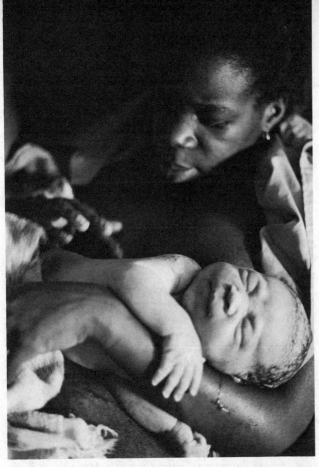

Suzanne Arms

ways of becoming attached to your baby and her/him to you. "Bonding" in humans is an ongoing process.

Right after the birth, practitioners evaluate your baby's heart rate, respiration, muscle tone, color and reflexes. Their conclusions are often expressed in the one- and five-minute Apgar score (from one to ten). Most infants score between seven and ten. Your practitioner will have oxygen and suctioning equipment at hand in case the baby needs help breathing, which is vital since lack of oxygen can cause brain damage. Gentle suctioning of the nose and throat is done if needed. It must always be carefully done to prevent injury to delicate tissues. The baby will be wet-looking, covered with a waxy substance called vernix and usually not very bloody. Her/his head may be oddly shaped temporarily, having been molded during its passage through your vagina.

Your baby may or may not nurse right away.* Some do, and know exactly what to do. (They have been sucking *in utero*.) Others aren't quite ready yet or need a little guidance. Babies born to unsedated and/or unanesthetized mothers often have strong sucking reflexes. This is a good time to let your baby suckle even if you don't plan to breastfeed later. Babies need to nurse in order to receive important antibodies and nutrients from your colostrum. If the baby doesn't seem to want to nurse right away, or if hospital staff objects, remember that *you are in charge and can make it hap-*

---

*When you have received drugs, your baby may not want to nurse, or be able to, until the drugs wear off.

---

*pen.** Sucking is important for you, too. It stimulates oxytocin, which makes your uterus contract to expel the placenta and stay contracted afterwards. It also slows down the bleeding.

You are still connected to your baby by the umbilical cord, attached to the placenta inside you. Physicians in hospitals used to cut the cord as soon as the baby breathed or cried; many still do. But now many practitioners wait five or ten minutes until the cord has stopped pulsating and all the blood has gone out of it into the baby. This enables the baby's circulatory system to get going on its own and provides extra blood supply, including iron. Then they clamp the cord in two places, cutting it between clamps a few inches from the navel. Sometimes partners cut the cord. In a week or so, the bit of cord left on the baby's navel dries up and falls off.

DELIVERY OF THE PLACENTA

After a short interval the cord lengthens, you may feel a contraction, have a rush of blood and expel the placenta. You may not feel a contraction and be told to push. Contractions usually come sooner when you are sitting up or squatting. It is extremely important to have the placenta totally out, which completes the birth cycle. Until this happens, blood vessels remain open and women are especially vulnerable to infection and hemorrhage. Once the entire placenta is born, blood vessels close down. The pregnancy cycle reverses itself; your uterus clamps down and begins to shrink. Breastfeeding helps this process. Expulsion of the placenta usually happens within ten minutes to a half-hour or so; sometimes it takes longer. If all else is normal, it's reasonable to wait, watchfully. Usually the placenta comes out by itself, helped along by your baby suckling or by someone else sucking on your nipples. If the placenta doesn't come out, your practitioner may give you a shot of Pitocin, pull gently on the cord (controlled traction) or extract it manually (if, for example, there is hemorrhage, and it must come out quickly). If you are at home and have problems at this point, you may have to go to the hospital.

THE FIRST FEW HOURS AFTER THE BABY IS BORN

Mother and Baby

It is best if your baby stays with you and your partner for as long as you want after birth. Parents and child

---

*It is important for you to have discussed breastfeeding with your practitioner (and your pediatrician, if possible) in advance, and to have made sure that you can reach her/him after the baby is born, so that any hospital orders preventing you from being with your baby can be changed.

sleep and wake together, get to know each other, and the baby nurses whenever s/he wants.

While parents and baby stay together at home, in freestanding birth centers and some hospital rooms, it is more difficult in most hospitals. (Definitely make your wishes known beforehand.)

There is no medical reason to separate healthy mothers and babies after birth. It is your right to keep your baby with you; s/he belongs to you. Babies with minor and even major health problems benefit from being close to their parents; they also may need medical observation at the same time.

The First Hour or Two

Practitioners will do a complete physical exam of your baby. It is not necessary that they do it right away (unless there is an obvious problem). In the hospital ask to have it done in your presence so that you can see exactly what is happening, and ask any questions you may have.

Silver Nitrate Drops and Vitamin K

In most hospitals, nurses routinely put silver nitrate drops into babies' eyes after birth—one drop in each eye—to prevent infection from their mothers' vaginal organisms. (The gonococcal bacteria, if left unattended, can lead to blindness. [See Chapter 14, "Sexually Transmitted Diseases."]) Tetracycline and erythromycin are alternatives to silver nitrate.* Careless insertion of silver nitrate may cause babies' eyes to swell up after birth (so can long-labor pushing or heredity). Home birth attendants leave the decision up to parents as to whether or not they want the baby to receive drops. If you refuse the silver nitrate, pay close attention to your baby's eyes during the first week or so to make sure that they remain clear and don't look infected. If they do become runny and/or swollen, with lashes stuck together, your baby must get medical care, must receive antibiotics and often has to remain in the hospital five days until cultures come back negative.

Babies born in hospitals may also receive Vitamin-K injections after birth to prevent a rare (one in 2,000) disorder known as hemorrhagic disease of the newborn (when the blood doesn't have enough clotting factor). Twenty-five years ago these injections became mandatory in hospitals to counteract the anticlotting effects of many drugs, which sometimes caused jaundice. In out-of-hospital births, Vitamin-K injections may or may not be given. If it has been a traumatic birth with excessive head-molding, Vitamin K is necessary. You can give Vitamin K orally to the baby, but it's not clear that it works as well, and it tastes bad. Ask your practitioner about silver nitrate and Vitamin K. You have a legal right to refuse both treatments.

Where You Are After You Give Birth Affects How You Feel

The comfort of being at home cannot be overestimated, being in my own bed aferward, familiar cracks in the ceiling, my family all around.

After a normal delivery in a freestanding birthing center, most women go home within twelve to twenty-four hours. The usual stay in a hospital is two to four days, though a few hospitals now let new mothers leave earlier. If you want to leave soon after the birth, make arrangements with your practitioner and the hospital.

We had planned a home birth but, because of an unexpectedly long labor, wound up delivering in the hospital instead. Our disappointment, however, was tempered by our doctor's promise that if everything went okay, we could return home right after the birth. Megan was born that day at noon, and by five P.M. I was back at home taking a much needed shower, while Peter and my mother and his parents prepared supper and admired the baby. Then we all sat down to a celebration birthday supper, complete with cake and champagne and Megan in the middle of the table in her basket. By nine P.M. Peter and I were asleep in bed with Megan snuggled between us. The next day, the midwife came, checked me and the baby and answered my barrage of questions. Later in the day, friends came bringing food and baby presents. I remember those days as among the happiest in my life.

You may want to stay in the hospital a few days, especially if you have other children at home or no household help.

I have five kids at home. I look on this as my only vacation this year!

Some hospitals have "rooming in," where your baby stays with you all the time; they may have "modified rooming in," where your baby stays with you whenever you want, or just during the day, and then goes back to the central nursery whenever you are tired or at night. (One nurse-midwife found that mothers who kept their babies with them were more rested than mothers whose babies stayed in the nursery!) But many hospitals still separate mothers and babies routinely, sometimes for twelve to twenty-four hours at first and then most of the time except for feedings; nurses place babies in warming cribs, take them to central nurseries and bring them to mothers for feedings every four hours. Most newborns and mothers find it difficult to

---

*Most states have a law requiring silver nitrate; some physicians and hospitals may feel they cannot administer antibiotic alternatives without changes in the law.

Less Usual Presentations

In the above description of labor, we have assumed the baby's position in the uterus to be the most common—*left occipito anterior* (L.O.A.). This means that the baby is head down in the uterus, lying on its left side, with the occiput, or back part of the skull, toward the mother's front. It is the most efficient way for a baby to slip past the pubic bone and into the birth canal.

Another position is head first but faced the opposite way, with the baby's face toward the mother's front. This is called *posterior presentation*. It can mean a longer labor, since the baby may try to turn around during labor in order to be born in the more favorable way, facing the mother's back. With a posterior baby, you may experience labor pains in your back. Feel free to take labor positions most comfortable for you.

Some babies present buttocks down or feet (footling) or hands first. They are in *breech* position, which can mean a long back-labor. Sometimes you can turn a breech baby around yourself from the thirtieth week of pregnancy on (see p. 350). They may turn themselves during labor or may not turn at all. A *skilled* practitioner may be able to turn them from the outside (external cephalic version).* If your practitioner has delivered many breech babies successfully and if your pelvis is big enough and the baby small enough, you'll be able to birth her/him vaginally. *Squat: it widens your pelvic outlet significantly!* A danger in breech birth is that after the baby is delivered the head will be trapped, and the baby will try to breathe and will suffocate. Knowledgeable practitioners wrap the baby's emerging body in warm blankets to keep cold air from shocking her/him into taking a breathful of mucus; they also insert a finger into the woman's vagina, clearing a passageway for air. Footling breeches are usually delivered by Cesarean (unless they are the second of twins, when the cervix has opened wide enough). These days most obstetricians in training rarely if ever learn the necessary skills to perform external cephalic versions or to help deliver breech babies vaginally; they perform Cesareans instead.

Some babies lie horizontally (*transverse lie*) and their heads never engage. They must be born by Cesarean.

adapt to hospital routines. In addition to the stress of being in a strange, sterile environment, hospital rules

*See Brigitte Jordan, "External Cephalic Version," *Women and Health*, Vol. 7, Nos. 3/4 (Fall/Winter 1982), pp. 83–102, for a historical, cross-cultural and physiological description of this procedure.

can interfere with the natural process of recovery and with getting to know your baby.

I had my first baby in the hospital. For the next four days I hardly slept. My roommate was nice, but she liked the TV on all the time. Then there were the nurses who came in every couple of hours to take my temperature or give me a laxative or scold me for nursing "too long" on one side. During visiting hours and at night, they took the baby to the nursery, and I would fantasize that she was the one I heard crying. I felt tense and depressed most of the time.

There are good reasons for going home as soon as possible. Babies in hospital nurseries are at significant risk for infection.* There's an advantage to immediate hands-on practice in taking care of your baby, especially if it's your first.

SOME SIGNS OF ABNORMAL LABOR AND DELIVERY

If complications should arise during labor, your body will usually give you some warnings. It is, of course, of vital importance that you be aware of them and make your practitioner aware of them. When you are awake and not medicated, you will have a much clearer sense of what is going on. Also, some complications are set into motion by anesthesia.

Here are a few signals that should warn you to notify your practitioner immediately.

Continuous and Severe Lower Abdominal Pain, Often Accompanied by Uterine Tenderness

This is different from the pain of normal labor contractions, which comes on with increasing intensity and then gradually disappears completely until the next contraction—a pain which comes and goes.

An Abnormal Presentation or Prolapse of Cord, Placenta or Extremity

If any of these occurs, an experienced practitioner must decide if a Cesarean is required. Prolapsed cord (when

*Central nurseries used to be considered sanctuaries where babies were kept safe from infections, chilling, mucus problems and overexhaustion from medicated or operative deliveries. Yet in large nurseries, infants receive intermittent and often impersonal care, a poor substitute for mothering. Some nurseries breed *Staphylococcus aureus*, *Streptococcus* and *Salmonella* (which cause "nonsocomial" infections—infections acquired in a hospital). These clearly iatrogenic—hospital-caused—illnesses can be serious, sometimes resulting in infant death. (See Ruth Lubic, "The Impact of Technology on Health Care—The Childbearing Center: A Case for Technology's Appropriate Use," *Journal of Nurse-Midwifery*, Vol. 24, No. 1 [January/February 1979], pp. 6–10.)

the cord falls into the vagina and there is the danger that it might be compressed, thereby cutting off oxygen to the baby) and placenta previa (placenta first instead of baby first) generally call for a Cesarean section.*

Excessive Vaginal Bleeding

There are a number of reasons for this, such as cervical laceration, placenta abruptio (when the placenta suddenly becomes detached from the uterus) or delivery before the cervix is fully dilated. It is normal, however, to have a bloody mucus discharge just before complete dilation, especially when the cervix is opening up very quickly.

Abnormally Slow Dilation of the Cervix

When contractions are severe and the cervix is still not dilating regularly, then the ineffective contractions may be creating undue stress on the fetus, the mother or both. This is a particularly hard condition to diagnose, since pain is subjective and many labors last much longer than others. This is part of the "dystocia" category discussed in "Cesarean Section" (p. 384). Many midwifery techniques (see pp. 336–39) can help this type of labor. However, sometimes even then there will be little or no cervical dilation.

Abnormality in Fetal Heartbeat

This condition is a sign that the baby may be in trouble. Fetal heartbeat should be checked regularly throughout labor.

Any Adverse Change in Condition of Mother or Baby

If the pattern of heartbeat and/or blood pressure changes, if the woman develops a fever or if some other difficulty arises, it is essential that an experienced doctor or midwife be present to interpret the signs.

PREMATURE LABOR AND DELIVERY

A premature baby is one who is born during or before the thirty-seventh week of pregnancy. Until recently a baby of five and a half pounds or less was considered premature, but now doctors are more concerned with the maturity and functional development of the baby than with her or his birth weight.

We know little about the cause of prematurity in nearly half the cases. Poor health, inadequate nutrition, stress and heavy smoking all increase one's chances of having a premature delivery.* Some specific causes of premature labor are infectious diseases (such as syphilis), toxemia of pregnancy, diabetes, thyroid disturbances, fetal abnormalities, placental abnormalities (placenta previa, placenta abruptio, etc.) and multiple pregnancies—twins or triplets. Some of these problems can be avoided through adequate nutrition and health care. Statistics show that poorer women and young teenagers receive poorer and less prenatal care and are more likely to deliver prematurely than middle-class women.

Premature labor proceeds like normal, full-term labor. It may be a little slower owing to weaker contractions or more rapid because the baby is smaller. *Premature babies are extremely susceptible to the dangerous effects of the drugs used during labor*, so if you are prepared to handle labor without drugs you will be doing your baby a great service.

The smaller and more feeble the baby, the more s/he needs immediate care. In the U.S., most premature babies are placed in oxygen-, temperature- and humidity-controlled incubators, kept in intensive care nurseries and protected from every possible source of infection, since they are very susceptible and infection is common in hospitals. Increasingly, mothers are spending more time with their babies in these nurseries, some of which are set up for parents, others not. Be assertive about staying with your baby as much as possible—your presence, your voice, your touch, your love will help her/him thrive. Some doctors are exploring the advantages of keeping older or larger premature babies in incubators close to their mothers' bedsides, so that mothers can take them out to cuddle and hold close.† These babies grow and develop much more quickly than those who are left more to themselves in incubators. Mothers turn out to be the most watchful attendants, and if anything seems to be going wrong, they quickly signal nurses or doctors.

It is best to feed your baby breast milk.[28] The antibodies in colostrum fight the very infections to which the premature baby can succumb. You can pump your own milk with an electric or hand breast pump (some hospitals have them handy) if your baby must stay in an incubator, and feed it to her/him. (See p. 400 for more).

---

*Seventy percent of deaths of newborn babies in the United States are due to low birth weight. This is a tragedy, since we can prevent much prematurity by good nutrition, competent prenatal medical care and adequate birth control for those who may be unable to carry a fetus to term (e.g., young teenagers whose bodies are not yet developed enough).[27]

†Michel Odent, at his clinic in Pithiviers, France, is one. See *Birth Reborn*. Also see Robert B. Berg, "'Early' Discharge of Low-Birth-Weight Infants," *Journal of the American Medical Association*, Vol. 210, No. 10 (December 8, 1969), pp. 1892–96.

---

*Michel Odent, in *Birth Reborn*, discusses the possibility of vaginal birth if only a bit of the placenta covers the cervical opening.

You may not be prepared yet for delivery and motherhood; you may feel uncertain and anxious, constantly worried about your baby. Find people with whom you and your partner can talk. All hospital staff should be aware of your feelings, encourage you to spend as much time with your baby as you want, explain the reasons for all hospital procedures and answer all your questions as completely as possible.*

OBSTETRICAL ROUTINES, PROCEDURES AND DRUGS

The mechanism of labor is both powerful and delicately balanced. Each part and process has a function in helping the baby be born well. Our attendants must respect the process and not interrupt it, hinder it or speed it up (unless absolutely necessary). Contractions massage the baby to squeeze excess fluid out of its lungs, amniotic fluid equalizes pressure and cushions the baby's head, membranes hold the waters in, the perineum has a chance to stretch slowly. Like any other animal, we need a calm environment for labor to proceed at its own pace, and we tense up when we are afraid, causing labor to slow down. Like elephants and dolphins, we labor best with females like ourselves nearby.

Occasionally things go wrong and we need medical intervention. We are fortunate it is being refined. At the same time we must be aware that most commonplace drugs and hospital procedures have never been scientifically proven beneficial for healthy mothers and infants.[29] Most of the time medical obstetrics interferes with our bodies in outrageous ways, as if male doctors over the course of the past century had sat down and systematically figured out how to interrupt each natural step of the labor process, one by one.† It is a credit to our basic health and resilience that, despite such assaults, we and our babies emerge so healthy. It is sad that so many of us expect intervention as the norm and rely on it for safety and pain relief when it is not always safe and we can deal with pain in so many other ways. It makes no sense for us to accept routine tampering with our bodies, our strengths and the safety of our children. It makes sense to learn as much as we can so that we use medical resources during labor only when we really need them.*

DRUGS AND INTERVENTIONS IN HOSPITAL BIRTH

Like a snowball rolling down the hill, as one unphysiological practice is employed...another frequently becomes necessary to counteract some of the disadvantages, large or small, inherent in the previous procedure.[30]

During prenatal visits with your physician or midwife, go over each intervention, medication and procedure described in this section. Find out what procedures and drugs are in common use at the hospital, the preferred drug dosages and the choices you will be able (allowed) to make. If you have preferences, discuss them thoroughly beforehand, write them down and send copies to your physician or midwife, to the hospital and to the head of nursing.

Once you arrive at the hospital, you have a right to know the names and risks of anything done or given to you, and to refuse them. (See "Our Rights as Patients" p. 584, for more).

"Prepping" (Shaving Pubic Hair)†

This is totally unnecessary. It is just one part of the male medical ritual of depolluting, purifying women.‡ (We heard one doctor say, "I like my women clean.") Prepping desexes us, makes us look like little girls again. Doctors believe that pubic hair contains germs and prepping decreases the risk of infection. In fact, prepping *increases* the risk of infection, when surface skin cells are scaped off and sometimes razors nick skin. As hair grows back, it is itchy and uncomfortable.

Many hospitals don't prep anymore, or offer the procedure as an option.

Enemas

Enemas used to be routine, but many hospitals don't give them anymore. They are not necessary. Women often have a natural diarrhea before labor begins or

---

*See Resources: Sherri Nance, *Premature Babies: A Handbook for Parents*, for a sensitive discussion about all aspects of prematurity.

†Michel Odent, throughout *Birth Reborn*, speaks of modern obstetric practice as "the systematic elimination of the mother from the childbearing process." Sally Inch's *Birthrights* gives a detailed description of the effects of drugs and interventions. Doris Haire wrote *The Cultural Warping of Childbirth* out of a concern that obstetrical practices and drugs are causing retardation, brain dysfunction and learning disabilities in our children.

*See Resources: *Home Birth, A Practitioner's Guide to Birth Outside the Hospital*, by Sagov, et al., for discussions of the ways in which women in labor, their partners and practitioners mutually decide about whether or not to use interventions and drugs, balancing medical necessity with personal values.

†Two British studies conclude that routine prepping and enemas constitute "unjustified assaults" on women, and that there is no evidence of benefit. (M. L. Romney, "Predelivery Shaving: An Unjustified Assault?" *Journal of Obstetrics and Gynecology*, 1: pp. 33–35, 1980; also M. L. Romney and G. Gordon, "Is Your Enema Really Necessary?" *British Medical Journal*, 282: pp. 1269–71, April 18, 1981.

‡See Ann Oakley's *Subject Women*.

during labor. You can request an enema if you think it will make you feel better or if feces in your rectum seem to be holding up your labor; often enemas stimulate labor. But if you are in active labor already, it can make your contractions stronger and more uncomfortable, which in turn may make you ask for drugs, thereby setting off the chain of procedures related to their use. One "medical" reason for giving enemas is to prevent contamination of the perineum by feces. Yet enemas result in watery feces which may be less "clean" than natural diarrhea.

Making Women Lie Down

This increases the length of labor and the risk of distress to the baby while decreasing the strength and efficiency of contractions.[31] When you lie down you press on your inferior vena cava (a major vein), which soon decreases blood flow and oxygen supply to the fetus. Since it is often more uncomfortable to lie still than to be upright and/or moving around, you may become more tense, which causes your labor to slow down even more and makes you feel more pain. At this point you may ask for drugs or your labor may "need" medical intervention, when in fact what you *really* need is a change of position, movement, a shower or bath to relax you, and loving, holding, touching.

Rupturing the Amniotic Sac (Membrane)—Amniotomy

Many physicians routinely rupture membranes early in labor, or if they think your labor isn't progressing fast enough, by puncturing the sac (through your cervix) with a small hook something like a crochet hook. It doesn't hurt; you can feel the waters rushing out. The baby's head then moves down to press against your cervix, perhaps releasing more oxytocin and thereby causing stronger contractions. Early amniotomy, though more convenient for the doctor, does not usually benefit baby or mother.[32] The stronger contractions can place pressure on the placenta or umbilical cord as the baby pushes against it; if the cord is wrapped around the baby's neck or is very short, it can also be affected by such pressure, which may cut off the flow of blood which contains oxygen. In addition, the baby's body and head are no longer cushioned by amniotic fluid. Stronger contractions may be more difficult for you to handle; you are also more prone to infection. The medical answer: possibly drugs to weaken (counteract) strong contractions, Pitocin to speed up labor because of the risk of infection, fetal monitors to check the baby's heartbeat and occasionally Cesareans because these interventions have endangered your baby's life.

Sometimes when a woman is dilated about eight centimeters and the baby's head has descended down far enough, a practitioner may decide to rupture the membranes to speed that phase of labor. If your practitioner suspects fetal distress s/he may rupture the membranes to check the amniotic fluid for the presence of meconium (not a completely reliable indicator). (Some practitioners use an amnioscope, a rod with a light and mirror on it, to "see" the color of the fluid without having to rupture the membranes, a less invasive procedure.)

Intravenous Solution (IV)

Many hospitals automatically set up an IV for every woman early in labor. A nurse will introduce a hollow tube into a vein in your hand or arm and affix it with adhesive tape so that fluids can flow (be infused) into your bloodstream. The IV is used 1. "just in case" something goes wrong and emergency anesthesia becomes necessary, or to try to prevent hypotension (lowered blood pressure) from epidural anesthesia; 2. to nourish us with a glucose solution and prevent us from becoming depleted and dehydrated when we are not allowed to eat or drink during labor; 3. to introduce oxytocin (now almost routine in many teaching hospitals in order to speed up labor); 4. to teach students about IVs.

There is no reason for IVs to be used in normal labors; instead you should be able to drink fruit juices, water, honeyed teas. They *are* useful, however, when you can't keep anything down and vomit a lot (rare), or when you have become extremely dehydrated.

IVs make it difficult for you to move around (immobility can slow down your labor). They can be uncomfortable and make you feel awkward and passive. They may make you anxious. If you must have an IV, ask the nurses to put it securely into the arm or hand you use the least. Ask for an IV pole so you can continue to move around. Ask someone else to push it. You must be sure to urinate often, at least once an hour or more, as fluids accumulate and a full bladder can hinder your baby's descent. Be as active as you can. (You can even take a shower with an IV.)

Elective Induction and Acceleration of Labor

When labor does not begin within a given amount of time or moves "too slowly" (each physician and hospital has a particular policy), many physicians will induce or accelerate ("augment") it. When there is no reason for induction other than the physician's or the woman's convenience, it is known as "elective induction." In 1978, the FDA came out against the practice of elective induction by Pitocin (see below), yet often physicians get around this ban by performing amniotomy to start labor or by "stripping" the membranes.

The first step in induced or accelerated labor involves artificial rupture of the membranes with attendant risks (see above). Sometimes the physician will "strip" rather than rupture the membranes: during an internal examination in the hospital or even during a routine office visit, if s/he feels the baby is "ready," s/he uses a finger to separate the amnion (bag of waters) from the uterine wall. No one knows exactly why this causes labor to begin. When obstetricians strip the membranes, they often do it without informed consent. It is an unnecessary, invasive and risky procedure, for if there is an unrecognized placenta previa (a placenta nearer to the cervix than the baby is), the placenta could be stripped away from the uterus, with harmful and possibly catastrophic effect to the baby, or, if the baby is not ready, a premature birth may result.

To start or speed up labor, physicians have used a drug called Pitocin, or "Pit," to substitute for oxytocin, a hormone present in natural labor. It is safest to administer Pitocin through an intravenous drip, because then the dosage can be more easily controlled than if it is injected or given orally. *(Refuse these last two procedures!)* Control of the dose is essential because Pitocin can cause very strong contractions, creating potential dangers for both the baby and the woman. Prostaglandins are also being used experimentally to induce and augment labor.

Induction and acceleration involve considerable risks.* Many physicians' estimates of fetal maturity are off by three to seven weeks.[33] Without knowing the baby's age we can't know if s/he is ready to endure the stresses of labor and delivery and extrauterine life. Some induced babies born too soon have hyaline membrane disease (immaturity of the lungs) and respiratory disease syndrome (RDS). Pitocin may cause jaundice in the newborn. Induction is sometimes begun before a woman's cervix is ready ("ripe")—before a certain amount of dilation and effacement—so that her uterus doesn't respond strongly enough to Pitocin and the baby must be born by Cesarean. Artificially provoked uterine contractions can be much more violent and prolonged than natural ones, and they may interfere with blood flow to the uterus and placenta, causing fetal distress. Such contractions also can cause uterine rupture and hypertension. Even with the smallest dose some women have prolonged contractions which close up the cervix. Most women experience these unnatural contractions as more painful than natural ones because they don't follow a wavelike course but reach high intensity instantly and remain intense for a long period. If you are unprepared (and even when you are prepared) you may become discouraged by the pain and rely upon an epidural, with its accompanying risks, to reduce pain.

*See Timothy Chard and Michael Richards, *Benefits and Hazards of the New Obstetrics,* for a discussion of the controversy surrounding induction and acceleration.

Induction or acceleration may be appropriate when there is some question about the baby's survival and/or when the mother has toxemia, hemolytic disease (Rh factor) or maternal diabetes. Yet these complications are now usually regarded as indications for a Cesarean section, since the use of Pitocin may further compromise the baby.

If you are being induced, or if the physician is accelerating your labor, make sure of four things. 1. Be as certain as possible that your baby is mature enough to be born. 2. Nurses and physicians must start you with the *smallest* dose of Pitocin. There's no way beforehand to gauge the sensitivity of your uterus to Pitocin. 3. You must have expert medical assistance; the baby's heart must be constantly monitored. 4. You must have good labor support, someone near you to help you with your relaxation and your breathing.

My doctor decided to induce my labor.

At the hospital I got some injections of what I thought was Pitocin. My labor was very intense and unexpectedly short—four hours. My daughter had to be delivered by forceps because her heartbeat was slowing down and I couldn't push her out quickly enough. I was told her life had been endangered because my contractions were too strong and the placenta had separated from the uterine wall too early. My doctors were heroes! They had saved her life.

Three years later, seven months pregnant, I asked my doctor a casual question about my first labor and delivery. He began reading my record to me. He read about injections of Pitocin and Demerol.

Amazed, I said, "That's not my labor. That's someone else's record."

It turns out that the Pitocin stimulated my labor too strongly so that indeed it wasn't natural and was dangerous, and then they gave me Demerol to slow everything down. My strong contractions made the placenta separate early. I'm sure that the Demerol slowed my daughter's heartbeat and oxygen intake. It also explains why she was so sleepy the first three days and didn't immediately nurse.

In other words, the dangers would not have happened if I hadn't been induced and then slowed down. My doctors gave me the feeling that they were responsible for saving my daughter's life, and if they hadn't been there...Now I know they were responsible for the dangers to my daughter's life—if not completely, at least in great part. Induction complicated my labor and delivery.

Fetal Monitors

Fetal monitors are machines which electronically record the baby's heart rate during labor. There are two basic kinds of monitors: external (noninvasive) and internal (invasive). The most accurate external monitor is applied by temporarily sticking gummy elec-

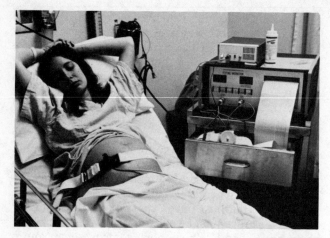

Sam Sweezy/Stock Boston

trodes onto the laboring woman's abdomen. The electrodes pick up and record the fetal heartbeat. In addition, two straps, about two to three inches wide, are placed around the woman's abdomen. The upper belt holds the tocodynamometer, which records the intensity of the uterine contractions, and the lower strap holds an ultrasonic transducer (ultrasound), which monitors and records the fetal heart rate.

Internal fetal monitors are now almost routine in many hospitals.* Electrodes connected to wires within a plastic tube are introduced into the woman's vagina and attached directly to the baby's presenting part (usually the scalp) by means of metal clips or screws. (No one has bothered to find out if this causes pain to the baby; it certainly seems as if it must!) The wires coming out of the vagina are held in place by an elastic strap around the woman's thigh. These electrodes measure the baby's heartbeat. The woman's contractions are measured either by a catheter designed for that purpose, introduced into her uterus through her vagina, or by the external tocodynamometer strap described above. A printout shows the baby's heartbeat, which is also audible. The woman will probably have a blood pressure cuff, and often an IV.

Though the monitor may be useful in some truly high-risk situations and necessary when labor is induced or accelerated or the woman anesthetized, it entails many discomforts and risks to women and babies.[34] 1. Ultrasound has never been proven safe. 2.

Many women say that the straps and the pressure of the transducer are uncomfortable. 3. Ironically, fetal stress picked up by the monitor may be a product of invasive hospital routines/procedures, including the monitor itself. Since women with a monitor cannot move around much, if at all, labor may slow down or stop. 4. Machines get old and break down. They often interpret normal signs as pathological or indicate normality when something is really wrong. The machine may lose the baby's heartbeat when s/he moves, or the electrode may slip out of the baby's scalp. 5. Hospital personnel tend to pay *less* attention to women with monitors. Also, partners and attendants may direct their attention and support away from the woman and pay attention mainly to the machine. 6. Hospital personnel may interpret machine data incorrectly. Incomplete understanding of the range and fluctuation in fetal heart rate during and between contractions has led to unnecessary forceps and, these days, unnecessary Cesarean deliveries. 7. Women and babies run a much greater risk of infection with the internal monitor. Infection frequently occurs when the uterine catheter is used. The baby's scalp may bleed because of the way the screw has been attached. Postdelivery rashes are common where the electrode was attached (85 percent in one study), and scalp abscess is not uncommon (20 percent). 8. Monitoring has contributed to the recent rise in C-sections, an added risk for mother and baby.

Routine use of fetal monitors has not significantly decreased the newborn death rate nor the number of brain-damaged children. Several randomized controlled clinical trials demonstrated that the use of fetal monitoring, as compared with supervision of labor by nurses with stethoscopes, did not improve Apgar scores or decrease neonatal mortality. David Banta recommends that electronic fetal monitoring "should be limited to specific high-risk groups as part of carefully designed evaluative trials of efficacy,"[35] and Havercamp and Orleans add that fetal blood scalp sampling should be used along with EFM to avoid false positive diagnoses of fetal distress.[36] This procedure, in fact, is the *only* way to verify distress recorded by the monitor; it analyzes the acidity of the baby's blood. Not all hospitals which use fetal monitors have the capability to interpret blood acidity ranges. In addition, "the technique is difficult, awkward, uncomfortable for women and technically difficult even with considerable experience."[37] It involves another puncture in the baby's scalp.

*While the monitor has been thoroughly studied from many perspectives, many studies do not make clear that a monitor becomes *essential* if a woman has epidural anesthesia. Because it is known that fetal distress gradually begins to increase as the epidural is used, mandatory use of the monitor is the only responsible way to employ this type of anesthesia. Not incidentally, the "two-hour limit" for second-stage labor also arose from the combination use of the epidural and monitor, since it is at about two hours at most that fetal distress begins to show almost routinely. Given the combined risks of the monitor and the epidural, this "option" for women must be questioned seriously.

Episiotomy

Episiotomy is the most frequently performed obstetric operation in the West. It is one of the most intense and dramatic ways in which the territory of women's bodies is appropriated, the only operation performed on the body of a healthy woman without her consent. It represents obstetrical power:

AN EPISIOTOMY

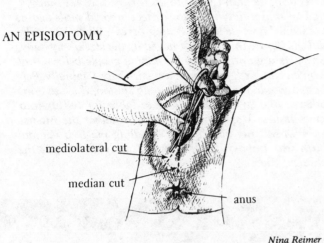

mediolateral cut

median cut

anus

Nina Reimer

Babies can't get out unless they are cut out. It prevents women from experiencing birth as a sexual event, and is a form of ritual genital mutilation.[38]

An episiotomy is an incision through skin and muscles in the perineum, the area between the vagina and the anus, to enlarge the opening through which the baby will pass. The procedure is necessary only in rare cases of fetal distress, when the baby must come out quickly and the woman's tissues just won't stretch any more.

Doctors believe that episiotomies will prevent perineal tears extending to the anus (third-degree lacerations); that they prevent damage to the baby's head; that they keep the pelvic floor from becoming too stretched and guard against uterine prolapse, cystocele and rectocele (when the uterus falls into the vagina, when the bladder or rectum protrude into or through the vaginal walls). Yet the available data reveal that episiotomy doesn't accomplish the above goals.[39]

There is no justification for routine episiotomy,* yet many physicians continue to perform it routinely. They rarely learn those midwifery techniques which can prevent or minimize tearing. For instance, in most births you will have little if any tearing when you are upright, sitting or squatting to breathe or push your baby out, resting between contractions; when your practitioner helps you to control your pushing, open up and relax; when s/he carefully massages, softens and supports your perineum using warm oils and wet compresses.

Some physicians believe that they are performing a service to the woman's partner.

*When a woman is in the lithotomy position (on her back with legs raised) she literally has to push uphill, against gravity, thus putting enormous strain on her perineum, and "necessitating" an episiotomy. Once she sits up, or squats, that strain is lessened.

I saw my doctor at the checkup six weeks after my baby was born. Full of male pride, he told me during my pelvic exam, "I did a beautiful job sewing you up. You're as tight as a virgin; your husband should thank me."

Many women find intercourse extremely painful after being stitched up too tightly. Stitches are often itchy and extremely painful for several weeks as they heal. Some women are allergic to the stitches; others have had stitches which didn't dissolve. While there are no studies to prove it, many women report permanently impaired sexual sensation after episiotomies.*

You have a legal right to refuse episiotomy.

Forceps†

Instead of the woman pushing the baby out, in a forceps delivery the physician pulls the baby out with a double-bladed instrument. In general, forceps resemble hinged salad tongs, except that the "blades" are longer and curved to fit the shape of the baby's head. The doctor introduces each blade into the vagina separately and places them on the side of the baby's head, usually over the ear but sometimes at the temples. Then s/he attaches the two blades together outside the vagina.

The usual reasons for a forceps delivery are:

1. to speed up second-stage labor if there is severe fetal distress; if anesthesia or positioning prevent the mother from pushing out her baby (very common);

2. if the umbilical cord is wrapped tightly around the baby's neck or if the cord prolapses;‡

3. in case of unusual presentation;

4. to shorten a "long" second-stage labor. Many physicians over the past few decades have used forceps in *uncomplicated* labors to shorten the pushing phase, which they believe to be exhausting to the mother and possibly dangerous to the baby. Yet this phase of labor can normally go from one half-hour to three hours or more. *Unless there is some indication that the baby is having trouble getting out, doctors have no medical reason for introducing forceps.* Forceps have caused serious fetal damage. Many midwifery techniques should be tried first.

Today Cesarean sections are replacing forceps in

*See also Sheila Kitzinger, *Episiotomy: Physical and Emotional Aspects* and *Some Women's Experiences of Episiotomy*, London: The National Childbirth Trust, 1981.

†In European countries, midwives and some doctors use the vacuum extractor, a suction device which attaches to (covers part of) the baby's head in the uterus and helps draw the baby lower as the mother bears down, too. It allows the mother to be active and is minimally invasive and much safer than forceps.

‡The positioning of the cord around the neck is common and occurs in 25 to 30 percent of deliveries (C.E. McLennan with collaboration of E. C. Sandberg, *Synopsis of Obstetrics*, 8th ed. St. Louis: C. V. Mosby Co., 1970, p. 166). Usually the practitioner can loosen it and slip it over the baby's head.

most situations—one reason for the spectacular rise in C-sections. You may "choose" to have a Cesarean rather than a forceps delivery; on the other hand, you may prefer forceps to a Cesarean operation.

CESAREAN SECTION

Cesarean section appears to be a sometimes useful and needed technique presently utilized in an undocumented, unclarified and uncontrolled manner.[40]

Cesarean sections are life-saving operations when women have certain problems before or during labor—severe pre-eclampsia, serious diabetes, transverse lie of the baby, failure of the baby to descend at all, cord prolapse, placenta previa, baby much too large, active herpes lesions, sudden unexplained fetal distress.

She had been head down for three months before the birth but somehow she turned, put her foot through the amniotic sac, tore off the placenta and the uterus collapsed. My contractions were very painful and came every three minutes. Then I started bleeding. We watched her heart rate go down on the monitor. The doctor said a Cesarean was necessary. They tried a spinal three times; it didn't take. My husband was going through hell; he couldn't do anything. Finally I was given general anesthesia. I came to three hours later. I'd lost a lot of blood.

Afterwards every day I asked the doctors and nurses if there was anything I could have done to make it less traumatic, more normal. I got the facts. There was nothing I could have done. I kept reliving it, asking my husband lots of questions like a child. The hospital people were wonderful.

Not having seen her born really hurts. They gave her to my husband to hold right after. It took me three days to unwrap her and look at her naked and see that she was really all right.

It was so quick and different than we'd planned. So much happens in such a short time; there's no time to process it. I wish there had been some way to prepare for it. It was good that it was done; it saved my life and hers.

Please let women know that in regard to Cesareans there is a "gray area" between the life-or-death emergency situation and the absolutely unnecessary operation. In my case, I had been in extremely painful labor for hours and hours, with back-to-back long-lasting contractions (unexpected because my first labor had been intense, but short and manageable). David held me, massaged me; I walked, stood, squatted, took baths. Now, I'm no martyr, but I think I could have stood it if there had been any progress, but there was very little. Most discouraging, the baby's head wasn't engaged. After nine hours I said to my doctor, "I need a Cesarean."Not one to jump into a

C-section, he didn't want to do it right away. Finally, I had an epidural. When it took effect, I could smile again. We waited a while longer—no progress. When he finally did the Cesarean, he was amazed by the size of my baby. She was a giant! I know that some people believe that women can birth just about any-size baby vaginally. Perhaps I would have been able to do so, too, if I had done other things and been willing to labor for twenty-four more hours. Maybe not. I wonder whether the intense pain wasn't my body's way of telling me that vaginal birth was impossible this time. I am glad I made the choice I did.

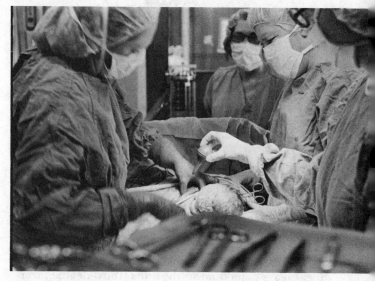

CESAREAN BIRTH   *Vaughn Sills*

Cesareans must be performed in hospitals with proper drugs and anesthesia techniques, antibiotics and blood transfusion equipment. Nurses will shave your pubic hair and insert a catheter into your urethra to empty your bladder. If you are awake for the operation, nurses may place a screen below your shoulders so that you don't see it, though sometimes you can see in a mirror. They will wash you down with an antiseptic solution. You'll have either regional (spinal or epidural) or general anesthesia. With general anesthesia you should receive as small a dose as possible (epidural doses will be greater than for labor-pain relief). When your abdomen has become numb or when you are unconscious, the physician makes a small horizontal cut in your abdominal wall, low down near the line of your pubic hair. (Sometimes a vertical cut will be necessary to get the baby out quickly.) The physician then cuts horizontally through the uterine muscle and eases the baby out. If you are awake, ask to see the baby being born. The baby's nose and mouth will be suctioned with a mucus catheter. When s/he is breathing well, you or your partner can hold her/him.

The physician then removes the placenta and sews you up, layer by layer.

Almost every woman needs to believe that her Cesarean was necessary. However, in response to the tremendous increase in Cesareans over the past decade, two major investigatory studies suggest that 33 to 75 percent of Cesareans were *not* necessary, having been performed as a result of current medical procedures and attitudes alone.[41]

With Deb, my first baby, around the time of my due date my doctor told me that he'd had a dream about me which worried him: that the baby was okay now, but the head would be too big to fit through my pelvis and there would be trouble. He wanted to do a Cesarean right away. I made him wait two weeks; I didn't think he was giving me half a chance. But I was not allowed to go into labor, and he did his Cesarean. Three years later, after a smooth labor at home with a midwife attending, I gave birth to Emily, whose head was much bigger than Deb's had been.

A childbirth educator from C/SEC (see Resources) tells a more typical story:

A woman phoned me today. She had given birth to her first child eight weeks ago. After being in labor for only four hours she had dilated from four to nine centimeters. Suddenly they transported her to the delivery room, and yelled at her to push even though she didn't feel the urge to push and told them so. But they pressured her and, half-sitting up, holding her legs (a typical Lamaze position), she pushed for twenty-six minutes—she has it on record. At the end of that time her cervix was swollen—of course it swells when you push like that—and they told her that she wouldn't be able to deliver vaginally. Within fifteen minutes she'd had a Cesarean. Reason given: "Failure to progress."

The above-mentioned studies conclude that Cesareans, being major operations, carry two to four times greater risk of death than vaginal deliveries.* They cause postoperative infections in 33 percent of women. They frequently cause respiratory distress problems in both premature and full-term babies and psychological damage to the mother, if not to the family unit as a whole. In addition, anesthesia exposures during Cesareans may leave large numbers of babies with delayed motor development and other neurological defects.

What is happening, and why? In 1968, the average Cesarean rate was 5 percent. In 1981, the national average had risen to 17 to 20 percent, and in some teaching hospitals it now goes as high as 25 to 40 percent (in some months). Factors responsible for the

increase—some statistically measurable, others not—include:

1. *Physicians' practice of defensive medicine.* The most common cause of Cesareans today is not fetal distress or maternal distress but obstetrician distress.[42] Physicians think that if they do a Cesarean and a baby is born "less than perfect" they have covered themselves legally. In fact, more suits have been instigated for malpractice associated with Cesarean surgery than for failure to perform it.

2. *"Once a Cesarean, always a Cesarean."* This dictum accounts for 30 percent of all Cesareans. Repeat Cesareans are elective surgery, not obligatory. *In fact, many women—perhaps the majority—can have vaginal births after Cesarean (VBACs).* They need information, encouragement, self-confidence and support to do so.* A woman who had two VBACs tells this story:

One day in the supermarket I started to talk with a woman who was looking at my youngest child with such longing. She said, "I so much want to have more kids, but I had a Cesarean and I'll never go through that again." There was such pain in her eyes. I said, "I'm here to tell you that you don't have to!" and told her my story. You could see that she started to light up; then she sort of flickered out. "But my doctor said women who have Cesareans can't deliver vaginally." She agreed to find out why she'd had it in the first place. At least she now had some hope. No one had ever allowed her to hope before.

Most often the condition which makes a Cesarean necessary in one birth, if it was necessary at all, won't exist in the next. Physicians claim uterine rupture is a risk,† but ruptures occur so rarely that women must weigh this fact against the many known risks of abdominal surgery. VBACs are far safer in most cases. ACOG's March 1982 pronouncement that women who meet certain criteria can have "trial" labors will enable only a few women to have vaginal births after Cesareans, as long as the medical climate remains negative.‡

3. *Obstetrical training.* Physicians and residents are not trained in normal obstetrics, and now don't even learn skills such as external cephalic version (gently turning breech babies around) or delivering breeches

---

*Studies of maternal mortality are continuing at the CDC (Center for Disease Control).

*See Resources: Nancy Wainer Cohen and Lois Estner's book *Silent Knife: Vaginal Birth After Cesarean and Cesarean Prevention*; also Elizabeth Shearer, "Education for Vaginal Birth After Cesarean," in *Birth: Issues in Perinatal Care and Education*, Vol. 9:1, Spring 1982, pp. 31–34.

†Ruptures occurred (rarely) in the past when incisions made vertically in the upper half of the uterus didn't heal properly, and when modern surgical techniques and emergency medicines were not available to minimize risks.

‡Conditions: the mother must have the shorter horizontal scar; the baby must be properly positioned, head down; the baby must be no more than eight pounds, eight ounces; the pregnancy must have been completely normal; the mother's condition must be monitored.

vaginally. In addition, at the same time that the birth rate has come down, obstetrics/gynecology is growing as a surgical specialty; new residents need training, and have to perform a certain number of procedures in order to meet a quota.

4. *Belief that Cesareans mean "better babies."** Infant mortality and morbidity rates *have* declined in recent years, but not primarily because of obstetrical intervention. In fact, C-section babies are often distressed. The existence of neonatal intensive care units has been largely responsible for keeping alive low-birth-weight and premature babies who otherwise would have died.

5. *Changing indications for Cesarean sections.* Women's bodies haven't changed, but physicians' eagerness to perform Cesareans has led them to expand the meaning of the word *dystocia.* Physicians tell women that their pelvis is too small (cephalopelvic disproportion) or their labor is too slow (failure to progress in labor), and call both "dystocia," when in fact if women could labor naturally, moving around and squatting, they could deliver normally in most cases. Dystocia has been called a "wastebasket" term. It accounts for 43 percent of all Cesareans and 30 percent of the increase in Cesarean sections from 1970 to 1978.

Now that physicians are less experienced in delivering them, the number of Cesarean deliveries for *breech* babies continues to increase, and now accounts for 12 percent of the Cesarean rate. Cesareans can mean healthier births for very large or very small breech babies but, in general, many more breech babies could be delivered vaginally just as safely if practitioners learned how to do it and encouraged women to squat for delivery. Cesareans are also replacing forceps deliveries.

6. *Economic incentives.* Many third-party insurance payments will reimburse most of the cost of a Cesarean, while only a small portion of a vaginal delivery is covered. Anesthesiologists, obstetricians and hospitals also receive more money for Cesareans.

7. *Obstetrical practice and technology.* Fetal monitors, induction, oxytocin challenge tests, epidurals, amniotomies and women laboring on their backs all cause problems which then necessitate intervention, which is rapidly translated into Cesareans.

8. *Physician attitudes* underlying these factors, while not statistically measurable, can point up why Cesareans are so dear to the medical heart. This discussion was heard among a compendium of doctors:

What's so great about delivery from below?...You don't want the baby squeezed out like toothpaste in a tube?...You might say we're helping women to do what nature hasn't evolved her to do for herself.

---

*Despite the evidence that C-section babies are not necessarily "better," at least two cases of forced Cesarean section have occurred where physicians got court orders, claiming that failure to accept a Cesarean section was evidence of "child abuse."

By and large, I think American obstetrics has become so preoccupied with apparatus and with possible fetal injury that the mothers are increasingly being considered solely vehicles. In many cases small and uncertain gain for the infant is being purchased at the price of a small but grave risk to the mother.[43]

Several organizations have sprung up over the past decade, two among them being Cesarean/Support, Education and Concern (C/SEC) and the Cesarean Prevention Movement. C/SEC aims to inform women and families about Cesareans and to humanize medical attitudes and policies. CPM grew out of C/SEC. Its founders, all of whom had had Cesareans, realized that their Cesareans had been medically unnecessary, and that in the future most of them could labor naturally and deliver vaginally. These convictions were reinforced by the experiences of hundreds of women who contacted them. As a result, CPM's goals are to educate women and practitioners in order to decrease the number of women having a first (primary) Cesarean and to increase the number of women having VBACs. Both organizations have brought about positive changes in hospital Cesarean practices, both advocate VBACs and have positively affected women's attitudes about themselves and their capabilities. Throughout the country, women are forming or joining VBAC classes, in which they talk about their previous experiences, fears and hopes, and learn concrete ways of preparing physically and emotionally for the births

VAGINAL BIRTH AFTER CESAREAN *Suzanne Arms*

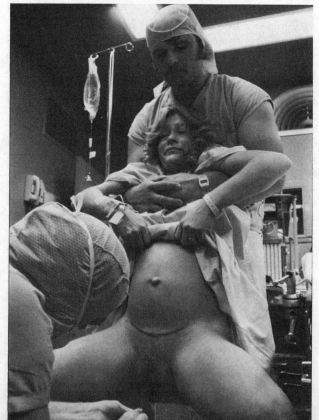

of their next babies. They learn how to prevent unnecessary Cesareans (see the box "What You Can Do to," p. 371, and Cohen and Estner's book *Silent Knife*.)

Drugs

Every single drug given to the mother during labor crosses the placenta and reaches her baby, some in greater amounts and with greater rapidity than others. If the baby is premature, smaller than average or in poor health, the consequences can be particularly dangerous. Even a normal baby can suffer from the effects of maternal medication.

No drug has been proven safe for mothers and babies. Obstetric drugs used routinely for labor and delivery have not been approved for that purpose by the FDA, and thus they assume the status of experimental drugs.[44]

Some infants whose mothers received analgesia and anesthesia during labor and delivery have had retarded muscular, visual and neural development in the first four weeks of life.[45] This doesn't mean all babies will be so affected, nor will the babies affected be permanently retarded in development; but four weeks is a long time in the life of a newborn infant.

Anesthetized mothers often feel quite separate from their newborns:

I was really doped up when my baby was delivered and barely got to see that she was alive before she was whisked away to the nursery. When I finally woke up and she was able to be brought to me, I remember thinking, Is this really my baby? Do I really want to take her home with me? It took me a while to feel connected to her.

We mothers sometimes suffer more from the after-effects of the drugs used in our labor than we might have from the labor itself. The problem is compounded because along with each drug often come two or three other procedures designed by the hospital to reduce, as much as possible, the risk of the medication used.

Analgesics decrease our overall perception of pain, and *anesthesia* removes our sensation of pain altogether by creating loss of consciousness, "sleep"or a temporary loss of feeling in the specific area affected.

Analgesia

Tranquilizers

As soon as labor becomes intense, you may be offered a tranquilizer or narcotic "to take the edge off your contractions." Tranquilizers are given primarily for anxiety; they are not pain-killers. They can sharply reduce your ability to cope with your labor. You may fall asleep until the contraction reaches its peak, and then wake, panic and actually experience more pain than you would have without the drug. Though a small amount can help you sleep and wake refreshed, a glass of wine can have the same effect. Tranquilizers may have a depressant effect on some newborn functions. For example, Valium reduces a newborn's body temperature, muscle tone and ability to suckle. Other tranquilizers may cause labor to slow down or even cease altogether.[46]

Narcotics

Narcotics can seriously depress fetal respiration and make babies less able to suck, sleepy, dopey and not responsive to their environment. Even small amounts of Demerol (meperidine) affect your baby's responsiveness.

Barbiturates

Barbiturates, derivatives of barbituric acid, have been used to produce sleep. Nembutal and Seconal fall into this category, as do Luminal, Sodium Amytal and Barbital, to name a few. These drugs, dangerous to the fetus, cross through the placenta readily and depress fetal respiration and responsiveness.*

Barbiturates early in labor are often given in combination with a small amount of *scopolamine*. Scopolamine, sometimes called "Twilight Sleep," is an amnesiac and a hallucinogen that has the effect of making you forget what you experienced during labor, even though it does not stop your sensations at the time, and you may later feel you have lived through a forgotten torture. Like other hallucinogens, scopolamine can cause some women to become physically violent and others to become stuporous or to talk uninhibitedly. They often must be tied into bed and constantly watched so as not to cause themselves physical damage by thrashing about wildly during contractions.

Scopolamine both prolongs the second stage of labor and increases the Cesarean-section rate. The combination of scopolamine and Demerol causes severe neonatal (newborn) depression. There is no reason for its continued use and yet it is still given in many areas. Try to avoid any practitioner or hospital which uses it.

Most women receiving analgesics are instructed not to walk around during labor as they may become dizzy or faint.

---

*T. Berry Brazelton determined that barbiturates taken by the woman lodge in the baby's midbrain for up to a week after delivery. See "Effect of Maternal Medication on the Neonate and His Behavior," *Journal of Pediatrics*, Vol. 58, No. 4 (1961).

General Anesthetic Agents Inhaled by the Mother

Inhalation gases are administered with each contraction. The point is to breathe in the right amount of the vapor just in time to have it working during the peak of the contraction. These drugs slow down labor, serve as depressants to the newborn's responsiveness and have potentially fatal complications if too much is inhaled. *Ether* can retard labor and may provoke vomiting, excessive uterine relaxation and bleeding in the mother.[47] *Nitrous oxide* can delay for *months* the development of the baby's motor skills—attempts to sit, stand and move around. In view of these serious risks, it is appalling to note that inhalation anesthesia was still being used in one-third of U.S. deliveries in 1977.

Anesthesia

General anesthesia puts the woman completely to sleep. It should not be used during labor because it slows it down and has a severely depressant effect on the baby. Furthermore, injudicious use of general anesthesia for delivery can lead to the woman's (and sometimes the baby's) death.

Physicians who want their patients to be totally unaware of the obstetrical procedures used during the last minutes of labor will often give them general anesthesia. Sometimes it is used during a Cesarean section. But physicians are using it less than in previous years because of the risks involved and because newer technology has been developed.

Regional anesthesia: If the physician decides s/he wants a numbing effect only during delivery to perform an episiotomy or to use forceps s/he may give the mother a *pudendal block.** The pudendal block anesthetizes only the vulva, or external female organs, by injections of novocaine. Even this relatively minor anesthetic can cause a "persistent decrease in oxygen saturation in the newborn during the first 30 minutes of postpartum observation."[48]

Another form of anesthesia, the *paracervical block*, is in use.† Many anesthesiologists consider it dangerous to both fetus and mother. Complications such as convulsions and severe hypotension are common, and

---

*Pudendal block anesthesia is named for the pudendum, or external female genitalia. Pudendum in Latin means "that of which one ought to be ashamed." Obviously we can't imagine a more inappropriate name!

†It is used mainly by obstetricians rather than anesthesiologists. The only possible excuse for its continuance is the unavailability of better anesthesia technology and of better-trained anesthesiologists. The FDA Subcommittee on Anesthetic and Life Support Drugs considered placing warnings on the drug bupivacaine and then declined to do so. If this is the procedure presented to you, consider trying to find another physician or another hospital. (Some Lamaze programs actually encourage the use of this procedure because the physicans who "accept" Lamaze use it.)

it has led to a significant number of fetal deaths. Since the anesthetic is injected into the area around the cervix, there is the possibility that it will accidentally be injected into the presenting part of the baby. Moreover, the injection site is very close to the main artery of the uterus, which increases the chance of its being absorbed rapidly by the placenta and depressing the fetus.

Spinal anesthesia is used just during delivery to anesthetize the entire birth area (from belly to toes). The anesthesiologist injects spinals, or subarachnoid blocks, into the subarachnoid space around the spinal column. Spinals totally stop labor, all motor functions and our urge to bear down, so instead of our pushing the baby out, the obstetrician must use forceps. Aftereffects may include headache (usually the result of an overly large needle which causes spinal fluid to leak, though this problem is rare now), stiff neck and backache. Misadministration of the spinal has resulted in failure of heart and lung function and even death. Spinals can and should be avoided, except when necessary for an emergency delivery.

If everything has gone normally and no drugs have been administered up until this point, the actual delivery is the worst time to give anesthesia. In fact, the perineum usually becomes numb at delivery—a natural anesthesia. And, if you have learned how to "breathe" or push your baby out in a comfortable position, you are able to experience fully the satisfaction of delivery without an anesthetic to cut off sensation and make your recovery that much more difficult.

Two forms of *continuous regional anesthesia* are given to the woman during active labor and continuously readministered until delivery. They require the services of a trained anesthesiologist, not available twenty-four hours a day in most hospitals.

For most of us, the end of active labor, from eight centimeters to ten centimeters of dilation is intense. During this time you may feel like or be pressured into taking some medication "to tide you over." But "transition" is for the great majority of women the shortest part of labor. So when you consider anesthesia, you need to weigh the possible risks and aftereffects of the technique against your ability to cope. This anesthesia will in almost every case last as you push the baby out, eliminating sensations of giving birth. It may in fact prolong your labor, requiring further intervention.

The caudal requires an injection into the sacral canal at the base of the back. For a continuous caudal (given from about eight centimeters of dilation), a catheter is introduced into the lower back and the anesthetic is injected into the catheter in measured doses. A caudal requires a significantly larger dose of anesthetic than does either a spinal or an epidural (explained below), and it therefore carries a greater risk to both mother and baby. Furthermore, the failure rate for caudals is higher than for epidurals, owing to the greater chance of improper needle placement. Maternal hypotension (sudden drop in blood pressure)* and subsequent lack of oxygen to the baby is a potential problem that the anesthesiologist must carefully guard against.

Epidural anesthesia† can be administered to laboring women at any time. For this reason, many obstetricians and anesthesiologists, and some new mothers as well, would have us believe that the epidural is the answer to our labor problems. Increasingly, as older types of pain relief are found to be hazardous, to choose a hospital birth is to choose the epidural. Fewer and fewer physicians know how to manage labor without this drug and its related interventions.

Epidurals can be useful when a woman has serious respiratory disease as the drug involved reduces the work the lungs have to do. It may make it easier for a diabetic woman, for it reduces the demands on her metabolism. It can slow down precipitate labor and also moderate a premature urge to push, as with a footling breech. It is used increasingly in Cesarean operations instead of general anesthesia.

Epidurals have been assumed to be safer than caudals for mother and baby because a different type of anesthesia is used. However, like caudals, they often cause maternal hypotension. Transverse arrest (the baby's getting stuck in a sideways position in the uterus) is another possible complication of epidurals, as they can cause the uterine muscles to relax too much.

Behavioral changes in newborns whose mothers received epidural anesthesia include decreased rooting activity (a basic food-searching survival technique) and muscular floppiness.[49] Esther Conway and Yvonne Brackbill also found negative behavior changes after continuous regional anesthesia, but they concluded that the effects on the baby were less than those suffered by babies whose mothers had received high doses of labor medication or general anesthesia.[50]

Epidurals are administered like a continuous caudal through a tiny catheter placed in the back by a needle. An injection is made in the middle of the woman's back and the catheter moved into her epidural space (not into the spinal column), the space around the base of the spinal cord. The anesthetic is dripped in in measured doses. An experienced anesthesiologist must administer the anesthetic, since a mistake in placement can lead to serious consequences for the mother—in the extreme, paralysis or death.

When administered properly, epidurals will eliminate the sensations of labor in most cases and, unlike the standard spinal, numb only the area immediately around the perineum and lower uterus, belly to knees. However, when you choose epidurals you also invite a number of interlocking procedures, most of which increase the risks of the method. (These procedures are done for caudals, too.) These include:

1. An intravenous hydrating solution attached to one arm.

2. Blood pressure gauging. Your blood pressure will probably be checked every fifteen to thirty minutes, since a drop in blood pressure is common and can have serious effects on the fetus as well as on the mother. You will probably have to wear a blood pressure cuff continuously on the other arm.

3. Artificial rupture of the membranes (bag of waters). If your membranes have not already ruptured by themselves your doctor will probably rupture them before you are given an epidural or caudal. This is routine, but it is also done to make sure that the baby's head is firmly positioned in the birth outlet and to prepare for the attachment of an internal fetal monitor.

4. Most doctors give Pitocin to women receiving continuous regional anesthesia, to start again or speed up contractions stopped or slowed down by the anesthetic. Ruptured membranes plus Pitocin create very strong uterine contractions which *must* be monitored, since the baby is at risk of distress; you cannot feel their strength, and your uterus might rupture.[51] Some hospitals now measure the dosage by machine so that this is much less likely to happen.

5. A fetal monitor, with all its attendant risks. It is especially important during continuous anesthesia (caudal or epidural) to check the baby's heart rate, since fetal distress rises with the length of time the anesthesia is administered.

6. Much higher (three to four times) incidence of forceps delivery. As the urge for and coordination of pushing are decreased, many babies remain in an occiput, transverse or posterior position. The mother can't push her baby out and ends up "needing" forceps.

7. A Cesarean section. With epidurals there is a higher Cesarean rate. Because the monitor is used almost routinely these days and the epidural is usually administered early in labor, it is difficult to separate the influence of the epidural from the monitor in increasing the C-section rate. "Failure to progress in labor," the prime indication for C-sections, is often the direct iatrogenic result of a labor slowed down by epidural anesthesia.

---

*If the woman becomes hypotensive she should turn (or be turned) on her side immediately to take pressure off the *inferior vena cava*, the major source of blood returning to the heart. Hypotension can be contained or prevented in most cases by this maneuver and by the generous use of an intravenous solution started well in advance. Some effects of hypotension on the mother may be shocklike symptoms, altered pulse rate, nausea and vomiting. Its effects on the fetus are slowed heart rate, decreased flow of blood through the placenta and insufficient oxygen intake. These effects tend to show up immediately.

†In August 1983, the FDA said that bupivacaine, commonly used for epidurals, should not be used at its highest dosage level (0.75) for obstetrical purposes, as over the past two years, sixteen women had died of cardiac arrest when high concentrations were accidentally injected into veins instead of just under the skin. *Boston Globe*, Wednesday, August 24, 1983, p. 17.

AFTERWARD

Your baby is born. You have done all in your power to give her/him the healthiest and safest birth possible. You may feel delighted with the labor and birth—high, fulfilled, ecstatic and immensely close to your partner and your baby.

Birth is such a powerful event that to participate in it often isn't enough. We relive the birth of our child many times over during the following days, weeks and months, thinking and talking about it, feeling it in our heart. This reenactment is a natural and sometimes essential means of understanding what has happened. When we have experienced birth in the setting of our choice, with no or few complications, we relive the event in a clear, happy way. But when our experience was altered by unexpected complications and medical interventions, we may have conflicting feelings—joy *and* disappointment, confidence *and* a sense of inadequacy. We may feel confusion and less satisfaction.

All that we learned before the birth of our child can help us afterward to assimilate its complexities and depths. Even with our knowledge we are sometimes unable to find a language adequate and powerful enough either to express our wonder and sense of accomplishment or our frustration, anger and outrage.

When our experiences have been negative, the memories haunt us. Unhappiness may be right on the surface, easily accessible, taking the form of grief, anger, of having been violated. We may think, *I* didn't have my baby; the system had it for me. Or we may bury our strongest emotions, denying how terrible the experience was because to admit it would bring us to the edge of such deep anger that we don't know how to handle it or whom to blame. We excuse and defend physicians and institutions, describing bad experiences as good ones. We become defensive: "Yes, others don't need these unnecessary, even barbaric procedures, but in my case it was necessary." We apologize for being selfish and wanting something different: "It doesn't matter. After all, my baby is fine and that's all that counts. But why am I crying?" We feel ashamed of not having had that "natural" birth we'd prepared for. (Often other mothers make us feel badly, too, by subtly implying that we were at fault.) Or we feel distant from the baby.

My next memory was waking up the next morning. "You have a beautiful daughter," they said. "Where is she? Give her to me. She's mine!" They brought her. I wasn't even glad to see her. I wasn't sure she was mine.

And worst of all, inappropriately, we blame ourselves—"My body just didn't work right"—instead of seeing clearly how the system undermines our knowledge and self-sufficiency; instead of saying to ourselves, as one mother did, "Whatever the luck of the draw for your labor, be assured that you have done the best you could on that day for your baby."

If you were dissatisfied with your experience, it can be healing to reflect on it and come to terms with it. Question what happened, talk about it, send for your hospital records and check them against your memories of the event. Understand the choices you made and why you made them. Allow yourself to feel the deep range of your emotions. A good friend or an experienced counselor may help you to go through this process; perhaps a group of women might be more helpful.

After you explore your feelings and get your questions answered, you will then be able to move on, to think of doing things differently next time if you plan to have more children. Sometimes it takes many years to understand fully what happened, a process which can be difficult but enormously strengthening. For some of us, it has been the beginning of activist work to change childbearing conditions.

Even now, seventeen years after my daughter's birth, I am still learning how dangerous the medical techniques used were for her. I didn't know that my doctors, the "best in town," were as ignorant as I. As for "natural" maternal feelings, well, I just didn't have them. Move around during labor? I lay flat on my back, never dreaming another position was possible. Insist on keeping her with me after she was born? I held her for a moment, felt her breath on my hand and let them take her away. (Though I kept repeating over and over, like a song to the white walls of the recovery room, "I have a daughter! A daughter! A daughter!" and I felt like a child at Christmas who had been given a marvelous present.) Sometimes I blame myself, but not for long. My tears still turn to anger as they have for years; both fuel my determination to help other women find alternatives to conventional obstetrical care. When I am lucky enough to be present at the births of my friends' children, the simplicity and joy of these births affirm and vindicate all of us who work toward loving and informed care for all childbearing women.

NOTES

1. Judith Dickson Luce. "Birthing Women and Midwife," in *Birth Control and Controlling Birth: Women Centered Perspectives*, Helen B. Holmes, Betty Hoskins, Michael Gross, eds. Clifton, NJ: The Humana Press, 1980, p. 240.

2. Dorothy Wertz. "Man-Midwifery," in *Birth Control and Controlling Birth*, p. 147.

3. Barbara Ehrenreich and Deirdre English. *Witches, Midwives and Nurses*. Old Westbury, NY: The Feminist Press, 1973, p. 41.

4. Dorothy Wertz. *Man-Midwifery*, p. 149.

5. Mary Roth Walsh. *Doctors Wanted—No Women Need Apply: Sexual Barriers in the Medical Profession 1835–1975*. New Haven: Yale University Press, 1977.

6. Dorothy Wertz. *Man-Midwifery*, p. 153.

7. Barbara Ehrenreich and Deirdre English. *Witches, Midwives and Nurses*, p. 30.

8. G. J. Barker-Benfield. *The Horrors of the Half-Known Life: Mate Attitudes Toward Women and Sexuality in 19th-Century America*. New York: Harper and Row, Inc., 1977.

9. Diana Scully. *Men Who Control Women's Health: The Miseducation of Obstetrician-Gynecologists*. Boston: Houghton-Mifflin, 1980; Michelle Harrison. *Women in Residence*. New York: Penguin Books, 1983; Gena Corea. *The Hidden Malpractice: How American Medicine Mistreats Women*. New York: Jove/HBJ, 1978.

10. Richard and Dorothy Wertz. *Lying In: A History of Childbirth in America*. New York: Schocken Books, 1979, Chapter 7; Neal Devitt. "Hospital Birth vs. Home Birth, The Scientific Facts, Past and Present," Chapter 37, *Compulsory Hospitalization: Freedom of Choice in Childbirth*, Vol 2, Stewart and Stewart, eds. Marble Hill, MO: NAPSAC Publications, 1979.

11. G. J. Barker-Benfield. *The Horrors of the Half-Known Life*, p. 63.

12. Neal Devitt. "Hospital Birth vs. Home Birth," pp. 487–92.

13. *Ibid.*, pp. 493–94.

14. Joseph B. DeLee. "The Prophylactic Forceps Operation," *American Journal of Obstetrics and Gynecology* 1 (1920), pp. 32–44.

15. Frederick Leboyer. *Birth Without Violence*. New York: Alfred A. Knopf, Inc., 1975, pp. 24–26.

16. Stanley Sagov, et al. "The Issue of Safety" Chapter 2 in *Home Birth, a Practitioner's Guide to Birth Outside the Hospital*, Rockville, MD: Aspen Systems Corporation, 1983.

17. Roslynn Lindheim. "Birthing Centers and Hospices: Reclaiming Birth and Death," *American Review of Public Health*, 2 (1981), pp. 1–29.

18. Michelle Harrison. *Woman in Residence*, p. 17.

19. Ellen Switzer and Joan Kline. "Pregnancy and Childbirth 1982: New Options," *Family Circle Magazine*, March 16, 1982.

20. Ina May Gaskin. "Practicing Midwifery—A Talk by Ina May Gaskin," *Childbirth Alternative Quarterly* (Summer 1981), p. 4.

21. Barbara Katz Rothman. *In Labor: Women and Power in the Birthplace*. New York: W. W. Norton Co., Inc., 1982, p. 290.

22. C. D. Kimball, C. M. Chang, S. M. Huang and J. C. Houck. "Immunoreactive Endorphin Peptides and Prolactin in Umbilical Vein and Maternal Blood," *American Journal of Obstetrics and Gynecology* Vol. 140, No. 2 (May 15, 1981), pp. 157–64; Michel Odent. "The Evolution of Obstetrics at Pithiviers," *Birth and the Family Journal*, 8:1 (Spring 1981), pp. 7–15.

23. Nancy Wainer Cohen. *Birth, A Commentary*, available from the Boston Women's Health Book Collective.

24. Constance Beynon. "The Normal Second Stage of Labor: A Plea for Reform in Its Conduct," *Journal of Obstetrics and Gynecology of the British Empire*, Vol. 64, No. 6 (December 1957), pp. 815–20.

25. Roberto Caldeyro-Barcia. "The Influence of Maternal Bearing-Down Efforts During the Second Stage and Fetal Well-Being," *Birth and the Family Journal* (Spring 1979). Available as a reprint from *Birth*, 110 El Camino Real, Berkeley, CA 94705.

26. Barbara Katz Rothman. *In Labor*, p. 20.

27. National Institutes of Health. Department of Health and Welfare Publication No. 77–1079, 1977.

28. V. Crosse, et al. "The Value of Human Milk Compared with Other Feeds for Premature Infants," discussed in Doris Haire and John Haire, *Implementing Family-Centered Maternity Care*, pp. V, 42–43, ICEA publication (see Resources).

29. Obstetrical practices in the United States, 1978, Washington, DC, April 17, 1978, 95th Congress, 2nd session, U.S. Senate, Committee on Human Resources, U.S. Government Printing Office.

30. Doris Haire. *The Cultural Warping of Childbirth*, p. 32. Available from ICEA (see Resources).

31. Susan R. McKay. "Maternal Position During Labor and Birth: A Reassessment," *JOG Nursing* (September/October 1980), pp. 288–91.

32. S. Gabbe, B. Ettinger, R. Freeman and C. Martin. "Umbilical Cord Compression Associated with Amniotomy," *American Journal of Obstetrics and Gynecology* (October 1, 1976), pp. 353–55.

33. National Institutes of Health. *Cesarean Childbirth*, Publication No. 82-2067, October 1981, pp. 31–318.

34. Antenatal diagnosis, Bethesda, Maryland, 1979, National Institutes of Health Consensus Development Conference, NIH Publication No. 79-1973; A. D. Haverkamp, M. Orleans, S. Langendoerfer, et al. "A controlled trial of the differential effects of intrapartum fetal monitoring," *American Journal of Obstetrics and Gynecology* 134:399 (1979); A. D. Haverkamp, H. E. Thompson, J. G. McFee, et al. "The evaluation of continuous fetal heart rate monitoring in high-risk pregnancy," *American Journal of Obstetrics and Gynecology* 125:310 (1976).

35. David Banta. "Risks and Benefits of EFM," *Birth Control and Controlling Birth*, p. 191.

36. Albert Havercamp and Miriam Orleans. "An Assessment of Electronic Fetal Monitoring," *Women and Health*, Vol. 7, Nos. 3/4 (1982), p. 132.

37. A. Havercamp and M. Orleans, "An Assessment of Electronic Fetal Monitoring," p. 119.

38. Sheila Kitzinger's talk at Boston College, Autumn 1981.

39. D. Banta and S. Thacker. "The Risks and Benefits of Episiotomy: A Review," *Birth*, Vol. 9:1 (Spring 1982), pp. 25–30.

40. Helen Marieskind. *An Evaluation of Cesarean Section in the United States*, a report submitted to the Department of Health, Education and Welfare, June 1979, National Institutes of Health, Report of the Task Force; *Cesarean Childbirth*, NIH Publication No. 82-2067, October 1981, p. 25. Also see Jeanne Guillemin, "Babies by Cesarean: Who Chooses, Who Controls?" The Hastings Center Report, 11:3, June 1981, pp. 15–18.

41. National Institutes of Health. *Cesarean Childbirth*. Helen Marieskind, *An Evaluation of Cesarean Section*.

42. Dr. Gerald Stober, quoted in Christopher Norwood, *At Highest Risk*. New York: Penguin Books, 1980, p. 227.

43. Dr. I. Kaiser, quoted in Helen Marieskind, *An Evaluation of Cesarean Section*, pp. 114–15.

44. Doris Haire. "Research on Drugs Used in Pregnancy and Obstetrics," presented to the Subcommittee on Investigations and Oversights of the House Committee on Science and Technology, Washington, DC, July 30, 1981. Available from the Boston Women's Health Book Collective. Also, "Use of Drugs for Unapproved Indications: Your Legal Responsibility," *FDA Drug Bulletin*, October 1972.

45. In Doris Haire and John Haire. *Implementing Family-Centered Maternity Care*, pp. iii–10; from W. Bowes, Y. Brackbill, E. Conway and A. Steinschneider, *The Effects of Obstetrical Medication on Fetus and Infant*, Monograph of the Society of Research in Child Development, Vol. 35, No. 4 (1970), University of Chicago Press. Control groups showed that this effect was directly related to the obstetrical medication used. Furthermore, R. Kron, M. Stein and K. Goddard show, in "Newborn Sucking Behavior Affected by Obstetrical Sedation" (*Pediatrics*, 37 [1966], pp. 1012–16), that newborn sucking behavior may be depressed for as long as four days after delivery by barbiturates used routinely on the laboring mother.

46. John J. Bonica. *Principles and Practice of Obstetric Analgesia and Anesthesia*, Vols. 1 and 2. Philadelphia: F. A. Davis Co., 1972, p. 268.

47. Charles E. McLennan with collaboration of Eugene C. Sandberg. *Synopsis of Obstetrics*, 8th Ed. St. Louis: C. V. Mosby Co., 1970, p. 176.

48. Doris Haire and John Haire. *Implementing Family-Centered Maternity Care with a Central Nursery*, pp. iii–13.

49. John Scanlon. "Obstetric Anesthesia as a Neonatal Risk Factor in Normal Labor and Delivery," *Clinics in Perinatology*, Vol. 1, No. 2 (September 1974), p. 479.

50. *Ibid.*, p. 478.

51. E. Daw. "Oxytocin-Induced Rupture of the Primigravid Uterus," *Journal of Obstetrics and Gynecology of the British Empire*, Vol. 80 (April 1973), pp. 374–75. The uterus of a first-time mother ruptured due to excessive contractions caused by oxytocin and the rupture was not discovered until after the baby had died, since the strength of the contractions was masked by the epidural anesthesia and the fetal heart was monitored only intermittently.

RESOURCES

Books

Arditti, Rita, Renate Duelli Klein and Shelley Minden, eds. *Test Tube Women*. Boston: Pandora Press, Routledge and Kegan Paul, 1984. This book's many varied articles provide a strong feminist insight into new reproductive technologies and other issues, such as testing during pregnancy.

Arms, Suzanne. *Immaculate Deception: A New Look at Women and Childbirth in America*. New York: Bantam Books, 1977. The first systematic exposure of the abuse of technology and intervention in normal childbirth and of how women have lost their power over normal childbearing to male doctors. A beautiful tribute to midwives. Passionate, angry and powerful.

Ashford, Janet Isaacs, ed. *The Whole Birth Catalog*. Trumansburg, NY: The Crossing Press, 1983. An essential resource. It directs women to every group, idea and product available, and provides detailed descriptions of books and journals. Fun to read.

Balaskas, Arthur, and Janet Balaskas. *New Life*, Rev. Ed. London: Sidgewick and Jackson, 1983. An exercise book which stresses relaxation, squatting and changing positions during labor. Excellent drawings of the pelvis.

Baldwin, Rahima. *Special Delivery*. Millbrae, CA: Les Femmes Publishing, 1979. Positive discussions and descriptions of normal pregnancy, labor and birth. Useful information if you are planning a home birth.

Barker-Benfield, G. J. *The Horrors of the Half-Known Life: Male Attitudes Toward Women and Sexuality in 19th-Century America*. New York: Harper and Row Publishers, Inc. (Harper Colophon Books), 1977. If you want to understand the origins of male attitudes in America, read this dense, witty description of the nineteenth-century medical and moral climate.

Bing, Elizabeth, and Libby Colman. *Making Love During Pregnancy*. New York: Bantam Books, 1982. Sensitive discussion and drawings.

Borg, Susan O., and Judith Lasker. *When Pregnancy Fails: Families Coping with Miscarriage, Stillbirth and Infant Death*. Boston: Beacon Press, 1981. A useful, compassionate discussion for parents who need guidance and support, and for professionals who want to better understand the impact of loss on parents.

Brewer, Gail Sforza, and Tom Brewer, M.D. *What Every Pregnant Woman Should Know: The Truth About Diet and Drugs in Pregnancy*. New York: Penguin Books, 1979. Convincing arguments for the relationship between good prenatal nutrition and newborn health.

———, and Janice Presser Greene. *Right from the Start*. Emmaus, PA: Rodale Press, 1981. A guide for pregnant women and new mothers. It asks penetrating questions and supplies useful information.

Cassidy-Brinn, Ginny, Francie Horner and Carol Downer. *Women-Centered Pregnancy and Birth*. San Francisco: Cleis Press, 1984.

Chard, Timothy, and Martin Richards. *Benefits and Hazards of the New Obstetrics*. Philadelphia: J. B. Lippincott, 1977. Researchers and practitioners discuss the pros and cons of using medical technology for childbirth.

Cohen, Nancy Wainer, and Lois Estner. *Silent Knife: Cesarean Prevention and Vaginal Birth After Cesarean*. South Hadley, MA: J. F. Bergin, 1983. Discusses in an upbeat way how to prevent Cesareans, how to have a vaginal birth after a Cesarean and how to create positive attitudes toward childbearing. Well researched, containing many women's poignant stories.

Corrucini, Carol G., and Patricia E. Cruskie. *Nutrition During Lactation and Pregnancy*. California State Department of Health, 1975. Special concerns for diets of Mexicans, blacks, Chinese, Japanese, Filipinos, Native Americans and vegetarians.

Davis, Elizabeth. *A Guide to Midwifery, Heart and Hands*. New York: Bantam Books, 1983. About setting up a midwifery practice. It describes pregnancy, labor and birth from a midwife's point of view, and is strong on emotional aspects of childbearing. Good practical information.

Dick-Read, Grantly. *Childbirth Without Fear*, 4th Rev. Ed. New York: Harper and Row Publishers, Inc., 1978. The English doctor who originated "natural childbirth" stresses education and relaxation rather than activity and breathing, and talks about the fear-tension-pain syndrome. Idealized, reactionary view of women as mothers.

Edwards, Margot and Mary Waldorf, *Reclaiming Birth: History and Heroines of American Childbirth Reform*, Trumansburg, New York: The Crossing Press, 1984. A women-centered empowering book. It weaves together the life and work stories of these women with a clear and critical assessment of the movement's successes and failures.

Ehrenreich, Barbara. *For Her Own Good: 150 Years of the Experts' Advice to Women*. New York: Anchor Books, 1979. No other book makes modern women's manipulation by succeeding generations of male experts so credible or so devastating. It exposes the unscientific basis of "scientific" expertise used to control women. Indispensable for an understanding of how women's role becomes defined in modern industrial society.

———, and Deirdre English. *Witches, Midwives and Nurses*. Old Westbury, NY: The Feminist Press, 1973. This powerful booklet gives a brief history of how male doctors seized control of healing and then of birthing.

Gaskin, Ina May. *Spiritual Midwifery*, Rev. Ed. Summertown, TN: The Book Publishing Co., 1978. From The Farm midwifery service, story upon story about childbirth, followed by practical midwifery information. (The Farm provides an excellent model for an alternative birthing arrangement, and their statistics are fantastic, with very low Cesarean, mortality and morbidity rates.) The book's language is a little dated.

Goldbeck, Nikki. *As You Eat So Your Baby Grows*. Woodstock, NY: Ceres Press, 1977. A lot of basic nutrition information discussed in a simple, understandable way.

Haire, Doris. *Cultural Warping of Childbirth*. Available from ICEA Bookcenter, P.O. Box 20048, Minneapolis, MN 55420. A classic, short review of cross-cultural childbearing practices.

Harrison, Michelle. *Woman in Residence*. New York: Penguin Books, 1983. A chance to see what actually occurs in hospitals and among doctors and medical students as they give gynecological and obstetric "care" to women. Written from the truly caring viewpoint of a conscientious woman doctor.

Hazell, Lester. *Commonsense Childbirth*. New York: Berkeley Medallion, 1976. Good reading. A complete, sensible approach to childbirth. The author has had four children and conveys what it feels like to lose a child. An excellent critique of childbirth problems caused by the medical profession and an encouraging view of home birth.

Holmes, Helen B., Betty Hoskins, Michael Gross, eds. *Birth Control and Controlling Birth: Women-Centered Perspectives*. Clifton, NJ: The Humana Press, 1980. A collection of papers presented at and the ensuing round-table discussions from the Ethical Issues in Human Reproduction Technology: Analysis by Women (EIRTAW) Conference, held in June 1979. Rich, lively reading.

Hosken, Fran P. *The Universal Childbirth Picture Book*, 2nd Ed., illustrated by Marcia L. Williams. Lexington, MA: Women's International Network News, 1983. The pictures have been helpful to many women. Available in French and Spanish. An Arabic edition forthcoming.

Inch, Sally. *Birthrights*. New York: Pantheon Books, 1984. A clear, systematic description of the few advantages and the many disadvantages of current obstetrical practices and drugs. A valuable, factual tool for parents and childbirth educators.

Ingelman-Sundberg, Axel, Mirjam Furuhjelm, Claes Wirsen and Lennart Nillson. *A Child Is Born*. New York: Dell Publishing Co., Inc., 1977. Classic. Fine, detailed color photographs of the growth of the fetus, and a photo story of a Swedish couple's pregnancy and birth experience.

Jordan, Brigitte. *Birth in Four Cultures*. St. Albans, VT: Eden Press Women's Publications, 1978. An anthropologist who understands birth compares U.S. customs with those of Sweden, Holland and the Yucatan. She helps make clear that those practices we call "scientific" are actually birthing rituals.

Kay, Margarita Artschwager. *Anthropology of Human Birth*. Philadelphia, PA: F. A. Davis Co., 1982. A marvelous, informative collection of articles on birthing practices in the U.S. and throughout the world.

Kitzinger, Sheila. *The Experience of Childbirth*. New York: Penguin Books, 1978. One of the best. English childbirth educator and anthropologist Kitzinger combines Read, Lamaze and Method Acting to prepare women for birth. The book incorporates the psychological and physical aspects of childbearing.

———, and John Davis, eds. *The Place of Birth*. New York: Oxford University Press, 1978. Drawn from meetings among British (and some American) health care providers, it raises critical current issues such as the safety of home vs. hospital birth, routine obstetrical intervention, father participation, etc.

Lang, Raven. *Birth Book*. Palo Alto, CA: Genesis Press, 1972. About home deliveries. Moving personal descriptions of birth by mothers and fathers. Good photographs. It gives the reader a good idea of what the early 1970s felt like in California.

Marieskind, Helen. *An Evaluation of Cesarean Section in the United States for the Department of Health, Education and Welfare*. Washington, DC: Department of Health, Education and Welfare, June 1979. This excellent report examines the factors causing the increased U.S. Cesarean rate.

Myles, Margaret F. *Textbook for Midwives*, 9th Ed. New York: Churchill Livingston, 1981. The English midwives' bible. Quite medically oriented.

Nance, Sherri. *Premature Babies, A Handbook for Parents*. Filled with helpful factual information and many personal anecdotes. A true self-help book; the women who worked on it compiled this information because they couldn't find it anywhere else.

Newland, Kathleen. *Worldwatch Paper 47, Infant Mortality and the Health of Societies*. Worldwatch Institute, 1776 Massachusetts Avenue NW, Washington, DC 20036, December 1981. A summary of the relationship between the infant mortality rate of a country and the amount of money that country has. It stresses the need for a more humane distribution of resources, and documents education of mothers as the most important factor in predicting good outcome.

Noble, Elizabeth. *Essential Exercises for the Childbearing Year*, 2nd Ed. Boston: Houghton Mifflin, 1982. Easy to understand, informative, well-illustrated. Includes detailed discussions of the pelvic floor, and of the physiological reasons for doing specific exercises.

Oakley, Ann. *Women Confined: Towards a Sociology of Childbirth*. New York: Schocken Books, 1980. A strong analysis of childbirth as a complex life event and a critique of the socialization of women and the medicalization of childbirth.

Odent, Michel. *Birth Reborn*. New York: Pantheon Books, 1984. A fascinating description of his maternity clinic in Pithiviers, France, a gentle, calm birth environment in which women are encouraged to "listen to their bodies" during labor and birth, supported mainly by midwives. Odent describes the evolution, practices and philosophy of Pithiviers. This book is a useful guide for practitioners who are seeking to "demedicalize" their point of view.

Peterson, Gayle. *Birthing Normally: A Personal Growth Approach to Childbirth*. Berkeley, CA: Mindbody Press, 1981.

How women's attitudes and emotions affect their pregnancies and births.

Romalis, Shelly, ed. *Childbirth: Alternatives to Medical Control.* Austin, TX: University of Texas Press, 1981. A series of essays focusing upon the issue of male and medical control of childbirth. An excellent discussion of physician training, father-physician relationships and the Lamaze method.

Rothman, Barbara Katz. *In Labor: Women and Power in the Birthplace.* New York: W. W. Norton and Co., Inc., 1982. Combines her own personal childbirth experiences with a critique of obstetrics in the U.S. today. Rothman contrasts the medical model of birth with the midwifery model.

Sagov, Stanley, Richard Feinbloom, Peggy Spindell and Archie Brodsky. *Home Birth: A Practitioner's Guide to Birth Outside the Hospital.* Rockville, MD: Aspen Systems Corp., 1983. An extremely detailed, useful description of how this particular family practice group handles pregnancy, labor and birth. Sensitive discussions of the midwife-physician relationship and of home birth. An essential book for medical students, doctors and midwives. Also an enormously reassuring guide for parents.

Scully, Diana. *Men Who Control Women's Health: The Miseducation of Obstetrician-Gynecologists.* Boston: Houghton Mifflin, 1980. A fascinating behind-the-scenes study of obstetrical training, including analyses of gynecology texts, observations of operating rooms and teaching hospital clinics, interviews with medical students. It shows how inadequate residency training is and how it too often conflicts with women's needs.

Shaw, Nancy Stoller. *Forced Labor.* New York: Pergamon Press, Inc., 1974. A powerful sociological analysis of how women from different classes are treated by doctors and nurses during pregnancy and childbirth.

Stewart, David, and Lee Stewart, eds. *Compulsory Hospitalization: Freedom of Choice in Childbirth?; The Five Standards for Safe Childbearing; Safe Alternatives in Childbirth; 21st Century Obstetrics Now!* NAPSAC Publications, P.O. Box 267, Marble Hill, MO 63764. The proceedings from several NAPSAC conferences. A multitude of interesting and useful articles.

U.S. Department of Health and Human Services. *Cesarean Childbirth.* Bethesda, MD: National Institutes of Health, NIH Publication No. 82-2067, October 1981. An assessment of Cesarean birth in the U.S. A task force studied the increase in Cesarean rates; effects of Cesareans on mothers, infants and families; economic factors related to the rising Cesarean rate; legal and ethical considerations; and whether or not Cesareans improve "outcome." A useful (and somewhat depressing) compilation of facts which stresses the inadequacy of the information we do have and urges more study.

Varney, Helen. *Nurse-Midwifery.* Boston: Blackwell Scientific Publications, 1980. An excellent, detailed nurse-midwifery text. The first text written specifically for the education of American nurse-midwives.

Wertz, Richard, and Dorothy Wertz. *Lying-In: A History of Childbirth in America.* New York: Schocken Books, 1979. The only complete social, legal and cultural history of childbirth in the U.S. up to the 1970s. Many little-known facts.

Williams, Phyllis. *Nourishing Your Unborn Child*, Rev. Ed. New York: Avon Books, 1982. Basic information on good nutrition, including scores of recipes.

Young, Diony. *Changing Childbirth: Family Birth in the Hospital.* Rochester, NY: Childbirth Graphics Ltd., 1982. An optimistic, realistic book about every facet of birth in hospitals, from family needs to obstetrical practices to provider strategies for implementing change. A little dense, filled with facts, not to be read through at a sitting. But come to it with a particular need for information and your questions will be answered at length.

——, and Charles Mahan. *Unnecessary Cesareans: Ways to Avoid Them.* Available from ICEA Bookcenter, P.O. Box 20048, Minneapolis, MN 55420, 1982. Small, but extremely useful handbook.

Periodicals

Birth: Issues in Prenatal Care and Education
110 El Camino Real
Berkeley, CA 94705

Cesarean Prevention Clarion
P.O. Box 152
Syracuse, NY 13210

Journal of Nurse-Midwifery
Elsevier Science Publishing Co., Inc.
52 Vanderbilt Avenue
New York, NY 10017

Mothering
P.O. Box 2208
Albuquerque, NM 87103

NAPSAC News
P.O. Box 267
Marble Hill, MO 63764

The Practicing Midwife
156 Drakes Lane
Summertown, TN 38483

Women and Health
The Haworth Press
28 E. 22nd Street
New York, NY 10010

Catalogs

For *Bookmarks*, a catalog of recommended readings prepared by the ICEA, contact:

ICEA Bookcenter
P.O. Box 20048
Minneapolis, MN 55240
(800) 328-4815
(800) 752-4249 (Minnesota residents)

A similar catalog of readings entitled *Imprints* is available from:

Birth and Life Book Store
7001 Alonzo Avenue NW
P.O. Box 70625
Seattle, WA 98107
(206) 789-4444

Associations Concerned with Childbirth Education and Childbearing Resource Centers

American College of Nurse-Midwives, 1522 K Street NW, Suite 1120, Washington, DC 20005, (202) 347-5445. The professional organization for nurse-midwives in the United States. It administers national certification examinations, accredits nurse-midwifery educational programs, provides membership services, produces publications for its members and the public and holds an annual convention.

American Foundation for Maternal and Child Health, Inc., 30 Beekman Place, New York, NY 10022. Concerned with protection against abuses of drugs, interventions and obstetric procedures which could cause damage to the fetus, infant or child in later life.

Association for Childbirth at Home International (ACHI), P.O. Box 39498, Los Angeles, CA 90039, (213) 667-0839. Founded in 1972. It trains childbirth educators and is developing midwifery training programs to comply with state laws throughout the U.S., and provides pamphlets and reprints.

Birth Day, Box 388, Cambridge, MA 02138. A group devoted to helping parents who want to have a home birth. They offer childbirth classes to people planning to have their babies at home, in birthing centers and in hospitals.

Cesarean Prevention Movement (CPM), P.O. Box 152, Syracuse, NY 13210. CPM has as its goal the reduction of the primary Cesarean rate and the increase of vaginal births after Cesareans (VBACs). It puts out a feisty newspaper, the *Cesarean Prevention Clarion*.

Cesareans/Support, Education and Concern (C/SEC), 22 Forest Road, Framingham, MA 01701, (617) 877-8266. C/SEC serves parents and professionals who want information and support in relation to Cesarean childbirth, Cesarean prevention and VBACs. It has been instrumental in humanizing Cesareans.

Home-Oriented Maternity Experience (HOME), P.O. Box 450, Germantown, MD 20874. It provides education and support for couples having a home birth, offers a series of classes and puts out a quarterly newspaper. Founded in 1974. HOME has published an excellent comprehensive guide to home birth.

Informed Homebirth, Inc., P.O. Box 788, Boulder, CO 80306. It offers classes to prepare parents for home birth, holds intensive midwifery classes and provides tapes for people planning a home birth.

International Association of Parents and Professionals for Safe Alternatives in Childbirth (NAPSAC), P.O. Box 267, Marble Hill, MO 63764. NAPSAC's goals are to promote education about the principles of natural childbirth; to act as a forum facilitating cooperation among parents, childbirth educators and medical professionals; to encourage and aid in the implementation of family-centered maternity care in hospitals; to assist in the establishment of maternity and childbearing centers; to help establish safe home birth programs; and to provide educational op-

portunities to parents and parents-to-be that will enable them to assume more personal responsibility for pregnancy, childbearing, infant care and child-rearing. NAPSAC is openly antiabortion.

International Childbirth Education Association (ICEA), P.O. Box 20048, Minneapolis, MN 55240, (612) 854-8660. ICEA is an interdisciplinary organization, founded in 1960, which represents a federation of groups and individuals, both parents and professionals, who share an interest in childbirth education and family-centered maternity care. There are regional chapters.

La Leche League International, Inc., Box 1209, 9616 Minneapolis Avenue, Franklin Park, IL, (312) 455-7730. It provides all kinds of information and support about breastfeeding. There are chapters in many cities.

Maternity Center Association, 48 East 92nd Street, New York, NY 10128, (212) 369-7300. Founded in 1918, it began training public health nurses in midwifery in 1931. It established the MCA Childbearing Center in New York City in 1975, the country's first freestanding birth center. This organization offers excellent publications, such as the *Birth Atlas*, and conducts all sorts of classes, conferences and seminars. Its general director, Ruth Watson Lubic, has worked long and hard to improve maternity care.

Midwives Alliance of North America (MANA), c/o Concord Midwifery Service, 30 South Main Street, Concord, NH 03301. MANA was created to expand communication and support among North American (and Canadian) midwives; to form an identifiable and cohesive organization representing the professional midwife on a regional, national and international basis; to promote guidelines for the education and training of midwives and to assist in development of midwifery educational programs; to promote guidelines for basic competency of practicing midwives; to promote midwifery as a quality health-care option for women and their families; to promote research in the field of midwifery care; to establish channels for communication and cooperation between midwives and other professional and non-professional groups concerned with the health of women and their families.

National Association of Childbearing Centers (NACC) (formerly Cooperative Birth Center Network [CBCN]), Box 1, Route 1, Perkiomenville, PA 18074, (215) 234-8068. Begun in 1981. It is working on the public and policy levels in government, industry and the health professions. NACC is dedicated to developing closer ties within the rapidly growing national childbirth center movement and to promoting an understanding of the birth center concept. NACC constituents are operating birth centers, individuals and groups interested in establishing childbirth centers, and consumers of maternity care.

Traditional Midwife Center International, % Linda Holmes, 64 Cambridge Street, East Orange, NJ 07018. A networking organization, of collecting and preserving documents and artifacts pertaining to midwives and traditional birthing practices throughout the world.

20

POSTPARTUM

By Dennie Wolf and Mary Crowe

With special thanks to Robbie Pfeufer

This chapter in previous editions was written by Paula Doress, Vilunya Diskin, Esther Rome and Marty Ruedi.

BECOMING A MOTHER

The months after having a baby are a mix, a real mix. Some days you love it. Imagine having the chance and time to roll on the bed and drink in the smell of a baby and find the tiny daily changes in a body your body made. Other days you're on a bus with a wet baby and a stroller that's rolling down the aisle. You look at the neat, childless people in the other seats and you feel messy, clumsy, alone and in the way. I remember Mondays when I could barely shuffle between my part-time job and the sitter's, with the baby wailing in the car seat. Then Wednesday would roll around, she'd wake up laughing with her arms out, we'd sail through the morning and I'd come to work thinking, This isn't easy. But, God, does it matter!

Celebration and change surround the birth of a baby. But the new life isn't just the baby's—it's yours, too. Being a mother can bring deep pleasure, intimacy and skill.

But in this culture, at this time, motherhood also challenges our well-being. As mothers, many of us assume the role of the "all-time giver," and bury our own needs for adult company, nurturance, sexuality. Increasing numbers of us are under the chronic stress that comes from balancing the roles of mother, worker and lover.

Suzanne Arms

We neglect our own physical and mental health, even those of us who wanted children and who have the protection of enough income, help and closeness with friends or lovers. The strain is even greater for low-income and single mothers and for women who do not fit the motherhood "ideal" (like lesbian women or women who do not want their babies).

Motherhood can be a time of insight. Birth and nursing give us a new respect for our bodies. Caring for, playing with and cuddling children, we discover new dimensions to loving. Many of us wake up, as never before, to the politics of being women and caregivers. As we move between homes and workplaces, our own lives teach us the changes in housing, health care, wages and work structures that families need. Hours spent caring for others make us more concerned about what sexism, racial prejudice and nuclear weapons mean for the future.

When we move into the first year of motherhood prepared and aware, we can wrestle with the issues and take hold of the possibilities. In this chapter we present the stories, wisdom and strategies of many new mothers: women who had difficult and easy postpartum experiences, women who became mothers alone or with partners, women with male and female partners, first- and many-time mothers, mothers who worked at home and mothers who chose or had to take on or continue outside work.*

THE POSTPARTUM EXPERIENCE

Many women describe three phases of postpartum experience. During the first days after delivery, we deal with the emotional and physical effects of having given

*In this chapter we have focused on the experience of birth mothers and do not discuss adoptive mothers' or stepmothers' transition to motherhood. We believe that the experience of assuming the social role of motherhood is much the same for any woman who becomes a primary caretaker, regardless of the circumstances.

birth. Over the next few months we learn what it means to be parents and adjust to life with a baby. Eventually, after daily life becomes more settled (usually in the second half of the postpartum year), we begin to face some of the long-term issues motherhood raises for us.

This doesn't mean, however, that you will experience postpartum in terms of defined phases or that postpartum ends when a year is up. You will probably have some of these feelings at various times and at various levels of intensity for years to come. Postpartum, like birth, is a very individual experience.

THE FIRST PHASE: TRANSITION TO PARENTHOOD

During the first few days postpartum we make the transition from pregnancy to motherhood. This is a time of enormous change; physically our bodies recover from birth and begin to nourish the baby; emotionally we may feel everything from exhilaration to exhaustion, uncertainty and sadness. Our birth experience may also affect how we feel, as may our readiness to become mothers and whether or not we have support from partner, family and friends.

Feelings About the Birth

If the birth has gone well and the baby is healthy, you may feel incredibly high, tremendously relieved and proud of what you have just accomplished.

Even though I'd had a long and difficult labor, I felt ecstatic after the baby was born. I wanted to leap out of bed and run around the room to celebrate. Then, after a couple of hours, fatigue caught up with me and I began to feel utterly exhausted. Every muscle and bone ached. Still, I didn't mind somehow. It was a good kind of tiredness—the kind that comes when you've been pushed to the limits of your capabilities. Along with the weariness came new, quieter feelings of peace, happiness, tenderness for my baby and a connection to all womankind!

But you may have other feelings, too, especially if the birth did not live up to your expectations, or if you encountered unexpected intervention or complications.

We had planned a birth with no intervention, and I had an emergency Cesarean instead. Even though I was relieved that everything was okay and thrilled with my baby, I had the nagging sense that I had failed somehow. Later I got over feeling that it was my fault, but I still felt cheated out of the birth experience we had hoped and planned for. Sometimes I still can't help feeling a little jealous when I hear women talk about their wonderful birth experiences.

In the days following delivery you may think about the birth a lot, want to talk about it in detail and try to resolve your feelings about it. You may relive it over and over, perhaps fantasizing different outcomes for parts you feel ambivalent about. (See p. 405 for more.)

The "Baby Blues": Early Postpartum Depression

Within a few days after birth, you may experience the "baby blues." They can appear as anything from a fleeting sense of inexplicable sadness to a full-blown depression which temporarily incapacitates you. You may cry unexpectedly, feel worried about your lack of maternal feelings or frightened by the reality of the sudden responsibility thrust upon you. Many of us have vivid dreams and fantasies.

The birth of my baby was wonderful, but the next day I kept having the sense that something was missing, that I'd lost something in the process. Looking at my soft, flat belly, I finally realized what it was: I missed being pregnant. For days afterwards I found myself wanting to feel the baby kick. Even though I had a real, live baby to deal with, I felt hollow inside. It took a while to accept the fact that this baby was the same one I'd carried for so long.

Immediately after the birth of my baby I felt high and exhilarated. But that night I got sad. I cried all night long. During the next few days I lay on my bed thinking of how I would kill myself. I couldn't sleep at all. I tried to tell the nurses I was depressed and all they gave me were sleeping pills. I felt like I'd never feel anything again but this incredible despair. I had nightmares. The one I remember best is where I would be feeding the baby. I would fall asleep and the baby would fall off the bed and be killed. I don't know why I had these dreams and impulses. I have a happy marriage and it was a wanted pregnancy.

Almost everyone has these feelings to some extent; postpartum blues often appear just as your milk comes in. Hormonal changes may be at least partly responsible for sudden shifts in mood, and depression can be heightened by being physically run down, anemic or exhausted from being woken repeatedly at night.

Usually these feelings last only a day or two. If you are insecure about your ability to care for or relate to your baby, your confidence will grow as you get to know her/him better. In addition, talking with other mothers about fears and anxieties can help you feel less alone. With a caring partner, friends or family, the "baby blues" are less likely to occur and easier to handle.

When depression lasts more than a few days it is usually caused by a combination of social and physical factors. For a discussion of more serious postpartum depression, see the box on p. 406.

Physical Changes After Birth—Taking Care of Ourselves

For me, physical recovery was no big deal. Because I had an easy birth and no episiotomy, I healed very fast and felt back to normal within a few days. The only thing that bothered me was sore nipples (for the first couple of days) and night sweats, which lasted about a week. Otherwise I felt terrific. Maybe I was just high from the birth, but I seemed to have a lot more energy then than I do now, several months later.

For at least two weeks after the birth I was very uncomfortable. In addition to feeling the episiotomy stitches, my whole pelvic area ached, and it hurt to stand for more than a few minutes. I couldn't sit for a week! Even after I got home, I found I couldn't do anything. I hated the feeling of being helpless. Because I was in so much pain, I was very touchy and found it hard to respond to my husband or to the visitors who came to see me and the baby.

Our bodies undergo enormous changes after birth—a pregnancy in reverse. Your uterus will become firm, contracting often, reducing in size so that by the tenth day after delivery you will no longer be able to feel it above the pubic bone. Breastfeeding your baby speeds up this involution process by releasing the hormones you need to trigger uterine contractions and keep them going. (Sometimes milk not coming in can be a sign of retained placenta.) These postdelivery contractions of the uterus are often strong and may startle you, especially following a second or subsequent child, but they will ease within a few days. Drinking raspberry tea and resting with a heating pad on your belly will help.

In another dramatic change your blood volume is reduced by 30 percent during the first two weeks postpartum. Under any other condition this loss would be felt as exhaustion, but many women are exhilarated instead.[1] If you do feel very tired or weak, you may be anemic. Be sure to eat enough iron-rich foods and/or continue taking iron and vitamin supplements.

As the uterine tissue breaks down, it is expelled in a discharge called lochia, similar to a heavy menstrual flow, which usually lasts from two to four weeks after birth. If bleeding is unusually heavy or suddenly resumes after this time, or if the lochia smells bad (a sign of infection), talk with your doctor or midwife. The immediate postpartum period is a time when infection can occur easily. Be on the lookout for signs—excessive bleeding, fever—that something might be wrong.

Many women find that after delivery, their pelvic floor and abdominal walls are very slack. Kegel ex-

ercises (see p. 333) immediately after birth, followed by gentle abdominal exercises and leg lifts, will help restore your muscle tone.

It may take a while for your bowels to start up and become regular. Drinking a lot of liquids keeps bowel movements soft and helps prevent urinary tract infections as well. Eat bran and stewed prunes. Relax and let your body take over. As long as you don't strain, you won't dislodge your recovering organs (a common fear), tear your stitches or aggravate hemorrhoids (varicose veins of the anus) which sometimes appear during pregnancy or the second stage of labor. If you have them, wipe with toilet paper soaked in water or witch hazel after each bowel movement, and take frequent sitz baths (one and a half inches of water with a strong brew of comfry tea to promote healing).

During the first twenty-four hours after delivery, apply ice packs to the perineum, labia, anus, etc., to reduce swelling. After twenty-four hours, try warm sitz baths (see above). Some midwives recommend honey or Vitamin E to heal stitches and tears; others prefer keeping the area dry and exposing it to infrared light for a few minutes at a time. Most also recommend waiting two weeks before taking tub baths (showers are fine, however).

As your tissues rid themselves of excess fluids stored up during pregnancy, you may drink, urinate and perspire more than usual. The sudden loss of estrogen can also cause night sweats, which may last for several weeks after birth. (These are similar to night sweats at menopause.) Some women also experience "hot flashes" during nursing, as their milk lets down.

When you nurse your baby from birth onward, without the hospital-enforced twelve-to-twenty-four-hour wait and according to the baby's demand for food, engorgement (painful swelling of breasts) will probably not occur. If you are not nursing regularly, your breasts may become markedly engorged when your milk first comes in, during the second or third day after delivery. Nursing frequently (to keep the breasts empty); applying heat in the form of hot showers, compresses or heating pad; and massaging the breasts (to promote circulation and letdown) should relieve engorgement quickly. Some women also recommend ice packs for pain. Whatever you do, don't stop nursing!

Some hospitals routinely give new mothers shots of DES or androgen (male hormone) to suppress their milk supply.* *We do not recommend these shots.* If you do plan to breastfeed, be sure to tell your practitioner and the hospital staff so they'll know *not* to give the shots. If you do not nurse your baby, binding your breasts tightly will ease discomfort when your milk

---

*DES may soon be banned for this purpose. Even if you are given the shots to suppress your milk, you can nurse. Just put your baby to your breasts regularly and persistently, and the suckling will cause your milk to come in. However, the hormones will reach the baby. Mothers are also at risk from DES (breast cancer, thromboembolism.) (See p. 497.)

comes in and will inhibit the supply. Before making the decision not to breastfeed, we hope you will consider the advantages carefully (see below).

After a normal delivery you will probably be out of bed within a few hours. Getting on your feet soon after birth means fewer bladder and bowel problems and a quicker recovery of energy. Getting up earlier can also reduce the hospital stay. Some hospitals, as well as birthing centers, now encourage the new mother to leave within twenty-four hours of a normal birth. This doesn't mean, however, that you should resume normal activities right away. It is very important to take care of yourself during these early days after birth. Resuming strenuous activity too soon can prolong the healing process and leave you feeling exhausted a week or two later. Even when you are feeling terrific, keep visitors to a minimum and let other people take care of household chores and any other children you may have. If you are alone at home, ask friends, relatives or neighbors to run errands and bring in meals. Your hospital may also provide homemaker services or social services. For at least six weeks, you should set aside extra time for rest and exercise.

Our friends set up a great system. Each night for the first week they would bring over a pot of something to eat. But they liked to stay and eat with us. We had to be their hosts! Finally, we asked them just to bring the food and let us eat by ourselves. We were too tired for company.

Recovery After a Cesarean Birth

If you had a Cesarean birth, you may feel sick and weak for a day or so, as well as very sore around the incision. You will probably have an intravenous feeding tube (IV) and a catheter (to drain the bladder) for twenty-four to forty-eight hours. Many women find the catheter very uncomfortable, so ask if it can be removed earlier. Also ask that the IV be placed so that it doesn't interfere with nursing the baby. If you had general anesthesia during the operation, your lungs will have accumulated fluid which must be coughed up. The "hut" or "chest" breathing exercises you may have learned in childbirth classes can help you to do this without too much discomfort. Many women also experience gas pains and/or constipation. Eating light, easily digested foods for the first few days will help.

After a Cesarean, you will be on your feet within a day. Walking may be painful, but it helps you to get your digestive system going and avoid blood clots in your legs (thrombosis). Within a few days you can begin exercises (see E. Noble, *Essential Exercises for the Childbearing Years*, listed in Resources) which speed healing and restore muscle tone, but you should avoid heavy lifting and strenuous exercise for at least six weeks.

Because you have had major surgery, you may be in the hospital for several days, so it's important that you feel cared for during your hospital stay. Ask for whatever makes you feel better, whether it's frequent visits from your partner, family and friends, food from home or a massage when you're feeling tired and sore. Some hospitals allow partners to stay overnight (you may have to provide your own sleeping bag on the floor).

On the second day, I insisted on getting up and taking a shower. Washing my hair was a big step toward recuperation. It made me feel that I was taking charge of my body again. Exercising helped, too—I started stretching my legs and doing ankle rotations immediately.

When you are feeling well enough, have adequate help at home and feel uncomfortable in the hospital, ask if you can leave early. (Perhaps you could return as an outpatient to have your stitches removed.)

FEEDING YOUR BABY

Most of us working on this book breastfed our babies because we wanted to and were proud that we could provide the best possible nourishment for our children. Even after returning to work, many of us found ways to continue breastfeeding. Both the advertising industry and hospitals continue to promote formula, even though research shows that breast milk is the best food for infants. Women who choose to breastfeed

George Malave/Stock Boston

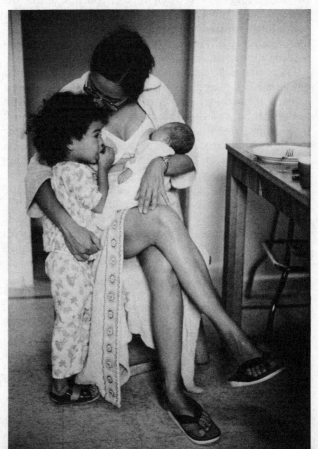

may have trouble finding information and support for their decision, or be pressured by family or doctors into stopping because they think that the baby isn't getting "enough" milk. Also, because our society tells us (in subtle and not so subtle ways) that breasts are sex symbols and bodies are sex objects, we may feel embarrassed or uncomfortable about using our breasts to feed our babies. We hear that nursing "spoils our figures" or ties us down so that we can't resume work or other activities. These myths serve to discourage women from making the choice to breastfeed.

Research shows that there are many good reasons to breastfeed and almost no reasons not to.[2] Human milk (unlike cow's milk) is ideally suited to a baby's needs. It provides exactly the right balance of nutrients, which adapt to your baby's changing requirements. Even babies who can tolerate no other food digest breast milk easily. In addition, breastfeeding helps to strengthen the infant's resistance to infection and disease, something no formula can do. Colostrum, the liquid in a new mother's breasts before the milk actually comes in, is especially high in antibodies that protect the tiny newborn against staphylococcus infections, polio virus, Coxsackie B virus, infant diarrhea and E. coli infections, the very germs to which infants are usually most susceptible. Breastfeeding also gives our babies a natural immunity to almost all common childhood diseases for at least six months, and often until we stop breastfeeding completely.*

In general, breastfed babies have fewer problems with allergies, constipation, indigestion, skin disorders and future tooth decay than bottle-fed babies. Breastfeeding is even thought to encourage better development of the dental arch, preventing the need for orthodonture later on.[3] For all these reasons, the American Academy of Pediatrics officially endorses breastfeeding as the preferred way of feeding babies.†

There are practical advantages, too. Formula must be prepared for each feeding in sterilized bottles. Breast milk is economical and always available at the right temperature, and there are no bottles to carry around! In addition, the milk supply adjusts to the baby's needs; the more the baby nurses, the more milk the breasts produce. As the baby weans, the milk supply tapers off.

Women who breastfeed tend to get back into shape earlier than those who don't. From right after birth, breastfeeding helps your body to expel excess fluids and tissue. Because the body burns about 1000 calories a day to produce breast milk, nursing mothers tend

to lose weight gained during pregnancy gradually during the first few months postpartum.

Finally, breastfeeding can be relaxing and sensual, close and satisfying. Some women become sexually aroused and even have orgasms while breastfeeding. This is because oxytocin, the hormone that triggers orgasm (and labor), is also responsible for the letdown of milk when stimulated by the baby's suckling. The breastfeeding mother and her baby have an intimate and interdependent relationship; many women feel extraordinarily close to their babies while nursing.

If you decide to breastfeed your baby, it is a good idea to have access to advice from experienced, successful nursing mothers. The La Leche League provides just this kind of advice, plus literature and support groups. Breastfeeding is a learned skill that takes determination and practice, especially since we don't grow up among a lot of women who do it. You can solve most breastfeeding problems with patience and the right kind of support.*

Some women choose formula so that others can feed their babies, and because it is easy to tell exactly how much milk the baby is getting. Occasionally women who want to breastfeed have severe difficulties which lead them to switch to partial or complete bottlefeeding at some point. If you decide to bottlefeed for these or other reasons, be assured that you can still have a close relationship with your baby. Whether you feed babies by breast or bottle, they like to be held close and cuddled during feedings. This physical closeness is important to the baby's emotional health, for it satisfies her/his need for touching and sucking, which is especially strong in the early months.

Breastfeeding Under Special Circumstances

There is no reason why women who have had Cesarean births cannot breastfeed their babies, though it may be a little more difficult getting started if the mother is uncomfortable after surgery and/or the baby is sleepy from drugs used during delivery. Some Cesarean mothers choose not to take painkilling drugs after surgery which will pass through their milk to the baby.

Mothers of premature babies and twins usually can and should nurse their babies.† If your baby is too

---

*Because of immunities in breast milk, some women delay having their babies inoculated against diseases until they stop breastfeeding. You might discuss this with your practitioner.

†There are serious disadvantages to formula use. An estimated 5,000 babies die annually in the U.S. due to formula abuse in some hospitals which actively promote its use, especially among poor women. Other health scandals in this country and abroad have involved deaths of babies who received contaminated or improperly mixed formula.

*Some common problems include difficulty with letting down milk and maintaining an adequate milk supply when the baby grows quickly. If you do have problems, we recommend consulting nursing mothers or supportive groups (such as La Leche) rather than relying on pediatricians for advice. Few physicians are experienced and/or supportive enough of breastfeeding to be really helpful; many actively discourage women from breastfeeding if the slightest problem arises.

†Research shows that the milk of mothers of premature babies contains more protein than that of mothers with full-term babies. (La Leche Information Sheet. No. 13, December 1980, available from La Leche League International. See Resources for address.)

small and weak to suck, you can express milk to be fed to her/him via a tube until s/he is strong enough to nurse. Even if you are separated from your baby by a prolonged hospitalization, you can usually make arrangements to breastfeed part time (see below).

With few exceptions, mothers with illnesses requiring medication can and should continue to nurse. If you are taking drugs that will pass through your milk to the baby, you and your practitioner can often make substitutions, lower the dosage or eliminate the drug. Make it clear to your practitioner that you want to continue to breastfeed your baby.

If for some reason you must stop breastfeeding (or choose not to initially), you may be able to reactivate your milk supply later by allowing your baby to suckle frequently. It may take some time for your milk to come in, and the process can be frustrating and difficult. Some determined women have resumed nursing weeks or even months after stopping completely. Occasionally, mothers of adopted children have even managed to breastfeed their babies successfully.

The La Leche League (see Resources) has documented examples of all the cases mentioned above, and can provide invaluable information, advice, literature and encouragement through a difficult period.

Sharing Feedings

If you plan to return to work, want time for yourself or feel it's important for your partner or other members of the family to feed the baby, it is possible to establish a part-time breastfeeding arrangement, especially after the first couple of months. You can express milk (by hand or breast pump), chill or freeze it (if it is not to be used within a few hours) and leave it for others to give to the baby. Alternatively, you may be able to find another nursing mother who would be willing to nurse your baby while you are out.

If you must miss feedings on a regular basis, be sure to express milk at the appropriate feeding times to keep up your milk supply. Remember, breastfeeding is a matter of supply and demand. We know of airline stewardesses who express milk while they are traveling and breastfeed their babies on the days that they are home.

Some women find that expressing milk is a real inconvenience. Others have trouble expressing enough milk to keep up an adequate supply. In these cases, you may nurse only once or twice a day, giving your baby juice or formula in between, or switch entirely to bottlefeeding. The point is to reach a compromise that you feel good about for yourself and your baby.

Breastfeeding and Contraception

When you are totally breastfeeding your baby (i.e., no supplementary formula or solid food), your menstrual periods usually do not return for seven to fifteen months after birth, because the hormones which stimulate milk production also inhibit menstruation. Breastfeeding, however, is *not* a reliable form of contraception after four to five weeks postpartum. It is possible (though rare) to ovulate and conceive before getting a period. Once you have resumed menstruation, you are even more likely to become pregnant. In choosing a form of birth control, avoid the IUD because of increased risk of pelvic inflammatory disease. Recently, the American Academy of Pediatrics cautioned that extended use of combination pills may affect your milk supply and/or the length of time you are able to nurse.[4] We have serious reservations about oral contraceptives. Also, since steroids can get into the milk supply, there may be as yet undiscovered effects on the baby. (See Chapter 13, "Birth Control.")

Tips for Successful Breastfeeding

In order to establish and maintain a good milk supply, you must take care of yourself. This means eating high-protein foods (a pregnancy diet plus 300 to 500 calories). Be sure to include foods rich in Vitamins B and C, iron and calcium.* If you have been taking prenatal supplements, keep taking them until your practitioner advises otherwise. Don't try to lose weight at this time. The ten or so extra pounds you retained after birth will help your body sustain milk production during the first few months. In addition, sudden weight loss can be harmful: if your body is forced to mobilize its fat supplies, your milk may contain higher amounts of some of the potentially hazardous chemicals found in our environment and food supplies.[5]

Be sure to drink plenty of fluids. A good rule of thumb is to drink a big glass of juice, milk or water every time you nurse. Keep one by your bedside at night, too.

Getting enough rest is *very* important. It is difficult for your body to produce increasing amounts of milk when you are tired and run down. If you feel your milk supplies are inadequate, try to cut down on outside activities and rest whenever possible. Some women also recommend supplemental brewers' yeast (which contains high amounts of B-vitamins) or a glass or two of dark imported beer (which contains yeast). You can also drink teas made from blessed thistle, camomile, fennel or fenugreek seed thirty minutes before nursing.

Remember, whatever you eat or drink will be passed on to your baby via your milk. For this reason, it is wise to avoid caffeine and drugs† (including over-the-

---

*Women who cannot drink milk because of a lactose intolerance can add lactase (a milk-digesting enzyme) to ordinary milk, making it digestible. This product is available in drugstores and goes under the trade name of Lact-Aid.

†Before taking any drugs, consult your practitioner as to whether they are safe for nursing mothers. Contact the La Leche League for a list of drugs to avoid while nursing.

counter remedies). Also, don't take more than a drink or two.

Some Problems You May Encounter

Sore Nipples

Some women have sore nipples during the first few days of breastfeeding. While hospitals often advise women to nurse only five minutes on each breast at four-hour intervals, many women find that nursing more frequently actually works better because the breasts don't become engorged (see below) and the baby sucks less vigorously at the nipple. If your nipples do become sore, exposing them to sunlight and air whenever possible will help, as will sparing applications of Vitamin-E oil, lanolin or calendula cream. Other ointments contain ingredients that could be toxic to the baby.

Engorgement

When your milk comes in on the second or third day, your breasts may feel full, heavy and painful to the touch. In some cases, they are so full you may have to express a little milk by hand before the baby can grasp the nipple. Frequent nursing on demand often prevents engorgement, but if it occurs, hot showers or hot compresses made with comfrey applied before nursing will usually remedy the situation within a day or so. By that time, your body will have adjusted its supply to the baby's demand for food.

Sore Breasts

If you have swelling, redness or a painful lump in one area of your breast, you may have a plugged duct, which can be caused by poor letdown, engorgement, infrequent nursing, tight clothing and/or stress and fatigue. Hot compresses, massaging the area and increased nursing will usually ease the discomfort. If the swelling is accompanied by fever and a tired, run-down, achy feeling (like flu), you probably have a breast infection (mastitis). In that case, contact your practitioner or midwife and make sure to get more rest. Some people recommend taking two to four capsules of echinacia root, or putting garlic (a natural antibiotic) under the tongue overnight.[6] If the condition does not improve in twenty-four hours, you may need medication. Rarely, a breast infection develops into an abscess that may have to be surgically drained. In most cases, however, early treatment will prevent this.

THE SECOND PHASE: ADJUSTING TO LIFE WITH A BABY

During the first few months after birth we learn what it means to have a baby in our lives. Many women describe early postpartum as a period of fragmentation and disorganization.

During those early weeks I felt like I was disappearing. I seemed to exist only in terms of other people's needs. Sometimes I wasn't sure where the baby ended and I began. I felt that I had lost my old self and was too tired, physically and emotionally, to find her again. But I was also discovering a new part of myself that I hadn't known about before: unexpectedly intense feelings for my new baby, a resurgence of love for my mother, connection with other women. I went from despair to overwhelming feelings of tenderness, all within the space of an hour.

During this time we have to find ways of coping with the changes this upheaval brings about.

Fatigue

Of all the stresses associated with postpartum, fatigue is the one mentioned by almost all parents. At some point most of us "crash" under the pressure of night after night of interrupted sleep—some for only a short while, others for months, especially when there are other children at home and/or little outside help.

For the first week after the birth I was flying. I seemed to have plenty of energy for everything—my new baby, my husband, even the constant stream of visitors who filled the house. Then, one day, it just caught up with me. Suddenly I could hardly get through the day with two or three naps. By nine A.M. I was exhausted. In addition, my perineum, which was nearly healed, suddenly began to ache and feel sore again. My body was clearly sending me a message. When I slowed down and began to take care of myself, I felt better, but I never did recapture that initial high of those days after the birth.

The first six months of my third baby's life are a blur to me. Constantly tired and irritable, I somehow got through each day, but it certainly was no fun for us all. The older children (three and six) suffered from not getting enough attention. Because the baby was breastfeeding six times a day there was almost no time to take the kids out or even get through the daily housekeeping. I still feel spread thin most of the time.

Some physical discomforts also contribute to fatigue. Common ones which last two to three weeks after birth are sweating (especially at night), loss of appetite, thirst (due to loss of fluids and nursing) and constipation. If you continue to lose sleep, you build up a backlog of REM* sleep loss, which can lead to emotional and physical disturbances. Your partner may also suffer the effects of sleep deprivation.

Some women get enough REM sleep even though the baby disrupts their usual sleep pattern. However, if you sleep most soundly in your sixth or seventh hour of sleep, have someone else feed the baby during the night, early in the morning or in the afternoon, so that once a day you can sleep for a longer stretch than the few hours between feedings. Keep housework to a minimum and ask for help with it and any other children you may have. If possible, nap whenever the baby naps.

Sexuality

Some of us have little or no interest in sex for a while after childbirth. Others resume sexual activity fairly quickly. We each need to set our own pace.

Low sexual interest can result from having your life shaken up, feeling exhausted, having to take care of your new baby, a mate and possibly other children. You may need to be nurtured and cared for, too.

All that first year, our old forms of go-to-it sexuality were just too much. I was too tired and I'd fall asleep in the first five minutes, leaving Jack frustrated, even angry. Other times I'd have the nursing and holding of the baby on my mind and intercourse seemed rough and crude. Also, I think that by the end of a day I had had a lot of skin-to-skin rubbing and touching and didn't feel sexually hungry at all. But Jack hadn't had much at all. The unevenness of it all was driving us nuts. After months and months of snarling, we just had to invent "middle ways" of being physical with one another. I think I picked it up from watching each of us with the baby—the nuzzling and the snuggling that goes on with no expectation of orgasm, just affection.

Low sexual interest can have physical causes. If you had an episiotomy or tear in the perineum during birth, the area may be sore for several weeks. Your vagina may feel dry, lacking its normal lubrication because of lowered estrogen levels (more common in nursing mothers).

If the vaginal area feels okay and the bleeding (lochia) has stopped, there is no medical risk in having intercourse. Masters and Johnson report that many women resume sexual intercourse within three weeks following delivery.[7] The "taboo" period varies from culture to culture. U.S. physicians advise no intercourse for six weeks to prevent infection; however, this rule originated in the days before antibiotics. If you sleep with one person regularly, you probably already share the same germs.

If intercourse is uncomfortable, use an unscented lubricant such as K-Y Jelly or a clear vegetable oil.* Be aware that some nursing mothers also experience painful cramps during and after intercourse.

As soon as you are ready to have intercourse again, you must use reliable birth control, even if you haven't had a period yet. Your old diaphragm will not fit. You can use condoms with lots of foam or jelly until you get a new diaphragm fitted. (For a discussion of other methods, see "Breastfeeding and Contraception," p. 401, and Chapter 13, "Birth Control.")

Learning How to Be Mothers

We may have grown up believing that because we are women, we are supposed to know how to care for a baby. Yet it is really experience that teaches us to be good mothers, including our own experiences babysitting or watching our mothers care for younger brothers and sisters. In the beginning we may be uneasy and afraid to trust our own good sense, especially with a first baby. Talking with other mothers about our feelings and fears can give us the confidence to try different things.

The first month was awful. I loved my baby but felt apprehensive about my ability to satisfy this totally dependent tiny creature. Every time she cried I could feel myself tense up and panic. What should I do? Can I make her stop—can I help her?

After the first month I got the hang of it, partly because I had such an easy child. She slept a lot, and when she was awake she was responsive—she'd look at me alertly and smile. Gradually my love for her overcame my panic. I relaxed, stopped thinking so much about my inadequacies and was just myself. It was pretty clear from her responses that I was doing something right.

I didn't know how to change a diaper any more than my husband did. In fact, I may have been more nervous about it, since I was "supposed" to know how. I learned to do it because I had to learn, and my husband learned, too.

Don't expect to love being a mother all the time. For instance, when your baby sleeps a lot, wakes up for feedings, smiles at you and goes back to sleep again, the baby business is a breeze. But when a baby is colicky (a catchword to describe baby discomfort, fussiness, crankiness) and cries sixteen hours out of twenty-four (that is not an exaggeration; one couple we know just went through forty-eight hours of constant wailing), your physical and mental powers may be stretched to their limits. There is nothing quite so

---

*REM (rapid eye movements) are associated with dreaming, which occurs during the deepest phase of sleep, and is believed to be necessary for physical and psychological replenishment.

*Avoid estrogen creams and/or pills recommended by some physicians, as the long-term effects of hormones on you and the baby are unknown.

jarring to the nerves as your own baby's cries. Watching the baby writhe in discomfort or pain fills a new parent with feelings of impotence, guilt and understandable anger. No amount of preparation can really equip you to withstand this calmly. But just realize that most babies are colicky for only a few hours each day—often in the late afternoon and evening—and usually outgrow it by around four months.

At around two weeks old she started crying from ten or eleven P.M. until six in the morning. We tried everything—walking, rocking, massage—but nothing seemed to help. Underneath I was sure it was my fault. One night, in desperation, Mark started dancing around the floor with her. I was so tired and they looked so funny that I started to laugh. Mark began to laugh, too, and the baby was so surprised that she stopped crying for a minute. It was enough to break the tension. After that, it seemed to get gradually better. I stopped blaming myself and realized that this was something she just had to go through, and all we could do was be there with her. After a few hard weeks she tapered off.

In many cases, colic is thought to be due to the immature digestive system of the baby.* Sometimes, however, an allergy to a protein in cow's milk is responsible. If you are breastfeeding, you can try to avoid dairy products for a week to see if it helps. Some vegetables (onions, garlic, cabbage, broccoli, cauliflower, brussels sprouts) and occasionally wheat can also cause gas pains in breastfed babies. It's a good idea to avoid any foods to which you are allergic, as the baby may also be sensitive to these substances. If you are bottlefeeding, you might try changing the formula.

You can try massaging your colicky baby's tummy, getting in a warm bath with her/him (heat often has a soothing effect) and offering weak solutions of camomile or spearmint tea. In very extreme cases, your practitioner may prescribe a drug (such as Donnatal) for your baby. Beyond that, the only advice we can offer is to have lots of people around to hold and walk the baby so you can get away for a period each day.

Whether your baby is "easy" or "colicky," getting along with her/him may take some time and work.

Other Changes

Living with a new baby means changing our lives in many ways. We discover we are on twenty-four hour call.

---

*During the 1950s, colic was usually thought to be caused by maternal hostility to the baby. Some doctors still believe this. If your pediatrician questions your feelings about motherhood, switch to another topic. What you need is practical help, not psychoanalysis.

I was used to getting out of the house in five minutes when I wanted to go somewhere. Now it can take me an hour to get organized for even a simple expedition. By the time I've gathered up the diapers, blankets and rattles, fed and changed the baby and put her in the snuggly, sometimes it's almost too late to go. And if I ever want to go out alone, I've learned I need to start phoning babysitters a week in advance.

Many babies are unpredictable in their sleeping and eating habits for the first few weeks. Some breastfed babies continue to nurse frequently and wake at night for months. We may be overwhelmed by the constant demands of baby care and find it difficult to get on with the rest of our lives.

I had been told that most babies ate every three or four hours and slept the rest of the time. Not mine! She wanted to nurse every two hours and sometimes more often than that. Sometimes she would sleep for an hour, sometimes for fifteen minutes. I loved her, but I also felt consumed by her needs. It was hard to adjust to the fact that I couldn't get anything finished, whether it was an article I was reading or folding the laundry. At the end of the day I would realize I hadn't accomplished anything. Once I accepted the fact that I was not going to function at my old efficient rate (at least for a while) and stopped feeling guilty about what I wasn't getting done, I felt freer to enjoy the time I was spending with my baby.

Some of us are reluctant or resentful about giving up activities we used to take for granted; for others, it's a holiday if we can stay at home for a while. Though it may seem like forever when you are living it, this phase passes. Within a few months, when the baby is older and on a more predictable schedule, you'll have more flexibility.

Isolation

For many of us, life with a new baby means coping with the monotony and isolation of long hours spent alone with an infant. This is particularly true after the first weeks when you do not work outside the home, the excitement of the birth event has worn off, friends and family are no longer coming around to visit and your partner has returned to work. There may be day after day without adult company.

You can get very nutty from being alone at home. I get so that I invent errands. I go outside just to buy a loaf of bread, just to see people. I notice that the streets are full of people like me, mothers with babies in strollers or carriages. I stand behind them in line and see how they try to engage in a bit of conversation because they want someone to talk to, just like me.

It is only in Western, modernized cultures that women are expected to "go it alone" with children. In other cultures, postpartum mothers live among mothers, aunts, sisters and cousins and are able to draw on their time, interest and wisdom.[8] Many of us feel more connected with our own mothers after giving birth, but when we are geographically or psychologically separated, we may overlook them as an important source of help and affection.

In fact, research into postpartum depression suggests that one of the most important protections a woman can have is a network of social relations.

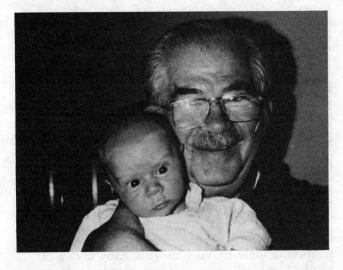

Nancy Hawley

For single mothers especially, family and friends are, as one woman put it, "better than vitamins, more than money."

When Alison was still a baby, I was in pretty hard shape. I didn't have work; I'd dropped out of school. The man I was living with was having a real bout with drinking. It would have been worse if it hadn't been for one of my brothers. He'd come down to the cottage after high school in the afternoon. We'd just hang out together. He adored both of my kids. I think he really took the hard parts out of being a mother alone.

When Willie was just a few months old, I joined a playgroup with several other mothers in the area. While the group was formed to get the babies together, its real function was as a support group for the mothers. It was reassuring to hear that someone else's baby was colicky and had been up all night and trade information and suggestions as to what we could do. It was also a help to share some of my ambivalent feelings about motherhood and discover that I wasn't the only one. I came to look on the playgroup as an oasis in what was otherwise a somewhat lonely existence.

If it's important to us, we can and should maintain our friendships with people who don't have children. But it may mean taking the initiative.

Before we had a baby, we used to go to dinner a lot with some friends. For a couple of months after the baby, they went on calling us on the spur of the moment. We couldn't get organized fast enough to find a sitter and go. They stopped calling. I missed them, so I called up and asked them to our house. Of course, the baby cried on and off, and they were put off. I could see what was happening, so I just said, "This isn't working. How about you call us way in advance, we'll be able to plan, and we can go."

There are other ways of avoiding isolation. Small babies are *very* portable, especially if you have a baby carrier (a frontpack or backpack) or stroller. As long as they are fed and changed regularly, babies make surprisingly good companions for almost any outing.

After a week, I was going crazy being alone at home with the baby. So I borrowed a baby carrier and just took her everyplace with me. I learned how to nurse in public without being obtrusive, and discovered she would sleep anywhere—in the carrier, on the floor of a friend's house, in a shopping cart, even in restaurants and movie theaters. Being mobile made me feel less confined and kept me in touch with the world.

Feelings During Postpartum

Once the full impact of living with a baby hits us, many internal and conflicting feelings, thoughts and fears may surface: I am supposed to be fulfilled because now I am a mother, but I feel ambivalent; I have to go back to work and fear losing touch with my baby; I have to be around all the time just to meet my baby's needs, so I don't have time for my other interests; I've lost my independence; I feel scared and inadequate— I need mothering myself.

All the time I was pregnant, people took care of me. But after the baby was born, she became the focus of everyone's attention, and I was reduced to the role of caretaker. I remember going shopping with the baby in the snuggly, and people would come up and say, "What a lovely baby," and never even look me in the eye. I was proud of my baby, but I felt a nonperson myself. I wanted to say, "I'm the one who cleans up the messes and gets up at night. Pay attention to me, too!"

We may feel angry at ourselves, our partner or our babies when we are particularly exhausted or isolated, or when we are not the perfect, nurturing, endlessly patient mothers we expected to be. Anger does not fit in with our fantasies about motherhood. But acknowledgment is the first step in dealing with our feelings.

405

I am a psychiatric nurse and therefore was aware of how angry thoughts about a baby postpartum are a normal part of the adjustment process. But I was unprepared for the enormous amount of anger I felt. I was angry about everything, it seemed. First, we had so carefully planned the conception (scientifically) of a baby girl, and I gave birth to a boy; then my sister-in-law, who had given birth six weeks before me, used the name I had reserved for my child for her baby. Then I realized how much my son resembled my father, who thirty years ago had rejected me. I also heavily identified with my oldest child about his displacement as kingpin. When I attempted to share childcare with my husband, who worked at home, I found myself at the mercy of two schedules, the baby's and his. It wasn't until six months later that I knew that my anger was dissipating. It was a full two years before I felt myself again. During this time I had obsessive fantasies about hurting the baby, how fragile he was, how easily I could drop him, how maybe I would forget him and leave the house, et cetera. I hated myself for such thoughts, but they persisted. It wasn't until I finally accepted the fact that a "nice woman like me" could have such anger that the fantasies abated. Postpartum for me was learning to deal with more anger than I've ever felt in my entire life. It felt like one long temper tantrum—unscreamed.

Postpartum Depression

The six or eight months after Peter was born were hard. My physical energy started to return when he slept through the night and more when he stopped needing a ten P.M. feeding. But my mental and emotional energy seemed to have disappeared for good. It was all I could do to get through a day. I took long naps and cried often. I got jealous about women my husband saw at work. I was out of touch about the me who had been an interesting, active and humorous person. Love him as I did, in some moods I resented Peter for even existing. To most people I pretended to be a "happy, young mother," but I was quite depressed. I didn't know about postpartum depression, so I blamed what I was feeling on my own failure to be a good mother. I think I also blamed my husband, as though he could have made me feel better. He was worried about his job and resentful that I was too low to give him any comfort. He accused me of having a child and now "not wanting one." (He didn't know about postpartum depression either.)

A lot of things contributed to my feeling better. I began admitting to friends how bad I was feeling; I began a cooperative playgroup with four other mothers. Most important, I went to a women's health group and learned that many women are depressed for several months after childbirth. All of a sudden I knew it wasn't my fault. I wasn't a bad person for what I was feeling.

Postpartum Depression

In modern technological societies, almost every mother (as many as 95 percent)* experiences periods (not just moments) of fear and depression. Almost a third suffer recurring depression. Up to two women out of each thousand experience depression which is deep and disabling enough to require hospitalization. Clearly we need information about postpartum depression in order to act to prevent it, to identify it, to cope with it in ways that will reduce its lasting effects.

Types of Postpartum Depression

Not all postpartum depression is the same. The range includes:

1. *The "baby blues"*: A several-day period of feeling weepy, frightened, uncertain or lonely, which typically occurs within a week to ten days after birth. In this type of depression the bleakness and fears do not persist, and can be dispelled with rest, relief from another caregiver, comfort given by a relative, lover or friend. Your interest in living and caring for your baby, your sleep patterns and appetites are undisturbed.

2. *Mild depression*: In this form of depression, bouts of feeling unable, lonely or frightened reappear, and may make it difficult to eat, sleep, make love, work. The feelings may be provoked by a specific incident, such as your baby crying all night or a talk with a childless friend who seems so much more energetic and interesting. Depression may descend when you are run down or under pressure (when you have guests or a job interview). Periods of depression last up to several days or a week. However, rest, time away from the house and childcare, or talking with someone who knows what it is like to care for an infant can break through the depression.

3. *Chronic depression*: If you suffer a serious postpartum depression the bouts of anxiety are frequent and last over weeks, even months. Under these circumstances, activities as basic as cooking, dressing and caring for your child seem impossible. This kind of depression is disabling—women suffering from it cannot get out of bed or out of their homes. The depression is not brought on by specific events but is the lasting result of feeling helpless. If you (or a woman you know) are suffering these feelings, it is very important to seek outside help from someone

*Estimates of the number of women affected and the seriousness of their depressions vary depending on the orientation of the researchers and the interview techniques they use. These figures are taken from Ann Oakley's *Women Confined* (New York: Schocken Books, 1980).

whom you trust—a family practitioner, a therapist, a spiritual healer.

What Causes Postpartum Depression?

Forty years ago most people believed that women who suffered more than the "baby blues" were mentally ill or unconsciously rejecting the normal responsibilities of motherhood. Today these explanations are being challenged, as it becomes clear that two different types of stress may be at the root of postpartum depression.[9]

Physical-stress theories say that the dramatic reduction in estrogen and progesterone in the postpartum period triggers depression.[10] They suggest that postpartum depression is similar to premenstrual depression, and note that some women are more sensitive than others to these hormonal swings. The hormonal changes of the postbirth period are also apparently similar to what occurs when people are in other high-stress situations, such as combat.

Although these biochemical theories do shift the blame from the individual woman, their major drawback is the implication that postpartum depression can be completely cured chemically with the help of mood-altering drugs. These drugs may treat the *symptoms* of depression temporarily and make a depressed woman feel better able to face the routines of childcare, but they do not cure depressions which are caused by nonchemical factors such as isolation, poverty or stress. (For the risk of these drugs, see Chapter 3, "Alcohol, Mood-Altering Drugs and Smoking.")

Other studies demonstrate that it is a woman's life situation that makes her vulnerable to deep depression in the months that follow a birth. Ann Oakley's studies of postpartum mothers living in London demonstrated that ninety-eight of the 102 women interviewed experienced recurrent depression. Oakley was able to point to the conditions which influence postpartum depression: 1. the amount a woman's partner participates in the process of having and caring for the child; 2. how realistic her picture of motherhood is; 3. whether she has and can hang onto interests outside of childcare; 4. how much she can call on a network of friends and relations for help and advice; 5. whether she lives in housing that cuts her off from other adults; and 6. whether she had little control over what happened during pregnancy and birth (see p. 390). Oakley's work confirms the findings of American research during the 1960s.[11] Apparently, whenever motherhood brings isolation and a loss of control, many of us mourn these losses through depression.

Who Is Most Likely to Suffer from Depression?

Some women are only briefly depressed following a birth, but a few end up in hospitals. Why are some of us so much more vulnerable than others? There are a number of factors which predict who will be hardest hit by postpartum depression. You are more likely to be depressed: 1. if you are having your first baby or you have been through the postpartum-depression experience before; 2. if moving and changes of lifestyle have created either geographic or emotional gaps between you and your family; 3. if your own family history includes the death of either of your parents when you were young, memories of desertion, sexual abuse, physical abuse or traumatic divorce which make you anxious about becoming a parent. Other factors affecting depression are: 4. your own physical health; 5. your own mental health (it helps to have a history of being able to handle stress or knowing others who can); and 6. your partner's willingness to share the pleasures and responsibilities of childcare.

One study found that 60 percent of women with a number of the situations described above developed mild or chronic depression.[12] If your history and circumstances put you at risk, you can act before your baby is born to make yourself less vulnerable. Reach out to friends or relatives who care about you. Lay the groundwork for sharing parenthood with your partner.

Coping with Depression

What if you are already in the middle of postpartum depression? Mothers who have been through it themselves make the following suggestions:

- Find out if the hospital, birthing center, a nearby women's center or a church sponsors a discussion group for new parents. Try it. If it helps, make long-term childcare plans so that you can go on attending.
- Talk with a friend about what troubles you.
- Take time for yourself *each day.*
- Go outdoors, with or without the baby, any time the weather permits. Make an effort to talk with other adults you meet—parents with children, the mail-carrier, neighbors.
- Do a little housework each day so that it does not defeat you by piling up. Better yet, do it with a friend, one day at her/his house, another day at yours.

- Locate another adult who can give you the "long view," someone who has raised children and who can tell you what it was like, what was hard, what made a difference. Houses and apartments everywhere are full of women who know a great deal about surviving and enjoying motherhood. They rarely talk about it because they think no one has any use for what they have learned.
- Take care of yourself. Find some kind of exercise you enjoy and do it as regularly as you can. Pay attention to pleasure. Wear something you like in the middle of the day. At the store, buy one food you love to eat. Try learning something new.

If your mood still does not change, you may need outside help. Signs which indicate you need help:

- You have lost interest in doing anything on your own behalf.
- You have become dependent on alcohol or drugs.
- You have attempted suicide.
- You have abused your child/children.
- You and your partner have serious, constant difficulties coping with the changes brought by parenthood; these difficulties include long, insulting arguments, physical abuse, affairs that threaten your ability to stay together, desertion.
- As a single person, you find yourself so desperate for affection that you become involved in a series of brief relationships which drain your energy and self-esteem without providing the affection or comfort you hoped for.

If you seek outside help, it is essential to find a counselor or therapist willing to look outside as well as within you to find the cause of your depression. In a culture like our own, which tends to devalue people who spend time caring for others, you may have to search for someone who will take your depression seriously. You also want a person who will help you learn to be assertive and constructive about making the changes in your life that may protect you from later depressions. Do not hesitate to ask other women if they can recommend anyone. Ask for recommendations through parent groups, women's centers, a nurse practitioner or pediatrician you like. After getting this kind of private help, your first-hand knowledge of postpartum feelings can enable you to reach out to other mothers as an individual or as a part of community action (see p. 415).

Celebrating the Pleasures

I had heard about the negatives—the fatigue, the loneliness, loss of self. But nobody told me about the wonderful parts: holding my baby close to me, seeing her first smile, watching her grow and become more responsive day by day. How can I describe the way I felt when she stroked my breast while nursing, or looked into my eyes or arched her eyebrows like an opera singer? This was the deepest connection I'd felt to anybody. Sometimes the intensity almost frightened me. For the first time I cared about somebody else more than myself, and I would do anything to nurture and protect her.

We are surviving. Just. Why don't they give Croix de Guerres to people who can go without more than two hours total daily sleep for five weeks? I thought babies ate at six-ten-two-six-ten-two—mine does. He also eats at five-seven-nine-eleven and four-eight-twelve. I am getting rather used to going around with my breasts hanging out. They are either drying from the last feed or getting ready for the next one. But the love—I never knew, never imagined that I would love him like this. This incredible feeling of boundless, endless love—a wish to protect his innocence from ever being hurt or wounded or scratched. And that awful, horrible, mad feeling in the first week that you'll never be able to keep anything so precious and so vulnerable alive.

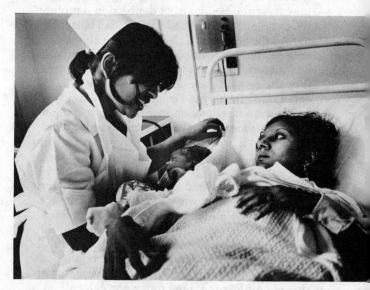

Suzanne Arms

THE THIRD PHASE: LONG-TERM ISSUES

For many of us there is a special quality to the later postpartum period (usually the period between six and twelve months after birth). It is often a time when chaos, fatigue and uncertainty ebb away and a tide of confidence and energy washes in. This is partly because our babies begin to sleep through the night, eat solid food, take predictable naps in the morning and afternoon. But this return to normal also comes from our own practicing, experimenting and learning during that first chaotic half-year.

I was getting together all the stuff I needed to take Pablo out—you know, the blanket, the diapers, the toys. I did it very smoothly, thinking all the time about the different buses we had to take. "This is it," I said to myself. "Being a mother is under my skin, in my brain, part of the way I pick things up and put them down."

No matter how much smoother daily life becomes, parenthood alters practically all of our "old" ways.

Partnership: Jealousy, Sex Roles and Intimacy

When I think back on it, adding a baby was like sending our relationship through a wringer and planting a garden smack in its middle—both at once.

Throughout the first year, adult caresses or conversations often lose out to a cry from the crib. Our partner becomes less a lover or a companion than "the other babysitter." Earlier in this chapter, we talked about practical issues in sexuality and childcare which come up during the first months. Some deeper or more complicated issues arise as the people in a couple relationship undergo a gradual shift to parenthood. This is not an easy transition. First, whether we have children at eighteen or thirty-eight, we have to balance being a parent with all the other concerns of our lives, whether it's finishing high school, finding work or caring for our own parents.

For both lesbian and heterosexual couples, one of the most difficult issues is jealousy, or competition for affection. Often there just isn't enough energy, time and affection for everyone.

When I nursed at night, the sight of me holding my full breast to this sleepy little baby used to drive Les nuts. When I'd get back into bed, he'd be wild to make love, fast and hard. It got to be quite a thing because I'd come back to bed feeling mild and sleepy. Les wanted to screw and I wanted to snuggle. We fought over it a lot until we realized we had to make time for some sex that was hard and fast and some that was cozy. A couple of months past the worst of it, we began to joke about "hard" and "soft" sex.

Second, we become parents in a culture that is riddled with strong, even irrational beliefs about men's and women's roles in child-rearing. The belief that mothers do their part by caring for children while fathers do theirs by contributing income affects our own behavior and shapes the social institutions all around us.* It requires hard work and self-awareness for men and women in heterosexual couples to stay friends and lovers as they become parents.[13]

Parents who adopt conventional sex roles may be jealous when each of their daily lives contains completely different people, routines, tasks and rewards.

There I was at home, by choice and liking it, except for this. Every day there were hundreds of small things—great ones like the baby rolling over or playing while I worked. Terrible ones like him choking or falling out of the infant seat. All these things were big to me. But when Marty came home, he'd listen for a minute, then start winding his watch or sorting the mail. I got to feeling like a housekeeper and he seemed more and more to be the invited guest.

It's one of those "grass-is-greener" things—I envied, sometimes even hated Sam when he went out to work. I don't know what I was imagining—that he hung around talking, went out to lunch, did interesting things. One time he was watching me bathe Annie in the sink. He asked if he could do it—he stood there, soaping her back over and over like he couldn't get enough of it, and he talked about how he hated to leave us in the morning and how he worried he would be closed out, left looking in at what she and I had together.

To My Husband

I mothered you,
then weaned you,
so we could parent
together.
Children grow so tellingly.
And who will dare
share this startling
gut
tenderness
when my son (soon)
moves on beyond where I
can pull him on my lap
and smell his hair;
I've lost the smell of your
grown-up hair.
Will this parenting lose us
each other?

We have to find ways of breaking through the barriers set up by jealousy, emotional fatigue and sex-role isolation. Many of us have found that our most powerful solution is to share the responsibilities of parenthood more equally. To share parenthood, both partners have to contribute time, work and caring. In

---

*The process of becoming parents can bring out traditional sex-role behavior. In early motherhood, women tend to act more passive, to become more emotionally expressive and more responsive to the needs of others. In becoming fathers, some men feel they should assert their authority, control their emotions and act rationally.

some arrangements, the adults split days at home fifty-fifty. In other situations, the one parent who does the most daily parenting asks her or his partner for limited but important commitments of time and interest which go beyond occasional "babysitting."

When Laurie was born I was bound and determined to do it all—be a full-time mother, a full-time, perfect housekeeper. I spent that first year rushing like a mad-woman from one duty to the next. I ended up feeling either like the good mother and the wicked wife or the wicked mother and the perfect wife. When I had Peter, my second, I said, "Hey, these kids are ending up with a six-thirty sweetheart, not a father, and I'm tired and lonely. There are two parents here; why am I in this alone?" When I asked Mike to help, he started taking Thursday afternoons off—out of back-vacation time. I still had the kids most of the time, but the idea that he would do that made a big difference between us.

Realistically, not all partners can take time off. In that case, the one who is away most can do whatever *is* possible: bathe the baby in the evening, put the baby to bed, make dinner.*

*For a more detailed discussion of the issues and "how-tos" of shared parenting, see Chapter 6 of *Ourselves and Our Children*, Boston Women's Health Book Collective (New York: Random House, 1978).

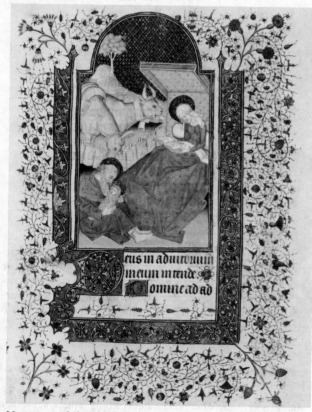

Mary rests while Joseph cares for baby
Book of Hours (French, 15th century), Walters Art Gallery, Baltimore, MD

Postpartum: The Second Time Around

For many of us, postpartum is a very different experience the second time around. Some aspects are much easier; having been through it all before, we know what to expect and are comfortable with many of the practical and emotional issues of childcare and parenthood. At the same time, incorporating a second child into our existing family can be difficult and stressful, especially if our children are closely spaced and/or we lack a partner, family or friends to turn to for support and help.

I started having children in my late thirties so I wanted them close together. My second child was born seventeen months after the first. In some ways I enjoyed the whole experience more. As a second-time mother I was more relaxed and less anxious about every little thing, and my second baby was more easygoing than my first. But that first year was also very hard. I was exhausted just trying to take care of two babies in diapers. In addition, my oldest child was jealous and needed a lot of extra attention which I couldn't always give. Having two babies on different feeding and nap schedules made life chaotic at times. I was much less mobile with two babies. Going to the grocery store could take all morning. What I found the hardest was having no time to myself. Someone always was wanting something. Unfortunately, my husband was not much help—his job required a lot of traveling and he was gone at least half of the time.
Now—a year and a half later—things are much easier. The kids go to family daycare three days a week and I've been able to go back to work part time and resume some of the interests and friendships that I had given up. I finally feel like my life, which was out of whack for so long, is beginning to have a rhythm again. I feel like a survivor. I'm proud of my kids and myself for having made it through.

THE HEALTH AND WELL-BEING OF MOTHERS

There are plenty of manuals on health care for infants. But almost nowhere is there a discussion of the health problems women encounter because they are mothers.

The Stress That Comes of Being a Mother

Caring for infants and young children is rewarding but *hard* work. If you have a child between one and three, you are doing something for or with that child about every five minutes, for as long as she or he is awake. While studies of stress have tended to ignore women at home with young children, research on factory workers shows that the result of routine work is fatigue, loss of concentration and appetite and eventual loss of self-esteem. In M. Howell's studies of childcare workers, she found that *six hours* marked the limit of an adult's patience and endurance when working closely with young children.[14] To avoid being worn down, we have to find ways of providing breaks, "recesses," even vacations. This is especially true for those of us who are on our own whether by choice, through separation from a partner or because our partners are uninvolved;* it is vital that women at home organize to provide "breaks" for each other through trading childcare hours, playgroups, or sharing the cost of hiring a sitter.

Mothers experience a second type of stress. Everything from myths to current research has made us believe that a woman must always put her family's needs before her own.

Getting ready to leave in the morning is a good example. It doesn't only mean me getting breakfast. It means being sure that each of the kids has what they need: the oldest one needs lunch money, the middle one needs boxes for art class, the baby needs eardrops and the right blanket for daycare. But it also means to me that everybody should go away feeling loved and safe and ready. If one of them cries, I get to work feeling sad and like I messed up.

Researchers have repeatedly found that almost twice as many women as men suffer recurrent or serious depression. Until recently this fact has been hard to explain, because men have been thought of as suffering higher levels of stress. Currently, we are coming to see that what men suffer are periods of high stress (e.g., job pressures, illness, etc.). What women, and especially mothers, experience is *chronic stress*, the continuing feeling that we must respond to what others ask of us, that we should, but rarely do, meet everyone's needs. All this may help make us vulnerable to depression during the postpartum months and throughout our years as mothers.

I have this dream that keeps coming back, since just a couple of months after my second baby was born. In it, I am caught in a wall, so that I am part of what is keeping the room from falling in on itself. In the room there are a lot of people—mostly family—eating and drinking. I want to come out, but they can't or don't hear me. I want to leave the wall, but I am caught and it seems like I am invisible to them.

*Many married women who are entirely responsible for the daily care of children live lives similar to those of single women, though they may have more money. Women who have distant or uninvolved partners may benefit from talking to single mothers about how they cope.

For as long as we nominate ourselves as what one mother called the "universal shock absorber," we are bound to fall short. We have to give some of the responsibility to others, whether through shared parenthood, community living or asking older children to pitch in.*

Who Cares for the Caregiver?

It usually feels right to be completely absorbed by a newborn baby. Once routines and basic skills are (more or less) in hand, however, it is essential to balance this preoccupation with an interest in caring for ourselves.

One day when I was leaning over to put Ben in the crib, I realized I had no idea what clothes I had on. I stayed there with my eyes half closed, not looking, trying to figure it out. I couldn't. I tried to remember brushing my teeth and I couldn't. I knew what shoes I had on, only because I only wore one pair ever.

Research on maternal health is beginning to show that we look after the physical and mental health of our children but skimp on our own well-being.† We insist that our children sit down and eat a nutritious meal while we eat leftovers. We send children out to play, to get exercise, sunlight and fresh air, while we stay inside and clean the living room. After the stitches heal, past the six-week postpartum checkup, medical programs usually ignore maternal health in favor of children's.

We may well spend fifty additional years—or more—in the bodies which gave us the children we so carefully watch over. We have to stand back from the ideals of self-sacrifice and monitor our own health just as we do our children's: tooth for tooth, vitamin for vitamin.

Part of the difficulty lies with the medical system. The dollar and hour costs are high for young families. Moreover, the practice of separating pediatric from adult care means that one bus or car ride and waiting period accomplishes only individual, not family, care. We need medical facilities with practitioners for adults and children, lab facilities under the same roof, nutrition and mental-health workers available, staffed playrooms so that mothers can take their time during their appointments.

*For a detailed discussion of the sources and effects of stress in low-income women, see *Families and Stress*, D. Belle, ed. (New York: Russell Sage Foundation, 1982). Women of all income levels can learn a great deal from this book about how the ongoing responsibilities of childcare may affect their well-being.
†Studies by John Eckenrode and his colleagues at the Harvard School of Public Health indicate that mothers do sacrifice their health care in favor of seeing that children are taken care of. It appears that in the days following stressful situations, children make more visits to clinics but mothers' visits drop off.

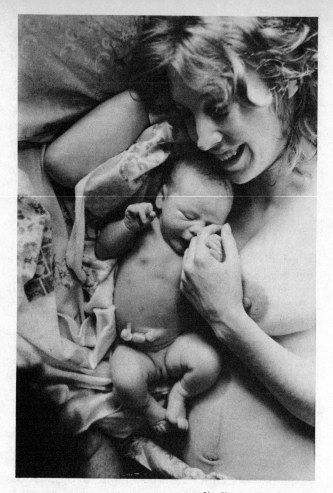

Modern Theories of Attachment: What Is the Cost to Mothers?

Anytime we leave our babies and feel a guilty, sinking sensation, we are responding to a cultural myth which states that any mother who loves her child would never leave that child if she had a choice. There is *no* question that children need the love and care adults can offer. Yet current beliefs about "the child's tie to his [sic] mother" cause many women to spend their child-rearing years leading lives that are narrower and guiltier than is healthy for any active adult.

Between 1930 and 1950 scientists observed how traumatic it was for infant monkeys to be reared without their mothers. Researchers began to ask the same sort of question about human infants and mothers: in the "natural laboratories" provided by World War Two and hospitalizations, they observed children's mourning and depression when separated from their parents.[15] They reasoned that the fuss an eight- or nine-month-old makes when approached by strangers signals the appearance of a very special tie to a particular human caregiver, the mother. In the end, what emerged was a "theory of attachment" which says that between six and nine months of age children become deeply attached to their mothers. After that time any prolonged or regular separation from the mother causes feelings of desertion which affect a child's ability to form relationships in later life.*

Pediatricians and conservative political groups have used these ideas to argue against mothers working outside the home, publicly funded daycare, part-time jobs or schooling that would open up alternatives to women with young children. But when we look closely at these arguments which challenge our options, this is what we find:

1. The original research was done in very severe circumstances. Sharing care with a partner, a sitter or relative is simply not the same as wartime or hospital separation.

2. In many, many cultures older children, aunts, even grandfathers assume major caregiving roles. Children are not harmed by being lovingly cared for by more than one person or by a person who is not the mother. Many families in this culture provide loving environments for children while single mothers go about the business of working and living.

3. When it has mattered economically or strategically, white middle-class families, as well as the federal government, thought it fine for women to be separated from young children. When women joined the workforce during World War Two, the government built large daycare centers where children could even eat supper with their mothers, then spend the night.[16]

In light of these facts, if we can make decent child-care arrangements, we won't go to work, a night course or an exercise class feeling as if we had "abandoned" a child. When our children have problems, we will not automatically think, Oh, if only I had stayed at home.

Being Workers and Mothers

The real personal decisions and compromises involved in going to work while you have a baby at home are enough for any woman. Sometimes the baby is sick, some days she cries when you leave, other times you love her to bits. But the tangle of guilts and shouldn'ts and dangers that have come to surround making that decision has just got to be cut away.

For many of us the prospect of working when we have very young children is complicated both practically and emotionally. We have to find childcare and juggle the double demands of home and workplace. We love and miss our children; we are afraid of being replaced in their affections; we want to know that other caregivers will care deeply, too.

These kinds of anxieties and questions are normal signs of caring. *However, the deep doubts and guilt that many of us feel in making and carrying out the decision*

*Some positive results from this work should not be ignored. This research has convinced hospitals to let parents stay with sick children and prompted orphanages to seek adoption for children as early as possible.

to work are not a necessary part of being a working mother. These doubts are our response to being raised as females in a culture which insists that nurturing, and especially childcare, is "women's work." Since nearly 60 percent of women with children under school age are in the workforce,[17] it is time to question the equation between motherhood and constant childcare.

CHILDCARE

For many of us the thought of childcare brings up images of too many children in a crowded, messy room looked after by overworked, poorly paid women. Reliable, affordable, high-quality childcare is hard to find.

There is a big difference between what childcare in this country could be and what it has been forced to become because it lacks social support. The federal government has consistently refused to plan for or provide significant financial support to a national childcare program, giving as a major reason the desire to keep families "intact" and provide for the emotional needs of young children. The net result has been that, for the most part, it has been impossible to build the thoughtfully designed, well-equipped, well-staffed childcare centers which we need. Many centers become shoestring operations in living rooms, basements and YMCAs. Wages of about 8,500 dollars a year for full-time work make it difficult to build a group of committed, experienced, skilled childcare workers.

Based on these circumstances, many of us fear that group childcare will hurt our children, that they may be ignored, unloved, bored. Our fears trap us: "If I can't afford a private sitter, then I belong at home." Some women can afford this choice. Others must go on welfare, borrow money, become dependent on support payments. Yet dropping out of the job market for several years can have both economic and personal costs (loss of seniority, benefits, personal identity). In order to make our decisions, we have to shake off some myths about childcare.

Myths About Childcare

- *Childcare means institutional daycare.* If you decide to work, you have some choices about the kinds of alternative care arrangements to make. Depending on income and circumstances, you can call upon extended family, trade hours with other parents, form playgroups and parent cooperatives, use private or publicly funded daycare.*

*Because we do not have the space to discuss the advantages and disadvantages of the different types of daycare here, we suggest that you talk with other parents about their experiences and/or consult one of the following resources: *Ourselves and Our Children*, by the Boston Women's Health Book Collective (Random House, 1978); *Family Day Care*, by Alice Collins and Eunice Watson (Beacon Press, 1976); *The Penguin Book of Playgroups*, by Joyce Lucas and Vivienne McKennell (Penguin Books, 1974).

- *Group care for a young child can be harmful.* The experiences of other countries like China, Sweden and Israel demonstrate that children raised in group care situations grow into normal adults. Studies done in the U.S. clearly show that children who experience group care, even from infancy, are just as affectionate, bright and emotionally healthy as children who have been raised totally at home. In fact, children who spend time in daycare may be more creative and independent than children who stay home.[18]
- *It is selfish for a woman to "sacrifice" her child so that she can work.* Contrary to the arguments of the political right, increasing numbers of us are not "choosing" to work. We are doing what we must to keep our families financially afloat. Only 29 percent of married women have partners with an income over 15,000 dollars annually, while it costs about 24,000 dollars a year to support a four-person family. Additionally, half of us—one out of every two women—will be separated from a partner while we still have the responsibility for child support.* Single women and lesbian couples have to face the fact that women earn only 59 cents where men would earn one dollar. Most women who have children on their own have no choice but to work or receive welfare.
- *Children are the losers when mothers work.* A great deal of child development research states that mothers who play with and talk to their babies have children who speak earlier, are more imaginative, seem brighter. This research makes us believe that we always ought to be on hand. It does matter that children's environments are interesting and that people care enough to help them practice skills, play, experiment. But that responsiveness can come from many different kinds of people. *Other* caregivers can give them experiences which we could never offer. For example, children who have additional caretakers learn to turn to other adults, to get along with other children (if they are being cared for in group situations), to understand more fully the many roles women take on. Instead of asking, "What do children lose when mothers work?" we must ask, "What are the costs—to children, women and society—when women who want and need to work stay at home 'for the sake of the children'?"

Finding and Using Childcare

All mothers need to find childcare sooner or later, whether it is for an afternoon off or for daily eight-to-six care. Here are some brief suggestions which may

*Even though fathers are often legally responsible for contributing to child support, only 34.6 percent of mothers receive payments and only 68.2 percent of these receive the agreed-upon amount. (See "Child Support and Alimony," Bureau of the Census, No. 112, September 1981, p. 23.)

make this task more manageable. (See Resources for books and other material which can be of further help.)

Planning Ahead

To get a head start on childcare, try to think during pregnancy what your childcare needs are most likely to be during the first year: will you be looking for occasional babysitting, part-time care, full-time care? If you work, find out what your employer provides in terms of maternity leave. Talk with your employer about your plans for returning to work. Find out from your employer or other workers about maternity leave (will it cost you seniority, vacation days, benefits?), taking sick days when your baby is sick, exemptions for working parents (some factories will give parents preference among shifts).

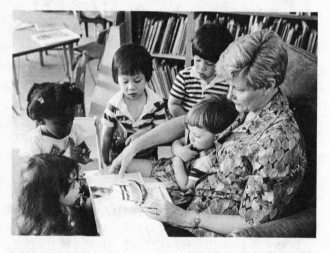

Elizabeth Crews/Stock Boston

Talk with other people you know who have babies. Ask them what their childcare needs were, how they met them, how they found good sitters, daycare centers or other forms of childcare. Visit some childcare facilities: an infant daycare center; a local babysitter; a family daycare home. Talk to several people's favorite babysitters to find out what makes caring for someone else's child pleasant or difficult. These visits and conversations will give you a feel for the kind of childcare you'll want to use.

Childcare arrangements will help, but they are not a substitute for working out the sharing of care with your partner, another family or friends. When children are sick, when your usual arrangements fall through, at night, on vacations, in emergencies, you will need people to help out.

When to Start Daycare and How Often to Use It

Some experienced parents suggest that you stay at home with your new baby for at least three or four months, if you can. This will let you get back on your feet and permit you to get to know your infant (babies begin to be much more responsive to faces, voices, games about that time). If you can afford it, use childcare at least occasionally before your baby is eight or nine months old, the age at which many infants become very frightened of strangers. Approach the task of finding childcare with the understanding that children of different ages require different kinds of care. The quiet, calm care which was perfect for the first four months may be boring and frustrating for a child who is learning to walk.

There is the possibility of too much childcare. Five days a week from seven A.M. to six P.M. is a long time for anyone to be away from home. We believe that children need private time with people they know and love. Part of planning childcare is providing time for parent and child to be together. If your schedule demands you find care for such extended periods, plan times in the morning and evening when you can focus your attention and affection on your child. Alternatively, consider if a family member or friend can pick up your child early on some days.

Finding Quality Childcare

What each of us wants from childcare varies, but there are some basics:

- Caregivers must be responsive to children, even when children are tired or cranky. They must care enough to notice when children are unhappy, sick or needing new activities. Children are growing human beings and need more than just watching.
- The physical space should not be overcrowded, dirty or chaotic. It should include areas for resting, quiet play, active play.
- The experience should have variety: indoor and outdoor time; rest periods and playtimes. Even small babies need this kind of variety to counteract monotony.
- Other children involved should be healthy, free of infectious diseases or behavior disorders that the caregiver or the other children cannot handle.
- You should be able to find out what goes on during childcare hours, should be free to observe and to talk with caregivers about things which concern you and them.
- The environment should be safe: no detergents within reach, no open doors to the street, no stairways without protective gates.

Beyond these basics, choosing childcare is a matter of what you feel comfortable with, can find, can afford.

But whatever situation you choose, you must trust the caregiver.

As much as you want the childcare you choose to be perfect and trouble-free, it is a human arrangement and requires attention, planning, looking after. Get to know the person(s) taking care of your child. Tell her/him what you know about your child. Ask them what they notice. If you have a feeling that something is not right, look into it. Talk to the caregiver(s), observe, ask other parents. If you are still concerned that the care is less than what you want, get together with other parents to try and change the situation or find something else if you can. Try not to communicate your doubts to your child. Unless you have no choice, don't go for a stopgap situation just "to tide you over." Multiple changes are hard on children and on parents.

Returning to Work

Most of us make plans for returning to work while we are still pregnant. After a baby is born, we may feel different about work than we expected. Some of us won't be ready or interested in returning to work after the usual eight- to ten-week maternity leave; others may be restless long before our scheduled time at home is up.

I went back to work six weeks after my daughter was born. I remember the midwife saying to me, "You have your whole life to work; your baby will only be little for a short time. Why don't you just enjoy your stay at home with her for a while?" She even suggested talking with my employer, but I was afraid of losing my job. I think now that I was overaccommodating. I wish I had waited longer before going back. Every morning when we are struggling to get out of the house by eight, I think, Wouldn't it be wonderful to be able to stay home with my baby today? I really missed something by not waiting at least a few more weeks.

Designing Work Options

Given the limits of the job market, women have been inventive when faced with the demands of wage-earning and childcare. Some women have found jobs to do at home: computer programing, editing, catering, family daycare, illustrating, typing. Some have also learned to use existing work structures, such as factory shifts, so that they can share childcare with a partner. In some cases, women have found, created, talked employers into part-time jobs which permit them to keep a foot "in both worlds." Women have also helped in the design of newer options: *"flex-time,"* an arrangement which permits workers to come in quite early in the morning or much later in the day, as long as they work their assigned number of hours; and *job-sharing*, which occurs when two people, both interested in part-time employment, share a single position.[19]

Though all working mothers need these options, few of us currently have them. To get them and to help make them available to other mothers, we have to pursue them everywhere—in union elections, in new contracts, by lobbying the benefits office at corporations where we work and by personally requesting them from supervisors and employers.

Inventing a Different Kind of Motherhood

There is nothing quite like the first year of being a mother to wake you up to what it's like to be stuffed into a role or a way of being that's too small. Inside your head you know that you are different, bigger, stronger, wiser. On the outside, people look at you like you're another one of those stroller-pushers.

Having female reproductive organs need not and should not determine how we spend what could be some of the fullest years of our lives. To open up the possibility of combining motherhood and selfhood, nurturance and sexuality, working and child-rearing, we need these changes in society:[20]

1. Timely help for pregnant women who do not have a working system of human support; who have been laid off from work; whose births may be problematic.

2. A new definition of prenatal classes which includes discussion of events past the birth, helping couples to think ahead to the role divisions and separations that may occur postpartum or by helping single mothers to plan for childcare.

3. Postpartum health care which includes the mother's (and father's) health as well as that of the baby. Women's groups could form around postpartum issues (infant care, working, social stress, couple relations). Women should be encouraged to think about designing their days so that their own health care (exercise, sitting down to meals, rest) is a part of their routine. Local health clinics could offer group counseling, and six-week checkups for mothers would include more than routine checks of stitches, weight, etc.

4. A postpartum hotline staffed by both experienced mothers and new mothers could operate twenty-four hours a day and offer both the opportunity to obtain concrete woman-to-woman advice and suggestions about where to turn for help with more serious problems.

5. A government-subsidized service in which women would be paid to visit new mothers, teach the how-tos of baby care, discuss the difficult issues that arise in the postpartum weeks and months and help women to explore their immediate community in order to locate childcare, other new mothers and other resources. At the very least, every well-baby clinic and doctor's office ought to have a bulletin board where these resources are listed.

6. Paid maternity and paternity leave for new parents, with full pay provided by all places of employment, as in Sweden and China; subsidized daycare so that there are enough places for the families who want them and so that daycare workers can be paid decently and work shorter hours under the kinds of physical conditions that will permit them to be responsive and inventive caregivers.

7. Daycare to be provided by *all* places of employment (as well as through at-large community centers) so that mothers can return to work if they want or need to. Employers must come to see this benefit as similar to offering health insurance and must cease arguing that it makes women more expensive to hire than men. Employment-based centers should encourage women to nurse and parents to eat meals with their children.

8. Awareness on the part of architects and planners that families with children have special needs that can and should be met: ramps so that we can ease strollers off sidewalks, parks with enclosed areas, common spaces with open carpeted areas where babies can play—maybe beside the washers and dryers in apartment basements.

9. Changes in the work structure so that part-time work becomes more widely available and better paid; tightening of the laws regarding equal pay for comparable work so that women's contributions to family incomes can be more substantial.

10. Paid consumer and citizen involvement by women in planning, monitoring and delivery of health care and community services, especially those which are meant to touch the lives of mothers and children, such as local clinics, public hospitals and mental-health facilities, park and recreation departments, housing authorities.

To see the problem as larger than ourselves helps.

One day I thought about all the mothers in all the households: apartment buildings, one- and two-family houses, farmhouses, mobile homes, rented rooms. I thought of us at home alone with our children. I thought how if we were all to come out from inside those walls and see how many of us there were, talk about all we knew and what we needed, we would see how large the problem was and we would take action.

Beyond imagining, we have to act. Now, as in the past, we have to offer each other what we need as mothers—childcare, advice, time to talk. We also have to work together in larger, more public groups to change the institutions and attitudes which often make parenthood difficult: whether it is an advertising industry with its one-dimensional portrayals of mothers, health-care facilities that fail to offer family care, congressmen who will not vote to fund daycare, universities that deny part-time study. We also have to act from our awareness of the many threats to our children's lives. We have many examples of mothers taking courageous public stands for their children's welfare: the mothers in Chile who help other families search for missing members, the mothers who demonstrate at the Pentagon against military buildup and nuclear arms, the mothers of Viet Nam veterans who counsel parents with draft-age sons, women of color who put long hours into fighting for decent education for all children.

NOTES

1. Reva Rubin. "Puerperal Change," in *Maternal Health Nursing*, Nancy A. Lytle, ed. Dubuque, IA: William C. Brown, 1967.

2. La Leche League International. "Breastfeeding, the Best Beginning," Publication No. 150, 1981; La Leche League International. "The Womanly Art of Breastfeeding," Publication No. 315, 3rd ed., July 1981.

3. La Leche League International. "The Womanly Art of Breastfeeding," Publication No. 315, 3rd ed., July 1981.

Jerry Berndt/Stock Boston

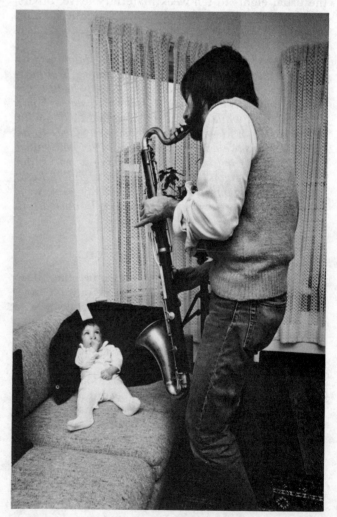

4. "OCs Said to Be Safe for Breastfeeding Mothers," *OB/GYN NEWS*, October 15, 1981.

5. Gail Brewer. "The Pregnancy After Thirty Workbook." Emmaus, PA: Rodale Press, 1978.

6. "Herbal remedies in pregnancy, and during and after birth," pamphlets available from *Birthday*, Cambridge, MA: M. Crowe, 1980.

7. William H. Masters and Virginia E. Johnson. *Human Sexual Response*, Boston: Little Brown and Co., 1966, p. 163.

8. Sheila Kitzinger. *Women as Mothers*. New York: Random House, Inc., 1978.

9. For an excellent discussion of challenges to older theories of postpartum depression, read Ann Oakley, *Women Confined*, New York: Schocken Books, 1980.

10. For a discussion of these physical-stress or hormonal theories, see D. A. Hamburg, R. H. Moos and I. D. Yalon, "Studies of distress in the menstrual cycle and the postpartum period," in *Endocrinology and Human Behavior*, R. P. Michael, ed., London: Oxford University Press, 1968. See also J. A. Hamilton, *Postpartum Psychiatric Illness*, St. Louis: C. V. Mosby Co., 1962, quoted in H. F. Butts, "Psychodynamic and endocrine factors in postpartum psychosis," *Journal of the National Medical Association*, Vol. 60, No. 3 (May 1968), pp. 224–27; see the chapter on postpartum depression in Maggie Scarf's *Unfinished Business: Pressure Points in the Lives of Women*, New York: Ballantine Books, Inc., 1980.

11. See R. E. Gordon, E. E. Kapostins and K. K. Gordon, "Factors in postpartum emotional adjustment," *Obstetrics and Gynecology*, Vol. 25, No. 2 (February 1965), pp. 158–66; and V. Larsen, et al., *Attitudes and stresses affecting perinatal adjustment*, final report, National Institute of Mental Health, Grant No. MH-01381–01-02.

12. R. E. Gordon, et al., "Factors in postpartum emotional adjustment," pp. 158–66.

13. Rhona Rapoport, Robert N. Rapoport and Z. Strelitz. *Mothers, Fathers and Society*. New York: Random House, Inc., 1980.

14. M. Howell. *Helping Ourselves: Families and the Human Network*. Boston, MA: Beacon Press, 1975.

15. This research includes Harlow's work with monkeys (H. Harlow, *Learning to Love*, New York: Ballantine Books, Inc., 1971); the work of Spitz on hospitalized children (R. Spitz and K. M. Wolff, "Anaclitic depression," *Psychoanalytic Study of the Child* Vol. 2 [1946], pp. 313–42); and John Bowlby's work on separation and attachment (J. Bowlby, *Attachment and Loss*, New York: Basic Books, 1969).

16. Perhaps the most striking example of this brief, all-out approach to daycare for working women is the story of the Kaiser aluminum plants during World War Two. See M. S. Steinfels's account in *Who's Minding the Children: The History and Politics of Day Care in America*, New York: Simon and Schuster, 1973.

17. U.S. Bureau of Census data, 1979.

18. See also Lois Hoffman and F. E. Nye. *Working Mothers*. San Francisco: Jossey-Bass, Inc., 1974; and the *New York Times*, December 13, 1981.

19. For a discussion of the work options women can invent see Chapter 8 in Boston Women's Health Book Collective: *Ourselves and Our Children*, New York: Random House, 1978. See especially Chapter 8, "Society's Impact on Families."

20. *Ibid.*

RESOURCES

Motherhood

Boston Women's Health Book Collective. *Ourselves and Our Children*. New York: Random House, Inc., 1978.

Ciaramitaro, Barbara. *Help for Depressed Mothers*. Available from the author, 214 Gibson Street, P.O. Box 808, Talent, OR 97540.

Delliquardi, Lyn, and Kati Breckenridge. *Mother Care*. New York: Pocket Books, 1978.

Donovan, B. *The Caesarean Birth Experience*. Boston: Beacon Press, 1978, Chapters 12–14.

Freidland, R., and L. Kort, eds. *The Mothers' Book: Shared Experiences*. Boston: Houghton Mifflin Co., 1981.

Grossman, F. K., L. Eichler and S. Winickoff. *Pregnancy, Birth, and Parenthood*. San Francisco: Jossey-Bass, Inc., 1980.

Howell, M. *Helping Ourselves: Families and the Human Network*. Boston: Beacon Press, 1975.

Kitzinger, Sheila. *The Complete Book of Pregnancy and Childbirth*. New York: Alfred A. Knopf, Inc., 1981.

Kitzinger, Sheila. *Women as Mothers*. New York: Random House, Inc., 1978.

McBride, A. B. *The Growth and Development of Mothers*. New York: Harper and Row Publishers, Inc., 1978.

Olds, S. W. *The Working Parents' Survival Guide*. New York: Bantam Books, 1983.

Nutrition and Exercise

Brewer, Gail. *The Pregnancy After Thirty Workbook*. Emmaus, PA: Rodale Press, 1978.

Davis, A. *Let's Have Healthy Children*. New York: New American Library, 1978.

Noble, E. *Essential Exercises for the Childbearing Years*. Boston: Houghton Mifflin Co., 1976.

Breastfeeding

Eiger, Marvin, and Sally Wendkos Olds. *The Complete Book of Breastfeeding*. New York: Bantam Books and Workman Publishing Co., 1972.

Guyer, R. L., and M. W. Freivogel. *Why Breast Feed?* Alliance for Perinatal Research and Services, Inc. Send $2.00 to Alliance for Perinatal Research and Services, P.O. Box 6358, Alexandria, VA 22306.

Kippley, Sheila. *Breastfeeding and Natural Child-Spacing: The Ecology of Natural Mothering*. New York: Penguin Books, 1975.

La Leche League International. *The Womanly Art of Breast-Feeding*, rev. ed. Franklin Park, IL: La Leche League International, 1981.

Pryor, K. *Nursing Your Baby*. New York: Harper and Row Publishers, Inc., 1973.

Raphael, D. *The Tender Gift: Breastfeeding*. New York: Schocken Books, 1976.

Baby Care

Boston Children's Medical Center and R. Feinbloom. *Pregnancy, Birth, and the Newborn Baby* and *Your Baby from Birth to Age 5*. New York: Dell Publishing Co., Inc., 1978.

Brazelton, T. B. *Infants and Mothers*. New York: Dell Publishing Co., Inc., 1969.

Howell, M. *Healing at Home: A Guide to Health Care for Children*.

Leach, P. *Your Baby and Child from Birth to Age 5*. New York: Alfred A. Knopf, Inc., 1978.

Spock, B. *Baby and Child Care*. New York: Pocket Books, 1977.

Childcare

Breithart, Vicki. *The Day Care Book*. New York: Alfred A. Knopf, Inc., 1974.

Collins, Alice H., and Eunice L. Watson. *Family Day Care: A Practical Guide for Parents, Caregivers and Professionals*. Boston: Beacon Press, 1976.

Evans, E. Belle, and George E. Saia. *Day Care for Infants*. Boston: Beacon Press, 1972.

Keyserling, Mary Dublin. *Windows on Day Care: A Report Based on Findings of the National Council of Jewish Women*, 1972.

Steinfels, Margaret O'Brien. *Who's Minding the Children: The History and Politics of Day Care in America*. New York: Simon and Schuster, 1973. Excellent.

The following booklet is available from Child Care Resource Center, 24 Thorndike Street, Cambridge, MA 02142:

Arvin, Sassen, and the Corporations and Child Care Research Project. *Corporations and Child Care*.

Organizations

COPE (Coping with the Overall Pregnancy Experience), 37 Clarendon Street, Boston, MA 02116. A Boston-based organization which provides a variety of support services for new parents.

La Leche League International, 9616 Minneapolis Avenue, Franklin Park, IL 60131. An international organization of nursing mothers which runs monthly support groups in many communities.

21

INFERTILITY AND PREGNANCY LOSS

By Diane Clapp, with Norma Swenson

With special thanks to Resolve, Inc.

This chapter in previous editions was called "Some Exceptions to the Normal Childbearing Experience" and was written by Jane Pincus and Barbara Eck Menning.

Many of us have childbearing problems which cause us difficulty and emotional pain. After years of using birth control and being voluntarily childless, we are confronted with the reality that when we consciously decide to have children, we are unable to conceive or unable to carry a pregnancy. The following is a description of a totally unexpected miscarriage in the thirteenth week:

My husband held me and we cried together. It is not hard to remember what we were feeling. The deepest and most obvious was the sense of loss. Almost as strong was the fear. We did not understand what was happening and why—why it was happening to us. Did this mean something was wrong with one of us? Did this mean we could never have children? Had I done something wrong during the early months to cause the miscarriage? We were also frightened by the amount and look of what was pouring out of me....It was terribly bloody. It wasn't bad enough that we were losing our baby, but in the midst of all that pain we had to stay strong enough to deal with all that blood. Why hadn't anyone given us any preparation? Since no one had ever told us about miscarriage, we had no tools to deal with it while it was happening.

We can learn to deal with potential problems and actual crises in two ways. First we will want to have a general awareness that things may go wrong. We can tuck away such information to be used if necessary. The knowledge itself can't hurt us, but if it upsets us, we can hold dialogues with ourselves, our partners or our friends. Secondly, if we do suspect we can't conceive, if we miscarry or have another problem, we will want more specific information to answer our questions: What is happening? What shall I do? Where shall I get help? How shall I cope? What is my next step? What other questions shall I ask?

I was told by a doctor that he does not discuss miscarriage so that he will not frighten women who (he thinks) are not going to have them.

This kind of attitude insults our intelligence and undermines our emotional strength. We and our doctors are practicing sound preventive medicine when we ask our questions as strongly as we can and they answer them respectfully and to the best of their knowledge.

We can also seek out the physiological causes of our problems by reading all the available literature, learning about diagnostic procedures and available treatments, asking for test results and insisting on further tests if we are not satisfied.

We can develop emotional strengths to cope with what we are living through. Crises may produce feelings of isolation, fear, anger, grief, guilt and helplessness, as well as obsessions and fantasies. During such times we need sympathetic support from our partners, our friends and others who have had similar experiences. We need to be able to reach out to others.

This chapter is meant to be a first tool to help us acquire some of the information we need.

INFERTILITY

Infertility is defined by most doctors as the inability to conceive after a year or more of sexual relations without contraception. The category includes women who conceive but can't maintain a pregnancy long enough for the fetus to become viable (able to live outside the mother). You have the right to consider yourself infertile whenever you begin to feel concerned about your failure to become pregnant. Infertility may be a temporary or permanent state, depending on your problem and on the available treatments. Many people are surprised to learn that infertility is fairly common. *Between 15 and 20 percent* of couples in the United States are infertile. In 35 percent of these cases, male factors are responsible; in 35 percent, female factors are responsible; in 30 percent, combined factors are responsible.

Infertility appears to be on the rise. It now affects over 10 million people. Some major factors which have led to this increase are: the rise in STD-caused infections which may lead to permanent damage to the reproductive system; widespread use of the Pill, which causes ovulatory problems; the IUD, which contributes to infertility by causing PID (pelvic inflammatory disease) after insertion; women's decision to delay childbearing into their thirties, when fertility decreases slightly; and the increase in environmental and industrial toxic products, which can affect both men's and women's reproductive systems. A badly done abortion, or one which has not been properly followed up, can cause infections which, if not treated, in turn affect fertility.

Though up until now one myth has held that infertility is the woman's problem, it has become clear that the man and woman must be diagnosed and treated together. If the man has the problem, then treatment of the woman alone has no value and usually involves many needless, painful and expensive tests. A man, because of his anatomy, is easier to diagnose: semen analysis is one of the logical tests to perform first.

Another myth is that infertility is not treatable. *In fact, 50 percent of infertile people treated are able to achieve a pregnancy!*

When you seek help for infertility, it is crucial to have a good relationship with your doctor. Find someone who specializes in infertility. The best infertility specialists are reproductive endocrinologists, who are obstetrician-gynecologists with two additional years of training in the field of infertility. If you don't have confidence in your doctor's methods, go elsewhere. Get a second opinion; that is your right.

It's important that your doctor be respectful of your body, mind and feelings; aware of your pain and strong emotions; and available to you when you need him or her. It's the responsibility of your nurse and doctor to explain words and procedures so that you can fully understand—it may take you a while, because you are learning a new language and may be under stress. It is often helpful to make a written list of questions to take with you to each appointment, and bring your partner or a friend with you.

You may need help from your partner, close friends or an infertility support group to obtain the necessary tests and diagnostic procedures you have learned about. Become as familiar with your own body's functions as you can.

EMOTIONAL RESPONSES TO INFERTILITY

Infertility is a life crisis. It is usually unexpected; often we don't know how to cope with the feelings raised by the experience of discovering we are infertile. There is an initial reaction of shock and denial.

I, like every other woman in this society, always believed that I would have children without any problems—as many as I wished, and when I decided it was the right time. Unfortunately, after four years of trial and error, tests, operations, et cetera, my husband and I are realizing that life does not always happen the way we plan it. I have found it quite hard dealing not only with our infertility problem but also with the reactions of people around me.

I'm sick of people telling me to "relax," "stop thinking it out," "adopt and you'll get pregnant," and all the other wonderful clichés that, although said to be comforting, ring of insensitivity. Friends and family can never possibly know the pain that I feel inside, the anger and resentment I feel every time I see a woman walking down the street with a big belly. How could they understand? How can anyone capable of having children understand?

Often it seems as if your life is on hold, as you postpone changing jobs, going back to school, etc., because "six months from now you will be pregnant."

I quit teaching five years ago to become pregnant. When that did not happen, everyone wanted to know what I could possibly be doing at home all day if I didn't have kids. Neither a mother nor a career woman, I stayed in limbo because I kept thinking, Maybe it will happen this month! I was drifting, and it is hard to believe so much time has gone by with just this single purpose in mind.

When women you know have children, it may be hard for you to relate to them. Feelings of envy, jealousy and "why them and not me" are common. Because holidays are so child-centered, they can become stressful, lonely and depressing times for you. You may feel isolated from friends and your mate. You may each react differently to the infertility crisis.

My husband is disappointed with our failure to conceive, but he could easily accept a child-free life. He says he understands my feelings and sympathizes, but doesn't care to hear any more about the subject. His view is "Play the cards dealt you"—you go on about your business no matter what. His disappointment is mitigated by involvement in a job he likes and other alternatives. I have not found a satisfactory alternative.

Anger is a common feeling, but it is hard to know where and toward whom to direct it. We tend to look for a reason for our infertility. We may feel that something we did in the past caused our present inability to conceive. Some people irrationally think that past abortions (even though properly performed), masturbation, unusual sex practices, etc., have caused this form of "punishment." They do not cause infertility, but our minds can trick us into believing it and make us feel terribly guilty.

Depression, sadness and despair are common.

What infertility seemed to do to me was to force a kind of confrontation with lifelessness or death. The fact that there would be no children meant that I was the last line of offense against death. Nobody to carry on who was living. The solution: disconnect. So I numbed out. I invested back into work, *which in the culture has been* man's *traditional way to combat mortality. If your work lives on, you haven't been wasting your time; there's a purpose to your life.*

Yes, I'm tired. I'm tired of an empty, longing, aching heart that yearns to hold a little baby of my own. Oh, I've tried everything. I've tried praying, relaxing, furthering my education, working hard at my career, social clubs, church work, service work, slimnastics, cross-stitch—you name it, I've tried it. And I still cannot get rid of that aching, yearning, longing emptiness that can only be known by barren women.

I grew up surrounded by the idea that if you were willing to work or study hard and always did your best, nothing was beyond your grasp. Generally I have found this to be true. The theory fell apart when I began to deal with my infertility problems. Not only did I become very depressed, but without the help of a friend of mine who shares the same problem I seriously doubt whether my marriage would have remained intact.

It is only through a great deal of pain and anguish that I have begun to accept the idea that I may never have children. After the initial shock wore off, my husband and I became closer than ever.

I wish that more doctors dealing with infertility would address themselves to the feelings of their patients instead of leaving them floundering, looking for their own resources.

CAUSES OF INFERTILITY

Fertility is based on several physiological events and their timing. Your partner must produce sperm of sufficient quantity, quality and motility (ability to swim). You must produce a healthy ovum. Sperm must be deposited in your vagina and move upward through cervical mucus to meet the ovum while it is still in the tube. (Timing of sexual relations is important, since an ovum may live as little as twelve or twenty-four

hours, a sperm as little as one or two days.) Once the sperm and ovum have united, the resulting group of cells must implant properly in the uterine lining and proceed to grow. The usual order of tests done in an infertility checkup is based on an organized attempt to check all the links in this chain of events.

A man may be infertile because of:

1. Problems of production and maturation of the sperm. These can be caused by previous infection, especially after puberty, such as mumps; undescended testicles; chemical and environmental factors; drugs; occupational hazards. Taking hot saunas and baths can cause overly high temperatures in the scrotal sac, an effect which lasts a few months. In addition, a varicocele (a varicose vein in the scrotum) can affect sperm production.

2. Problems with the movement (motility) of the sperm. These may be due to chronic prostitis and abnormally low or very thick semen. In addition, certain drugs used to treat emotional disorders can affect sperm motility.

3. Problems of conduction can result from scar tissue in the delicate passageways through which the sperm travel; this may be caused by infections or untreated STD. (Intentional blockage is accomplished by vasectomy.)

4. Inability to deposit the sperm into the cervix can be caused by sexual dysfunction, such as impotence or premature ejaculation, as well as by structural problems in the penis: for example, when the opening is either on the top or underside of the penis instead of at the tip. Spinal cord injuries and various neurological diseases can also contribute to this problem.

5. Other factors affecting male fertility are poor nutrition and poor general health. Researchers recommend that men eat well and increase their intake of zinc, Vitamin C and Vitamin E.

A woman may be infertile because of:

1. Mechanical barriers which prevent the union of the sperm and ovum, caused by scarring on the tubes or ovaries from previous PID or from certain IUDs (particularly the Dalkon Shield). There is a 9 percent higher risk of developing PID if a woman is using an IUD and this risk is increased sixfold if she has a Dalkon Shield. Untreated STD, such as gonorrhea, can also cause scarring and tubal blockage.

2. Endometriosis (see p. 500) can cause scarring and tubal blockage.

3. Endocrine problems. Failure to ovulate regularly or irregular menstrual periods may be due to a malfunction of the ovaries, pituitary, hypothalamus, thyroid or adrenal glands. Normally, several specific hormones are secreted at specific times in the menstrual cycle. If any one of these is not produced, or produced in insufficient quantity, the whole cycle can be thrown off. In addition, when ovulation is unpredictable the chances of conception are decreased, as women cannot count on a consistent cycle with a known

fertile time. Women often develop amenorrhea (absence of menstrual periods) following the use of birth control pills, which can result in infertility. Women who have irregular periods or who are older when they start their first menstrual periods seem to be more prone to this so-called "post-Pill syndrome."

4. Structural problems in the uterus or cervix due to congenital problems or DES exposure *in utero* can cause infertility by preventing conception or affecting the normal growth and expansion of the uterus during pregnancy. If the cervix is affected, miscarriage may result.

5. Cervical mucus of an incorrect consistency or pH (an expression of acidity and alkalinity) can act as a barrier to the normal movement of the sperm up into the vagina.

6. Other factors, such as genetic abnormalities, extreme weight loss or weight gain, excessive exercise, poor nutrition and environmental and industrial toxins, may affect a woman's fertility. Infections, such as those caused by T-mycoplasma and chlamydia, can cause infertility by changing the quality of cervical mucus and possibly causing early miscarriage.

Infertility also takes the form of repeated miscarriage or stillbirths. In these instances conception is not the problem; there is an inability to carry a pregnancy to live birth.

A couple may have a combination of problems which results in infertility. Some shared causes are: 1. *Immunological response.* You or your partner may have sperm antibodies which tend to destroy the sperm's action by immobilizing them or causing them to clump. 2. *Simple lack of knowledge.* Neither of you may know when you are fertile, how often to have intercourse during this time or what to do during intercourse to make pregnancy more possible.

Finally, for 10 percent of infertile couples, physicians cannot specifically diagnose any cause for their infertility ("normal infertility"). These couples are told everything is "normal" and they can do nothing but wait. This finding can be one of the hardest to cope with—the idea that there is nothing that can be done. You may be told that your problems are all in your head. This kind of attitude is not helpful at all. Often you may be victims of a condition whose cause or cure has yet to be discovered. We must all press for more research.

Masters and Johnson stated that one out of five couples who attended their infertility clinic over a twenty-four-year period conceived within three months with no treatment other than use of this basic information: if your menstrual cycle is regular, whether it be long or short, you will probably ovulate fourteen days (give or take twenty-four hours either way) before the beginning of your next period. In other words, you should try to become pregnant on the thirteenth, fourteenth and fifteenth days before your next period. During these three days, spacing your lovemaking is important (see

"Fertility Observation," p. 235). A man's sperm production decreases if he makes love too often, so you should have intercourse no more than once every thirty or thirty-six hours to keep active sperm in your genital tract during that period of time. It is wise to have intercourse two days before this three-day period to stimulate your partner's sperm production.

If your uterus is not tilted back, the most effective position for intercourse will be with your partner above and facing you, and a folded pillow under your hips to raise them. (If your uterus is tilted back, use three or four pillows.) Use no artificial lubricant, such as jellies or creams, and never douche afterward. If lubrication is necessary, saliva is the safest choice. He should penetrate as deeply as possible, and when he reaches orgasm he should stop thrusting and hold quite still, deep in your vagina. Approximately 60 to 70 percent of the sperm are contained in the first part of the ejaculate. Since it usually takes about twenty minutes for sperm to travel through the cervical mucus up to the uterus and fallopian tubes, it is a good idea to stay on your back with your knees elevated for about thirty minutes.*

Though these methods may at times seem too mechanical and may make you tense, try to keep in your minds and hearts your good feelings for each other.

If your menstrual cycle is very irregular, determine the time you ovulate by using a basal temperature chart, monitoring the type and amount of your cervical mucus (see "Fertility Observation," p. 422) and asking a fertility awareness group or your doctor for more help if you need it.

Many couples know that infertility and planned sex really affect their sexual life. Spontaneity in lovemaking decreases. You have to plan your sex life around your menstrual cycle; it becomes less an act of loving and pleasure and more a medically necessary response. Recording the time of your sexual relations on a temperature chart may make you feel like nothing is private or sacred in your life anymore!

I started with the temperature charts. This was quite taxing for me, and mentally depressing. I felt very regulated and calculating, both with my own body and in my relationship with my husband. I need not say what it did to our natural sexual impulses. But a child at all cost—this was how we felt.

My husband woke me every morning at six A.M. so that I could take my temperature. Afterward, he charted it. I needed his involvement.

From the chart you can determine if you are ovulating or not and can time your sex to coincide. If you

---

*Some women recommend douching with baking soda thirty minutes before intercourse to change the consistency of cervical mucus and make it less viscous, so that sperm encounter less resistance.

are ovulating normally, from the time of your last period until ovulation you'll have a fluctuating, low temperature (around 98 degrees or less). About the time of ovulation there's usually a sharp dip followed by a rise of half a degree or more. Some cycles show just a rise with no preceding dip. The higher plateau (usually around 98.4 degrees) is maintained until the day before your next period, when it drops again. Your doctor will give you a chart, or you can get one from your nearest Planned Parenthood Association.

You must wait at least two cycles to begin to interpret the chart with any degree of accuracy.

DIAGNOSIS

A complete infertility workup with all the diagnostic tests can take four or five menstrual cycles. Many of the tests have to be scheduled at specific times in your cycle and can't be combined. An infertility workup is expensive, and unfortunately medical insurance coverage in most cases is poor. The tests for women are invasive, painful, often undignified and emotionally exhausting.

Though the sequence of diagnostic studies will vary with both doctors and individuals, it will include some or all of the following:

1. *A general physical and medical history of both man and woman.*

2. *A pelvic examination of the woman.* Your reproductive tract, breasts and general development will be checked. You will want to tell your doctor about your menstrual history, including the onset and pattern of your menstrual periods; about any previous pregnancies, episodes of STD or abortions; about your use of birth control; about your sexual relations (frequency, position and related feelings); about where you live and what your job is, for environmental toxins may have affected you.

3. *A basal temperature chart.* You will take your temperature daily with a special thermometer and record it on the chart given to you.

4. *Semen analysis.* Your partner will ejaculate a sample of semen into a clean container. It must be kept at body temperature and examined as soon as possible under a microscope to determine the sperm count and motility. A count over 20 million sperm per cc is considered in the normal range; below 10 million per cc is considered poor. Yet men with low sperm counts *can* impregnate. The sperm must be able to swim in a forward motion and at least 60 percent should be normal in size and shape.

Repeat the semen analysis at least one more time, since a man's sperm can fluctuate in count and motility for many reasons. If the semen analysis is abnormal, your partner should pursue his own diagnosis before you have further tests done.

Any diagnosis of infertility can make things difficult for both man and woman.

My husband's sperm count was very low; we were both crushed. I don't think my husband believed it was actually happening. In fact, he often talked in the third person, not truly accepting the results. I love him and therefore hurt for him. I didn't know what to say. I couldn't say the typical, "Oh, it's all right" because we both knew it really wasn't all right. For some reason, I found I could handle a problem with myself but found it very difficult to handle my reaction to his problem. I was even more concerned that he couldn't handle his problem. Then we started seeing doctors for him.

If all male factors are normal, study of the woman will continue. You may need to have a

5. *Postcoital test (Sims-Hühner test).* Just before you expect to ovulate you will make love with your partner and within several hours will arrive at your doctor's office without washing or douching. The doctor will take a small amount of mucus from your vagina and cervix to be studied for the number of live, active sperm. A normal test result shows that sperm have the ability to penetrate cervical mucus and live in this environment. This test may be combined with another, also done at this time in your cycle, called

6. *Tubal insufflation (Rubin test).* A gas, carbon dioxide, is blown under carefully monitored pressure into your uterus through the cervix. Normally it will escape out the tubes into the surrounding cavity, causing shoulder pain when you sit up. (It is eventually absorbed into your body.) If the gas doesn't pass readily, pressure will be increased within safe limits. If the results are abnormal, it may be repeated or confirmed by X-ray studies. The Rubin test indicates that blockages exist but can't tell where they are located. As a result this test is now often being replaced by the

7. *Utero-tubogram,* also called *hysterosalpingogram,* which allows for direct visualization of the tubes and provides a permanent record that can be used for comparison if future X-rays are needed. Doctors usually perform this procedure in the first part of the cycle, before ovulation, to prevent possible X-ray exposure of a fertilized egg if conception has occurred.* It involves injecting a harmless dye into the vagina and uterus. The dye should pass up through the uterus to the tubes and out into the abdominal cavity. A series of X-rays are taken during this process. The dye then passes out into the surrounding cavity and your body reabsorbs it. This test can be painful, especially if pressure is used to get the dye to pass through the tubes. Practitioners may give you local cervical anesthesia or an oral medication to help you relax before this test.

*Remember that whenever you have X-rays, you are irradiating all future eggs.

423

8. *Blood levels of the hormones* estrogen, progesterone and prolactin as well as urine tests will be done to determine if your hormone levels are normal and whether ovulation has occurred.

9. *An endometrial biopsy* is another test to determine whether you are ovulating. It can be done any time from a week after ovulation is suspected to the first day of your period.* The doctor inserts a small instrument into your uterus after partially dilating your cervix (this will cause some unpleasant cramping), scrapes a tiny piece of tissue from the lining of the uterus (endometrium) and sends it to be examined microscopically. Tissue formed while progesterone is being produced (after ovulation) is different from tissue formed under the influence of estrogen (before ovulation) or in the absence of hormonal influence. Hormonal levels in urine and blood serum can also be helpful in diagnosis of ovulation and the total hormone picture.

10. If s/he finds no problem, your doctor may want to do a *culdoscopy* or *laparoscopy*, hospital procedures which allow direct visualization of the tubes, ovaries, exterior of the uterus and the surrounding cavities. In culdoscopy, a small incision is made in the back wall of your vagina; in laparoscopy, an incision is made near your navel. Both tests are done under general or spinal anesthesia and can yield a great deal of information.†

When you are going through these tests, once again your sex life comes under "scientific scrutiny."

We were supposed to make love at seven o'clock in the morning and then I had to run to my doctor's for the postcoital test. Who feels like making love at seven in the morning during a busy week anyway?

You also become a "public" figure. Relatives ask you, "Well, has it happened yet?" Or, worse, they don't say anything, but they look at you and sigh a lot. People you hardly know may comment on your problem. Hopefully, during these times you can support each other and learn to keep both your sense of humor and your sense of the awesomeness and privacy of sexuality.

TREATMENT

In 90 percent of cases a reason is found for the infertility. Your doctor should talk with you both and outline a plan for treatment.

*Doctors differ greatly in their thinking on the timing. Many think that taking such a minute piece of tissue presents no danger to a new conceptus. Others avoid possible hazard to a pregnancy by having the woman come in on the day her temperature drops, or even at the time her period starts. Some doctors advise using a condom during relations in this cycle so there will be no worry over a possible pregnancy.

†Some doctors prefer to do these procedures first; others do them as a last resort.

In general, male problems respond poorly to medical treatment. However, various hormones, also used to treat female infertility (clomiphene citrate, HCG [human chorionic gonadotropin], HMG [human menopausal gonadotropin]), are now being tried with good success in the male. A varicocele can be corrected surgically, with a rise in sperm count and motility usually seen three months after surgery. The stress of waiting to hear the results can take its toll on couples. Insemination with your mate's sperm is sometimes used if the count is low, in the hopes that with proper placement at the time of insemination chances of conception will be increased. If infection is causing a decrease in sperm motility, it may be corrected by treatment with antibiotics.

For women, treatment for endocrine disorders currently offers the highest degree of success. Doctors use a variety of drugs to correct hormonal imbalances, to help induce ovulation and to correct problems in the luteal phase (after ovulation).

The main drugs used to induce ovulation are clomiphene citrate; HCG, a hormone extracted from the human placenta; and HMG (trade name Pergonal), extracted from the urine of menopausal women.

Clomiphene citrate was introduced in the 1960s and is a commonly used infertility drug. It is taken orally on the fifth to the tenth day of the cycle. It appears to act directly upon the hypothalamus in the brain and causes it to produce more of the hormones FSH (follicle-stimulating hormone) and LH (luteinizing hormone), which then stimulate the ovary to ripen and release an egg. About 80 percent of women will ovulate with the help of this drug, and about 50 percent will become pregnant, with a 5 to 10 percent incidence of multiple births. Some women experience breast tenderness, hot flashes, headaches, blurred vision and throbbing feelings in the ovaries at the time of ovulation while on clomiphene citrate. A potential complication is hyperstimulation of the ovary which, if undetected, may result in ovarian damage. Ideally, women on this medication should have a checkup at the end of each cycle to be sure this complication isn't developing.

HCG is often combined with clomiphene citrate and given intramuscularly near the time of expected ovulation. It acts like LH on the ovary and helps the developing egg ripen and release.

HMG is a very potent hormone used to induce ovulation, and should only be prescribed by an infertility specialist. Treatment with HMG involves frequent injections of the drug and often daily visits to a laboratory where blood and urine are examined for estrogen levels. Some doctors also use ultrasound to monitor the development of the ovarian follicle(s).* By monitoring these levels carefully, the danger of multiple eggs being released from the ovary and consequent

*The effect of ultrasound on the ovary is unknown.

multiple births is reduced. Ovarian hyperstimulation is also a possible complication of use of this drug.

Bromocriptine is another drug used to treat female infertility due to high levels of the hormone prolactin in the blood. In breastfeeding mothers, prolactin levels are normally elevated. Occasionally this hormone is elevated in the infertile woman as well. It appears that high prolactin levels can disturb normal ovulatory patterns. In such cases, bromocriptine is taken orally until prolactin levels fall and normal ovulation results.

Problems in the luteal phase of the cycle may be treated with any or all of the following: clomiphene citrate, HCG and natural progesterone. Natural progesterone is available in vaginal suppositories or given via intramuscular injections. You usually insert the suppositories twice daily, starting after ovulation. Synthetic forms of progesterone are not advised, as they can be harmful to fetal development in an unsuspected pregnancy.

Surgical techniques can often correct cervical weakness and various structural problems of the uterus. Microsurgery is a special type of surgery used to repair tubes and to remove adhesions. Laser surgery using the carbon dioxide laser is also being used, often in combination with microsurgery, to remove scar tissue or endometrial adhesions. Endometriosis can be treated surgically and/or with oral medications. Cervical mucus problems, depending on their cause, are treated with hormones or a form of steroid (not a common treatment; effects are fluid retention and masking of other infections). Special douches can help if the mucus is overly acid.

Women often have a combination of problems, and their treatment may involve a combination of several medications, many of which are expensive. It is important to understand how these drugs work, how they affect you and how long you should use them. (See p. 36 for more information on the informed use of drugs.)

Shared infertility problems are usually treated by separate doctors. The man goes to a urologist and the woman to a gynecologist or infertility specialist. *Your doctors must communicate with each other.* For any couple with a shared problem, the potential to achieve pregnancy is improved dramatically if even one member of the couple can be treated and helped. If both of you can be helped, then your chances are excellent.

In all cases, there is a 5 percent spontaneous cure rate (a cure without any treatment whatever). Often, after many years of trying, pregnancy will finally occur. We do not understand these spontaneous cures well, but the fact that they do happen is a source of hope when all else fails.

In "inconclusive" infertility there are usually no clear-cut medical reasons. It can be difficult for you and your doctor to know when to stop the tests, to put away the thermometer or to stop various treatments. Your feelings of hopefulness may give way to depression, often a painful process. In the case of "conclusive" or "absolute" infertility, you have the facts from the doctor. You must now adjust to that reality and re-examine your life. You may feel as if "the death of all your babies" has occurred. You may feel grief for the loss of a part of womanhood or manhood, for the parts of you that don't work or have been cut out of you. If you deny or repress this feeling of grief, you prolong the process of its resolution. Somewhere inside you are dealing with the experience. You have the choice of living it as consciously and directly as you can or suppressing these very natural but painful emotions. Sometimes the pain of infertility is never completely resolved but is accepted as a familiar ache which may recur, unpredictably, throughout life. Grieving often takes a long time.* To do your "grief work," the support of friends, family and other people who have experienced infertility can be helpful.

In July of last year I underwent hysterectomy at the age of twenty-nine. Needless to say, I was crushed with grief. I never had the chance to have a baby and then all hope was snatched away. In my case it had to be done—fibroid tumors had practically destroyed my uterus (there were twenty-one, to be exact). I was very bitter for a while, but now I am healing. That is not to say I don't hurt sometimes; I think a pain this deep will always come back from time to time.

After learning of my untreatable infertility five years ago, I experienced the usual shock and denial. Unfortunately, I pushed down all other stages and feelings by submerging myself in work. Eventually we adopted a son and all seemed right with the world. I thought I had everything together, as I rarely thought of my infertility and was very active.

Last fall, for no obviously apparent reason, my infertility again became a prominent concern, and all the feelings I had submerged five years ago resurfaced. After four unstable months I ended up in severe, crippling depression.

Only with the help of counseling have I been able to begin to work through the feelings and to come out of my depressed state.

I share this only in the hope of helping someone else not to fall into the trap of thinking they have worked through to resolution their infertility, when in reality they have only dealt with the problem on an intellectual level. The pain of the past four months has been as intense as when I first learned of the diagnosis of infertility. I feel that somehow I failed myself because five years ago I was too frightened of the pain to face it. The truth is, it has to be faced sooner or later, and hopefully all the way to resolution.

*Some people immediately block this feeling of grief by planning to adopt. The adoption is more likely to be happy and successful if you can "work out" the grief.

It was relieving to meet and talk openly with other couples experiencing infertility. Each of us had our own specific difficulties but our feelings and reactions were quite similar. After the initial nervousness that accompanied our first two meetings, I began to feel much more accepting and able to deal with the previous two and a half years that had given us two pregnancies and two miscarriages. My almost constant obsession with pregnancy was lifted. I began to feel in touch with myself and somewhat alive again.

MISCARRIAGE

Another form of infertility results from problems in carrying a pregnancy the full nine months. One in six pregnancies ends in miscarriage, 75 percent of these before twelve weeks. Miscarriage, then, is a fairly common event. We want to be at least minimally prepared to know how it feels and what to expect. Miscarriage is both a physical event for a woman and a serious emotional crisis which may be shared by both of you or experienced by each of you in very different ways. Miscarriages are usually unexpected the first time. They most often come at the joyful time of early pregnancy, and thus are all the more of a shock.

When I found out I was pregnant, I danced around the house. My pregnancy was an easy one....My body was slowly and pleasantly changing. Because it was a conscious and well-thought-out decision to have a child, I felt free to revel in my pregnancy and motherhood. It was a special time. I mention all of this because having a miscarriage has to do with the loss of something so deeply ingrained for so long that it is partially by understanding the depth of the joy that one can understand the depth of the loss.

The term for miscarriage before twenty-six weeks is *spontaneous abortion*. If it is a *threatened abortion*, the cervix is still closed but the woman is experiencing cramps and bleeding or staining. Often bed rest is advised, and your doctor may order specific blood tests to check your hormone levels. In *inevitable abortion*, bleeding becomes heavy, cramps increase and the cervix begins to dilate. The fetus, amniotic sac and placenta, along with a lot of blood, may be expelled completely intact. You'll probably know when this is happening. It's very important to say here that if you are not in a hospital you must do the difficult task of collecting fetus and afterbirth, putting them in a clean container and taking them to a laboratory for examination. This will yield important information as to why you miscarried. Ask that specialized as well as routine tests be done, such as cultures for infection and genetic overview of tissues. If tests show you have lost a "blighted pregnancy" (where egg and sperm together have failed to divide correctly) then you can

try to be more at ease, knowing that this has been a random event and that the chances of it happening again are as small as before. If a study of the fetal tissue shows genetic abnormalities or suggests that you had an illness or infection, you'll work with your doctor on how to proceed. If the fetal tissue is normal, you may learn that your hormone levels were insufficient or that a weak cervix was at fault. Both of these conditions can be treated.

An *incomplete abortion* means that only part of the "products of conception" has been passed. Part remains within, and bleeding will continue. Usually a doctor will do a dilation and curettage (D and C) to clean out your uterus so that it will heal. A *complete abortion* means that everything in your uterus has been expelled. You will continue to bleed, but less and less. If you think you are bleeding too long, consult your doctor. (A D and C may be necessary.)

You may also experience a *missed abortion*. In this case, a fetus dies in the uterus but is not expelled. It can remain within for several months. Signs are lack of menstrual periods coupled with cessation of signs of pregnancy; sometimes there is spotting. Treatment is either a D and C or induction of labor.

Some possible causes for miscarriage are structural problems of the uterus, infection, weak cervical muscles, hormonal imbalances, environmental and industrial toxins, blood incompatibility between mother who is Rh negative and fetus who is Rh positive (there is now a drug, Rhogam, which can be given to women to prevent this reaction) and genetic error. Some research shows that 50 to 60 percent of all first-trimester miscarriages are caused by genetic abnormalities in the fetus. These miscarriages can be "nature's way" of screening out problems.

Try to learn why you had a miscarriage. Some of the diagnostic procedures outlined above for infertility will be useful here. Ask to see the pathology report, and ask that all terminology be explained fully. If you are not satisfied with the explanation, ask if there are other tests that can be done. It is your right to learn as much as possible about your miscarriage.

One miscarriage does not mean you are infertile. There is a 70 percent chance that you will have a successful pregnancy even after two miscarriages. However, if you have two or more in a row you may want to begin investigating. Plan with your doctor to check out each detail of your next pregnancy as it progresses, including possible reasons for any spotting or cramps, definite ways to deal with contingencies, tests to be made as they become necessary and so forth. You will need encouragement in this project from your partner, friends and/or a support group, possibly one geared to childbearing problems.

The time following a miscarriage is difficult. Physically, your body may still feel pregnant for a while, your breasts full and tender, your stomach enlarged. You may continue spotting for several weeks. If you have increased flow or odd- or foul-smelling discharge or a fever, contact your doctor. It is usually safe to have sexual intercourse after four to six weeks when your cervix is closed and there is less risk of infection.

You may not believe what is happening. During the miscarriage, feelings of helplessness may develop as cramping and bleeding increase. Many women fear that they may bleed to death. Having to go to the hospital may intensify your anxiety and fear.

We went home from the hospital dazed and tired. I was weak and enormously sad. I don't know that I've ever experienced such deep emotional pain. The loss was so great and so complete in the way that only death is. For the first few days I couldn't talk to anyone, but at the same time it was painful to be alone. I would just cry and cry without stopping. One of the clearest reminders that I was no longer pregnant was all the speedy changes my body went through. Within two days my breasts, which had grown quite swollen, were back to their normal size. My stomach, which had grown hard, was now soft again. My body was no longer preparing for the birth of a child. It was simple and blatant. Tiredness was replaced with weakness. And then there was the bleeding. My body would not let me forget. I knew things would improve once we could make love again and would be even better when we were full of hope. But it seemed so far away.

You will almost always feel grief and anger. You will need family and friends.

Most people didn't know how to give me support, and perhaps I didn't really know how to ask for it. People were more comfortable talking about the physical and not the emotional side of miscarriage. I needed to talk about both. It was also difficult for my husband, because people could at least ask how my body was doing. Unfortunately, he would sometimes be completely bypassed when someone called to talk with us, despite the fact that he, too, was in deep emotional pain.

Feelings of grief are often complicated by guilt, which can cause tension between you and your partner. You may wonder if either of you did something "wrong" (too much activity, too much sex, not enough good food, etc.). You will be blaming each other unnecessarily, for such factors rarely cause miscarriage. Dispelling the tension will take a while, longer for some than for others. It is best if you acknowledge and talk out your feelings. The effects of the miscarriage can last for months. On the date when the baby would have been born, there is usually a resurgence of grief.

If you experience more than three miscarriages, it is important to see a doctor who specializes in this problem. You will need one who is skilled and also compassionate and understanding of the losses you have experienced, and of how very precious these preg-

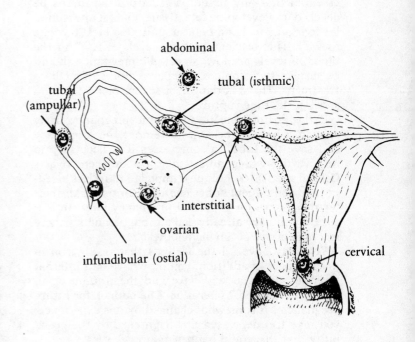

Nina Reimer

ECTOPIC PREGNANCY

nancies were to you. Such doctors are rare. Your helplessness and hopelessness may increase if you begin or return to treatments for your infertility and start working on becoming pregnant again.

ECTOPIC PREGNANCY

Ectopic pregnancy is another form of infertility. Pregnancy loss results because the fertilized egg starts developing in the tube instead of in the uterus. Between 5 and 10 percent of women who have had previous tubal surgery may experience ectopic pregnancy, but it can happen to any woman. Ectopic pregnancies are on the rise because of the increased incidence of PID and use of IUDs, which can result in scar formation on the tubes or inflammation of the uterine lining, which then "resists" implantation of the fertilized egg. If you're old enough to bear a child, have had intercourse and feel abdominal pains you don't understand, it's possible you have an ectopic pregnancy.

Because all the hormonal changes are similar to those of a normal early pregnancy, you can have all the early signs of pregnancy, such as fatigue, nausea, missed period and breast tenderness. As the pregnancy progresses, causing pressure in the tube, symptoms such as stabbing pain, cramps or a dull ache may become severe. In addition, you may or may not have menstrual-type bleeding. Ectopic pregnancy is sometimes misdiagnosed as an early spontaneous abortion. It is essential that any tissue passed from the uterus be checked for developing fetal tissue, that an ultrasound be done and/or that a beta subunit blood test be done as well. This test can pick up levels of HCG in the blood. If levels are low, an ectopic pregnancy should be suspected. Ectopic pregnancy requires immediate treatment. There is danger of severe blood loss and shock if the tube ruptures.

If the doctor detects an ectopic pregnancy early enough, s/he may be able to remove the pregnancy and save the tube. In some cases it is necessary to remove the whole tube and/or the adjacent ovary. Careful surgical technique is important; the less bleeding and consequent adhesions and scar tissue, the better the chance for a normal pregnancy later. In any case, if you have already had a tubal pregnancy there is a higher risk of having another.

You may have all the feelings that result from a miscarriage. In addition, you may have had internal bleeding, and you will have had the trauma of an emergency surgical operation. The outlook for future pregnancies is somewhat changed by this experience: you may feel depressed and frightened by the possibility that this could happen again.

STILLBIRTH

Stillbirth is fortunately a rare occurrence. But if it happens to you, statistics mean nothing. Usually it is the result of the baby's oxygen supply failing before it can be safely born or failure of its lungs or heart to oxygenate its system after the cord is cut.

Your body knows nothing about stillbirth. It is elaborately prepared for the close contact and physical nurturing of a baby. Your breasts are filled with milk, never to be used. (In some cultures, women who lose babies at birth frequently hire out as wet nurses to nurture other babies in place of the ones they have lost. The wet nurse is an esteemed person in these cultures.) You and members of your family are also prepared for the event of a new baby.

Some considerations are in order if you suffer a stillbirth, beginning with the moment the death is expected or confirmed. If the baby's death takes place before labor and delivery, delivery in the quickest and least hazardous way possible is desirable. You should have the chance to decide if you want to go into labor spontaneously. Your partner should be present as long as either of you wish. Once the baby is delivered, birth attendants should handle her/him in a reverent manner, and must be especially careful when autopsy is indicated to find the cause of death. You will need to decide if you want to see the baby, either immediately afterward or later on. It can help you accept the tragic

reality of what has happened. Above all, if possible, you and your family must be allowed your grief in privacy if you need and want it. You may want a room away from the nursery; hospital personnel should be told that you have lost your baby. You may need to withdraw at first and not confront a reality which may be too much to bear. There may be a period of numbness. If you ask for help in grieving, we hope those around you will offer it intelligently and humanely. Platitudes such as "You'll have another baby before you know it" or "Think of your wonderful children at home" have no place in this situation. You are experiencing the death of this particular child—no other actual or potential children have any relevance. Perhaps the best help others can offer is sympathetic listening and close physical comforting.

It is important for you to understand exactly what happened to the baby. Most likely, whatever happened was totally beyond your control or the doctor's. (If you do suspect malpractice by your doctor, seek legal counsel quickly and have the facts analyzed.)

There is a tremendous sense of void and of loneliness following any pregnancy loss. Society has few ways of dealing with this particular type of loss and as a result you may feel alone in your grief.

ALTERNATIVES FOR INFERTILE COUPLES

Donor Insemination

Once it has been determined that you are infertile, you will wish to examine the possibilities and alternatives for the future. You may once again find yourself asking, "Do I really want to be a parent?" Take this time to redefine your goals and get on with living your life. If male infertility or a transmittable genetic disease is the problem, donor insemination is a possibility. (For more information, see the section on donor insemination in Chapter 17, "New Reproductive Technologies.")

In Vitro Fertilization

In vitro fertilization is another alternative for some infertile women. More and more medical centers are offering this technique. At present, success rates for a successful ovulation, induction, fertilization, implantation and then a viable pregnancy are about 20 percent. The cost is 4,000 to 5,000 dollars per ovulatory cycle and you may need to undergo the treatment for several cycles. Insurance coverage is very poor. Obviously, *in vitro* fertilization is not a solution for the lower- or middle-income couple struggling with infertility. (For more information, see the section on *in vitro* fertilization in Chapter 17, "New Reproductive Technologies.")

Adoption

Adoption (an institution which has been undergoing significant change) may be an alternative for many infertile couples. But as the number of available children decreases, adoption becomes more difficult. It is most difficult to adopt Caucasian babies; many states have a five- to seven-year waiting list. Many white couples consider adoption of children of color, infants or children from other countries, special-needs children and older children, as the waiting periods are much shorter.

The adoption process raises many negative feelings, often surprisingly similar to the ones experienced during the first stages of coping with infertility. Feelings of powerlessness, anger and frustration are common, especially during the time of the so-called "home study," when the social worker is working actively with you. You may feel that s/he is evaluating and "testing" you on your potential as a parent. The home study can be lengthy and expensive (anywhere from 500 to 1,500 dollars) and often puts a strain once again on your relationship with your partner. Families and friends may not be as supportive as you would like, and you may go through periods of anxiety.

My husband and I found out we might become prospective parents in April. That gave us about seven to eight weeks to think about this. I had many things going through my mind. So many things could happen in the interim. The birth mother could still change her mind. I wondered what the child would be like. The baby's looks, personality, health—everything is unknown....

I thought a lot about bonding. I wondered what I'd feel like when someone put an infant in my arms saying, "Congratulations! You are a mother. This is your child." Who is this stranger? How am I supposed to love someone I do not even know? How am I supposed to feel? I believe these are healthy feelings, but still it is frightening to think about....

I believe couples facing adoption go through the same feelings that biological parents go through—the fears, insecurities, the great change of lifestyle. The only problem is that you do not have nine months to work your feelings through. It is like being told you are eight months pregnant.

The majority of adoptions today take place through social agencies, but there are still many "family" adoptions (people adopt a relative's child) and "private" adoptions, where a physician or lawyer arranges things. There is also an underground market for adoptions, where white babies are sold for extravagant sums (as much as 10,000 dollars each). Other countries' adoption policies vary considerably, from much more liberal laws than ours to more extremely restrictive.

It is helpful to talk with other adoptive parents and to join an adoption group (see Resources). Adoption should not feel second best; it should be a positive decision which you are comfortable with and excited about. When you decide to adopt, you will feel "pregnant," as excitement, anxiety, vulnerability and joy infuse your daily life until the child is placed in your home. Like all new mothers, you will make the transition from being childless to having a child with a variety of responses. And, like any new family, you will all need the support of friends and family.

Adoption poses a number of problems which prospective adoptive parents need to think about in advance. At first, like many parents, you may be totally focused on the baby as a baby, getting to know her/him and learning how to cope. The future seems far away, and the child as an adult seems remote. But as adopted children start to grow up and reach their teens, they may have very powerful feelings about being adopted which they do not always express.

In recent years, more and more adoptees have begun speaking out about their experiences, demanding access to information about their origins and searching for—and sometimes finding—their birth parents. Many now believe it is a human right, if not a constitutional right, to be able to know one's biological origins. (Constitutional challenges by adoptees to the sealed-record laws are now underway.) National organizations have been formed which support and assist searching adoptees. They also fight for changes in the laws and in the practices of social agencies which keep this knowledge secret. In many cases adoptive parents have become involved in helping their adoptive children with the search, as they have come to understand how important this knowledge and these experiences are to their children.

At the same time, the original parents, "birth parents" as they call themselves today, especially birth mothers, have also begun to speak out about their experiences, describing in many cases the abuse that constituted the adoption experience for them, including coercion by misleading information and by circumstances they could not control to give up their babies against their will. As one said, "If the adoptees hadn't come out of the closet, we birth mothers probably never would have." Birth parents, too, have formed national organizations for support, for help in searching for their adult children and with their efforts to change the adoption laws. Birth mothers tell us they never forget (contrary to what many social workers insist), that they passionately desire to know about their children's welfare and to see them if possible. They tell us that they did not surrender their children because they *didn't* care about them or love them (as adoptive parents and social workers sometimes suggest to adoptees) but because they *did*. They surrendered them because they believed, as they had been told, that their children would have a better life with other parents. Many birth mothers can never begin to heal from their "surrender" experience until they have been reunited with their children. (See p. 287 for more.)

Some adoptive parents and some of the larger social agencies in conservative areas have banded together and tried to stop this searching. They presume to speak for all adoptees and birth parents who, they claim, prefer the anonymity of the present situation. These groups are powerful and well-organized and have spent hundreds of thousands of dollars to lobby legislatures all across the country to require records to be sealed tighter than ever. They have no good answers to the powerful feelings the adoptees and birth mothers express, but appeal instead to conservative adoptive parents and members of the social work profession to preserve the status quo (see Appendix).

Very few studies have been done to verify the assumptions and the dogma on which the practice of adoption social work is carried out. These underlying assumptions usually are based on either traditional religious moral beliefs or Freudian psychoanalytic beliefs. The few studies which have been done demonstrate that these beliefs deny or neglect the true feelings and experiences of all those involved in the adoption process. We need to challenge the traditional assumptions and practices of social workers which have labeled certain feelings and desires "abnormal" and have distorted the experiences and needs of adoptees, birth mothers and adoptive parents alike.

The leadership in the social work profession today has begun to change; the emerging feeling seems to be that it is no longer possible for agencies to guarantee adoptive parents that they will never meet or hear from birth parents, or that adoptees will never be able to know their biological parents. As one social worker said, "We have forgotten who our real client is in all this controversy. It is the adoptee, and the needs of the adoptee, that should be uppermost in our thinking and planning."

Those who are involved in the movement to open records to separated family members are also proposing something called "open adoption," in which the contract between adoptee, birth parents and adoptive parents would not be closed at adoption but would remain open, allowing for visiting and communication, even though legal custody would, of course, remain with the adoptive parents. "Just knowing that she is all right, doing well, would have been such a relief," one birth mother said.

Loyalty to their adoptive parents often prevents many adoptees from expressing a desire to know their birth parents. Many adoptive parents fear that they will somehow "lose" their children and so become childless once again. Birth mothers or fathers fear rejection, not being "good enough" to measure up to their children's expectations, just as they once felt "not

good enough" to become the parents of their offspring. Nothing can really alleviate these fears the way going through the experience of a reunion can, but no one is ready in exactly the same way or at exactly the same time as anyone else. Searching is not for everyone. Some never search and never express the desire. Many remain in this position for years until something happens to release in them the desire to know.

Reunions may be brief or temporary or may grow into more long-lasting relationships. Sometimes there are painful rejections on one side or another. But most who have been through it agree that any knowledge at all is better than no knowledge, even if the mother is found in a mental hospital, or the father dead, or the son a murderer, as some have found. "When I saw how much it meant to her, I wished we had done something about it sooner," one adoptive mother said.

As a potential adoptive parent, you owe it to yourself and your future adopted child to investigate these controversies and hear the issues from all sides, but particularly from the adoptees. One important proposal to investigate is the idea of a separate legal contract, to be signed at the time of the adoption, in which you would agree to provide information to the agency from time to time about the child's progress, and in which the agency would agree to act as a go-between between you and the birth parents. In this way the agony of searching (often without success) would not be necessary, and adoptees could meet their birth parents easily as soon as they were ready. Birth mothers would be spared the torment of silence and lack of knowledge. And if we are to believe the adoptees, the relationship with the adoptive parents usually improves, if there is any change at all.

APPENDIX

In most states the legal status of an adoptee is different from that of all other persons in society, no matter how old the adoptee is. Usually, the original birth certificate is sealed permanently and a new, falsified certificate is issued by the state as if the adoptive parents had actually given birth to the child. Originally designed primarily to protect "privacy"—that is, to protect children from the "stigma of illegitimacy" as well as to protect the birth parents from the "stigma" of being "unwed mothers" or "unwed parents"—this practice results in an adopted person being barred *forever* from knowing his or her biological origins. But since the child's adoptive status is usually known anyway, his/her "illegitimacy" is already presumed. While the law in a few states has been changed to make it possible for adoptees to petition the court to open the sealed record for a "good purpose" (usually medical information), most adult adoptees are still in a sort of permanent "chattel" relationship to the state, since the state possesses crucial information about them which it will not reveal, even to their adoptive parents.

The notion that the birth mother is somehow being protected by these laws has also been challenged by the birth mothers themselves, many of whom say, "We renounce any desire for anonymity; we never asked for it, especially not from our own children." Temporary efforts to solve these problems, until and unless laws can be changed, are 1. reunion registries, which have been proposed even at the federal level, to match up persons seeking one another, so that only those who were seeking *mutually* could find one another; 2. open records, which could be made available to the adoptee at any point, or only at majority; 3. agencies playing a go-between role at the mutual request of parties involved.

RESOURCES*

Readings

Amelar, Richard D., M.D., Lawrence Dubin, M.D., and Patrick C. Walsh, M.D. *Male Infertility.* Philadelphia: W. B. Saunders Co., 1977.

Borg, Susan, and Judith Lasker. *When Pregnancy Fails: Families Coping with Miscarriage, Stillbirth and Infant Death.* Boston: Beacon Press, 1981.

Corson, Stephen L., M.D. *Conquering Infertility.* Norwalk, CT: Appleton-Century Crofts, 1983.

Graham, Katrina Maxtone. *An Adopted Woman.* New York: Remi Books, 205 E. 78th Street, New York, NY 10021. A moving and very detailed account of the author's search and her battle against the agency which placed her.

MacNamara, Joan. *The Adoption Advisor.* New York: Hawthorne Books, Inc., 1975.

Martin, Cynthia D. *Beating the Adoption Game.* La Jolla, CA: Oak Tree Publications, 1980.

Menning, Barbara Eck. *Infertility: A Guide for the Childless Couple.* Englewood Cliffs, NJ: Prentice-Hall, Inc., 1977.

Plumez, Jacqueline Hornar. *Successful Adoption.* New York: Harmony Books, 1982.

Organizations

American Adoption Congress
P.O. Box 23641
Washington, DC 20024

DES Action National Offices
Long Island Jewish Hillside Medical Center
New Hyde Park, NY 11040

Endometriosis Association
c/o Bread and Roses Women's Health Center
238 West Wisconsin Avenue
Milwaukee, WI 53202

National Association for the Childless
Birmingham Settlement
318 Summer Lane
Birmingham, England B19 3RL

Open Door Society
Check telephone book for local listing. Provides a newsletter and adoptive-parent group.

Resolve, Inc.
National Headquarters
P.O. Box 474
Belmont, MA 02178

A self-help organization which provides telephone counseling, doctor referrals, support groups, literature; it has chapters in over forty states.

*Please see the Resources for Chapter 15, "If You Think You Are Pregnant: Finding Out and Deciding What to Do," for more information about adoption.

V
WOMEN
GROWING OLDER

22

WOMEN GROWING OLDER

By Paula Brown Doress, with Norma Meras Swenson, Robin Cohen, Mickey Friedman, Lois Harris and Kathleen MacPherson

With special thanks to Edith Fletcher, Ruth Hubbard, Barbara Krentzman, Lucile Longview Schuck, Anna Shenke, Anne Smith (all members of the Older Women's Group) and to Marian Saunders and Diana Siegal.

Menopause by Louise Corbett

With special thanks to Tish Anisimov, Davi Birnbaum, Lorraine Doherty, Ruth Hubbard, Kathleen MacPherson, Audrey Michaud, Josephine Polk-Matthews and Diana Siegal (all members of the Menopause Collective)

The "Menopause" chapter in previous editions was written by Meg Hickey, Irene Davidson, Pamela Berger and Judy Norsigian.

...My birthday started with my standing wet on the hilltop watching lightning zag straight down to the earth—moving from north to west—then work in the studio—then a friend with gifts, then two loved sculptor apprentices with flowers and a salad fresh with surprises and green and fruits like flowers....

And when well-wishers hoping to please me referred to this birthday as my 29th, I asserted my conviction that 78 was far more wonderful than 29![1]

Several groups of women participated in discussions about this chapter, which covers the decades in a woman's life from the forties through the eighties and beyond. The Menopause Collective wrote the section on menopause. An older women's group, ages fifty-two to seventy-eight, meeting over the course of a year, talked about their lives, provided important resources, pinpointed issues and contributed to the writing and editing. A midlife group, ages thirty-nine to fifty-six, met with us in a series of sessions and became a support group for each other; they also met with the older women's group a number of times to gain perspectives on their own lives and those of their parents.

Women experience so many changes—physical, social, economic and emotional—during these decades that we can't do justice to them in a short chapter. Yet, because older women's concerns are so often overlooked, even in feminist books, it is important to begin.*

*Readers are invited to contribute experiences, ideas and poetry to the Midlife and Older Women Book Project, 28 Leamington Road, Brighton, MA 02135, for a new book being written in cooperation with the Boston Women's Health Book Collective by some of the authors of this chapter.

THE CONTEXT IN WHICH WE GROW OLDER

Age and Ageism

Someday each of us will be old if we live long enough. Most of us want to live a long life, yet our ageist culture values neither aging nor being old, and separates people by age and generation.

Ageism is systematic discrimination against persons because of their chronological age. It permeates our thinking in subtle and unconscious ways so that the discrimination against elders which goes on in every one of our social institutions appears to be "just the way things are"—until we name and confront it.

Ageism has several sources. First, our society denies the reality of infirmity and death, especially because many of us secretly cherish a belief in our own immortality. Infirmity threatens our national ideology of rugged independence. We isolate the aging and infirm to avoid acknowledging our ultimate interdependence and our own fears of infirmity and death. This massive denial discourages us from planning for our later years.

Second, isolation of elders and dismissal of their skills and wisdom is particularly prevalent in times of rapid social and technological change, when we may forget that we can still learn a lot about living from those who have a greater reservoir of life experience.

Finally, a major source of ageism in our profit-oriented system is the devaluing of all those who don't "produce"—the old, the young, and their caregivers.

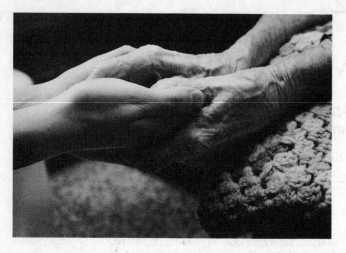

Bonnie Burt

For instance, some elders are pushed aside before we are ready to retire on the assumption that, once past a certain age, we can make no significant contribution.

Aging tends to exaggerate or deepen class differences. Wealthy elders are often able to maintain their economic position, while low-income persons inevitably grow poorer if they become ill and can't get paid work anymore. (This is especially true for women.)

Even as we ourselves age, we discriminate against older people.

I had always said, "Oh, I want to be with people of all ages, or with young people," but in fact I was avoiding being with people my own age—which would mean admitting I'm an old person—and missing out on a lot because of it!

I signed up for a weekend of hiking through the Elderhostels,* and that changed my mind. Everyone was so alert. We were all in sports clothes and we didn't have our hair waved just right. We're not Amazons by any means, just people interested in vigorous outdoor activity. [a woman in her seventies]

Midlife and elder women have taken action against stereotyped media images which foster ageism. The Gray Panthers and the Older Women's League conduct "media watches," and many individuals are keeping alert.

Every time I see a positive image of an older woman on TV, I write a complimentary letter to the sponsor of the program. And when I see something offensive, I let them know that, too.

*Elderhostels (see Resources for the address) is an adult education program for older people. Courses are given on a weekly basis with living arrangements in dormitories, usually in the summer. Many elders are also taking courses for credit and enrolled in degree programs. Further education is one of the greatest unmet needs of elders.

There have been successes: e.g., the images of midlife and older women depicted in medical journal ads have improved noticeably in the past decade.

Ageism, not age itself, is what limits elders. The fact that I can do things at seventy that when I was sixty would have been frowned upon as inappropriate for an older woman shows how absurd ageism is, and how much difference changing social attitudes can make. Every time we speak out, we change attitudes. Affirming ourselves is something that's in the air now. That makes a lot more things possible.

The Feminization of Aging

The single most significant fact about our aging as women is that the population of older persons is overwhelmingly female. Women live, on the average, eight years longer than men. And more people are living longer than ever before.*

RATIO OF WOMEN TO MEN IN THREE AGE GROUPS

Up to Age 45   ♀ ♀ ♀   ♂ ♂ ♂

Numbers are approximately equal—women 51 percent, men 49 percent. At age forty-five, the gap first begins to widen.

Over 65   ♀ ♀ ♀   ♂ ♂

By age sixty-five, women comprise 59 percent and men 41 percent. Women over sixty-five are the fastest-growing segment of the U.S. population. Between 1960 and 1970, the number of women over sixty-five increased twice as fast as the number of men over sixty-five.

Over 75   ♀ ♀ ♀   ♂

Women's longevity rates continue to outstrip those of men. Women's life expectancy is eighty-one; men's is 71.8. Women are two-thirds of the over-seventy-five population.[2]

The problems which arise with aging—chronic illness, insufficient economic resources, caregiving or needing care, surviving one's relatives and closest friends—are predominantly women's problems. Yet the researchers and policy makers have mainly been men who overlook older women's special concerns.

*People over sixty-five now make up 10 percent of the population of the United States and, if the trend continues, will be 25 percent of the population by 2020.

Because we are statistically "invisible," the resulting programs don't address our needs.

A positive side of our growing numbers is our potentially greater clout as a political constituency. Women over forty now make up more than 20 percent of the U.S. population. The government and the press are paying more attention to us. We need to take advantage of this attention to create, demand and fight for programs that will be responsive to midlife and older women's needs.*

Married or single, we must take friendships with women more seriously, for it is women who will most likely sustain us when we are older. Large numbers of women outlive their husbands, often by a decade or two, and a significant number even outlive their eldest sons.

I was brought up to believe that the people in my biological family were the most important people in my world. I'm still very attached to immediate family members but I have consciously extended my family to include my "sisters" in the women's community. [a woman in her fifties]

My loneliest times were during my marriage. I came out as a lesbian and my life with women has been a revelation. But so many women I meet don't understand my problems as a single parent and are younger than

*Write to us for a summary of "Concerns of Older Women," from the 1981 White House Conference on Aging. This report is often omitted when male speakers report on the conference. Make a copy and bring it to discuss at such meetings.

The Older Women's League is an important new national organization to advocate for older women's concerns. (See Resources.)

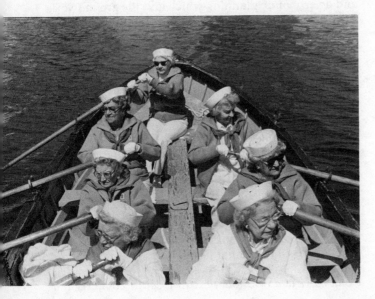

me. Coming to an older woman's meeting has made me realize that I want to meet more women my own age. [a woman in her forties]

I had never particularly liked women. When I was younger I remember thinking that men were where it was at; they were smart and they did things. I've rethought that a few times, especially after my experiences with death, divorce, major problems with children. We all have to deal with loss because we women are the ones who care for men when they are ill, and they are the ones who go first. It's given me a tremendous compassion for other women. [a woman in her sixties]

Ageism and Sexism—The Double-Edged Sword

The ageism we face is compounded by sexism and a double standard which considers women old at an earlier age than men.[3]

It was hard for me to tell the man I have been going out with how old I am. When I told him, I felt terrible, as if I were telling him I had some socially disgraceful disease. You can't imagine! [She is sixty-two; her friend is sixty.]

In fact, women have greater vitality. In terms of life expectancy, it can be argued that women are "younger" than men of the same age.

This double standard for aging leads us to accept the view that while older men are craggy, women are wrinkled; gray hair, distinguished on a man, shows that a woman is "over the hill"; maturity makes a man sexually attractive, a woman grandmotherly.

I'm never going to be a "gray-haired old lady," never! People don't listen to what you say anyway because you are a woman, but if you are an old woman, forget it. I'm going to dye my hair until I die.

Our culture sees the sexuality of midlife women and elders as a source of humor—grotesque, threatening or inappropriate. Such a prejudice arises in part from falsely equating sexuality with reproductive capacity.

Poverty

After a lifetime of being either unpaid or underpaid, it is no accident that older women are considerably poorer than older men.* The poverty rate for women over sixty-five is more than *double* that for men over sixty-five. The median income in 1980 for an older

*New studies of poverty in the 1970s and 1980s find that the new poor are single women with children.[4]

A RECENT POLL SHOWS THAT FOR MOST OLDER AMERICANS PROBLEMS OF POVERTY, LONELINESS, AND FEAR OF CRIME ARE A MYTH.

THERE ARE HOWEVER FOUR GROUPS THAT REPORT A DISMAL EXISTENCE.

THEY ARE: HISPANICS, BLACKS, PEOPLE MAKING UNDER $10,000 A YEAR,

AND WOMEN.

HEY! SOUNDS LIKE EVERYBODY'S HAPPY.

from "Sylvia" by Nicole Hollander

With women the majority of the older population, with the median income of married couples over sixty-two under 10,000 dollars, with blacks and Hispanics at least 10 percent of the aged population, it is truly amazing that this poll (reported in *The New York Times*, June 3, 1982) could designate these four groups as *exceptions*.
Nicole Hollander

white woman living alone was 3,087 dollars; for an older black woman living alone it was 2,385 dollars.[5] While many older women lack basic necessities, many more are faced with being poorer than when we were younger, struggling to get by on limited funds.

- There is neither compensation, recognition nor pension eligibility for women whose work is homemaking. When we return to the workforce later in life, we often must take jobs which pay extremely low wages.* Many midlife and older women find themselves unemployable for lack of "recent" experience.†
- Due to sex discrimination, women earn less and receive less income from retirement plans.
- Women often work in the kinds of marginal jobs and industries which are not unionized and do not provide benefits such as pensions.
- Many women are not in the paid labor force for enough years or for the particular years required for pension eligibility. The majority of women workers are employed from age seventeen to twenty-five, leave to raise a family and return to work sometime between thirty-five and forty-four. Yet employees are not eligible to join pension plans in most companies until age twenty-five, while in other companies new employees over forty-five are excluded.[8]
- Widowed or divorced women may find themselves ineligible for their husband's pensions. Many companies offer employees a choice of higher benefits in their lifetime or a reduced rate if spread over both spouses' lifetimes, and many husbands choose the former. Only 5 percent of widows collect on a deceased spouse's benefits. Widows are the majority of the elderly poor.[9]

Economic Planning

Many of the women in the elder women's group talked about how important it is to take ourselves seriously and do economic planning which lays the groundwork for having choices in our later years. Often we have to learn about money for the first time. The middle years—approximately forty-five to sixty-four—are critical for women economically. If we have not worked for pay before, in these key years we can work for pay, establish a retirement fund and plan for our older years as well.

I want to earn as much money as possible now before the potentials and the opportunities are completely gone. So I'm working harder, not necessarily because I want to but because I feel the time is getting shorter. [a woman in her fifties with grown children]

I'm envious of people who can plan for the future—I know it's wise. But I'm blocking out thinking about getting older because I can't deal with any more than the present. If I tried to put away money for the future I would have to do without the tiny creature comforts and

*Among women over forty-five, 48 percent work in retail sales, unskilled or semiskilled factory work, private household work and other service jobs; 28 percent do clerical work. While men's earnings peak in the middle years, women may have difficulty establishing or maintaining employability.[6]

†The requirement of "recent" experience, as Tish Sommers (of the Older Women's League) points out, is not overtly sexist or ageist, but its effect is to exclude older women. If we are unable to find work during our middle years, we are also ineligible for most income supports and services which are designed for mothers with children under eighteen or elders over sixty-five. In response to this abysmal situation, the Displaced Homemakers programs, started by two such women, offer counseling, job training and placement. (See Resources.)[7]

little delights of life which I want now. [a woman in her forties who is divorced and the sole support of her children]

Because we all are growing older, we all have a stake in supporting older women's demands and concerns. We have to work on upgrading women's jobs and salaries as well as learning to plan for ourselves. Many social changes that would help older women to participate more fully in the workplace are similar to those needed by younger women with children: caregiving services for children and sick family members, better access to health care, flexibility in jobs.

I developed a new material for sculpting after my husband died. No one knew about it until a few years ago when I was invited to come to the university as a visiting artist. So I started my teaching career at seventy-two. I had two classes for fifty students and taught one day a week for three years. Oh, how I loved it! It was wonderful! Then they restructured the school and got rid of all the part-time teachers, and I couldn't possibly undertake to do a full-time teaching load, so I had to stop teaching.

Working a nine-to-five job is not the only way of being "productive." We know that we contribute to society whether we are working for pay, raising children or grandchildren, caring for a sick family member or working in our communities as volunteers. Whatever our differences, we must stand together as we fight for the changes that will recognize and reward our contributions to our families and communities.

THE MIDDLE YEARS

Exploration, Growth and Expansion

Midlife, the years approximately between forty-five and sixty-five, is more a life stage than a particular chronological period. Midlife often announces itself with a surge of new energy, perhaps simply restlessness, or with a growing recognition that we are coming to the end of familiar roles and ways of living. We take stock of our lives, desire to use our time and our abilities in new and different ways.

One day after twenty-odd years of marriage and three children I asked myself, "Who am I? What am I doing? Where am I going?" The only answer I could come up with was "I am a wife and mother." That was only part of me—not all of me. When I was younger I used to have fairly clear edges, but over the years being the mother and wife with unmatched fervor made those edges fuzzy.

I loved my work as a nurse. I'd never married or had children. I always denied that I experienced sexism until,

when I was thirty-eight, a new male nurse was promoted to head of my service. That left me fuming. I used my life savings and then some to go back to college and then medical school. I've never been sorry.

I just want more! More time free of kids to focus on my work; more time to myself; more passion in my marriage, or from somewhere else! [a woman in her forties]

This surge of energy may come with release from two decades of child-rearing. Even while we miss our children, we can use freed-up time for refocusing—to acquire new skills, refine old ones, spend more time with people, get a job, work harder at our present job, enjoy time for reflection. It feels, as one woman puts it, like "getting ourselves back."

I am writing to assure women of middle age or beyond that it is not too late to attend school and begin a career, or to switch careers.

All my life I had wanted to be a nurse but instead was a secretary. Finally, at age fifty-seven, when the youngest of our children graduated from college, I took a year from the workaday world to attend school and become a licensed practical nurse.

I made the highest grade in our class on the state board exam. I am not telling this to be boastful but to encourage others who might think they are too old to learn.

Seven years later, at age sixty-five, I am happily employed as an LPN—my lifelong dream.

I returned to college for several reasons—as a response to a suddenly very empty house (three sons going away to school at once) and a major change (we had just moved to the country from a large city), to increase my knowledge of rural social work and to finish a degree begun thirty years earlier. I wanted to prepare for what I dimly perceived might be the beginning of a new chapter—and what turned out to be a whole new edition!

The unexpected results were that I rediscovered my own intelligence and found skills I had been unaware of. I connected with much younger women and forged relationships that have continued long after graduation. I encouraged several contemporaries to jump in and try it! In my fieldwork in human services, I came in contact with various local and state decision-makers, and immediately found the door wide open for getting involved with community issues. This in turn enabled me to start an independent practice, working with and for elders and their families. I will never have to retire, and as my professional focus and confidence deepen and grow, I learn valuable lessons from those elders who are not only my clients but my teachers.

We may experience a change in our perspective—a heightened awareness of the passage of time and of the value of the time we have left.

Now is the time to do the things I've always wanted to do. I'm no longer thinking in terms of "someday," but "soon." [a fifty-year-old woman]

It was a shock when a friend of ours, a middle-aged man, died suddenly. It got me thinking that I don't know how many years Dan and I have left together. I've been working hard and had some successes. Work is still very important to me, but I no longer want it to absorb my whole life. Now that we're in our forties, I want to spend time together and have fun.

When I was fifty I was the oldest person in my community and quite conscious of being older. I thought (this seems ridiculous now that I am seventy-six) that I certainly had to plan ahead because I wouldn't have much time left. In the next five or ten years I wanted to go to Africa and travel a lot before I died.

Enjoy now as much as you can because there is almost never a tomorrow the exact way you would like to have it. [an eighty-five-year-old woman reflecting on her past choices]

Losses During the Middle Years

In addition to growth and expansion, the middle years can bring a number of painful losses which, coming in quick succession, feel like "a crescendo of losses." Statistically, many of the important losses that women face cluster in the forty-five to fifty-five-year period. We mourn these losses and often don't know how to express our feelings or to whom.

Some losses undermine our image of ourselves as young, healthy, even immortal, as when diseases attack the very wholeness of our bodies. Breast cancer strikes one out of eleven women, mostly between forty-seven and fifty-three, bringing the threat of surgery or even death. Forty percent of women are estimated to have had a hysterectomy by age 40.* The rest of us lose our fertility at menopause at the average age of fifty. Our children leave home at about the same time that our fertility ends. Other important relationships may end or change: our husbands may die—the average age of widowhood for women is fifty-six.[10] Or they "pass on—to a younger woman." Our parents may become ill or die. If we have to care for them or for our husbands, we may have to give up or postpone long-awaited changes or adventures. All these situations may leave us with less money and/or no health insurance and cause considerable stress.

Changes in Body Image

Not as serious as threats to our health, but sometimes causing painful feelings of loss, are the surface signs of aging which eventually require us to develop a new body image. As we notice the changes or observe that others respond to us differently, we may keenly feel the loss of our youthful looks, in which we have been taught that much of our value resides.

When I walk down the street with my daughter now, I notice that when male heads turn in our direction they are looking at her. My pride in her blossoming young womanhood is bittersweet, because I miss getting that attention myself.

Employers may unfairly dismiss us as incompetent and useless if we don't present a contemporary (read "youthful") image, and deny us opportunities if we "look our age" or have "let ourselves go" by refusing to diet or dye our hair. In our social groups and relationships youthful appearance may be overly valued.

A few months ago I let my white hair re-emerge after some years of dyeing it. I thought it was more authentic. The man I am seeing now is about my age [sixty-two]. He said that because he doesn't have white hair, he would like me to continue coloring my hair. After thinking it over, I decided that I prefer it colored, too.

Most lesbians' culture is youth-oriented, and I feel better with my hair brown rather than gray. People don't look at me as though I'm old. [a fifty-two-year-old woman]

Some of us feel more confident when we can delay the outward signs of aging by using makeup and hair dyes.* Yet a growing number of us believe that our years and experience entitle us to wear our graying hair, wrinkles or extra pounds—badges of mature womanliness—with pride. Being older provides a time to experiment with different colors, unconventional styles and new ways of presenting ourselves.

I look in the mirror and am always a little surprised that, with my graying hair and some new wrinkles, I don't feel what I'm "supposed" to be feeling.

If I were not constantly bombarded from reading, media and society in general with reminders that now that I'm fifty-three I'm supposed to be in crisis, withdrawing, feeling depressed, isolated, incapable or ashamed, these ideas wouldn't occur to me. I am simply building on what was before, seeking out new opportunities. I am, as always, energetic and involved.

---

*Fifty percent of women have had a hysterectomy by age sixty-five. (See p. 511.)

*See Chapter 7, "Environmental and Occupational Health," for a discussion of carcinogens in cosmetics, especially most commercial hair dyes.[11]

I like being heavier. I take up more space. People listen to me more.

Grandmother Rocking

Last night I dreamed of an old lover
I had not seen him in forty years.
When I awoke,
I saw him on the street,
his hair was white,
his back stooped.
How could I say hello?
He would have puzzled all day
about who the young girl was
who smiled at him.
So I let him go on his way.
                           —Eve Merriam

When Our Children Grow Up and Leave

At this time most of us feel the satisfaction of a job well done, or at least over.* Many women look forward to this time as a release from constant responsibility.† Yet we feel sadness, for we no longer have a daily relationship with our child(ren), some of whom had become close friends and confidants.

Divorced or single mothers of dependent children receiving child-support payments or welfare may face economic dislocation when children leave home.‡

When child-raising has been our main work and we haven't planned what to do next, we may be at loose ends. Identity crises have less to do with the "emptied nest" and more to do with the question, "What am I going to do with myself now?"

As we develop our own skills and interests, we can acknowledge missing our children, yet be glad of the extra time for our other pursuits.

The "Dependency Squeeze" of the Middle Years

Just when we are gearing up to focus on what *we* want, perhaps for the first time, new family demands may actually increase, with pressures for attention from both older and younger generations.

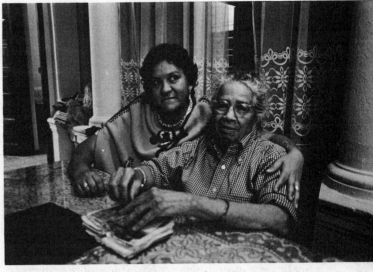

Sarah Putnam

As a single parent with young children and aging parents having health problems, I am pulled between two sets of needs. The pressures are most intense on Sundays when I "should" visit my parents. (They get home-care services on weekdays but none on weekends.) At the same time, since I work every day and go to school two nights a week, I want to do something wholesome and "outdoorsy" with my children. When Monday morning dawns I haven't had a day to sleep late, peruse the Sunday papers, bake bread or go for a walk with a friend—and when I try to take one I end up feeling guilty all the next week.

A further complication is that our mates or lovers may resent attention to aging parents just when children have left.

Because of financial pressures, some adult children are coming back home to live.* Some mothers wearily resume old parental roles and feel used and abused.

"I can't tell you how many times they have borrowed our car and wrecked it. Does that ring a bell?"
"Are you kidding? Why do you think my car has all those different-color fenders?"

Other mothers, feeling newly independent, are better able to create new kinds of relationships.

After my children were grown and wanted to return home, I made it clear they were welcome only as equal adults bearing their share of the responsibilities of the home, not in a mother-child role.

---

*Child-raising is such a major part of so many women's lives that we cannot possibly do it justice here. For a whole chapter on parents' feelings when their children leave home, see *Ourselves and Our Children: A Book by and for Women* (see Resources).

†In Lillian Rubin's study of middle-aged women, at least one-quarter of the women expressed relief when the last child left home.[12]

‡Fourteen million women who are divorced, separated, widowed or who lose AFDC benefits when their children leave home are in particularly difficult situations and often have trouble finding work. Government services have been created seemingly without these women in mind. (See "Displaced Homemakers" in Resources section.)

*The stress of this return is sending some parents to therapists. (Roberta J. Apfel, M.D., lecture on depression, Beth Israel Hospital, Boston, Spring 1982.)

441

You may have a respite between child-rearing and the caregiving demands of the middle and later years.

One of the main reasons that I'm taking an extended trip is that I feel I have this golden moment when Deborah doesn't have a baby she needs help with and my parents are still well.

Often we don't have many choices. Yet even as we attempt to meet many demands on our time and energy, we are entitled to make some time for ourselves.

Loss of People We Love

As we watch our parents and relatives age, we begin to prepare ourselves for their deaths.

Two of my favorite uncles died a few years ago. Now my favorite aunt at seventy has cancer of the pancreas, and a third uncle has just had his second heart attack. I wept and wept about these real and threatened deaths of people who are like stalwart, familiar trees in the landscape of my childhood. I shouted, "No, I can't stand this; not my favorite aunt!" I know that it's inevitable. I dread my mother's phone calls now because every time she announces another illness, another death. Such present and imminent loss makes me value everyone I love, and life itself.

My aunt said that every winter when she goes down to Florida a few more of her friends there have died. I said I can't imagine what that would be like; she said, "Well, that's just the way it is."

My mother now suffers both from a chronic and a progressive disease in an advanced state, and from some of the debilitating effects of being in poor health and approaching eighty. She seems to be gradually fading away, her hair becoming whiter, her skin paler.

In my own life at the same time I have been going through a difficult transition—the end of a fifteen-year marriage—and experiencing some physical changes of midlife. For a while I equated them with my potential decay and imminent death, as a parallel to my mother's decline. My periods had become prolonged and heavy, I was anemic, looking pale (like my mother), and my hair was graying. I chipped a tooth twice in one month and began to worry about whether this meant my bones were becoming fragile. The bleeding got worse; I wore a pad for weeks each month because tampons were insufficient; it felt like a diaper, which is what my mother has to wear. My gynecologist recommended a hysterectomy. I felt totally sexless, listless and lifeless. Now I see that some of these changes were transitory health problems which I got help for, and others simply the normal changes of middle age, with depression and stress exaggerating my feelings and fears.

Some of my relatives had criticized the decision to place my mother in a nursing home. Part of my identification with her decline came from guilt that I could go on and live and even enjoy my life when my mother was in such poor health.

One night during that time I dreamed of my own death. Instead of fear, I felt peace and completion. My work on earth had been accomplished. My only sadness was regret at not being able to attend my daughter's wedding. I transformed myself into a beautiful rainbow—nature's chuppah [Jewish wedding canopy]—and protected the festivities from bad weather. I could feel that my daughter recognized the rainbow as my gift to her.

When I awoke I was at peace with saying goodbye to my mother when the time came. I knew she would no more want to take me with her, scary as it is to die alone, than I would want my daughter's life to end with my death.

Widowhood

Three out of four women will be widows. Of 12 million widowed persons in the U.S., 10 million are women,[13] and many more millions of women have lost "unofficial" partners, male and female, whom they had been loving or living with. A widowed woman lives, on the average, eighteen years after the death of a spouse. Chances of remarriage are low and decrease with age, because three out of four elderly men are married* but only one out of three elderly women is.

The stress of widowhood is enormous, one of the most difficult life situations women live through. *Widows are particularly vulnerable to disease and often lose health insurance coverage just when it is most needed.* Grief is compounded when we:

- have found our main identity in being a wife;
- are isolated and lonely after the initial mourning period;
- find that most of our friends are in couples;
- have to seek new friends as a formerly married person;
- have to seek paid employment for the first time in decades;
- need a crash course in financial planning.

We must negotiate all this while we are still numb with the shock of loss.†

We need people to call us up, visit, bring food, invite us to do things, shovel the car out, and leave us alone when that's what we want. Yet some may pull back, especially after the initial formalized mourning pe-

---

*The majority who have lost their wives remarry. Those who remain single have higher death and illness rates. It is thought that women adjust better to widowhood despite the stresses because of our greater ability to make and keep friends.[14]

†The full impact of our loss may come months or even a year later. For some women it takes up to two years to feel pleasure and enjoy life again. Be wary of doctors who try to medicate away our normal grieving, or label it pathological if it takes "too long."

riod, embarrassed or frightened by our grieving or our neediness. Many women have found special support and understanding from other widows. (See Resources, "Widowed Persons' Service" for widow-to-widow groups.) Ultimately we can build new lives.

When I was widowed at forty-nine, with five children ages twelve to twenty-two, my whole life was in turmoil. I had to cope not only with my own grief and insecurities but also those of his distraught parents and our children. I couldn't sleep nights for fear of the future. Would the children's lives be ruined, their educations shot; would I ever get over the emptiness on the other side of the bed? I developed giant hives, a swollen toe the doctor couldn't account for, lost fifteen pounds—even the dog developed allergies. Sleepless at night, I felt inadequate and aimless by day. Something had to be done, and I finally realized I was the only one who could do it.

I resolved to think objectively about each thing I felt unable to cope with. I started by reading the insurance policies in the long reaches of the night when I couldn't sleep—I slept exhausted trying to make sense of the legalese. I read library books on the stock market and investments. I read Consumer Reports *on cars. I encouraged my children to get jobs and fill up their free time with income-producing activities. My twelve-year-old began babysitting and keeping track of her income and expenditures. The day she reached $1000 was a triumph for her. They all gained some sense of security from knowing they could produce their own clothes and spending money, even save some toward college tuition. They were too busy to get into teenage trouble. I rented our summer cottage instead of selling it—a stroke of genius, as it provided us in June and September a place to renew ourselves physically and emotionally. I made a list of the things I could have fun at without a man, and did them. I took a part-time job. I set my life in order again—a very different order, but my own. I developed a new self-confidence and* joie de vivre. *It took about three years.*

When my husband died five years after our divorce, I experienced, with the utter finality of his death, the absolute end of our relationship. Suddenly the years of separation were obliterated and I mourned deeply the loss of my husband, the father of my children, and the ending of the whole life we had shared.

My husband died after a seven-year period when his health had been deteriorating and I had been his primary caretaker. My mother died within six weeks of his death. So, in addition to losing a husband and a mother, I lost a part of myself, my role as a helping, caring person.

I went out to my mother's farm and sat out there for six weeks. I did a lot of different things, but I spent a lot of time writing about what I had left now that I no longer had that identity: who am I?

And what I had left was that I was a woman and I was growing older, and that was the beginning of both my feminism and my understanding of the concept of aging. That became a new identity for me.

A lot of us women are not reared to believe that we can make something of what we are. I had been my parents' child and my husband's wife and my children's mother. Now I had the opportunity to be a person in my own right.

Coping with a Series of Losses

This process is one of our most difficult midlife tasks.

A psychiatrist gave me Valium when I was in my forties. I took it or Equanil regularly or fairly frequently for about five to ten years. Now I think that tranquilizers suppressed or sent underground the pains of that period (divorce, death of mother, betrayal by a lover). These pains still surface with agonizing strength. Maybe if I had fully faced them and "digested" them at the time they happened, this would not be the case.

When devastating losses occur in a cluster, we feel stunned and very much alone. Don't expect too much of yourself at this time. One of the best things you can do for yourself is accept your feelings as normal and not try to carry the load without help. Watch out for doctors who want to medicate away legitimate feelings of sadness and rage. It is a sign of strength to be able to acknowledge feelings of despair, anger, guilt, emptiness, fear, relief, anxiety, confusion. There is no right time or right way to grieve.* Each of us has her own unique rhythm. Talking with women who have "been there" often helps, as does reminiscing, writing or keeping a journal.

It takes enormous energy to rebuild your life. Don't exhaust yourself trying to take care of the emotional needs of others. Take special care of yourself. You will probably need more rest than usual. Go slowly—give yourself time to heal, to regain your trust in the world and in your own capacities.

MENOPAUSE

Prevailing Social Views

Stereotypical thinking about menopausal women includes many myths (many created and perpetuated by doctors and psychiatrists).

The first thing that comes to my mind about menopause is FALLACIES: menopause is blamed for every

---

*In the professional literature one often finds unhelpful prescriptive statements, like the assertion that if grieving lasts more than six months or a year it is pathological.

mood change and unexplained feeling, the way menstruation is with younger women; also descrimination and derision—"she must be going through the change."

Helene Deutsch, a disciple of Freud, referred to menopause as women's "partial death." Mastering psychological reaction to menopause was, she said, "one of the most difficult tasks of a woman's life."[15] It would be more accurate to say that our most difficult task is mastering reaction to the cultural stereotype of menopausal women, a process which is complicated and made even more difficult by the fact that we cannot help internalizing that image to some degree.

The "raging hormones" myth describes menopausal women as so incapacitated by hormone fluctuations that they are incapable of rational thought and behavior, and should certainly not hold any kind of responsible position.* A more recent myth, part of the "superwoman" mystique, suggests that the usefully busy woman will hardly notice menopause at all. Neither extreme is accurate or helpful to women.

Particularly damaging is the myth linking menopause and depression. In the first half of this century, doctors and families hospitalized thousands of women for a "disorder" called "involutional melancholia," a "mental disease" which supposedly occurred during or just after menopause. Some of us remember aunts, great-aunts or grandmothers who went into mental hospitals at menopause, some never to emerge again. Though contemporary studies fail to demonstrate that depression among midlife women is associated with menopause, the fear of going crazy at menopause is still part of our culture.[17] Yet involutional melancholia is not a disease but a myth.†

Even when a menopausal woman feels comfortable with herself, her family and others around her may resent her independence, mood swings or irritability, perhaps even fear these as signs of her growing older. They may urge drugs, surgery or psychotherapy on her rather than being willing to live with her through the changes.

Misogyny taints much of the medical literature. A well-known gynecologist/writer has referred to menopause as "a living decay,"[19] and another ob/gyn has said (in a federally sponsored symposium) that menopausal women are a "caricature of their younger selves at their emotional worst."[20] According to another doctor (and author of a best-selling book), the menopausal woman is "not really a man but no longer a functional woman," and after menopause will "just be marking time until she follows her glands into oblivion."[21] After helping to create the above stereotypes, doctors reinforce them by treating menopause as a deficiency disease to be managed with estrogen replacement "therapies," tranquilizers or surgery. In our efforts to counter such myths, we may unwittingly suggest that we can sail through menopause without even noticing its physical discomforts and emotional changes, not to mention the social realities facing midlife women. If we overlook the changes of menopause, we run the risk of trivializing our experience. Menopause is an important physical and emotional life transition, and we are different after we have gone through it. We can be strengthened and empowered by acknowledging the reality of our experiences and giving one another support during this transition.

Medical Definitions and Our Definition of Menopause

Definitions of menopause vary in medical literature, with little consensus on when it begins and ends and disagreement about its definitive signs. Texts refer to the "climacteric" as a fifteen-year period (from forty to fifty-five or forty-five to sixty) in the transition between reproductive ability and its ending: "The [female] climacteric is the gradual process of ovarian failure which normally precedes and extends beyond the last menses and within which menopause is only an event."[22] Menopause refers specifically only to the cessation of menses (menstrual periods). The current most widely used definition of menopause is a retrospective analysis—two years after the last menstrual period.[23]

Such textbook definitions fail to take into account the social and cultural context in which we live through menopause, our understanding of it and our varied emotional reactions. Going through menopause is experiencing the whole period which begins when we first have menstrual irregularities until menstruation finally stops completely and our bodies adjust to changes in estrogen production.

No one definition will satisfy every woman or cover all the varying aspects of menopause as we individually experience them.

I think of menopause as the psychological and emotional shifting of gears we experience when our hormone production changes, preparing us for a new stage of life.

Menopause is a slow turning in life. Your insides are changing but you remain the same person. Some people

---

*Nineteenth-century doctors taught (and practiced on) the belief that the uterus was a source of disease and hysteria, especially once reproduction was over. Male doctors used myths about menopause to keep women out of medicine by casting doubt on their emotional stability.[16]

†Involutional melancholia has been dropped from the current edition of the *Diagnostic and Statistical Manual of Mental Disorders*. However, even up to the present time, women are subjected to treatments to cure depression presumably associated with menopause. "Over 70% of the population in mental hospitals is female....Over 70% of those undergoing electro-shock therapy are women, and more than 70% of those persons whose behavior is modified and controlled by therapy are women."[18]

battle with this period as if trying to stop it. Some accept it and go through it more easily.

It's the end of periods and birth control. What a relief!

In the past twenty years, research into menopause has at last increased, partly because of the increased visibility of midlife women. Unfortunately, drug companies have done most of the research,[24] basing it on women who seek medical treatment rather than taking random samplings of the population at large. Women-initiated research might choose more relevant issues based on our own experiences.

Physical Changes

Although medical and popular literature often discuss numerous menopause "symptoms," only three signs can be directly attributed to changes in estrogen production: 1. changes in menstrual cycle, 2. hot flashes and sweats ("vasomotor instability") and 3. vaginal changes (decrease of moisture and elasticity in the vagina, sometimes called "atrophy").[25]

Menstrual Changes

For most women the first signs of approaching menopause are changes in the menstrual cycle. Some of us menstruate more frequently than before, others skip periods or find that they are more widely spaced. We may have shorter periods with lighter bleeding or longer and/or heavier bleeding, sometimes with clots and "flooding."

The last time I flew in an airplane I perceived that I was flooding (though bolstered by a tampon and two pads) and rushed down the aisle to the bathrooms. Blood flowed down my stockings and into my shoes. More dripped onto the carpet. Both bathrooms were occupied, of course. I waited, breathing deeply and resisting the very strong urge to kick in both doors.

Because very heavy or extended bleeding is such a frightening, disruptive and debilitating symptom, we can easily be pressured into taking drastic action, such as unnecessary surgery. (See the section on hysterectomy in Chapter 23, "Some Common and Uncommon Health and Medical Problems.") MDs think of heavy and irregular bleeding as a possible sign of cancer,[26] but this is only true in a small minority of cases.* It is a possibility, so do check it out by asking for an endometrial biopsy, an office procedure. (See the sec-

*Only 6 percent of women develop uterine or ovarian cancer during the menopausal years, forty-five to fifty-four. The risk of cancer increases as we pass menopause, climbing to 14 percent for ages sixty to sixty-four, the years of highest risk. [27] The risk is substantially increased if we have taken ERT, however. [28] (See the section on cancer in Chapter 23.)

tion on uterine cancer in Chapter 23.) Because the training of MDs focuses so heavily on pathology and so little on the normal processes of women's bodies, many MDs have not learned that heavy, irregular or extended bleeding may simply reflect hormonal instability in women approaching menopause. Many women choose hysterectomy simply because of the disruption that the flooding causes in work and social life. However, many women are learning to cope by talking with other women who have this problem and by discovering new ways to decrease the flow, such as nonmedical approaches and alternative healing methods. If you want to consider these techniques, you should know that the most serious health risk you face, once cancer has been ruled out, is that of becoming anemic. Have your hemoglobin checked regularly and take iron if yours is low.*

Premenstrual symptoms may intensify or change, too, or begin to be noticeable for the first time.

The worst discomfort for me has been a great increase in premenstrual tension, extreme nervousness, breast soreness, headaches and insomnia for a week to ten days before my period.

One woman in five has no changes in her menstrual cycle at all until menstruation suddenly stops.[29]

It is hard to tell exactly when menstruation stops for good; periods may stop for several months, then start up again, and such fluctuations can last for a year or longer. Midlife women with irregular periods are at risk of pregnancy until they have been period-free for twenty-four months.

Hot Flashes

The sign most commonly associated with menopause is hot flashes (or flushes). Some women describe it as a sensation of heat in the face or moving through or across the upper half of the body. Sweating may follow, and sometimes you may experience a feeling like suffocation. Chills frequently precede or follow. Hot flashes vary in intensity, duration and frequency. They can be aggravated by stress and diet. Some women get hot flashes when their bodies become overheated—during a heat wave, for example—when the thermostat is set too high, when they eat highly spiced food or drink coffee or alcohol.

During hot flashes, blood vessels dilate and constrict irregularly and unpredictably. No one knows exactly why this occurs. When ovarian estrogen production declines, the pituitary gland (located in the head) sends signals for the production of more estrogen. One theory is that hot flashes may be the body's attempt to respond.

*You should not take iron unless a test shows you are anemic; you may take too much. (See p. 521 for guidance on iron supplements.)

Hot flashes may begin when menstruation is still regular or just beginning to fluctuate and continue after your periods end. Some women never experience them, while others have them off and on as late as their eighties. Many women are not bothered by their hot flashes. Some flashes are so mild that at first the woman experiencing them may think the room is too hot, there are too many blankets on the bed or the weather has changed. Some of us, however, are incapacitated by them. The sweating that follows can be so profuse that we need a complete change of clothes or bedclothes. Some women wake up five or six times a night or more, so that sleep may be seriously disturbed.

Some of us are embarrassed by hot flashes and particularly by their unpredictability, an embarrassment due in large part to the negative status of the aging woman as well as to the taboos, still prevalent, about "noticing" menstruation and menopause. Though you may feel hot or sweaty, most onlookers fail to notice what is usually a very slight change in coloring. Check your face in the mirror the next time you have a flash and you'll probably be reassured. Many of us find hot flashes less burdensome after we discuss them (and menopause in general) with other women. Some women carry folding fans to cool themselves, making themselves more comfortable and at the same time showing others that menopause is a perfectly normal occurrence.

Vaginal Changes

Changed estrogen levels may produce changes in the vagina. (See p. 451).

Ovarian Function

When our ovaries no longer produce enough hormones to trigger the release of eggs or to build up menstrual blood and tissues on the inside wall of the uterus, both ovulation and menstruation eventually stop. *Contrary to popular and medical myth, these changes in ovarian function do not mean that our bodies or our ovaries stop producing estrogen.* Long before the ovaries slow down, alternative sources of estrogen production are functioning in the fatty tissues of the body and in the adrenal glands, and the ovaries themselves usually continue to secrete small amounts of estrogen for ten years or longer after periods cease.

Adrenal Glands

Throughout life our adrenal glands help us cope with stress and maintain our resistance to disease.* As es-

*Many researchers believe that resistance to cancer (the factor that permits some people, exposed to the same carcinogens as the rest of the population, to avoid cancer) is related to adrenal function. (See "Cancer," p. 522.)

trogen from our ovaries begins to decline (beginning about age twenty-five), our adrenal glands gradually take over until they become our major source of estrogen after menopause. This is accomplished by converting a secretion called *androstenadione* into *estrone* (a nonovarian type of estrogen) in our blood and body fat. Exercising speeds this conversion process, and having a little fat on our bones makes it easier. While all living is stressful, we can make the adrenals' job easier by eating a healthy diet (including enough Vitamins C and B) and getting adequate exercise and rest. Also, you may want to try relaxation practices and other ways of minimizing the effects of stress. (See Chapter 5, "Health and Healing: Alternatives to Medical Care.") At this time in our lives comfortable habits, such as drinking coffee and alcohol and eating sweets, may actually become additional stresses on the adrenals, especially since the protection once provided by ovarian estrogen to heart, digestive organs, lungs, bones and skin must now come from the adrenals.

Other Changes

Some women cry more easily, feel irritable at times, are less patient or feel disorganized. Some of these emotional changes may be related to hormonal fluctuations. They may, however, also be a response to a culture which devalues older women or to the traumatic events which so often occur in midlife.

I definitely feel emotionally different. I am more assertive, my tolerance of people is lower, I get hurt and at times am confused about my feelings.

In what used to be a two-handkerchief movie, I may have to use four.

Minor physical changes also occur during these years, more or less at the same time as menopause. Our hair may turn gray, we may grow more facial hair, need reading glasses, gain weight. It is difficult to distinguish between signs of menopause and signs of aging; menopause itself is a sign of the aging of the female reproductive system. It is a common myth that all changes in midlife women are caused by menopause, with the implication that a woman's reproductive cycle is the major factor in her life and that once it stops, she is a changed person. In fact, men as well as women go through many of the changes, proof that they are not caused primarily by "estrogen deficiency."

Medical Approaches to Menopause

There is no growth without change. Menopause is a crucial stage in our psychic maturation.

I welcomed the end of my menstrual periods because for years I had experienced premenstrual tension and heavy bleeding. The hot flashes were not a bad tradeoff if I could be free of periods at last. I have not had a period for four years; I feel healthier than ever, have an active and joyful sex life with no "dry vagina" problems, and do a lot of physical activities. This is definitely the best period of my life. [a fifty-one-year-old woman]

The Medical Scenario

To illustrate the "medicalization" of menopause, here is a sequence of medical events which can overtake a woman in midlife. This scenario describes extreme medical intervention, but variations of this scenario are unfortunately all too common. At the beginning of menopause, the midlife woman may have irregular or heavy bleeding which she reports to her doctor. The doctor does a D and C for diagnostic purposes, which may also reduce the bleeding temporarily. She is relieved to find out that her uterus is healthy. However, as the year passes, she may have more irregular or heavy bleeding. Her doctor advises another D and C; she follows his advice. Again, she finds nothing untoward, and there may be temporary relief.

More time elapses. Heavy or irregular bleeding returns and the woman may become anemic. The doctor now recommends hysterectomy. At this point, the woman is frightened by her symptoms, confused about the exact state of her uterus and in all likelihood intimidated by what she feels is the doctor's superior knowledge of her body. So she has the hysterectomy, convinced by the physician to have her ovaries out, too, "in case" of future cancer. Since hormone levels commonly fluctuate after the operation, she may become depressed. For this, too, the doctor offers medical remedies: tranquilizers and estrogen, which can be "safely" administered since there is no longer a risk of uterine cancer. She may be referred to a psychiatrist. If the woman is anxious about the risk of breast cancer, either because she already is in a high-risk group or because she is taking estrogen, she may easily succumb to the suggestion of a "prophylactic" mastectomy. And here this scenario ends: little more can be done to this unfortunate woman's body, gynecologically speaking. Paradoxically, she may feel grateful, not realizing that she has had dangerous and unnecessary medical "care."

Though some practitioners are beginning to consider menopause a normal part of a woman's life and are learning about wholistic approaches, many doctors still think of menopause as a disease and offer medical solutions far more often than necessary.

The medical approach "protects" us from the normal discomforts and changes of outlook which accompany menopause and other transitions of the aging process. It leads us to believe that these changes are so painful or dangerous that we cannot get through them without drugs and/or surgery; that nonmedical alternatives are ineffective, or that we are incapable of applying them systematically enough to benefit us. Many doctors do to menopausal women what they do to women in childbirth: they intervene in advance to prevent us from really *living* the experience of change.

Seeking Medical Treatment

Though many women are bothered by menopausal signs, most of us do not require treatment. It is only when these symptoms seriously interfere with our daily lives, when we have tried some nonmedical alternatives and they haven't worked, that we may consider getting medical help from a practitioner who will respectfully discuss the options.

Estrogen Replacement Therapy

Since the 1940s, doctors, influenced by aggressive drug industry promotions and prestigious fellow physicians, have given hormone "therapy," also known as estrogen replacement therapy (ERT), for menopausal "symptoms." Massive advertising campaigns conducted in the seventies made Premarin into the fifth most popular drug in the U.S.; by 1975, 6 million women were taking it.[30] Articles and books celebrated ERT in the most extravagant terms, claiming that it prevented hot flashes, vaginal dryness, cancer, heart trouble and depression; that it reversed aging, unwrinkled the skin, heightened sexual desire and stopped osteoporosis.* Without adequate study, physicians prescribed it freely.

I had been using estrogen for about six months when I found it was making me depressed, so I stopped taking it. This was a rather brave thing for me to do at the time, because the doctor had been telling me it would "keep me young" for the rest of my life.

When it was first developed, ERT seemed to offer a miraculous cure for the "disease" of menopause. Since then, five studies published between 1975 and 1976 show unmistakably that ERT is associated with a five-to fifteen-times' increased risk of endometrial cancer (cancer of the lining of the uterus), especially among women who have taken estrogen for more than a year.[31] An expert advisory group to the National Institutes of Health reported also that most of the claims made for ERT were inflated or incorrect.[32] In 1979, the FDA

---

*Osteoporosis is a disease of postmenopausal women in which the bones become thin and brittle and break easily, sometimes spontaneously. (See p. 461 for more on osteoporosis.)

issued regulations requiring all estrogen products to contain an insert describing the risks of ERT.* It lists only two possible benefits: relief of hot flashes and of vaginal dryness, both of which are linked to loss of ovarian estrogen. The package insert (in such small print that many midlife women can't read it) warns that women with a history of cancer, breast cysts, blood clots or arteriosclerosis should not take estrogen; neither should women with kidney, liver or heart disease. Thus millions of women have been the unwitting subjects of a mass experiment which the passage of time revealed to be life-threatening for some.[33] Prescriptions for menopausal estrogens fell drastically, but then leveled off as drug companies, public-relations firms and physicians scrambled to minimize the findings, uncover new ways of proving estrogen "safe" from cancer risks and find still other uses for it.[34]

Women considering ERT should be aware of the following additional considerations:

1. There is currently controversy about the role of ERT, the Pill and DES in connection with breast cancer. Some studies show increased risk of breast cancer in women who have taken DES and the Pill and in some groups of women on ERT. This must be of special concern to midlife women, since three out of four breast cancers occur after age fifty and the peak period for breast cancer coincides with menopause.†

2. Taking ERT interferes with, covers up, distorts and delays the body's natural adjustment to decreased estrogen levels, a transition which most women can pass through without major difficulty.

3. ERT is only effective against osteoporosis or the other "problems" of menopause for a few years. (See below.)

4. Taking estrogens can exacerbate any tendency toward uterine fibroids (already more common near menopause) and accelerate their growth, which can lead to other complications and thus increase the risk of hysterectomy.

5. Taking hormones can create vitamin deficiencies.[35]

6. Because of the risk of endometrial or breast cancer with estrogen use, many surgeons are more eager than ever to recommend prophylactic hysterectomies, oophorectomies and mastectomies in order to be able to offer estrogen "risk free."

7. Finally, being on hormones means that you rely on chemical substances whose effects need to be carefully monitored and may not be fully known for years, so that you need to be under the care of expert physicians, which may involve frequent and expensive office visits.[36]

*Only after consumer lawsuits successfully opposed the objections of the drug industry and the American College of Obstetricians and Gynecologists (ACOG).

†Brian MacMahon, a leading cancer epidemiologist, calculates that long-term use of menopausal estrogens (seven to ten years) increases the risk of breast cancer *two times* over what it is for women who do not take them (personal communication). Given that the current general risk of breast cancer is one in eleven, this means that *approximately one in six women who take estrogens at menopause may develop breast cancer*, already the leading killer of women between ages forty-seven and fifty-three.

Cumulative Effects of Estrogen

Some women born between 1920 and 1930 have been exposed to one form of hormone after another since their youth. These women were given DES at a time when doctors prescribed it more or less routinely to prevent miscarriage and to dry up milk after birth, often without telling women what they were taking. Some in the 1960s and 1970s took DES as a "morning-after pill" intended to prevent pregnancy after unprotected intercourse.

When the birth control pill first went on the market (at far greater dosages than were later found necessary or safe), members of this age group took it for long intervals, before studies resulted in warnings about its risks. As they grew older, many of these same women were given estrogen for "symptoms" associated with menopause.

It is not known what the cumulative effect of so much estrogen over so many years may be on women now in their fifties and sixties. They, perhaps more than any other group of women, have reason to examine the literature about the effects of estrogen. If this has been your experience, you may want to be in touch with one or more of the DES and menopause self-help groups. Many of them have information which your doctor may not have. Do everything you can to get your medical records. (See "Our Rights as Patients," p. 584.)

When and How to Use ERT

If you are seriously troubled by hot flashes, and the nonmedical approaches (see below) don't work for you, you may want to consider ERT in as small a dose and for as short a time as possible. Choose a doctor who is expert in this and not responsible to a drug company. (See "Our Rights as Patients," p. 584.) Keep a careful record of your medications and any unusual bleeding, discharge or breast swelling. Be sure to get a checkup from your doctor at least every three to six months while you are on ERT. Some women who have taken estrogen for short periods of time (two to three months) and then discontinued it feel relief from hot flashes; others report that the flashes have returned in full force or even stronger.*

*Some researchers think that if the estrogen is tapered off gradually, this problem can be minimized.

I was placed on Premarin after surgical menopause. The medication was stopped after six months and severe night sweats began within a month. After three months of trying to wait them out, I went back on Premarin; then it was stopped again. The hot flashes then came at infrequent intervals and were easy to tolerate.

You may prefer to put up with the flashes, knowing that they are temporary and cause no permanent damage to your health.

The hot flashes go on and on, but I endure, can even say, "Hello, hot flash, my old friend..."

ERT also alleviates vaginal dryness. It has been suggested that estrogen creams or suppositories applied to the vagina are not as risky as orally ingested estrogen.[37] Unfortunately, the body absorbs the estrogen through the vaginal walls, and though it bypasses the liver, which metabolizes hormones, the overall risks are probably similar. (See p. 452 for self-help approaches to vaginal dryness.)

Progesterone Treatments

Doctors sometimes prescribe the hormone progestin, a synthetic progesterone (see below for risks), or Depo-Provera, an injectable progesterone (see Chapter 13, "Birth Control," for risks) to control excessively heavy or prolonged menstrual bleeding. Some women decide to take these in an attempt to avoid hysterectomy, but they don't always work.

Estrogen and Progestin Combined

While we question estrogen use altogether and emphasize nonmedical alternatives, researchers and clinicians today continue to search for "safe" estrogen supplements. A current crop of studies seeks to show that estrogen may be administered with less or even no risk of endometrial cancer when combined with progesterone. However, not only do clinicians disagree over dosages, sequences of administration and types of hormones, but there is some evidence that the combination may produce other, even more serious effects, such as heart disease and stroke.[38] If women are again to be subjects of experiments with hormones, we must at least be fully aware of the risks we run.*

Nonmedical Approaches

Nonmedical methods of dealing with menopause include exercise, diet, vitamin supplements, herbal ther-

*If you choose this route, make sure your physician is closely monitored by researchers who are responsible not to a drug company but to a public board.

apy and various other techniques. These are much more under our control than medical approaches, and we may experience many kinds of benefits.

Eating well is essential. In addition to a good diet, many midlife women find vitamins and minerals helpful. Vitamin C, Vitamin D and calcium are essential for bone formation. Vitamin-A deficiency has been associated with heavy menstrual bleeding; supplements in moderate doses may help.* Magnesium can help relaxation. Some women find that Vitamin E reduces leg cramps, and others note that it modifies or reduces hot flashes. (Avoid Vitamin E in large doses if you have high blood pressure.)† Some women find that Vitamin-B complex reduces edema, and others that it helps joint pains and eases stress. (See also "Eating Well, p. 454.)

Some women use herbal teas to reduce or control heavy menstrual bleeding and to reduce the discomfort of hot flashes and headaches. Since instructions vary or lack specificity about which herbs to use, how strong these teas should be and how much you should drink, consult an herbalist or wholistic practitioner who knows about herbs. If you want to try these yourself, consult several books. Pay particular attention to any cautions, because some herbs can be harmful in large amounts.

Relaxation techniques, such as meditation, giving and getting massages and yoga, can reduce stress and depression. Sex, including masturbation, can be relaxing and also helps prevent insomnia and vaginal dryness. Many women find these approaches, as well as acupuncture, helpful for head and neck aches, tension and lower back pain and especially for menstrual problems like heavy bleeding.

Finally, and most importantly, daily moderate exercise is essential for good health throughout menopause. (See Chapter 4, "Women in Motion," for strategies on how to start exercising even if you've been mostly sedentary for years.) *In fact, exercise, especially aerobic exercise, can produce in midlife many (if not all) of the things that the estrogen literature of the early seventies claimed would follow estrogen intake, including (for some women) reduction of hot flashes!*

During my vacation I hiked eight to ten miles a day in good, fresh country air. I cannot recall a single hot flash during that time, although I had them both before and after the trip. Perhaps I was tired enough to sleep without being aware of the flashes, but I don't think that was the case—I never felt healthier.

*Vitamin A in high doses can be toxic. Try increasing foods containing carotene, with low-dose Vitamin A (no more than 10,000 IUs daily) first.
†Water-soluble Vitamin E, taken in moderate doses, is unlikely to affect blood pressure.

A few years ago when I was going through change of life I started having joint aches and swelling of hands in the morning. I increased the amount of exercise and took some mineral supplements and Vitamin E, and the condition disappeared within a few weeks.

While these are all useful hints, they are not magic, and in most cases they are not enough by themselves. An equally important part of any nonmedical approach is to avoid or cut down your consumption of certain substances which tend to aggravate menopausal signs: alcohol, caffeine, sugar, chocolate, white-flour products, nutritional yeast, etc., as well as many prescription drugs: tranquilizers, sleeping pills, antidepressants, etc.

Support Groups for Menopausal Women

Women have always relied on one another for information and understanding. The networks of support groups that have proliferated in recent years are an especially important source of strength for midlife women. In these groups we get emotional support, increased understanding of our particular experience of menopause, and "body" information. Best of all, we reduce the sense of isolation so many of us have known as we recognize the social, economic and political context of our common condition.

I had never been in any kind of support group before. I thought it would be a discussion group and everyone would be an expert except me, and I'd be embarrassed because I wasn't an expert on anything. But that's not the way this group worked. There's a lot of mutual help; people really listen to each other and laugh a lot. Now I don't worry about menopause or growing older the way I used to.

Validated by the new knowledge that I had the same powerful physical and emotional experiences as all women, I was proud to have gone through menopause and some difficult life changes at the same time. For instance, creating a new life for myself after my divorce, I love my friends and know they have gone through similar challenges.

MATURE WOMEN AND SEXUALITY

Sexuality continues throughout a woman's life. Some women first become fully aware of their sexuality in their middle years, and have unexpectedly powerful sexual feelings.

I was shocked by being so horny after I was divorced, because it's not only sexual, it's aggressive. Certainly not

what my mother taught me. It took me a long time to understand that I could lust. [a fifty-year-old woman]

I'm no longer worried about pregnancy; the children are gone; my energy is released. I have a new surge of interest in sex. But at the same time the culture is saying, "You are not attractive as a woman; act your age; be dignified," which means to me, be dead sexually. It's a terrible bind for a middle-aged woman. I say, acknowledge, applaud, enjoy sexuality! Get rid of the stereotypes! Change the image of women to include middle-aged beauty and sexuality! [a woman in her fifties]

If you are sexually involved with men, keep using some form of birth control until you haven't had a period for two years. Birth control pills and the IUD are not recommended for midlife women.* Some midlife women consider the chances of pregnancy to be so low that they are willing to rely on abortion as a backup. But when you are certain you do not want to have a child and would not consider abortion, continue to use birth control.

Many older women who would like to be sexually active with men lack the opportunity, especially since with each year of age there are fewer men in their age range.†

I have a great interest in sex, still, and a great desire for it. But what makes it most poignant that I don't have the right partner is that I am capable of giving now to a degree that I never achieved when I was young. [a divorced woman in her sixties]

Even married, we may not be as sexually active as we might like if our partners lose interest in sex.

Our society admires older men who have relationships with women much younger than themselves but makes older women with younger partners the butt of jokes and derision. Yet some of us have younger men as partners.

It's hard to read the younger-man/older-woman thing. We have to send out signals if a sexual relationship is what we want. I've had a problem if the man is the same age as my son, though after thinking about it I've decided it's okay for me. What really bothers me is my vanity—exposing a middle-aged body to a beautiful younger man.

The joy of making love with a young man who is so full of energy and straightforward is wonderful.

*For discussion of the Pill, see pp. 237–47. IUDs should be avoided by midlife women because they may trigger or exacerbate the heavy bleeding and flooding that sometimes precede menopause.

†A Duke University study showed that of older men interested in sex 87 percent were sexually active, while among interested older women only 60 percent were sexually active.[39] The implication in this study is that women can only be "sexually active" with men.

Some midlife or older women are for the first time considering or having sexual relationships with women:

Women and men have been socialized so utterly differently, and we have grown so different in the last decades, too, that if we restrict ourselves to heterosexual relationships, it's going to get harder and harder as we get older. I'm married, and though my husband is considerably older than I, he's still very active. But if this relationship comes to an end—which would mean his death, because we're never going to separate—my sexual satisfactions would surely have to come either from myself or from other women. I can't imagine forming another relationship with a man. [a sixty-year-old woman]

Others of us have been lesbian for many years. (See "Older Lesbians," p. 154.)

Many of us would rather not have sex at all, or prefer to limit our sexual expression to masturbation and fantasy rather than changing our sexual orientation or a lifetime pattern of being involved in one special relationship.

I frankly don't need it, and I don't miss it at all. I had a very, very full sex life—and I was mad about my husband, which is a nice way to be. When he died it was a real shock, but that's twenty-five years ago now. I've run around with a few men since, but nobody that I really wanted to connect with. You have to have a certain desire toward a person, and I haven't discovered another person that I had that desire for in twenty-five years now. I'm used to my life the way it is now, and I don't think that my life is incomplete. [a seventy-three-year-old woman]

Many single older women miss not just sex but touching, gentleness, closeness and the excitement of romance.

Some of you say you have husbands at home that won't go anyplace. I have buried three husbands, and I wish I had one to sit home with me now. [a woman in her sixties]

It's the intimacy that I miss more than the actual sex act. Shared jokes—you know. I'm finding this with a number of women as well as with men, but the whole romantic aspect of my life seems to have gone by. I miss that. [a woman in her seventies]

Sex and Aging: Physiological Changes

We are physically able to enjoy sex more. With sexual experience we develop a large, complex venous system in the pelvic area which enhances our capacity for sexual tension and improves orgasmic intensity, frequency and pleasure.*

Elder women who seek any form of sexual expression, whether pleasuring ourselves or making love with others, face changes, too.

Vaginal Changes

Changed estrogen levels may produce changes in the vagina. Thinning of the vaginal walls, loss of elasticity, flattening out of ridges, foreshortening or narrowing of the vagina and especially dryness or itching may make intercourse less comfortable or even painful. These conditions may lead to irritation and increased susceptibility to infection. It is not clear whether these vaginal changes are caused by the changed estrogen levels of menopause or simply by aging. Some women never have this problem. Since there have not been many studies of this condition, no one knows how many women are troubled by it. Doctors, with their gift for nomenclature, call it "vaginal atrophy" and describe it in medical texts as occurring five or more years after

---

*Sexual activity with a partner or ourselves and pregnancy also contribute to the complexity of the pelvic venous system.[40]

Julie Harper

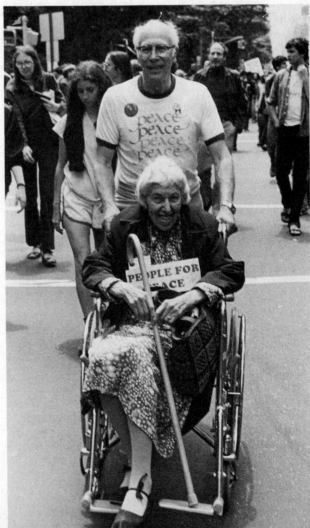

menstruation ceases. Yet many women experience vaginal changes earlier in menopause, and others at age sixty or later. In addition, little is known about how long such a condition lasts, how troublesome it may become or how easily it can be corrected.[41]

Many "experts" recommend "regular intercourse" to maintain easy vaginal lubrication.

I asked a woman gynecologist with an excellent reputation, "Does it have to be intercourse? What about widows, or divorced women, or lesbians, or women whose husbands aren't too interested in sex or are ill?" And I couldn't get a straight answer from her, even though I kept trying.

The fact is that we can maintain and improve our ability to lubricate through any type of arousing sexual activity.[42] There is nothing unhealthy about losing interest in genital sexual activity; we are not sex machines obligated to keep our bodies perpetually in condition for potential partners. There is also no evidence that vaginal dryness is irreversible.

I had a problem with dryness when I started having sexual intercourse again after a few years. In a month or two, my vagina began to get wet faster. [a woman in her sixties]

You may take longer to become amply lubricated.[43] Sometimes lubrication does not take place at all: saliva, K-Y Jelly or a vegetable oil can reduce dryness. Itching can be relieved by applying bancha tea or Vitamin-E oil topically to the pubic and vaginal area. Sexual activity, masturbation and Kegel exercises (p. 333) all help maintain vaginal muscle tone.

Slower Arousal Time

The slower arousal time of older women and men has compensations.

When Jay used to lose his erection I would think that I had failed as a woman because I couldn't keep him aroused. But now I see that it can mean more time to play around and a chance to start over again so that lovemaking lasts longer. [a woman in her forties]

Drugs and Disease

Drugs and disease can affect sexual behavior. Some drugs may affect sexual function or interest. Medication for high blood pressure can prevent erections, as can too much alcohol. (The depressive effect of alcohol becomes more pronounced as people get older.) Diabetes can make erections difficult for a man; its effect on the sexuality of women is not well understood.[44] L-dopa, prescribed for Parkinson's disease, may increase sexual interest. Ask your practitioner about the

effects on sexual interest, arousal or functioning of any medications which are prescribed for you or your partner.

Changing Attitudes and Communication

Women now in their older years must shed years of training to act on the knowledge that there are alternatives to intercourse and that they can initiate sex. The physiological changes of aging invite both men and women to break through old patterns, assumptions, misunderstandings and miscommunications. Men may misinterpret their slowness to arousal as a sign that their sexual capacities are eroding, and in panic seek out other (younger) women. Women may fear that their aging bodies' diminished "attractiveness" has slowed their partner's arousal, or interpret their own lack of lubrication as loss of attraction to their partner. It is important for both partners in a relationship, whether heterosexual or lesbian, to realize that changes are normal and to talk together to find out what is pleasurable. Such communication may be difficult at first and requires practice. You may want to get some help.

If one or both of you have some physical difficulty, see p. 182. Do what pleases you and your partner, even if it seems unusual or strange. Chances are, if you like it, other couples do, too. A greater capacity for empathy and loving, developed through the years of living, can make sex better. A seventy-year-old woman, recalling a love affair at fifty, says:

My immense pleasure and response were for him an incredible high, and that made me feel so marvelous. It was not just the physical part but our delight in each other that was so enormously exciting. It was a circular or spiral effect, because I had not realized that another person could enjoy my passion. Before this, I had experienced my passion and my partner would experience his passion. But this was different. And of course it's very much that way in a lesbian love affair, that delight in the other woman's total experience, the total emotional response. Danny took great pride in that just as a woman does with another woman. He thought it was marvelous that I was multiple-orgasmic. After he died, I was in a state of shock for over a year. The mutuality we shared was rare with a man. My subsequent love affairs have all been with women.

Some people continue to be sexually active in their seventies, eighties and even nineties.

I am seventy-four years old and have been married for fifty-two years. We are fortunate to have good mental as well as physical health. This is not entirely a matter of luck. We have worked at it. Our good times have been more numerous than our bad times. The medical profession has only recently discovered the healing power of laughter. In our fifty-two years together we have had a lot of laughs. A sense of humor is as important as food, especially within the confines of marriage. For us the sharing that comes with having a warm and loving sex life over so many years deepens our joy in one another.

AGING AND PREVENTIVE HEALTH—SPECIAL ISSUES

While many people equate getting old with getting sick, the truth is more complex. Aging brings physical changes, most of which have little to do with sickness.

At sixty I am more vigorous and healthy than I was twenty years ago. My eighty-five-year-old mother shows me that by the eighties certain things in your body do start to give way, but even though she gets around less easily, she's certainly what I'd call healthy.

In our fifties and beyond, a lifetime of exposure to occupational health hazards may have caused a debilitating disease.* Yet while disease and chronic ill health are among the realities of the older years for many of us, they are not the only reality. And social factors can disable us more than is necessary: isolation from family and friends; caregiving for relatives and family without outside help; poor medical care, due to high cost, lack of insurance coverage, inadequate medical understanding of aging and maldistribution of doctors. Poverty is a special health issue for older women. Money worries due to being on a small, limited income and the fears of cutbacks to Social Security, Medicare and other government programs add greatly to the unhealthy stresses of daily living. Inadequate income also makes it harder to take care of our bodies in simple but crucial daily ways. It is difficult, for instance, to get enough exercise if we don't feel safe on the streets or have little access to indoor exercise facilities. A worsening economic situation and drastic cuts in social programs make it more difficult each month for thousands of older women to get adequate calories, let alone vitamins and special diets. Some already subsist partly on pet food. Many are starving.[46] Some are homeless or without adequate heat. Having insufficient money also severely restricts our access to medical care, especially in a time of reduced government aid. Four million American women between forty-five and sixty-five have no health insurance.[47] Without a major turnaround in social priorities and policies, the health of great numbers of older women will worsen drastically over the next few years,

with more emergency hospitalization for anemia, dehydration and hypothermia* and collapse and deaths from all causes.

Here we will address special issues† for all older women as we seek to keep as healthy as possible.

Throughout our life we can take active steps to maintain good health and lessen the impact of illnesses or chronic conditions when we are older. We can rethink the ways in which we take care of ourselves and acquire new habits which will serve us well for the rest of our lives. We can stop smoking, exercise more, eat as well as possible, reduce our dependence on caffeine, sugar, alcohol, tranquilizers. Currently there is growing evidence that many of the changes of aging, even those once thought biologically inevitable, are preventable and even reversible with changes like these.[48]

The point is not simply to live longer but to have the highest possible quality of life as long as we live.

By reading many books and articles on women, mental health, nutrition and exercise I began to see that my life could and should change. The changes did not come easily. My husband resisted. After all, I was rocking the boat in which we had become quite comfortable. I took up Tae Kwon Do [Eastern self-defense]. To my amazement, after a few months of kicking and hitting an imaginary opponent, my chronic insomnia and stiff neck disappeared. Gone also were the painful attacks of gastritis. I began feeling more energetic. Encouraged, I decided to put into practice some of the nutritional advice which I'd been reading. I stopped eating white sugar in any form. No more of my favorite cream-filled doughnuts. No more processed food, including white bread, noodles and spaghetti: in came more fresh vegetables and grains. Out went sleeping pills, aspirin and other medications: in came vitamins. It was not an overnight sensation. After all, I was trying to undo the damage done over forty-some years.

That was more than five years ago. Today, all the ailments I mentioned earlier are completely gone. No more of that headachy feeling from constipation—I count my blessings every day for being freed from this debilitating condition from which I suffered for so long. No more pains in my legs from varicose veins (some of my friends had surgery for this). No more stiff neck from internalized stress and tension. If you never suffered from chronic insomnia, you don't know the joy of being able to sleep all night, every night. All these things which I thought I would have to live with the rest of my life are gone.

*Hypothermia is a condition in which the body temperature drops drastically. Older people are more vulnerable to cold.

†Many of the more serious health problems which affect midlife and older women appear elsewhere in this book because they affect younger women, too: hypertension, cancer, arthritis, heart disease, diabetes, arteriosclerosis. The troubling but not life-threatening problems—visual impairments, hearing loss, difficulties in walking—along with osteoporosis, which primarily affects women over sixty, are discussed on pp. 458–62.

*One study of 1,100 persons over fifty in Ohio found that a main factor influencing health was occupation, past or present. "Those persons who have, or had, low-income occupations (and the disadvantages that go along with a lifetime of low income) were in poor health much more frequently than those with middle-income or high-income jobs."[45]

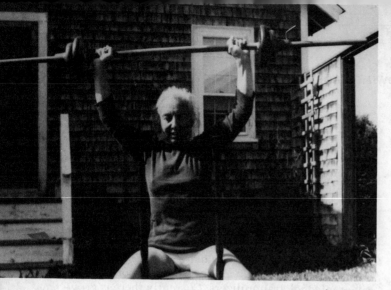

Deborah Wald

Exercise

Exercise becomes increasingly important. Women begin to lose bone mass at around age thirty-five, yet this may be largely due to inactivity. Weight-bearing exercise increases bone density. Runners, for example, tend to have high thigh-bone densities.[49] Heavier women are less vulnerable to osteoporosis (see p. 461), possibly because their bones carry more weight.

Many of the benefits of exercise for older women are already evident. Exercise can lower blood pressure and reduce atherosclerosis, risks of heart attack and stroke, arthritis, emphysema and osteoporosis. It is central in finding and keeping a comfortable weight. It helps us sleep, improves bowel functioning, often relieves depression and generally makes most people feel better.

My grandmother in her early nineties noticed that when she moved around more, her memory improved.

There seems now to be clinical evidence that after exercise blood rushes to the skin, bringing with it extra nutrients, and the skin's temperature rises as well. The collagen content then increases and skin actually thickens and becomes more elastic and less wrinkled. Delightfully, it is never too late to start exercising, and there are forms of exercise which fit almost any kind of physical limitation. A few tips: start slowly; watch less TV, or exercise while you watch; better yet, exercise with a friend for company and support; try walking, yoga or swimming; take an exercise class to help you overcome sedentary habits. Review Chapter 4, "Women in Motion," for other ideas.

Eating Well

While the same basic principles of healthy eating apply throughout life, nutritional requirements change somewhat with age. You need fewer calories (unless you are working or exercising hard), but the same nutrients and more of certain ones. See Chapter 2, "Food,"

for all but the following few items of special interest to older women, and for sources of nutrients listed below.

Note: Some of the hints here and in Chapter 2 become less easy to follow in our older years, especially when we can't easily get out to shop or are on a small fixed income and cannot afford to buy fresh foods. If we have dentures or problems with teeth or gums, small changes in diet may be all we can manage—but even cutting down on junk foods can help a lot. If you put off cooking because you are just preparing meals for yourself, try designating one day per week as cooking day. Fix several dishes, including a main dish and a soup you like, and then eat them on alternate days, or freeze some in individual portions for later.

Since we absorb nutrients less well as we age and require fewer calories altogether, we may need supplements. (See the discussion of menopause on pp. 443–47.)

However, try to get as much of the nutrients you need from your food. See p. 17 in Chapter 2 for the advantages and risks of supplements. Though the particular balance needed by women over thirty-five sounds complicated, resources like the *Department of Agriculture Handbook* No. 456 and *Laurel's Kitchen* (see Resources section of Chapter 2, "Food") can help you figure out whether you are eating well or what to change.

Protein

Since we don't absorb as much protein as we age, try to make protein foods a higher proportion of what you eat. However, be sure to balance with a sufficient amount of complex carbohydrates (whole grains, etc.; see p. 12).

Calcium, Magnesium and Phosphorus—A Balance of Nutrients

For postmenopausal women, calcium is an essential nutrient, as it prevents the bone loss that can lead to osteoporosis.* Unfortunately, women over thirty-five absorb calcium less easily,[50] so we must make a special effort to get more exercise (this is indispensible to helping our bodies absorb calcium), eat a calcium-rich diet, learn about the other nutrients that aid or inhibit calcium absorption and get the right balance of such nutrients.

- Phosphorus intake should equal but not exceed calcium. If phosphorus is too high, the parathyroid

*Calcium supplements can help us be sure we are getting the recommended 1,500 to 2,000 milligrams, but we need to balance this with about 750 to 1,000 milligrams of magnesium. Dolomite has often been recommended as containing the proper amounts of calcium and magnesium, but recently there have been reports of harmful trace minerals, such as arsenic and lead, found in dolomite, so until this controversy is resolved it is better to buy calcium and magnesium supplements separately in a two to one ratio.

Weight and Weight Gain at Midlife and Later

As older women we are probably more preoccupied with food, eating and dieting than any other group in society, with the possible exception of teenage girls. One out of two of us puts on weight at midlife because our metabolism is slowing down and we no longer need as many calories to sustain us. Often, too, we are more sedentary than before, with fewer people in the household, fewer chores, less physical mobility, less exercise. If we continue the same food intake and get no more exercise (or even less) than before, we will tend to gain weight. In fact, women on the average gain almost ten pounds between thirty-five and forty-five and two more between forty-five and fifty-five. *There is good evidence that this weight has an important function*: the conversion of androgens into estrogen in our body fat is one of the three sources of estrogen after menopause. Some fat, therefore, is crucial: women who are very thin have a higher rate of osteoporosis. It is also true that above a certain level, too many pounds can contribute to ill health—diabetes and high blood pressure in particular. There is controversy today, however, over what constitutes "too many pounds" (see Chapter 2, "Food"). It may be that physicians and actuarial tables have set the ideal weights too low.

Consider the several factors below in assessing your weight. If all these factors and their total combination are within the normal range and you feel well, your weight is probably fine.

1. Are you getting a reasonable amount of regular exercise?

2. Are you eating well?

3. Is your weight stable or changing slowly? Sudden weight gain or loss is dangerous at any age and more so as we grow older. If you plan to lose weight, do it slowly, as a result of long-term, permanent changes in eating and exercise patterns.

4. Is your blood pressure within normal range? After menopause, blood pressure tends to rise with increases in weight.

5. Is your blood sugar well within the normal range? As your weight increases, the likelihood of getting adult diabetes increases, and the disease often signals itself by slight rises in blood sugar.

6. How is your lung power and control? The lungs have been overlooked until recently as an indicator of general health. The simple, risk-free, pulmonary function test is a good indicator and predictor of long-term health and longevity (for women better than for men). Usually done in a doctor's office as part of a general checkup, it measures lung power and control as you exhale. Yoga is a good way to build lung capacity.

7. Are your cholesterol readings normal? High cholesterol, by itself, is only an indicator of possible problems if it is a particular type of cholesterol. A special test measures lipid density, high-density lipoproteins (HDL) in high concentrations being a prognosticator of good circulatory health, and low-density lipoproteins (LDL) in high concentrations being an indicator of possible problems.* The test is expensive but worth asking for if questions have been raised about your health in relation to your weight.

8. Do you have signs of arthritis or osteoporosis? Either one can indicate that you need to change your diet and exercise patterns. Women who are overweight are more prone to osteoarthritis, while women who are underweight are at higher risk for osteoporosis.

---

glands are stimulated to draw calcium from the bones. Most American women who eat meat and drink cola drinks probably have overly high phosphorus levels which inhibit calcium absorption. If you avoid milk because of its fat, replace it not with soda but with skim or part skim milk or milk products. If your body can't tolerate dairy products (lactose intolerance) refer to Chapter 2, "Food," for nondairy sources of calcium. Lactose intolerance may increase with age.

- Magnesium intake should be half of calcium intake. If your magnesium level drops lower, calcium will be lost. There is some evidence that the older we are, the more magnesium we need (around 450 to 500 milligrams daily), especially when we are under stress.[51] Magnesium can help muscles and nerves relax—and is safer than tranquilizers.

- You need Vitamin D, 400 to 800 IUs a day for calcium and phosphorus absorption.

Fiber

The fiber in vegetables, fruit, whole grains and bran helps with constipation (exercise helps, too). Fiber and oats may also lower cholesterol levels.

Fats

Aging makes us less able to resist the damaging effects of all fats. See Chapter 2, "Food," for which fats to eat and how to cut back.

*See "Hypertension, Heart Diseases and Circulatory Diseases," p. 540, for more.

Potassium

Plentiful in fresh fruits and vegetables, potassium becomes especially useful to women at midlife because it helps 1. heart action, which may be less effective during the estrogen transition;[52] 2. the elimination of fluid build-up, which continues cyclically for many postmenopausal women because of other sources of estrogen; 3. to balance sodium, which we may now have in greater quantities than we need; and 4. to lower blood pressure (along with a low-sodium diet). Coffee, tea, alcohol and too much sodium deplete potassium.

GETTING MEDICAL CARE

Despite the larger role that each of us can play in our own health care, at times we have to turn to the medical system. As midlife and older women, we face some special obstacles to good care.

Older women cannot count on the medical profession. Few doctors are interested in them. Their physical and emotional discomforts are often characterized as post-menopausal syndrome, until they have lived too long for this to be an even faintly reasonable diagnosis. After that they are assigned the category of senility.[53]

Inadequate Research

Medical research until very recently paid little attention to aging women's health concerns. Even today, medical literature focuses on menopause as the primary midlife health issue as though reproductive organs were the center of a woman's life. Failing to acknowledge women as workers outside the home, researchers have not studied occupational health issues for older women. Since the practitioner or clinic you visit may not have adequate information about the diseases and their prevention or the physical changes which affect older women in particular, you may have to educate the practitioners who treat you.

Physicians' Attitudes

The medical profession and other health personnel share the culture's negative attitudes toward the old. In a medical context this can take the form of active avoidance and dislike or a less obvious pattern of paternalism....Physicians, like the lay public, are personally ambivalent and frightened by aging and death.[54]

The basic ageism which shapes many physicians' attitudes toward older patients is compounded by sexism. The medical world seems to hold the underlying prejudice that once we can no longer have children, we have outlived our usefulness. Physicians and medical personnel dismiss older women's complaints and health problems as neurotic or imaginary far more

than men's, and at earlier ages. They have been heard to call aging women "old bags" and other insulting names. When such attitudes affect the quality of our medical care, they endanger our health.*

Inappropriate Sources of Care

At present, no one medical specialty specifically addresses aging.† Most ob/gyns are not particularly interested in women past menopause, especially when we have had a hysterectomy or refuse estrogen replacement therapy. Internists, family practitioners, primary-care physicians and well-informed GPs are often more appropriate physicians for older women— *when they have a positive attitude and enough information about aging.* Today interest in aging is growing and there are a number of geriatric centers and clinics, though these are mostly located near large medical centers.‡

Limits of the Medical Approach to Chronic Conditions

Many of the conditions we suffer from in the older years are not subject to outright "cure." Chronic diseases do not respond to the daring surgery or high-technology interventions which physicians are trained to prefer. The ordinariness of diet, braces, physical therapy and aspirin is boring, and doctors often give us less attention when these are what we need. Medical treatments that do help in some chronic conditions are often expensive,§ time-consuming and painful; sometimes they are dangerous and ineffective. This is another reason to look into nonmedical approaches to healing. (See Chapter 5 for alternatives.)

Misdiagnosis and Failure to Treat Reversible Conditions

Especially when we are past sixty, doctors tend to blame all our physical and emotional problems on "aging" and don't look for treatable disorders. They'll interpret emotional or mental confusion as "senility" when these may be signs of poor nutrition, treatable

---

*These attitudes and practices are less blatant toward women who have ample financial resources and private physicians.

†Of 2,000 doctors surveyed, 76.5 percent said training in geriatric medicine would help doctors give better care to elderly patients. Over half reported that at least one-fourth of their patients are sixty-five or older.[55]

‡There is a lively controversy today in medical schools and among health providers about whether geriatrics should be a medical specialty in its own right or whether geriatric training should be integrated with other medical specialties.

§Medicare and many private health insurance plans do not adequately cover care for chronic conditions unless they require institutionalization.

physical malfunctions, grief or responses to inappropriate medication. Time after time physicians offer older women tranquilizers, sedatives, antidepressants and hormones instead of looking for what's really wrong. As one nurse put it: "When a man complains of dizziness he gets a workup; an older woman gets Valium." We ourselves may play into this pessimism about whether we can actually get better.

I was afraid when I broke my wrist that it would take ages if ever to heal, and so I hesitated to do a more "aggressive" type of therapy for it. Now it's much better, and I'm going to begin that therapy. My fear and a stereotype of being old held me back.

Overprescription of Drugs

Many older people take several medications daily for various chronic conditions, often prescribed by different physicians. Most physicians don't realize that people over sixty are more sensitive to many drugs and should take lower doses of them if they take them at all.*

I can't tolerate any of the drugs I've been given for pain. When I take medication there's something in my system that feels dislocated, as if all my internal furniture has been piled up in the middle of the room or something. So I just live with the pain in my hands and get help with certain jobs.

Some drugs can cause depression (for which we may be offered more drugs) or mental confusion, though symptoms often stop when the medication is stopped.†

Practitioners frequently neglect the crucial step of finding out what medications a woman is taking before prescribing others. Elders have had so many bad reactions to taking too many medications that this "condition" has been given a name, "polypharmacy."[57] Bring to your medical appointments a list of all the medications you are taking. A woman we know asked her doctor to review all her medications. As the doctor reviewed the list he began to cut down the dosage of most of them and cut a few out completely.

In nursing homes, many elders are literally "tranquilized" into quiet and compliance. If you believe that you or a relative or friend are being inappropriately or excessively medicated, do all you can to change the situation.

I went to visit a ninety-four-year-old friend who lives in a nursing home. She was recently diagnosed as having various ailments which require anywhere from three to ten pills a day. She was never told what the pills were or what they were for. When the nurse came to her room to give her the pills, my friend looked her squarely in the eye and said, "The doctor only knows my body and how it works for a short time. I know it for ninety-four years, and nothing is going in it until I know what it is!"

Making changes means, for many of us, turning around decades of a certain kind of dependency on doctors. It may involve changing their stereotype of us, asking more questions, going in with a friend for support and advocacy, learning all we can about our health problems and making informed decisions,* seeking second opinions more aggressively, checking the negative effects of all medications, looking for nonmedical alternatives, refusing unnecessary surgery. Physicians who are taken aback when younger women use these tactics may be even more surprised, and even hostile, when their long-time patients ("their girls") begin to change. It takes courage to break old patterns, especially when you are feeling sick or frightened. Probably the most helpful thing you can do is to join or create a self-help or self-health group of women your age—even two or three people—to talk openly about your body changes and go to doctor appointments together to help each other get the best care you can. You can provide transportation and emotional support for each other when undergoing treatments which may be painful or scary.

The system itself must change, too, especially in research and medical training. Insurance, Medicare and Medicaid must pay for preventive measures, and for the devices—eyeglasses, hearing aids, canes, etc.—which help us deal with the daily limitations of chronic diseases and aging. Proud of the years we have lived and the contributions we have made to society, we must insist on health and medical care which enable us to live our lives as fully as possible.

THE OLDER YEARS
Pleasures and Potentials

In our older years we may feel entitled to do what pleases and satisfies us, to slow down, to let go the strain of former obligations, to express our thoughts and feelings more strongly than ever before.

---

*In older people, the ratio of fat to muscle is higher. The higher the fat, the longer drugs stay in the body. Because of this, the next day's dosage may be added to that still retained in the body from previous days, and the older person will become overmedicated.

†Drugs which are especially problematic for elders are reserpine, methyldopa, digitalis, procainamide, beta-blocking agents, all barbiturates, alcohol and tranquilizers.[56]

*Since we do not want to settle for mediocre or uninformed health care (especially when we have limited time and/or money or live in a rural area where choices in medical care are few), our best bet is learning as much as we can from women's health organizations, books and courses. If we are informed, we can tell health practitioners when we think their care or knowledge is inadequate. When we do so, we should be prepared to offer constructive and specific resources—books, articles, audiovisual materials—or know where they can be found.

Old age, because of its time perspective, can be a period of emotional and sensory awareness and enjoyment. I savor life more often. When I draw an iris, I see that iris more vividly than I did when my physical sight was better. When I read a book now, I read it more slowly. Several books I have reread, one I have just finished reading the third time.

Elemental things of life have assumed greater importance. I spend more time looking at sunsets. I am more aware of the importance to myself and others of touching (both physical and emotional), of communication, of tenderness.

Space and time for quiet reflection is more available for me now. In a strange way, impossible to put into words, I am experiencing a unity beyond space and time.

Sometimes I feel guilty to be happy when there are so many things wrong in the world and I'm not doing something about making joy possible for others. Yet the universe is going to have to get along without me sometime and so I don't have to change everything. Many of my companions are interested in a better, more compassionate world; I don't have to rush to do it all. [a seventy-eight-year-old woman]

...I know myself better and have more time to pursue my own interests. I enjoy less tempestuous relationships with children and grandchildren. I enjoy a personal growth not possible in my busier years. [a seventy-three-year-old woman]

Physical Impairments and Chronic Conditions

Some of us, however, miss these possible pleasures due to illness (often linked to low income) or to the loss of certain capacities.* The majority of women over sixty-five have some chronic health problem or condition which may limit activity over a period of time.[58] We should never automatically assume that *any* of these are the inevitable result of aging; instead we must investigate what we can do. Be suspicious of any practitioner who dismisses most complaints with "What do you expect at your age?" Many problems are as treatable now as they are at any age.

When we do have to give up a degree of independence or a cherished activity because we can't see, hear or move around as well as before, we may need time to get used to our limits and find alternative ways to manage.

Not to be able to drive (during day or night) may affect our independence, forcing us to give up cherished activities and even social relationships.

I loved my job and would have been happy to work for several years more, but it was getting more and more difficult commuting back and forth because my vision was so impaired. Driving back home in the dusk was

scary. I felt as though I had my nose right up against the windshield.

Organized around the nuclear family and the individual automobile, this society magnifies the isolation of older women, so many of whom live alone. (In protest, one Gray Panther member came to a hearing with great difficulty to demonstrate that the lowest step of the elders' bus was not wheelchair-accessible.) To live in more interdependent ways—sharing a house, organizing carpools—might be better for us. We must work for more and improved public transportation, and communities in which it is safe to walk around.

Eyes

Our eyes have less elasticity by midlife. If you are farsighted, you probably will need stronger glasses, or perhaps glasses for the first time. Some nearsighted people can give up glasses, except for driving or other distance viewing; others may require bifocals. We may have trouble adjusting to them or feel embarrassed about wearing them.

If you experience sudden flashing light and black spots, get medical attention at once. These could be symptoms of a detached retina—an emergency. In our seventies and eighties or even earlier, cataracts (cloudy lenses) may develop. While there isn't much evidence yet that these specific conditions can be prevented and not much is known about cause, eye repair is one of the few areas where medicine's heroics really pay off, restoring sight or improving it. Until cataracts are "ready" for surgery, however, the impaired vision can be limiting and discouraging. A second opinion is a particularly good idea for eye surgery, since some doctors will urge operations when they aren't necessary, or sooner (or later) than is appropriate. If you are having cataract surgery, also investigate postsurgery options in advance. A recent improvement is the possibility of *implants* placed at the time of surgery, rather than contact lenses or new glasses afterwards. Be sure your *ophthalmologist* (a medical doctor who specializes in eye diseases) is experienced in this procedure.

Glaucoma is a chronic eye disease, usually appearing at midlife or later, in which the pressure of fluid inside the eye becomes too great. This excess pressure can damage the optic nerve and cause blindness if untreated. Because it affects women more than men and rarely causes early pain or symptoms, be sure your medical exams regularly include a test for glaucoma after age forty-five.

Tests, done with a *tonometer*, are quick and painless, but some are more accurate than others. *Optometrists*, who measure eye function, can perform some tonometry only in certain states. Ophthalmologists have the most accurate diagnostic equipment and skills.

If detected early, some mild glaucoma can be treated effectively with drops taken regularly. More severe

---

*Recent research has shown that mental capacity stays the same or may increase; only the speed of reaction time decreases.

glaucoma requires surgical treatment with regular follow-up, since there are no permanent cures.

Feet

If you've always been active, you probably take your feet for granted. If you begin to notice aches and pain, not just when walking but when you rest as well, this may be part of skeletal or bone changes. (See "Osteoporosis," p. 461, and the section on arthritis in Chapter 23, "Some Common and Uncommon Health and Medical Problems.") But it is more likely to mean that you simply need more regular exercise to avoid stiffness. Some people swear they notice the effects of sugar and caffeine in their bones, especially their hands and feet.

Foot problems you already have may get worse as you age, especially if you have put on weight. Well-designed shoes with a firm, supportive arch may prevent fatigue as well as bunions* and other foot problems.

Most of us notice an increase in corns, calluses and other dry, scaly, hard skin on toes, heels and soles. Toenails often become much thicker, harder and sometimes yellower. This may be a sign of a fungus, so check with your practitioner. Soaking your feet regularly, an old-fashioned custom, is vastly preferable to harsh chemicals or carving off dead skin with a razor blade. After a long soak, try a pumice stone to work off the excess skin. You can bleach yellow toenails, if they bother you, with ordinary household bleach, diluted, or cover them with opaque nail polish.

Caring for our feet, especially cutting our own toenails, may gradually become a near-impossible chore, especially if we cannot bend as well as we used to and must ask others to help us. It can be frustrating to need others for such simple acts. Insurance plans do not cover routine care by podiatrists, yet they will pay for care of problems and infections caused by neglect of routine foot care.†

You can do foot exercises with a friend or by yourself: rise on your toes, walk on them; flex heels and ankles, pick up a pencil with your toes, etc.

Before going to sleep at night, give each foot a slight massage. It will warm your feet and help you to get to sleep more quickly, and the stretch may help you to maintain enough flexibility to care for your own feet. Find a "foot partner," massage each other's feet and help each other with grooming tasks.

Hearing

Hearing is a function we take for granted until we suddenly notice that we are missing what is being said

---

*Bunions are extremely painful, sudden misalignments of the cartilage under the tendon of the big toe. They can be caused by inadequate exercise and poor shoes, or sometimes from the stress of sudden exercise, like running, without adequate preparation. Surgical treatment is not always successful.

†Medicare covers only acute conditions and will not pay for any type of preventive care.

"Why a lip reading class?" my friends ask. The reason is a gradually increasing hearing loss I have had for several years. Unless I'm in a room with good acoustics and with people who speak clearly, I have trouble following the conversation.

In the meantime, here I am in the lip reading class of our community education program, learning a lot about how to face up to hearing difficulties. The mutual support of the group is reassuring.

While there's no magic cure, hearing aids, signing and lip reading can help. Lip reading is hard work. Many sounds can't be seen, so we are learning to be aware of other body clues and are improving our visual skills in general.

We are also planning strategies for better community understanding: distributing a leaflet titled "Tips for Talking to the Hard of Hearing" and doing a skit demonstrating some of the problems and issues.

Tips for Talking with a Person with a Hearing Difficulty

1. Don't talk from another room or from behind her.
2. Reduce background noise. Turn off radio or TV if possible.
3. See that the light falls on your face, so she can use visual clues.
4. Get her attention before speaking.
5. Face her directly, and on the same level if possible.
6. Keep your hands away from your face. Avoid speaking while you are smoking or eating.
7. Don't shout. Speak naturally but slowly and distinctly—and continue that way without dropping your voice.
8. She may not hear or understand something you say. If so, try saying it in a different way rather than repeating.
9. Recognize that she will hear less well if tired or ill.
10. Be patient. Even hints of irritation or impatience hurt.
11. Be an attentive listener. It's probably easier for her to talk than to listen.

Hearing aids of many different types exist, but unfortunately there are hucksters who make their money from misleading older people with hearing loss. If you are considering a hearing aid, do some reading first (see Resources).

or must ask people to repeat more often than feels comfortable.

Every once in a while I miss out on parts of a conversation or don't understand what I am hearing. When this happens, I discover to my later discomfort that, occasionally, I act as if I did hear—bright smile, nod of agreement. When this happens I feel so separate from people that I'm with.

Being hard of hearing is an invisible handicap. No one knows unless you tell them. You have a right to ask people to speak in a manner that enables you to understand.

One of the most important things a hard-of-hearing person can do for herself, I have discovered, is to be very assertive. Tell each person you talk with to speak louder or more clearly, and force yourself to keep reminding that person if she forgets.

Common as it is, hearing loss is not an inevitable accompaniment of aging, though it does seem to run in some families. The enormous increase in the volume and range of noise accompanying industrialization has contributed significantly to hearing loss in the present generation of over-sixty-fives, especially among factory workers and urban dwellers.

It is crucial to obtain an accurate diagnosis of the cause of hearing loss, because treatment varies depending on whether one has nerve or conduction deafness. Conduction deafness, unlike nerve deafness, can often be corrected with surgery.

Urinary Incontinence and Urinary Tract Infections

Starting around the time of menopause, some women begin to notice a slight loss of urine as they cough, sneeze, laugh or exert themselves during strenuous activity. The tissues around the urethra begin to thin out just as the vagina does, in response to reduced estrogen, sometimes making bladder control more difficult. Women who already have a history of this problem may find it getting worse. Kegel exercises (p. 333) and sit-ups or leg lifts to strengthen the abdominal muscles may help control this problem.

As we age, the environment in the vagina and urethra becomes less acid; therefore more of us are vulnerable to urinary tract or bladder infections. Cutting back on white flour, sugar and caffeine products; drinking more clear fluids and fresh-fruit unsweetened citrus juices (especially plain cranberry); and adding Vitamin C and magnesium sources may help (see the discussion of cystitis, p. 506).

Memory Loss and Confusion

It is frightening to become aware that simple everyday tasks have become a problem, or to notice a decline in your capacity for sound judgment. If you observe either an increasing confusion or loss of memory in yourself, a friend or family member, don't assume "That's it! It's all downhill from here."

What does it mean to have memory lapses? We may simply be slowing down, our memory declining just as vision or hearing do, so that we will have to work a little harder at remembering and give ourselves more time. As we get older we have more memories, so retrieving a particular memory may be more difficult.[59] When we are depressed and haven't had a chance to express grief or other emotions, preoccupation with these feelings can interfere with memory.

As one who copes with considerable memory loss at age sixty-eight, my major aid is list-making. Knowing that I may well forget an idea or "to-do," I write it down immediately. As a result, I am far better organized than at any earlier time of my life and accomplish more.

Though we experience memory lapses throughout our lives, we worry about them more when we are older. It isn't helpful when younger persons say that they also forget things because it trivializes the fear older women experience.

We can exercise memory or prevent memory loss through "mindfulness," paying attention to everyday tasks, making small (and large) decisions for ourselves.

Severe memory loss and confusion are often diagnosed as "senility" (sometimes called "dementia"). There can be several reversible causes (whose physical signs or symptoms may not be obvious): drug toxicity (from overmedication or drug-interaction), dehydration, hormonal disorders, vitamin deficiency, chemical or mineral imbalance, hypothermia,* anemia or other blood disorders, fever or an acute infection, depression or grief, endocrine or metabolic disorders. A small stroke, a traumatic event or accident, a series of losses or an abrupt relocation can also trigger acute confusion and disorientation.

More precise means of diagnosis have recently identified Alzheimer's disease (*not* reversible), as a major cause of severe and permanent memory loss, confusion and depression. It is now believed that Alzheimer's disease accounts for 55 percent of all diagnosed "senility."† Be sure to get a prompt and thorough assessment from your practitioner (a second opinion is often necessary) to avoid inappropriate labeling of senility.

---

*See footnote on p. 453.

†To keep abreast of changes in the field, contact the Alzheimer's Disease and Related Disorders Association (see Resources).

For the small percentage of elders who are correctly diagnosed with some kind of organic brain disease, drug and other therapies are available. Memory-enhancing drugs have proved helpful to some.

Depression

Please do not listen to doctors or others who imply that being depressed is typical of aging, because it need not be. If you lose your appetite, don't feel sexual, sleep too much or can't sleep and can't enjoy anything, if such symptoms continue for over a month and if talking to friends doesn't help much, you may need professional help. Fees are prohibitive for most older persons. Unfortunately, Medicare does not cover psychotherapy without a diagnosis of severe psychopathology, which you may not want to have on your record since this can be used to disqualify your judgment in legal matters or prevent you from getting needed insurance coverage.

It is deplorable, yet still true, that many mental-health professionals do not care to work with elders.* (They think it's depressing!) *You* may have to persist to find one who trusts your ability to grow.

Medication can sometimes help, but it should be taken with *extreme caution* because elders experience more and greater effects from psychoactive drugs, and some drugs may even cause or deepen depressions. *Medication should never be given alone, only in conjunction with psychotherapy and not as a substitute for it.*

Osteoporosis

Normally a woman's bone mass peaks at age thirty-five, after which she tends to lose about 1 percent of bone mass every year (10 percent per decade). At sixty-five the loss declines to 3 or 4 percent every ten years.[61] In osteoporosis, which may start in earlier years but usually does not show up until much later, bones become thin and brittle as the amount of bone mass decreases more severely. While many have thought it a "normal" condition of aging, osteoporosis is in great part preventable.

Contributing Factors

Lack of important nutrients is a significant factor in two-thirds of cases. Osteoporosis may occur after both artificially induced menopause (surgical removal of ovaries or radiation therapy that makes the ovaries nonfunctional) or natural menopause; this suggests that changing estrogen levels are at least *in part* responsible. Some long-term steroid medications, such as cortisone for arthritis, also contribute to osteoporosis (see footnote describing "iatrogenesis," p. 556). The profile of a woman most at risk for osteoporosis includes the following characteristics: white, aged sixty and over, small-boned, slender and sedentary. Usually she has exercised very little, taken in insufficient calcium during her growing years and breastfed several children in her teens and early twenties. Often she also smokes and drinks alcohol excessively.

Symptoms

During its early stages, osteoporosis produces no symptoms, or only mild ones such as backaches or back-muscle spasms. An older woman may be unaware she has osteoporosis until she fractures her spine, hip or wrist in a simple fall. Repeated fractures are common once the process starts. A possible sign in postmenopausal women is pain in the upper or lower spine lasting for several days and then stopping, which may be caused by disintegrated vertebrae which collapse spontaneously. In a more advanced form, these "compression fractures" in the upper spine cause a condition commonly called "dowager's hump"; the resulting shortened chest area may make digesting food more difficult.

Diagnosis

Although routine X-rays may show signs of osteoporosis, they also show reduced bone mass caused by other conditions,* so they do not make a definitive diagnosis of osteoporosis possible. If either you or your health practitioner suspect early osteoporosis, it's best if you can go to a metabolic bone disease service, usually only found in a large urban medical-research center. More sensitive and precise diagnostic methods, not yet widely available, are dual photon absorptionometry and quantitative CT scanning of the spine.[62]

Treatment

Predictably, physicians emphasize treatment of existing osteoporosis, usually once a dramatic fracture occurs, and neglect early prevention.† They usually prescribe, after the fact, the very activities that might have prevented the condition from developing in the first place—replacement calcium, Vitamin-C and -D supplements, weight-bearing exercises such as walking, special back-exercise regimens and physical therapy. But they may also want to combine such treatment with estrogen replacement therapy and sodium fluoride.

---

*See Robert Butler's chapter, "Emotional Problems and Mental Illness in Old Age" in *Why Survive?* (listed in Resources) for a critique of psychiatry's failure to treat elders.[60] Also consult the numerous books on psychiatry's abuses of women.

*Osteomalasia (rickets), when the bones are soft; an endocrine disorder such as hypothyroidism, diabetes mellitus, hypoglycemia and Cushing's syndrome; any of the four bone marrow tumors: plasma cell myeloma, Ewing's tumor, reticulum cell sarcoma and Hodgkin's disease of the bone.

†For the first time, a medical organization—the American Society for Bone and Mineral Research—has formally addressed osteoporosis prevention, announcing guidelines which stress adequate calcium intake, regular weight-bearing exercise and avoidance of smoking.

461

Estrogen Replacement Therapy and Sodium Fluoride—Controversial Medical Treatments

In recent years the emphasis of medical research and practice has shifted to prevention of osteoporosis through medical intervention with ERT and/or sodium fluoride. These treatments are still controversial,* so be sure to consider the risks of ERT as discussed on pp. 443–44 and those of sodium fluoride (see below). We believe there is adequate evidence that self-help alternatives are as effective and subject us to no risk.

Recent research reports that rapid bone loss following premature menopause can be prevented for up to eight years by taking ERT; yet after eight years the positive effect ceases, and bone loss actually increases.[63] Such findings suggest that women who experience this problem should try weight-bearing exercise and an improved calcium-rich diet before seeking medical treatment. ERT also offers protection against osteoporosis to women who go through a natural menopause, but there are risks.†

Sodium fluoride in measured doses[65] seems to increase bone mass so that there is less chance of fracture. However, the quality of the new fluoride-induced bone cells is questionable, and the other effects of fluoride are debilitating enough—inflamed joints, recurrent vomiting, anemia in 40 percent of women in one study,[66] gastric and joint pain and ankle edema in another[67]—to warrant its use only in severe cases and only under careful research controls.

Coping with and Overcoming Impairments and Chronic Conditions— Some Examples

Four years ago, at age eighty-one, I got diabetes. It has impaired my living condition, but it doesn't get me down. In fact, I have always had the feeling that the more we have to fight and overcome, the stronger we are. Obstacles are here to be overcome. That's part of life, and it gives us a good feeling that we are not just little ants, we are fighters.

It's not only the physical impairment which has to worry you and the doctor. It is also your state of mind. The healthy mind creates the healthy body, and the healthy body creates the healthy mind. Sometimes a frail body can draw its strength from a courageous mind.

I coped with some of my feelings of loss about my diminished hearing by developing a new interest in foreign movies. I was missing a lot at the theater* and in American movies, but when I go to a foreign movie I can read the subtitles so I don't miss a thing—and I'm expanding my horizons! [a seventy-eight-year-old woman]

For a number of years I have been living with Paget's disease in my right hip.† The doctor gave me the feeling that there were a limited number of steps "programed" for that hip and that I should give up many of the activities I enjoyed.

Fortunately others, professionals and lay friends, suggested I continue more or less as I was, testing limits and letting discomfort be the determining factor in what I did. When camping, I found I could take some of the easier hikes and avoid the strenuous ones. I had difficulty climbing stairs at a railroad station, so I found I could navigate them by putting both feet on a step before I went to another. If I had pain when I got up after sitting engrossed with a book, I consoled myself with the awareness that this, too, would pass as I limbered up. I accepted these limits to my flexibility and found I could live within them. Then, several weeks ago, I found that I didn't have to accept them as completely. It all began with borrowing a bicycle and relearning how to ride one. It took some getting used to, but I found out how to take advantage of my strong left hip and soon was braving traffic and riding, once more, with confidence. I experienced a new freedom, a new sense of my body's resources.

Then I learned from a hiking book that all my life I had been walking incorrectly. Soon I began changing, using a more productive method. I began to feel more grounded and, at the same time, freer. [a woman in her seventies]

CAREGIVING AND ALTERNATIVE LIVING ARRANGEMENTS

Caregiving—A Gap in Our Delivery of Health and Medical Services

Approximately 1.5 million chronically disabled people over fifty-five are confined to their homes in the U.S. RNs provide only 18 percent of nursing care, such as

---

*In April 1984, a National Institute for Health Consensus Development Conference recommended use of estrogen to prevent osteoporosis despite the known risks.

†In a research study at the University of Washington in Seattle, nearly 1,000 women who had taken estrogen for six or more years reduced the risk of fractures by 50 to 60 percent.[64]

*Signing is a way to make cultural events accessible to persons with hearing loss. If you are planning a cultural event, be sure to find someone who will sign.

†Paget's disease is a disease characterized by a softening and bowing of bones, which thickens and enlarges the deformed bones but leaves them structurally weak. Several million Americans may have it, but most do not require specific treatment. Some of those who have it require little attention, but in others the disease produces deformities and a wide range of complications.

bandaging, giving injections, etc. Household members provide 80 percent of the home care their ailing relatives receive (bathing, dressing, feeding).

It is the plight of thousands of women (and some men), upon whom the health system depends, to care for the aged, the chronically ill, and the disabled. They are the invisible laborers without whom neither the health system nor the patient could survive.[68]

Women are nine or ten times more likely than men to care for an aging spouse or parent or spouse's parent. We often marry men who are older than we are; we maintain our health and live longer than they do. When caregiving is work we want to do, respected by our family and community, it can be rewarding. Too often, however, others simply expect it of us.

We planned for my husband—I was going to be the person who sustained him until his death. We never worked out who would care for me. It's an unseen social service that women do; if the wife dies first, he finds another woman.

Traditionally, women have cared for family members in their own homes. In modern times some of this care has shifted to nursing homes, where it is also carried out by women, paid at the lowest wage levels. However, a variety of services have been developed to help people remain in their homes, due to a growing awareness that it is best to avoid institutionalizing persons in need of care whenever possible. Unfortunately, though such services are not only desirable but cost-effective, they are not uniformly available and are often threatened by cuts in already meager government support. Thus family-provided care most often still means woman-provided care, in isolation, without pay or needed respite or support services, without the security of job-retraining, a pension or even health insurance when the person we care for dies.

For three years, I was confined caring for a sick husband twenty-four hours a day. Then my doctor said I had to send him to a nursing home because my blood pressure was rising.

We rushed my husband to the hospital with a stroke, and it was a medical miracle. Now I'm not so sure it was a blessing. He is not always rational and cannot be left alone. Naturally, I had to give up my job. Financially, we are in terrible shape, but disaster will strike when he dies. I am fifty-seven and won't be eligible for anything. I can't see any way out.[69]

For a growing number of us, caregiving demands conflict with our jobs. (Nearly half of all married women, and even more single women, ages forty to fifty-nine, are in the labor force.) Clearly, we need services which would make continued employment possible, such as day centers or home-care workers. Short-term nursing-home placement—even for a weekend—would help relieve the pressure on a woman carrying a full-time job along with the second job of caregiving.* Some social service organizations are pioneering support groups for caregivers. (See Resources.)

When We Need Care

What if we had a different cultural perspective on dependency? What if instead of a Declaration of Independence we had a Declaration of Interdependence?

Women learn to accept and even expect that others will be dependent on us. Yet we fear becoming dependent ourselves.

After my recent eye surgery it took me ages to work up a head of steam to get back the energy level that I normally work at. I'm afraid that if I really got sick and couldn't work, there would be no one to help. [a fifty-five-year-old divorced woman with grown children]

I have a great abhorrence for the ghettos of nursing homes. I would rather struggle with overcoming physical difficulties in my own house than be put in the hands of people that I'm paying and then having to please them so they'll be nice to me. [a woman in her seventies]

Chronic illness or a disability which occurs late in life may be a blow to our pride and our habits of self-sufficiency. It raises the question of who will be there to care for us and whether we feel we can accept care. On the other hand, we may feel perfectly entitled to receiving from others what we have given for many decades.

Learning to accept being cared for without resentment or loss of pride is one of the tasks of our later years. It helps when those caring for us can do so without taking over our lives or taking away all our choices.

The interdependency between my children and me is healthy. If I needed to be taken care of at some point, unless they change radically, I might be able to tolerate that. [a sixty-five-year-old widow who helps with the care of her grandchildren on occasion]

Making Plans

It is a good idea to plan beforehand with family members or friends the kind of care and living situation we want when we are no longer able to manage alone—ideally neither regimented nor paternalistic, offering a wide range of challenges, providing com-

---

*Some of us may want to care for a sick family member ourselves. When we do we should receive a salary and credit toward a pension. We may need a variety of services when the person we care for dies.

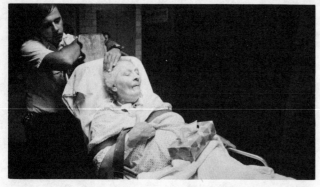

Michael Weisbrot/Stock Boston

munity, privacy and as much freedom as possible, where being old is only a *part* of who we are.

Nursing Homes

We ourselves, or our relatives, may have to go into nursing homes when we come to need fairly constant nursing care. (Only a small percentage of elders, 5 to 8 percent, live in nursing homes, but 68 percent of those who do are women.)[70]

Nursing-home care is often poor, putting profits ahead of quality care, paying workers little, skimping on patient needs. Often, in the interest of "efficiency," the routines are set up to serve only the sickest residents, depriving healthier residents of a chance to use their full capacities. Having other people or pets to care for may sustain attentiveness and memory. Lacking any meaningful decisions to make, residents become confused and disoriented.[71] Physical and mental abilities deteriorate when we have neither mental stimulation nor chances to exercise and carry out simple tasks on our own.

We are critical of many aspects of nursing-home care—the skyrocketing costs, impersonal care, medicalization of everyday life and lack of privacy and choices for residents. Economic incentives have favored nursing-home care over other care alternatives, resulting in a situation where over half of nursing-home residents could, with adequate social support, manage to live in the community, while many who desperately need nursing-home care are placed on interminable waiting lists.* Because nursing-home care is essential for some, we must work to improve quality of life and care and innovate in ways that give residents more control.

Some recent innovations include regular visits from preschool children, waist-high garden plots for persons in wheelchairs, and private rooms for sexual activity, a right won after residents at a rest home instituted a lawsuit to obtain it.†

*See Christine Bishop, Alonzo Plough and Thomas R. Wille-main, "Nursing-Home Levels of Care: Problems and Alternatives," *Health Care Financing Review*, Fall 1980.

†See Resources for pamphlets on how to choose a nursing home and how to help your family member with a move to a nursing home.

Support Services and Strategies for Living Independently or in Alternative Housing and Care Arrangements

As we grow older, it becomes more difficult to separate health, housing and socioeconomic needs into neat compartments. Those of us who live with chronic conditions know that we need concerned persons nearby to help us with everyday tasks that have become difficult. This can contribute more to our well-being and ability to live in the community than doctor visits or medical interventions.

Despite vast differences in our well-being, living conditions and income levels, most of us want to be self-sufficient as long as possible.

A variety of services can help us, as individuals or couples, to stay in our own homes even when we need occasional nursing services or help with everyday tasks. Meals on Wheels is a program that delivers hot lunches to elders, usually five days a week. Visiting nurses, physical therapists and home-care health aides may be available to perform needed services in the home. Home care in the form of health aides or homemakers is a highly beneficial and cost-effective program, yet it is not consistently available and is continually threatened with cuts. Lifelines, an emergency response system, permits older persons with potentially life-threatening conditions to live alone.* Some changes to work for to make continued living in one's home a reality are 1. converting part of a home to an accessory apartment for additional income and closer neighbors; 2. convincing banks to support home equity conversion. (This means that people who fully own a home which has appreciated in value, but do not have the cash to pay living expenses or upkeep, can turn to banks for a "reverse mortgage." Banks then own an increasingly greater share of the home and provide cash needed for living.) At some point for many of us, living alone is no longer feasible. We may experience physical changes, reduced energy or fewer resources; we may have problems that require having others nearby; we may be lonely. Yet we probably will not need twenty-four-hour care or medical services on a daily basis. Until recently, government reimbursement and financing policies encouraged institutionalization. However, there is a growing movement for alternatives, particularly in housing, often at its most innovative in rural areas where limiting red tape is at a minimum.

Living with others is not only cost-effective but care-effective, because housemates can participate in looking out for one another rather than paying others to do so. Cooperatives, intergenerational living with relatives or friends, congregate housing, turning part of

*We wear a button and press it if we need help. It also goes off automatically if we become unconscious. The button is attached to a device in our telephone which transmits a signal to a hospital or other receiving station to send emergency help.

a house into an accessory apartment, small group homes—these are all new patterns of living together.* Total privacy is surely impossible, but we gain dignity, companionship and security. Many elders have the strength, will and independence of spirit to make the changes required for new living arrangements.

Congregate Housing

For the past year and a half, I have shared an apartment with four other persons, a man and three women, all of us older. I had some questions before I came in: Would I still have privacy? Would I be able to get along with persons I had not even met before? The answer to both is "Yes."

The technical name for this particular kind of living is congregate housing, but I am beginning to think of us as a "family of choice." We care for one another, celebrate special days and meals together. We have our differences, too, which we settle ourselves, growing in our decision skills. I think it would be impossible to make it work if those of us with few health problems had to take care of those who had more. One woman in our apartment, legally blind, needs a homemaker to help with shopping, cleaning, bathing, et cetera. Without home-care assistance, the responsibility would be too much for the others. But we can and do help each other in important little ways.

Privately Run Retirement Homes

These may be appropriate alternatives for elders who do not need nursing care or case management but prefer not to be alone. In the words of a geriatric social worker describing her community:

Two women from Maine triumphed over midlife crises by going into a whole new field of endeavor. After being turned down by eight banks, they finally obtained funds for renovating an enormous old house in a small rural village. They provide room, board and laundry for a group of fourteen elders, most of whom have lived in the area for many years. Using the fruits of a large organic garden and orchard, bartering surplus seedlings for fish and other commodities, they acquired such a good reputation for their food that they were asked to cater weddings and parties. These activities in turn have enabled them to keep their costs—and their rents—fairly low, and give the residents the option of participating in the food preparation or festivities.

A huge wraparound porch and a fine piano brought in (and played daily) by one of the residents are other assets that add to the lively atmosphere. During harvest season, neighbors come in to help prepare fruits and vegetables for canning, freezing and preserving. One guest—a former log driver, now ninety-three—has cut and stacked four cords of wood for the past three years! Their latest venture, paid for in less than a year, is a heated swimming pool, in constant use by those who live there and other elders who are encouraged to swim by their doctors; local schools and families also come for swimming lessons and recreation.

We are impressed by the variety and innovativeness of support services for elders and their caregivers in other countries.

- The Scandinavian countries provide service buses to bring cleaning and laundry, hairdressing supplies, books and hot food to elders who wish to remain in their homes. Homemakers and personal care attendants are provided to those who need them. An alternative is the service house, where all such services are available on the premises to those who live there. The state pays family caregivers.
- In New Zealand, low-interest loans, services and subsidies are available to families who wish to care for elderly relatives at home.
- In England, clusters of about twenty apartments for elders are staffed by a state-employed "helper" who gets people to doctor appointments and so on. Respite care, short-term placement in nursing homes, is available to give caregivers a breather. Caregivers are organized in an advocacy organization.

Many of these services or equally creative ones are available or potentially available to elders in this country. However, our programs exist as a patchwork of innovations in a crazy quilt of cutbacks and threatened cutbacks. For instance, chronically scarce funding, often awarded to innovative pilot programs, is not renewed after they succeed and are no longer "new."* As a nation, we have not deliberately decided (as have the Scandinavian countries) to make the older years a good time of life, free from financial worry and deprivation. As an ever greater percent of the electorate enters the older years, we develop a growing base of support for such a national commitment.

DEATH

At all ages we struggle with the reality of death. We lose our parents; as parents we may lose infants or

---

*One private agency near Boston funded through a private foundation maintains an application and interview process, brings together people whose needs fit each other, encourages them to learn as much as possible about each other and try a weekend or a week together, and helps them, should they wish, to write their own contract.[72]

*We are grateful to Andrew Dibner of the Boston University Gerontology Center, who made this observation after a several-months' fact-finding tour of European caregiving facilities and options.

children. People we love die. If we become terminally ill at any age, we have to cope with our imminent deaths. But the impetus to accept this reality for ourselves comes for most of us as we grow older.

We have the fear that if a person faces death that means she does not participate in life. Actually, it works the other way. The more we acknowledge and recognize death, the more we can live in the present. [a fifty-two-year-old woman]

I am more aware of a mystery and beauty in life since I have accepted death as a personal eventuality for me. Before then, I had thought of death out there; now I know that I am going to die. That has released me for more vivid living. I reach out more. Almost everything reminds me of its connections with other things; my present is many-textured. I do not look to the future with dread. It has to be shorter than my past but it does not have to be less rich. [a seventy-eight-year-old woman]

Some of us continue to feel ambivalent and scared about acknowledging death, or have difficulty coming to grips with the reality of it for ourselves.

Intellectually I'm very glib about it, but in my gut I can't accept that one day I won't be here. [a seventy-four-year-old woman]

In our culture, discussion of death has been taboo until the last few years. Modern medical science often distorts our ideas of death. Many doctors view it as an adversary, an evil, a visible defeat. They often use every medical means possible to prolong life for its own sake without considering its quality or whether there is any hope of recovery, and without taking into account the ill person's wishes.

In response to the excessive medicalization of death, terminally ill people, their friends and relatives and concerned professionals have created *hospices*,* a humane alternative to general hospital or nursing-home care. More than a place, hospice is an idea and a service. The thing we fear most when we are seriously ill is prolonged and unmanageable pain. Hospice workers assist people to manage pain, to die at home or in special places neither home nor hospital. The patient and family together are the focus of attention. Hospices offer support, understanding and respite to everyone involved. Bereavement counseling may continue for a substantial period beyond the family member's death.†

---

*At this writing these special places exist in only six or seven localities. More are being started. See Resources.

†We need to work for federal and state legislation to permit the creation and continued existence of free-standing hospices, as alternatives to hospital death. Competition from profit-making chains and from hospitals now threatens survival of community hospices (see Chapter 24).

Taking Control of Our Own Death

We know we cannot control whether we die, so we often jump to the conclusion that there is *nothing* we can do about it—no control, no choice.

Yet we do have elements of control. Many of us can choose our place of death—at home or in a hospital or hospice. As long as we are able, we can fight for medical care that allows us to keep our dignity, instead of accepting care which is inappropriate for extreme pain and terminal illness. Only we can authorize a precise disposal of our property, donate vitally needed organs like kidneys and corneas for transplant if we wish, and perform the little details that insure an easier burden for relatives and friends.

Though legal, medical and theological controversies abound, many of us would like to participate fully in the decision about when and how we will die. The right to control our deaths is part of our basic right to have control over our bodies and our lives.

I have been searching for a doctor who would let me participate not just in my health care but in my own death, too. [a woman in her seventies]

We want to be able to define for ourselves what we consider a tolerable quality of life, a worthwhile existence.

I've had a lot of things done to my body and I'm seventy-three. I've made up my mind that enough has been done to me. If something bad happens, something major, I'm not sure I want to be repaired again. No more tampering with my body! I don't want to live to be one hundred if I'm all botched up.

An elderly friend of mine had had one stroke and was on strong medication to prevent another. One day recently, despite a warning sign, she did not call her doctor. "He'd just put me back in the hospital." The next day she died peacefully in her bed, having remained active to the very end. I call that a good death.

We may actively decide we want to avoid a long, drawn-out period of illness and dependency, to avoid a medicalized death in which life is prolonged by artificial means and/or to choose the occasion and means of our death. We can make a *living will** when we are well, stating what we want and do not want; however, there's no guarantee that these written wishes will be honored.

Laws vary from state to state. In many states it is not legal to decide how or when we want to die. To

---

*Sample copies and other information available from *Concern for Dying* (see Resources).

466

protect loved ones from possible prosecution as accessories, some dying persons have chosen to go off by themselves when taking a fatal substance. We may even have to forego some of the talking and planning we might want to do in order to protect our loved ones from legal harassment.

I have for years kept a precious bottle somewhere. I talked with my daughter about it and she asked me, "Please, if you are ever ready to do this, tell me first." But I said I couldn't do that because I would be laying too heavy a burden on her; she would certainly feel that it was her job to dissuade me. [a woman in her sixties]

An important way to gain the power to choose our own deaths is by working to change the laws and social attitudes related to death and dying and by challenging legal, medical and religious control. Some organizations exist to help us raise these issues publicly and deal with them personally.

Claiming the right to control the ending of our lives in no way minimizes the seriousness or the finality of the decision, nor the pain and grief of those we leave behind. Yet the issues are complex. It is certainly more appropriate for the dying person rather than any outside authority to weigh all the factors involved.

SURVIVAL SKILLS

Many women are still going strong at seventy or seventy-five and beyond. We want to end this chapter with their voices as they tell of the "survival skills" which keep them active, creative, involved and feeling good about themselves and their lives.*

*Most of the older women we spoke with in preparing this chapter enjoy reasonably good health and adequate economic situations. Though this is not the case for large numbers of women, these experiences highlight the *potential* for the older years; a potential (the birthright of every person) denied to so many of us because of inadequate food, housing, care, transportation, health and medical care and the constant worry about how to pay for all of these.

Photography class at Freedom House, Roxbury, MA

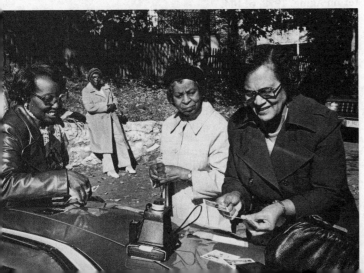

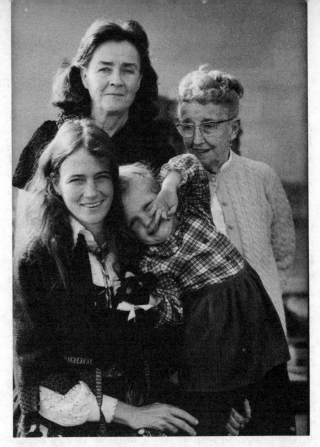

Peter Simon

In our mothers' time, the only acceptable role for a woman over sixty was a homebody, puttering around in the kitchen, not going out anywhere. We still have that image we can follow. If you don't question it, you may find that you are following a stereotype instead of your own true path. You have to go out and look for what really meets your needs. For myself, I look for activities that I can shape as well as contribute to and that get me out of the house. I enjoy my work visiting elders who can't go out; it makes me feel that I am contributing to others. My women's support group meets my needs as an older woman and is something that I can help define.

It is important to challenge the stereotypes of elders as rigid, unable to form new relationships or to experience change and growth.*

There's a discrepancy between my image of an older person in her seventies and the way I feel. In fact, there's no connection. My concept of a grandmother was of someone who didn't do much. But I became a grandmother at forty-seven. I started a vigorous exercise program at forty-three, and am still running every day at seventy-six and love it.

*Professionals, researchers and practitioners have contributed to the stereotyping of elders by perpetuating the "disengagement theory"—the idea that elders gradually withdraw from life by divesting themselves of important roles and commitments as an appropriate adjustment to aging and approaching death. It would be more appropriate to say that "disengagement" is an inappropriate giving-in to ageism and the impoverishment of many elders. We have learned from the many lively, vital, elder women we spoke with that it is possible to live fully for as long as we live.

467

The seventies have been the best decade of my life. From what I have seen with my friends, it is either the best or the worst. My creative work as an artist is what keeps me alive; my friends keep me happy and contented. If I had to give up people I would never have another happy day, but I would stay alive if I could work. [a seventy-seven-year-old woman]

It is not so different to be over eighty, except that accidents and illness can make a change. If I had not broken my hip I would probably still be very active today, but I wouldn't have the insight I have. Being confined gives me more time for reflection.

I know I have grown in the last ten years, even at my age. I have become more optimistic. A lot of young people seem to be drawn to me. I don't know if I give more now than I used to, or have more composure and insight. That sounds funny, but it is a fact.

I had to concentrate on getting well, and this makes you rather self-centered. Sometimes I catch myself thinking, I am too busy with my body. What about exercising my mind? That's why I think that intermingling with different kinds of people, young and old, is very important. The segregation of the aged is absolutely ridiculous, cruel, unproductive and costly. [an eighty-five-year-old woman]

Staying in Touch with Our Inner Selves—Nourishing the Spirit

Staying in touch with ourselves helps us reach out to others, cope with the hard things in our lives and keep on growing. There are many ways that we can stay in touch with ourselves—writing in a journal, reading a book, exercising, meditating, walking in the woods, a long hot shower or bath, camping. For some of us, being connected with a spiritual community helps, too.

Last week, at age seventy-three, I sat in a group of older women discussing religion and spirituality and was reminded of our midweek prayer meetings sixty years ago, except that no woman there was witnessing to the teachings of her childhood church indoctrination but was describing instead her "spirituality." The world's religions have all been founded by men and promote their beliefs, not to mention their reverence of dominance. I don't choose to have men control my moral and spiritual values. In looking within myself for what I value most, I discover I put honesty first, nurturing next, then striving for peace and justice in human relationships and cherishing our earth and universe. I nourish my spirit through music, nature study and meditation but mostly through relatedness to people I love.

A thought has come to me in the last few years. I doubt that when I die my life will be over—my life with all its loving and caring and striving. Can it be that all my

loved ones—mother, sister, other relatives—can all this love be gone? Nothing in nature disappears. Out of our bones, our skeletons, new life comes in some other way.

Support Groups for Older Women

Friendship is valuable not merely for happiness and mental well-being but for physical health and survival as well.[73] Since aging in this country too often means increasing isolation, the middle and older years are a good time to create a support and friendship network if you don't already have one. A study at Yale found that, regardless of age, persons with strong social bonds (marriage, friends, group or organizational affiliations) had a mortality rate 2.5 percent lower than those who were relatively isolated. The other important finding was that friendship and support from *any* of these sources contributed to survival.

I am open to the new adventure of meeting people. Once I was congratulated for having been one of the founders of the Boston Gray Panthers. I had to answer that I didn't deserve any thanks. The Gray Panthers deserve thanks from me. Those relationships and that connection mean so much that I am just plain grateful.

It is never too late to form a support group.

NOTES

1. Personal communication from Jean Tock, sculptor.
2. *Growing Numbers, Growing Force: A Report from the White House Mini-Conference on Older Women.* The Older Women's League, 3800 Harrison Street, Oakland, CA 94611, 1980, pp. 38–39.
3. Susan Sontag. "The Double Standard of Aging," *Saturday Review of the Society*, Vol. 95, No. 39 (September 23, 1972), pp. 29–38.
4. Barbara Ehrenreich and Karin Stallard. "The Nouveau Poor," *Ms.*, August 1982, pp. 217–24.
5. *Growing Numbers, Growing Force*, p. 38.
6. Marilyn R. Block, et al. *Uncharted Territory: Issues and Concerns of Women Over Forty.* University of Maryland, Center on Aging, 1978, p. 144.
7. Tish Sommers. "Employment Problems of Older Women," available from the Older Women's League (see note 2 above), pp. 3–4.
8. Marilyn R. Block, et al., *Uncharted Territory*, pp. 157–58.
9. Report of the National Commission on Social Security Reform, 1981. *Note:* This is a report that was prepared in the last days of the Carter administration and came out in early 1981. It was not widely circulated and was superseded by a subsequent report by the Reagan administration. The 1981 report contains important information for women. It is not easy to get but it is possible to obtain a copy if you persist.
10. Phyllis Silverman. *Helping Women Cope with Grief.* Beverly Hills, CA: Sage Publications, 1981, p. 39.

11. *HHS News*, U.S. Department of Health and Human Services, October 31, 1980; *HEW News*, October 15, 1979.

12. Lillian Rubin. *Women of a Certain Age*. New York: Harper and Row Publishers, Inc., 1979.

13. Phyllis Silverman, *Helping Women Cope with Grief*, p. 39.

14. Knud J. Helsing, Moyses Szklo and George W. Comstock. "Factors Associated with Mortality After Widowhood," *American Journal of Public Health*, Vol. 71 (1981), pp. 802–9.

15. Helene Deutsch. *The Psychology of Women: A Psychoanalytic Interpretation*, Vol. II. New York: Grune and Stratton, 1944.

16. Mary Roth Walsh. *Doctors Wanted: No Women Need Apply! Sexual Barriers in the Medical Profession*. New Haven: Yale University Press, 1977.

17. Myrna Weissman. "The Myth of Involutional Melancholia," *Journal of the American Medical Association*, Vol. 242, No. 8 (August 1979), pp. 24–31.

18. Janice G. Raymond. "Medicine as Patriarchal Religion," *Journal of Medicine and Philosophy*, Vol. 7 (1982), pp. 197–216.

19. Robert Wilson. *Feminine Forever*. New York: M. Evans and Co., Inc., 1966.

20. David Reuben. *Everything You Always Wanted to Know About Sex*. New York: David McKay Co., Inc., 1969.

21. *Ibid*.

22. Patricia Kaufert. "The Perimenopausal Woman and Her Use of Health Services," *Maturitas*, Vol. 2, No 3 (October 1980), pp. 191–205.

23. Sandra Ritz. "Growing Older Through Menopause," *Medical Self-Care*, Vol. 15 (winter 1981), pp. 14–19.

24. Rosetta Reitz. *Menopause: A Positive Approach*. New York: Penguin Books, 1982; Barbara Seaman and Gideon Seaman. *Women and the Crisis in Sex Hormones*. New York: Bantam Books, 1977; *Consumer Reports*, November 1976, p. 642.

25. Vidal S. Clay. "Menopause," in *Women's Health and Medical Guide*, Patricia Cooper, ed. Des Moines, IA: Meredith Corp., 1981.

26. *Ibid*.; see also Patricia Kaufert, "The Perimenopausal Woman."

27. Surveillance, epidemiology and end results, incidence and mortality data, 1973–1977, U.S. Department of Health and Human Services, Public Health Service, National Institutes of Health publication #81-2330.

28. Donald Smith, et al. "Association of Exogenous Estrogen and Endometrial Cancer," *New England Journal of Medicine*, Vol. 293 (December 4, 1975), pp. 1164–67.

29. Vidal S. Clay, "Menopause."

30. Barbara Seaman and Gideon Seaman, *Women and the Crisis in Sex Hormones*.

31. Kenneth J. Ryan. "Cancer Risks and Estrogen Use in the Menopause," an editorial in *New England Journal of Medicine*, Vol. 293 (1975), p. 1200.

32. Barbara Seaman and Gideon Seaman, *Women and the Crisis in Sex Hormones*.

33. S.M. Wolfe, testimony of Public Citizens' Health Research Group, Washington, DC, August 1, 1979.

34. Sharon Lieberman. "New Discovery: Public Relations Cures Cancer," *Majority Report*, February 1977; see also S. Lieberman, "But You'll Make Such a Lovely Corpse," *Majority Report*, February 19–March 5, 1977.

35. Barbara Seaman and Gideon Seaman, *Women and the Crisis in Sex Hormones*.

36. Lila Wallis. "Can Hormone Therapy of the Menopausal Syndrome Be Made Safe?" Proceedings of the Women in Medicine Conference, Cornell Medical School, 1981, pp. 89–92.

38. Barbara Seaman and Gideon Seaman, *Women and the Crisis in Sex Hormones*.

38. Paul C. MacDonald. "Estrogen Plus Progestin in Postmenopausal Women," *New England Journal of Medicine* (December 31, 1981).

39. Quoted in Marilyn R. Block, et al., *Uncharted Territory*, p. 43.

40. Mary Jane Sherfey. *The Nature and Evolution of Female Sexuality*. New York: Vintage Books, 1972, p. 102.

41. Jane Brody. "Personal Health: Sex in the Elderly," *The New York Times*, July 5, 1978.

42. Alice Lake. *Our Own Years: What Women Over 35 Should Know About Themselves*. New York: Random House, Inc., 1979, p. 98.

43. Robert Butler and Myrna Lewis. *Sex After Sixty*. N. Miami, FL: Merit Publications, 1976, pp. 92–93.

44. "How Your Health Affects Your Sex Life," *Family Circle*, June 8, 1982.

45. Robert C. Atchley. "Later Adulthood in Oxford Township." Summary of one-year data, Scripps Foundation Gerontology Foundation, Miami University, Oxford, OH, 1975.

46. Loretta Schwartz-Nobel. *Starvation in the Shadow of Plenty*. G.P. Putnam's Sons, 1980.

47. *Growing Numbers, Growing Force*.

48. S.V. Saxon and M.H. Etlen. *Physical Change and Aging: A Guide for the Helping Professions*. New York: The Tiresiav Press, 1978; see also *Journal of the American Medical Association*, Vol. 247, No. 8 (February 26, 1982), pp. 1106–12.

49. J.F. Aloia, et al. "Old Runners Overtake the Aging Process," *Medical World News* (April 30, 1979).

50. G. Donald Whedon. "Osteoporosis," an editorial in the *New England Journal of Medicine*, Vol. 305, No. 7 (August 13, 1981), pp. 397–99.

51. Warren E.C. Wacker. *Magnesium and Man*. Cambridge, MA: Harvard University Press, 1980.

52. World Health Organization recommendations as quoted by Maggie Lettvin, personal communication, May 9, 1983 (see Resources).

53. Robert Butler. *Why Survive: Being Old in America*. New York: Harper-Colophon, 1975.

54. *Ibid*., p. 178.

55. *Medical World News* (September 13, 1982), p. 70.

56. Alex Comfort. *A Good Age*. New York: Crown Publishers, Inc., 1976, p. 62. For a more complete list see *Health Facts*, Vol. VII, No. 34 (March 1982), p. 7.

57. *Beware*, a film about the dangers of overmedication for elders. Adelphi University Center on Aging, Garden City, NY 11530.

58. Robert Butler, *Why Survive?* p. 179.

59. Alice Lake. *Our Own Years*, pp. 215–16.

60. Robert Butler, *Why Survive?* pp. 231–35.

61. Donald G. Whedon, "Osteoporosis," pp. 397–99.

62. *Ibid*.

63. R. Lindsay, et al. "Bone Response to Termination of Estrogen Treatment," *Lancet*, Vol. 1 (1978), pp. 1325–27.

64. Noel S. Weiss, et al. "Decreased Risk of Fractures of the Hip and Lower Forearm with Postmenopausal Use of Estrogen," *New England Journal of Medicine*, Vol. 303, No. 21 (November 20, 1980), pp. 1195–98.

65. B. Lawrence Riggs, et al. "Effect of the Fluoride/Calcium Regimen on Vertebral Fracture Occurrence in

Postmenopausal Osteoporosis," *New England Journal of Medicine*, Vol. 306, No. 8 (February 25, 1982), pp. 446–50.

66. *Ibid.*

67. Joseph Lane. "Postmenopausal Osteoporosis: The Orthopedic Approach." *The Female Patient*, Vol. 6 (November 1981), pp. 43–51.

68. Elinor Polansky. "Take Him Home, Mrs. Smith," *Healthright*, Vol. II, No. 2 (winter 1975–1976).

69. Tish Sommers. "A Feminist View of Death." Presented at Drake University Law School, Des Moines, Iowa, March 27, 1976.

70. *Older Women—The Economics of Aging.* The Women's Studies Program and Policy Center at George Washington University in conjunction with the Women's Research and Education Institute of the Congresswomen's Caucus. First printing October 1980; second printing January 1981, Washington, DC.

71. Ellen J. Langer and Judith Rodin. "The Effects of Choice and Enhanced Personal Responsibility for the Aged: A Field Experiment in an Institutional Setting," *Journal of Personality and Social Psychology*, Vol. 34, No. 2 (1976), pp. 191–98.

72. *Planning and Developing a Shared Living Project*, a guide for community groups, prepared by Action for Boston Community Development, Inc., and Concerned Boston Citizens for Elder Affairs: Housing Alternatives Committee, Boston, MA, 1980, pp. 4, 5.

73. Lisa Berkman and S. Leonard Syme, cited in *Boston Globe*, February 3, 1982. Judy Foreman, "Friends: As Vital as Family."

RESOURCES

Books

Anderson, Beverly, and Adeline McConnel. *Single After 50: How to Have the Time of Your Life.* New York: McGraw-Hill, Inc., 1981. Not a feminist book, but full of useful tips fo heterosexual women and men. Lively and empowering.

Block, Marilyn R., Janice L. Davidson and Jean D. Grambs. *Women Over Forty: Visions and Realities.* New York: Springer Publishing Co., Inc., 1981.

Bluh, Bonnie. *The "Old" Speak Out.* New York: Horizon Press, 1979. Interviews with women and men in their sixties, seventies, eighties, nineties and even past a hundred tell of the joys and pleasures as well as the struggles of the older years.

Boston Women's Health Book Collective. *Ourselves and Our Children: A Book By and For Women.* New York: Random House, Inc., 1978. See especially chapters entitled "The Teenage Years" and "Being Parents of Grownups."

Butler, Robert N. *Why Survive? Being Old in America.* New York: Harper-Colophon, 1975. Essential reading. Includes an excellent directory of organizations and government programs.

———, and Myrna I. Lewis. *Sex After Sixty: A Guide for Men and Women in Their Later Years.* New York: Harper and Row Publishers, Inc., 1976. Available in large-print edition.

Caine, Lynn. *Widow.* New York: Bantam Books, 1974. A moving account of one woman's experience.

Christenson, Alice, and David Rankin. *Easy Does It: Yoga for People Over 60.* Saraswati Studio, Inc., 12429 Cedar Road, Cleveland, OH 44106.

Clay, Vidal. *Women: Menopause and Middle Age.* Pittsburgh: Know, Inc., 1977.

Cunningham, Imogen. *After Ninety.* Seattle: University of Washington Press, 1977. Photographs of people over ninety along with interviews with those who knew and worked with Cunningham.

Geba, Bruno. *Vitality Training for Older Adults.* New York: Random House, Inc., 1974. A therapist working with elderly in nursing homes advocates massage because many residents of nursing homes are starved for touch. Includes resources for political action.

Gordon, Mary. *Final Payments.* New York: Ballantine Books, Inc., 1978. This novel paints a powerful portrait of the isolation of caregivers. It's a story about a young woman of thirty re-entering the world of paid work and social relationships after caring for her father for ten years.

Hare, Nancy L., and Peter V. Rabins. *The 36-Hour Day.* Baltimore: Johns Hopkins University Press, 1981. A family guide to caring for persons with Alzheimer's and related dementing illnesses and memory loss in later life.

Harlow, Jan. *Good Age Cookbook: Recipes from the Institute for Creative Aging.* Boston: Houghton Mifflin Co., 1979.

Hunter, Laura R. *The Rest of My Life.* Growing Pains Press, 22 Fifth Street, Suite 204, Stamford, CT 06905.

Kübler-Ross, Elisabeth. *On Death and Dying.* New York: Macmillan Publishing Co., Inc., 1969.

Lake, Alice. *Our Own Years: What Women Over 35 Should Know About Themselves.* New York: Random House, Inc., 1979. Highly recommended.

Markson, Elizabeth, ed. *Older Women: Issues and Prospects.* Lexington, MA: Lexington Press, 1983. Academic in tone, but filled with useful information. The article on sexuality is especially useful.

Myerhoff, Barbara. *Number Our Days.* New York: Simon and Schuster, 1978. Warm and personal account of elderly Jews in California by an anthropologist.

Neugarten, Beatrice L., ed. *Middle Age and Aging.* Chicago: University of Chicago Press, 1968.

Notelovitz, Morris, and Marsha Ware. *Stand Tall! The Informed Woman's Guide to Osteoporosis.* Triad Publishing Co., Box 13096, Gainesville, FL 32604, 1982. $6.95. An excellent self-help resource.

Olson, Laura Katz. *The Political Economy of Aging.* New York: Columbia University Press, 1982.

Porcino, Jane. *Growing Older, Getting Better: A Handbook for Women in the Second Half of Life.* Reading, MA: Addison-Wesley, 1983. Highly recommended.

Pym, Barbara. *Quartet in Autumn.* New York: Harper and Row Publishers, Inc., 1977. Available in large-print edition by G.K. Hall, 1979. Novel about two women and two men who work together in an office and their plans and concerns with the transition of retirement.

Rathbone-McCuan, Eloise, and Tedi Dunne. *The Surviving Majority: Older Women and Their Health.* American Public Health Association, 1981. Order from E. Rathbone-McCuan, University of Vermont School of Social Work, 451 Waterman Building, Burlington, VT 05405. $5.00

Reitz, Rosetta. *Menopause: A Positive Approach.* New York: Penguin Books, 1979. An excellent self-help resource.

Robertson, John A. *The Rights of the Critically Ill.* Order from C.L.U.M., 47 Winter Street, Boston, MA 02108. $3.75 plus

67¢ handling. A detailed straightforward guide covering crucial topics, such as hospices, relevant statutes and living wills.

Robey, Harriet. *There's Dance in the Old Dame Yet*. Boston: Atlantic-Little Brown, 1982.

Rose, Louisa, ed. *The Menopause Book*. New York: Hawthorne Books, Inc., 1977.

Rubin, Lillian. *Women of a Certain Age: The Midlife Search for Self*. New York: Harper and Row Publishers, Inc., 1979.

Sarton, May. *As We Are Now*. New York: W.W. Norton and Co., Inc., 1982. A novel about a woman placed without her consent in a badly run boarding home for elders. She takes control of her fate in a shocking ending.

———. *Kinds of Love*. New York: W.W. Norton and Co., Inc., 1980. A novel about the friendship between two older women and their bonds with each other, with family and others in their community. Celebrates caring and connection.

———. *A Reckoning*. New York: W.W. Norton and Co., Inc., 1981. A novel about a woman with terminal cancer who takes control of her death and ultimately finds it "a ripening"—one of the most interesting parts of her life.

Scott-Maxwell, Florida. *The Measure of My Days*. New York: Alfred A. Knopf, 1968.

Shields, Laurie. *Displaced Homemakers: Organizing for a New Life*. New York: McGraw-Hill, Inc., 1981.

Silverman, Phyllis. *Helping Women Cope with Grief*. Beverly Hills, CA: Sage, 1981.

———. *Mutual Help Groups: Organization and Development*. Beverly Hills, CA: Sage, 1980.

Skeist, Robert J. *To Your Good Health!* Chicago: Chicago Review Press, 1980. A practical guide for older people. Large print.

Slagle, Kate Walsh. *Live with Loss*. Englewood Cliffs, NJ: Prentice-Hall, Inc., 1982. Practical, compassionate techniques for coping with many kinds of loss and moving through grief to growth.

Thomas, Sherry. *We Didn't Have Much, But We Sure Had Plenty: Stories of Rural Women*. Garden City, NY: Doubleday/Anchor Books, 1981.

Voda, Ann M., Myra Dinnerstein and Sheryl R. O'Donnell, eds. *Changing Perspectives on Menopause*. Austin, TX: University of Texas Press, 1982.

Wilkinson, Carol Wetzel, with Graham Rowles and Betty Maxwell. *Aging in Rural America: A Comprehensive Annotated bibliography, 1975–1981*. Gerontology Center, West Virginia University, Morgantown, WV 26506, 1982.

Wolf, Deborah Coleman. *Growing Older: Lesbians and Gay Men*. Berkeley, CA: University of California Press, 1982.

Women as Elders/Nos Ainées, special issue of *Resources for Feminist Research/Documentation Sur La Recherche Feministe: A Canadian Journal for Feminist Scholarship*, Vol. 11, No. 2 (July 1982) (bilingual). Order from Ontario Institute for Studies in Education, 252 Bloor Street W., Toronto, Ontario, Canada, M5S1V6. $5.00 for the special issue.

Worden, J.W., and William Proctor. *Personal Death Awareness*. Englewood Cliffs, NJ: Prentice-Hall, Inc., 1976.

Periodicals

Broomstick. A bimonthly (six issues per year) newsletter by, for and about women over forty, sponsored by Options for Women Over Forty, 3543 18th Street, San Francisco, CA 94110, (415) 431-6944.

Hot Flash. A newsletter for midlife and older women. An outgrowth of "Health Issues of Older Women: A Projection to the Year 2000," one of three conferences funded by the Administration on Aging in 1980, sponsored jointly by the National Action Forum For Older Women at Stony Brook, which also publishes *Forum*, a newsletter for older women. Vol. 1, No. 1, contains a questionnaire, several articles and an order form for complete conference proceedings and videotapes. Write to The School of Allied Health Professionals at SUNY Stony Brook, Health Sciences Center, SUNY, Stony Brook, NY 11794.

Membership Organizations and Sources of Printed Information and Referrals

Alzheimer's Disease and Related Disorders Association, Inc.
National Headquarters: c/o Mary McLaughlin
360 North Michigan Avenue, Suite 601
Chicago, IL 60601
(312) 853-3060

American Association of Retired Persons
Program Dept.
1909 K Street NW
Washington, DC 20049
(202) 872-4922

Members receive their magazine, *Modern Maturity*. AARP has many subdivisions, including a women's division and a health division. The Institute for Lifetime Learning helps older persons pursue educational and/or career changes.

American Health Care Association
1200 15th Street NW
Washington, DC 20005
(202) 833-2050

"Thinking About a Nursing Home: A Consumer's Guide for Choosing a Long-Term Care Facility" includes a checklist of questions to ask.

Elderhostel
100 Boylston Street, Suite 200
Boston, MA 02116
(617) 426-7788

Short-term, intensive campus-based educational experiences for older adults. Most programs take place during the summer. Publishes three seasonal catalogs.

Gray Panthers—National Office
3635 Chestnut Street
Philadelphia, PA 19104
(215) 382-3300

An intergenerational membership organization. Advocates for concerns of elders and other social change issues. Their bimonthly newsletter, *Network*, is available for $12.00 annually, $15.00 for organizations, libraries and foreign subscriptions.

National Self-Help Clearinghouse
33 W. 42nd Street, Room 1222
New York, NY 10036

Write to them for the self-help clearinghouse in your area. They also publish a bimonthly newsletter, *The Self-Help Reporter*.

National Women's Health Network

Their committees on midlife women's health and older women's health are jointly planning a conference for 1984, and volunteers are welcome. Call the national office. They regret they cannot answer individual health queries at this time.

Older Women's League—Educational Fund
3800 Harrison Street
Oakland, CA 94611
(415) 658-0141

Ask for their literature list of provocative and carefully researched "Gray Papers." Highly recommended.

Older Women's League—National Office
1325 G Street NW, Lower Level B
Washington, DC 20005
(202) 783-6686

Advocates for women's legislative concerns; a membership organization, nationally and locally. Members receive their newsletter.

Public Affairs Pamphlets Catalog
381 Park Avenue
New York, NY 10016

See especially pamphlet #559, "Partners in Coping: Groups for Self and Mutual Help."

SAGE: Senior Actualization and Growth Explorations
2455 Hilgard Avenue
Berkeley, CA 94709

A growth center for people over sixty-five, founded by a psychiatrist in 1974. Its premise: "Old age can and should be a rich, creative culmination." Use of wholistic health techniques such as massage and biofeedback.

Special Resources on Selected Issues

Death and Dying

Concern for Dying
250 West 57th Street
New York, NY 10019
(212) 246-6962

An educational organization that publishes a newsletter and will send you a living-will form.

National Hospice Organization
1311-A Dolly Madison Boulevard
McLean, VA 22101
(703) 356-6770

Publishes a national directory.

Hearing Aids

Marshall, Patricia. "Making Sure Hearing Aids Help," *FDA Consumer*, June 1976. Order from U.S. Government Printing Office, Washington, DC 20402, HEW Publication No. (FDA) 76-4003. Makes connections between aging and hearing loss.

Rudick, Joan, and Richard Bimont. "Tuning In on Hearing Aids," *FDA Consumer*, May 1980. Order from U.S. Government Printing Office, HHS Publication No. (FDA) 80-4024.

Lesbian and Gay Issues

Senior Action in a Gay Environment (SAGE)
208 West 13th Street
New York, NY 10011
(212) 741-2247

The oldest organization providing services to older lesbians and gay men. Services are available in N.Y.C. only, but the organization maintains a list of groups around the country and provides information for starting groups dealing with lesbian and gay aging. Newsletter available.

Menopause

Menopause: A Self-Care Manual, 1981, and *La Menopausia* (Spanish edition), 1981. Order from Santa Fe Health Education Project, Box 577, Santa Fe, NM 87501. $4.20 each includes postage. Bulk rates available.

"*Menopause: A Natural Process*," rev. ed. 1982, 27 pages. Order from San Francisco Women's Health Center, Box 14367, San Francisco, CA 94114. $2.00 plus postage.

Research on the Menopause. World Health Organization, Technical Report Series No. 670, Geneva, Switzerland, 1981. 120 pages. Available from WHO Publications Center USA, 49 Sheridan Avenue, Albany, NY 12210. Price upon request.

Nursing Homes

Brody, Elaine M. *Long-Term Care of Older People: A Practical Guide*. Human Sciences Press, 1977.

Moss, Frank E. and Val Hammadreus. *Too Old, Too Sick, Too Bad: Nursing Homes in America*. Aspen Systems Corporation, 1600 Research Boulevard, Rockville, MD 20850.

National Citizens' Coalition for Nursing Home Reform, 1424 16th Street NW, Suite 204, Washington, DC 20036. (202) 797-8227. A coalition of ninety-nine member groups and hundreds of individuals, including nursing home residents and their families, committed to improving the quality of life and care for long-term-care residents.

Vladek, Bruce. *Unloving Care: The Nursing Home Tragedy*. Basic Books, 1980.

Widowhood

Widowed Persons' Service, K Street NW, Washington, DC 20049. Recently bereaved persons can write for information describing services, help in locating a group in their area, referral, etc., as well as a free copy of the pamphlet "On Being Alone." Organizations wishing bulk orders of the pamphlet can write to NRTA-AARP, Widowed Persons' Services, Box 199, Long Beach, CA 90801.

VI
SOME COMMON
AND UNCOMMON HEALTH
AND MEDICAL PROBLEMS

23

SOME COMMON AND UNCOMMON HEALTH AND MEDICAL PROBLEMS

All sections below are by Mary Crowe, except where otherwise indicated. Most sections are based on work by Sarah Berndt, Edith Butler-Hallstein, Alice Downey, Susan Keady, Sandra Malasky and Betty Mitchell (all of the New Hampshire Feminist Health Center).

With special thanks to Norma Swenson, Judy Norsigian, Nora Coffee, Carol Englander, Craig Henderson, Jeanne Hubbuch, William Kaden, Rose Kushner, Charlotte Mayerson, Maryann Napoli, Gina Prenowitz and Leslie Walleigh

This chapter in previous editions was called "Common Medical Problems and Practices" and was written by Terry Thorsos, Judy Norsigian, Meg Hickey and Norma Swenson.

This chapter could have been a book in itself. We've had to choose only those health problems which affect large numbers of women or for which it is difficult to get reliable information elsewhere. Please be aware that information is constantly changing, and make use of the resources listed at the end of the chapter.

The entries in this chapter suggest nonmedical alternatives when possible—self-help techniques especially, and nonmedical practitioners. (See p. 57 for guidelines on choosing alternative practitioners.) Often, however, you will go to a doctor, nurse, clinic or hospital for treatment of the health problems discussed here. Please see Chapter 24, "The Politics of Women and Medical Care," for a discussion of the U.S. medical system and suggestions for choosing and using medical care.

GYNECOLOGICAL EXAMS, TESTS AND PROCEDURES

Medical practitioners consider a number of exams, tests and procedures to be part of good routine medical care. However, these procedures can sometimes be invasive, upsetting and even unnecessary.* The following suggestions may help you decide whether and when you need these tests.

Before giving your consent for any of the procedures and/or tests described below, ask your physician the following questions:

1. Why does s/he think you need the procedure?

2. What are the benefits of the procedure over others?

3. How is it done?

4. What are you likely to feel during and after the procedure?

5. What are the risks involved?

6. What are the negative effects, including effects on future fertility?

7. What may happen if you have no procedure done?

8. How experienced and skilled is the practitioner in doing this procedure? For instance, how many does s/he perform in a year?

While no health practitioner can guarantee the outcome of any exams, tests or procedures, s/he has a responsibility to give you all the available information. If you have doubts or feel you need more information, seek another opinion.

The Physical Examination and Basic Tests

During any physical exam, a practitioner should take the time to explain exactly what s/he is doing and why. This enables us to learn more about our bodies and ask questions if we are unsure about anything. If your

*Some doctors order tests just to try to protect themselves against possible lawsuit.

practitioner seems rushed or impatient, consider finding someone else. Bring a friend along to act as your advocate if that is what you want. With a practitioner who is respectful, gentle and informative, you will be able to relax more easily during the exam.

As part of a general examination, we should expect:
- questions about full family and personal medical history;
- an examination of the head (including eyes, nose and throat), skin and nails;
- a breast examination, with instructions in breast self-exam;
- listening to the heart and lungs with the stethoscope placed in several positions and a breath exhalation test;
- a blood pressure and pulse check;
- a hematocrit for hemoglobin count and a CBC (complete blood count);
- a blood-sugar check if you have a family history of diabetes;
- a gonorrhea test and a blood test for syphilis;
- a urinalysis (this also can be used to check thyroid function);
- a weight check (see Chapter 2, "Food");
- a Pap test;
- an abdominal exam;
- a pelvic exam, including a rectal exam (especially if you are over thirty-five).

Examination of Organs

The practitioner should examine your abdomen by touch (palpate) for any signs of liver or spleen enlargement and check your back for any pain or tenderness in the area of the kidneys.

Pelvic Examination

This should include an examination of your external genitals (vulva), an internal exam using a speculum,

Jean Raisler

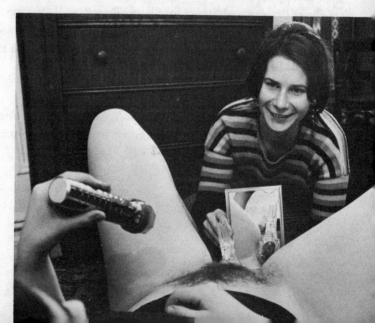

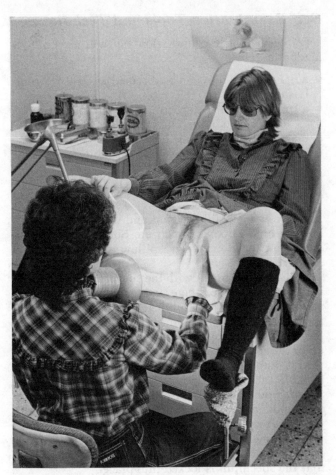

Virginia Coudron

infection, lesions, discoloration, damage or growths. S/he will take a Pap smear for abnormal cervical cell growth (a possible precursor of cancer), a culture for gonorrhea and sometimes a smear of discharge to examine under a microscope.

Some women experience pressure in the bladder or rectum with a speculum in place. Relaxing your muscles as much as possible may help. If not, ask the practitioner to readjust the speculum or try a different size.

Some practitioners keep a hand mirror available. If you wish to see your cervix, ask for help in positioning the mirror and light source. This is an opportunity to learn how and what to look for when examining your cervix in a self-exam.

After removing the speculum the practitioner will put on a clean plastic glove and insert two fingers of one hand into your vagina while placing the other hand on your lower abdomen. By pressing down on the abdomen and manipulating with the fingers in your vagina, s/he can locate and determine the size, shape and consistency of the uterus, ovaries and tubes. S/he can also locate any unusual growths, tenderness or pain.

Palpation of the uterus is usually painless, but palpation of the ovaries sometimes causes discomfort. The ovaries are difficult to find and often the twinge of pain you feel is the only way the practitioner is aware that s/he is touching your ovaries.

The bimanual examination will be more comfortable for you and easier for the practitioner if you are able to relax your neck, abdomen and back muscles and breathe slowly and deeply, exhaling completely.

To do the rectovaginal exam the practitioner will insert one finger into the rectum and one into the vagina in order to obtain more information on the tone and alignment of the pelvic organs as well as the ovaries, tubes and ligaments of the uterus. This exam can

Peggy Clark

a bimanual internal exam and a rectovaginal examination. If you have been doing regular self-exams (see p. 478), you will be more familiar with pelvic exams and can tell the practitioner of any changes you have noticed or simply help her/him understand what is normal for you. If it's your first exam, *say so*. Ask the practitioner to go slowly and explain what s/he is doing. Be sure to empty your bladder before the exam.

When examining the vulva, the practitioner will first check visually for irritations, discoloration, swelling, bumps, skin lesions, size and adhesions of the clitoris, hair distribution, lice and unusual vaginal discharge. S/he will then check internally with a finger for any Bartholin's gland cysts or pus coming from the Skene's glands. S/he will ask if you ever lose urine when you laugh or cough (urinary incontinence is a sign of uterine prolapse, rectocele or cystocele).

Then the practitioner will insert a speculum into the vagina to hold the walls apart. (The speculum should be warmed metal or plastic, and gently inserted.) S/he will examine your vaginal walls for lesions, inflammation or unusual discharge and will check your cervix (now visible) for unusual discharge, signs of

BIMANUAL PELVIC EXAM

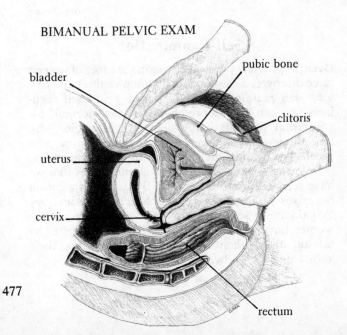

bladder

pubic bone

clitoris

uterus

cervix

rectum

also help detect rectal lesions and test the tone of the rectal sphincter muscles. If you are over thirty-five, the practitioner should also check for masses or blood in the rectum (sometimes an early sign of colon cancer). Some women find the rectovaginal exam unpleasant; others don't mind it. You may feel as if you are having a bowel movement as the practitioner withdraws his/her finger from your rectum. Don't worry—you won't.

Some practitioners are much more sensitive and skilled in internal exams than others; some women find it easier to relax than others. You can do Kegel exercises (see p. 333) and practice inserting a tampon or speculum before an internal to help you practice relaxation.

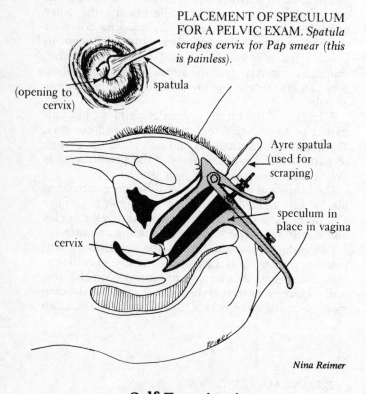

PLACEMENT OF SPECULUM FOR A PELVIC EXAM. *Spatula scrapes cervix for Pap smear (this is painless).*

(opening to cervix)

spatula

Ayre spatula (used for scraping)

speculum in place in vagina

cervix

Nina Reimer

Self-Examination

Over the past few years an increasing number of women have discovered the benefits of doing vaginal and cervical self-examination. By examining yourself regularly you can learn more about what is "normal" for you; what your discharges look like; the color, size and shape of your cervix; and the changes in your mucus during different stages of your menstrual cycles.

Doing self-exam, we see parts of our bodies that we have learned to ignore or fear. By using a speculum ourselves we use a small part of medical technology to gain back some control over our bodies. Many women have taken self-examination a step further by talking about their experiences and sharing their knowledge with other women in self-help groups.

Self-Examination Tools and Techniques

For cervical self-examination you will need only a few basic items:

- a light source that can be directed, such as a strong flashlight;
- a speculum (plastic speculums are inexpensive and easier to get than metal; you can get one at a pharmacy which carries medical supplies);
- a lubricant such as K-Y Jelly or Lubifax, or warm water;
- a mirror with a long handle;
- antiseptic soap or alcohol.

Find a comfortable setting and get into a relaxed position on the floor or couch, etc. Some women prefer sitting on the floor with a pillow at their back for support.

Familiarize yourself with the speculum and then lie back with your knees bent and your feet placed wide apart. You may want to lubricate the speculum (see above). Hold the speculum in a closed position with the handle pointing upward. Some women prefer to place the speculum into the vagina sideways and then turn it. Experiment until you discover the most comfortable variation for you.

Once you have fully inserted the speculum, grasp the handle and firmly pull its shorter section toward you. This opens the blades of the speculum inside your vagina. Now hold the speculum steady and push down on the outside section until you hear a click; this means that the speculum is locked into place.

For some women placing the speculum and finding the cervix may take some effort. Breathe deeply and manipulate the speculum gently while looking into the mirror. Focus the light source on the mirror to help you see better. (A friend can help with this.) With the speculum in the correct position you will be able to see both the folds in the vaginal walls and your cervix, which looks pink, bulbish and wet. (If you are pregnant your cervix will have a bluish tint and if you are menopausal or nursing it may be quite pale.) Depending on where you are in your menstrual cycle, your secretions may be white and creamy or clear and stretchy. By learning what is "normal" for you, you will more easily be able to identify any changes that may indicate ovulation, an infection or pregnancy.

Some women prefer to remove the speculum while it is still in its open position, and others close the blades first. Clean it afterwards with antiseptic soap or alcohol and store it for later use.

Pap Smear

The Pap smear is a method for distinguishing normal from abnormal cells of the vagina, uterus and cervix. It is most accurate in detecting cervical abnormalities. Since the recommended treatments for various kinds of abnormal cells detected by Pap smears remain controversial among practitioners, it will help to understand some basic facts about Pap tests and our treatment options (see p. 527).

To take a Pap smear a practitioner will, during the speculum exam, use a Pap stick or cotton swab to take one or more samples of cervical tissue from the outside of the cervix and just inside the cervical canal. You may feel a slight scraping sensation. S/he places the gathered cells on a glass slide and "fixes" them to prevent them from deteriorating. A good cell sample is essential for an accurate test. The slide goes to a cytology laboratory for analysis.

Dilation and Curettage (D and C)

A D and C is often used to find the cause of uterine bleeding or to treat it, especially in emergencies. It is also used to diagnose uterine fibroids, endometrial polyps and uterine cancer. In addition, it may be part of a diagnostic workup for cervical cancer. It is often performed to prevent infection following an incomplete abortion or after delivery, if part of the placenta is left in the uterus. The diagnostic D and C is rapidly being replaced by vacuum (Vabra) aspiration or endometrial biopsy (see p. 480).

DILATOR AND CURETTE, INSTRUMENTS FOR A D&C

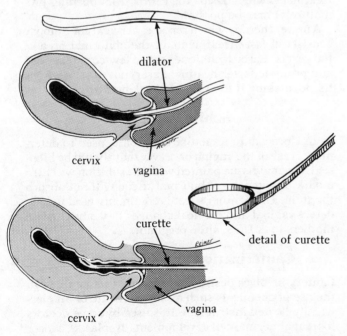

Nina Reimer

Many physicians still prefer to do a D and C in a hospital using general anesthesia, which creates total relaxation of the pelvic muscles and allows a more accurate pelvic exam. When such accuracy isn't nec-

essary it can be performed on an outpatient basis using local anesthesia, thereby minimizing the risks and expense, which are both greater with general anesthesia.

D and C sometimes involves enlarging (dilating) the opening of the cervix by inserting a series of tapered rods that become progressively wider in diameter. Increasingly, laminaria (long stems of kelp) are inserted 24 hours before the D and C to dilate the cervix gradually and painlessly. The practitioner then inserts a long, thin metal instrument with a spoon-shaped end (curette) through the cervix into the uterus to scrape out some of the uterine lining. (The doctor sometimes takes a tissue sample from the cervical canal.) The procedure should take five to fifteen minutes.

Most women have some bleeding following a D and C and may also pass small clots and/or have cramps for a couple of days. The risks include infection, hemorrhage, perforation of the uterus or surrounding internal organs and complications related to the anesthesia used.

Vabra Aspiration

A newer alternative to the D and C for diagnostic purposes is Vabra or endometrial aspiration, which involves inserting a small cannula into the cervix and removing the uterine lining by means of low-pressure suction. This procedure can be done in an office with local anesthesia, thus eliminating the risks of general anesthesia. It usually causes the same mild to moderate cramping as the D and C. Some physicians recommend Vabra aspiration as part of a gynecological exam for all women at risk for endometrial cancer.

Cervical and Endometrial Biopsy

In a biopsy, a sample of tissue is removed to be examined under a microscope as an aid in diagnosis.

CERVICAL BIOPSY

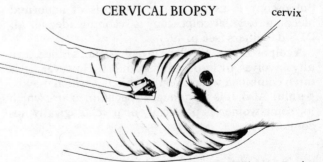

Christine Bondante

A *cervical biopsy* is done on abnormal areas of the cervix which appear through visual examination with or without Schiller's solutions or through the use of a colposcope (see p. 480: "Colposcopy"). An instrument which looks like a paper punch removes the tissue sample from one or more sites on the cervix.

The biopsy may be done on an outpatient basis and generally without the use of anesthesia. Most women experience some cramping during the biopsy and spotting afterwards.

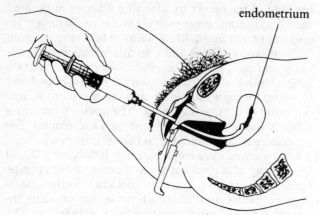

endometrium

ENDOMETRIAL BIOPSY *Christine Bondante*

In an *endometrial biopsy* (which can also be done on an outpatient basis with local anesthesia, if necessary), usually a scraping instrument (curette) is inserted through the cervix to obtain a sample of the uterine lining. The procedure may be part of an infertility workup. It has a fairly high accuracy rate when used to diagnose cancer of the uterine lining (endometrium) but the Vabra technique is generally thought to be more accurate for this purpose.

Colposcopy

This procedure involves the use of a colposcope, a lighted magnifying instrument resembling a small mounted pair of binoculars, to examine the vaginal walls and cervix for abnormal cells. It is more accurate than a Pap smear since it can identify the specific areas where the abnormal cells are located. A biopsy can then be taken from those areas for accurate diagnosis. Colposcopy is useful in the diagnosis of abnormal bleeding. Regular colposcopy is recommended for all DES daughters (see p. 497).

A colposcopy, easily done in a physician's office, usually involves little or no discomfort. However, it is often combined with a cervical biopsy, which may be painful. Also, it is a prolonged speculum exam, which for some women is physically or psychologically uncomfortable.

Conization or Cone Biopsy

Conization, used for both diagnosis and treatment, removes a cone-shaped section of the cervix. It is often recommended when a woman has severe dysplasia or cancerous cells confined to the cervix. A diagnostic conization may turn out to be therapeutic if it removes all the abnormal tissue.

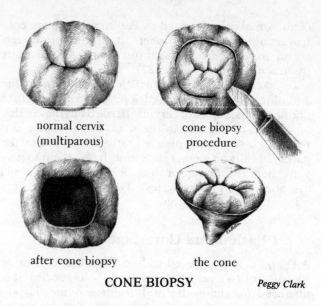

normal cervix
(multiparous)

cone biopsy
procedure

after cone biopsy

the cone

CONE BIOPSY *Peggy Clark*

A major surgical procedure, conization is done in a hospital under general anesthesia. Though the edges of the cervical area from which the cone is taken are sutured or cauterized, bleeding and infection are fairly common short-term complications. The removal of too many mucus-secreting glands may affect fertility by causing a decrease in cervical mucus. Sometimes pregnant women suffer a miscarriage after conization because of removal of muscle tissue, though "circlage" treatment (which keeps the cervix from opening prematurely) may be possible.

A newer therapy which replaces cervical cone biopsy consists of *laser* treatments of the abnormal area of the cervix. Laser techniques cause few complications and promote faster healing. Laser, however, destroys tissue, making it unavailable for laboratory analysis.

Schiller's Test

In this procedure an iodine solution is used to determine areas of the vagina or cervix that should be biopsied. Normal tissue painted with the solution will turn a dark brown color. Abnormal tissue will not absorb the stain. The Schiller's test is commonly used to help detect vaginal and cervical changes in women whose mothers took DES while pregnant.

Cauterization and Cryotherapy

Cautery involves destroying abnormal tissue through the use of chemicals such as silver nitrate or an electrically-heated instrument. It is used by some doctors to treat abnormal cell development (dysplasia), cancer *in situ* or cervical erosion (a reddened area which develops around the cervical opening). Sometimes cautery is used to treat chronic cervicitis, vaginal or vulvar warts and endometriosis involving the cervix or vagina. Cautery can be done in a doctor's office, preferably right after your menstrual period. The practitioner inserts a speculum and applies the cautery tip to the affected area.* After treatment a scab forms, allowing healthy new tissue to grow. The scab falls off in a week or so, and complete healing takes seven or eight weeks. Side effects include swelling of the cervix, profuse discharge for two or three weeks and, rarely, infection or infertility if the cervical glands are damaged.

Cryotherapy, often called cryosurgery and sometimes "cold cautery," involves the use of liquid nitrogen to destroy abnormal tissue by freezing. It can be done in an office and takes only a few minutes. Cryotherapy causes much less damage to the cervical opening than cauterization. It may, however, cause a profuse watery discharge and temporary changes in the cervical mucus. It does not seem to cause infertility. Unfortunately, many doctors do not have cryotherapy equipment in their offices.

After either cauterization or cryotherapy, you should not douche, use tampons or have sexual intercourse for ten to fourteen days while your cervix heals. Until healing is complete, Pap smears will be inaccurate and difficult to interpret. *Note:* Cautery occasionally causes scarring, which makes all future Pap smears difficult to interpret.

Carbon Dioxide Laser

Laser is a new technique, sometimes used as an alternative treatment to cone biopsy, cauterization or cryotherapy. Done on an outpatient basis in the hospital, it involves using a laser beam to destroy cells in a small area and results in little or no damage to the surrounding cells. Laser treatment causes little or no bleeding and the treated area heals quickly. This technique is so new and expensive that it is currently available only at certain large hospitals or medical centers. As more doctors are trained in its use and the equipment becomes more widely available, laser treatment may replace the older methods.

After a laser treatment, a Pap smear may show atypical cells for four to six weeks. You should, however, have two follow-up smears at three-month intervals and two more at six-month intervals before returning to your regular Pap smear schedule.

Laparoscopy

The laparoscope is a lighted tubelike instrument which, when inserted through a small incision made below the navel, allows the physician to see the uterus, tubes and ovaries.

Laparoscopy is useful in the diagnosis of ovarian cysts, ectopic pregnancy, infertility caused by blocked tubes, unexplained pelvic pain or masses, endometriosis, and in the recovery of an IUD which has perforated the uterus. It is also used in some female sterilization techniques. Laparoscopy is usually done in a hospital under either general or local anesthesia. Before inserting the laparoscope, the practitioner will inflate your abdomen with carbon dioxide to move the intestines out of the way and expose the pelvic organs to better view. With local anesthesia, you may experience an uncomfortable pressure or fullness. You may feel some pain under your ribs for the first few days after a laparoscopy as your body gradually absorbs the excess gas.

Anesthesia

It is as important to understand the type of anesthesia that you will receive as the type of surgery you will undergo. Before surgery you should ask the person who will be administering the anesthesia the following questions:

1. What type of anesthesia will be administered?
2. Why has s/he chosen this type or combination?
3. How will the anesthesia be given?
4. How may you feel after the surgery?
5. What are the possible risks and benefits of this type of anesthesia as compared to others?*

Be sure to tell the person who will be administering your anesthesia about any allergies to medication, prior anesthesia reactions, current medications you may be taking and information about your past and current health.

Anesthesia works by blocking pain. There are three types of anesthesia: *general*, in which you are unconscious; *regional* or *conduction* (including spinal and epidural), in which you are awake but numb in a specific region, usually the lower half (or a zone) of your body; and *local*, in which you are awake and only the area being operated on is numbed. General anesthesia makes you unaware of pain by working on the part of the brain that recognizes pain. Conduction and local anesthesia block the signals sent to the spinal cord and brain from the site which is anesthetized.

General anesthesia is administered by needle into a vein (intravenous), by inhalation or by a combination of both. When you get intravenous anesthesia, you will probably first be medicated with sodium pentothal (to induce deep sleep).† If you receive inhalation anesthesia, you will inhale it in gaseous form directly into the lungs via a tube inserted down your throat. Most types of anesthesia are administered after you are given medication to help you relax, which makes the procedure easier for the anesthesiologist and for you. If you are given gaseous anesthesia (such as halothane

---

*No anesthesia is needed, since normally there are no nerve endings in the cervix.

*Anesthesia capability varies from hospital to hospital as well as from one anesthesiologist or anesthetist to another. Not all facilities offer a choice.

†However, you are not truly "asleep," and you may hear or even remember conversations of those around you.

or nitrous oxide), adequate oxygen must be mixed with the gas, as general anesthesia lowers blood pressure and respiration rate. You may experience nausea, confusion or dizziness for several hours or days after having either type of general anesthesia. Rarely (about once in 10,000 to 20,000 cases) there is a death or paralysis as a direct result of the anesthesia.

Spinal anesthesia (usually preceded by a local anesthetic) is injected into the spinal canal through the membrane which covers the spinal cord. You will feel numb in the legs, pelvis and possibly higher, depending on what anesthesia is needed for your surgery. Spinal anesthesia is most often used for operations within the abdominal cavity.

Anesthetic effects from spinals may last longer than those from general anesthesia. About one woman in twenty will get a postoperative headache which may last for several days, because of small losses of spinal fluid from the injection site. Lying flat on your back for eight to sixteen hours after surgery without lifting your head may help relieve your symptoms. You can also ask for a patch to be put over the hole (a "patch procedure") so that it doesn't leak.*

Epidural or caudal anesthesia is injected continuously into the space near the base of the spinal column but not into the canal itself. It works by bathing the nerve endings leading to large areas of the body such as the perineum and legs with anesthetic solution, and is frequently used in childbirth. For more on epidural and caudal anesthesia (similar to epidural, sometimes used for rectal and genital surgery), see Chapter 19, "Childbirth." Always ask whether regional rather than general anesthesia is possible in your case, especially if you have a history of respiratory problems.

In *local anesthesia* a solution or jelly which numbs the nerve endings is applied to the mucous membranes, followed by an injection which blocks specific nerves (e.g., an injection of lidocaine given by the dentist).

Surgery

There are many different types of surgeons, calling themselves (and each other) by different names. General surgeons are a good choice *only* when they have special training for the procedures they perform.

Because there is a great deal of unnecessary surgery performed on women, we need to exercise great caution when deciding on an operation. Many public health researchers are convinced that excess surgery results from excess surgeons, since the U.S. has both the most surgeons and the highest rates of surgery in the world. An important part of surgical training is learning to persuade patients to agree to an operation. Because virtually all surgical procedures are reimbursed by insurance and graded according to their complexity, surgeons have strong financial incentives to perform

a lot of surgery, especially the more difficult operations. Hospitals similarly benefit from concentrations of elective (i.e., nonemergency) complex surgeries. And, precisely because surgery has become so common, many people have internalized the surgical mentality ("When in doubt, cut it out.") and are easily convinced that an operation is necessary.

Before giving your consent to surgery, you may want to take the following steps:

1. Get a second or even third opinion, preferably from a physician in a different specialty or who is *not* one of your doctor's close colleagues. (Many insurance policies and Blue Cross/Blue Shield programs will pay for this second opinion.) Try to find a doctor who is interested in helping you avoid surgery where possible. For example, internists may suggest nonsurgical alternatives not offered by ob/gyns and general surgeons. Such doctors are sometimes called "conservative," meaning that they don't resort to invasive measures unless they believe that it is absolutely necessary to do so. Procedures most frequently found unnecessary after a second opinion are hysterectomy, knee surgery, vein stripping, prostate removal, D and C, cataract extraction, breast surgery and gallbladder removal.* (See also "Our Rights as Patients," p. 584.)

2. Ask your surgeon about studies which show improved *outcome* for the procedure in your case. For example, careful studies have shown that much coronary bypass surgery is useless and sometimes even shortens life, yet the popularity of this procedure is constantly increasing. (See the section on heart diseases, pp. 542–45.)

3. Ask also about the surgery's potential risks and negative effects.

4. Investigate in a self-help group or on your own what alternatives, medical and nonmedical, can be tried before or instead of surgery. Medical researchers themselves now suggest that at least seven common operations may no longer be necessary or may soon be replaced by other, less invasive, treatments: hysterectomy, tonsillectomy, cholecystectomy, appendectomy, cardiac revascularization, gastrectomy and radical mastectomy.†

5. Ask whether the surgery has been widely performed, where and on how many people; check with your insurer to see if it is known and reimbursable. Since there is *no* regulatory or legal authority anywhere controlling surgery, new experimental procedures are constantly being launched without adequate testing and evaluation.

6. Ask specifically about mortality and morbidity rates in the institution where the surgery will be performed. (Call your state Department of Public Health

---

*This complication has become less common since the introduction of finer-gauge needles.

*This conclusion is the result of second-opinion monitoring programs set up by insurance companies, Medicaid/Medicare and Blue Cross/Blue Shield.

†See U.S. Department of Health Resources Utilization Statistics, 1978, National Center for Health Statistics.

or Health Systems Agency.) Some hospitals have more careful criteria and much better outcomes than others for certain procedures.

7. Carefully investigate the training and affiliations of the surgeon you are considering. Ask how often s/he performs the proposed procedure.

8. Ask if you can avoid general anesthesia (one of the major risks of most surgery) and hospitalization (a major source of postoperative infections) by having the surgery done as an outpatient or office procedure.

9. Talk all this over with your family and trusted friends.

10. Take the time you need to make a careful decision.

Before and After Surgery

Because surgery badly depletes the body of nutrients, you will need to eat a diet high in protein, vitamins and minerals to replenish these losses. You may also want to take supplements of Vitamins A, B, C and D, as well as zinc and iron. (See also the section on hospitalization, p. 582.)

INFESTATIONS

Crabs, or Pubic Lice

Phthirus pubis is a roundish, crablike body louse that lives in pubic hair and occasionally in the hair of the chest, armpits, eyelashes and eyebrows. You can "catch" them by intimate physical contact with someone who has them, or from bedding, towels or clothes that person has used. They are bloodsuckers and can carry such diseases as typhus. The main symptom of crabs is an intolerable itching in the genital or other affected area; they are easily diagnosed because they are visible without a microscope.

Though it may be difficult, try not to scratch. Scratching can transfer lice to uninfected parts of the body. Excessive scratching around the urinary opening can even lead to urinary tract infections.

Practitioners usually prescribe Kwell for crabs. This drug should be used with caution (see the section on scabies, below). Vonce, R.I.D. and A-200 Pyrinate are safe nonprescription drugs which are almost as effective as Kwell for crabs. Do not use any of these drugs in or around your eyes. If you have crabs in your eyebrows use an ophthalmic petroleum jelly.

Alternatively, you can try a very hot sauna, a treatment routinely used in Scandinavia. Either way, it's important that all intimate contacts, including lovers, family members and friends, be treated as well.

After treatment you should use clean clothing, towels and bed linen. Crabs will die within twenty-four hours after separation from the human body, but the eggs will live about six days. Previously used bedclothes. towels, etc., are safe after a week without use. Anything dry-cleaned or washed in boiling water can be used immediately.

As with scabies, the itch may persist for some time after treatment, especially if your skin is very irritated from scratching. Soothing skin preparations, such as aloe vera, can ease the symptoms and help your skin to heal faster.

The first time I got crabs I felt embarrassed and humiliated. I'd gone to visit my boyfriend at college and when I came home I began to itch. I couldn't believe that he would give me something like that—especially since I'd mistakenly associated crabs with people who didn't wash enough. I didn't know what to do so I just ignored them as long as possible. When the itching became really intolerable I went to a clinic. Once I learned how crabs are transmitted and that they are both very common and easy to cure, I felt a lot better. The next time I went to visit my boyfriend I took a bottle of A-200 with me. Turns out he hadn't known what to do either!

Scabies

Scabies are tiny parasitic mites that burrow under the superficial layers of the skin, depositing eggs and feces and causing intense irritation. Symptoms usually include intense itching (often worse at night) and red, raised bumps or ridges on the skin, which may be found on the hands (especially between the fingers), on or under the breasts, or around the waist or wrists, genitals or buttocks. Scratching the area can break the skin, causing secondary bacterial infections.

Scabies is highly contagious. You can get it through sexual contact as well as from infested bed linen, towels, clothing and occasionally even furniture. If you've never had scabies, it may take a month or more for the skin reaction to develop. During this time you can pass it to someone else without knowing you have it. Once you've had scabies, however, your skin will react much more quickly, often within a day after reinfestation.

Diagnosing scabies can be tricky because it is easily confused with poison ivy, eczema, allergies and other skin conditions. Sometimes physicians will prescribe medication for scabies before they know what you really have. Because these medications can cause allergic reactions, do not apply them until you have a definite diagnosis (specially made by examining a small scraping of the irritated area under a microscope).

The most common and effective treatment is a lotion called Kwell,* available by prescription only. Apply after a hot bath or shower (avoiding face, eyes and mucous membranes), leave on for twelve hours and carefully rinse off. If you need a second treatment, wait two weeks before reapplying.

An alternative to Kwell, often prescribed for preg-

*This drug should be used very carefully. Its active ingredient, lindane, is a potent pesticide which penetrates the skin and can cause allergic reactions. In addition, lindane has been found to cause tumors in laboratory animals. Pregnant women, infants and children should not use this drug.

nant women, is Eurax, whose active ingredient is crotamiton. It should be rubbed into the skin and reapplied after twenty-four hours.

An old-fashioned treatment using sulfur is making a comeback in popularity among dermatologists. It is especially recommended for treating infants, young children and pregnant women for scabies. It is considered less irritating than other chemicals that kill scabies, it seems to be less toxic and it seems to work.

The one disadvantage to the sulfur treatment is cosmetic. It smells like rotten eggs and can stain clothing.

For the adventurous, the recommended mixture is 6 percent sulfur, 3 percent balsam of Peru and the rest petroleum jelly. The mixture is put on the infected areas and left on for twenty-four hours with a new application each night for three consecutive nights. Some pharmacists will mix the ingredients for you.

Treatment is important for any friends, lovers or family members with whom you've had intimate contact. You should also wash any clothing, towels, bedclothes, furniture covers, etc., in very hot water and dry at the hottest possible temperature.

Even after treatment, you may continue to itch for several days or weeks. This doesn't mean you still have scabies; more likely your skin is still hypersensitive and needs some time for the irritation to die down. A soothing lotion (containing calamine or aloe vera) will ease the symptoms. If the itching is really intolerable, an antihistamine may help.

CERVIX

Cervicitis

Cervicitis is a term used loosely to describe an inflammation or infection of the cervix. Cervicitis is often related to other infections, such as common vaginal infections, STDs or PID. It can also result from a break in the tissue of the cervix caused by an IUD insertion, abortion or childbirth. Untreated, chronic cervicitis can cause fertility problems by blocking the passage of sperm or altering the cervical mucus.

Depending upon the severity and length of infection, you may notice an increased vaginal discharge, pain with intercourse, an aching sensation in the lower abdomen and/or the need to urinate more frequently. Severe infections may also bring fever.

Diagnosis

When you touch your cervix, it may feel warmer and larger than usual. Movement of your cervix with your finger may also be uncomfortable. If you examine yourself with a speculum, your cervix will look red and slightly swollen and you may observe a discharge. If only the cervical canal is affected, your cervix will look normal but you may see a yellowish discharge coming from within the cervical opening.

If you go to a practitioner for an internal exam, be sure to tell her/him whether or not your discharge is normal. (Sometimes physicians mistake scar tissue and normal discharge for cervicitis.) A culture and wet mount will determine if the cause of the infection is bacteria or an STD. In some cases, a Pap smear will also be taken to rule out the possibility of cervical cancer.

Medical Treatments

If tests show that an STD such as gonorrhea, syphilis or chlamydia is responsible for the infection, you will get oral or injected antibiotics. For mild cervicitis caused by other infections or injury, physicians usually prescribe vaginal creams containing sulfa, antibiotics or iodine-based gels. For more severe cases, some physicians recommend cryosurgery or electrocautery. While these treatments work well when all other methods have failed, use them only as a last resort, as they can be painful and it will take about six weeks for your cervix to return to normal.

Self-Help Treatments

When symptoms are mild and not related to PID or serious STDs, the following remedies may help: goldenseal douche (a quarter of a teaspoon to one quart of water two times a day for two to three weeks), Vitamin-C douche (500 milligrams in one quart of water daily for three to four weeks) or vinegar douche (see p. 518). For more information on herbal remedies, see Resources.

To speed healing and strengthen the immune system and for future prevention, you may want to try oral doses of Vitamin C (500 to 1,000 milligrams a day), zinc (twenty-five milligrams a day) and Vitamin E (400 milligrams a day). You can also apply Vitamin E directly to your cervix with your finger. You can use slippery elm as a douche or paste applied directly to the cervix in a diaphragm or on the end of a tampon.

No matter what treatment you use, try to combine it with extra rest and good nutrition.

Cervical Erosion

Cervical erosion refers to a large or small sore (benign lesion) that may develop on the cervix beside the cervical opening. It is usually pinkish red and sometimes rough-looking. Approximately 95 percent of all women of childbearing age have cervical erosion at some point, which can be caused by injury to the cervix from childbirth, infection, an IUD or the friction of intercourse (for some women).

Cervical erosion has few symptoms and causes little discomfort. The commonest symptom is a whitish discharge (leukorrhea) which may have an unpleasant odor. When the erosion is irritated, a bloody discharge may also appear. Usually the erosion is not discovered unless the woman has a pelvic exam. If you look at your cervix with a speculum, you may see a red and rough-looking area which feels slightly indented to the touch.

Diagnosis

The first step in diagnosis is a Pap smear. If abnormal cells are present, some of the cervical tissue is removed and examined under a microscope (a biopsy). A biopsy will distinguish cervical erosion from cervical cancer. There is controversy over the best approach to cervical erosion. Most physicians think it does no harm and should be left alone, and others think that if cervical erosion is not treated, it may become chronic and possibly lead to cervical cancer.* It is also thought that untreated cervical erosion may affect a woman's fertility. You can monitor your erosion with regular self-exams and consult a practitioner if it seems to be enlarging.

Medical Treatments

For mild erosion, most practitioners prescribe a sulfa cream (e.g., Sultrin Vaginal Cream, AVC Cream or Vagitrol) to be applied well up inside the vagina, usually twice a day. However, these treatments may not help unless you have an infection (see "Cervicitis," p. 484).

If the erosion is severe, your physician may suggest cauterization or cryotherapy. Always get a Pap smear before undergoing these treatments; if the erosion is benign, you may save yourself unnecessary treatment. In addition, it is very difficult to interpret abnormal Pap smears accurately after these procedures.

Self-Help Treatments

For mild erosion, use the methods suggested for cervicitis. Some women find that not using tampons during their periods helps to reduce erosions.

Cervical Eversion

A practitioner may confuse cervical erosion with cervical eversion and suggest unnecessary treatment. Cervical eversion is a common condition in which the tissue which lines the cervical canal grows on the outer vaginal portion of the cervix, making it red with a bumpy-looking texture but smooth to the touch. It has almost a bandlike appearance. Eversion requires no treatment unless accompanied by infection. Those of us whose mothers took DES during pregnancy are more likely to have eversion. We may also develop it as a result of cervical injury during abortion, childbirth, etc.

Most women do not have any symptoms; in those who do, the most frequent sign is a slightly increased nonirritating vaginal discharge.

*However, there is no evidence that this actually happens.

Cervical Polyps

Cervical polyps appear as bright red tubelike protrusions out of the cervical opening, either alone or in clusters. They consist of excess cervical tissue which "heaps up" within the cervical canal. Polyps, which are very common, are often formed as the body attempts to heal itself after a cervical infection by growing new tissues, or during pregnancy when hormonal changes stimulate excess cervical tissues to grow. "Contact" bleeding following intercourse, douching or self-exam is often the only symptom. Polyps sometimes bleed during pregnancy. Most contain many blood vessels with a fragile outer wall.

Medical Treatments

Polyps do not necessarily require treatment. When they are small and there is little or no contact bleeding you can usually just keep track of them with regular self-exams. You may want to have them removed if your symptoms change or the polyp begins to grow. Cervical polyps are rarely cancerous. Occasionally, however, they look like cervical cancer and produce similar symptoms. In that case you can have a Pap smear and biopsy to tell for sure.

A polyp can be removed in a doctor's office, usually under local anesthesia. The practitioner usually twists the polyp off and seals the base with an electric cautery needle. If your polyp is very large or if you have multiple polyps, you may have to go to the hospital for removal. Sometimes polyps recur after removal. In that case a D and C may be necessary to remove them permanently.

Cervical Leukoplakia

Leukoplakia, a white patch of tissue which forms on mucous membranes (inside the cheek, vagina, cervix, etc.), is our body's attempt to seal off an area that contains abnormal cells. Most common in women over forty, it is sometimes associated with vaginal discharge or bleeding. If you see leukoplakia on the cervix, have the patch rubbed firmly during a Pap test. If your Pap test is normal but the area of whiteness is still present, most practitioners suggest removing it or biopsying it, as leukoplakia is thought by some doctors to be a precancerous growth. However, most women with leukoplakia never develop cancer.

Cervical Intraepithelial Neoplasia (Cervical Dysplasia) (CIN)

"Dysplasia" means abnormal cell growth; cervical dysplasia or cervical intraepithelial neoplasia (CIN) is the term used to describe abnormal cells on or near the cervix. In most cases there are no symptoms, and it is detected by a routine Pap smear.

485

CIN is *not* cancer and does not develop into cancer in most cases. CIN occurs along a continuum: at one end the cells are all normal, while at the far-distant other end lies invasive cancer. The several stages or classes of CIN along the continuum can be difficult to distinguish; one stage or class blurs into the next, and different laboratories or physicians may "place" a given cell sample differently. Diagnosis is therefore often difficult, and treatment decisions can be controversial and hard to make. *Some* women with CIN will develop more severe changes (and at varying speeds), while most women's cells will return to normal. There is no way to determine in advance which will happen. Therefore, all cases of diagnosed CIN are treated and/or watched closely with repeated Pap smears and other diagnostic tests.

Because we can't see CIN and we don't know what is going on, we often feel anxious when we are diagnosed as having it. There is no need to panic when a Pap smear comes back abnormal. Most cell changes like CIN are very slow. Some physicians may want to rush you into treatment. Because the diagnostic tests are not always accurate, and because physicians vary in their diagnoses and preferred treatments, it is good to get the opinion of a second physician and a different laboratory about your condition. Most diagnosed cases of CIN are mild, and the cells return to normal spontaneously. We can monitor any changes by more frequent Pap smears or other diagnostic tests.

The results of Pap smears and other diagnostic tests are classified according to how much of the surface tissue (epithelium) of the cervix is affected and the kind and degree of cell changes that exist. There are three different classification systems currently in use.

Below is a chart which compares all three systems, showing where they are the same or different. The three systems are named "Dysplasia," "Cervical Intraepithelial Neoplasia" (CIN), or the "Class System." The chart shows the continuum from normal healthy cells at the far left to invasive cancer at the far right.

Prevention

1. Studies show that using a barrier method of contraception (such as the condom or diaphragm) rather than oral contraceptives (the Pill) or an IUD may help to prevent CIN or cancer. One study showed that for women who had already been diagnosed as having CIN, use of condoms was associated with a return to normal cervical cells.* It is important to monitor your condition with repeated Pap smears or other tests in addition to employing preventive efforts.

2. Some sexually transmitted infections and diseases can contribute to abnormal cervical changes. (See Chapter 14, "Sexually Transmitted Diseases," for methods of prevention.)

3. Eating foods high in Vitamin C and/or taking supplements may help prevent CIN or cervical cancer. After a diagnosis of cervical abnormality, taking folic acid (ten milligrams per day) and Vitamin C (a hundred milligrams per day) may help reverse the condition.†

*A.C. Richardson and J.B. Lyon. "The Effect of Condom Use on Squamous Cell Cervical Intraepithelial Neoplasia," *American Journal of Obstetrics and Gynecology*, Vol. 140, No. 8 (August 15, 1981), pp. 909–13.

†A hundred milligrams per day should prevent any major deficiency of Vitamin C, but many women will want to take more if they are often exposed to conditions which destroy it.

Comparison of Pap Smear Classification Systems*

			Precursors				
				Dysplasia			
Dysplasia	Benign	Atypia	Mild	Moderate	Severe	CIS†	Invasive Cancer
CIN	Benign	Atypia	CIN I	CIN II		CIN III	Invasive Cancer
Class	Class I	Class II	II–III‡	Class III		Class IV	Class V

Sources: Comparisons of CIN and dysplasia systems are based on a similar diagram in *Dysplasia Training for Clinicians*, the syllabus used in an OFP-sponsored training workshop held in Los Angeles, April 4–5, 1981.

Correlations with the Class system are based on descriptive terminology found in *Office Gynecology*, by Robert Glass, M.D. (Williams and Wilkins, 1976), and on consultation with Norma Jacek, M.D., and Sadja Greenwood, M.D.

*Provided to all participants in the workshops sponsored by the California Office of Family Planning, "Secrets Your Pap Smear Reports Never Told You" (Berkeley, 1982).

†Cancer *in situ* or localized cancer.

‡The shaded portion indicates variation in interpretation of the extent to which CIN I and mild dysplasia are comparable to Class II.

4. Because there is evidence linking herpes to CIN and cancer, if you have herpes it is especially important that you have an annual or even twice-yearly Pap smear. While this can't prevent cell changes, it can help you to catch them early and seek appropriate treatment.

5. We must insist on more research into the connection between occupationally induced abnormalities and CIN and cancer, as well as the role of male partners in CIN and cancer.

Who Is at Risk of CIN (Dysplasia) or Cervical Cancer?

We don't yet know the causes of the cellular abnormalities that we call CIN and cervical cancer. However, certain factors may put you at higher risk for these conditions.

1. If you have sexually transmitted infections such as herpes, chlamydia, trichomoniasis and condyloma,* you are at a higher risk for CIN.

2. Recent studies suggest that a protein substance in sperm may cause cellular changes in certain susceptible women. Women whose partners develop cancer of the penis are also at greater risk.

3. Being exposed to synthetic hormones (such as DES or the Pill) may increase your chances of developing CIN or cancer.

4. Recent studies have linked cervical cancer with smoking.

5. If you began intercourse at an early age, your risks may be greater. Physical changes in the types of cells which line the vagina occur especially during our teens: more vulnerable softer cells are gradually replaced by tougher (squamocolumnar) cells. If we began intercourse before those changes were mostly complete, our cells are more vulnerable to whatever may cause cellular changes.

6. If either or both you and your partner had multiple sexual partners, your risks of developing abnormal cervical cells may be somewhat greater. Barrier contraceptives (condoms or the diaphragm) may reduce such risks. This pattern has sometimes been used to "blame" women for sexual activity which "caused" their cellular changes. First, we do not know what causes such changes. Second—and often ignored— the number of sexual partners of a woman's *mate* (not the woman herself) may affect the degree to which she is at risk of cervical abnormalities.† Third, some women who have only had one partner have developed cellular changes. Last, *neither* early age at first intercourse nor many partners *causes* cellular abnormalities. Blaming the victim of such abnormalities certainly won't cure them.

7. If you or your partner work at jobs which involve contact with carcinogenic substances (such as those in the mining, textile, metal or chemical industries), you may be at higher risk for cervical abnormalities.

8. Finally, women in a low socioeconomic bracket who do not have access to healthful living and working conditions have a much higher incidence of CIN and cancers, and are more likely to develop such problems at an earlier age than middle-class women. This may also be related to the greater occupational hazards confronted by poorer women and/or their partners as well as their lack of access to good nutrition.

**DES Daughters and CIN
by Kris Brown**

The type of cancer, squamous cell, which CIN *may* develop into should not be confused with clear cell cancer, which is linked to DES exposure. It is not known at this point whether DES daughters are or will be at a higher risk for CIN or squamous cell cancer. Still more research is needed.

DES daughters who have been diagnosed to have dysplasia should be aware of two issues:

1. One study of a small number of DES daughters who had cryosurgery showed results of cervical stenosis (narrowing of the cervical canal, which can affect menstruation and childbirth) in varying degrees of severity. Non-DES-exposed women in the same study did not experience these side effects from cryosurgery.

2. Metaplasia, a normal process whereby tissue changes from one form to another, may be present in a larger area in DES-exposed than in non-DES-exposed women. Why is this important? Some people feel that the changed tissue may be more vulnerable to precancerous or cancerous change and pathologists may mistakenly interpret the change as abnormal (dysplasia or CIN). Such misdiagnosis can lead to unnecessary treatment and the possible harmful effects of cervical stenosis.

Diagnosis

The first step is the Pap smear. If you have an abnormal result, have a second smear to confirm the diagnosis. If the follow-up Pap smear indicates mild

---

*The human papillomavirus (HPV), which causes condyloma warts, can also cause invisible flat lesions on the cervix. These lesions, which can show up as abnormal Pap smears or can be seen with a colposcope, are probably more common among women than the visible condyloma warts. Increasingly, evidence suggests that both forms of HPV infection are trigger factors to the onset of cervical cancer. This link to cervical cancer actually appears stronger for HPV than for herpes or other STDs.

†J.D. Buckley, et al. "Case-Control Study of the Husbands of Women with Dysplasia or Carcinoma of the Cervix Uteri," *Lancet*, Vol. 2 (November 1981), pp. 1010–15.

CIN, physicians usually recommend a "wait and see" approach, with another Pap smear to monitor changes in six weeks to three months. If the results show more than mild CIN, most physicians suggest an office procedure called colposcopy, which often includes a tissue (punch) biopsy. Both Pap smears and colposcopies may be repeated for diagnostic monitoring.

Medical Treatments

Like the condition of CIN, treatments vary from very mild to more serious. What you want is to get appropriate treatment for the condition you have and to avoid unnecessary or inappropriate treatment or surgeries. Different physicians may have varying "preferred" treatments for each diagnosis. This is why second- and even third-physicians' opinions may be important in deciding on your treatment.

It is important that procedures such as colposcopies, punch biopsies and cones be done by physicians who have special training, skills and experience. The mildest treatment is the "wait and see" approach with repeat Pap smears and/or colposcopies (see p. 480) and punch biopsies. Regular condom use may also help. The next step up the treatment ladder is cryotherapy, an office procedure in which suspicious cells are frozen and then slough off, allowing new healthy cells to replace them (see p. 480). A carbon dioxide laser (see p. 481) may be used instead of cryotherapy, especially when the abnormal area is too large or advanced to be treated with cryotherapy.

When repeated Pap smears or colposcopies confirm severe dysplasia or cancer *in situ* (CIS, or localized cancer) *or* if the abnormal area extends into the cervical canal (and therefore cannot be reached for colposcopy or cryotherapy), a cone biopsy (conization or conical) is often recommended. The cone-shaped piece of tissue removed by this surgery in the hospital is examined to insure that all borders of the abnormal area were removed. If the abnormal area extends beyond the edge of the removed cone, the physician may recommend either a second conization (to remove a larger area) or a hysterectomy (removal of the cervix and uterus). Hysterectomy is also generally recommended as the appropriate treatment for invasive cancer (see p. 537). It involves major surgery and some risks.

Some of these treatments can be uncomfortable and occasionally somewhat painful. After a cone or punch biopsy, cryotherapy or laser treatment, do not use tampons, douche or have intercourse. (This minimizes pain and the risk of infection.) Some women experience cramping, tenderness, bleeding and/or discharges.

A cone biopsy involves some risk of future infertility because it may weaken the cervix. A hysterectomy permanently ends a woman's reproductive capacity. Both surgeries can be appropriate and save women's lives. However, if such a treatment is recommended, it is important to seek a second or even third opinion on whether it is appropriate and what other treatment options may be available, especially for severe CIN or cancer *in situ*.

BENIGN BREAST CONDITIONS

In adolescence, when our breasts first begin to develop, we usually feel both pleased and awkward. We worry about whether they will be too big or too small, attractive or unattractive. At this age, we sometimes walk hunched over, clutching schoolbooks to our chests in the hopes that no one will notice our newly maturing breasts. Other times we may stuff tissues into "training" bras and wear tight sweaters. Our self-images quickly become tied up with our own and others' reactions to our breasts. These reactions can be as confusing and contradictory for grown women as they are for teenagers. Many of us discover that our breasts can be intensely pleasurable to us as well as to those who look at us or with whom we make love. A few women can even experience orgasm from breast stimulation alone. At other times, however, we may be embarrassed or inconvenienced by our breasts. In addition, many of us develop fears concerning our breasts—from the simple fear of "sagging" to the often overwhelming fear of disease and loss of a breast.

These feelings, both positive and negative, are reinforced by our society's obsessive fixation on breasts. Provocative images of bared breasts are on billboards and magazines everywhere. They are used to sell everything from cars to whiskey. They can also be a factor in getting or keeping jobs. Many men feel free to whistle or stare at our breasts or even to touch them uninvited. Some women may resent or pity us because of our "size." What should be a short-lived adolescent confusion over growing up is prolonged into a lifelong concern with breast size and shape. This sexual context often makes it difficult for us to think about our breasts as functioning parts of our bodies that need health care. It also makes breast problems particularly disturbing.

Wide Range of Normal Breasts

Women have breasts of all sizes and shapes—large, small, firm, saggy, lumpy. One woman's breast may be different in size or shape from her other breast. Nipples may be prominent or inverted. The areola (the area surrounding the nipple) may be large or small, darker or lighter, and usually has little bumps just under the skin. Sometimes there are long hairs near the edge of the areola.

These individual differences, along with the changes caused by age and menstrual cycles, often produce needless anxiety. Unfortunately, we do not usually have sufficient information about what is normal, either in

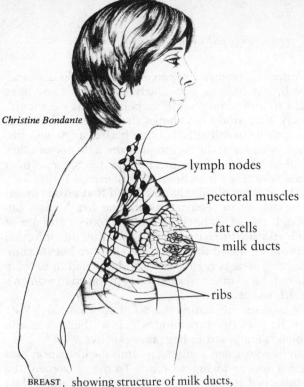

Christine Bondante

BREAST, showing structure of milk ducts, lymph nodes, and fat cells

— lymph nodes

— pectoral muscles

— fat cells
— milk ducts

— ribs

appearance or function, to be able to tell when something is abnormal and requires further attention. This lack of information often results in a fear that every change or pain is a symptom of cancer, when in fact *most conditions causing change, lumps or pain are not cancer.* The following are some of the common *benign* (noncancerous) conditions.

Fibrocystic Condition

(This is also called, or includes, cystic mastitis, mastodynia, mastasia, sclerosing adenosis and ductal dysplasia.) At least half of us experience some swelling, discomfort or lumpiness in our breasts which comes and goes with our periods. During ovulation and just before menstruation, hormone levels change, often causing the breast cells to retain fluid. Cysts (small sacs filled with fluid or semifluid materials) often develop. If you examine your breasts during these times, you may find a series of rather sore lumps in one or both breasts, especially in the areas nearest the arms. Most lumps will usually decrease or disappear within a day or two of the start of your period.

Some women have this fibrocystic (also called cystic) condition from their very first period. Others develop it in their twenties or thirties. The condition may continue—some months slightly better, others worse—until it disappears around menopause. For a few women, the condition is progressive, increasing slowly over the years from a monthly mild soreness to a constant state of sharp pain and lumpiness. Many of us, especially as we get older, find that while the pain and fullness still come and go with our periods, some of the lumps have become permanent. These lumps may or may not shrink after menopause.

"Condition" or "Disease" Controversy

Until recently, most doctors referred to this hormonally-induced, cyclical pain and lumpiness as a "disease," partly because they thought it was abnormal and partly because insurance will often pay for the treatment of "diseases" but not "conditions." Now an increasing number of physicians and laywomen argue that this inaccurate terminology causes needless anxiety in millions of women about a normal aspect of the menstrual cycle that is no more a disease than menstruation, menopause or pregnancy. (Nursing a baby can be uncomfortable and complications can occur, but we do not call it "lactative disease.") Referring to it as a disease can also lead to overtreatment.

Though traditional medical opinion has been that a fibrocystic condition increases your chances of getting breast cancer, now some newer studies, plus reinterpretation of old data, cast serious doubt on that conclusion.* Most women who have benign lumps do *not* develop cancer.

Fibroadenomas

If you are in your teens or twenties and find a lump that does not fluctuate with your period, it is most likely a fibroadenoma. Fibroadenomas rarely develop in women past their thirties. Those which appear early may last throughout life. Women may develop one or more fibroadenomas in one or both breasts. The cause of these growths is unknown, though some research suggests that they may be related to fat consumption. Occasionally a fibroadenoma will grow large enough to interfere with circulation or to distort the breast's shape. Such fibroadenomas are usually removed surgically. Sometimes the fibroadenoma will grow back, though not necessarily as large as previously. These growths sometimes shrink at menopause, an indication that they may be a normal occurrence. (Cancer rarely, if ever, shrinks.) The main problem with fibroadenomas is that they often "feel" like cancer. The younger you are, the more likely your doctor will assume that any lump you may have is a fibroadenoma and not a cancer, but since there is no way to be certain except by physical examination, you and your doctor will probably want a needle or surgical biopsy. At present, nothing specifically links fibroadenomas with an increased risk of breast cancer.

Breast Self-Exam

Breast self-exam is a technique by which you examine your own breasts for suspicious lumps. It is recommended by most physicians as a method for the early detection of cancer.

*S. Love, et al. "Fibrocystic Disease of the Breast: A Non-Disease?" *New England Journal of Medicine*, Vol. 307 (October 14, 1982), pp. 1010–14.

Prevention of Breast Cancer

At this point there is no known way to be sure that you will never get breast cancer, but there are ways in which you can protect yourself against environmental factors which may cause or encourage the disease. You can also strengthen your immune system to fight it. It is logical that the younger you are when you make any changes aimed at prevention, the more likely they are to be effective. (Remember that breast cancer may develop for as long as twenty years before it shows up.)

Cutting down on the fat in your diet is probably the single most important thing you can do. High incidence rates of breast cancer are apparently related to diets high in fat, and in the standard American diet fats (meats and dairy products) make up 40 percent of the total calories. The American Cancer Society, the National Cancer Institute and the National Academy of Sciences have all issued guidelines and recommendations concerning the high-fat diet and cancer. Try to substitute foods high in fiber (fruit, vegetables and whole-grain cereals) for fatty foods.

The breast is highly vulnerable to cell damage through X-rays. If possible, avoid unnecessary X-rays, especially during puberty or pregnancy. You can protect the breast with breast shields during X-rays of the lower back. For dental X-rays, a lead apron and collar should be provided to protect the body. X-rays of the arms and legs are less dangerous. (See also p. 524.)

For a while, after someone I knew got breast cancer, I checked my breasts regularly. But it was so confusing. Sometimes there were lumps and sometimes there weren't. At first, every time I'd find one, I'd run to the doctor and he'd say, "Oh, it's nothing. Don't worry. You're too young to have breast cancer." So I quit examining my breasts. I'll probably start again when I'm older.

I just feel so uncomfortable touching myself there.

I'm afraid of what I'll find. . . . I can't stand the thought of having my breast removed.

I seem to go by spurts and spells. For several months, I'll be very conscientious and examine my breasts carefully after each period. Then something comes up and I'll skip a month. Then I guess I just forget and several months or even a year will go by before I get around to doing it again. But I never seem to be able to make it a habit. I feel guilty and then get angry with myself. Why can't I find time for something so important? Why do I have so little self-discipline? Then I think about what will happen if I get breast cancer. I probably won't find it in time and it will be my fault if I die of it.

American women (60 percent or more) do not practice breast self-exam regularly, although many have tried to and almost all of us believe that we should. Study after study has shown that women who begin the routine usually discontinue it after a few months. Those who learn the technique from a doctor or other medical personnel are more likely to continue than those who learn it from another source.

The authors of this chapter found that no one in our group of seven regularly examined her breasts (although two of us have had mastectomies and are at high risk for breast cancer). Extending our informal survey, we found that almost no one we knew examined her breasts regularly. Most had tried to develop the habit and many were actively involved in women's health issues.

Why does this issue raise so many emotions? Why is it hard to do something which we believe in and which is supposed to help save our lives?

In most women's minds, a lump means cancer and cancer means losing a breast. To many women, the prospect of losing a breast is more frightening than the possibility of death from cancer.

If more people knew that most cases of breast cancer need no longer be treated with mastectomy, women might not avoid the practice so much or delay seeking treatment when they do find a lump. (See also "Early Detection Controversy," p. 531.)

What to Do if You Find a Lump

There are no adequate words to describe the panicky anxiety that follows the discovery of a distinct lump which wasn't there before. Cancer is the first thought which flashes into our minds, along with a lot of wild, confused thoughts about "why this should be happening to me." Some women rush immediately to the nearest doctor. Others remain quiet about their lumps, afraid to go to the doctor for fear it is cancer. They can't face the thought either of having the disease or of having to undergo a mastectomy, often mistakenly assuming that it is the only treatment course.

It is important to remember that 80 to 90 percent of all lumps are not cancer. One possible first step in finding out is self-screening.

Self-Screening

There are some self-screening techniques which can help you distinguish between lumps more likely to be benign and those which probably require medical evaluation. The following steps may be especially helpful to women with lumpy breasts for whom it would be both impractical and very costly to see a doctor whenever lumps appear.

First, if you are still having periods and have no previous history of either lumps or cancer, observe whether the lump disappears or fluctuates in size during your monthly cycle—a sure sign that it is not malignant. It is common medical practice, especially for younger women, for a doctor to recommend first watching the lump for a month or two. *There is no evidence that this will make any difference in length of life, even if the lump does prove cancerous.** Do not feel the lump every day or you may not be able to tell if there is any change. The best times to check are during the three or four days before and, for comparison, three or four days after the first day of your period.

You can also try changing your diet. Many women have found that they can reduce or totally eliminate certain noncancerous lumps this way. Though not yet proven conclusively, many medical studies have supported links between diet and benign breast conditions.

Here are some suggestions on diet and vitamin supplements that often help reduce breast lumps:

1. Avoid fatty and fried foods.

2. Reduce salt in your diet.

3. Eliminate foods and beverages containing caffeine—coffee, tea, most colas, chocolate and many brands of aspirin and cold remedies.

4. Don't smoke.†

5. You may want to try daily supplements:

- Vitamin E: 400 to 800 IUs (already widely prescribed by many physicians for fibrocystic conditions);
- Vitamin B$_6$: 100 to 200 milligrams;
- evening primrose oil: two to four grams.

While dietary changes bring lump reduction in some women within just one cycle, others must continue the diet for up to six months to get improvement. If after two months the lump has not definitely decreased, you will probably want to proceed to medical screening.

Medical Evaluation of a Lump

Once you have decided that your lump needs professional screening, the proper selection of a physician or medical facility is essential. Although your lump will probably turn out to be benign, on the outside chance that it *is* cancer, it is best to go to a breast specialist who has considerable experience with both cancer and benign conditions, not necessarily a gynecologist. Even though you may have a good relationship with your own doctor, chances are high that s/he does not keep up with current research on diagnosis and treatment options. You may find that your "loyalty" to your doctor is locking you into diagnoses and

treatments which may be inappropriate for you. A local women's health center or the Cancer Information Service listed in Resources may help you find a sympathetic and more experienced physician. If you live in a small town, you may want to consider going to the nearest large city with a research or university hospital. The National Cancer Institute (see Resources) sponsors an increasing number of hospitals with breast-evaluation centers where you can have your lump evaluated by a team of specialists. The advantage of going to such a team is that they can be more flexible about diagnosis and treatment, as they are much more likely than local doctors to keep up with current research. Of course, a disadvantage is that you may have to travel far from your home. (See "Introduction to Cancer," p. 522.)

Avoid scheduling your appointment just before or during the first few days of your period or around ovulation. Your breasts may be more lumpy during these times, and the doctor may miss a more suspicious lump hidden by the general swelling.

The doctor should examine your breasts carefully as you raise your arms over your head and then lower them to your sides while you are sitting up and again while you are lying down. This procedure is very important, as a lump can sometimes be felt in only one of these positions. The examination may be uncomfortable but is generally not painful. The physician will make a professional, though inevitably somewhat subjective, judgment on whether the lump "feels" like cancer. Cancers are usually more irregular, harder and less freely moving than benign growths, but *only a biopsy* (a procedure to remove part or all of a lump and examine some cells under a microscope for evidence of cancer) *can tell for sure, even if a mammogram is also done.* (See the section on mammography, p. 493.)

Needle Aspiration—The First Step

Needle aspirations, when possible, are the best first procedure for suspicious lumps. Most lumps turn out to be benign fluid-filled cysts, and it is simple for the doctor to test for these with an aspiration, an office procedure. The aspiration avoids the problems of minor surgery associated with a surgical biopsy, and it is quicker and less painful as well. The physician inserts a fine needle into the lump. Many physicians give a novocaine shot first; others don't. Some women feel that the novocaine shot is as painful as the procedure itself. If the lump is a cyst, fluid is drawn off and it collapses. Because most cysts (well over 95 percent) are benign, especially in younger women, many doctors do not send the fluid for laboratory testing (biopsy). If you are at high risk for breast cancer, you may want the fluid biopsied. Discuss this with the physician before the aspiration, as it may be too late to request the test afterwards. If the cyst grows back rapidly, a surgical biopsy is probably called for, as

---

*Many oncologists and other expert researchers have agreed with this statement, especially since we have so little evidence of treatment benefit. Certainly, if this active watching makes you anxious, seek a biopsy as soon as possible.

†One study found that all the women who got no relief from eliminating salt and caffeine were also smokers. The women who then quit smoking subsequently found their lumps noticeably reduced.

rapid regrowth is sometimes a sign that the lump is cancerous.

If the lump does not yield fluid when it is aspirated, it may still be a cyst or other benign growth, but a biopsy is needed to be certain.

The use of aspiration as the first step in evaluating a lump is increasing but is not yet routine everywhere. Since most lumps turn out to be cysts, aspiration as a first step saves much time, expense and anxiety. If your doctor does not suggest an aspiration at first, you may want to request one. A few lumps, however, are buried so deeply within a generally lumpy or large breast or may "feel" so much like cancer that some doctors will recommend a surgical biopsy first rather than an aspiration. Others may want to try a "needle biopsy" first (see below).

Biopsy

This procedure involves removing all or part of a lump and examining it for cancer. Biopsies can be either incisional (removing only part of the lump, either through surgery or with a needle) or excisional (removing all of the lump through surgery). The most common type of incisional biopsies are needle biopsies called Tro-car or Tru-cut biopsies. These can be done as simple in-office procedures. After applying a small amount of anesthesia to the breast (similar to the novocaine which dentists use), the doctor inserts a corkscrew-shaped needle which carves out a small part of the lump. The withdrawn sample of breast tissue is sent to a laboratory for cancer testing. Besides leaving less of a scar, this needle biopsy technique is less expensive and time-consuming than a surgical biopsy.

However, the results of any incisional biopsy (needle or surgical) can only be completely trusted if they are positive, that is, if cancer is found. This is because lumps are occasionally heterogeneous—part cancerous and part benign. There is always the possibility that an incisional biopsy may miss the malignant part.

Still, a needle biopsy may be a good second step for a woman under thirty with no significant risk factors. Cancer is extremely rare in these younger women and their lumps, even those which do not fluctuate with their periods or yield fluid when aspirated, almost always turn out to be benign. Such a young woman may decide that she is satisfied with the incisional needle biopsy, especially if the results show that the lump is a fibroadenoma. To date, this type of lump has not been found to be heterogeneous.

Attitudes toward biopsies vary enormously among physicians. Some physicians biopsy everything just to be sure. Others avoid the procedure. Some, if they think the lump doesn't "feel" like cancer, take a cautious "wait and see" attitude, which is appropriate at times, or a "don't bother yourself about it" attitude, which may be too casual and is insulting as well. If the lump has not been aspirated, ask if that might not be a reasonable prebiopsy procedure. Try to find a doctor who will explain why this particular lump of yours should or should not be biopsied. This will put you in a better position to decide if you would feel comfortable with the doctor's possible recommendation regarding treatment in case of cancer.

If you choose to have a biopsy, you then need to decide on the type of biopsy and whether to have it with general or local anesthesia.

If a woman tends to develop a lot of lumps, it is much easier to check them with a needle biopsy than to cut each one out completely. Frequent surgical excisional biopsies can leave the breast scarred and distorted, and can build up confusing scar tissue within the breast. However, the age when women develop the most lumps is in their thirties and forties. Although most of these lumps are benign, the incidence of breast cancer rises steeply after age forty. Consequently there is increasing risk that a needle biopsy will miss a cancer after age forty, even though such instances are rare.

Anesthesia

Needle biopsies are almost always done with local anesthesia. Surgical biopsies—which may be excisional or incisional—can be done with either local or general anesthesia. Some women consider it too stressful to be awake during the biopsy and thus prefer general anesthesia. Others choose a local because they prefer being awake and/or because they are concerned about the serious health hazards of general anesthesia (see p. 481).

You may meet resistance if you want local anesthesia. Many surgeons recommend the general out of habit, because they think people are too frightened by the idea of a local, because insurance is more likely to pay, or simply because they themselves are uncomfortable with a person who is conscious.

About 10 percent of the time, the size or depth of the lump or a very large or lumpy breast makes the surgery more complicated, and general anesthesia may be required.

Before the Biopsy

We do not advise the one-step biopsy, in which you sign a release allowing a mastectomy before you even know whether or not your lump is cancerous. In this procedure, the doctor removes the lump and examines it by the frozen section method while you are still under general anesthesia. For this test, the lump is frozen immediately upon removal. Technicians cut a thin slice of the lump and examine it under the microscope for signs of cancer. The results of a frozen section (always tentative) are usually available within twenty minutes. If cancer is found, your doctor proceeds with a mastectomy. The major problem with the one-step is that occasionally the quick-frozen section test is inaccurate, and women's breasts have been removed when they did not have cancer. Even if you do have cancer, the one-step gives you no time to consider your options. For example, mastectomy might be an inappropriate treatment for your type of cancer. You can prevent any misdiagnoses or unwanted treatments more easily when the biopsy is separated from any other treatment and the permanent section is used as the determining test for cancer. The permanent section takes several days but is more accurate and gives additional information about the type of cancer which may be helpful in deciding what further treatments, if any, to take. The National Cancer Institute specifically advises against the one-step biopsy (followed immediately by a mastectomy), although many doctors still practice it.

Before the biopsy, you may want to ask the surgeon to cut so as to leave the smallest possible scar. Sometimes doctors are not careful about this, because they assume the breast will be removed later during a mastectomy. (However, you may not choose mastectomy even if you do have cancer.) Depending on the size and location of the lump, the incision can sometimes be made along natural wrinkle lines or along the edge of the areola, or under the arm. Any scar, discoloration or distortion left by the biopsy usually becomes less noticeable over time, though this varies significantly from one woman to another.

Be sure that estrogen and progesterone (ER and PR) receptor assays are planned. These tests, which indicate how much a tumor is influenced by the hormones estrogen and progesterone, must be done *immediately* after the lump is removed. The information can make a big difference in treatment decisions (see below). ER

and PR assays are not yet routine everywhere, so don't assume they will be done automatically, or that the physicians involved understand the crucial nature of the time factor.

"Prophylactic" Mastectomies

Prophylactic ("preventive") mastectomies are being performed in increasing numbers on women who do not have breast cancer but are considered to be at "high risk" for the disease (see p. 494). Unfortunately, the type of surgery used in most prophylactic operations (the subcutaneous mastectomy) does not guarantee that the woman will avoid breast cancer. In the subcutaneous mastectomy, approximately 80 to 95 percent of the breast tissue is removed, leaving the skin, nipple and some underlying fat intact. A silicon or saline implant is generally inserted at the same time to replace the breast tissue and give a more normal appearance. Complications run about 50 percent. Some women will develop cancer in the small amount of remaining breast tissue. Keeping this in mind, any woman who is considering a prophylactic mastectomy should probably consider having a simple mastectomy rather than the more cosmetic subcutaneous mastectomy. However, even this will not provide complete assurance. It is always possible that an undetected cancer had already developed in the breast and was present in other parts of the body before the mastectomy.

A few women request prophylactic mastectomies but more frequently doctors suggest it. Yet even women labeled at "high risk", the usual candidates for prophylactic mastectomies, are just as likely not to develop breast cancer as they are to develop it.* Prophylactic mastectomy is a particularly suspect recommendation when the only risk factor is a mild fibrocystic condition which may respond to dietary changes.

Only when medical science can predict with total accuracy who will get breast cancer might prophylactic mastectomy become more generally appropriate. Until then, think extremely carefully if a doctor recommends it to you.

Mammograms

Before the biopsy, the doctor may want you to have a mammogram (an X-ray of the breast to detect cancer). Many physicians use this additional test to help them determine whether a surgical biopsy is necessary. However, the use of mammography for routine screening of women with no symptoms, despite its increasing popularity among doctors, is very controversial.

Biopsy—When to Consider It

1. If you are worried about anything different you may notice in your breasts—whether a doctor thinks it is necessary or not. Many women have good instincts about which changes, especially lumps, are harmless and which are dangerous. One cancer specialist said he always listens to his patients' intuitions, as they are often correct.

2. If a doctor thinks from her/his experience that the particular lump is suspicious or feels like cancer. (See also the sections on needle aspirations [p. 491] and mammography [below].)

3. If other symptoms which may indicate cancer are present. These include hard, swollen lymph glands in the armpit area, a skin rash on the breast, nipple discharge or dimpling or puckering of the skin around the nipple. (These symptoms are usually caused by other conditions but should be examined, especially when they accompany a lump.)

4. If you are at "high risk" for breast cancer and have found a lump. (See "The High Risk Controversy," p. 494.)

---

*This is further evidence that the risk factors which doctors have traditionally used to try to predict breast cancer are incorrect.

The "High-Risk" Controversy

It is extremely important to inquire carefully about the basis for any "high risk" label assigned you by your doctor. Few doctors have adequate training in epidemiology or genetics, and most are too busy to keep up with today's sophisticated risk studies. Inappropriate labeling may lead to unnecessary, dangerous and expensive tests and procedures, as well as the emotional stress of believing you are in greater danger of developing breast cancer than the average woman.

Recently, the American Cancer Society re-evaluated its list of factors believed to be associated with an increased or "high" risk of developing breast cancer. In 75 percent of cases *none* of the risk factors predicted the disease.* In thousands of other cases, women believed to be at risk for one or more of these reasons never develop the disease. While the American Cancer Society and many of its physician leadership have concluded that all women are therefore at "high risk," in reality only a few factors are truly known to increase one's risk, and even these cannot *predict* breast cancer. For example, only if a mother or sister had a confirmed diagnosis of breast cancer *before age forty* does a woman's risk increase significantly, more so if the cancer was in both breasts. Exposure to radiation, DES and meno-pausal estrogens in increasingly large doses will almost certainly increase one's risk, since the body's response to these substances is clearly dose-related. A previous personal history of breast cancer increases the likelihood of discovering new cancer (not a metastasis) in the other breast (by about 1 percent per year, or 15 to 20 percent over a lifetime).

But other than these factors, we conclude that all women are roughly at equal risk. (No woman has higher than a 20 percent risk of developing breast cancer.) Since breast cancer tends to be discovered in the 40-to-60 age range all of us will face that risk equally if we live to that age. Most of the rest of the factors are connected in some way with higher socioeconomic status, which in the U.S. generally means access to the American diet—high in fats and sugars, low in fresh vegetables, fruits and whole grains—and American sedentary habits—riding in vehicles, sitting at work and at home, and not exercising.

As the incidence of breast cancer continues to rise, a more constructive way for us to think about our risks is to disregard the outmoded and misleading studies of the past and think about our future by taking prevention seriously. (See p. 490, "Prevention of Breast Cancer," and p. 524, "A Program to Reduce the Risk of Cancer." See also Chapter 7, "Environmental and Occupational Health.")

Advantages and Disadvantages of Mammography

Mammograms do offer important advantages, such as detecting some cancers which aren't yet palpable (easily felt), serving as a map or guide to surgeons and providing a "baseline" against which later mammograms can be compared to see if any unusual changes have taken place in recent years. There are also serious drawbacks to the procedure, including misdiagnoses, both through missing cancers which are there and mistakenly identifying benign lumps as cancerous. In addition, there exists a small but definite possibility of mammography causing a breast cancer.

There have been cases where false positives (mistaken diagnoses of cancer) from mammograms combined with false positives from quick-frozen section biopsy tests (see previous section) resulted in the removal of breasts from women who didn't have cancer. Remember that mammograms only indicate *possible* cancerous areas. A *permanent section test* (surgical biopsy) on a sample of that area is required to confirm the diagnosis of cancer (see "Biopsy" p. 492).

Currently, different medical organizations offer con-flicting recommendations for the use of mammography, thus making it difficult for a woman to decide what is best for her to do.

Who Should Have Mammograms?

If you are over fifty years old or if you have already had one or more breast cancers detected, the advantages of mammography probably outweigh the risks. If you have had cancer, the chances that you will develop either a recurrence or a separate new cancer are much greater than the chances that a mammogram itself will precipitate a cancer.

For women over fifty, one major study found that death rates from breast cancer were about 30 percent lower for those who had a mammogram each year. This single study represents most of the evidence for the assumption that breast cancer is curable if it is "caught early enough." However, this same study did not show any advantage in annual mammograms for women under fifty.* While the exact reasons for these age differences are unknown, they are probably related to the changes in breast tissue caused by menopause and the general aging process.

But what should you do if you are under fifty and

*"New Alert Raised on Breast Cancer," *The New York Times*, Oct. 18, 1982.

*Studies replicating this result are not available thus far.

your doctor recommends a mammogram? There is no easy answer to this, but it is important to ask why this procedure, whose usefulness for your age group has not been demonstrated, is being recommended. Then consider those reasons in light of the advantages and disadvantages of mammography. Do not feel that you must have the mammogram just because the doctor wants you to. After considering all factors, you may decide to go ahead with the test, but the decision should be a cooperative one between you and your doctor.

The two issues of importance concerning mammography and younger women are effectiveness and safety. No study of women under fifty has yet shown reduced death rates from breast cancer for those who have had mammograms. This may be because the breast tissue of premenopausal women is denser and does not show up as well in a mammogram. Overall, mammography has a false-positive rate (indicating cancer where there is none) of about 7 percent. Estimates of false negatives (missing a cancer which is present) vary from 4 to 30 percent. These false positives and false negatives are more common among premenopausal women. Despite this, the number of younger women receiving mammograms is rising constantly. The average age for a first mammogram has decreased steadily over the past decade.

Taking a test which may not be very effective would not be so bad (except for financial and emotional reasons) if there were no dangers involved. However, this is not the case with mammography. While the attendant risks may be small, there is at present no way to predict which women will turn out to be vulnerable to them. The major problem is that mammograms use radiation and radiation can cause cancer. This is rather ironic, because radiation is also used to *treat* cancer. High doses of radiation (as released by a bomb) can cause cancer to develop within a few months. Low doses (as in mammography and other medical X-rays) may be just as dangerous, although they may not work as rapidly. Since cancer cells tend to be more susceptible to radiation than normal cells, radiation is often used to treat cancer. Radiation can kill a human cell, damage it or leave it unaffected. However, cells which are damaged rather than killed by the radiation may themselves progress into cancer in anywhere from two to twenty years. While not everyone who is exposed to low radiation doses develops cancer, there is no known safe level of exposure, and the effects are definitely cumulative. Thus the woman who has one chest X-ray or mammogram is less likely to develop cancer than a woman who has had many diagnostic X-rays. Still, there is no guarantee that even one exposure will not result in cancer.

There is also strong evidence that the breasts of younger women may be more susceptible to radiation damage than those of older women. In addition, any woman who starts annual or frequent mammograms at twenty-five or thirty-five is clearly increasing the amount of radiation exposure over her lifetime, thus increasing her chances of breast cancer. If a radiation-induced cancer takes twenty years to develop, a fifty-five-year-old woman might develop breast cancer at seventy-five, but a twenty-five- or thirty-five-year-old woman may develop it at forty-five or fifty-five.

With all this evidence in mind, we must strongly discourage routine or baseline mammography for symptom-free women under fifty until its effectiveness for this group has been demonstrated and the extent of its danger is better known.

If your doctor suggests a mammogram because you have a lump which "feels" like cancer, you may want to consider having some sort of biopsy before a mammogram (see previous section). If the lump is suspicious enough to warrant a mammogram, then, in most cases, it is suspicious enough to warrant a biopsy regardless of the mammogram's results, since mammograms tend to be inaccurate for younger women. This assumes that a needle aspiration has not revealed the lump to be a cyst and that it does not fluctuate with your period. If the biopsy reveals the lump to be benign, as most lumps are, you will have avoided unnecessary exposure to radiation.

The decision to have or not to have a mammogram is more complex if you are under fifty and have no suspicious lumps but are considered to be at "high risk" for breast cancer. (See the section on risk controversy, p. 494.) Many doctors argue that "high-risk" women have the most to gain from mammography—they are more likely to have cancers that mammography can detect. But it may also be that they have the most to lose from it. Perhaps being at "high risk" means greater vulnerability, less resistance than other people to carcinogens such as radiation. Should this be the case, then "high-risk" women would be advised to avoid mammography more than average women. At this time, neither interpretation of "high risk" is proven.

Currently, the very concept of "high risk" is being questioned. One recent study suggested that all women are at equal risk of developing breast cancer. The researchers, however, concluded that all women were therefore at "high risk," and thus should have regular mammograms before age fifty! But even if all women under fifty were at equal risk of developing breast cancer, we must remember that no studies have yet shown any advantage of mammography in detecting the disease or reducing its death rate for women under fifty.

You may decide that you prefer to take the risk of having one or more mammograms during your younger years, but doctors recommending the technique should make it clear to you that mammography's usefulness in your case has not been proven and that the procedure is potentially dangerous for you.

Many physicians feel that the danger of induced cancer is much less from today's mammograms, which use considerably less radiation than those of twenty years ago. Definite progress has been made in this area. There is more frequent monitoring of equipment for radiation leakage or improper settings. Standards are stricter, and operators are better trained.* Researchers are hopeful that certain research, especially some studies currently under way in Scandinavia, will provide evidence that mammography can reduce breast cancer rates in younger women.

Even if mammography does turn out to be effective for younger as well as older women, this usefulness may still be bought at the price of inducing cancer in some women in order to save others. This is no boon to any woman who may die from radiation-induced breast cancer. For this reason, we believe that researchers should emphasize developing truly safe screening methods. Some progress in that direction has taken place but much more is needed.†

Results of Biopsies

Waiting for the results of a biopsy can be an excruciating experience. Ask when the results will be ready and whether the doctor's office will call or you should call them. If you haven't heard by the appointed day, call. If the results are *negative*, that means you do not have cancer. *Positive* results mean that cancer was found. (See "Breast Cancer," p. 529.)

If the Results Are Negative

Most likely (in 80 to 90 percent of all biopsies) the tests will be negative. If you are premenopausal, the doctor is likely to say that the lump is just "fibrocystic," a term that has unfortunately become a catchall term for noncancerous lumps in younger women. You may be so relieved that you don't have cancer that you don't want to bother with any more medical terms. However, you should ask the doctor exactly what "fibrocystic" means in terms of *your* lump. You need to know the precise name, whether this type tends to recur and whether it is ever related to cancer. Your doctor may not know or be willing to share this information, so you may have to be very persistent.

You have a right to obtain and examine a copy of all your medical records, and it is a good idea to get a copy of the biopsy test results. The information may

---

*Recent studies reveal that many poor-quality radiation services persist outside university centers.

†This progress is seen in the experimental (and currently not very accurate) tests for breast cancer such as sonography (employing sound waves), thermography (measuring heat patterns in the breast), diaphanography (using bright light) and monoclonal antibodies (injecting special small cells designed to find and highlight cancer in the body). These techniques have no known dangers. If improved, they will represent real breakthroughs in the detection of breast cancer.

> ### Mammography—Breast X-Rays
> 1. Recommended for follow-up of women of any age who already have breast cancer.
> 2. Shown effective in reducing breast cancer death rates only for women over fifty.
> 3. Effectiveness for women under fifty is unproven. Research continues.
> 4. Problems with mammography:
>
> - The radiation used may cause cancer.
> - There are frequent misdiagnoses (false positives and negatives); in a few cases unnecessary mastectomies were performed.*
> - There is an increasing ability to detect "minimal cancers"—a type that does not tend to spread or be life-threatening. This may result in unnecessary treatments which further distort the "cure" and "survival" rates.
>
> 5. Advantages of mammography:
>
> - It detects some cancers before they can be felt.
> - It serves as a map or guide to the surgeon.
> - Baseline mammograms may be compared with later mammograms for suspicious changes.

be helpful in years to come as new data become available as to which, if any, types of lumps are associated with cancer. Having your own copy helps when getting second opinions or changing doctors. It also provides protection against the common problem of loss of medical records.

DES

A DES daughter with cancer:

It's not something that just happened. I've got cancer, and at least I'm alive. But I feel that it never should have happened. It could have been prevented. It should have been prevented. And that is very difficult to live with.

---

*Study of the national screening program sponsored jointly by the National Cancer Institute of the National Institutes of Health and the American Cancer Society found a group of thirty-seven women who had mastectomies when they did not have cancer. To date, these women have not been notified of the mistaken diagnoses. Consequently they are living with all the fears of recurrence and death which are common to people with cancer. In addition, they and their families and friends mistakenly give credit to mammograms for discovering their cancers "early enough" and to mastectomy for "curing" them. (See Susan Rennie in Cancer Resources.) The analysts involved stopped this program partly because they believed that routine screening could create as many cancers as might be detected, and that overtreatment dangers would continue.

Overview

DES is a synthetic form of estrogen that was prescribed for 3 to 6 million women in the United States between 1941 and 1971. DES stands for the chemical name diethylstilbestrol, but it has been manufactured under more than 200 brand names* and given out throughout the U.S. and in many other parts of the world† in pills, injections and suppositories.

Despite the fact that studies as early as the 1930s showed estrogens to be carcinogenic in laboratory animals, the FDA approved DES in 1942 for lactation suppression and treatment of menopausal symptoms and vaginitis.

In 1947, the FDA extended approval of DES in even higher doses for use during pregnancy, even though there had been no studies to examine potential effects on the fetus or on women. Doctors commonly prescribed DES if a woman had a history of miscarriage, diabetes, high blood pressure or slight bleeding during pregnancy. Some researchers and drug companies strongly recommended DES as a preventive measure even before there were signs of trouble.

Although studies showed conclusively as early as 1953 that DES was ineffective in preventing miscarriage, the FDA did not warn against using it in pregnancy until 1971, after its link to cancer was established. During the intervening eighteen years, millions were needlessly exposed. Even afterwards, it was and still is prescribed for nonpregnant women—for menopausal problems, to suppress lactation, for morning-after contraception, for acne and in advanced cases of breast cancer.

*A partial list of DES-type drugs is published by the National Cancer Institute, NIH Publication No. 81-118 (March 1980).

Here are some of the names under which DES and similar hormones have been sold: Amperone, AVC cream with Dienestrol, Benzestrol, Chlorotrianisene, Comestrol, Cyren A., Cyren B., Delvinal, DES, DesPlex, Di-Erone, Diestryl, Dibestil, Dienestrol, Dienestrol cream, Dienoestrol, Diethylstilbestrol Dipalmitate, Diethylstilbestrol Diphosphate, Diethylstilbestrol Diproprionate, Diethylstilbenediol, Digestil, Domestrol, Estan, Estilben, Estrobene, Estrobene DP, Estrosyn, Fonatol, Gynben, Gyneben, Hexestrol, Hexoestrol, H-Bestrol, Menocrin, Meprane, Mestilbol, Methallenestril, Metystil, Microest, Mikarol, Mikarol forti, Milestrol, Monomestrol, Neo-Oestranol I, Neo-Oestranol II, Nulabort, Oestrogenine, Oestromenin, Oestromon, Orestol, Pabestrol D., Palestrol, Progravidium, Restrol, Stil-Rol, Stilbal, Stilbestrol, Stilbestronate, Stilbetin, Stilbinol, Stilboestroform, Stilboestrol, Stilboestrol DP, Stilestrate, Stilpalmitate, Stilphostrol, Stilronate, Stilrone, Stils, Synestrin, Synestrol, Synthoestrin, Tace, Teserene, Tylandril, Tylosterone, Vallestril, Willestrol.

†There is evidence that DES has been used in the following countries: England, France, Spain, the Netherlands, Israel, the Philippines, Australia, Japan, Belgium, Czechoslovakia, the Ivory Coast, West Germany, Italy, some South American countries, Mexico and Latin America. In some of these, particularly Mexico and Latin American countries, DES is still being used.

Who Is Exposed and How to Find Out

Several million people (mothers, daughters and sons) have been exposed to DES, most without knowing it. If you were born after 1940, ask your mother if she had problems with any of her pregnancies or if she remembers taking anything when she was pregnant with you. (It is generally believed that DES was most widely used between 1947 and 1965 when "wonder drugs" were so popular.)

I didn't remember taking anything besides vitamins during my pregnancy, but when my daughter asked me, we checked, and there it was on the medical record.

If a woman doesn't know whether she took DES, she can check with the doctor she saw at that time. However, many doctors no longer have their medical records, and some refuse to give the information. You may find something in the medical records at the hospital where the birth took place.

Any woman who is not sure whether her mother took DES can get a special exam (see below) from a medical-care provider knowledgeable about DES exposure.

Medical Problems and Medical Care

DES Daughters

Clear cell adenocarcinoma of the vagina and cervix is the type of cancer linked to DES exposure. It was reported only a few times in women under thirty-five before it was discovered in DES daughters. It cannot be overemphasized that although the risk is low, between one in 700 and one in 7,000 DES daughters will develop this cancer. Clear cell cancer has been found in girls and women between the ages of seven and thirty-two, with the peak at ages fifteen to twenty-two. It has an 80 to 85 percent survival rate.* Regular exams using special techniques can find this cancer early so that it can be treated. Clear cell cancer is fast-growing and, in the early stages, sometimes symptomless. The most common treatment is hysterectomy with partial vaginectomy, which can be followed by reconstructive surgery.

Adenosis is the presence in the vagina of a type of cell (columnar cell) not usually found there. Many who are DES daughters (and a few who aren't) have adenosis. The columnar cells may produce a lot of mucus, which can be mistaken for vaginal infection. Adenosis is a clue that a woman may have been exposed to DES; however, some DES daughters over thirty no longer have adenosis. Adenosis does not need treatment, but does need to be watched regularly for any changes.

*A.L. Herbst and H.A. Berne. *Developmental Effects of Diethylstilbestrol (DES) in Pregnancy*. New York: Thieme-Stratton, 1981, p. 66.

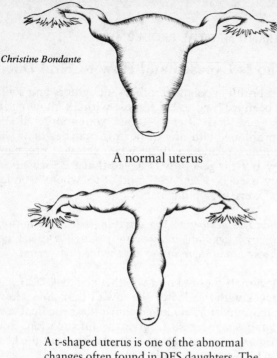

Christine Bondante

A normal uterus

A t-shaped uterus is one of the abnormal changes often found in DES daughters. The uterus may also be smaller than normal. The unusual size and shape may contribute to pregnancy problems for DES daughters, most notably pre-term labor.

Structural changes, such as cervical "collars" or "hoods," are also common among DES daughters. They do not need treatment and may disappear after age thirty. DES daughters are also more likely than others to have a T-shaped uterus. Some structural changes may contribute to pregnancy problems (see below).

Metaplasia is a normal process whereby tissue changes from one form to another. While all women have areas of cells undergoing metaplasia around their cervix, this area of changing tissue may be larger in DES daughters with adenosis. This metaplasia raises two concerns: first, some suspect that this area may be more vulnerable to precancerous or cancerous changes.* Second, pathologists may mistakenly interpret the change as abnormal (dysplasia). Such misdiagnosis can lead to unnecessary treatment with possibly harmful effects.

Dysplasia. Most researchers do not find dysplasia (see p. 485) to be more common among DES daughters. However, DES daughters who do have dysplasia may want to approach treatment recommendations with caution.†

*H.G. Hillemanns, et al. "The Stilbestrol-Adenosis-Carcinoma Syndrome," *Obstetrical and Gynecological Survey*, Vol. 34, No. 11 (1979), p. 814.

†One study of a small number of DES daughters found that cryosurgery (a common treatment of freezing the affected tissue) resulted in sometimes serious aftereffects in these women that did not occur in nonexposed women. (G. Schmidt, et al. "Reproductive History of Women Exposed to Diethylstilbestrol *in utero*," *Fertility and Sterility*, Vol. 33 (January 1980), p. 21; and G. Schmidt, "Cervical Stenosis Following Minor Gynecological Procedures on DES-Exposed Women," *Obstetrics and Gynecology*, Vol. 56, No. 33 (September 1980), p. 334.

Squamous cell carcinoma, usually of the cervix, is a slow-growing cancer which is sometimes preceded by dysplasia. Research is needed to ascertain whether DES daughters will be at a higher risk for this cancer in later years.

Pregnancy problems are more common in DES daughters, partially due to abnormalities in the uterus and/or cervix. They may have trouble conceiving or carrying a first pregnancy to term due to miscarriage, premature delivery and tubal pregnancy (pregnancy in the fallopian tube instead of in the uterus). Early in pregnancy, watching for signs of a tubal pregnancy may help prevent serious problems. Later on, a pregnant DES daughter should receive "high risk" obstetrical care.

When I got pregnant, I found out that the doctor who was doing my DES exams didn't know anything about pregnancy problems for DES daughters. So I brought him seven articles that DES Action gave me. We both read them and, as a result, he checked my cervix at every prenatal visit. It took fifteen seconds and took away tons of anxiety.

Other problems, such as endometriosis, menstrual irregularities and pelvic inflammatory disease (PID), have been reported by many DES daughters. There is as yet no research on whether these problems are more significant among DES-exposed women.

Contraception for DES daughters poses some special considerations. *Birth control pills* may be inadvisable due to the possible effects of further estrogen exposure on someone who is already at increased risk of a hormone-related cancer.* *IUDs* for DES daughters are questionable because of the possible cervical and uterine abnormalities. Barrier methods are often the overall safest choice.

The DES Exam

DES-caused changes do not usually show up in regular pelvic examinations or Pap smears. Starting with your first period or any signs of trouble (discharge or bleeding), see a medical care provider experienced in DES screening. Ask whether the person who examines you is following other DES daughters and if s/he is familiar with the techniques described below.

A DES exam consists of:

- a careful visual inspection of the vagina and cervix for physical abnormalities;
- a gentle palpation of the walls of the vagina;
- a four-sided (quadrant) Pap test of the cervix *and* vagina;

*See DES Task Force, "Summary Report," 1978. NIH publication 82–1688, reprinted in October 1981.

- iodine staining of the vagina and cervix (normal tissue stains brown, adenosis tissue does not stain). (See "Schiller's Test," p. 480.)

The clinician may also do further tests or refer you to a special doctor or special clinic for more tests. These may include biopsy (p. 492) and colposcopy (p. 480).

DES Mothers

Some of the few studies available suggest that DES mothers have an increased incidence of breast cancer and cancer of the uterus, cervix or ovaries and of non-cancerous tumors of the uterus. Most studies agree that there is a time lag of ten to twenty years between taking DES and developing a related disease.

If you are a DES mother, get a professional breast exam every year in addition to performing monthly breast self-examination.

DES Sons

Ongoing studies report several areas of concern for DES sons: underdeveloped testes, benign (noncancerous) cysts on the epididymis (the part of the testicle which stores mature sperm), undescended testicles (which may increase the risk of testicular cancer) and sperm and semen abnormalities (which may cause fertility problems). Concerned sons can be examined by a urologist and DES sons can practice regular self-examination of the testes.

Emotional Issues

Not surprisingly, some DES mothers feel guilty when they find out that something they took may have harmed their children. Some find it difficult to tell them, though it is essential to do so. Many mothers describe relief after telling their children and talking about the health care they need.

Some DES daughters and sons are angry that something over which they had no control may seriously affect their health. Others fear medical problems. However, many also describe how good it feels to gather information which helps them get quality medical care.

I read about the report on DES and its link to cancer back in 1971. I cut the article out of the paper and stuck it in my bureau drawer. Five years later my daughter was fourteen and I knew I had to do something soon. So I found a doctor who knew about DES and how to do the exam, and I finally told my daughter. What a relief!

It really helped me to talk with other DES daughters. We compared notes and I went back to my next medical appointment with a list of questions and a friend for moral support. We had a long discussion with the doctor, who was surprised at how much we knew.

DES, which has caused me so much pain, has at least allowed me new and needed understandings. I know to keep myself informed. I would like to work with my doctors. I know that they haven't always read the medical journals. I know that they cannot care about the outcome of my case nearly as much as I do.

Although we know much more about DES than we did ten years ago, daughters, sons and mothers face unanswered questions about their future health. More research is needed in all areas. Furthermore, some doctors still do not know about the DES exam, special pregnancy problems and other recent medical findings; their ignorance can result in serious overtreatment or undertreatment. Finally, we need to tell the DES story so that people who have been exposed can receive the medical care they need, and so that we can help prevent similar medical mistakes from happening in the future.

DES Action

DES Action is the consumer-oriented group dedicated to providing information about DES to the public and to the medical world. It is a national nonprofit organization composed of DES-exposed individuals, medical care providers and others who want to help

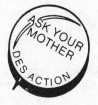

DES Action

499

educate people about DES. There are thirty-two local DES Action groups in twenty-seven states. DES Action provides general information about DES, referrals to knowledgeable physicians and support for DES-exposed people. Its quarterly newsletter, the *DES Action VOICE*, contains medical, legal and personal articles (see Resources).

For information about DES, send a business-size stamped, self-addressed envelope to DES Action, Long Island Jewish Hospital, New Hyde Park, NY 11040.

ENDOMETRIOSIS

Endometriosis, which can be an extremely painful disease, occurs when some of the tissue which usually lines the uterus (endometrium) grows in other parts of the body. This "normal tissue in an abnormal location," sometimes referred to as growths, nodules, tumors or lesions, most commonly develops in the pelvic area—on the ovaries, external surface of the uterus, ligaments or fallopian tubes. Growths occasionally occur on the bladder, intestines or even distant parts of the body—in the arm, lung or head.

These abnormally located growths build up and bleed at the time of the menstrual period. They respond to the hormonal influences of the cycle just as the uterine lining does. Since this build-up has no way to leave the body as menstrual flow does, it may cause internal bleeding, inflammation and formation of cysts and scar tissue.

Endometriosis may cause severe pelvic pain around menstruation, ovulation and/or sexual activity; excessive or irregular menstrual flow; a higher than average rate of miscarriage; infertility; and other severe health problems, including ruptured ovarian cysts (sometimes called "chocolate cysts"); adhesions; increased risk of ectopic pregnancy and general debilitation. And yet some women experience no symptoms except perhaps infertility. The disease may not even be discovered until they have surgery for another problem.

I experienced the first symptoms of endometriosis (in my case, very severe pain when having a bowel movement) when I was nineteen years old. About five years later I began to have the same kind of pain at midcycle and during my periods. I mentioned this to several doctors, and they seemed unconcerned. A year or two later I began to have premenstrual spotting, which increased in duration as time progressed. I went to at least four different doctors. No one even mentioned endometriosis....At the age of thirty I had new symptoms: chronic, low-level pelvic pain and pain on intercourse, in addition to pain on pelvic examination. At this time the word "endometriosis" was first mentioned, and a diagnosis by laparoscopy followed a few months later. [a thirty-three-year-old woman]

A particularly difficult aspect of the disease for many women is that it is chronic. In one survey, 60 percent of 200 women said that they were unable to carry on normal work and activities, usually for one to three days at a time and sometimes for weeks or even months, not including the time lost for surgery. One woman calculated that three days lost to pain each month for twenty years added up to a staggering two years of her life. While most people would not make light of two years lost to illness, the recurring nature of this condition—the fact that it comes and goes with the menstrual period and gets better and worse—means that women often don't get recognition and sympathy for the difficulties it causes.

The biggest problem is looking very healthy. People don't seem to understand pain and sickness unless they can see physical evidence. This makes you feel absolutely desperate. [a twenty-four-year-old woman]

Causes

How the tissue mislocation occurs is still a mystery. Since the growths sometimes appear in scar tissue from previous pelvic surgery, one theory is that surgery may spread endometriosis or that the trauma of surgery somehow causes it. Another theory proposes that remnants of a woman's own prenatal tissue later develop into endometriosis, and another that menstrual blood and tissue flow back through the fallopian tubes into the pelvic cavity to develop on some organ, muscle or ligament. (This is called retrograde flow, or tubal reflux.) Hormonal, immunological or chemical factors may also contribute to the disease's development. There is some evidence of a correlation between primary dysmenorrhea symptoms (see p. 214) and endometriosis. Preliminary findings from a survey done by the Endometriosis Association (see the box on p. 502) show that 97 percent of women with endometriosis also reported symptoms of primary dysmenorrhea. This, coupled with some women's reports that antiprostaglandins (drugs used for primary dysmenorrhea) relieve some of their symptoms, suggests that the intense cramps and excessive prostaglandin production associated with dysmenorrhea may be related to endometriosis.

The endometrial growths themselves may produce prostaglandins which initiate the disease. More research is needed to look into the connection between these two conditions and to see whether antiprostaglandins are an appropriate treatment. Antiprostaglandins are relatively safe compared to the drugs and treatments now used for endometriosis. Meanwhile, young women with severe menstrual cramps should not dismiss them as a "normal" aspect of early womanhood. Instead, they should watch for other signs of endometriosis.

Myths impede both diagnosis and treatment of

endometriosis. The medical literature labels it "the career woman's disease" and describes the typical endometriosis sufferer as an upwardly striving, white, educated, egocentric woman in her late twenties or early thirties who has postponed pregnancy in favor of her career. This anachronistic view probably exists because these are the women who tend to have the financial resources, education, sense of entitlement and private doctors necessary to obtain a correct diagnosis. However, women of color do develop the disease, though the medical system has historically overlooked that fact. Also, it is *not* true that the disease typically begins in the late twenties and early thirties. Many young women have symptoms of endometriosis by their late teens or early twenties. Contrary to medical myth, early pregnancy—even teenage pregnancy—does not confer immunity to the disease. Too many women have blamed themselves, thinking, It's my fault because I did not become pregnant early.

Another myth is that menstrual pain is primarily psychological. Many doctors still don't take it seriously, which makes them slow to diagnose endometriosis.

Diagnosis

Though physicians can sometimes diagnose endometriosis by pelvic exam or external examination by hands (palpation), most usually advise laparoscopy for a definitive diagnosis when they see growths on the vagina or vulva. Since laparoscopy, a surgical procedure, entails some risks, you and your doctor should carefully consider your history of symptoms. Endometriosis is sometimes confused with other disorders and diseases (for example, PID, ectopic pregnancy, cysts, cancer, appendicitis or diverticulitis) which have similar symptoms.

Treatments

Choosing a treatment is rarely simple. A number of factors may enter into your decision, among them your age, location of the endometriosis and its severity, the extent of your desire for pregnancy, past experiences with hormones and family history.

The aim in treating endometriosis is to stop the ovary from working and producing estrogen, and also to stop menstruation. While doctors often recommend pregnancy as a "treatment," it is certainly a dubious one. It is, of course, best to have a child because you want to, not to cure a disease. Pregnancy is not a cure anyway, though it may offer temporary relief. And it is not always possible to become pregnant, as women with endometriosis have higher than average infertility. If you have the disease and know you want a child, be aware that delay may make pregnancy less likely if the disease advances. *Hormonal* treatments exist.

Danazol (a derivative of the male hormone testosterone, marketed as Danocrine in the United States or Cyclomen in Canada) is the current medical favorite. It produces a pseudomenopause and can purportedly dissolve small implants. One drawback is that it can cost as much as 150 dollars or more a month, or 900 dollars to 1,350 dollars for a typical six-to-nine-month treatment period, a cost which may be prohibitive for a woman without insurance coverage. Furthermore, the Endometriosis Association did a survey of 180 women taking danazol, and fully half experienced either no relief or a recurrence of symptoms immediately or within a short time of discontinuing the drug.

Birth control pills and progestagen (synthetic progesterone such as Provera or Depo-Provera), which produce a pseudopregnancy, are much less common forms of hormonal treatment.

If you have a mild case of endometriosis, you may want to consider hormonal treatment rather than undergo surgery. It can also be a way to "buy time" for pregnancy. On the other hand, some studies report a higher pregnancy rate following surgery.

Surgery to treat endometriosis includes a wide range of treatments, from "conservative" (scraping, cutting or cauterizing the growths) to "radical" (hysterectomy, with or without removal of the ovaries). Surgery for endometriosis is common and perhaps not always necessary. Some doctors believe that surgery should be performed only where specifically indicated, such as in the presence of a large (greater than five centimeters) collection of growths or when it is thought that infertility is caused by endometrial adhesions.

The hardest part in deciding treatment is picking the lesser of two evils. [a twenty-eight-year-old woman]

In the words of a thirty-three-year-old woman describing eleven years of intensifying symptoms:

Doctors seemed unsympathetic about the fact that by this point I was in almost constant pain. They suggested that I try to get pregnant; I mentioned that intercourse was now quite painful. They shrugged and suggested a few drinks or a few aspirins a day.

Some women, searching for cure and relief from pain (sometimes they have to use prescription pain-killers for extended periods of time) have turned to alternative forms of healing—visualization, meditation, acupuncture, chiropractic, homeopathy, herbs and nutritional therapies among them. The Endometriosis Association currently has too few reports to evaluate these methods but requests that women with endometriosis write them about their experiences.

The Endometriosis Association keeps careful records of these reports as well as reports on medical treatments. In gathering and sharing information, we work to build mutual support so that women will not feel isolated. Together we hope to encourage researchers to build on what we have learned, to find better solutions and cures and to recognize endometriosis as the serious health problem that it is.

> The Endometriosis Association, founded in January 1980, is a national self-help organization with three major goals: supporting and helping women with endometriosis, educating the medical community and public about the disease and conducting research.
>
> The Association offers information/support meetings, crisis telephone services, a newsletter, an informational brochure and other literature, and access to a small library of selected materials.
>
> The "mother" chapter and national headquarters are located in Milwaukee, Wisconsin; other chapters and groups are scattered around the country.
>
> Since 1981 the Association has been gathering information from hundreds of women who have had endometriosis. Each woman completes an extensive questionnaire covering her experiences with the disease and the medical system. Data from the questionnaires is available to members through an internal data bank and is computerized at the Medical College of Wisconsin so that health professionals and others may have access to it.
>
> For additional information, including locations of chapters, please send five dollars to the Endometriosis Association, c/o Bread and Roses Women's Health Center, 238 W. Wisconsin Avenue, #700, Milwaukee, WI 53203.

PELVIC INFLAMMATORY DISEASE (PID)

I obtained a copy of my medical records and discovered that I had been complaining of the same problem—pain in my lower right abdomen—for a couple of years.

I tried several different doctors, none of whom took it seriously or were very sympathetic. If anything, they made me feel unclean, almost to the point of being ashamed. I had severe menstrual irregularities, fevers, bleeding between periods, bleeding after intercourse, pains and general malaise. Several times I was treated with antibiotics, which brought only some temporary relief. Never was the issue resolved as to what was causing this. Never were my sexual partners or practices mentioned.

Pelvic inflammatory disease (PID) is a general term for an infection that affects the fallopian tubes (sal-

pingitis), ovaries (oophoritis), both tubes and ovaries (salpingo-oophoritis) and/or uterus (endometritis). It is primarily caused by sexually transmitted diseases (see Chapter 14). "Annually, nearly one million women in the United States suffer from PID and its sequelae. They account for more than 2.5 million physician visits, 250,000 hospital admissions and nearly 150,000 surgical procedures."* These statistics probably greatly underestimate the amount and consequences of PID now occurring. This is primarily because so much PID is undiagnosed.

Symptoms

PID symptoms vary. They may be so mild that you hardly notice them, but the primary symptom is pain. For instance, you may be aware of tightness or pressure in the reproductive organs or an occasional dull ache in the lower abdomen. On the other hand, the pain may be so strong that you have to go to a hospital emergency room. You may feel pain in the middle of your lower abdomen. This is the most effective time to treat PID, for the infection has not yet spread from the uterus to the tubes. However, most women seek treatment only after they feel pain on one or both sides of the lower abdomen, which means that the tube(s) has already been affected (salpingitis).

You may have some, most or none of these other symptoms:

- sudden high fever or low-grade fever which can come and go;
- chills;
- lower back or leg pain;
- frequency, burning or inability to empty bladder when urinating;
- abnormal or foul discharge from the vagina or urethra;
- pain or bleeding during or after intercourse;
- irregular bleeding or spotting;
- increased menstrual cramps;
- increased pain during ovulation;
- inflammation or infection of the cervix—this can manifest itself as a number-two or -three Pap smear;
- swollen abdomen;
- swollen lymph nodes;
- lack of appetite;
- nausea or vomiting;
- pain around the kidneys or liver;
- acnelike rashes on the back, chest, neck or face;
- feelings of weakness, tiredness, depression;
- diminished desire to have sex.

The intensity and extent of the symptoms depend upon which microorganisms are causing the PID, where

*James W. Curran, M.D. "Economic Consequences of Pelvic Inflammatory Disease in the United States," *American Journal of Obstetrics and Gynecology*, Vol. 138, No. 7, Part 2 (December 1, 1980) pp. 848–51.

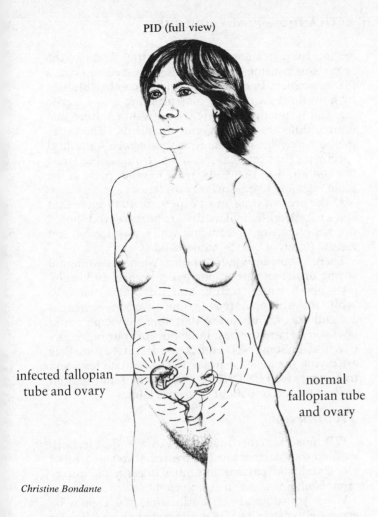

PID (full view)

Christine Bondante

infected fallopian tube and ovary

normal fallopian tube and ovary

PID can cause a sharp pain at the most infected site and/or can cause pain throughout all or part of the abdomen.

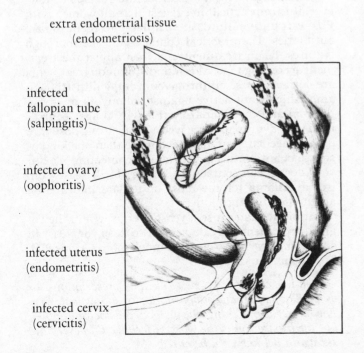

extra endometrial tissue (endometriosis)

infected fallopian tube (salpingitis)

infected ovary (oophoritis)

infected uterus (endometritis)

infected cervix (cervicitis)

they are (uterus, tubes, lining of the abdomen, etc.), how long you have had it, what if any antibiotics you have taken for it and your general health—i.e., how much stress you are under and how well you take care of yourself. Doctors characterize PID as acute, chronic or "silent" (when a woman doesn't notice her symptoms). Another way of categorizing PID is in terms of increasing severity—as endometritis, salpingitis or peritonitis (inflammation of the lining of the abdomen).

Complications

PID complications can be very serious. If untreated, PID can turn into peritonitis, a life-threatening condition, and also cause other serious infections, such as tubo-ovarian abscess. It can affect the bowels and the liver (perihepatitis syndrome). Ectopic pregnancy can result from tubes having been damaged in an earlier PID episode or clogged by infection at the time of conception.

PID can cause chronic pain from adhesions or lingering infection; infertility; ectopic pregnancy; early miscarriage; infection in a woman's or her newborn infant's eyes, pharynx and lungs; some forms of arthritis; and death. Pregnant women with chlamydial infections may be at a higher risk for stillbirth or neonatal death.[*]

Most PID is caused by the microorganisms responsible for STDs. These may enter the body during sexual contact with an infected man or woman[†] and also during an IUD insertion, abortion, miscarriage, childbirth, surgery, procedures involving the uterus such as endometrial biopsy, hysterosalpingogram (X-ray of the reproductive tract) or donor insemination when there has not been careful screening for all STDs. It is not uncommon for male sexual partners of women with PID to have no or few symptoms but to be carrying the organisms which can cause it,[‡] so they must be tested and treated as well and should use a condom.

My husband had no symptoms at all although I had been suffering from chronic PID for years. Neither of us could figure out how I got sick. It took us a long time to find a doctor who cultured both of us for organisms. I finally got over it when we both started getting tested and treated according to what organisms were found: chlamydia, mycoplasma, staph, strep.

Doctors may lead women with chronic PID to believe that they are at fault for not responding to an-

[*]David H. Martin, M.D., et al. "Prematurity and Perinatal Mortality in Pregnancies Complicated by Maternal Chlamydia Trachomatis Infections," *Journal of the American Medical Association*, Vol. 247, No. 11 (March 19, 1982).

[†]The incidence of PID is very low among lesbians.

[‡]Attila Toth, M.D., and Martin L. Lesser, Ph.D. "Asymptomatic Bacteriospermia in Fertile and Infertile Men," *Fertility and Sterility*, Vol. 36, No. 1 (July 1981) pp. 89–91.

tibiotic treatment when in fact it is their sexual partners who need treatment also.

You are at higher risk for developing PID if you are exposed to infected mucus—especially infected semen—during menstruation and ovulation when your cervix is more open. Certain bacteria can attach themselves to moving sperm and get into the uterus and fallopian tubes.* (Birth control pills seem to create dense cervical mucus which prevents sperm from entering the uterus and so reduces the risk of developing PID.) Women using IUDs are also at much higher risk, as sexually transmitted organisms can travel through the cervix (left open by an IUD tail). In the past, it was assumed that gonorrhea caused most PID. However, chlamydia, mycoplasma and a number of aerobic and anerobic microorganisms (those which need oxygen and those which don't) are being found more and more frequently in cervical, endometrial and tubal cultures taken from women with PID.† These organisms may reside in the genital tract for years.

Diagnosis

It would be ideal if, when you got PID, you could know right away exactly which organisms were causing it so you could get the appropriate antibiotics. But such exactness is rarely possible because pinpointing the organisms often takes a few (or many) tests and in most places tests are unavailable; if they are being done they are liable to be inaccurate and expensive (though it may cost less to get a culture done in the first place than to go to doctor after doctor). Even when you can find a doctor and lab which cultures for mycoplasma and chlamydia, you often cannot trust a negative culture result; these organisms are difficult to culture. Sometimes the organisms infecting the uterus and fallopian tubes will not show up in a cervical culture. Although some doctors rely on blood tests, especially sedimentation rates and white blood cell count, to indicate whether or not you have an infection at all, these are not reliable for diagnosing PID.‡ Sometimes an endometrial biopsy can be useful if hard-to-culture organisms are suspected and not found in a cervical or vaginal culture. However, such a biopsy can further spread organisms from the cervix and vagina to the uterus. X-rays and ultrasound are usually useless in revealing the presence of PID.

If you have PID and a male sexual partner, he must get a test done, too. Frequently, men are diagnosed as

having NGU (nongonococcal urethritis). Some of the organisms causing these infections in men can cause PID in women. In men, the specimen can be obtained by a urethral swab or by masturbating into a sterile jar, and it must immediately be put into culture mediums (different for different organisms). The latter method may be important, because men's urethral specimens (like cervical specimens from women) may not contain the organisms living in other parts of the male reproductive or urinary systems.

At the present time, most experts seem to agree that since your health and fertility are at stake, you should not delay getting treatments while waiting for test results (often of questionable validity).

There is currently a lot of discussion, research and strong disagreement among gynecologists and urologists about cause, testing and treatment methods. While these arguments are going on among researchers and doctors, be aware that your pelvic pain and how you feel are the best indicators of your reproductive health. Some STD clinics and fertility specialists are giving the most accurate and up-to-date tests and treatments for PID. Call VD hotlines and information centers to find out about tests and clinics.

Treatments

PID must be treated just as STDs are; that is, both you and your partner must be treated. If you are treated alone and your partner continues to carry the microorganism(s), you will be reinfected.

When you do start on antibiotics, you cannot be accurately cultured again until you have been off them for at least a couple of weeks. Taking the wrong drugs can make organisms more difficult to get rid of. However, it is impractical to suggest that all women with PID wait until cultures are available to them to take antibiotics. The practical course is to take thorough cultures, begin treatment and then adjust the treatment according to what is found. Common treatments are tetracyclines, erythromycin, ampicillin (though ampicillin is not active against chlamydia or mycoplasma) and metronidazole (Flagyl). Longer courses than ten days (up to three weeks) and strong doses are usually needed. You may need more than one kind or course of antibiotics to get rid of the infection. You or your doctor can contact the Centers for Disease Control in Atlanta for the most up-to-date information about effective antibiotics.

Antibiotics can cause a yeast overgrowth in the vagina. Treatment may be needed to keep the yeast in check while trying to cure the much more serious PID. Try yogurt for yeast.

*Attila Toth, M.D., William M. O'Leary, Ph.D., and William J. Ledger, M.D. "Evidence for Microbial Transfer by the Spermatozoa," *American Journal of Obstetrics and Gynecology*, Vol. 59, No. 5 (May 1982), pp. 556–59.

†Richard L. Sweet, M.D. "Antibiotic Options for Acute GYN Infections," *Modern Medicine* (June 1981), pp. 73–80.

‡Lennart Jacobson, M.D. "Differential Diagnosis of Acute Pelvic Inflammatory Disease," *American Journal of Obstetrics and Gynecology*, Vol. 138, No. 7, Part 2 (December 1, 1980), pp. 1006–11.

I felt like crying today as I filled my prescriptions for ampicillin for PID and suppositories for subsequent yeast. The money is one thing, the visits to the doctor another, but the frustration is the worst. I feel like I'd never have sex again if I knew I'd be cured.

According to the Centers for Disease Control, hospitalization should be strongly considered when 1. the diagnosis is uncertain, 2. surgical emergencies such as appendicitis and ectopic pregnancy must be excluded, 3. a pelvic abscess is suspected, 4. severe illness precludes outpatient management, 5. the woman is pregnant, 6. the woman is unable to follow or tolerate an outpatient regimen, 7. the woman has failed to respond to outpatient therapy or 8. clinic follow-up after forty-eight to seventy-two hours following the start of antibiotic treatment cannot be arranged. Many experts recommend that *all* women with PID be hospitalized for treatment.* Unfortunately, many physicians do not follow these recommendations.

Most women are hospitalized for PID or possible PID only for fertility testing or when they have acute attacks. It can be hard to find a doctor who will hospitalize you if you are single (and therefore presumed to be uninterested in pregnancy) or if you have subacute, chronic PID which oral antibiotics have not cleared up. In the hospital you can get intravenous (IV) antibiotics which provide a sufficient concentration of medication in your body to fight the infection. When antibiotic treatment is not successful even then, it is probably because the antibiotics were not the correct ones for the infection and/or you were reinfected because your sexual partner was not treated successfully. IV antibiotics may also fail because of problems such as pelvic abscess, septic pelvic thrombophlebitis or an incorrect diagnosis. Instead of cystitis accompanying or preceding PID, you may be told that you have chronic cystitis caused by trauma to the urethra during intercourse and to try intercourse in another position; instead of having a sexually transmitted infection, you may be told that you have infected yourself with organisms from your colon by wiping yourself from back to front; you may be told that you have a spastic colon or that you have an emotional, not a physical, problem.

You and your doctor may decide you should have surgery to try to restore fertility by opening closed, scarred tubes (tuboplasty). You may have adhesions, fibrous bands of scar tissue caused by infections. These can bind your internal organs together, causing pain and infertility. In this case, you may decide to have a laparotomy to cut them out. Remember that surgery itself can cause adhesions. Remember, also, that physicians sometimes attribute pain solely to adhesions and fail to recognize the presence of infection.

You may be urged to have a hysterectomy if the doctor thinks PID has ruined your pelvic organs beyond repair. Also, emergency hysterectomies are done

in some cases of acute PID. It seems possible that with more thorough culturing and correct antibiotics, many of these hysterectomies could be avoided. Some women elect to have hysterectomies in order to get over persistent, debilitating PID.

Personal Issues

Many of us have felt guilt and anger about our own or our partner's sexual experiences which have led to the constant physical problems and pain of PID. We are also angry at a medical system which is not prepared to deal adequately with the growing numbers of women getting STDs, more and more of whom are coming down with PID. Asymptomatic sexual partners may not want to have tests and treatments or not understand that we need to avoid intercourse with them. They may look for other people to have sex with, which may feel like punishment to us, and which puts us in further danger of exposure. Unfortunately, instead of expressing our anger outwardly we may just become depressed. It is also enormously frustrating to deal with a doctor or an entire clinic which either does not have the facilities or refuses to culture for chlamydia and mycoplasma. Many doctors do not recognize that we are sexually active, and they disapprove of us for contracting what is so often a sex-related disease or doubt the severity and significance of our pelvic symptoms. Finding ourselves so untrusted, belittled and judged by the medical world adds to the physical and emotional pain we suffer from PID.

It feels like a dirty trick was played on me, doctor after doctor telling me my pain was not in my pelvis but in my head. How many times did I conscientiously and politely ask about getting a mycoplasma test? Even though there was a lab doing these tests in the same hospital (a major university teaching hospital), my doctors wouldn't do the tests because they didn't believe in them. I am still mad and sad and bitter. It took months and a lot of pain before I found a doctor who would do a mycoplasma test. It was positive; mycoplasma was probably a cause of my PID.

There are many things you can do to help heal yourself while you wait for test results to come back and antibiotics to take hold and work. Very hot baths and heat applied directly to the lower abdomen help relieve pain and bring disease-fighting blood and drugs to your pelvis. A heating pad can be your best friend at this time. Close your eyes and visualize your reproductive organs as healthy, pink, oxygenated and relaxed. Do not use tampons or douche; to do so may force microorganisms up into your uterus. Do not reuse a douche bag which may be harboring infectious organisms. Have intercourse *only* when you feel completely well through an entire monthly cycle and your partners have had negative tests for *all* STDs. Some-

*U.S. Department of Health and Human Services, Public Health Service, Centers for Disease Control, Center for Prevention Services, Venereal Disease Control Division. "Sexually Transmitted Diseases Treatment Guidelines, 1982," *Morbidity and Mortality Weekly Report Supplement*, Vol. 31, No. 2S (August 20, 1982), pp. 435–45.

505

times it takes months to feel better after PID. Some women have short bouts of PID months after the initial infection is cleared up, particularly if they abandon their daily health routines or are under too much stress. Acupuncture may help control pain and rebalance energy. You can soak cotton cloth in castor oil, place it on the abdomen, cover it with plastic to prevent greasiness and then cover it with a heating pad or hot water bottle to bring a maximum amount of heat to the pelvic area. Ginger root compresses and taro root poultices may relieve pain, help eliminate accumulated toxins, keep the area loose and freer from adhesions and dissolve already formed adhesions. (These are strong medicines and best used with the guidance of a wholistic health practitioner.) A garlic clove peeled, crushed and wrapped in sterile gauze, tied with dental floss (leave a long string to pull it out with), and used as a homemade tampon for four days (changed daily) can help relieve vaginitis and cervicitis. A number of herbs and teas are useful against infection of the reproductive and urinary tracts. Raspberry leaf tea strengthens the reproductive system. Eliminate sugar and cut down on dairy products (to lessen mucus production); take plenty of Vitamins C, A, D and B-complex and zinc and other minerals. Eat wholesome, fresh foods; avoid stress as much as possible. Eliminate alcohol, tobacco and other drugs which lower your resistance to disease, and reduce coffee consumption. You may be unusually tired and run down. Get plenty of sleep. Complete bed rest is recommended, but difficult to achieve.

To prevent PID, follow these guidelines:

Prevention of PID is like prevention of STDs, since so much PID is caused by sexually transmitted organisms. Birth control foams, creams and jellies kill some bacteria that can enter the vagina during intercourse. Don't have intercourse without using a barrier method (condom, diaphragm) of birth control, especially when your cervix is more open than usual. Have your male partners use condoms, particularly if either of you have more than one sexual partner. Do not use IUDs for birth control.

Be aware that PID is increasing at an incredible rate. You may have to be an unsupported advocate for yourself and your friends until a time when more doctors begin testing and treating women and their partners accurately.

URINARY TRACT INFECTIONS (UTIs)

Urinary tract infections are so common that most of us get at least one at some point in our lives. They are usually caused by bacteria, such as Escherichia coli (*E. coli*), which travel from the colon to the urethra and bladder (and occasionally to the kidneys). Tricho-

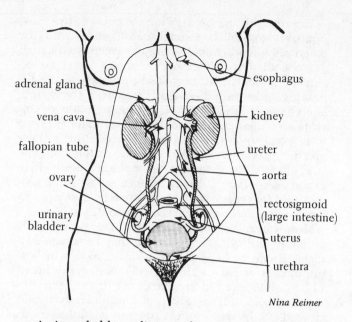

Nina Reimer

moniasis and chlamydia can also cause UTIs; low resistance, poor diet, stress and damage to the urethra from childbirth, surgery, catheterization, etc., can predispose you to getting them. Often a sudden increase in sexual activity triggers symptoms ("honeymoon cystitis"). Pregnant women are especially susceptible (pressure of the growing fetus keeps some urine in the bladder and ureters, allowing bacteria to grow), as are postmenopausal women (because of hormonal changes). Very occasionally, UTI is caused by an anatomical abnormality or a prolapsed (fallen) urethra or bladder, most common in older women or women who have had many children.

Cystitis (inflammation or infection of the bladder) is by far the most common UTI in women. While the symptoms can be frightening, cystitis in itself is not usually serious. If you suddenly have to urinate every few minutes and it burns like crazy even though almost nothing comes out, you probably have cystitis. There may also be blood in the urine (hematuria) and pus in the urine (pyuria). You may have pain just above your pubic bone, and sometimes there is a peculiar, heavy urine odor when you first urinate in the morning.

It is also possible to get mild temporary symptoms (such as urinary frequency) without actually having an infection, simply because of drinking too much coffee or tea (which are diuretics), premenstrual syndrome, food allergies, anxiety or irritation to the area from bubble baths, soaps or douches. As long as you are in good health and not pregnant, you can usually treat mild symptoms yourself for forty-eight hours before consulting a practitioner.* Cystitis often disappears without treatment. If it persists more than

*See the box below, and "Cystitis: The Complete Self-Help Guide," by Angela Kilmartin (listed in Resources).

Preventing Urinary Tract Infections, Treating Mild Infections and Avoiding Reinfections

1. Drink lots of fluid every day. Try to drink a glass of water every two or three hours. (For active infection, drink enough to pour out a good stream of urine every hour. It really helps!)

2. Urinate frequently and try to empty your bladder completely each time. Never try to hold your urine once your bladder feels full.

3. Keep the bacteria in your bowels and anus away from your urethra by wiping yourself from front to back after urinating or having a bowel movement. Wash your genitals from front to back with plain water or very mild soap at least once a day.

4. Any sexual activity that irritates the urethra, puts pressure on the bladder or spreads bacteria from the anus to the vagina or urethra can contribute to cystitis. Make sure that you and your lover have clean hands and genitals before sex, and wash after contact with the anal area before touching the vagina or urethra. To prevent irritation to the urethra, try to avoid prolonged direct clitoral stimulation and pressure on the urethral area during oral-genital sex or masturbation. Make sure your vagina is well lubricated before intercourse. Rear-entry positions and prolonged vigorous intercourse tend to put additional stress on the urethra and bladder. Emptying your bladder before and immediately after sex is a good idea. If you tend to get cystitis after sex despite these precautions, you may want to ask your practitioner for preventive tablets (i.e., sulfa, ampicillin, nitrofurantoin); a single dose of a tablet after sex has been shown effective in preventing infections and is usually not associated with the same negative effects as prolonged courses of antibiotics.

5. Some birth control methods can contribute to or aggravate a urinary tract infection. Women taking oral contraceptives have a higher rate of cystitis than those not on the Pill. Some diaphragm users find that the rim pressing against the urethra can contribute to infection. (A different-size diaphragm or one with a different type of rim may solve this problem.) Contraceptive foams or vaginal suppositories may irritate the urethra. Dry condoms may put pressure on the urethra, or the dyes or lubricants may cause irritation.

6. If you use sanitary napkins during your period, the blood on the pad provides a convenient bridge for bacteria from your anus to travel to your urethra. Change pads frequently and wash your genitals twice a day when you are menstruating. Some women also find that tampons or sponges put pressure on the urethra.

7. Tight jeans, bicycling or horseback riding may cause trauma to the urethra. When you engage in sports that can provoke cystitis in you, wear loose clothing and try to drink extra water.

8. Caffeine and alcohol irritate the bladder. If you don't want to stop using them, try to drink less of them and drink enough water to dilute them.

9. Some women find that routine use of cranberry juice (preferably the kind without sugar) or Vitamin C to make their urine more acid helps to prevent urinary tract problems. (If you have an infection, try combining 500 milligrams of Vitamin C and cranberry juice four times a day; you can substitute fresh cranberries in plain yogurt for the juice.) Whole grains, meats, nuts and many fruits also help to acidify the urine. Avoid strong spices (curry, cayenne, chili, black pepper).

10. Diets high in refined sugars and starches (white flour, white rice, pasta, etc.) may predispose some women to urinary tract infections.

11. Women use a wide variety of herbal remedies to prevent or treat urinary tract infections. Drinking teas made of uva ursi, horsetail or shavegrass, cornsilk, cleavers, comfrey, lemon balm or goldenseal may be beneficial to the bladder. You may want to consult a herbalist.

12. Keep up your resistance by eating and resting well and finding ways to reduce stress in your life as much as possible.

13. Vitamin B_6 and magnesium-calcium supplements help to relieve spasm of the urethra which can predispose to cystitis. This is especially helpful for women who need to have their urethras dilated repeatedly.

14. If you have an infection, soak in a hot tub two or three times a day; try a hot water bottle or heating pad on your abdomen and back.

forty-eight hours, recurs frequently or is ever accompanied by chills, fever, vomiting or pain in the kidneys, consult a practitioner. These symptoms suggest that infection has spread to the kidneys (pyelonephritis), a serious problem which requires medical treatment. Some researchers estimate that 30 to 50 percent of women with cystitis symptoms also have "silent" kidney infections. Consult your practitioner if cystitis symptoms are accompanied by any of the following: blood or pus in the urine, pain on urination during pregnancy, diabetes or chronic illnesses, a history of kidney infection or diseases or abnormalities of the urinary tract. Untreated chronic infections can lead to serious complications, such as high blood pressure or premature births (if they occur during pregnancy).

Diagnosis

When cystitis does not respond to self-help treatments within forty-eight hours or recurs frequently, get a urine test. An ordinary urinalysis is not sufficient to test for cystitis—make sure your practitioner takes a "clean voided specimen."* Your urine will be examined for evidence of blood and pus and a culture will be taken. Sometimes, even when you have symptoms, the culture may come back negative (i.e., not show a cause for the infection). False-negative cultures may be due to mishandling or overly dilute urine; you may also get a false negative if your cystitis is caused by something other than bacterial infection (such as anxiety or stress). On the other hand, a negative culture accompanied by white cells in the urine (called "acute urethral syndrome") may indicate a chlamydial infection. (See Chapter 14, "Sexually Transmitted Diseases.") Sometimes women have bacteria in their urine (bacteriuria) without symptoms. If bacteriuria shows up during a routine urine test, you should be treated to prevent kidney infection and other complications.†

A sensitivity test, which shows what kind of antibiotics to use, is usually not necessary unless you have had many infections or severe symptoms indicating pyelonephritis. Women who have had pyelonephritis repeatedly may be tested for abnormalities of the urinary tract. The usual test is an IVP (intravenous pyelogram) in which a dye injected into the bloodstream collects in the kidneys, showing any blockages or obstructions on an X-ray.

Treatments

For symptoms which are severe or indicate a kidney infection, medications are usually started immediately. For milder infections, many practitioners prefer to wait for culture results before prescribing a drug.

Most urinary tract infections respond rapidly to a variety of antibiotics. Drugs commonly used include antibiotics such as ampicillin, nitrofurantoin, tetracycline or sulfonamides (Gantrisin). (Women who may be G6PD-deficient should not take sulfonamides; see "Hereditary and Other Types of Anemias," p. 521.) The medication may be given in a single large dose or may be spread out over ten to fourteen days. If symptoms

persist for more than two days after you start taking drugs, see your practitioner again.

Antibiotics often cause diarrhea and vaginal yeast infections. Eating plain yogurt or taking acidophilus in capsules, liquid or granule form helps to prevent this diarrhea by replacing the normal bacteria in your intestines killed by the drugs. See p. 518 for information on preventing and relieving vaginal infections.

For pain with UTIs, there is a prescription drug called Pyridium, a local anesthetic that relieves pain but does not treat the infection itself. It dyes the urine a bright orange, which will permanently stain clothing. Pyridium can cause nausea, dizziness and possibly allergic reactions. Self-help remedies are probably better.

Have a follow-up urine exam when you finish taking the drugs (a culture if you have repeated UTIs) to be certain the organism is gone.

Sometimes chronic cystitis will involve the Skene's glands (at the opening of the urethra). In such cases you may think you are cured, then the glands are squeezed (as in intercourse, for example) and release some pus, which starts the cystitis symptoms all over again. Sometimes the Skene's glands are removed (meatotomy) to solve this problem, though specialists disagree about the need for this operation. (Recovery takes about a month.)

Your practitioner may recommend other surgical procedures, such as stretching the urethral opening and/or making a slit in the urethra to help drainage (internal urethrotomy). Ask for documentation of their effectiveness. Surgery is often recommended to correct a prolapsed bladder or urethra, which can be connected with chronic urinary tract infections. Kegel exercises (see p. 333) can avoid the need for this surgery and help prevent future infections.

Even with drugs and/or surgery, many women continue to have recurrent urinary tract infections. Sometimes these treatments just don't work—especially over the long term. It especially helps to address the factors (such as diet, stress and lowered resistance) which make us vulnerable to repeated infections.

UTERUS AND OVARIES
Abnormal Uterine Bleeding

Abnormal uterine bleeding is a term used to describe a variety of unusual bleeding patterns. We may have unusually light or very heavy periods, bleeding or spotting between periods, cycles that vary widely in length. Abnormal bleeding is frequently due to hormonal changes and is most common in teenagers just beginning to menstruate or women just entering menopause. Many women in their thirties experience light spotting at the time of ovulation, due to the sudden drop in estrogen. Doctors use a particular term, "dysfunctional uterine bleeding," to describe abnormal bleeding due to a menstrual cycle in which ovu-

---

*Wash the area carefully, urinate a little, then collect the rest of your urine in a sterile jar.

†Some women who have cystitis symptoms without the presence of bacteria in the urine have interstitial cystitis, a frequently misdiagnosed and mistreated disorder. See *Ms* magazine, June 1983, p. 101, or contact the collective.

lation did not occur—an anovulatory cycle. Women who don't ovulate regularly may have late periods and very heavy bleeding due to a build-up of estrogen. Other possible causes of prolonged, heavy or irregular bleeding include the IUD, birth control pills, pelvic inflammatory disease, ectopic pregnancy, polyps, fibroids, endometriosis and cervical or uterine cancer. (See the sections on each of these conditions for information on their treatments.)

In postmenopausal women, abnormal bleeding may be caused by estrogen replacement therapy, vaginitis or overgrowth of the endometrial tissues (endometrial hyperplasia), or cancer.

Sometimes, even after extensive testing, no clear-cut reason for bleeding is found.

Self-Help Treatments

If you are premenopausal, you may be able to stabilize your menstrual flow by reducing stress and changing your diet. Cutting down on animal fat and adding fiber helps to restore normal hormonal balance by lowering cholesterol (which is converted to estrogen in your body). In addition, supplements of Vitamin A, E and C with bioflavinoids, as well as zinc, copper and iodine, can help regulate heavy bleeding. Consult a wholistic nutritionist, if available, to advise you on dosage. Acupuncture can also help to restore hormonal balance. If you are bleeding heavily, increase your iron intake to prevent anemia (see p. 521).

Medical Treatments

If you are premenopausal and having light, irregular bleeding, your practitioner may suggest waiting a month or two to see if your system rights itself. (Sometimes stress can contribute to hormonal imbalances.) If abnormal bleeding persists, however, and diagnostic tests indicate a hormonal disturbance and/or anovulatory cycles, most practitioners recommend hormone treatments (usually combination birth control pills or intermittent Provera) to help restore normal menstrual cycles. If you want to avoid taking hormones and the bleeding isn't too heavy, you may want to continue self-help measures while observing the amount of bleeding carefully. If you do choose hormone therapy, find a physician who has skill and experience in it, as mistakes in dosage, duration or estrogen/progesterone balance can lead to an unnecessary D and C or even a hysterectomy. If you are ovulating and the bleeding is related to the post-ovulation phase of your cycle (see the discussion of menstruation in "Stages in the Reproductive Cycle," p. 209) or if you are anovulatory and wish to become pregnant, you may consider taking Clomid, a powerful fertility drug that stimulates ovulation. Clomid is associated with certain risks, such as the formation of multiple ovarian cysts.

Pelvic Relaxation and Uterine Prolapse

Pelvic relaxation is a condition in which the muscles of the pelvic floor become slack and no longer adequately support the pelvic organs. In severe cases, the ligaments and tissues which hold the uterus in place may also weaken enough to allow the uterus to "fall" or "prolapse" into the vagina. Women sometimes experience pelvic relaxation and/or uterine prolapse after one or more very difficult births, but the tendency can also be inherited. Uterine prolapse is often accompanied by a falling of the bladder (cystocele) and rectum (rectocele) as well.

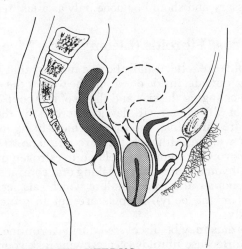

PROLAPSED UTERUS   *Christine Bondante*

Often the first sign of pelvic relaxation is a tendency to leak urine when you cough or sneeze or laugh suddenly. If your uterus has fallen into your vagina you may have a dull, heavy sensation in your vagina or feel like something is "falling out." These symptoms are usually worse after standing for long periods.

Prevention and Self-Help Treatments

The best way to prevent pelvic relaxation and uterine prolapse is to do regular Kegel exercises and leg lifts which strengthen the muscles of the pelvic floor and lower abdomen (see Chapter 19, "Childbirth"). One way of determining whether your pelvic muscles are in good shape is to try starting and stopping the flow of urine when you go to the bathroom. If you can't stop the flow, you need to do more Kegels. Some practitioners recommend doing up to a hundred a day, especially during pregnancy when the pelvic muscles are under particular stress. You may also strengthen a slightly prolapsed uterus by relaxing in the knee-chest position (kneeling with your chest on the floor and your bottom in the air) several times a day. Some women find that certain yoga positions, such as the shoulder and head stands, relieve discomfort from a prolapsed uterus.

Medical Treatments

Medical intervention is usually not necessary for pelvic relaxation or even mild uterine prolapse. If the prolapse is severe enough to cause discomfort, you can have a pessary (a rubber device which fits around the cervix and helps to prop up the uterus) inserted. The disadvantages include difficulty in obtaining a proper fit, possible irritation or infection and the need to remove and clean the pessary frequently. A surgical procedure called a "suspension operation" can lift and reattach a descended uterus, and often a fallen bladder or rectum as well. Many physicians recommend hysterectomy for prolapsed uterus but it is frequently unnecessary and should be done only as a last resort.

Uterine Fibroids (Lieomyomas, Myomas)

Fibroids are solid, usually benign tumors* that appear on the outside, inside or within the wall of the uterus, often changing the size and shape of it. About 20 percent of all women will develop fibroids by the time they are thirty-five, and they are more likely to affect black women. Although they are of unknown cause, these growths seem to be related to estrogen production: if you are pregnant or taking oral contraceptives or menopausal estrogens (all of which raise estrogen levels in the body), fibroids are apt to grow more quickly.

Fibroids may be discovered during a routine pelvic exam. Because fibroids keep growing, ask your practitioner how many you have and how big they are. If they have grown no further when you have a second exam six months later, a yearly checkup will be sufficient.

Small fibroids are usually symptom-free. However, very large or numerous fibroids may cause pain, bleeding between periods or excessive menstrual flow. (Since they usually do not cause abnormal bleeding, if you do have fibroids and abnormal bleeding, be sure to be carefully checked for other causes.) Depending on their size and location, fibroids can also cause abdominal or back pain and urinary problems. Large fibroids can make it difficult to conceive or to sustain a full-term pregnancy.

Self-Help Treatments

You may be able to reduce large fibroids by eliminating your intake of synthetic estrogen (found in birth control pills) and stopping estrogen therapy (ERT). Yoga exercises may ease feelings of heaviness and pressure. If your fibroids cause heavy bleeding, see the

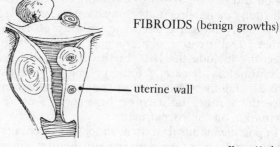

FIBROIDS (benign growths)

uterine wall

Karen Norberg

nutritional therapy section in "Abnormal Uterine Bleeding" (p. 508). Visualization techniques may be helpful in dealing with fibroids.

Medical Treatments

In many cases no treatment is necessary, but if you have excessive bleeding, pain, urinary difficulties or problems with pregnancy, you may want to have the fibroids removed. *Very* occasionally this can be done during a D and C, but usually a myomectomy (which removes fibroids and leaves the uterus intact) is necessary.* This is major surgery with a higher complication rate than hysterectomy. Myomectomy may cause internal scarring, which can lead to painful intercourse, backaches and abnormal uterine bleeding. If you are pregnant, myomectomy can cause miscarriage. In approximately 10 percent of cases, the fibroids will return.

Many physicians recommend hysterectomy as a treatment for fibroids in women who are past childbearing age or who do not want more children. This surgery may be unnecessary, particularly for women nearing menopause, when the natural decline in estrogen levels usually shrinks fibroids. Alternative treatments include radiation and birth control pills, but these are considered controversial and can cause serious complications. If your doctor suggests any of these treatments, be sure to get a second opinion.

If you have suspicious bleeding or menstrual flow that seems irregular it may be caused by endometrial polyps. A health practitioner very often will discover a polyp during a regularly scheduled examination. A D and C may be done to remove polyps, and further tests may be suggested to insure that the specimen is not malignant. Sometimes polyps can be removed in the doctor's office. (They are almost never malignant.)

---

*The word "tumor" is very scary to most of us. It is part of an older language of illness that was used by many of our grandparents, both patients and doctors, to disguise the mention of cancer. Actually, tumors are growths of cells which serve no purpose. Over 90 percent of all tumors are benign and harmless.

*A new technique, called "hysteroscopic resection," in which the fibroid is shaved off, is reportedly safer and has fewer complications than myomectomy. It is experimental, however, and should be done only by an experienced endoscopist. Before having this procedure, you will have to sign an experimental consent form. (See "Our Rights as Patients," p. 584.)

Ovarian Cysts

Ovarian cysts are relatively common and often don't cause any symptoms or discomfort. A cyst usually develops when a follicle has grown large—as one or more do every month during ovulation—but has failed to rupture and release an egg. Most of these cysts fill with fluid; others become solid, usually benign tumors. Cysts may be accompanied by symptoms such as a disturbance in the normal menstrual cycle, an unfamiliar pain or discomfort in your lower abdomen at any point during the cycle, pain during intercourse and unexplained abdominal swelling. Found by a routine bimanual pelvic exam, cysts usually disappear by themselves, though some types may have to be removed.

To determine whether a cyst requires treatment, wait a cycle or two for it to disappear. If it persists, a practitioner may use ultrasound, X-ray, culdoscopy or laparoscopy to learn about the cyst. A tissue sample will reveal if it is benign or malignant. Practitioners disagree about the necessity of removing benign cysts, though most agree that cysts remaining after suppression with oral contraceptives should be treated.

If your physician advises removal of the ovary along with the benign cyst, get a second opinion. This conventional practice is, in many cases, unnecessary. Ovaries perform many functions, even after menopause.

Recurrent cysts may indicate a hormonal imbalance or life stresses. Changing your diet, learning how to reduce stress, and acupuncture may also help to get your system back in balance.

HYSTERECTOMY AND OOPHORECTOMY

Of all adult women today, 62 percent will have had a hysterectomy (removal of the uterus) or oophorectomy (removal of the ovaries) by the time they are seventy. The operations are frequently done together, with oophorectomy done routinely as "part" of hysterectomy, when in fact it is often not necessary.* Today, the vast majority of hysterectomies and oophorectomies are elective—that is, performed by choice and not as an emergency or lifesaving procedure.† Several careful

*Some women do not know whether they have had their ovaries removed. Others agreed to the removal without realizing that it is an *elective* procedure or without realizing the disadvantages. If you are uncertain about the extent of your surgery, obtain a copy of your medical record from the hospital. Also *write* to your surgeon (keeping a copy of your letter) and ask for a reply in writing.

†The elective nature of many hysterectomies is highlighted by the fact that different groups of women have different rates of hysterectomy. The U.S. has twice the rate of England and Sweden. Doctors' wives, for example, have more hysterectomies proportionately than any other group. Traditionally, women of color have had twice as many hysterectomies as white women (often a form of sterilization abuse, also a problem for poor white women [see p. 256]); recently the rate for young white women

studies have shown that at least 30 to 50 percent of these operations are clearly unnecessary and another 10 percent or more can probably be avoided by using alternative therapy.* The incidence of this surgery rose by 25 percent between 1971 and 1975, dropping off at the 1971 level by 1980. But the rise was fastest for younger women: between 1970 and 1978, 3.5 million women under forty-five had hysterectomies.† In 1980, half of the 649,000 hysterectomies were done on women under forty-five, and half of those included oophorectomies. Every woman faces the possibility that these procedures will be recommended.

Both procedures are considered major surgery; we are only beginning to understand their long-term effects on our health, sexuality and life expectancy. Certainly, they have saved lives and restored health for many women. But they also involve significant risks—both immediate and long-term—that we need to be aware of. There is now tremendous controversy over hysterectomy and oophorectomy within the medical profession and the women's community as the rates of unnecessary procedures and the risks become more widely publicized.

Why are so many women having so many more hysterectomies and oophorectomies? More are being done for conditions that would not have "required" surgery ten years ago. Too often surgeons recommend them (and women agree to them) as an easy solution to routine gynecological problems, a way of preventing cancer and a permanent method of birth control. A growing number of gynecologists also recommend the procedure for sterilization ("hysterilization"). Dr. Ralph C. Wright, a Connecticut gynecologist and perhaps the most outspoken advocate of routine hysterectomy, gives another and more dangerous argument:

>...The uterus has but one function: reproduction. After the last planned pregnancy, the uterus becomes a useless, bleeding, symptom-producing, potentially cancer bearing organ and therefore should be removed. If, in addition, both ovaries are removed...another common source of inoperable malignancy is eliminated.‡

Physicians frequently attribute the sudden spurt of pelvic surgery to the apparent increase in endometriosis, uterine bleeding, pelvic infections and endometrial cancer. (Ironically, the increased use of estrogen replacement therapy [ERT] may have partially caused the increased rate of endometrial can-

has risen sharply. The highest rate of hysterectomies is found in the South and West, where gynecologist-surgeons tend to cluster in large numbers.

*See S. Ruzek in Resources for Chapter 24, "The Politics of Women and Medical Care." See also p. 512, "When Is Hysterectomy Necessary?" and p. 512 on indications for oophorectomy.

†See C. Easterday, et al., and N. Lauerson in Resources. (The latter is listed in General Resources.)

‡For more information on Dr. Wright's article, see Resources. The removal of ovaries as a form of cancer prevention is a particularly spurious argument, since ovarian cancer is rare.

When Is Hysterectomy Necessary?

A number of life-threatening conditions require hysterectomy, including:

1. invasive cancer of the uterus, cervix, vagina, fallopian tubes and/or ovaries (8 to 12 percent of hysterectomies are performed to treat cancer);

2. severe, uncontrollable infection (PID);

3. severe, uncontrollable bleeding;

4. life-threatening blockage of the bladder or intestines by the uterus or growth in the uterus;

5. sudden dropping (prolapse) of the uterus out of the vagina;

6. conditions associated with rare but serious complications during childbirth, including rupture of the uterus.

If you have any of these conditions, hysterectomy may not only save your life but free you from significant pain and discomfort.

Some conditions which are not life-threatening but may justify hysterectomy include:

1. precancerous changes of the endometrium (hyperplasia);

2. severe, recurring pelvic infections (see the sections on STDs and IUDs in Chapter 13, "Birth Control");

3. extensive endometriosis, causing debilitating pain and/or involving other organs;

4. fibroid tumors which are extensive, large, involve other organs or cause debilitating bleeding;

5. pelvic relaxation (uterine prolapse).

Depending on their severity, many of these conditions can be treated without resorting to major surgery.* Fortunately, new diagnostic techniques, such as sonography, Pap smears and laparoscopy, make it possible to avoid or delay many hysterectomies that might have been done in the past. Unfortunately, most surgeons do not make frequent enough use of such techniques, believing that there is no advantage to saving a uterus, especially if a woman is past her child-bearing years.

Hysterectomies are frequently performed unnecessarily for the following reasons:

1. small fibroids which are not causing problems;

2. abortion (during the first and second trimesters);

3. sterilization;

4. cervicitis;

5. mild dysfunctional uterine bleeding;

6. pelvic congestion (menstrual irregularities and low back pain).

These problems can usually be treated with cheaper and safer alternative therapies. If your doctor insists on hysterectomy for one of these, consider changing physicians.

---

cer—and also unmanageable fibroids which indicate hysterectomy.) The surgery increase may also be connected with the increased availability of health care via more health insurance and more federal monies going into the medical system. In some cases, poorer women are now more able to get needed (or needless) surgery.

Ob/gyns and surgeons have powerful economic incentives to perform hysterectomies and oophorectomies. They are more profitable than less complicated, often less dangerous procedures, and provide a source of income to compensate for the declining birth rate and resulting loss of obstetrical fees. Surgeons' fees and hospital fees for the procedures are expensive—the average cost of a hysterectomy varies from 3,000 to 6,000 dollars (approximately five times the cost of a tubal ligation). Health care analysts believe it is no accident that hysterectomies occur far less frequently under prepaid insurance plans (such as HMOs) than under indemnity plans such as Blue Shield. Most hysterectomies and oophorectomies are performed as part of a private practice, where the surgeon and woman alone make decisions, often consulting no other physician.* Why are women willing to risk their lives in surgery? What factors should they consider?

*See Diana Scully's study of ob/gyn training, "Men Who Control Women's Health: The Mis-Education of Obstetrician-Gyne-

Risks and Complications of Hysterectomy and Oophorectomy

Surgeons recommending hysterectomy seldom tell us that the rate of death from hysterectomy is fairly high, between one and two women in 1,000;† that as a sterilization method, hysterectomy has ten to twenty times the complication rate of tubal ligation with its contraceptive failure rate of 1 to 2.2 percent. Women unknowingly play an enormous gambling game, assuming that we will not suffer from complications of anesthesia or surgery or from serious aftereffects.

Forty to 50 percent of all women who have hysterectomies have surgical complications, including:

1. *Infection.* Most can be treated successfully with antibiotics, but some infections can be severe or even uncontrollable and may result in death. Many surgeons now order antibiotics routinely before surgery.

2. *Urinary tract complications.* Almost half of the women who have hysterectomies will have a kidney

cologists," for an important analysis of how these decisions are made. (This study is listed in Resources for Chapter 24, "The Politics of Women and Medical Care.")

*See individual sections for alternative treatment, also Lauersen's *Listen to Your Body.*

†This works out to between 600 and 1,200 women annually, some of whose hysterectomies were unnecessary. (See C. Easterday, et al., in Resources.)

or bladder infection following surgery. In most cases the problem is not serious, but sometimes additional surgery is necessary. In radical hysterectomy, sensory nerves may be cut (sometimes unnecessarily) and women can lose both the sensation of having to urinate and control over bladder functions.*

3. *Hemorrhage.* More than one in ten women require transfusions, some due to undetected preexisting anemia.

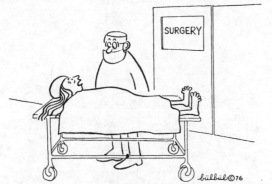

I hope you can justify this hysterectomy to my women's health group.

Less common surgical complications include:

1. *Bowel problems,* which can occur if there is damage to the intestines during surgery; 2 percent of all women who have a hysterectomy need further surgery to remove scar tissue from the bowel.

2. *Blood clots,* which are rare but always dangerous because of the possibility of the clot traveling to the lungs or brain, which can be fatal.

3. *Death or paralysis from anesthesia.*

4. *Postsurgical complications* can include abnormal bleeding, postsurgical infection, improper healing that can cause narrowing of the vagina and heavy discharge.

Long-Term Risks

One recent study suggests that if you are premenopausal at the time of hysterectomy, you have a three times greater risk of later developing coronary heart disease. (The risk appears to be the same whether or not your ovaries are removed.) According to this study there are more deaths from coronary heart disease following hysterectomy than deaths from uterine cancer.†

Even if your ovaries are *not* removed, there is a slight chance of sudden or premature menopause.‡ Most

*Injury to the ureters or urinary tract occurs in 2 to 5 percent of every 1,000 cases. (See C. Easterday et al., in Resources.)

†See B. Centerwall in Resources.

‡This is usually due to the decreased supply of blood to the ovaries, which causes them to lose their ability to produce hormones—either immediately or over a period of time. (See K. Knutsen, also N. Newton and E. Baron, in Resources.)

physicians assure us that we can avoid these risks and symptoms by taking oral estrogen therapy (ERT), which has its own risks. (See the sections on ERT, p. 447, and menopause, p. 443.)

Hormonal responses vary from one woman to the next, for reasons not yet established. Some women suffer severe hot flashes and lack of lubrication. Others are more fortunate.

After my hysterectomy-oophorectomy, I went home with my prescription for estrogen to await the worst. I started to read a lot about ERT being harmful to women. The reasons for not taking ERT seemed to be a lot stronger than my fears of menopause, so I quit the program cold turkey. Lubrication was a problem at first after discontinuing the estrogen. We kept the tube of K-Y Jelly on the night table. My own glands took over and lubrication is rarely a problem now.

Some women continue on ERT while still others may wish to follow the more gradual reduction suggested by Susanne Morgan (see Resources; see also "Vaginal Changes," p. 451).

Hysterectomy, Oophorectomy and Sexuality

Many women are concerned about the effect that hysterectomy with or without oophorectomy will have on sexual response. Physicians and popular literature tend to be blandly reassuring and state that any sexual difficulties we may experience are "all in our heads." Only recently has the physiological basis of women's sexuality begun to be understood. In fact, from 33 to 46 percent of women have difficulty becoming aroused and reaching orgasm after this surgery.* Moreover, we now know why these changes occur.

First, many women experience orgasm primarily when the penis or a lover's fingers push against the cervix and uterus, causing uterine contractions and increased stimulation of the abdominal lining (peritoneum). Without the uterus or cervix, there may be much less of this kind of sensation.

Second, if the ovaries are removed, ovarian *androgens* which affect sexuality may be greatly reduced, thus lowering sexual response. *These hormones cannot be replaced by ERT.*† Even when the ovaries are not removed, this hormonal change may occur because the surgery may interfere with the blood supply.

I had a hysterectomy two years ago at the age of forty-five. I went from being fully aroused and fully orgasmic to having a complete loss of libido, sexual enjoyment and

*L. Zussman, S. Zussman, R. Sunley and E. Bjornson. "Sexual Response after Hysterectomy-Oophorectomy: Recent Studies and Reconsideration of Psychogenesis," *American Journal of Obstetrics and Gynecology,* Vol. 40, No. 7 (August 1, 1981), pp. 725–29.

†For replacement options, see below.

Hysterectomy Procedures

These are the common procedures for hysterectomy. Rather than simply accepting the *name* of the procedure your surgeon proposes, ask for a complete description with diagram.

- *Total hysterectomy*, sometimes called *complete hysterectomy*. The surgeon removes the uterus and cervix, leaving the fallopian tubes and ovaries. You will continue to ovulate but will no longer have menstrual periods; instead the egg is absorbed by the body into the pelvic cavity.

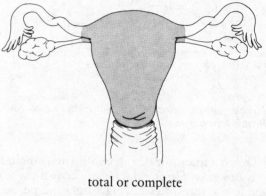

supracervical

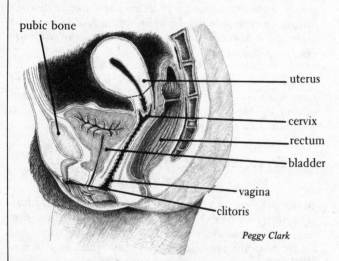

Peggy Clark

PARTIAL HYSTERECTOMY (*uterus tipped to show line of surgical incision; ovary hidden*). *After surgery the cervix and the stump of the uterus remain, requiring regular Pap tests.*

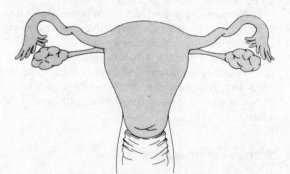

total or complete

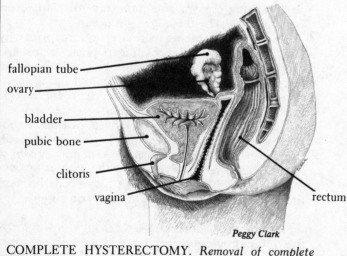

Peggy Clark

COMPLETE HYSTERECTOMY. *Removal of complete uterus, including cervix (ovaries and tubes are attached to top of vagina).*

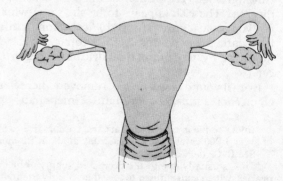

total with bilateral salpingo-oophorectomy

radical   *Christine Bondante*

514

● *Total hysterectomy with bilateral salpingo-oophorectomy*. The surgeon removes the uterus, cervix, fallopian tubes (*salpingo*) and both ovaries (*oophor*).* "Bilateral" means both sides, though sometimes one ovary may be left if it is not diseased. In rare cases (usually to treat widespread cancer), the surgeon will remove the upper part of the vagina and perhaps lymph nodes in the pelvic area. This is sometimes called *radical hysterectomy*.

Abdominal vs. Vaginal Hysterectomy

Removal of your uterus can be done either through an abdominal incision or through the vagina. The surgeon will have to recommend an abdominal incision if your ovaries are to be removed, if there is a large tumor in your uterus or if you have chronic pelvic disease. (Surgeons usually prefer an abdominal approach because it enables them to see the pelvic cavity more completely. However, in an abdominal hysterectomy they are more likely to remove healthy ovaries because they are more accessible.) The incision is made either horizontally across the top pubic hairline (called a "bikini" incision) or vertically between the navel and pubic hairline. Vertical incisions (across the grain of the muscle) tend to heal more slowly. Discuss with your doctor whether you can avoid one.

Vaginal hysterectomy, useful in cases of prolapsed uterus (when the uterus bulges into the vagina; see p. 512) and for a number of other conditions, has the advantage of a shorter recovery period and faster healing. In addition, because the incision is made inside the vagina, you will have no visible scar. However, since vaginal hysterectomies are performed less frequently and require greater skill, it is important to find a surgeon who does this procedure regularly. Mistakes during surgery can result in permanent urinary tract difficulties. Other disadvantages include a possible shortening of the vagina which can result in painful intercourse afterwards, and possible temporary severe back pain as a result of being placed in a lithotomy position (head down, bottom up) during surgery.

A new, large and well-researched study by the Centers for Disease Control suggests that the 50 percent complication rate of abdominal hysterectomy may be anywhere from two to four times higher than that of vaginal hysterectomy. The exception: women who have had previous Ce-

sareans have a nearly 65 percent complication rate after vaginal hysterectomy.

Oophorectomy: Reasons and Risks

Oophorectomy means removal of the ovary—either one (unilateral) or both (bilateral); the fallopian tube(s) may be removed as well. When both ovaries are removed, a hysterectomy is usually performed at the same time. Common reasons for oophorectomy include ectopic pregnancy, endometriosis, benign or malignant tumors or cysts on the ovary and pelvic inflammatory disease.* An enlarged postmenopausal ovary may be cancerous and urgently requires a checkup.

If only one ovary is removed and not your uterus, you will continue to be fertile and have menstrual periods. If both ovaries are removed, however, you will experience surgical menopause. Even if one or both ovaries are retained, you may experience symptoms of hormonal loss because of loss of blood supply to the ovaries.

Many surgeons routinely remove the ovaries of women during hysterectomy, whether or not the ovaries are diseased,† if the woman is past forty-five or so. For decades, this practice has been one of the most controversial in gynecology. Those in favor argue that oophorectomy prevents the possibility of future ovarian cancer, which strikes one in 100 women over forty and has a cure rate of only 10 to 20 percent. On the other side, studies show that the actual risk of developing ovarian cancer following hysterectomy is very small (about one in 1,000). Other physicians think the cancer risk is insignificant compared to the risks involved in losing ovarian function: circulatory disease, premature osteoporosis and sudden menopause, all of which raise the difficult question of ERT. (See the sections on ERT, p. 447, and menopause, p. 443.)

Oophorectomy affects the hormonal balance of both postmenopausal and premenopausal women, since the ovaries usually continue to produce significant amounts of hormones after menopause. (See p. 512, "Risks and Complications of Hysterectomy and Oophorectomy.")

---

*See P. Braun and K. Knutsen in Resources. Rarely, ovaries were removed in cases of cancer of the uterus, breast, cervix or abdominal cavity because ovarian secretions are known to increase the chances of developing recurrent cancer in these areas. This strategy is now outmoded and has been replaced by chemotherapy. (See the section on cancer.)

†The terms "diseased" and "healthy" are frequently used carelessly by surgeons when referring to ovaries. Given the rarity of ovarian cancer, ask carefully in advance whether an ovary with a cyst or mild fibrous involvement would be removed as "diseased."

---

*Very occasionally a physician will leave the cervix, but because this procedure carries the risk of infection or cancer in the cervix, it is considered largely outmoded.

orgasms immediately after the surgery. I went to doctors, all of whom denied ever having seen a woman with this problem before and told me it was psychological. Before surgery my husband and I were having intercourse aproximately three to five times a week, simply because we have an open and loving relationship. Now I find that I have to work at becoming at all interested in intercourse. And I no longer have the orgasm that comes from pressure on the cervix, though I still have a feeble orgasm from clitoral stimulation.

Third, vaginal lubrication tends to lessen after oophorectomy.

Fourth, local effects of surgery may occasionally cause problems. If your vagina has been shortened (see the section on vaginal hysterectomy, p. 515), intercourse may be uncomfortable. Scar tissue in the pelvis or at the top of the vagina from either the vaginal or abdominal procedure can also cause painful intercourse.

Some of us will find sex unchanged or more enjoyable after hysterectomy. In the words of a woman who had a hysterectomy because of huge fibroids:

I had terrible cramps all my life and genuine feelings of utter depression during my periods. My ovaries were not removed and my libido was not affected. My sexual response, if anything, improved. I also had for the first time no fear of unwanted pregnancy and more general good health.

Sex may be better when the operation helps to relieve a painful condition such as infection, endometriosis or heavy bleeding.

Many women do experience genuine loss of sexual desire or response or both, so you must weigh the benefits of surgery against the sexual risk which is *not* "all in the head" and cannot necessarily be predicted in advance.

One self-help group (at the Elizabeth Blackwell Women's Health Center in Philadelphia) exchanged information about what increased their desire and ability to orgasm. Their suggestions included:

- More strong and deliberate "turning on" by themselves or their partner, through humanely erotic (not pornographic) reading, pictures, films; through verbal lovemaking; through massage, "sexy" clothing, candlelight, change of location or partners or techniques, dancing, (play) wrestling and activities which physically move the pelvic area.
- More effort in intercourse to push the penis hard against the far end of the vagina in order to stimulate the peritoneum. Deep penetration is helped by the female-astride position or the man-on-top position with the woman's legs on the man's shoulders and pillows under her hips.
- Use of coconut oil or K-Y Jelly to lubricate the clitoris and vagina.

- More experimentation with oral sex or delicate manipulation of the clitoris.
- Learning to use penetration with fingers first (gentle internal stimulation to prepare for intercourse with a penis); this helps lubrication occur more rapidly.
- Relearning a new pace for lovemaking, moving more slowly, respecting the fact that arousal may take longer.
- Trying the testosterone pellet (see below) to restore the ability to become aroused.

Androgen replacement therapy is at least partially effective in restoring sexual response. When testosterone (one of the androgens) is administered orally or through injection in a dosage sufficient to restore libido, "masculinizing" effects may occur, such as lowered voice, acne and facial hair. However, another way of administering testosterone, with greatly lowered side effects, is through a small slow-release pellet inserted under the skin in the hip region by a simple office procedure every six months.* This procedure is quite readily available to British women, but American women have difficulty finding a physician familiar with it. One woman who has received this kind of therapy says:

In the last week we've made love oftener than in the past two months. It's a great feeling! We've giggled and rolled on the floor like a couple of kids. Previously, I'd shied away from any physical contact that would end up in bed. My body is much more sensitive, though I don't have the same deep internal orgasms as before. Sometimes I think if I'd had the help of hormones a few years ago, I'd never have appreciated the feelings I have now. I know there will still be times when I am depressed and longing for the deep orgasms I once had, but I'll be able to remember the three years when I had no feelings at all and it won't seem bad.

We have our doubts regarding *any* hormone therapy. Keep looking for new information about them.

Even if you were prepared for hysterectomy and did not expect to feel depressed, you may cry frequently and unexpectedly in the first few days or weeks after surgery. This may be due to sudden hormonal changes. Many women are upset. Losing any part of ourselves, especially a part that is so uniquely feminine, is bound to have an impact. You may feel robbed. If you are premenopausal you may bitterly resent the fact that you cannot have children. Acknowledging feelings of anger and grief after losing a part of yourself or losing some of your sexual responsiveness is an important part of the recovery process.

---

*Margaret H. Thom and J.W. Studd. "Hormone Implantation,"*British Medical Journal*, March 22, 1980, p. 848; also, Thom and Studd, "Ovarian Failure and Ageing," *Clinics in Endocrinology and Metabolism*, Vol. 10, No. 1 (March 1981), p. 105. The latter article has a long and useful bibliography.

Thousands of women like me must confront the depression that comes with the loss of their sex lives and the anger they feel when they finally find out that this loss was a side effect of surgery that may have been unnecessary to begin with.

We or our caregivers may or may not recognize post-hysterectomy depression promptly. Many gynecologists recommend psychiatric help and prescribe tranquilizers (or other habit-forming drugs) but almost never encourage treatment of underlying physical or sexual conditions caused by the surgery.* Tranquilizers taken together with estrogen therapy may produce negative effects, yet many physicians routinely prescribe both.

If you are depressed, try to find a women's support group where you can talk about your feelings in a supportive atmosphere. If you can't find a group through a local women's health center, consider starting a postsurgery group of your own. (For information on support groups you can contact, see Resources.)

Some women feel only relief following hysterectomy or hysterectomy/oophorectomy, especially when the operation eliminates a serious health problem or chronic, disabling pain.

For information on recovering after these operations, see Susanne Morgan's book (particularly the chapter entitled "After Surgery"). (See Resources.)

Self-Help: Recovering from a Hysterectomy or Oophorectomy

After a hysterectomy you may be in the hospital for five to seven days, depending on the kind of procedure and the amount of anesthesia you had. For the first day or two you will probably have an IV and a catheter inserted. You will usually be given medication for pain and nausea. Within a day you will be on your feet and encouraged to do exercises to get your circulation and breathing back to normal. You may also be told to cough frequently (to clear your lungs). (Holding a pillow over an abdominal incision or crossing your legs if you had a vaginal incision will help to reduce pain.) When your bowels become active again (usually on the second day) you may also have gas pains to contend with. Walking, holding onto a pillow and rolling from side to side in bed and slow deep-breathing exercises will help. By the third or fourth day you can begin to have light solid foods as well as fluids.

After you go home, you will have light vaginal bleeding or oozing that gradually tapers off. You may also have hot flashes caused by estrogen loss. (Even if your ovaries were not removed, estrogen may be lost due

*Despite publication of the 1981 study by Zussman, et al. (see the footnote on p. 513), many surgeons continue to believe that all posthysterectomy problems are psychological/emotional in origin. Medical school texts and courses remain similarly unaffected.

to the disruption of blood flow to the ovaries during surgery.) You will probably continue to have some pain as well which pain-killers may not relieve entirely. Consult your practitioner if you have excessive pain accompanied by fever or discharge, as this may signal an infection.

Try to arrange for someone to take care of you for the first few days. For at least the first few weeks, ask family and friends for help with household chores and children.

Your practitioner may tell you to avoid tub baths, douches, driving, climbing or lifting heavy things for several weeks. If you have to drive or have small children at home who need to be carried, ask for suggestions as to how to do these tasks safely. Most practitioners also recommend waiting six to eight weeks before resuming intercourse and/or active sports. Some women return to these activities much earlier. Start with light exercise (such as walking) and gradually build up to your old routines. Visualizing yourself as healthy and active can speed the recovery process. Full recovery generally takes four to six weeks, but some women feel tired for as long as six months or even a year after surgery.

VAGINA AND VULVA
Vaginal Infections (Vaginitis)

All women secrete moisture and mucus from membranes which line the vagina. This discharge is clear or slightly milky and may be somewhat slippery. When dry, it may be yellowish. When a woman is sexually aroused this secretion increases. It normally causes no irritation or inflammation of the vagina or vulva. If you want to examine your own discharge, collect a sample from inside your vagina—with a washed finger, of course—and smear it on glass.

Many bacteria grow in the vagina of a normal, healthy woman. Some of them help to keep the vagina somewhat acid, which keeps yeast, fungi and other harmful organisms from multiplying out of proportion. These harmful organisms may secrete wastes which, in large amounts, irritate the vaginal walls and cause infections. At such times there may be an abnormal discharge, mild or severe itching and burning of the vulva, chafing of the thighs and, occasionally, frequent urination.

Some of the reasons for vaginal infections are a general lowered resistance (from stress, lack of sleep, bad diet, other infections in our bodies); too much douching; pregnancy; taking birth control pills, other hormones or antibiotics; diabetes or a prediabetic condition; cuts, abrasions and other irritations in the vagina (from childbirth, intercourse without enough lubrication, tampons or using an instrument in the vagina medically or for masturbation). Postmenopausal women are particularly susceptible. We can also get many of these infections during sex with a partner who has them (see Chapter 14, "Sexually Transmitted Diseases").

Prevention

1. Wash your vulva and anus regularly. Pat your vulva dry after bathing and try to keep it dry. Also, don't use other people's towels or washcloths. Avoid irritating sprays* and soaps (use special nonsoap cleansers for skin very sensitive to plain soap). Avoid talcum powder.†

2. Wear clean cotton underpants. Avoid nylon underwear and pantyhose since they retain moisture and heat, which help harmful bacteria to grow faster.

3. Avoid pants that are tight in the crotch and thighs.

4. Always wipe your anus from front to back (so that bacteria from the anus won't get into the vagina or urethra).

5. Make sure your sexual partners are clean. It is a good practice for a man to wash his penis daily, and especially before making love. Using a condom can provide added protection. If you or your male partner are being treated for a genital infection, make sure he wears a condom during intercourse. Better yet, avoid intercourse until the infection is cleared up.

6. Use a sterile, water-soluble jelly if lubrication is needed during intercourse (something like K-Y Jelly, for example, *not* Vaseline). Also, recent studies show that birth control jellies slow down the growth of trichomonads and possibly monilia. Using these jellies for lubrication and/or general prevention is a good idea, especially with a new partner you may not know very well.

7. Avoid sexual intercourse that is painful or abrasive to your vagina.

8. Cut down on coffee, alcohol, sugar and refined carbohydrates (diets high in sugars can radically change the normal pH of the vagina).

9. Applying unpasteurized plain yogurt (those containing lactobacilli) in the vagina replenishes "good" bacteria normally found in the vagina and often destroyed when we take antibiotics, and helps to prevent infections and cure mild symptoms.

10. If you are prone to vaginal infections, douching occasionally with plain water, a solution of one or two tablespoons of vinegar in one quart of warm water (mildly acidic) or a solution of baking soda and water may help prevent vaginal infections. Remember to douche with great caution (see below). You can also make your own boric acid vaginal suppositories (see below) and use one weekly as a preventive.

11. Take care of yourself. Not eating well nor resting enough makes you more susceptible to infection. Continue most of these practices even after you get an infection.

Medical vs. Alternative Treatments

The usual treatment for vaginitis is some form of antibiotic or sulfa drug, which kills infection-causing bacteria. In the process, however, these drugs disturb the delicate balance of bacteria in the vagina and may actually encourage some infections (such as those caused by yeast) by altering the vagina's normal acid/alkaline balance. Some of these drugs also have unpleasant or even dangerous side effects.

As an alternative to antibiotics for vaginitis, many women are turning to natural and herbal remedies which help to restore the normal vaginal flora and promote healing. For example, you can use herbs to make soothing douches, poultices or sitz baths. (You should not rely on these remedies, however, if you have a serious STD [see Chapter 14] or an infection that involves your uterus, tubes or ovaries.)

Note: There is no need for douching except as part of a treatment or prevention program. Be careful when douching. Too much pressure can force air or fluid into the uterus and abdominal cavity. Use lukewarm water, never have the bag more than two feet above your hips and never squeeze a bulb-type bag hard. Wait until the air is out of the tubing and the solution is running through before putting the nozzle into your vagina. Never douche if you are pregnant. If you experience vaginal pain and/or fever after douching, contact a practitioner or go to a hospital the same day. Alternatives to douching include inserting poultices or tampons soaked in herbal solutions and sitz baths.*

Yeast Infections (Also Called Candida, Monilia or Fungus)

Candida albicans, a yeast fungus, normally grows in harmless quantities in your rectum and vagina. When your system is out of balance, yeastlike organisms may grow profusely and cause a thick, white discharge which may look like cottage cheese and smell like baking bread. If a woman has a yeast infection when she gives birth, the baby will get yeast in its throat or digestive tract. This is called thrush and is treated orally with nystatin drops or gentian violet.

Candida grows best in a mildly acidic environment. The pH in the the vagina is normally more than mildly acidic (4.0 to 5.0), except when we take birth control

---

*"Feminine hygiene sprays" may irritate or cause an allergic reaction in the skin of the vulva. They are at best unnecessary and often harmful. The FDA has suggested and may soon require that all "feminine hygiene sprays" carry a warning on the label.

†Recent studies indicate that it may cause ovarian cancer. (See Brigham and Women's Hospital Study, reported in *Cancer*, July 15, 1982. See also D.L. Longo and R.C. Young, "Cosmetic Talc and Ovarian Cancer," *Lancet*, Vol. 2 [August 1979], pp. 349–351.)

*For more information on alternative remedies for vaginitis, send for "Home Remedies for Vaginitis," Santa Cruz Women's Health Center, 250 Locust Street, Santa Cruz, CA 95060. Send a stamped, self-addressed envelope and 50¢.

pills or some antibiotics, are pregnant, have diabetes and when we menstruate (when the pH rises to between 5.8 and 6.8, because blood is alkaline). Obviously, we often find ourselves with a vaginal pH favorable to monilia, so preventive measures are especially important.

Once monilia sets in, treatment usually consists of some form of nystatin, e.g., Mycostatin, taken as a suppository. Suppositories have fewer side effects than nystatin taken orally, and they can be used during pregnancy, but they may not be strong enough to cure severe yeast infections. Other methods of treating monilia include various prescription creams and pills.* You can paint the vagina, cervix and vulva with gentian violet. This is bright purple and it stains, so a sanitary pad must be worn. This messy procedure really helps, except in occasional cases when there is a severe reaction to gentian violet.

Self-Help Treatments

Some of us have had success with the following remedies: yogurt douche (daily); goldenseal-myrrh douche (simmer one tablespoon of each in three cups of water, then strain and cool); and garlic suppositories (peel but don't nick a clove of garlic, then wrap in gauze before inserting). Boric acid powder (600 milligrams in size 00 gelatin capsules inserted daily into the vagina for fourteen days) is perhaps the most effective nondrug method for stubborn cases. Yellow dock douche two to three times a week works well. Also, you can acidify your system by drinking eight ounces of unsweetened cranberry juice every day.

For a long time I felt as though I were on a merry-go-round. I would get a yeast infection, take Mycostatin for three weeks, clear up the infection and then find two weeks later that the itching and the thick, white discharge were back. Finally, once while on medication I also douched with Lactinex† and carefully watched my sugar intake. This worked for me and the monilia has not recurred in many months.

Trichomoniasis

Trichomonas vaginalis, or trich, is a one-celled parasite that can be found in both men and women. Many women have trich organisms in their vaginas, though often they are without symptoms. Usually women with

*New treatments include Monistat 7 (in cream or vaginal suppository form) once a night for seven nights (miconazole nitrate 2 percent); clotrimazole (Gyne-Lotrimin), dose: one 100-milligram tablet once a day for seven days, two 200-milligram tablets once a day for three days or three 500-milligram tablets for one day only. All are equally effective. (*Medical World News*, November 22, 1982.)

†This and similar products are sold over the counter and help to produce the lactic acid favorable to growth of the "friendly" bacilli.

trich have a thin, foamy vaginal discharge that is yellowish green or gray in color and has a foul odor. If another infection is present along with trichomoniasis, the discharge may be thicker and whiter. Trich is usually diagnosed by examining vaginal discharge under a microscope. It can also cause a urinary infection. It is most often contracted through intercourse (thus trichomoniasis can be considered an STD) but can also be passed on by moist objects such as towels, bathing suits, underwear, washcloths and toilet seats. Sometimes emotional stress can cause symptoms to flare up or recur.

The usual treatment for trich is oral doses of metronidazole (Flagyl). We think that women should use this drug with great caution, as metronidazole has caused gene mutations, birth defects and cancer in animal studies. Women with blood diseases, central nervous system disorders or peptic ulcers should *not* take this drug. Pregnant and nursing mothers should also avoid metronidazole, as it can pass through the placenta and breast milk to the baby. Many women who take this drug experience unpleasant effects such as nausea, headache, diarrhea, joint pain and numbness of arms or legs. In addition, anyone taking metronidazole should avoid alcohol, as the combination can make the effects of both worse.

In some cases, you can treat trich successfully with sulfa creams (low efficacy), Betadine or self-help remedies (see below). Unless you detect the infection early, however (and often even when you do), these treatments are not always as effective as Flagyl. If you have a stubborn case which has not responded to other treatments and decide to use Flagyl, ask for a single oral dose instead of the usual three-to-seven-day course of pills. Recent studies show that one dose has a 98 percent cure rate and far fewer negative effects.* Since men can also carry and transmit the infection, some practitioners believe male partners should be treated at the same time.

Nitrimidazole, which is available in England, is reported to be as effective as Flagyl. It may soon become available in the U.S.

Self-Help Treatments

1. Vinegar douches. Trich grows best in an alkaline environment so acidic douches may eliminate a trich infection if appied early enough. (See the section on preventing vaginitis, p. 518.)

2. Goldenseal-myrrh douche.

3. Chickweed douche: boil one quart of water, add three tablespoons of chickweed. Cover, let sit five to ten minutes, strain. Douche daily for a week.

4. Garlic suppositories inserted every twelve hours (see above).

*"Single Dose Metronidazole Effective in Trichomoniasis," *Obstetrics and Gynecology News* (March 1–14, 1982).

One trichomoniasis specialist advises that taking tub baths, wearing loose clothing (since exposure to air destroys parasites causing infection) and avoiding tampons, douches and vaginal sprays will help prevent recurrences.

Gardnerella (Formerly Called Hemophilus)

The *Hemophilus* bacterium is one of the most common causes of vaginitis. Like monilia, it thrives when the normal pH of the vagina is disturbed. You can get gardnerella through sexual intercourse, and less commonly from douche nozzles, toilet seats, washcloths and towels. The symptoms are similar to those of trich, though the discharge tends to be creamy white or grayish and especially foul-smelling (often "fishy") after intercourse. Although the bacterium is fairly easy to recognize on a "wet mount" (a mixture of vaginal secretions and saline solution observed under a microscope), it is sometimes diagnosed incorrectly. A culture is a more reliable test, especially if you have more than one infection, but it is expensive and not widely available.

The usual treatment is antibiotics (tetracycline or ampicillin—60 percent effective), sulfa cream or suppositories (black and Mediterranean women, see footnote on p. 270) (less than 30 percent effective) or Betadine gel. Some physicians prescribe Flagyl as the drug of choice (see "Trichomoniasis," p. 519). Gardnerella can be transmitted sexually, so your partner must also be treated, usually with antibiotics. Another effective antibiotic is cephradine (Anspor), a new cephalosporin; cost is about thirty dollars.

Self-Help Treatments

Self-help treatments include 1. acidifying your system by drinking eight ounces of unsweetened cranberry juice every day; 2. boric acid (600 milligrams in size 00 gelatin capsules—insert into the vagina for fourteen days); 3. alternate salt water and vinegar douches for a week; 4. yogurt douche; 5. garlic suppository and goldenseal or bayberry bark douches. 6. Some women find that taking extra Vitamins B and C also helps clear up infections. (The general recommendation for all of the above is once daily.)

Nonspecific Vaginitis

Other vaginal infections are called nonspecific vaginitis. The discharge may be white or yellow and possibly streaked with blood. Vaginal walls can be cloudy, puffy with fluid and covered by a thick, heavy coat of pus. Cystitislike symptoms may be the first sign (see p. 506). You may have lower back pain, cramps and swollen glands in the groin. It is usually treated with sulfa creams or suppositories (Vagitrol, Sultrin, AVC Cream) and occasionally with oral antibiotics. Other treatments are available for people allergic to sulfa.

Some researchers believe that most cases of nonspecific vaginitis are actually caused by *Hemophilus*. Others disagree. A wet smear or culture can usually determine the cause.

Self-Help Treatments

Self-help remedies are the same as for infections caused by *Hemophilus*, plus a douche of aloe vera liquid to soothe membranes and chlorophyll to increase the oxygen content of cells lining the vagina.

Vulvitis

Vulvitis, an inflammation of the vulva, is usually caused by irritation; a bacterial or fungal infection; injury or allergy to common commercial products such as soaps, powders, deodorants, sanitary napkins, synthetic underwear, pantyhose and medications. Vulvitis often accompanies other infections such as vaginitis or herpes. Stress, inadequate diet and poor hygiene can make you more susceptible to vulvitis. Women with diabetes may develop vulvitis because the sugar content of the cells is higher and the pH is higher in the vagina; these factors cause susceptibility to infection. Postmenopausal women often develop vulvitis because, as the hormonal levels drop, the vulvar tissues become thinner, dryer and less elastic, making them susceptible to irritation and infection.

Vulvitis symptoms include itching, redness and swelling. Sometimes fluid-filled blisters form which break open, ooze and crust over (these may resemble herpes). Scratching can cause further irritation, pus formation and scaling, as well as secondary infections. Sometimes, as a result of scratching, the skin whitens and thickens. In diabetic vulvitis the skin may look beefy red; in postmenopausal vulvitis, sores and red, irritated areas often appear.

Prevention

See the section on preventing vaginitis, p. 518.

Medical Treatments

If you have a vaginal infection or herpes, treating these problems will usually clear up the vulvitis as well.

Depending on the cause of vulvitis, your practitioner may prescribe antifungal creams. If itching is severe, s/he may prescribe cortisone cream or other soothing lotions. (Low-dose cortisone creams are good for a short period of time. Fluorinated ones cause thinning and atrophy of the skin if used for a long time.) Postmeno-pausal women may be given topical estrogen cream or ERT (estrogen replacement therapy) but should use both with extreme caution, since they have been implicated in various forms of cancer (see p. 447).

If the vulvitis persists or worsens, you may need a vulvar biopsy to rule out the possibility of cancer. This can be done in an office under local anesthetic.

Self-Help Treatments

Discontinue using any medications, soaps, powders, deodorants, toilet paper, etc., to which you may be sensitive. Keep your vulva clean, cool and dry. Hot boric acid compresses and hot sitz baths with comfrey tea are soothing. Use soft cotton or linen towels and underclothes to prevent chafing. Cold compresses made of plain, natural yogurt or cottage cheese also help relieve itching and soothe irritation. Calamine lotion also helps relieve itching. Aveeno colloidal oatmeal bath can be very soothing. Use a sterile, nonirritating lubricating cream such as K-Y Jelly during intercourse and other genital sex. Finally, try to eat well, get more rest and find ways of coping with stress.

ANEMIA

Anemia results from a shortage of red blood cells and/or a low hemoglobin content of these cells, and occurs four times as often among women as among men. (The hemoglobin molecule carries oxygen to every part of the body. When we are anemic, our tissues get less oxygen.) Often vague, symptoms may include chronic fatigue, irritability, dizziness, shortness of breath, headaches and bone pain. Dark-skinned women may look gray, light-skinned women very pale. Mild anemia may have no noticeable symptoms.

Iron-Deficiency Anemia

Iron-deficiency anemia is by far the most common form in women, often caused by heavy menstrual periods as well as bleeding associated with miscarriage, abortion, childbirth or surgery for fibroids. Pregnant women are especially prone to anemia because the fetus absorbs much of the iron the mother takes in.

Prevention and Treatments

The best preventive is an iron-rich diet. (See the chart on pp. 18–19.) Cooking foods in iron pots increases their iron content. If despite eating an iron-rich diet you are still anemic, you may want to take supplements. (Some practitioners recommend that pregnant women routinely take iron supplements.) Ferrous gluconate and chelated iron are the most eas-

ily absorbed forms of iron. They work best on an empty stomach, but if they cause nausea or cramps take them with food. Taking Vitamin C at the same time will increase absorption. Even so, some women find through subsequent hematocrits that they cannot absorb iron pills. In that case, try blackstrap molasses. Iron pills can cause tarry stools or constipation, which can be remedied by eating more whole grains, bran and fruit and drinking lots of water. Iron interferes with the absorption of Vitamin E. If you are taking Vitamin E supplements, be sure to take them at least six hours before the iron.

Vitamin-Deficiency Anemias

Pregnant women, women who have had many children, women on oral contraceptives and malnourished women can become anemic due to a lack of folic acid (an essential B-vitamin). You can prevent or treat this deficiency by eating whole grains and dark green vegetables and/or taking folic acid supplements. (One caution: too much folic acid may contribute to the development of breast cysts.) Vegetarians who eat no animal or dairy products sometimes suffer from pernicious anemia caused by lack of Vitamin B_{12} (present in all animal products). Symptoms may include burning or weakness in the legs. Adding brewers' yeast (which often contains B_{12}), a fortified cereal like Grape-Nuts, spirulina (a microalga) or fermented foods like miso, tempeh or fermented sprouts to the diet will help. Women who lack a protein called the "intrinsic factor," necessary for oral absorption of Vitamin B_{12}, will need monthly injections of this vitamin.

Hereditary and Other Types of Anemias

Some forms of anemia can be inherited. Sickle cell anemia is found in some people of African ancestry and thalassemia affects people of Mediterranean descent. Also, some African and Mediterranean (especially Italian) women inherit a deficiency in an enzyme called G6PD (glucose-6-phosphate-dehydrogenase), which causes them to develop hemolytic anemia (which may be fatal) if they take sulfa, aspirin or antimalarial drugs.

Finally, anemia can result from chronic illness such as kidney disease, thyroid disease, arthritis or cancer. Exposure to certain drugs, chemicals, metals or radiation can occasionally cause anemia.

Testing for Anemia

The hematocrit is a basic screening test for anemia. In this cheap and simple test, blood is taken from a prick on your finger and the percentage of red blood cells is measured. The normal hematocrit for a woman who is not pregnant is 37 to 47 percent. An annual test is a good idea; it will enable you to get an idea of changes from year to year. If your hematocrit is low, ask for a CBC (complete blood count), a lab test done on blood removed from a vein in your arm. In some cases other specialized expensive tests may be needed.

ARTHRITIS

Although arthritis encompasses over a hundred different joint diseases, women, who get arthritis twice as often as men, most often develop either osteoarthritis or rheumatoid arthritis. The former is a degenerative disease in which the cartilage, usually in the knees, hips, ankles or spine, gradually wears away. Common symptoms are swelling, redness and stiffness around the joints. Osteoarthritis, which is most common among older women (affecting about 25 percent), is not usually a crippling disease.

In rheumatoid arthritis, which affects about 3 percent of adult women, the body manufactures antibodies which attack the membranes covering the joints. In severe cases, the heart, lungs and kidneys can be affected. Symptoms include pain, swelling and redness in the fingers, knees, hips and back, fatigue, anemia, fever and weight loss. They may be mild or severe, spreading to many joints and getting worse over time. In severe cases, the joint supports (cartilage, ligaments and tendons) become inflamed and the joints themselves may begin to degenerate. A blood test can distinguish rheumatoid arthritis from other forms of the disease.

Prevention and Self-Help Treatments

(See *The Arthritis Helpbook* in Resources.) Exercise, relaxation and nutrition can both prevent and treat arthritis, sometimes reducing or eliminating the need for medical treatment. Regular exercise, such as yoga, walking or swimming, stretches, strengthens and preserves the joints. Daily rest is especially important when arthritis is severe. Some studies suggest that a diet low in fats can dramatically reduce pain, swelling and stiffness.* Since certain foods (such as beef, pork, milk, sugar, chocolate, MSG, pepper, alcohol and artificial preservatives) actually trigger attacks, eliminating them from your diet can be the key to preventing arthritic attacks. Some women find that regular consumption of alfalfa alone (in tea, sprout or pill form) prevents flare-ups. Acupuncture and Vitamin-C supplements may also be helpful.

Arthritis pain can also be related to stress and depression, making us less motivated to take care of ourselves and thus causing more pain, setting up a cycle that is difficult to break. Meditation, yoga, re-laxation exercises and biofeedback may help us break the stress-depression-pain cycle. Symptoms sometimes abate temporarily during pregnancy.

Medical Treatments

The most common treatment for mild arthritis is aspirin, which relieves both inflammation and pain. Too much aspirin, however, can cause stomach irritation and bleeding. (Taking aspirin with food reduces this irritation.) Other anti-inflammation drugs commonly prescribed for arthritis include Motrin, Nalfon, Naproxen and Sulindac. Ask about negative effects before taking any of these drugs.

For severe or crippling arthritis, your physician may recommend surgery to repair or replace damaged joints. Other treatments sometimes used for severe rheumatoid arthritis include gold-salt injections, antimalarial drugs, steroids and other powerful anti-inflammatory agents. These drugs, which can have dangerous side effects, should be recommended only when all other methods have failed.

INTRODUCTION TO CANCER

Most of us (about two-thirds) will never get cancer. Many who do are cancer-free years after their original diagnosis. Why does this illness hold so much terror for us? It is partly due to the constant media attention, treatments that seem almost as bad as the disease, and the uncertainty of cure (61 percent of those who do get cancer die within five years).* For women, there is the added factor that cancer often develops in our sexual or reproductive organs (breasts, ovaries, uterus). Since the conventional treatment, for example, in breast cancer, has been surgical removal, we may fear losing our attractiveness or "womanliness" in a society which so often locates a woman's identity in her physical attributes. We may also face the loss of certain sexual pleasures. (See the discussion of hysterectomy on p. 511, for example.)

Then there is the shame, the "What have I done to deserve this?" feeling which so often sweeps over someone who has cancer. And no wonder! All around us, the word "cancer" is used to describe any particularly immoral or illegal situation. Drugs and juvenile delinquency are "cancers" in our society. Watergate is the "cancer of democracy," not the "heart attack."

This fear and shame means that many of us avoid thinking about cancer even when we ourselves have it. Because of this avoidance, we do not always make the best medical decisions or live as full a life as possible.

---

*See *Clinical Research*, Vol. 27, No. 4 (1981).

*American Cancer Society. *Cancer Facts and Figures, 1984.*

What Is Cancer?

Through a process not completely understood, normal cells sometimes become abnormal and begin to grow out of control. These abnormal cells may spread (metastasize) throughout the body, taking over organs and preventing them from functioning. Some cancers are fast-growing, others are slow. Each type of cancer has its own particular pattern of growth, spread and probability of cure or survival time.

Who Gets Cancer?

While people of all ages can get cancer, it is most often found in older persons, as the disease can take as long as twenty years to reach a detectable state.

Over the past twenty-five years, the death rate from cancer has increased 34 percent among the black population and only 9 percent in the white population. The incidence (number of new cases) is also higher among blacks; in some cases (such as cervical cancer) the rate is twice as high for black women as for white women.* At least part of the reason for these differences must be the discrimination which causes many black people to be exposed more frequently to workplace and environmental carcinogens (cancer-causing substances) than whites, to have less access to high-quality medical care, nutritious food and decent living conditions.†

Women develop less cancer and die less frequently from it than men do; the gap (except for lung cancer) is widening.‡ At least part of this difference exists because until recently men consumed much more tobacco and alcohol and were more often exposed to workplace carcinogens. It may also be that as women we are better able to handle stress and thus keep our immune (disease-fighting) systems stronger. Or there may be something inherent in our immune or metabolic systems which increases our ability to fight cancer.

Terminology

The following terms are frequently misunderstood or misused, even by medical personnel. Ask for careful explanations—it is your right to know exactly what is going on.

Mortality (death) rates tell how many people died from cancer per 100,000 population per year.

Survival rates, generally given for five-, ten- and twenty-year periods, report how long people with specific kinds of cancer usually live. Survival rates are always calculated from the date the cancer was first diagnosed. These rates are most helpful when they are subdivided according to such factors as how far advanced the cancer was at first diagnosis, the type of treatment received, and the age, sex, race, socio-economic status and occupation of the people involved.

FIVE-YEAR SURVIVAL RATE PERCENTAGES (ADJUSTED FOR NORMAL LIFE SPANS) AMERICAN CANCER SOCIETY—1984

Type of Cancer	White		Black	
	Local- ized	Metas- tasized	Local- ized	Metas- tasized
Lung (male and female)	42	4	24	3
Colon/Rectum (male and female)	77	29	59	20
Breast*	88	50	79	35
Uterus/Cervix	82	41	78	35
Uterus/Internal (corpus or endometrial)	90	40	69	18
Ovary	81	20	81	19

Cure rates purport to tell how many people are completely cured of their cancers. However, cure rates are generally based on survival rates, resulting in the misleading impression that many people are "cured" who have merely survived for a specified (usually five-year) period. For example, physicians usually consider a five-year survival a cure in breast cancer, even though many women die of the disease in the sixth or seventh year.

Remission is sometimes used loosely to refer to any improvement, other times in a more technical sense with very strict criteria regarding amount of change in tumor size and blood tests. Some cancer therapies will produce technical "remission" of certain symptoms but do not increase cure or survival rates. Remission rates are usually given as percentages of persons "going into remission" after receiving various types of treatments.†

We should keep in mind that while statistics provide useful information, they can't really predict what will happen to us as individuals.

---

*Ibid.

†We were unable to find significant separate statistics for other minorities, nor is it clear if Hispanic peoples were counted as white in the above figures. (See also Chapter 24.)

‡From 1953 to 1978, there was a 25 percent increase in men's cancer death rates and a 7 percent decrease in women's. However, as women's smoking has increased, their lung cancer rate is also increasing, and will soon be the leading cause of cancer death in women. (See American Cancer Society, *Cancer Facts and Figures, 1984.*)

*While breast cancer is mistakenly thought to occur only in women, a small number of cases (less than 1 percent) occur in men.

†Long-term remission refers to a specific number of disease-free years and is preferred to "cure," as people with cancer are often considered to have their disease under control rather than to be entirely cured. It is the pessimists' (or realists') substitute for "cure."

Causes

Cancer rates increase with exposure to carcinogens (such as radiation, asbestos, some pesticides), smoking, alcohol or particular dietary habits (see below). Certain genes and viruses have caused cancer in laboratory animals and similar processes are suspected but not conclusively proven in some human cancers. Yet it is not clear how these substances cause cancer, or why everyone who develops the same kind of cancer does not respond in the same way, either to the disease or to treatments. There are also unexplained cases of spontaneous remission: approximately 7 to 8 percent of people with terminal cancer suddenly recover and live out their lives apparently free of the disease. These different responses show that our individual immune systems are very important factors.

It seems most likely that cancer is caused by a build-up of one or more factors to the point (different for each person) where the body's immune system can no longer handle the load. Thus smoking will not guarantee that you will get cancer, but it will increase your chances. (Smoking or smoking combined with heavy alcohol consumption accounts for 20 to 30 percent of all cancers.*) Add smoking to heavy drinking, repeated X-rays, constant stress,† exposure to pollution‡ or excessive overweight, and the risk of cancer goes up.

Both environmental and hereditary elements appear to cause cancer. Heredity refers to the traits and tendencies passed on to us by our parents in our genes, while environment includes all that we eat, breathe or come into contact with. Most researchers now believe that environment is responsible for the development of 85 to 95 percent of all cancers.

Prevention

While we can do many things to reduce our risk of cancer (such as stopping smoking, limiting X-rays), many other factors, such as air pollution and the many environmental carcinogens which bombard us in our daily lives, are not so clearly under our personal control. Even diet changes can be expensive and resisted by family, friends and physicians.

Thus cancer prevention means restructuring both our personal lives and the society at large so that a clean environment, safe jobs, healthy food and less stressful living become top priorities.

---

*Cancer Facts and Figures, 1984.

†See L. LeShan, You Can Fight for Your Life (listed in Resources), for more on stress and loss as they may affect cancer.

‡See Chapter 7, "Environmental and Occupational Health," for more on environmental and workplace carcinogens.

A Program to Reduce the Risk of Cancer

(In the list below, factors which seem to be especially related to breast cancer are marked with an asterisk.)

*1. Don't smoke, and avoid smoke-filled environments.

*2. Avoid X-rays whenever possible.

*3. Avoid estrogen replacement therapy at menopause and any other medication with estrogen such as the "morning-after pill" (DES). The relationship between oral contraceptives and breast cancer is very controversial. Some studies have shown that women who take birth control pills have a higher risk of breast cancer. Most newer studies do not confirm this risk, and instead indicate that the Pill may lower women's chances of developing uterine and ovarian cancers. To be on the safe side, women concerned about their risk of breast cancer may want to avoid oral contraceptives, especially since birth control pills pose other serious problems.

4. Minimize consumption of smoked, salted or pickled foods, such as bacon. Avoid additives, preservatives and refined flour.

*5. Keep fat consumption low—about 15 to 20 percent of total calories; reduce both saturated and unsaturated fats while making sure that both are supplied in the diet.

*6. Limit or eliminate alcohol.

*7. Research has shown that people who are overweight (more than 40 percent above the old "norms") get more cancer and die more frequently from it. In breast cancer, this may be related to ovarian estrogen levels. Many studies point to high levels of estrogen as a precipitating factor in breast cancer. There is evidence that fat tissue manufactures its own estrogen. While this process may be helpful during and after menopause as a natural form of "estrogen replacement therapy," it may also be dangerous to a woman who is very large or who already has elevated estrogen levels.

*8. Maintain frequent and regular bowel movements. Increasing exercise and dietary fiber may help.

*9. Avoid hair dyes made from petroleum bases.

10. Eat a diet high in organic whole grains, vegetables and fruits rich in bran and fiber.

11. Eat food high in beta carotene (a Vitamin-A precursor found in carrots and other yellow and dark leafy vegetables as well as some yellow fruits). Or take supplements of beta carotene. Be wary of large doses (greater than 10,000 to 15,000 IUs daily) of Vitamin A, as it can be toxic and is not a substitute for beta carotene.

*12. Eat foods high in selenium (brewers' yeast, eggs, garlic, onions, liver, asparagus, tuna, mushrooms, shrimp, kidney, whole grains and brown rice). Selenium can be toxic in high doses so be careful of any megatherapy or supplementation.

Costs

The total costs to the U.S. economy of cancer research and treatments is a high 15 to 20 billion dollars per year. Medical treatment for cancer can reach approximately 20,000 dollars for an individual, not including hidden costs like transportation, babysitters and loss of income.

Unfortunately, the profit motive affects how this country tackles cancer. Major research has emphasized high-profit treatments rather than prevention. (Chemotherapy, for instance, can cost 500 dollars per month.) These benefit hospitals, doctors and the pharmaceutical, insurance and medical-equipment companies, but have not yet brought significant progress in eliminating cancer. Government and industry do little to clean up the environment, the workplace or hazardous consumer products or to discourage the profitable dietary and smoking habits that contribute to cancer. In fact, the government subsidizes tobacco production. One cancer researcher remarked that a cure for cancer may never be found because too many people depend on it for a living.

What to Do if You Have Cancer

Inform yourself. The first thing to do is learn all you can. Unfortunately, there is no reliable cure for most cancers, and all the once-accepted theories and treatments in the field are now under question. It helps to be persistent and aggressive in seeking the most up-to-date information and to have someone you trust do it with or for you.

Resist the pressure to rush. Your doctor or your family may pressure you to begin treatment immediately. Yet most cancers have been developing for two to twenty years before being discovered. Several studies have shown that a short delay of three or four more weeks while you get adjusted to the idea, seek out information and get second or third opinions should not make any difference in the ultimate outcome of your disease. If you decide then to follow your doctor's original advice, you will feel much better about the decision. If you decide to take another course of action, you may have saved yourself unnecessary treatment or considerable regret at not having made your own choice.

Talk to others with cancer. Try joining (or starting) a group for people with cancer. Being with those who understand and have faced the same problems can provide the kind of practical information and emotional support which is simply not routinely available from those providing conventional medical cancer treatment.

Joining my cancer discussion group is one of the best things which has happened to me since my diagnosis.

In a group founded by those who have cancer rather than one started by professionals at a hospital or a service organization, you may feel freer to confront all aspects of your situation. These include critical evaluation of traditional and alternative therapies; the problems surrounding childcare, insurance, jobs and marital relations; and ways of coping with your own fears as well as those of family and friends. If you can't find or create such a group, talk with individuals—people in waiting rooms, people suggested by your doctor, friends or clergy. Don't hesitate to call persons you haven't met. Many people with cancer are glad to talk about their experiences.

Factors to Consider When Deciding on Conventional Medical Treatment (Surgery, Radiation and Chemotherapy)

Unfortunately, there has been little progress over the years in effective cancer treatment. Many doctors and hospitals have one preferred treatment which they will urge you to accept. Specialists tend to recommend their own approach; for example, surgeons promote surgery and radiologists radiation. Yet new research indicates that many factors—age, sex, previous health history, type and stage of cancer—can influence how well a treatment works. The data are changing rapidly and even those doctors who are familiar with the most recent research often can't agree on how to interpret the information. Ideally, you should have access to a team of specialists to be sure of getting the treatment most appropriate for your cancer and for you.

Because so many variations exist, we cannot give a comprehensive guide to cancer treatments. What we can do is discuss some of the issues and indicate what you need to know in order to make informed decisions. Where no one treatment has proved best, it often makes sense to choose the one which will disrupt your body and your life the least.

While everyone wants the benefits of the most current therapies, it is tragic to give false hope, waste limited finances or subject already ill persons to painful treatments unless there is good reason to believe that the treatment will pay off with either increased survival time or improved quality of life remaining. We urge anyone considering surgery, chemotherapy, radiation or any of the alternatives to study carefully what can be reasonably expected from the treatment in their particular case.*

There are other factors to consider. Choosing anything but the most conventional and locally available treatment often involves traveling quite a distance. This may separate you from loved ones and a familiar environment, important factors in the healing process.

*See also Chapter 24, "The Politics of Women and Medical Care," p. 555.

Also, most forms of treatment are very expensive, and pursuing a less available treatment may mean even more expense—for second-opinion medical visits, travel, noninsured costs. Many women (perhaps having internalized the culture's view of women as secondary) feel guilty about using their own or their family's money on themselves. In making this difficult decision, every woman deserves both the clearest, most current information and the strongest possible support from family and friends.

Surgery

Surgery has been the mainstay of cancer therapy for over a century. It helps with local control of the disease and seems to be effective in a few types of cancer (such as nonmelanoma skin cancers and cervical cancer). But surgery is not always the best treatment, and it takes the body a long time to recover from it. See p. 482 for some things to consider before consenting to surgery.

Surgery and Early Detection

Until very recently, most doctors believed that surgery would work if they caught the cancer before it had a chance to spread. For this reason, when possible they would cut a sizable area around the cancer to "be sure to get it all." They based this approach on the theory that cancer begins in one place (e.g., the lung or breast) and spreads from there.

However, over the past twenty years or more, cancer has been detected earlier and earlier with, in most cases, no corresponding drop in the death rate (see "Early Detection Controversy," p. 531). This has made many physicians question the entire notion of early detection. Now many doctors are beginning to view some cancers as systemic diseases which tend to show up first in certain areas but are already microscopically present throughout the body. There is evidence to support both theories, and the final answer may lie somewhere in between. However, the treatment you are offered will reflect the theory preferred by the doctor or hospital you go to.

Radiation and Chemotherapy

Radiation (via high-power X-rays or internal implants) and chemotherapy (chemicals taken by pill or injection) are supposed to kill cancer throughout the body in places that surgery can't reach. They themselves have carcinogenic (cancer-causing) potential, yet are theoretically more harmful to cancer cells than to normal cells. So far neither therapy has been very successful in curing or prolonging life in regard to the common cancers such as breast, colon and lung cancer, although they have reduced some cancer symptoms.

Negative effects common to both chemotherapy and radiation include nausea, fatigue and diarrhea. In addition, chemotherapy may also result in amenorrhea (cessation of menstruation, usually permanently), alopecia (hair loss, usually not permanently), heart damage and suppressed immune systems (seriously lowering resistance to infections). Radiation may cause skin burns, extreme sun sensitivity, weakened bones and sudden bone fractures, as well as "ulcers" (body sores that do not heal). Some drugs lessen these symptoms, but they may have their own negative effects. Marijuana often helps reduce the nausea and pain and is now legal in many states for people with cancer. Both forms of treatment involve repeated trips to a medical center or hospital.

Chemotherapy and radiation were formerly used only when cancer recurred in the same organ or metastasized elsewhere. Increasingly, doctors favoring the systemic theory of cancer recommend radiation and/or chemotherapy immediately after surgery even when there is no evidence of spread (e.g., breast lumpectomy with radiation). A few physicians try chemotherapy and radiation without surgery (if the cancer is too advanced for surgery).

We feel some concern that physicians are overusing chemotherapy and radiation in instances where there's no proven benefit—almost as though they were "miracle" cures. This is understandable. Most doctors genuinely want to help their cancer patients and are frustrated by the lack of a reliable cure. Most people with cancer feel more reassured when they and the doctor are doing *something*. Overtreatment is psychologically appealing on both sides; both want to hope that "this time" treatment will make the difference.

Popular articles about cancer often give the impression that chemotherapy is working wonders with all types of cancer. This image makes people more likely to accept treatment under the false notion that it will increase their survival time also. Actually it has shown significant results only in a few of the less common types.* Doctors often urge the therapy by quoting the statistics on these rare types of cancer without making it clear to the person that this treatment cannot be expected to be of benefit. This lack of informed consent raises false hopes. *It is important to check that chemotherapy has been proven effective for your type of cancer.*

It is also important to find out exactly *how much* increased survival time can be gained. Sometimes the percentages doctors or researchers give are mislead-

---

*Chemotherapy has produced dramatic increases in five-year survival rates in childhood leukemia, young-adult Hodgkin's disease and other lymphomas. A child treated for leukemia may gain many precious years of life. However, s/he may get another form of cancer later on, caused by the chemotherapy chemicals themselves. It may be inappropriate to call the leukemia treatment a "cure" in all cases. (See American Cancer Society, *Cancer Facts and Figures, 1984.*)

ing: what is called 50 or 100 percent increased survival time may mean only two or three more months, or it may mean two or three years more. See the questions below.

Many people question whether the possibility of longer survival times is worth the negative effects of these therapies. Others feel that even one more day of life is worth any price. Only you can make this difficult decision with the support of those who love you.

Questions You Need to Know the Answers to

An asterisk indicates those questions that doctors frequently do not or cannot give sufficient answers for. Press your doctor to find out and let you know, but also check books, medical journals and resource centers and speak to others who have had the same form of cancer as you.

*1. Exactly what form of cancer do I have? Is it slow- or fast-growing?

*2. What therapies are available?

*3. How effective is each therapy? What is the probability of cure? What definition of "cure" is used?

4. What benefits can I expect? Longer life? Reduced symptoms? Reduced pain, etc.?

*5. Can the therapy prolong life by months? By years?

*6. What percentage of people treated benefit from the therapy—25 percent? 50 percent? 75 percent? How is that benefit measured?

7. Will I be able to continue my regular activities during the therapy? What about sex? Working? Athletics?

8. Will the therapy require overnight stays in the hospital or can it be done on an outpatient basis?

9. What are the potential negative effects? How serious are they? What percentage of people get them? Are they permanent? Are there any drugs that will help alleviate these effects? Do these drugs themselves cause any negative effects? How long does any symptom usually last? How soon after receiving treatment are symptoms likely to begin? (For example, does nausea generally start immediately, within twenty minutes or several hours later?)

10. How long will the therapy last? Each session? How many sessions?

*11. How many people get recurrences after this treatment, and how soon?

*12. Are there survival, cure, mortality and remission rates for this therapy for my type of cancer, broken down by such factors as type of cancer, age, sex, race, socioeconomic status, occupation, geographical location, etc.?

13. What are the costs involved? Does insurance usually cover them?

*14. May I speak with some of your other patients?

Do you know of any local groups for people with cancer? Any groups for family members and friends?

Alternative Therapies

The medical establishment as a whole regards most alternatives to surgery, radiation and chemotherapy with great caution or outright hostility. Yet women are increasingly seeking out unconventional approaches because the conventional therapies have not significantly improved survival rates and have many disadvantages. To date, alternative therapies are most often used along with conventional ones or as a last resort for advanced cancers after conventional treatments have failed. A few physicians are willing to work with combined approaches.

What alternatives are available and what can we expect from them? This is not an easy question to answer because we don't have reliable statistics on survival, recurrence, and mortality for the alternative therapies.*

Alternative therapies are often reported in what is called anecdotal style: one particular person who was cured of cancer (or greatly helped) by a certain treatment tells her/his story. This style, which makes for inspirational reading, presents great problems. It is hard to confirm individual case histories. Even when it is determined that the person involved did use the treatment and recovered from cancer, there is still no proof that it was the treatment which caused the cure; some people have spontaneous remissions. The important issue is what percentage of people treated with a certain therapy recovers or improves and how that compares with other therapies. Physicians, while they decry the use of the anecdotal style regarding alternative approaches, often resort to it to convince people under their care. Also, it is frequently through looking at the unusual cures that we find ideas for new or improved treatments. By all means ask the same questions about these alternative therapies that you ask about conventional methods.

The following list of alternative cancer therapies is more detailed than the above description of surgery, radiation and chemotherapy because this information is often hard to find. Keep in mind that the alternatives have not been tested in large-scale, long-term trials.

---

*Supporters of nonconventional treatments contend that their therapies might show better results if 90 percent of their patients weren't already terminally ill, with immune systems suppressed by radiation and chemotherapy. Meanwhile, it is equally important to remember that the statistics we do have on conventional medical treatments do not themselves show significant improvements in overcoming cancer.

The Gerson Diet and Detoxification Therapy

Perhaps the most promising of the nontoxic alternatives is the Gerson diet and detoxification therapy. The diet consists of organically-grown fresh fruits and vegetables. It forbids salted, processed or refined foods and fat. Meat is not allowed in the early stages of treatment. In most cases, the therapy includes tablets and injections of various nutrients, especially potassium and pancreatic enzymes. The Gerson therapy, developed in Austria in the 1920s and 1930s, is one of the few alternatives for which there are records and reports of long-term survival rates. For more information, contact the Gerson Institute of California, run by Dr. Gerson's daughter (see Resources).

The therapy itself is very rigorous and should be followed precisely for at least a year and a half. It is not sufficient to merely eat more healthily.

Physicians and various health practitioners have developed other diet therapies. Most of them are similar to the Gerson diet, though there are some discrepancies, especially between raw and cooked foods. Most also include procedures for detoxification (removing wastes from the body through skin, bowels, etc.) and spinal adjustments (see "Chiropractic," p. 66). Many people who use these diets experience periods of nausea and headache and occasional pain and fever. The therapy's supporters attribute these to the removal of toxins which created the conditions for cancer. A similar and also promising approach is the metabolic therapy developed by Dr. William Kelley of the International Health Institute (see Resources).

Meganutrition Therapies

Two-time Nobel prizewinner Linus Pauling states that large daily doses of Vitamin C, as high as fifty grams, can aid in both preventing and treating cancer. A study in Scotland supported his claim, but many doctors have vehemently attacked Pauling because similar studies in the U.S. have shown no improvement. Pauling and his associates believe that the American studies are faulty because they are based on people who had already had chemotherapy (which represses the immune system and may inhibit the vitamin's action).

Other researchers have found evidence that megadoses of other nutrients, especially Vitamins A and B-complex, the previtamin beta carotene and trace minerals such as potassium and selenium, can help in the prevention and treatment of cancer. Carlton Fredericks' *Winning the Fight Against Breast Cancer, the Nutritional Approach* (see Resources) contains a good summary of this research.

Care must be taken with any of the megatherapies. Some vitamins, such as A and D, can be toxic at high levels. For this reason many doctors argue strongly against all megatherapies. Advocates, on the other hand, contend that what would be a toxic dose in a healthy person is needed by someone whose system is trying to deal with cancer.

Laetrile

The most controversial and probably best-known of all the unconventional therapies is laetrile therapy. Produced from apricot pits, laetrile releases a cyanide into the system. Like chemotherapy and radiation, it is toxic to the body. Thousands of people have credited laetrile with their recovery from cancer. (See above for the limits of anecdotal reporting, however.)

Opponents point out cases where people who might have received good results from the traditional therapies chose laetrile instead and succumbed to their disease. Despite a blanket condemnation of laetrile by the prestigious Sloan-Kettering research center, some studies at that very institute showed that laetrile delayed metastases of breast cancer in mice. (See Ralph W. Moss's *The Cancer Syndrome*, listed in Resources.) The case for or against the drug is still not resolved. It is illegal in many states.

Hydrazine Sulphate

Hydrazine sulphate is an inexpensive substance that several researchers have found to help control the process of cachexia, or wasting away, which is the actual cause of death in over 50 percent of cancer cases. The doctors studying it think that if the other bodily systems can remain healthy and not be drained by the cancer, then any cancer therapy, traditional or alternative, will have a better chance of working. Overdoses can cause serious side effects, but at the proper dosage level there are few or no adverse effects.

Pyschological/Spiritual Alternatives

Visualization, meditation and other psychological/spiritual approaches to cancer are gaining favor with both doctors and the general public. These emphasize people's self-healing capabilities and the ability of the mind to influence the body's recovery. (See also Chapter 5, "Health and Healing: Alternatives to Medical Care.")

The Simonton Technique

Probably the best-known of these is the Simonton visualization technique in which the person with cancer learns to picture her/his body's defense system cleansing the body of cancerous cells and replacing them with healthy cells. Some hospitals offer counselors who teach this and other aspects of the Simonton approach. While too new to have long-term survival statistics, this therapy appears to have been a major factor in the recovery of many people with cancer, including some for whom the conventional treatments had failed. (See O. Carl Simonton, et al., *Getting Well Again*, listed in Resources.)

Prayer

Many of us have found that prayer, meditation or other spiritual approaches can help to transform our experiences with serious illness from a terrifying, hopeless time into a period of personal growth and fuller enjoyment of life. Sometimes this spiritual healing includes "cure" and sometimes it does not.

Faith Healers and Psychics

If you are considering visiting a psychic or faith healer, try to find out as much as possible about the healer in advance. Making your own decision here is just as important as in any other type of treatment. Do not be rushed into a commitment by well-intentioned friends or deterred by ridicule from nonbelieving friends. We do caution anyone to avoid any faith or psychic healer who charges exorbitant fees or insists that you must "prove your faith" by refusing all other treatments.

Danger of Blaming the Victim

When using psychological/spiritual approaches such as the Simonton technique or faith healers, we need to be careful not to blame the victim for getting cancer—"she brought it on herself, all that repressed anger"—or condemning her if she doesn't get well—"she just isn't strong enough; she doesn't really want to get well; she doesn't have enough faith." Those of us who have cancer need the support and help, not the judgment, of our friends, families and health practitioners.

Problems in Getting Alternative Therapies

When a woman asks her doctor about nontraditional approaches, she often receives ridicule and warnings. Doctors often sincerely believe they are protecting their patients in this way, for medical journals expose them only to the negative side. Of course, there *are* people—in both conventional and alternative fields—who try to take advantage of the fear and desperation of some people with cancer. But doctors' warnings may also reflect the medical establishment's resistance to theories and treatments which do not follow the line of drugs, radiation and surgery.

In large part due to opposition from the medical world, alternative clinics are not well funded or widely available. A decision to go to one usually means added

and noninsured expenses for treatment, travel, childcare, housing, etc.

Friends and family who disapprove of therapies may withdraw emotional or financial support. Still, many women have found it worthwhile to push past these obstacles to find alternative sources of healing.

Some kinds of cancer are very painful near the end, while others aren't. Often women feel that it is a sign of weakness to take any medicine for the pain, or they are afraid of addiction. Occasionally doctors have these same inhibitions. If pain is preventing you from living as normally as possible and from enjoying the company of family and friends, you should feel no hesitation in asking for relief. Morphine and codeine are usually used, and there is an increasing acceptance of marijuana.

Remember that metastasis does not inevitably equal death. But if death does seem to be imminent, you can do much to insure that you live your remaining time as fully as possible.

I don't want to die, but since I accepted the fact that I probably will, I am more at peace. It's as if my energy had been used up denying the reality of my own impending death and, when I stopped struggling against the idea, I suddenly felt free. I could begin to think about living again, about what to do with the time I do have. I have my down days, when I ask, "Why me? Why can't I die twenty years from now? Why can't I live to see my children grow up, my grandchildren born?" But these days are fewer and fewer. In a sense, I'm lucky to know about my death in advance. I won't be like those who die unexpectedly with things left unsaid and undone. I've planned what I want to do, who I want to see. I've started working on projects that I had always wanted to do but was too busy for. I can't afford to travel or do much special, but then anything I do now seems special.

I am not dying of cancer; I am living with cancer. I try to deal with the problems caused by my cancer in my daily life, but my emphasis is on the living, not the dying.

BREAST CANCER

If you turned to this section first, we hope you will go to the beginning of the "Benign Breast Conditions" section (p. 488) and read from there. If you ever do have a breast cancer diagnosis following biopsy, you will be much better able to cope with it and to decide what to do next if you have done some reading and thinking beforehand.

Since breast lumps are so common and most of them are not dangerous, it is important for us to familiarize ourselves with ways of recognizing and dealing with them.

If the Biopsy Results Are Positive

No one who has not had the experience can understand the waves of shock, disbelief, fear and anger that overcome you after finding out you have cancer. This emotional trauma comes exactly when you need to focus all your energy on learning about your treatment options.

The usual first reaction is to do whatever your doctor suggests. This is appealing at a time when you may need to feel that you are being taken care of, but it has not always resulted in the best of care. While most doctors are well intentioned and believe in the treatments they offer, they tend to offer only one treatment—usually modified radical mastectomy. Physicians as a whole have been slow to accept new therapies even when numerous studies have demonstrated that the new approaches have the same or better effectiveness with fewer negative effects. Many are unwilling or unable to discuss all the available therapies. Only three states, Massachusetts, California and Minnesota, have laws which require that women be informed of all the medical options.

At this point, it is advisable to get second and third opinions before committing yourself to a course of treatment. The National Cancer Institute (see Resources) sponsors many centers where your case can be evaluated by a team of specialists. Oncologists (cancer specialists), surgeons and radiologists work together to prescribe the best combination of treatments for your individual situation. They are more likely to be up to date on research. This team approach helps to avoid the tendency of most physicians to promote their own specialty: surgeons urging surgery, radiologists presenting radiation as the best solution, etc. Such centers may also offer more treatment choices, possibly including experimental therapies (see "Our Rights as Patients, p. 584).

Remember, there is no rush. You can take several weeks or even a month to adjust and find out about your options. If you had an excisional biopsy, the main cancer is already out. If you only had an aspiration or incisional biopsy and are worried about any cancer remaining in the breast, you could have the remainder of the lump removed surgically. In some cases, this could be the end of the treatment. You can always decide later to have further treatment such as mastectomy, radiation or chemotherapy. Some doctors will try to rush you into a decision by stating that the biopsy may have "stirred up" the cancer and it is therefore important to proceed immediately with mastectomy. This is an outmoded theory.

There is a tendency to rush women into treatments before they have a chance to get second opinions and learn about all the available options. No one knows for sure how long you can safely wait before beginning treatments, and doctors' opinions on this issue may vary widely. The same doctor who tells one woman she must not wait even one or two weeks may later assure another woman that she needn't worry about the necessity of waiting four to six weeks for a hospital appointment to begin treatments. There is no evidence that this will make any difference in length of life even if the lump does prove cancerous (see p. 490).

The entire field of breast cancer medicine is changing rapidly as old, established theories and treatments are coming under question while newer techniques have not been used long enough to be completely evaluated. While we cannot tell you which therapy will be best for you, we can point out some directions to pursue and pitfalls to avoid.

A good place to begin is the reading list in Resources. We also recommend writing to the Breast Cancer Advisory Center (see Resources). This organization, founded by a woman with breast cancer, keeps one of the most current files on breast cancer treatments and doctors who are experienced with them.

Stages of Breast Cancer

There are several systems for staging cancer, but all are based on the three elements called TNM—*T*umor size, number of malignant *N*odes, and whether or not you have distant *M*etastases (cancer in other parts of your body). The following (clinical and histological) are the two most commonly used systems. Many people, including quite a few doctors, confuse or combine the two. The stage of the cancer is important because doctors usually base their recommendations for treatment on how well other women with cancer at the same stage and a similar personal history have responded to the treatments.

Clinical Stages*

When physicians think that a particular lump "feels" like cancer, they estimate the size of the suspected cancer by the apparent size of the lump and the "feel" of nearby lymph nodes and other organs. In addition, they may order blood tests and liver or bone scans to see if cancer exists beyond the breast. (These tests are often routine and do not necessarily mean that your cancer has spread.) Lymph nodes which seem to be involved are frequently merely inflamed or hardened but not cancerous. Likewise, nodes may be malignant but not palpable; that is, they cannot be felt. This estimated clinical stage must be confirmed by a biopsy and permanent section. *It is not wise or necessary to submit to a bone scan or other tests until there is a diagnosis of cancer obtained by surgical biopsy in permanent section.*

*For all stages (I to IV) see Craig Henderson, et al., "Cancer of the Breast—The Past Decade (Medical Progress)," Parts I and II, *The New England Journal of Medicine*, Vol. 302 (January 3, 1980), pp. 17–30; (January 10, 1980), pp. 78–90.

Stage I

A small lump (less than three-quarters of an inch or two centimeters) which is palpable and does not appear to have spread to either the lymph nodes under the arms or to more distant parts of the body. Eighty-five percent of women with Stage I cancer are still living five years after diagnosis.

Stage II

The tumor size (three-quarters of an inch to two inches or two to five centimeters) is larger than in Stage I. Nodes may or may not be palpable and there is no evidence of distant metastases. Sixty-six percent of women with Stage II cancer survive five years from diagnosis.

Stage III

The lump is large (greater than two inches or five centimeters) and the lymph nodes appear by palpation to be involved, although there is no evidence of more distant spread. Smaller tumors are included in this stage if they are attached to the chest wall or have invaded the skin. For women with Stage III cancer, the five-year survival rate is 41 percent.

Stage IV

This is the same as Stage III, except that there is evidence also that the cancer has metastasized and is growing in other parts of the body. At this stage, a cancer is not considered curable. Mastectomy is not useful unless the cancer has spread throughout most of the breast or the breast is infected and ulcerated. Ten percent of women with Stage IV cancer live five years after diagnosis.

Histological Stages

The histological stage is based on the number of cancerous lymph nodes. A surgeon removes a sample of about ten lymph nodes from the axilla (underarm area) nearest the breast with the malignancy. This is usually done during the main breast surgery—lumpectomy or mastectomy. Occasionally, the lymph node sample is done as a separate operation. General anesthesia is preferred for lymph node surgery because the operation can be painful and lengthy. Surgeons sometimes have to make several cuts before finding nodes and, in about 16 percent of all women, they are unable to find any.

Removing the nodes is not an attempt to cure or halt the spread of cancer. Its only purpose is to see if the cancer has gone beyond the breast but node status also predicts survival most accurately. Cancer in the nodes is an indication that undetected cancer *may* exist elsewhere in the body. Removing more than ten or so nodes may increase arm problems later. Some cancer experts also believe that the nodes serve a protective function, delaying or slowing metastases.

Histological Stages NSABP*		
Number of Cancerous Nodes	Percent Survival† 5 Years	10 Years
None	78.1	64.9
1–3	62.2	37.5
4 or more	32.0	13.4

Other factors relating to your type of cancer include the location of the tumor (central, lateral or medial); presence or absence of estrogen and progesterone receptors; and the grade of malignancy, including differentiation (whether or not cells still retain the characteristics of the normal breast cell rather than the embryonic appearance of the advanced cancer cell), plenomorphism (variety of cells in the same area) and mitotic rate (growth rate). Research on these and other aspects of tumors is in progress.

Early Detection Controversy

For years doctors assumed that breast cancer began in the breast and was confined there until it reached a certain size or condition, when it began to spread systematically—first to nearby areas, then to more distant parts of the body. According to this view, if it is found early enough, cancer is curable because the surgeon can "get it all."‡

The disturbing fact, however, is that breast cancer mortality rates have not declined significantly in the past half-century despite progressively earlier detection and treatment. Most of the medical profession has responded to this unexpected result by assuming that the solution is to discover the cancer still earlier. They emphasize improved detection techniques, especially mammography for cancers too small to feel.

In the past decade, many medical researchers, biostatisticians and interested laypersons have strongly questioned these assumptions. Considerable evidence now indicates that the period when cancer is confined to the breast is either nonexistent or so short that in many cases cancer exists elsewhere in the body before it is detectable in the breast. This *systemic theory* of cancer is now rapidly replacing the theory based on spread from a localized tumor. It is also becoming increasingly evident that different types of cancer behave very differently. Some data indicate that 25 per-

*National Surgical Adjuvant Breast Project.

†*Ibid.*

‡Almost all (90 percent) of lumps are discovered by women or their partners, either through breast self-exam or incidentally while washing, dressing, making love, etc. Today those lumps which do turn out to be malignant tend to be smaller and much less likely to be associated with disease in lymph nodes or other organs than the breast cancers doctors used to see regularly years ago. However, this earlier detection has not brought a corresponding improvement in survival or cure rates.

cent of women with breast cancer have a type which metastasizes rapidly right from the beginning. The remaining 75 percent are thought to have tumors which grow at varying rates, including a few very slow-growing ones which may never cause serious illness or death. Currently there is no way to predict who will develop which type of cancer, although postmenopausal women tend to have slower-growing breast cancers than premenopausal women.

For example, according to this new view of breast cancer, one common type of breast cancer may have a twelve-year course from the first abnormal cell to the resultant death. In year one or two, the very first cancer cells may circulate throughout the body, attaching themselves to other organs and beginning to grow while the tumor is forming in the breast. A strong immune system may be able to dispose of weaker or slower-growing metastases. By year three or four, the cancer may be visible on a mammogram. By year five or six, it can be felt by the woman or her doctor as a suspicious lump. In year seven or eight, metastases may begin to have their effect and the woman may notice that she does not feel as energetic or as well as she used to. By the tenth year, her health deteriorates significantly, and death comes in the twelfth year. Thus, for this common cancer, the time from first abnormal cell to death is twelve years.

If this woman's cancer is discovered in the sixth year after the first abnormal cell, she will be recorded as living six more years and will be included in five-year survival statistics. If it is detected by mammogram two years earlier (i.e., in the fourth year after the first abnormal cell), she will have eight years more and mammography and early detection will receive the credit for her increased survival. According to this new view of cancer, the early detection has not really made a difference, as the metastases (which are what kill, not the cancer in the breast) were present almost from the beginning.

What early detection has done in this case is increase the time that the woman was aware of her disease in addition to increasing the length of her treatments. If she is going to die anyway, proponents of this theory ask, what is the sense of her suffering two more years with the emotional drain of knowing she has cancer, or of living with a mastectomy or the possible effects of radiation or chemotherapy?

What is worse, they claim, is that this woman and thousands like her will be recorded as having lived two or three years longer due to early detection. This will inflate the statistics, making it appear that mammograms, chemotherapy, mastectomy, etc., improve survival rates when actually the disease has a course of about twelve years, and differences in survival only reflect where along that time line a particular woman's cancer is detected. Other breast cancers may have different time schedules—some very short, others so long that while the woman may eventually die of breast cancer twenty or thirty years after diagnosis, she has

by then lived as long as she could expect even without cancer. Or her cancer may still be there when she dies of some other cause.

Data to support this view is increasing, though it is not definitely proven yet. As we go to press, this theory is a more logical explanation for mortality and survival statistics than any other. If it should turn out that the *type* of cancer (fast- or slow-growing) is more important than *when* it is diagnosed, we will need to rethink our entire approach to cancer detection and treatment.

Those who now see breast cancer as a systemic disease of varying types conclude that earlier and earlier detection is not the definitive solution. In fact, they contend, the emphasis on early detection obscures a very serious problem—overtreatment of breast cancer. They warn that early detection without sufficient attention to cancer type has often led to overtreatment—in particular, to unnecessary mastectomy in cases of slow-growing cancers which would probably never have been life-threatening or in cases of fast-growing cancers which have already begun growing in other parts of the body long before the lump is found. (Until recently, all breast cancers were treated the same way, as if there were no differences in growth rates or other traits.)

What does this mean for us as women? Can we put off going to the doctor with an unusual lump? We can't know in advance whether our lump is benign or a fast- or slow-growing cancer. While the slow cancers may never be life-threatening and the fast ones may be beyond the help of current medical practices, there may also be a middle group of cancers for which early detection makes a difference. Consequently, until we have more compelling evidence, it is probably best to have any suspicious lump checked, although you may choose a period of self-screening first (see p. 490). You might want only a diagnosis, and then may want to look at some of the alternative therapies listed in the general section on cancer, starting on p. 527. If you know *for sure* that you would not choose any of the medical forms of cancer treatment currently available, then you may not even want to go for diagnosis.

If cancer is found, be as assertive as you can in demanding that the type of treatment you receive is appropriate for the type of cancer you have, and that it meets your needs.

More aggressive cancers may require more aggressive therapies, while slower, less invasive cancers may be best treated with more minimal therapies. There is already a trend in this direction, as more and more physicians adopt the systemic view of cancer.

For some of us, the systemic view has a special personal meaning. Those of us who have cancer have often blamed ourselves (or felt blamed by others) for not "finding it early enough," for not practicing breast self-exam faithfully or for not choosing to have periodic mammograms or regular medical checkups. Paying attention to breast changes and lumps is important, but we don't need to take on the extra burden of guilt for something that is out of our control, namely the type of cancer we have.

History of Breast Cancer Treatments and Current Treatment Controversy

For the better part of this century, almost everyone agreed that the Halsted radical mastectomy was *the* way to treat breast cancer. In 1960, over 90 percent of women in the U.S. who had surgery for breast cancer underwent this operation, which removes the entire breast plus the underlying muscles and the nearby lymph nodes. The Halsted radical leaves a woman with a sunken chest wall and usually a swollen, less mobile arm. Believing that cancer begins locally and then spreads in a predictable, gradual manner, physicians assumed that the more tissue they removed, the more likely that they would "get it all" and thus prevent the spread of the disease. Yet as the years went by, statistics failed to support this theory. Survival and mortality rates did not improve significantly.

Some doctors and laywomen began to question both the use of the radical mastectomy and the idea it was based on. They pointed to growing evidence that cancer may not begin locally and then spread in a predictable manner but may be microscopically present throughout the body from the very beginning of the disease (the systemic theory: see "Early Detection Controversy," p. 531). In a number of countries, including Canada, England and the Scandinavian countries, physicians were removing much less breast tissue than in the Halsted radical procedure and were getting almost identical survival rates. Slowly, American surgeons began to try these less extensive operations. In 1979, the National Cancer Institute declared that the Halsted was no longer the preferred treatment except in a few rare cases, and today the Halsted radical accounts for 5 percent or less of breast cancer operations.*

Still, most physicians have not retreated very far from the theory behind the Halsted radical. Now the most common treatment for breast cancer is the modified radical mastectomy, which removes the entire breast, some lymph nodes and some muscle (rather than all the underlying muscles and all the lymph nodes). This is less disfiguring and leads to fewer subsequent health problems. However, most of the above arguments against the Halsted also apply to the modified radical. Numerous studies have shown that this modified operation, like the Halsted before it, does not provide more protection than some of the even less extensive surgeries with radiation therapy.†

*National Cancer Institute, NIH Consensus Development Conference Summary, "The Treatment of Primary Breast Cancer: Management of Local Disease," Vol. 2, No. 5 (June 1979).

†U. Veronesi, et al. "Comparing Radical Mastectomy with Quadrantectomy, Axillary Dissection, and Radiotherapy in Patients with Small Cancers of the Breast," *The New England Journal of Medicine*, Vol. 305 (July 2, 1981), pp. 6–11.

Treatment Conflicts

Breast cancer treatment is one of the most controversial areas in medicine today. There are currently two main questions. First, how much surgery is necessary—must the surgeon remove just the lump, the lump plus some surrounding tissue or the entire breast? The second concerns the role of chemotherapy and radiation. Should these two therapies be used only after surgery has failed to halt the spread of the cancer? Or should one or both be employed immediately following surgery, even when there is no evidence of cancer anyplace else in the body? The trend is toward less extensive surgery with more chemotherapy and radiation, but the issues are by no means settled. All the controversy makes it difficult to sort out the competing claims.

In making their treatment decisions, women frequently feel caught between well-intentioned but competing factions with no way to determine what is best in their particular situation.

After I and the guy I live with had spent almost two hours with the surgeon, we came away convinced that simple mastectomy was the only sensible treatment. I so wanted to be sensible about it all. Then I went to Boston for a second opinion. I went up full of skepticism, feeling that they could never be as convincing as my New York surgeon, but that I must go through the motions to satisfy myself that I had heard the "other side" [in this case, for lumpectomy plus radiation]. It turned out that the "other side" was equally convincing, and I went back to New York feeling really torn. I felt like a statistic that was being wooed by both sides to show how successful their treatments were. "Good instincts," commented an oncologist friend. "That's precisely what it's all about." [This woman, after more research and much agonizing, went back to Boston for a lumpectomy plus radiation.]

The decision of what treatment to take is never easy. Sometimes one physician seems more reasonable. Sometimes your intuition will point strongly to a certain option. Sometimes one hospital is more conveniently located. Sometimes a friend's experience is influential. All these factors and more will enter into your final choice, which is often a compromise. In the end, each woman will make the decision in her own way, ideally with the most informed and friendly support possible.

Treatments

Most women receive a combination of the four types of conventional medical treatments—mastectomy, radiation, chemotherapy and hormone therapy. The *primary therapy* is the first treatment to the primary site of the cancer (the breast). *Adjuvant therapies* are any additional treatments following the primary treatment. Mastectomy is usually considered a primary treatment and chemotherapy an adjuvant.

Lumpectomy, mastectomy and radiation are *local therapies*, limited to the breast or other specific body area. In contrast, chemotherapy and hormone therapy are *systemic therapies* which circulate throughout the entire body, hopefully eliminating stray cancer cells which already exist in other parts of the body.

The goals of your various treatments depend on the stage of the cancer, its type and other factors such as your age and general health. Some treatments are intended to "cure," some to prolong life, some to produce remission of symptoms. Although these treatments may not result in increased survival time, quality of life may be improved. Other therapies primarily relieve pain or the side effects of the other treatments. *It is important that you ask your doctor to clearly explain the goal of each recommended treatment, its possible adverse effects and the most likely physical consequences of not taking the treatment.* Try to find out the statistical *five-, ten- and fifteen-year disease-free survival and mortality rates* for women with the same type and extent of disease (local, regional, metastatic), in the same menopausal status, who have selected the same treatment your doctor is recommending. You can then compare this information to results of other available treatments. (See questions in the general cancer section, p. 527.) All this will help you decide which treatments, if any, are best for your individual case.

Treatment Options for Local Disease (Usually Clinical Stages I and II)

The following *primary treatments* (surgery and radiation) are listed in order from least disfiguring and debilitating to most.

Procedures Which Remove Less than the Entire Breast

1. *Lumpectomy* (also called tylectomy, wide excision, segmental resection or partial mastectomy) removes the lump and a varying amount of surrounding tissue. Adverse effects include scarring and some disfiguring of the breast (though this may be only slightly more than that caused by the original biopsy), depending on the size of the lump and the size of the breast.

2. *Radiation therapy* is lumpectomy plus radiation. Therapy usually consists of radiation treatments to the breast five days a week for five weeks after the lump is removed. Radiation implants may also be placed in the breast for several days. Adverse effects include fatigue; muscle pain; dry, red, itchy skin; and extreme sun sensitivity. (Sun should be carefully avoided. A painful burn can occur even through a white blouse.) Occasionally (in 5 percent of women receiving the treatment) the radiation causes cracked ribs. An-

other 10 percent develop a lung ailment similar to bronchitis which lasts about a month, generally does not recur and is painful but not life-threatening.*

Quadrantectomy removes the quarter of the breast with the tumor and is usually followed by radiation. This surgery is performed mostly in Europe. Problems occur which are similar to those resulting from lumpectomy, but there is more breast disfigurement.

Procedures Which Remove the Entire Breast —Mastectomy

These are again listed from least to most disfiguring and debilitating.

1. *Simple mastectomy* (also called total mastectomy) removes the entire breast but leaves the chest muscles and lymph nodes. The adverse effects include the emotional trauma of losing a breast, scarring, and posture and balance problems related to the size and weight of the remaining breast.†

2. *Total mastectomy with auxiliary dissection* is the simple mastectomy plus a lymph node sample to stage the cancer. Adverse effects are the same as in simple mastectomy, with more scarring and occasional arm problems such as fatigue and swelling and the inability to raise the arm completely or to lift and carry heavy items, plus less overall resistance to infection.†

3. *Modified radical* removes the entire breast plus some muscle and lymph nodes. The negative effects are the same as for total mastectomy, except that arm problems are likely to be more frequent and severe, depending on the number of nodes and amount of muscle removed. The amount of muscle removed will also affect the appearance of the chest.†

4. *Radical mastectomy* (Halsted). As of 1979, this operation is not recommended by the National Cancer Institute (see p. 533). Adverse effects include all of the above. Arm problems tend to be severe and constant. The ribs and lungs, no longer protected by a layer of muscle, are more vulnerable to injury and illness.

There are variations within each surgical type and a multitude of different names for the same operation. Doctors also tend to use the terms differently. Thus one doctor's "modified radical" is another doctor's "total mastectomy plus lymph node sample." This makes it difficult to compare advice from different physicians. Sometimes the distinctions between procedures are blurred for insurance purposes. A few surgeons may cut (or report that they cut) a little bit more than

*Craig Henderson, et al. "Cancer of the Breast—The Past Decade (Medical Progress)," Parts I and II, *The New England Journal of Medicine*, Vol. 302 (January 3, 1980), pp. 17–30; (January 10, 1980), pp. 78–90.

†These procedures usually offer the option of reconstruction, however.

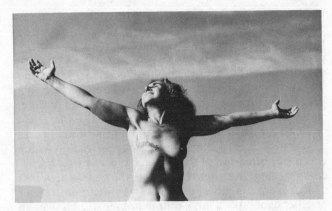

Woman with tatoo over mastectomy scar   *Hella Hammid*

the whole breast in order to qualify for the higher fees granted the more extensive surgery. In order to be sure you understand how much your surgeon intends to remove, *ask to see diagrams and photographs and have her/him explain why this particular surgery is being recommended for your type of cancer.*

Must I Have a Mastectomy?

In most cases, no. For Stages I and II breast cancer (which account for 90 percent of all cases), there appears to be no difference in long-term (fifteen- and thirty-year) survival rates for radical mastectomy, modified radical mastectomy, simple mastectomy and lumpectomy plus radiation.* Thus the least debilitating and disfiguring surgeries—lumpectomy plus radiation or simple mastectomy—seem to be enough. Studies on lumpectomy alone are not complete. It may turn out that it is as effective in many situations. All the other therapies have equivalent survival rates. Most surgeons, however, prefer some form of mastectomy because that is the operation they were originally taught and have experience with.

Doctors often try to dissuade women who want radiation therapy (lumpectomy plus radiation) by telling them that it is a new therapy and hasn't yet been proven over the long term. In fact, lumpectomy with radiation is new only in the U.S. In Canada and Europe, doctors have statistics showing that mastectomy and lumpectomy plus radiation have equivalent survival rates for twenty-five years from diagnosis.†

---

*A. Bluming. "Treatment of Primary Breast Cancer Without Mastectomy—A Review of the Literature," *Journal of the American Medical Association*, Vol. 72 (May 1982), pp. 820–28.

†M.V. Peters. "Wedge Resection With or Without Radiation in Early Breast Cancer," *International Journal of Radiation and Oncology, Biology and Physiology*, Vol. 2 (November–December 1977), pp. 1151–56. See also S. Mustakallio, "Conservative Treatment of Breast Carcinoma—Review of 25 Years Follow-Up," *Clinical Radiology*, Vol. 23 (1972), pp. 110–16.

If preserving your breast is not a central issue for you or reconstruction is an option, or if the lump is large and your breast small, mastectomy may be your best choice.

If lumpectomy plus radiation seems a reasonable choice for you, it's necessary to look for an experienced physician and a hospital with the needed equipment and staff experienced in the technique.

Treatment Options for Regional Disease

Regional disease refers to breast cancer which has extended to the lymph nodes. These adjuvant treatments are usually given in addition to one of the primary local therapies listed above for local disease.

1. *Chemotherapy* uses injections or tablets of anticancer drugs to reach malignant cells which are circulating or lodged throughout the body. Some of the chemotherapy agents have very serious side effects; others are mild. (See the discussion in the general cancer section, p. 525.)

Currently, only premenopausal women have shown much improved survival with chemotherapy. The gain is small—about 15 percent—but is statistically significant.* Postmenopausal women have fared as well without chemotherapy as with it. Many researchers think this is because the right combination of drugs has not yet been found for postmenopausal women. This may be the case, but postmenopausal women taking this therapy should know that the effectiveness of chemotherapy is unproven for their situation, and that they cannot necessarily expect the treatment to prolong their lives.

Therapy using a combination of drugs, especially the combination called CMF (Cyclophosphamide, Methotrexate and 5-Fluorouracil), has given better results than the use of single agents (one drug used alone).†

Tamoxifen, an antiestrogen drug, should be avoided by premenopausal women with ER − (estrogen-receptor)—negative readings, as one large trial showed that

---

*B. Fisher, et al. "Ten-Year Follow-Up Results of Patients With Carcinoma of the Breast in a Co-operative Clinical Trial Evaluating Surgical Adjuvant Chemotherapy," *Surgery, Gynecology and Obstetrics*, Vol. 140 (1975), pp. 528–34. See also B. Fisher, et al., "Disease-Free Survival at Intervals During and Following Completion of Adjuvant Chemotherapy: The NSABP Experience from Three Breast Cancer Protocols," *Cancer*, Vol. 48 (September 15, 1981).

†G. Bonadonna, et al. "Combination Chemotherapy as an Adjuvant Treatment in Operable Breast Cancer," *The New England Journal of Medicine*, Vol. 294, No. 8 (1976), pp. 405–10. See also B. Fisher, et al., "Ten-Year Follow-Up Results of Patients with Carcinoma of the Breast in a Co-operative Clinical Trial Evaluating Surgical Adjuvant Chemotherapy," *Surgery, Gynecology and Obstetrics*, Vol. 140 (1975), pp. 528–34; B. Fisher, et al., "Disease-Free Survival at Intervals During and Following Completion of Adjuvant Chemotherapy: The NSABP Experience from Three Breast Cancer Protocols," *Cancer*, Vol. 48 (September 15, 1981).

such premenopausal women receiving it actually had decreased survival times.*

How soon chemotherapy should begin and how long it should continue are still unknown. Some evidence indicates that any benefit that occurs happens early on. This evidence supports early chemotherapy after diagnosis and casts doubt on long courses of treatment.†

2. *Hormone Therapy.* The purpose of hormone therapy is to repress or eliminate estrogen in the body. It is useful only for women with estrogen-dependent cancers (also called ER+ or estrogen-positive, estrogen-rich or high-estrogen). Both surgery and drugs are used in hormone therapy.

Drugs. The antiestrogen drugs used most frequently, Tamoxifen and male hormones, often induce an early and sometimes permanent menopause. Some doctors include these drugs as part of chemotherapy, so you may not know that you are receiving them unless you ask.

Surgery. All the following are considered outmoded, as drugs can generally produce the same effects without the major problems associated with surgery. Some doctors try surgery when drugs and other treatments have not been successful:

Oophorectomy (surgical removal of the ovaries). This procedure is usually done only after chemical hormone therapy has been tried, but it is of almost no value in postmenopausal women or women under thirty-five. It sometimes helps in premenopausal women over age thirty-five.

Adrenalectomy (removal of the adrenals) or *hypothalectomy* (removal of the hypothalamus), other techniques to limit estrogen production.

Treatment Options for Metastatic Disease (Stage IV)

Once the cancer has metastasized, there is no known cure. All the above treatments are used in attempts to control the disease and prolong life. For example, radiation and chemotherapy may be used to relieve pain and shrink tumors. Mastectomy is probably unecessary unless the primary tumor is very large. A few women live beyond five or ten years with metastatic cancer.

What Are Your Chances? (The Prognosis of Breast Cancer)

Overall, the prognosis for breast cancer is not very encouraging. The mortality (death) rates presented in the literature are confusing. One group of researchers

*B. Fisher, et al. "Treatment of Primary Breast Cancer with Chemotherapy and Tamoxifen," *The New England Journal of Medicine*, Vol. 305 (1981), pp. 1–6.

†F.M. Schable. "Rationale for Adjuvant Chemotherapy," *Cancer*, Vol. 39 (1977), pp. 2875–82.

reports that one-third of women who get breast cancer die from it. This figure is based on the data reported to health authorities which show that each year approximately 100,000 new cases of breast cancer are diagnosed while about 33,000 women die from the disease. However, other researchers contend that this data is incomplete and often inaccurate, either because not all cancer deaths are reported or the cause of death may be listed as something other than breast cancer—such as pneumonia or heart disease—which was a complication of the breast cancer or breast cancer treatment. Studies that follow the course of breast cancer from diagnosis to death (whether from cancer or other causes) of a large number of individual women find that almost 80 percent of women who develop breast cancer eventually die from it. This rate has not changed significantly since the 1930s. However, some women live with the disease for as long as twenty or thirty years; while they do eventually die of breast cancer, their life spans have not been shortened. Many physicians no longer speak in terms of cure. Instead they refer to long-term remission or survival rates. According to this view, breast cancer, like diabetes or other chronic diseases, may be controlled but not yet cured.

Research has found that some groups of women do better than others. You are more likely to be among those with long-term survival if:

1. You are past menopause.

2. You have no malignant lymph nodes. This is the most important single predictor found so far. (See "Histological Stages," p. 531.)

3. Your cancer is estrogen dependent—has high levels of estrogen receptors. These ER-high (also called "positive") cancers tend to have fewer or later recurrences no matter what type of treatment is used. ER-high cancer is more common in postmenopausal women.

4. You have one of the following types of cancer and no positive nodes. These cancer cell types tend to grow and metastasize very slowly. They account for about 20 percent of all breast cancers.

- *in situ* cancer
- adenoid cystic-carcinoma
- colloid carcinoma
- comedo carcinoma
- medullary carcinoma
- papillary carcinoma
- tubular carcinoma

5. Your tumor cells are highly differentiated; that is, they retain the characteristics of normal breast cells rather than the embryonic appearance of advanced cancer cells.

Even with these indicators, it is difficult to make predictions for any specific woman. Some women (about 15 percent) with very good prognoses die quickly from the disease while a few (about 7 to 8 percent) of those whose conditions have been called terminal recover and live normal life spans. There are still many unknown factors. It may well be that an individual's particular immune system and general health as well as her emotional attitude may be as or more important than the treatment chosen.

Ongoing Studies

Each of the four studies noted below is in the process of comparing the survival, recurrence and metastases rates of large numbers of women with clinical Stages I and II breast cancers to determine if one kind of treatment is more effective than another. When finished, these studies may add new data or verify previous findings, thereby providing information for women faced with crucial treatment decisions. If you want information about the progress of the studies or would like to be a participant, contact the persons listed. Participants receive free travel, lodging and medical treatment. Each woman agrees to accept the researchers' assignment of which treatment she will receive, and be "followed up" (keep the researchers informed of her condition) for the rest of her life.

1. Comparison of modified radical to lumpectomy with radiation. Begun 1979. Preliminary results possibly ready 1984. Funded by NCI. Contact: Dr. Alan Lichter, (301) 496-5457.

2. Comparison of three therapies—modified radical, lumpectomy plus radiation and lumpectomy alone. All three therapies include lymph node sample for staging. Begun 1976. Preliminary results possibly available late 1984. Funded by NCI. Sponsored by NSABP.* Contact: Dr. Bernard Fisher, Dept. of Surgery, University of Pittsburgh, (412) 624-2671.

3. Comparison of results from various chemotherapies in both ER-positive and ER-negative Stages I and II breast cancers. Begun 1981. Preliminary results possibly available 1985. Contact: Mary Ketner, Executive Coordinator, Clinical Studies, University of Pittsburgh, (412) 624-2671.

4. Comparison of progress of women who eat a special low-fat diet (fat consumption limited to 20 percent of calories) compared to that of women who continue to consume their usual diet (average American diet consists of 40 percent fat). Begun 1983. Contact the National Cancer Institute (see Resources).

---

*National Surgical Adjuvant Breast Project.

While all cancers are frightening, breast cancer seems to hold the most terror for us as women. The available information is confusing and the experts often disagree. This makes it even more important that we become active participants in all stages of detection, treatment and decision-making. The information in this section is necessarily brief. You owe it to yourself to take the time to research all the available options and get additional opinions. If you have not read it already, we recommend turning to the general section on cancer next. It has more information on treatments (including alternatives to the accepted trio of surgery, radiation and chemotherapy). In this section, we have tried to make definite recommendations wherever possible, but so many areas are still unsettled that we can only indicate the issues involved and urge you to find out what new data have become available since the publication of this book.

Without

Without breasts
a woman's heart
rounds and softens her body,
bears her milk.

Without hair
a woman can fully
receive sunlight,
is crowned with the smoothness
of her scalp.

Without legs
a woman moves
with song and thought.

Without ears
she hears
what words
obscure.

Without eyes
she is not limited
by the confusion
of objects, color.

Without uterus, ovaries,
she spawns wisdom
with the turn of the moon.

Without her life's breath
a woman becomes earth,
the bearer of herb and seed,
rock and ground root.

Elana Klugman

Invasive Cancer of the Cervix

If severely abnormal cells have spread beyond the upper tissue layer (surface epithelium) of your cervix into the underlying connective tissues, you have invasive cervical cancer. A Pap smear followed by a biopsy can determine this. At first the spread is very shallow and may not involve the lymph or blood systems. In its early stages, cervical cancer is 100 percent curable.

Most physicians recommend a hysterectomy (removal of the uterus) with close follow-up. If the cancer has spread into the lymph or blood system, physicians usually suggest radiation or hysterectomy/oophorectomy. (Chemotherapy is not as effective as local radiation.) Sometimes a combination of the two is used.

Radiation treatment is given in two ways. If the tumor is large, you will be given external radiation daily over a period of several weeks. During treatment you will have to make daily trips to the medical center or hospital which, depending on how far away you live, can be exhausting and cause you considerable inconvenience. This is a time to ask family and friends to help with your other commitments and as traveling company and support. Negative effects of the radiation treatment include diarrhea, skin changes, rectal bleeding and fatigue. Since each person reacts to radiation differently, the amount may have to be increased or decreased depending on your response. The negative effects of the radiation therapy are thought to be short-lived. When the radiation treatment has reduced the size of the growth, internal radioactive materials are placed inside your uterus or in the upper portion of your vagina. You will be hospitalized and given general anesthesia for this procedure. The implants are left inside your body from one to three days while you are in the hospital. This type of treatment directs a greater amount of radiation to a smaller area. Radiation treatment for early invasive cancer has a 60 to 90 percent survival rate, depending on the size of the tumor and the amount of spread. (See p. 522 for a general discussion of cancer and survival rates.)

Surgical treatment for invasive cancer usually involves a radical hysterectomy.

You should be involved in your treatment and have the final say in all decisions concerning your cancer. If you have any doubts about treatments recommended by your physician, get a second and third opinion if you can.

Ovarian Cancer

Ovarian cancer is a malignant tumor of the ovaries. While it is less common than cervical or uterine cancer, ovarian cancer affects 17,000 new women a year in the U.S. The exact causes are still unknown, but it is clear that women who have never had children, postmenopausal women and women who have breast cancer or cancer of the intestines or rectum are at increased risk for ovarian cancer. Women who work in the electrical, textile and rubber industries, have received extensive pelvic radiation or live in urban areas seem to develop it more often than others. Women with a family history of ovarian cancer, women who are very overweight and those who have taken estrogen other than in the birth control pill also are prone

to develop this cancer.* Recent evidence suggests that the regular use of talcum powder on genitals and/or sanitary napkins increases the risk by as much as three times.†

Early signs are often vague. They include mild stomach upsets, gas and abdominal pain. Sometimes there is tenderness and pain from a build-up of fluid within the pelvic and abdominal cavity caused by irritated gland cells.

Diagnosis

Your practitioner may suspect ovarian cancer if during a pelvic exam your ovary feels enlarged or less mobile than normal, or if s/he feels unusual growths. Diagnostic tests may include ultrasound and X-rays of your stomach and bowel, and a CAT scan. You may also have a blood test to check for cancers which produce their own protein or hormonal substances. If you have surgery, a frozen section of cystic or solid tumor will indicate whether the entire ovary should be removed, as well as the need for further surgery.

Medical Treatments

The many types of ovarian cancer differ in their sensitivity to different types of therapy. Current medical options include radiation, chemotherapy and surgery, with a combination of chemotherapy and surgery appearing to be most effective. Radiation treatment is used in special circumstances, such as when your overall health makes major surgery risky. Because ovarian cancer is difficult to detect early, its cure rate is only 10 to 20 percent. See "Introduction to Cancer," p. 522, for more on treatments.

Cancer of the Uterus

Cancer of the lining of the uterus (endometrial cancer) is the most common pelvic cancer, affecting fourteen out of every 10,000 women yearly. Most women who develop this cancer are past menopause and in their fifties; 10 percent are still menstruating. If you are overweight, if you have diabetes, high blood pressure or a hormone imbalance which combines high estrogen levels with infrequent ovulation, or if you take synthetic estrogen, your risk of developing uterine cancer is increased. During the early 1970s there was a sharp rise in the incidence of uterine cancer due to increased use of estrogen therapy (ERT) to relieve

---

*While removal of the ovaries (oophorectomy) is frequently suggested in order to protect women who are at risk for ovarian cancer, the possible risks and effects of this operation do not justify it. (See "Hysterectomy and Oophorectomy," p. 511.)

†See Brigham and Woman's Hospital Study, reported in *Cancer*, July 15, 1982. See also D. L. Longo and R. C. Young, "Cosmetic Talc and Ovarian Cancer," *Lancet*, Vol. 2 (August 1979), pp. 349–51.

symptoms of menopause. (See pp. 447–48.) Bleeding after menopause is the most common symptom of uterine cancer. For women who are still menstruating, increased menstrual flow and bleeding between periods may be the only symptoms. Unfortunately, the Pap smear is unreliable in detecting the abnormal cells of uterine cancer. If you are premenopausal, your practitioner may suggest a D and C as the first step because it not only screens for cancer but frequently relieves abnormal bleeding from a variety of less serious causes. If you are postmenopausal, you will probably have an aspiration or endometrial biopsy (an office procedure), and if the biopsy is not conclusive, your practitioner may suggest a D and C. Before agreeing to a D and C, however, make sure that you have both considered the risks and discussed alternatives for diagnosis and treatment of abnormal bleeding (see p. 508).

Prevention and Self-Help Treatments

Since endometrial cancer appears to be influenced by factors such as obesity, hypertension or diabetes, controlling these conditions with self-help methods may prevent this type of cancer from developing or spreading.

Medical Treatments

Medical treatment for uterine cancer includes surgery, radiation and chemotherapy. There is wide disagreement about which is best. Outside the U.S. radiation is used frequently with good results. In this country radical hysterectomy is the most common treatment, sometimes with follow-up radiation after surgery if the tumor was large, if spread to lymph nodes was suspected or if the cellular changes were more excessive than usual. If you should have a return of the cancer after one of the above treatments, progesterone treatments may help slow its spread.

When uterine cancer is found early, the success rate of conventional treatments is very high.

DIABETES

Diabetes, a very common metabolic disorder more prevalent among women than men,* changes the way our bodies break down and use starches and sugars (glucose). Normally insulin, a hormone produced in the pancreas, helps to convert glucose to energy that can be used immediately or stored by our body cells. Eighty to 90 percent of diabetes is non-insulin-dependent diabetes (NIDD), in which the pancreas produces insulin but the body is not able to utilize it effectively.

Less common is insulin-dependent diabetes (IDD), where there is a deficiency or total lack of insulin which must be replaced by injection.

Untreated diabetes can cause heart and kidney disease, blindness, problems in pregnancy or childbirth and nerve and blood vessel damage, and can reduce our ability to fight infection. Insulin-dependent diabetics may face coma or death from either a lack of insulin (hyperglycemia, or high blood sugar) or an overdose of insulin (hypoglycemia, or low blood sugar).

Non-insulin-dependent diabetes, formerly called "maturity onset diabetes," most often occurs in people over forty. Symptoms usually develop slowly and may include weakness, headache, a vaguely sick feeling, extra hunger and thirst, more frequent urination, itching and minor skin or vaginal infections.

In contrast, insulin-dependent diabetes—formerly called "juvenile onset diabetes"—usually begins before the age of eighteen with severe and rapidly-developing symptoms. These include greatly increased hunger, thirst and urination and a sudden, dramatic loss of weight.

The underlying causes of diabetes are still being investigated. A diet high in sugar and simple carbohydrates may cause latent diabetes to become overt. NIDD seems to be closely associated with weight. Eighty-five percent of all NIDD diabetics are 20 percent above their so-called "ideal weight."* For reasons not yet understood, obesity seems to make cells less sensitive to insulin, with the result that even producing more insulin than normal isn't enough to keep up with the body's demand. NIDD often disappears with weight loss. It is not clear, however, that being overweight actually *causes* diabetes. Other nutritional factors, such as the effect of repeated dieting or the amount of sugar in the diet, may be involved. (See Chapter 2, "Food.") Diabetes is linked to hereditary factors. IDD may also be triggered by viral illnesses in those who are genetically susceptible to the disease.

Diagnosis

If a routine blood or urine test shows abnormally high levels of sugar, health workers will suspect diabetes whether or not there are symptoms. A common diagnostic test measures blood glucose before and after eating, and the results are compared. A similar test, the glucose tolerance test, may also be used.

We can use simple urine tests at home to monitor blood sugar levels. This can help us to prevent serious problems as well as evaluate the treatment we are using.

---

*The peak ages are forty-five to fifty-four, when women develop it twice as often as men, after which the rate declines slightly.

*Since these "ideal weight" figures are being revised upward, it is not certain what the implications will be for treatment of diabetes.

Prevention and Self-Help

While there is no cure for diabetes, the best way to prevent and control it is through diet and exercise. The vast majority of people with diabetes who are not totally dependent on insulin can control the disease through diet and exercise alone, while the remainder can usually substantially reduce the amount of insulin needed.*

The *traditional* diet for diabetes restricts carbohydrates (starches) and is therefore high in fat. Current research indicates that diets *high* in *complex* carbohydrates† and fiber not only help our bodies to handle glucose more effectively but also lower the risks of long-term complications such as heart disease, stroke, blindness, kidney disease and gangrene.

Some new studies have shown that certain starchy foods such as white potatoes and rice (brown or white) can raise blood sugar levels higher than very sweet foods such as bananas, ice cream and some candy bars. Foods which raise the blood sugar level a great deal are said to have a high "glycemic index." However, we should not exaggerate the importance of these findings, for example, to the point where we suggest that it's perfectly fine for diabetic persons to put maple syrup on their pancakes or substitute pastries for carrots, which have a high glycemic index. Even though it is probably true that the considerable fat content of some sweet foods (e.g., ice cream) causes a more gradual rise in blood sugar, it is also true that the fat itself may contribute to other problems (such as heart disease and certain cancers) which are far more serious than high blood sugar levels. The glycemic index can be a useful guide, but keep in mind other factors. (See "Diabetics and the Glycemic Index," by Bonnie Liebman, listed in Resources.)

In general, avoid saturated fats and sugar. It is also advisable to eat several small meals during the day rather than three large ones. Since animal studies on all the artificial sweeteners (whether FDA-approved or not) show some risks, it seems prudent to avoid them, certainly for routine use. *Note:* If you are taking insulin and want to change to a high-carbohydrate diet, do so gradually and inform your practitioner, as your insulin requirements will need to be adjusted.

Diets consisting largely of processed foods may also lack important minerals. If your diet is low in zinc, which helps the pancreas synthesize insulin, a supplement of thirty milligrams a day may be helpful. (Too much can be harmful.) You might also find out about chromium supplements (which help the cells absorb sugar) in an organic yeast-based form called the "glucose tolerance factor." The usual dose is 200 micrograms a day. (*Note:* Dosages vary according to individual needs and diet.)

In addition to diet, regular exercise (such as walking or jogging) further reduces the body's need for insulin and therefore helps to prevent as well as control the disease. Exercise can also help with weight loss in cases of weight-related NIDD.

Medical Treatments

Despite the evidence that diet and exercise are the safest, cheapest and most effective treatment for the majority of us who are not totally insulin-dependent, many physicians continue to prescribe insulin for all cases of NIDD. They focus their research on new types of insulin and new ways of administering it. Yet according to some researchers, only about one-quarter of people on insulin therapy are actually completely insulin-dependent.* Unnecessary insulin may cause heart disease and promote weight gain.† One study showed that those receiving insulin do not live as long as those using diet and exercise.

Hypoglycemic pills, an alternative to insulin (which make the cells more sensitive to insulin and thereby reduce the amount of glucose in the blood) are useful, especially for people who can't stay on a strict diet or for whom diet alone doesn't work.

Those of us who are completely insulin-dependent (IDD) must take insulin by injection, as it cannot be absorbed by mouth. The correct dosage depends on food intake, exercise and levels of glucose in the blood and urine. An insulin overdose can cause acute hypoglycemia, which can lead to coma and death. Some researchers think that many diabetes complications are actually caused by insulin overdoses.

HYPERTENSION, HEART DISEASES AND CIRCULATORY DISEASES

Hypertension

Hypertension (high blood pressure) is sometimes called "the silent killer" because it is often symptomless and, when untreated, can lead to heart disease and strokes, the leading killers of both men and women in the United

---

*Bonnie Liebman. "Food Over Pharmaceuticals," *Nutrition Action* (March 1982), p. 11.

†Complex carbohydrates include foods such as whole grains, beans and vegetables. Simple carbohydrates which contribute to diabetes include processed foods—white flour, white rice, pasta, cakes, cookies, etc. For more information, see Chapter 2, "Food."

*Bonnie Liebman. "Food Over Pharmaceuticals," *Nutrition Action* (March 1982), p. 11.

†"Insulin May Do Harm to Adult Diabetics," *Prevention*, April 1978.

States. Untreated, it can also affect the brain and eyes and cause serious problems during pregnancy.

About 20 percent of women of all ages in this country develop hypertension at some point in their lives. (Even children may do so.) No one yet knows how hypertension in women thirty-five and under affects life expectancy, an increasingly important question as larger numbers of women who are or have been taking oral contraceptives move into this age range. (About 25 percent of all women who use oral contraceptives develop hypertension.) In addition, blood pressure tends to rise naturally with age.

Women of color, especially blacks, seem to be more susceptible to hypertension than white women. This is probably due to a combination of environmental, dietary, stress and genetic factors.

Symptoms

Severe cases of hypertension may be accompanied by warning symptoms such as headache, dizziness, fainting spells, ringing in the ears and nosebleeds. However, you can develop hypertension without realizing it. The only way to get a sure diagnosis is to take periodic blood pressure readings. Sometimes special tests are necessary (see below).

Cause

Approximately 5 percent of all cases of high blood pressure are caused by glandular or hormonal abnormalities. But in the other 95 percent, no single obvious cause is found. This is called "essential hypertension." Causes other than oral contraceptives are still being investigated, including diet, properties of the water supply, victim's size, stress and heredity. Many of these factors may interact to cause hypertension.

Diet, and excess salt intake in particular, is thought to play a key role in causing hypertension. The average American diet contains ten to fifteen grams of sodium a day (about five to ten times as much salt as our bodies need). Meat and dairy products contain a fair amount of salt naturally, while canned and processed foods, fast foods, snacks and soft drinks have large amounts of salt added during processing.

Cadmium, a trace element found in white-flour products and in many water supplies, has been strongly linked to hypertension. Hypertension is much more common in areas where water is soft, perhaps because the acid in soft water extracts cadmium from the surrounding earth and rocks.

Research shows that those of us who are very overweight are at greater risk for developing hypertension. Nevertheless, there is no evidence that obesity itself causes hypertension. The stress associated with being fat in a "thin" society may well be a more important factor. While some studies show that losing weight can be as effective as diet or drugs in controlling hypertension, others indicate that regular exercise is much more important than the amount of weight loss.

Stress is also linked to hypertension. When we are under pressure or tense, blood pressure, breathing rate and heartbeat all tend to increase. When our lives are continually stressful, we have a greater chance of developing high blood pressure.

Finally, those of us with a family history of hypertension are at somewhat greater risk.

Diagnosis

Blood pressure is described by two numbers (for example, 120/70). The top number is the systolic pressure (the force of the blood in the arteries when the heart is pumping blood out). The bottom number is the diastolic pressure (the force of the blood in the arteries when the heart is filling with blood). In general, a systolic pressure of above 140 or a diastolic pressure above 90 are considered signs of hypertension.

Blood pressure varies with the time of day, activity and stress. Only a *consistent* elevation of the blood pressure means hypertension. At least three elevated blood pressure readings, taken days or weeks apart, should be obtained before hypertension is diagnosed and treated. Some researchers think that a diagnosis of mild or borderline hypertension should be delayed until consistent readings have been obtained over a period of years, since slightly elevated blood pressures fall by themselves within a few years in a majority of cases. Also, since women normally have higher blood pressure than men, the distinction between "normal" and "borderline hypertensive" is difficult to interpret. For example, it is normal for blood pressure to rise during pregnancy (temporarily) and after menopause, and to fluctuate more as part of the aging process. (Older women often need more than one blood pressure reading for an accurate diagnosis.)

Since the stress related to a medical exam or procedure may raise blood pressure, make an effort to check your blood pressure when you are not anxious—perhaps at home, at work or at a neighborhood health center. Large women should be sure to use a cuff big enough to fit around the arm; otherwise they may get a false inflated reading. Taking blood pressure is an easy skill to learn. (Kits with stethoscope and blood pressure cuffs are available in drugstores and many discount and department stores for forty dollars or less. Families and friends can share the cost and the equipment.) Checking blood pressure is a type of preventive health care we can provide for ourselves and each other. Increasingly, libraries, senior centers and shopping centers are also providing this screening service, but *don't* rely on coin-operated machines, which are not always adjusted properly and can give false readings.

Prevention and Self-Help Treatments

You can often prevent hypertension in a number of simple ways, and also lower mildly raised blood pressure—enough, in many cases, to eliminate the need for potentially risky drug treatments.

1. Diet is probably the single most important factor in preventing and treating mild hypertension. Gradually restrict salt intake by avoiding processed foods and eliminating salt during cooking and at the table. Replace white flour with whole grains whenever possible and make sure to include enough protein, potassium and calcium in your diet (see Chapter 2, "Food"). Eating garlic can also help to prevent or reduce slightly elevated blood pressure. Some people also recommend Vitamin-B and potassium supplements to help the body excrete excess fluids and sodium.

2. Avoid smoking. Studies show smoking contributes to heart disease. Also, keep alcohol consumption down to two ounces a day or less.

3. Get together with people in your community to investigate the water supply. If you find that it contains cadmium, try to eat less of this trace mineral in foods (especially white-flour products). A high salt level may call for changes in winter highway maintenance, or in wetlands development.

4. Avoid combination oral contraceptives and other estrogens. If you do take the Pill, insist on finding out your blood pressure both before and a few months *after* starting. If it is initially high, don't take the Pill; if it rises, switch to another contraceptive.

5. Regular aerobic exercise (such as fast walking, jogging or bicycling) often brings slightly elevated pressures down to normal.

6. Losing weight if you are very large can prevent or lower high blood pressure. It is most effective in conjunction with exercise. Crash dieting, however, is *not* recommended.

7. Try to reduce stress in your life. Biofeedback, meditation and relaxation therapies may help.

Medical Treatments

When the above methods do not work or hypertension becomes severe, you may need drugs. Diuretics (which eliminate water from the tissues) are the most commonly used. Other antihypertensive drugs reduce the amount of blood pumped from the heart or relax the blood vessels. Often a combination of the two is used. (See p. 36 for guidelines in taking drugs.) Also, hypertension drugs treat only the symptoms of the disease; they do not cure it. You will probably have to take medication for life. Be cautious when physicians recommend drug therapy without attempting less risky methods first. If your hypertension is severe, you will have to evaluate the risk of taking medication against the benefits of preventing a crippling or life-threatening stroke.*

Heart Diseases and Circulatory Diseases

Are Heart Diseases and Circulatory Diseases Women's Problems?

Most people typically think of men, not women, as having heart attacks. Most research on the subject, therefore, has been on men. Yet although men do suffer more heart attacks than women, heart disease is the most frequent cause of death in women over the age of fifty-five. In addition, a greater percentage of women who have heart attacks die from them. Until heart disease research focuses on women more adequately, the reason for this will probably remain unexplained.

Women are far more likely than men to have strokes. While overall stroke deaths have been declining since 1950, as we approach menopause our rates of death from cerebral vascular disease and stroke already surpass men's and continue to climb faster thereafter. Stroke is directly related to high blood pressure, which becomes much more common after menopause and is more chronic among women.

What Are These Diseases?

Atherosclerosis is a slowly developing disease process in which the passageway through the arteries becomes narrowed and roughened by fatty deposits called plaques. In the most common type of heart disease, called coronary artery disease or ischemic heart disease, the development of plaque blocks one or more of the arteries that supply the heart muscle with blood. When sufficient blood can no longer reach the heart, part of the heart dies from lack of oxygen and other nutrients. This is a "heart attack," or what physicians call a myocardial infarction (MI), coronary thrombosis or coronary occlusion. When the artery blockage is partial it may cause chest pain, a condition referred to as angina.

Atherosclerosis can also lead to a narrowing of the blood vessels which supply blood to the brain. Called a stroke, or cerebral hemorrhage, this leads to the death of that part of the brain.

Less common types of circulatory disease are congenital heart disease, phlebitis, hypertrophic disease, vulvular heart disease and cardiomyopathy. The causes

---

*Since no long-term studies show the percentage of persons with hypertension who can reduce their blood pressures through nondrug approaches, it is impossible to say how many people really require drugs. Most doctors have little interest in nondrug approaches. However, studies comparing people treated by drugs with others treated by diet alone do show comparable effects and a longer life span among the diet-treated group.

are similar for all and may lead to congestive heart failure or arrhythmia (irregular heart beats).

Who Is at Risk?

The more of the following risk factors a person has, the more likely she or he is to develop atherosclerosis and subsequent heart disease, circulatory problems or stroke. The first three (in that order) are the best-established risk factors at present.

- High blood pressure (hypertension).
- Smoking.
- Elevated serum (blood) cholesterol.*
- Diabetes.
- Taking oral contraceptives (particularly if the woman also smokes). (See Chapter 13, "Birth Control.").
- A family history of coronary artery disease *and* a husband with a history of heart attack.
- Over age fifty (heart attack is uncommon in women under the age of fifty). Most women are protected from serious heart and circulatory conditions while ovulating regularly, which is why deaths rise dramatically after menopause. The source of this protective effect is not clear.†
- Hysterectomy before age forty-five (see p. 513).
- Studies have indicated that certain "personality" factors (habitual impatience, hostility, high competitive drive, for instance) may predict heart attacks and can be minimized by stress-reduction techniques. However, these studies have been done almost exclusively on men.‡

Prevention

Considering the seriousness of these diseases, we are disturbed that so few resources are directed toward prevention as compared to emergency care and treatment. We are also concerned that very little is known about how to prevent heart disease and stroke specif-

*Cholesterol can be of two types: HDL (high-density lipoproteins) and LDL (low-density lipoproteins, including VLDL, or very-LDL). If you have elevated cholesterol, chances are it is of the LDL type which is associated with coronary heart disease and heart attack risk. Be sure to ask your doctor which type you have, since elevated HDL levels definitely protect against heart attack. Certain foods and activities definitely raise HDL levels. (See "Aging and Preventive Health;" p. 453.)

†However, preliminary studies of women taking menopausal estrogens appear to show that they receive some protection against fatal heart attacks. See *Health Facts* (September 1983), p. 5.

‡Many people speculate that when women are in the workforce as much as men, their heart attack rates will rise accordingly. So far, only one study shows this, and it only shows it for women married to blue-collar husbands or who have several children. (Smoking is much more prevalent among women from working-class backgrounds.) Another study shows *lower* cholesterol levels among working women, even when all other factors are controlled.

ically for women. The "experts" seem to assume that what is good for men must be good for women, too.

1. *Smoking.* The more you smoke, the more likely you are to have a heart attack. Women smokers who take oral contraceptives are especially at risk for both heart attack and stroke. We urge you to give up smoking. For particulars on women and smoking, see Chapter 3, "Alcohol, Mood-Altering Drugs and Smoking."

2. *Diet.* Diet is probably an important factor in preventing heart disease, although the scientific evidence is not absolute. Eating saturated fats tends to raise blood cholesterol (of the LDL type) so cutting back on these fats (see p. 15 in Chapter 2, "Food") will probably help prevent heart disease. However, the food industry has been capitalizing on the low-cholesterol issue by promoting highly processed hydrogenated foodstuffs as beneficial because they are "polyunsaturated." Many scientists now question the value of eating more polyunsaturates and are increasingly concerned about the negative health effects of highly processed foods.

Current medical advice to avoid foods high in cholesterol and saturated fats may pose special problems for women. In an effort to reduce fat intake, some women may eliminate or cut back on dairy products, which may be their main source of calcium. (Inadequate calcium is a factor in the development of osteoporosis and hypertension.) No prevention study we know of has included women, a serious flaw considering that hormonal factors are believed to affect the ways in which dietary cholesterol is converted into serum cholesterol, the type of cholesterol which is known to increase the risk of heart disease.

3. *High blood pressure.* Many experts feel that high blood pressure (hypertension) can be controlled by dietary and lifestyle changes (reducing salt and weight, stopping smoking and increasing calcium intake, exercise and relaxation) without resorting to drugs. Because of most drugs' potential negative effects, including earlier death, this effort is worthwhile. In some cases, however, drugs may become essential for reducing blood pressure so as to reduce the risk of both heart attack and stroke.

4. *Exercise.* Regular exercise is believed to reduce the risk of heart attack, can definitely lower blood pressure and, in some cases, raises beneficial HDL cholesterol levels (see Chapter 4, "Women in Motion").

5. *Weight.* Excess weight itself does not directly affect the heart, but it may increase blood pressure, cholesterol and blood-sugar levels, which increase the risk of heart disease and stroke. A combination of general weight reduction and exercise can be an important strategy for reducing the risk of cardiovascular and circulatory disease in some women.

Heart Attack

Recognizing the Signs of Heart Attack

Unfortunately, the first sign of heart disease can be sudden death from heart attack, especially for women. One-fourth of all people who have heart attacks had no previous "warning" or knowledge of heart disease, and 60 percent of heart-attack deaths occur before the person reaches the hospital.

Symptoms of Heart Attack

Do you have *one or more* of the following for more than two minutes:
1. Chest pain and shortness of breath?
2. Irregular pulse?
3. Sweating or dizziness?
4. Severe pain in your jaw, neck, shoulder or arm?

If so, seek medical attention immediately.

Some describe the pain as viselike or constricting, like a rope being pulled around their chest. Others describe the pain as feeling like a heavy weight crushing their chest. It is useful to know that chest pain can also come from conditions other than heart attack.* Heart pains that occur with exertion but go away with rest indicate angina, a condition which may not be immediately life-threatening but which should be evaluated by a physician.

Getting Help

If you, or anyone you are with, experience heart-attack symptoms, CALL A PHYSICIAN OR AMBULANCE OR GO TO A HOSPITAL IMMEDIATELY. DO NOT WAIT TO SEE IF THE SYMPTOMS GO AWAY! As women, we may be afraid of being seen as "hysterical" or feel that we will be ridiculed for going to the hospital unless we have something "really serious." To ignore heart-attack symptoms is to risk our lives.

Most cities have ambulances staffed by paramedics who are trained to administer cardiopulmonary resuscitation (CPR)* and to monitor the heart rate and rhythm and administer intravenous drugs on the order of physicians with whom they are in contact by radio. It is important to keep calm. Medical personnel often give the person an analgesic drug such as morphine to induce relaxation and relieve chest pain. Oxygen may also be given.

Most urban hospitals have special coronary care units where sudden changes in the rhythm of the heart can be detected immediately and treated, reducing both damage to the heart and the likelihood of death. Every effort should be made to seek emergency medical care from a well-equipped and well-staffed hospital.

Treatments

For women who have had a heart attack or who have been diagnosed as having coronary artery disease or angina, there are two approaches to treatment: medical and surgical. Within the medical and scientific communities, there is considerable controversy over the relative effectiveness of these two approaches.

Coronary bypass surgery, popular in recent years, is done primarily to relieve chest pain which persists in some people after a heart attack. Coronary bypass surgery involves removing a vein from the leg and attaching it to the coronary artery to "bypass" the obstructed area. Some people experience dramatic relief of pain and can lead physically active lives after surgery. There is no evidence, however, that surgery increases life expectancy.† Nonetheless, over 100,000 procedures are done each year in the U.S. at a cost of over 1.5 billion dollars.

Several excellent studies have shown that more conservative treatment is equal or superior to bypass surgery for most people.‡ This medical approach to treatment focuses on *heart conditioning*—a program of progressively more strenuous exercise combined with a low-fat diet, relaxation techniques and drug therapy. Blood pressure is lowered and participants are urged to stop smoking. (For some participants, any exercise at all is dangerous.)

Before having bypass surgery, even for seemingly intractable pain, a woman may want to consult with a cardiologist who specializes in the *medical* treatment

---

*Chest pain can also come from muscles in the chest, the lungs, the diaphragm, spine or organs in the upper abdomen. Often it is difficult even for practitioners to determine the pain's precise origin. Shooting pains that last a few seconds are common in young people, and a "catching" sensation at the end of a deep breath does not need attention. Chest-wall pain, rarely present at the same time as a heart attack, can often be identified by pressing a finger on the spot, which would increase the pain. Hyperventilation (too rapid breathing which changes the carbon dioxide balance in the blood) can cause both dizziness and chest pain.

*CPR is an emergency procedure combining mouth-to-mouth resuscitation and closed-chest heart massage. In some U.S. cities, CPR is credited with saving as many as 200 lives a year. To learn CPR, call your local chapter of the American Red Cross or American Heart Association.

†For an excellent discussion of the controversy with reference to the medical literature, see Marcia Millman's *The Unkindest Cut: Life in the Backrooms of Medicine*, pp. 215–52 (New York: William Morrow and Co., Inc., 1978). See also Office of Technology Assessment, U.S. Congress, "Assessing the Efficacy and Safety of Medical Technologies," GPO Stock No. 052-003-00593-O, September 1978.

‡For only one group, those with obstruction of the left main coronary artery, does surgery improve chances of survival.

of heart disease. If your family doctor or a clinic refers you to a heart surgeon who advises surgery, try to get a second opinion from a medically oriented cardiologist who is not part of your surgeon's immediate colleague network. This will insure that you get a truly different treatment perspective. A final note of caution: the death rates for heart surgery vary enormously from hospital to hospital. Generally, well-known university-affiliated medical centers with specialized coronary surgery teams have the best records. The more frequently the teams operate, the less often their patients die. *Never consider undergoing bypass surgery at a hospital where fewer than 200 bypass operations are performed each year.** (See the section on surgery, p. 482.)

Stroke

Because high blood pressure is easily detectable, stroke is among the most preventable of the causes of sudden death. Yet true prevention, as described above, must begin *before* high blood pressure appears.

Strokes may be very mild, so mild that you or your practitioner may not recognize them. They may cause only minor or temporary impairment. These are called *transient ischemic attacks*, or TIAs. When an artery bursts because of high blood pressure, either damaging part of the brain or impairing its function due to the pressure of pooled blood, the result is a *cerebral hemorrhage*. Depending on the type of stroke you have, if you survive you may experience speech loss, paralysis or other loss of mental and physical function. Rehabilitation and therapy sometimes achieve remarkable results by helping undamaged parts of the brain to "take over," but there is no way of reversing the brain damage itself, and frequently there is no improvement.

Signs of Stroke or TIA

These include intense, mounting headache lasting many hours; sudden or gradual blackout; dizziness or vision problems; sudden weakness or numbness in the face, arms, fingers, toes; slurring of speech; difficulty in walking. Any one or more of these symptoms call for action, even though they may happen over several hours. Go immediately to a hospital emergency room or call your regular physician (if s/he is unavailable,

leave a message to meet you there). While less can be done to save a life than in the case of heart attack, prompt treatment may reduce impairment, prevent another stroke (they tend to come in threes) and maximize future functioning.

SYSTEMIC LUPUS ERYTHEMATOSUS (SLE)

Systemic lupus erythematosus, a connective tissue disease characterized by inflammation, can affect different parts of the body, especially the skin, joints, blood and kidneys. Its cause is unknown, though certain predisposing traits may be inherited. (These may or may not result in the actual development of SLE.) Certain drugs (including birth control pills), stress, exposure to sun, infections and pregnancy can trigger SLE, though the mechanism is unknown. SLE is an autoimmune disorder, which means that the body's immune system becomes defective and produces antibodies against *normal* parts of the body, causing tissue injury. A hallmark of this disease is often unusual fatigue, a sign of generalized inflammation. As with arthritis, people with SLE have both flare-ups and remissions (symptom-free periods).

Close to a million women in the U.S. have SLE—*ten times more than the number of men affected*. Also, SLE is three times more common in blacks than in whites. These two factors may explain why knowledge of and research into SLE has been so inadequate.

Since SLE is so often misdiagnosed and therefore mistreated, it is important for women to learn about the characteristics and symptoms of SLE. Any four of the following could indicate the presence of SLE: 1. facial rash ("butterfly" across the cheeks); 2. other disclike lesions or rash marks ("discoid lupus"); 3. whitening of fingers after exposure to cold (Reynaud's phenomenon); 4. hair loss; 5. mouth or nasal ulcers; 6. arthritis *without* deformity; 7. inflammation of the lining of the lungs or heart (pleuritis or pericarditis), often indicated by shortness of breath and/or chest pains; 8. light-sensitivity; 9. convulsions; 10. anemia, low white-blood or platelet count; 11. presence of cells without nuclei (LE cells); 12. chronic false-positive tests for syphilis; and 13. excessive protein or cellular casts in the urine. You can detect the last few symptoms only through lab tests, which you should request if you think you have SLE. Other characteristics include fever, muscle weakness, joint pains and/or redness as well as the fatigue mentioned above. While many women with lupus have these symptoms, others simply don't feel well but can't put their finger on a specific problem.

Treatment for SLE will vary from woman to woman. Extra rest, a good diet and avoiding the sun will help somewhat. The following can provide effective relief

---

*This is the number of operations deemed necessary to maintain an adequate program of open-heart surgery by the ICHDR (Intersociety Commission for Heart Disease Resources), a national committee of leading cardiac surgeons and specialists. (See "Optimal Resources for Cardiac Surgery: Guidelines for Program Planning and Evaluation," Report of the Intersociety Commission for Heart Disease Resources, Circulation 52 [1975], A23–37.) As bypass surgery has become more popular, there has been a proliferation of poorly conceived and poorly planned units that provide less-than-optimal care.

from the SLE symptoms, though they sometimes cause other problems: anti-inflammatory drugs such as aspirin; antimalarial drugs (which can cause irreversible retina damage, so regular eye exams are necessary to detect this problem early on); and steroids (which can cause high blood pressure, ulcers, swelling and other negative effects—use with caution!). Gynecologists tend to know little about SLE, so it is wiser to consult an internist or other physician with special knowledge of autoimmune diseases (rheumatologist).

SLE is *not* usually life-threatening, although it can be extremely disabling. The ten-year survival rate is higher than 90 percent. Kidney involvement is the most serious complication and can require kidney dialysis as part of the treatment. Pregnancy is potentially problematic since women with SLE have a higher-than-average rate of miscarriages and often experience flare-ups after the birth.

Because symptoms are often invisible, vary a lot in severity and usually come and go (as with many chronic diseases), women with lupus are often accused of being hypochondriacs. Physician ignorance, job discrimination, lack of support from family and friends and the need to restrict activities are just some of the problems experienced by women with SLE.

Support groups are a key resource for women coping with lupus. If you have lupus, ask your doctor about other women who have this problem or contact the Lupus Foundation (see Resources).

When I first found out I had SLE ten years ago, I was immediately faced with many changes: I had to drop out of school, was hospitalized three times that summer, gave up running five miles a day and lost twenty pounds by fall. In the years that followed I learned to cope with my limitations and regain my strength. When my ninety-year-old grandmother complains about not being able to do what she used to, I sympathize. For me that happened at twenty-five. Today, after returning to complete a second graduate degree, I work full time. I control my illness by taking medication daily but I am still afraid to tell my employer and hate to miss days because of flare-ups. I maintain my health with regular exercise (I swim three-quarters of a mile a day), a good diet and rest. Acquaintances and even good friends don't always understand when I cancel plans, leave early or wear long sleeves in summer. But the other lupus patients in a support group I attend understand me; we speak the same language.

TOXIC SHOCK SYNDROME (TSS): A NEWLY RECOGNIZED DISEASE

Toxic shock syndrome (TSS) is a rare but serious disease which mainly strikes menstruating women under thirty who are using tampons. (Menstrual sponges, contraceptive sponges and diaphragms used during the menses have also been associated with TSS.) Although only a small number of menstruating women have gotten TSS (six to fifteen per 100,000 menstruating women), a few of them have died. An increasing number of non-tampon-related cases are showing up in postoperative (male and female) and postpartum patients in hospitals.

TSS is probably caused by a new strain of the bacterium *Staphylococcus aureus* (*S. aureus*), which infects some part of the body, often the vagina, and produces toxins (poisons) which go into the bloodstream, causing a bodily reaction. No one yet knows why some women with *S. aureus* bacteria in their vaginas get TSS and others don't. We wonder if a woman's vaginal secretions and the type of birth control she uses, which significantly affect the vaginal pH, are factors. Higher-absorbency tampons are more likely to be associated with TSS.

This disease is a syndrome, or group of symptoms. At present, only those people who have *all* the symptoms are officially counted as having TSS. However, there are reports of people with a few of the symptoms who may have a milder form of the same disease. The symptoms are:

- a high fever, usually over 102 degrees;
- vomiting;
- diarrhea;
- a sudden drop in blood pressure which may lead to shock;
- a sunburnlike rash which peels after a while. The rashes are easiest to see on a person's trunk and neck, and the peeling is obvious on the palms of the hands or the soles of the feet.

Treatments

If you get any of the aforementioned symptoms during your period and you are using a tampon, remove it immediately. Do not use tampons or any other internal method for catching menstrual blood until you get a culture showing that you have no *S. aureus* in your vagina. TSS can progress extremely rapidly, within hours. It's a good idea to get in touch right away with a medical person, preferably at a medical facility, who can keep track of what is happening to you. For a mild case, the most important thing is to drink lots of fluids and rest if possible.

TSS involving severe dehydration or very low blood pressure may require hospitalization. Although antibiotics do not seem to affect the symptoms once the disease has started, they can still significantly reduce the chance of recurrence. Since this type of *S. aureus* is penicillin- and ampicillin-resistant, beta-lactamase resistant antistaphylococcal antibiotics must be used.

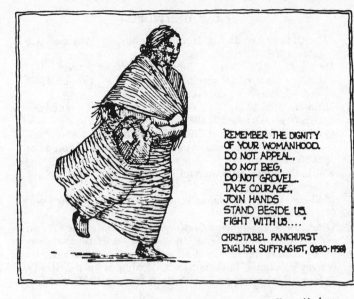

"REMEMBER THE DIGNITY
OF YOUR WOMANHOOD.
DO NOT APPEAL,
DO NOT BEG,
DO NOT GROVEL.
TAKE COURAGE,
JOIN HANDS
STAND BESIDE US,
FIGHT WITH US...."

CHRISTABEL PANKHURST
ENGLISH SUFFRAGIST, (1880-1958)

Karen Norberg

RESOURCES

General

See also periodicals and groups in "Women and the Medical System."

Ammer, Christine. *The A to Z of Women's Health: A Concise Encyclopedia.* Foreword by Mary Jane Gray, M.D. New York: Everest House, 1983.

Benson, Ralph C. *Handbook of Obstetrics and Gynecology.* Los Altos, CA: Lange Medical Publications, 1980.

Bunker, John, et al. *Costs, Risks, and Benefits of Surgery.* New York: Oxford University Press, 1977. An extensive study of U.S. surgical practices.

Federation of Feminist Women's Health Centers. *How to Stay Out of the Gynecologist's Office.* Illustrations by Suzann Gage. Culver City, CA: Peace Press, 1981.

———. *A New View of a Woman's Body.* Illustrations by Suzann Gage. New York: Simon and Schuster, 1981.

Gardner, Joy. *Healing Yourself,* 7th rev. ed. Available from Healing Yourself, Box 752, Vashon, WA 98070.

Gerras, Charles. *The Complete Book of Vitamins.* Emmaus, PA: Rodale Press, 1977.

Graedon, Joe. *People's Pharmacy.* New York: Avon Books, 1980.

Hirsh, Robert A., et al. *Health Care Delivery in Anesthesia.* Philadelphia: George F. Stickley Co., 1980.

Jones, Howard W., and Georgeanna Seegar. *Gynecology,* 3rd ed. Baltimore: Williams and Wilkins, 1982.

Lauersen, Niels, M.D., and Eileen Stukane. *Listen to Your Body.* New York: Simon and Schuster, 1982.

Lettvin, Maggie. *Maggie's Woman's Book.* Boston: Houghton Mifflin Co., 1980.

Madaras, Lynda, and Jane Patterson, M.D. *Womancare: A Gynecological Guide to Your Body.* New York: Avon Books, 1981.

Napoli, Maryann. *Health Facts.* Woodstock, NY: Overlook Press, 1982.

Padus, Emrika. *The Woman's Encyclopedia of Health and Natural Healing.* Emmaus, PA: Rodale Press, 1981.

Parvati, Jeannine. *Hygieia: A Woman's Herbal.* Berkeley, CA: Bookpeople, 1978.

Peters, Linda. "Women's Health Care: Approaches in Delivery to Physically Disabled Women," *Nurse-Practitioner* (January 1982), p. 34.

Philbrook, Marilyn McLean. *Medical Books for the Layperson: An Annotated Bibliography* (supplement). Boston: Trustees of Boston Public Library, 1978. $2.00.

Popenoe, Cris. *Wellness* (supplements four and five). Yes! Bookshop Guides, Yes! Bookshop, 1035 31st Street NW, Washington, DC 20007, (202) 338-2727. Extensive annotated listings of wholistic resources.

Prevention Magazine Editors. *The Prevention Guide to Surgery and Its Alternatives.* Emmaus, PA: Rodale Press, 1980. How to decide on surgery and surgeons, get second opinions, etc. Discusses alternatives and nutrition.

Shephard, Bruce D., M.D., and Carroll A. Shephard, R.N., Ph.D. *The Complete Guide to Women's Health.* Tampa, FL: Mariner Publishing Co., 1982.

Sonstegard, Lois, Karren Kowalski and Betty Jennings, eds. *Women's Health. Vol. I: Ambulatory Care.* New York: Grune and Stratton, 1982.

Stewart, Felicia, M.D., Felicia Guest, Gary Stewart, M.D., and Robert Hatcher, M.D. *My Body, My Health.* New York: John Wiley and Sons, Inc., 1979.

U.S. Congress, Office of Technology Assessment. "The Implications of Cost-Effectiveness Analysis of Medical Technology, Background Paper #4: The Management of Health Care Technology in Ten Countries," October 1980.

U.S. Department of Health, Education and Welfare/Public Health Service. *Healthy People: The Surgeon General's Report on Health Promotion and Disease Prevention.* DHEW (PHS) Pub. No. 79-55071, 1979.

Benign Breast Conditions

Love, Susan, et al. "Fibrocystic 'Disease' of the Breast—a Nondisease," *New England Journal of Medicine,* Vol. 307, No. 16 (October 14, 1982), pp. 1010–14.

Cervical Intraepithelial Neoplasia (CIN)

Clark, Adele, and Martina Reaves. "Cervical Dysplasia: The Ambiguous 'Condition,'" *Second Opinion* (September 1982).

Popkin, D.R. "Treatment of Cervical Intraepithelial Neoplasia with the Carbon Dioxide Laser," *American Journal of Obstetrics and Gynecology* (January 15, 1983).

Stafl, Adolf, and Richard Mattingly. "Cervical Intraepithelial Neoplasia," Chapter 31 in R.F. Mattingly, *Telinde's Operative Gynecology,* 5th ed. Philadelphia: J.B. Lippincott, 1977.

Wright, Cecil, et al. "Laser Surgery for Cervical Intraepithelial Neoplasia: Principles and Results," *American Journal of Obstetrics and Gynecology* (January 15, 1983).

DES

Books

Bichler, Joyce. *DES Daughter*. New York: Avon Books, 1981.

Herbst, Arthur, and Howard Bern. *Developmental Effects of Diethylstilbestrol (DES) in Pregnancy*. New York: Thieme-Stratton, 1981.

Meyers, Robert. *DES: The Bitter Pill*. New York: G.P. Putnam's Sons, 1983.

Orenberg, Cynthia. *DES: The Complete Story*. New York: St. Martin's Press, Inc., 1981.

Articles

Anderson, B., et al. "Development of DES-Associated Clear Cell Carcinoma: The Importance of Regular Screening," *Obstetrics and Gynecology*, Vol. 33, No. 3 (March 1979), pp. 293–99.

Dieckmann, W., et al. "Does the Administration of Diethylstilbestrol During Pregnancy Have Therapeutic Value?" *American Journal of Obstetrics and Gynecology*, Vol. 66, No. 5 (November 1953), pp. 1062–81.

Herbst, A.L., et al. "Adenocarcinoma of the Vagina: Association of Maternal Stilbestrol Therapy with Tumor Appearance in Young Women," *New England Journal of Medicine*, Vol. 284 (April 22, 1971), pp. 878–81.

———. "A Comparison of Pregnancy Experience in DES-Exposed and DES-Unexposed Daughters," *Journal of Reproductive Medicine*, Vol. 24, No. 2 (February 1980), pp. 62–69.

Kaufman, F. J., et al. "Upper Genital Tract Changes Associated with Exposure *in utero* to Diethylstilbestrol," *American Journal of Obstetrics and Gynecology*, Vol. 128 (May 1977), pp. 51–59.

Robboy, S. J., et al. "Cooperative Diethylstilbestrol Adenosis (DESAD) Project," *Obstetrics and Gynecology*, Vol. 53, No. 3 (March 1979), pp. 309–17.

Schmidt, G., et al. "Cervical Stenosis Following Minor Gynecologic Procedures on DES-Exposed Women," *Obstetrics and Gynecology*, Vol. 56, No. 3 (September 1980), pp. 333–35.

———. "Reproductive History of Women Exposed to Diethylstilbestrol *in utero*," *Fertility and Sterility*, Vol. 33 (January 1980), p. 21.

Smith, O.W. "Influence of Diethylstilbestrol on the Progress and Outcome of Pregnancy as Based on a Comparison of Treated and Untreated Primigravidas," *American Journal of Obstetrics and Gynecology*, Vol. 58, No. 5 (November 1949), pp. 994–1009.

Groups

DES Action, 2845 24th Street, San Francisco, CA 94117, and Long Island Jewish Hospital, New Hyde Park, NY 11040. Numerous resources available including pamphlets for DES daughters and DES sons (single copies free); "Community Organizing for Health: A DES Action Manual," by Pat Cody and Nancy Adess ($3.95); *Fertility and Pregnancy Guide for DES Daughters and Sons* ($6); "Ask Your Mother," a 20-minute slide show on case-finding geared toward nurses and nurse practitioners (sale, $110; rental, $50); *DES Action Voice*, a quarterly newsletter with legal and medical updates ($15 yearly).

Endometriosis

"The Disease We 'Catch' from Being Modern Women," *Self* (May 1980).

Dmowski, W.P. "Current Concepts in the Management of Endometriosis," *Obstetrics and Gynecology Annual: 1981*, Vol. 10, Ralph Wynn, ed.

"Endometriosis May Spread to Lungs, Adjacent Organs." *Ob-Gyn News* (October 1, 1980).

Goldstein, Donald, et al. "Adolescent Endometriosis." *Journal of Adolescent Health Care*, Vol. 1, No. 1 (September 1980), p. 37.

Keith, Carolyn. "Endometriosis." *WomenWise*, Vol. 6, No. 1 (Spring 1983).

Madaras, Lynda, and Jane Patterson. *Womancare*. New York: Avon Books, 1981.

Older, Julia. *A Woman's Guide to Endometriosis*. New York: Charles Scribner's Sons, Inc., 1984. An extremely thorough, clear discussion of all aspects of endometriosis.

Valverde, Clara. "Endometriosis: Healing with the Mind's Eye." *HealthSharing*, Vol. 2, No. 1 (Spring 1981), p. 13.

Pelvic Inflammatory Disease (PID)

Gregg, Sandee, and Judy Ismach. "Beyond 'VD,'" *Medical World News* (March 31, 1980).

Herbst, Arthur L. "Reproductive and Gynecologic Surgical Experience in Diethylstilbestrol-Exposed Daughters," *American Journal of Obstetrics and Gynecology*, Vol. 141, No. 8 (December 15, 1981).

Jacobson, Lennart. "Differential Diagnosis of Acute Pelvic Inflammatory Disease," *American Journal of Obstetrics and Gynecology*, Vol. 138, No. 7, Part 2 (December 1, 1980).

Lauersen, Niels, and Steven Whitney. *It's Your Body: A Woman's Guide to Gynecology*. New York: Grosset and Dunlap, 1977, pp. 156–58.

Senanayake, Pramilla, and Dorine G. Kramer. "Contraception and the Etiology of Pelvic Inflammatory Disease: New Perspectives," *American Journal of Obstetrics and Gynecology*, Vol. 138, No. 7, Part 2 (December 1, 1980).

Vancouver Women's Health Research Collective. "*PID: Pelvic Inflammatory Disease*." VWHRC, 1501 W. Broadway, Vancouver, B.C., Canada V6J 1W6, 1983. $2.00. A comprehensive, illustrated 34-page booklet with extensive bibliography. Very useful.

Urinary Tract Infections (UTIs)

Brooks, Beth, and Jackie Niemand. *A Woman's Guide to Treating and Preventing Bladder Infections*, Emma Goldman Clinic for Women, 715 N. Dodge Street, Iowa City, IA 52240, 1979.

Kilmartin, Angela. *Cystitis: The Complete Self-Help Guide*. New York: Warner Books, Inc., 1980.

O'Donnell, Mary, et al. *Lesbian Health Matters!* Santa Cruz Women's Health Collective, 250 Locust Street, Santa Cruz, CA 95060, 1979. Includes a section on the relationship between lesbian lovemaking and urinary tract infections, along with self-care suggestions.

Ritz, Sandra, and Anne Simon. "Bladder Infections: How to Get Off the Toilet," *Medical Self Care*, No. 12 (Spring 1981), pp. 9–14. Back issue available for $4.00 from *Medical Self Care*, Box 717, Inverness, CA 94937. Probably the most useful article available.

Sabath, Leon, and David Charles. "Urinary Tract Infections in the Female," *Obstetrics and Gynecology* (supplement), Vol. 55, No. 5 (May 1980), pp. 162S-69S. Describes diagnosis and medical management of urinary tract infections. Includes 57 medical references on the topic.

Hysterectomy and Oophorectomy

Books

Bunker, John, et al. *Costs, Risks, and Benefits of Surgery*. New York: Oxford University Press, 1977.

Centers for Disease Control. *Surgical Sterilization Surveillance: Hysterectomy in Women Aged 15–44, 1970–1975*. Issued September 1980.

Morgan, Susanne. *Coping with Hysterectomy*. New York: Dial Press, 1982.

Articles

Ananth, J. "Hysterectomy and Depression," *Obstetrics and Gynecology*, Vol. 52 (December 1978), p. 724.

Barber, H.R.K., E.A. Graber and T.H. Kwan. "Ovarian Cancer," *CA—A Cancer Journal for Clinicians*, Vol. 24 (November/December 1974).

Braun, P., and E. Druckman, eds. "Public Health Rounds at the Harvard School of Public Health: Elective Hysterectomy—Pro and Con," *New England Journal of Medicine*, Vol. 295 (July 29, 1976), pp. 264–68.

Burchell, R. Clay. "Decision Regarding Hysterectomy," *American Journal of Obstetrics and Gynecology*, Vol. 127 (January 15, 1977).

Centerwall, Brandon. "Pre-Menopausal Hysterectomy and Cardiovascular Disease," *American Journal of Obstetrics and Gynecology*, Vol. 139 (1981).

Cole, P., and J. Berlin. "Elective Hysterectomy," *American Journal of Obstetrics and Gynecology*, Vol. 129 (September 15, 1977), pp. 117–20.

Davies, Mary E. "A Consumer's Guide to Hysterectomy," *Medical Self-Care* (Summer 1983).

Easterday, Charles L., David Grimes and Joseph Riggs. "Hysterectomy in the United States," *Obstetrics and Gynecology*, Vol. 62 (August 1983), pp. 203–12.

Funt, Mark Ian, B. Benigno and J. Thompson. "Retain Ovaries During Premenopausal Hysterectomy," *American Journal of Obstetrics and Gynecology*, Vol. 129 (1977).

Hunter, D.S. "Oophorectomy and the Surgical Menopause," in *The Menopause*, pp. 212–13, R. J. Beard, ed. Baltimore: University Park Press, 1976.

Knutsen, K. "The Climacteric Following Supravaginal Hysterectomy," *Acta Obstetrica Gynecologica Scandinavia*, Vol. 3 (1951), pp. 9–24.

MMWR Morbidity and Mortality Weekly Report. U.S. Department of Health and Human Services/Public Health Service (April 24, 1981).

Newton, N., and E. Baron. "Reactions to Hysterectomy," *Primary Care*, Vol. 3 (December 1976), pp. 790–91.

Notman, Malkah T. "How Should You Advise Your Hysterectomy Patient," *Modern Medicine*, Vol. 15, No. 28 (February 1979).

Reid, D., and T.C. Barton. *Controversy in Obstetrics and Gynecology*. Philadelphia: W.B. Saunders, 1969, pp. 377 ff.

Rogers, Joann. "Rush to Surgery," *The New York Times Magazine*, September 21, 1975.

Rosenberg, Lynn, et al. "Early Menopause and the Risk of Myocardial Infarction," *American Journal of Obstetrics and Gynecology*, Vol. 139 (1981), p. 47.

Studd, J.W.W. and M. Thom. "Hormone Implantation," *British Medical Journal* (March 22, 1980), pp. 848–50.

Terz, Jose J., et al. "Incidence of Carcinoma in Retained Ovary," *American Journal of Surgery*, Vol. 113 (April 1967).

Thom, M., and J.W. Studd. "Ovarian Failure and Ageing," *Clinics in Endocrinology and Metabolism*, Vol. 10, No. 1 (March 1981), p. 105.

Wright, Ralph C. "Hysterectomy: Past, Present, and Future," *Obstetrics and Gynecology*, Vol. 3 (April 1969), pp. 560–63.

Zussman, L., S. Zussman, R. Sunley and E. Bjornson. "Sexual Response after Hysterectomy-Oophorectomy: Recent Studies and Reconsideration of Psychogenesis," *American Journal of Obstetrics and Gynecology*, Vol. 40, No. 7 (August 1, 1981), pp. 725–29.

Support Group

HERS (Hysterectomy Educational Resources and Services), 501 Woodbrook Avenue, Philadelphia, PA 19119. Counseling and support to women and their families when faced with adverse effects of the surgery or with elective surgery. Newsletter, $12 yearly.

Vaginal Infections (Vaginitis)

Bloomfield, Randall. "Vaginal Discharge: Which Culprit? Which Treatment?" *Modern Medicine* (September, 1981).

Hasselbring, Bobbie, "Every Woman's Guide to Vaginal Infections," *Medical Self-Care* (Summer 1983), p. 45.

Lossick, Joseph G. "Metronidazole," *New England Journal of Medicine*, Vol. 304, No. 12 (March 19, 1981).

O'Donnell, Mary, et al. *Lesbian Health Matters*. Santa Cruz Women's Health Center, 250 Locust Street, Santa Cruz, CA 95060, 1979.

Santa Cruz Women's Health Center. "Home Remedies for Vaginitis." Send 50¢ and a stamped, self-addressed envelope to Santa Cruz Women's Health Center (address above).

Van Sylke, K. Keller, et al. "Treatment of Vulvovaginal Candidiasis with Boric Acid Powder," *American Journal of Obstetrics and Gynecology* (September 15, 1981).

White, W., and P. J. Spencer-Phillips. "Recurrent Vaginitis and Oral Sex," *Lancet* (March 17, 1979).

Arthritis

Arthritis Information Clearinghouse, P.O. Box 34427, Bethesda, MD 20034. Provides information on professional, patient and public education materials on rheumatic diseases and related topics. Publishes a bulletin.

Benson, Herbert, M.D., with Miriam Z. Klipper. *The Relaxation Response*. New York: Avon Books, 1975. Send $2.20 to Avon Books, 250 West 55th Street, New York, NY 10019.

Dong, Collin H., and Jane Banks. *The Arthritic's Cookbook*. New York: Thomas Crowell/Harper and Row, 1973.

Hanson, Isabel. *Outwitting Arthritis*. Creative Arts Book Co., 833 Bancroft Way, Berkeley, CA 94710, 1980. For people with arthritis, this book comes as close as one can get to a written support group.

Krewer, Semyon. *The Arthritis Exercise Book*. New York: Simon and Schuster, 1981.

Lorig, Kate. "Arthritis Self Management," *Medical Self Care* (Winter 1981), p. 38.

———, and James Fries. *The Arthritis Helpbook*. Reading, MA: Addison-Wesley, 1980.

Cancer

Readings

American Cancer Society. "Report of the Cancer Related Check Up," *Ca—A Cancer Journal for Clinicians*, Vol. 30 (1980).

Antunes, Carlos, et al. "Endometrial Cancer and Estrogen Use: Report of a Large Case-Control Study," *New England Journal of Medicine*, Vol. 300, No. 1 (January 4, 1979).

Casagrande, J.K., et al. "Incessant Ovulation and Ovarian Cancer," *Lancet*, Vol. II (1979), p. 170.

Center for Medical Consumers and Health Care Information. "Breast Cancer," *Health Facts*, Vol. VIII, No. 44 (January 1983).

Consumer Reports. "Breast Cancer: The Retreat from Radical Surgery." New York: Consumers' Union of the U.S., Inc., January 1981. An excellent discussion of factors leading to new-option radiation therapy, also called lumpectomy plus radiation.

Cowan, K., and M. Lippman. "Steroid Receptors in Breast Cancer," *Archives of Internal Medicine*, Vol. 142 (February 1982), pp. 363–66.

Doll, R., and R. Pito. "The Causes of Cancer: Quantitative Estimates of Avoidable Risks of Cancer in the United States Today," *Journal of the National Cancer Institute*, Vol. 66 (1981), pp. 1191–1308.

Epstein, Samuel. *The Politics of Cancer*. New York: Anchor Books, 1979. Describes the cancer industry which makes millions of dollars in profits from research and treatments which have done little to help cancer patients.

Fisher, Bernard. "Breast Cancer Management: Alternatives to Radical Mastectomy, Sounding Board," *New England Journal of Medicine*, Vol. 301, No. 6 (August 9, 1979), pp. 326–28.

Fox, Maurice. "On the Diagnosis and Treatment of Early Breast Cancer," Special Communication. *Journal of the American Medical Association*, Vol. 241, No. 5 (February 2, 1979), pp. 489–94.

Fredericks, Carlton. *Winning the Fight Against Breast Cancer: The Nutritional Approach*. New York: Grosset and Dunlap, 1977.

Glassman, Judith. *Cancer Survivors and How They Did It*. New York: Dial Press, 1983. The author reports her investigations of the claims of various alternative therapies. Includes case histories of persons who received laetrile, Gerson therapy and others.

Gorbach, Sherwood L., and David R. Zimmerman. *The Doctors' Anti-Breast Cancer Diet*. New York: Simon and Schuster, 1984.

Gusberg, S. B. "The Changing Nature of Endometrial Cancer," *New England Journal of Medicine*, Vol. 302, No. 13 (March 27, 1980).

Guzick, David S. "Efficacy of Screening for Cervical Cancer: A Review," *American Journal of Public Health*, Vol. 68 (February 1978).

Henderson, Craig. *Breast Cancer Management: Progress and Prospects*. Wayne, NJ: Lederle Labs, 1982. A technical and thorough medical report by one of the top breast cancer researchers in the U.S.

Hoover, Robert, et al. "Stilboestrol (Diethylstilbestrol) and the Risk of Ovarian Cancer," *Lancet* (September 10, 1977), pp. 533–34.

Kaufman, et al. "Herpes Virus Antigens in Vulvar Carcinoma," *New England Journal of Medicine*, Vol. 305, No. 9 (August 27, 1981).

Kelly, Patricia T., and David E. Anderson. "Familial Breast Cancer: New Data Show Lower Risks for Some Sisters and Daughters," *Your Patient and Cancer* (May 1981).

Kushner, Rose. *Alternatives*. Available from the Kensington Press, c/o PBS, P.O. Box 643, Cambridge, MA 02139. From her own experience, Kushner writes about the archaic, insensitive treatment of women with breast cancer by physicians. The book includes report of treatments here and abroad.

Lake, Alice. "An Honest Report on Breast Cancer," *Redbook*, September 1981. A comprehensive and well-written overview of breast cancer.

LeShan, Lawrence. *You Can Fight for Your Life: Emotional Factors in the Treatment of Cancer*. New York: M. Evans and Co., 1977.

Lorde, Audrey. *Cancer Journals*. New York: Spinsters Ink, 1980. Important testimony of a lesbian feminist poet's personal and political reckoning with breast cancer and mastectomy.

Miller, A. B., and R.D. Bulbrook. "Special Report: The Epidemiology and Etiology of Breast Cancer," *New England Journal of Medicine*, Vol. 303, No. 21 (November 20, 1980), pp. 1246–48.

Morra, Marion, and Eve Potts. *Choices: Realistic Alternatives in Cancer Treatment*. New York: Avon Books, 1980. A clearly written guide to the traditional options available. Answers most questions concerning diagnosis and treatment.

Moss, Ralph W. *The Cancer Syndrome*. New York: Grove Press, Inc., 1980. Discusses the political climate that inhibits alternatives to the currently accepted cancer treatments, indicting both the National Cancer Institute and the American Cancer Society for irresponsibility.

The National Cancer Institute. *The Breast Cancer Digest: A Guide to Medical Care, Emotional Support, Educational Programs, and Resources*. Office of Cancer Communications, National Cancer Institute, Bethesda, MD 20205, 1979 (new edition forthcoming, 1984). Free.

National Women's Health Network. *Breast Cancer*, Resource Guide #1. National Women's Health Network, 224 Seventh Street SE, Washington, DC 20003, 1980.

Newell, Guy, and Neal Ellison, eds. *Nutrition and Cancer: Etiology and Treatment*. Volume 17 of *Progress in Cancer Research and Therapy*. New York: Raven Press, 1981.

Reid, Richard. "Genital Warts and Cervical Cancer, II: Is Human Papillomavirus Infection the Trigger to Cervical Carcinogenesis?" *Gynecologic Oncology*, Vol. 15 (1983), pp. 239–52.

———, et al. "Genital Warts and Cervical Cancer, I: Evidence of an Association Between Subclinical Papillomavirus Infection and Cervical Malignancy," *Cancer*, Vol. 50, No. 2 (July 15, 1982), pp. 377–87.

Rennie, Susan. "Mammography: X-Rated Film Rated," *Chrysalis*, No. 5 (1978), pp. 21–33.

Simonton, O. Carl, et al. *Getting Well Again: A Step-by-Step*

Self-Help Guide to Overcoming Cancer for Patients and Their Families. New York: Bantam Books, 1978. A discussion of methods by which the mind can influence the body both for health and toward disease.

"Special Report: Treatment of Primary Breast Cancer," *New England Journal of Medicine*, Vol. 301, No. 6 (August 9, 1979), p. 340.

"Suppression of Ovulation—by Pregnancy and Pill Use—Sharply Decreases Ovarian Cancer Risk" (digest), *Family Planning Perspectives*, Vol. 11, No. 6 (November/December 1979), pp. 363–65.

Walker, Alexander, and Hershel Jick. "Declining Rates of Endometrial Cancer," *Journal of Obstetrics and Gynecology*, Vol. 56, No. 6 (December 1980).

Organizations

The following organizations provide information and, in some cases, other services to persons interested in current cancer treatments. The first nine sources mainly present the view of established medical practices. On the other hand, resources ten to seventeen are either open to or actively promote alternative therapies. Addresses may change, so check with local cancer groups or a public library for new listings if you get no reply. Check phone directories for local offices of national organizations such as the American Cancer Society. Also check 800 Information for toll-free phone numbers.

American Cancer Society
777 Third Avenue
New York, NY 10017
(212) 371-2900

Breast Cancer Advisory Center
Rose Kushner, Director
Box 224
Kensington, MD 20895

Cancer Information Service, National Cancer Hotline: (800) 4CA-NCER (answered at all times except 12:00 midnight to 8:00 A.M.)
Also: (800) 555-1212
(and ask for their number in your area)

Encore
—(contact your local YWCA)

Food and Drug Administration
5600 Fishers Lane
Rockville, MD 20852
(202) 245-1144

Memorial Sloan-Kettering Cancer Center
1275 York Avenue
New York, NY 10021
(212) 794-7000

National Cancer Institute
9000 Rockville Pike
Bethesda, MD 20014
(301) 496-6641

Reach for Recovery
—(contact your local American Cancer Society)

RENU (Reconstruction Education for National Understanding)
(216) 444-2900

The following are open to or advocate alternative therapies:

Arlin J. Brown Information Center
P.O. Box 251
Fort Belvoir, VA 22060
(703) 451-8638

Cancer Control Society
2043 North Berendo Street
Los Angeles, CA 90027

Cancer Rehabilitation Center
7115 Brookshire
Dallas, TX
(214) 386-7610
(Simonton Technique)

Committee for Freedom of Choice in Cancer Therapy
146 Main Street, Suite 408
Los Altos, CA 94022
(415) 948-9476
(laetrile information)

Foundation for Alternative Cancer Therapies
P.O. Box HH
Old Chelsea Station
New York, NY 10011
(212) 741-2790

Gerson Institute of California
P.O. Box 430
Bonita, CA 92002
(diet)

Hippocrates Health Institute
25 Exeter Street
Boston, MA 02116
(617) 267-9525
(diet and related approaches)

International Health Institute
15048 Beltway
Dallas, TX 75234
(214) 233-0408
(Kelley therapy)

Metabolic Research Foundation
518 Zenith Drive
Glenview, IL 60025
(312) 299-7180
(diet and vitamin therapy)

American Cancer Society:
1. Local chapters have lists of places to purchase prostheses as well as types of prostheses on the market.
2. "Reach for Recovery"—a volunteer organization of women who have had mastectomies who will visit women in the hospital. Also available: a book of postmastectomy exercises. Contact through the local or closest American Cancer Society office.

RENU (Reconstructive Education for National Understanding):
Offers advice and support for women considering breast reconstruction. Call their twenty-four-hour answering service ([216] 444-2900); leave your name and number and someone will contact you, usually from your area.

ENCORE:
Support and exercise groups for women with mastecto-

mies. A YWCA-supported group. Contact through the local YWCA.

Diabetes

Biermand, June, and Barbara Toohey. *The Diabetics' Total Health Book*. J. P. Tarcher, Inc., 9110 Sunset Boulevard, Los Angeles, CA 90069, 1980.

Health Research Group. "Off Diabetes Pills" (Ralph Nader's report on hypoglycemic drugs). Send $3.50 to HRG, 2000 P Street NW, Suite 708, Washington, DC 20037.

Liebman, Bonnie. "Diabetics and the Glycemic Index," *Nutrition Action* (March 1982), pp. 8–11.

———. "Food Over Pharmaceuticals," *Nutrition Action* (March 1982), pp. 10–13.

"New Hope for Diabetics," *Diabetics Forecast* (May–June 1978).

"Insulin May Do Harm to Adult Diabetics," *Prevention*, April 1978.

Hypertension, Heart Diseases and Circulatory Diseases

Books and Pamphlets

The American Heart Association. *The Heartbook*. New York: E.P. Dutton, 1980. A comprehensive guide to all aspects of heart disease, prevention, etc.

Chobanian, Aram, and Lorraine Loviglio, with Patrick O'Reilly. *Boston University Medical Center's Heart Risk Book: A Practical Guide for Preventing Heart Disease*. New York: Bantam Books, 1982.

Eishelman, Ruthe, and Mary Winston, eds. *The American Heart Association Cookbook*. New York: Ballantine Books, Inc., 1979. Recipes and practical advice on cooking healthy food for the heart: low-fat, low-sugar and vegetarian meals.

Farquhar, John. *The American Way of Life Need Not Be Hazardous to Your Health*. New York: W.W. Norton and Co., Inc., 1979. A practical guide to behaviors that increase heart risks, and how to change them.

National Institutes of Health. *Coronary Artery Bypass Surgery* (Consensus Development 1980 Conference Summary, Vol. 3, No. 8). Office for Medical Applications of Research, NIH, Bldg. 1, Rm. 216, Bethesda, MD 20205.

U.S. Department of Health and Human Services. *Heart Attacks (Medicine for the Layman)*. NIH Publication No. 81–1803, reprinted August 1981 by the National Heart, Lung, and Blood Institute, Office of Information, NIH, Bethesda MD 20205.

Articles

Braunwald, E. "Coronary Artery Surgery at the Crossroads" (editorial), *The New England Journal of Medicine*, Vol. 297, No. 12 (September 22, 1977), pp. 661–63.

Dyerberg, J., et al. "Eicosapentanoic Acid and Prevention of Thrombosis and Atherosclerosis," *Lancet*, Vol. 1 (July 15, 1978), pp. 117–21.

Gotto, Antonio M., Jr. "Regression of Atherosclerosis," *American Journal of Medicine*, Vol. 70 (1981), pp. 989–91.

Haynes, Suzanne G., and Manning Feinleib. "Women, Work and Coronary Heart Disease: Prospective Findings from the Framingham Heart Study," *American Journal of Public Health*, Vol. 70, No. 2 (February 1980), pp. 133–41.

"Is Vitamin B$_6$ an Antithrombotic Agent?" (editorial), *Lancet*, Vol. 1 (June 13, 1981), pp. 1299–1300.

Lewis, Barry. "Dietary Prevention of Ischaemic Heart Disease—a Policy for the '80s," *British Medical Journal*, Vol. 2 (July 19, 1980), pp. 177–80.

Lewis, B., et al. "Towards an Improved Lipid Lowering Diet: Additive Effects of Changes in Nutrient Intake," *Lancet*, Vol. 1 (December 12, 1981), pp. 1310–13.

Lipinska, Isabella, and Victor Gurewich. "The Value of Measuring Percent High-Density Lipoprotein in Assessing Risk of Cardiovascular Disease," *Archives of Internal Medicine*, Vol. 142 (1982), pp. 469–72.

"Low Cholesterol Diets," *Medical World News* (June 7, 1982), pp. 142–43, 177.

Oliver, Michael F. "Risks of Correcting the Risks of Coronary Disease and Stroke With Drugs" (Sounding Board), *New England Journal of Medicine*, Vol. 306, No. 5 (February 4, 1982), pp. 297–98.

Petch, M.C. "The Progression of Coronary Artery Disease," *British Medical Journal*, Vol. 2 (October 24, 1981), pp. 1073–74.

Shekelle, Richard B., et al. "Diet, Serum Cholesterol, and Death from Coronary Heart Disease: The Western Electric Study," *New England Journal of Medicine*, Vol. 304, No. 2 (1981), pp. 65–70.

"Women, Work, and Coronary Heart Disease," *Lancet* (July 12, 1980), pp. 76–77.

Yaari, Shlomit, et al. "Association of Serum High Density Lipoprotein and Total Cholesterol with Total Cardiovascular and Cancer Mortality: In a 7-Year Prospective Study of 10,000 Men," *Lancet*, Vol. 1 (May 9, 1981), pp. 1011–14.

Systemic Lupus Erythematosis (SLE)

Aladjem, Henrietta. *Lupus: Hope Through Understanding*. Lupus Foundation of America, 11673 Holly Springs Drive, St. Louis, MO 63141, 1982.

Blau, S.P., and D. Schultz. *Lupus: The Body Against Itself*. New York: Doubleday Books, 1977.

Epstein W.V., and G. Clewly. *Living With SLE. A Handbook for Patients With Systemic Lupus Erythematosus*. San Francisco: University of California, Department of Medicine and Social Work, 1976.

Lupus Facts. Lupus Erythematosus Foundation, Boston, MA 02108.

Lupus News. A quarterly publication from the Lupus Foundation of America (address above).

Lupus and Pregnancy. Pennsylvania Lupus Foundation, P.O. Box 264, Wayne, PA 19087.

SLE. Arthritis Foundation, Atlanta, GA, 1978. Brochure, single copies free.

Toxic Shock Syndrome (TSS)

Centers for Disease Control, Atlanta, GA 30333.

International Toxic Shock Syndrome Network, P.O. Box 1248, Beverly Hills, CA 90213.

Robertson, Nan. "Toxic Shock," *The New York Times Magazine*, September 19, 1982.

Sweet, Richard. "Toxic Shock: Accurate Diagnosis and Aggressive Treatment," *Modern Medicine* (February 1983), p. 109.

VII
WOMEN
AND THE
MEDICAL SYSTEM

24

THE POLITICS OF WOMEN AND MEDICAL CARE

By Hilary Salk, Wendy Sanford, Norma Swenson and Judith Dickson Luce
Our Rights as Patients by Sherry Leibowitz and Joan Rachlin

With special thanks to David Banta, Gene Bishop, Mary Fillmore, Mary Howell, Judy Norsigian, Sheryl Ruzek and Karen Wolf

This chapter in previous editions was called "The American Health Care System" and "Choosing and Using Health and Medical Care" and was written by Barbara Perkins, Lucy Candib, Nancy Todd, Mary Stern and Norma Swenson.

THE AMERICAN MEDICAL CARE SYSTEM*

I've repeatedly described my symptoms to physicians—disconcerting symptoms to say the least: sudden menses cessation, elevated temperature, weight loss, anxiety, extreme fatigue, nausea, joint pain, vertigo—but the doctors have made only the catch-all diagnosis of "menopause," unsupported by any testing. They advised me to go into counseling, expecting me to "live with it," despite the fact that I have told them that the symptoms seem extreme, are increasing and have impaired and even curtailed my work, my studies, my personal relationships.

From a letter to the Women's Health Collective in Providence, R.I.:

I think you would have been proud of the way I handled the situation with the surgeon. Despite a fair amount of crying on my part (to top it all off, my husband was away when all this happened), I was able to demand a second opinion for my diverticulosis treatment, and the most conservative treatment possible. My surgeon was appalled when I balked at surgery Monday without what I felt was adequate time to discuss the situation or get another opinion. By Friday I was able to deal with him but it took about all I had. I really think that if it wasn't for my experience with the Women's Health Collective

*Space does not permit a discussion of women and dentistry, yet it appears that similar problems exist. See Paul I. Murphy and Rene C. Murphy, "The Perils and Pitfalls of Dentistry," *The New York Times Magazine*, April 29, 1979, pp. 110–11, 124–25.

and the support of my friends and family, I would have a temporary colostomy right now.

I, extremely well informed, well connected, verbally aggressive, have had to summon all my resources to get what I wanted in my treatment for breast cancer: medical care that was consistent with the findings of the latest literature and that took into account my needs as a woman.

As a young woman interested in one day having a family, I was never told that cimetidine "should not be used in pregnant patients or women of childbearing potential unless, in the judgment of the physician, the anticipated benefits outweigh the potential risks." I should have been informed of this and given the opportunity to make the decision myself in consultation with the doctor. This is one more indication of my rights and indeed my body being violated. My family raised me to trust doctors, but I no longer can do that.

In the words of a visiting nurse:

I learned to listen to patients, to speak their language, to let them set their own priorities for care, to teach them when they were ready. I also learned to evaluate the health care system through their eyes. Each day I confronted an irrelevant, noncaring, inadequate health care system, which refused to consider the personal, social, cultural and economic needs of the patient.

It is a sobering time for women using the medical system in this country. Although some women are satisfied with the medical care they get, many are not.* The women quoted above are only a few of the thousands speaking out about the physicians and other medical personnel in medical settings who have:

- not listened to them or believed what they said;
- withheld knowledge;
- lied to them;
- treated them without their consent;
- not warned of risks and negative effects of treatments;
- overcharged them;
- experimented on them or used them as "teaching material";
- treated them poorly because of their race, sexual preference, age or disability;
- offered them tranquilizers or moral advice instead of medical care or useful help from community resources (self-help groups, battered women's services, etc.);
- administered treatments which were unnecessarily mutilating and too extreme for their problem, or treatments which resulted in permanent disability or even death (*iatrogenesis*);†
- prescribed drugs which hooked them, sickened them, changed their entire lives;
- performed operations they later found were unnecessary, and removed organs that were in no way diseased;
- abused them sexually.

Why Focus on "Women and the Medical System"?

Women are part of the medical care system, either for ourselves or our children, spouses or aging parents, more than twice as often as men are. We are 85 percent of all "health care" workers in hospitals, and 75 percent in the system as a whole.‡ We carry out most

---

*We are basing the analysis in this chapter both on thousands of personal accounts and on the work of a wide range of people and groups: feminist writers and other investigative journalists; feminist, radical and progressive physicians; public health researchers; health workers and practitioners of all kinds; medical historians and medical sociologists; public interest groups and government specialists; as well as social and feminist critics of many different persuasions.

†*Iatrogenesis* is the process by which illness, impairment or death results from medical treatment. Some examples are cancers caused by DES, pelvic inflammatory disease (PID) or hysterectomy caused by an IUD, death or disability due to anesthesia accident (particularly when the surgery may not have been necessary), electrocution or burns from hospital equipment, infection from respirators, crippling or fatal strokes due to the birth control pill, addiction to tranquilizers and illness or death resulting from infant formula feeding in hospitals.

‡While ailing men do report many of the same problems with the medical care system as women, men use the system less. They do not, like women, have to consult physicians for normal events in the reproductive cycle, such as pregnancy. Men tend

doctors' orders—treatment regimens like special diets, medications and bed rest, etc.—either as unpaid workers at home or as paid workers. We teach about health both in the home and in the system—what is "good" and "not good" for you. At home we are usually the first to be told when someone doesn't feel well, and we help decide what to do next. Some health care analysts even call us "primary health care workers" or the "layperson on the team." Most "patient" communication for and about family members flows through women: we report signs and changes, symptoms, responses to treatments and medications. The system also depends on women: our direct reporting forms the basis of much of what medicine calls "scientific results," and our bodies provide the raw material for experimentation and research (e.g., the birth control pill), often without our knowledge and consent.[2]

Yet despite our overwhelming numbers and the tremendous responsibility we carry for people's health, we have almost no power to influence the medical system. Policy makers, usually male, have designed the system primarily for the convenience and financial gain of physicians, hospitals and the medical industries. *We believe that women, as the majority of consumers and workers, paid and unpaid, should have the major voice in health and medical care policy-making in this country.*

The last edition of *Our Bodies, Ourselves* expressed considerable optimism that women would be able to work together to change medical care. In fact, women of all ages have joined together in local communities and nationwide: the resulting Women's Health Movement has significantly changed the way many women look at medical care, and is successfully fighting in legislatures, hospital administrations and law courts for improvements. (See Chapter 25, "Organizing for Change: U.S.A.") Yet the abuses continue. The medical care system remains basically unresponsive, deeply entrenched as it is in American economic, political and social structures, and the influence of medicine* in people's lives continues to grow. For example, the insurance and drug industries continue to make unrestrained profits, and physicians are still the highest paid and among the least accountable of all U.S.

---

to come into the system only during crises. Many different studies have shown that medical care providers treat male patients with more respect than women and offer fewer tranquilizers and less moral advice.[1] Also, since only 10 percent of doctors are women, most women see male physicians, a situation which severely exaggerates male-female power imbalances.

*We use "medicine" to mean both the *tangible* personnel and institutions of the medical system like physicians and hospitals, and the discipline, field or profession of medicine. We also mean the *intangible* institution of beliefs, ideology and assumptions which influence or control our daily habits in ways most of us are not aware of (as do "the family" and "religion").

professionals.* Despite a few governmental programs—Health Systems Agencies (HSAs) and neighborhood health centers—the medical establishment† has the money and status to confound most citizen attempts to achieve community control.

Our critique of medicine has taken on a new dimension. We see basic errors in its fundamental assumptions about health and healing. Although conventional medical care may at times be just what we need, in many situations it may be bad for our health because it emphasizes drugs, surgery, psychotherapy (especially for women) and crisis action rather than prevention.‡ It is not enough to provide or improve medical care, to have more women physicians, to stop the abuses or to increase access to existing health and medical care for the poor and elderly—even though we support absolutely equal access to care for all classes and groups (see p. 585). We want to reclaim the knowledge and skills which the medical establishment has inappropriately taken over. We also want preventive and nonmedical healing methods to be available to all who need them. We are committed to exposing how the medical establishment works to suppress these alternatives (home birth and nurse-midwifery, for example), contrary to the spirit of the antitrust laws of this country.

Pessimistic as we are about the present system, we believe in the healing powers within all of us—our ability to help one another by listening, talking, caring, touching—and in the power of small groups as sources of information-sharing, support and healing. We still believe that we, as women, are the best experts on ourselves. The more we understand how vulnerable we become—both to disease and to dependency on experts—when isolated from one another, the more we see group experience and action as essential resources for health, from small consciousness-raising or self-help groups to large numbers of women organized for political action.

In this chapter we warn you of some of the dangers of this system and offer strategies to make it work for you as well as possible. We hope that you will feel entitled to demand more information about your health and medical needs, more able to distinguish when to turn to professionals, more empowered to take care of yourself and others when that is appropriate and more deeply convinced that good health is a fundamental right worth fighting for.

The Power of Medicine in Society

Why do most people have an almost religious belief in American medicine? Despite numerous bad or disappointing experiences, so many women say, "It must be my fault" or "I must just have had the wrong doctor," and fail to see that the system itself has serious faults. The institution and ideology of American medicine has penetrated so totally into the fabric of our lives over the past fifty years that most of us aren't even aware of its influence. Its power rests mainly on several widely held myths, which have in good part been created by an aggressive and highly successful public relations campaign of the wealthy AMA and other such groups.* Brought up as most of us were to "believe" in medicine, it is hard at first to realize how influenced (even at times manipulated) we have been by medical propaganda.

Myths and Facts

Myth: *American medical care is the best in the world.*
Fact: The U.S. spends more money on medical care, has more spectacular technology than any country on earth and has one of the highest ratios of doctors and hospitals to people. Yet it lags behind several European countries in infant mortality rates and life expectancy, two crucial basic indicators of health in the general population.[5] Clearly, we are not getting our money's worth.†

---

*Accountability in the case of the medical profession would mean that they be more responsive to our perceived needs and wishes in recognition of the fact that, as taxpayers, we support medical education, research, hospital construction and much of the medical care given in hospitals, nursing homes and clinics.[3] See also the footnote on p. 564 which discusses accountability.

†By "medical establishment" we mean the cluster of organized physician, hospital, drug and insurance groups like the AMA (American Medical Association), the ACOG (American College of Obstetricians and Gynecologists), the AHA (American Hospital Association) and the PMA (Pharmaceutical Manufacturers Association), which pay large sums to influence public opinion, legislation and policy on health and medical matters.

‡Women consume far more prescription drugs, undergo much more unnecessary surgery and are referred for psychotherapy much more often than men, though crisis care is medicine's model for both sexes. (See relevant chapters for details.)

*Misleading tactics have been applied by organized medicine and the drug industry in a variety of situations through their skilled manipulation of the media. Gullible reporters have announced breakthroughs and false reassurances for anything from reselling menopausal estrogens to claiming that the Pill is safe or "…no longer a menace" because it protects a certain subgroup of women from some cancers, etc.[4]

†Some physician apologists have claimed that black and minority groups "drag down" our international standing in infant mortality (a clear case of racism and blaming the victim); however, even some of the most racially homogeneous U.S. communities lag considerably below Europe's best.[6] See also Congressional Research Service, *Infant Mortality: A Report Prepared by the Congressional Research Service for the Use of the Subcommittee on Energy and Commerce, U.S. House of Representatives*, Washington, DC: U.S. Government Printing Office, June 1983; and National Center for Health Statistics, Division of Vital Statistics and Division of Analysis, *Provisional Infant Mortality Rates for the Total Population by State of Occurrence*: U.S., 1980–1982, Figure 3.

Myth: *Medical care has been responsible for the major improvements in world health.*

Fact: Many dread infectious diseases* were "conquered" in the past century, but this was most likely because of improved nutrition and sanitation, not medical care. *Their incidence rates were already falling* when medical treatments and vaccines were introduced. With the exception of smallpox, vaccines helped speed the decline of these diseases only minimally. *The disappearance of these diseases is the major source of our greater life expectancy in this century, leaving the chronic diseases, for which medicine has provided no cures.* Difficult as it is to believe, mortality from most of the chronic diseases, which are our leading causes of death today, has remained virtually unchanged throughout the century.[7]

Careful studies reveal that medical care has *not* been the most important factor in improving infant mortality rates. Factors such as education, income and race continue to be the most accurate predictors of whether infants live or die. *General improvements, especially in nutrition and fertility control, have contributed most to improvements in neonatal mortality rates.*[8]

Myth: *Medicine is a science.*

Fact: Medicine has prestige largely because it is associated with science in the public mind, and claims objectivity and neutrality. Much of the theory on which modern medical practice is based actually derives from the untested assumptions and prejudices of earlier generations of medical leaders. Even though medical schools vaunt their "scientific method," they never actually teach it.[9] Furthermore, the scientific method cannot be applied successfully to human beings, since it is rarely possible to experiment on them as one would on inanimate objects or substances.† (However, animal researchers sometimes produce useful results.)

Myth: *Medical treatments in current use have been proven safe and effective.*

Fact: Most accepted treatments, therapies and medical technologies today have never been *scientifically* evaluated in terms of benefit.‡ Fetal monitors and radical mastectomies are only two examples of technology coming into widespread use before being fully evaluated. Scientific evaluation (in the form of "ran-

domized" or "controlled" clinic trials [RCTs, CCTs]*) is difficult, time- and labor-consuming and expensive, and gets little funding from public sources. Most doctors have had no training in how to evaluate medical treatments and technology, and often base their recommendations simply on what they think may work. As we were told by an assistant professor of medicine at Harvard Medical School:

Too frequently practicing physicians indulge in "cookbook medicine": they open the latest medical journal and inflict the latest recipe on patients, assuring their patients that on the one hand they are receiving "the latest thing" and on the other hand that they are "not guinea pigs."...In fact, the practicing physician is often extending some scientist's last experiment into the community setting—and without obtaining the patient's informed consent! At the same time, the scientist who performed the original experiment five years ago and who wrote the paper two or three years ago has long abandoned that approach in favor of something with more promise for a real cure.

Fact: Most nonreproductive medical research is done only on men and the results are applied to women. Such a process is also far from "scientific." Despite the fact that women make up the greater number of patients, most research, in nutrition and drugs, for example, is conducted on men.[11] One result: women do not know the real benefits and risks of drugs they take.

Myth: *Medical care keeps us healthy.*

Fact: Although deep down many of us believe that medicine has created and sustained our health through the technological advances of the past fifty years, public health† studies show that our health is primarily the result of the food we eat, the water we drink, the air we breathe, the environment we live in, the work we do and the habits we form. These factors in turn result primarily from the education we have, the money we are able to earn and the other resources we are able to command. Still other factors contributing to good health and long life: control over one's personal life, influence over the larger forces that affect all our lives, loving friendships and a supportive community.

Drugs, surgery and medical technology (kidney dialysis machines or blood transfusions, for example)

---

*The diseases were typhoid, smallpox, scarlet fever, measles, whooping cough, diphtheria, influenza, tuberculosis, pneumonia, diseases of the digestive system and poliomyelitis.

†There are always physicians willing to try if allowed to, which is one reason why ethical review boards have been set up in many institutions to set standards which all investigators must abide by. (See "Our Rights as Patients," p. 584.)

‡"No class of [medical] technologies is adequately evaluated for either cost effectiveness or social and ethical implications." (Report from the Congressional Office of Technology Assessment. Quoted in *The Nation's Health*, November 1982. The report, "Strategies for Medical Technology Assessment," is available for $7.50 from the Government Printing Office, Washington, DC 20052. Refer to stock number 052-003-00887-4.)

*While there are other methods of evaluation, RCTs or CCTs are preferable. For these, very large numbers are required. Such trials also require that one group receiving treatment be compared with another (control) group receiving a different treatment or no treatment. This is the most difficult concept for the practicing physician, for whom the withholding of treatment is abhorrent. Without such evaluation, however, there is no way of *proving* that a certain type of medical treatment is effective, even if some people do seem to get better. "Only 10–20 percent of all procedures used in medical practice have been shown by Controlled Clinical Trials to be of benefit."[10]

†Public health, which is the study of diseases or conditions in groups of people, is to be distinguished from medicine, the study and treatment of disease in the individual. Epidemiology is the basic science of public health.

are invaluable tools, and many people would not be alive today without them. While few of us would want to live without these skills and emergency resources available to us and our families, it is fundamentally what *we* do or don't do, not what medicine does, which keeps us healthy.

By focusing on more profitable crisis-care after people get sick rather than using its tremendous resources to help us prevent illness before it happens, the medical establishment shows itself unwilling to consider what really can and must be done to keep people healthy. This is a political issue, not simply a medical one, although many medical spokespeople argue that medicine is apolitical, "scientific" or politically neutral. Because Americans spend increasing health dollars on treating symptoms, we have less to spend on preventing chronic diseases in the first place.* *To consider reallocating the money available would force all of us to confront our economic, political and social system as major contributors to our ill health.*

When we go to a physician, clinic or hospital, every one of these myths encourages us to *trust* professionals, to lean on their reassurances and to follow their orders. Especially when we are sick, it is difficult to be anything but trusting and compliant; being sick is frightening and we *need* to feel comforted. Since medical professionals offer false reassurances more often than we'd like to think, we *must* be as critical as we can, get all the information possible and ask friends and family to help us in doing this.

Poverty, Racism and Health

Poverty is the most basic cause of ill health and early death in our society. The poor, who are mostly women and children and disproportionately people of color, have more illnesses and die in greater numbers and earlier than people with more income and education.[12] Many of their health problems are diseases which result from attendant evils like malnutrition, workplace dangers, environmental pollution or excessive stress.

The medical system blames poor people for suffering the effects of poverty; for instance, accusing poor women of not taking proper care of themselves or their children, and seeing alcoholism and depression in working-class families as individual, preventable failures. Medicaid and Medicare programs, which offered the poor and elderly at least minimal access to medical care, have been cut drastically and would take decades to reinstate.† The very programs which reduce people's need for costly medical care—job training, food-assistance programs, health education to the

community—have been cut as well. The almost inevitable result will be increasing illness and death among the poor.* The United States, the richest country in the world, is the only modern industrial nation without a universal health service or a national health insurance program. Poor women are increasingly turned away from health facilities.[13]

Racism is a serious threat to health, and in some instances creates more barriers to obtaining needed care and to survival than does social class.[14] For example, even allowing for social class, black babies still die at a rate of 6,000 per year more than white babies living in the same geographic area, due mainly to low birth weight among black babies, which is almost entirely preventable.[15] In most communities, medicine's response to the widening "infant death gap" between those who are getting adequate nutrition and prenatal services and those who are not is to propose even more costly neonatal centers.† What's needed is not more expensive machines but a serious attempt to counter the effects of racism or class discrimination on the health of expectant mothers. Leadership for such an effort will not come from the medical establishment, which is heavily invested in technological and pharmacological solutions to problems, not social change.

Although people of color need medical care more often than white people do, they frequently get less. For example, black people are less likely to get the most modern specialty treatment and follow-up care for cancer, and do not survive as long after diagnosis. Similarly, even though hypertension is 82 percent higher among women of color, they do not receive any more treatment than white women.‡ Poor women and women of color often receive more abusive and damaging care than other women, and are more likely to be used as "teaching material" in hospitals,§ so that

cember 1982), p. 6. See also "Vast Reform Needed to Save Medicare, Study Says," by Robert Pear, *The New York Times*, November 30, 1983, for details on the probable bankruptcy of Medicare and the role of payments to doctors in that collapse.

*In Michigan, which has the highest unemployment rate in the country, the infant mortality rate in Detroit increased 3 percent from 12.8 per 1,000 in 1980 to 13.2 in 1981. (*The New York Times*, March 7, 1983.)

†Rhode Island's Women and Infant's Hospital, during the most economically depressed period in recent history, proposed building a 50-million-dollar hospital to include a high-technology neonatal intensive care unit to save low-birth-weight infants in distress. The proposal was at first denied, partly because the state health plan urges *deinstitutionalizing* wherever possible. Also, the Rhode Island Women's Health Collective showed at public hearings that such deaths are *preventable* when resources are spent on community-based nutrition and midwifery-care programs rather than expensive buildings and more high technology. Despite massive opposing testimony from citizens, the building program was approved.

‡See National Academy of Sciences, Institute of Medicine, Division of Health Care Services, "Health Care in a Context of Civil Rights: A Report of a Study," Washington, DC: U.S. Government Printing Office, #1804, 1981.

§See Rogers, et al., "Who Needs Medicaid?" *New England Journal of Medicine*, Vol. 307, No. 1 (1982), pp. 13–18.

*Prevention could reduce our illnesses by about half. (See Derek Bok, *op. cit.* p. 39)

†Nearly 50 percent of Medicaid recipients are categorized as minority" persons (National Health Law Program, Los Angeles, CA 90034). More than 80 percent of the federal cuts were in Medicare/Medicaid. See "The End of Cost Reimbursement" (Point of View), *Bulletin*, California Health Facilities Commission (De-

physicians in training can practice the craft they will use later on wealthy private patients.[16] Sterilization abuse is far more frequent. When clients do not speak English fluently, they are often treated as though they are stupid. Stereotypes so govern practitioners' responses that a minority or poor patient who has the same symptoms as a white middle-class person will receive a different diagnosis and different treatment. In the words of a woman depicted in the film *Taking Our Bodies Back*:*

It almost doesn't matter what I came in for, the place they send me is the "L" clinic ["L" is a code for sexually-transmitted diseases]. They say, "She's black, she's got bladder trouble or a vaginal infection, she must be a prostitute—send her to the 'L' clinic."

When poor women are badly treated, they don't have the money to sue. They may hesitate to complain assertively, fearing that then they will get no care at all, since "free" care may be cut off at any time. Paradoxically, when women decide not to return for care, their absence gives rise to the health administrators' accusation that "they just won't come," although services are available. Again, women are blamed. Poor women also have little access to the more costly nonmedical alternative practices.

Though we are more critical than ever of the present medical system, at the same time we are working for the right of every woman, regardless of race or income, to have access to that system. Above all, we want to promote those social programs which would reduce people's need for expensive medical interventions and work for the deeper societal changes which will help eliminate poverty and racism.

Medicalization and Social Control of Women's Lives

Everywhere one turns, medical professionals are claiming expertise in matters never before considered medical: in criminality, adolescence, overactivity in children, sex, diet, child abuse, exercise and aging. In this takeover, called *medicalization*, medical people become the "experts" on *normal* experiences or social problems.[17] Surely the most striking example of this process is the medicalization of women's lives.

Consider how often we are expected to go to physicians for normal life events. For our early sexual encounters we may expect to go to gynecologists for most birth control devices and perhaps even for advice about sex.† During pregnancy we are urged to see ob-

*For more information on this film, see Resources in Chapter 25, "Organizing for Change: U.S.A."

†Men do not go to urologists for their basic medical care; children are not segregated by sex when visiting pediatricians. Yet for decades many of us are expected to go to an obstetrician-gynecologist to obtain our basic care. We learn to do this without realizing that by doing so we begin to define ourselves and all our bodily needs in terms of our sex organs and reproductive capacities.

stetricians to be sure all is proceeding normally, and few of us have any alternative but the hospital for giving birth. (See Chapter 19, "Childbirth.") The medicalizing of childbirth has become so complete that it resembles treatment for a severe, life-threatening illness. When birth goes well, we are often grateful to the physician, and give her or him the credit for our success; when it goes badly, we are even more grateful for the interventions we believe saved us and our babies. And once the baby is born, we shift our gratitude and dependence to the pediatrician, so that even the first moments of mothering are conducted with an immediate sense of what our pediatrician thinks is right and proper.

When we are depressed or having difficulties in our personal relationships, we are encouraged to seek the advice and help of a psychiatrist instead of talking with friends. Women see psychiatrists in far greater numbers than men. (See Chapter 6, "Psychotherapy.")

Medicine has stepped up its treatment of menopause and of aging as diseases. In a sense, the medical world defines women as inherently defective throughout life, in that we "require" a physician's care for all our normal female functions.

Medical "care" offered often extends to value judgments about our behavior, as we hear how a good girl, a good wife, a good mother should behave.

After advising me on when to put in my diaphragm ("Dinner, dishes, diaphragm," he said), my ob/gyn went on to speak about the fairly serious postpartum depression I was experiencing. "I like to tell my new mothers to get out to the library once in a while to keep their minds alive, but basically to find their happiness in the fact that they are taking care of their husbands and raising a new generation."

When I told my doctor (foolishly) that I'm a lesbian, the whole visit turned into a moral lecture and he never really paid attention to my problem. I walked out when he recommended a psychiatrist.

These moral judgments carry a weighty power, though they are no more "scientific" than the judgments of a priest or rabbi.*

We don't question the role that the physician has taken in our lives because, for one thing, our exposure and acceptance began early. When we were little, our mothers took us regularly to "the doctor," an extremely busy and important person, who may have ignored what our mothers said, and certainly what we said, and had their own answers. It may have seemed that our mothers allowed doctors to do all kinds of embarrassing or uncomfortable things to us, and even

*See Janice Raymond, "Medicine as Patriarchal Religion," *The Journal of Medicine and Philosophy*, Vol. 7 (1982), pp. 197–216, for further explanation of this point.

that they did some of the same things themselves later on on the doctor's orders. Our mothers were very passive and compliant, in part because by the twentieth century male physicians had become the "authorities" on health. They had led a successful campaign during the late nineteenth and early twentieth centuries to eliminate midwives and sharply reduced the number of female physicians. For the first time in the history of the world, women were forbidden by law to be responsible for other women's childbirths, and were replaced almost exclusively by male physicians (see p. 592). When this happened, women lost both female role models and caregivers and also the support of a whole system of woman-to-woman guidance. (See "Women as Healers," p. 589.)

During the mid-twentieth century, the gradual further moving of childbirth out of the home and into the hospital continued the process of isolating women from one another. Perhaps we have yet to measure how deeply our self-confidence as women may have been damaged by the loss of midwives as role models and respected sources of information and female authority.

All these factors together have brought us into an extreme and enforced dependency on professional experts—usually male physicians or those trained by them.*

Through these many medical encounters in the course of our normal life experiences, physicians gradually initiate women into the medical belief system, warning us against listening to other women, belittling the advice of mothers, aunts, grandmothers and midwives—female lore—by calling it "old wives' tales." In this way, physicians prepare us to be their disciples. As we carry their message into our families and communities, we further contribute to the medicalization of society and a narrow, biological/technological perspective on the solution of human problems.†

It is difficult for most of us to recognize how "allopathic" medicine's proponents historically used women and women's central life experiences to initiate our entire society into a belief in and dependency on medicine. Despite much evidence to the contrary, most physicians believe sincerely that modern medicine has always helped women and that it deserves credit for society's overall health improvements since the turn of the century. Thus they tend to feel it is women's moral duty to teach children to place their faith in medicine.

---

*For more on this, see Barbara Ehrenreich and Deirdre English, *For Her Own Good*, listed in Resources in Chapter 25, "Organizing for Change: U.S.A."
†For a thorough analysis of medicalization and iatrogenesis, see Ivan Illich, *Medical Nemesis*, listed in Resources in Chapter 25.

Medicine as an Institution of Social Control

All societies establish institutions of social control, vested with the authority to define what is right or wrong, good or bad, sick or well. The schools, courts and churches all play a role in defining our morality, but perhaps none more thoroughly than medicine does today. When we "deviate"—fail to conform to norms of womanhood—we discover how powerful medicine is.* Consider the ugly pronouncements medical authorities have made over the years, in the name of "science," about so-called "inferior" groups of people like women and blacks, and the way these pseudo-scientific statements have been used to deprive these groups of social control and political power. For example, in the nineteenth century physicians claimed that to become a midwife or a doctor would "unsex" a woman: she would see things which would taint her moral character, cause her to "lose her standing as a 'lady'" and, because of the unusual physical and nervous excitement, "would damage her female organs irreparably and prevent her from fulfilling her social role as a wife and mother."[19] About blacks, a nineteenth-century physician wrote:

> ...the grown-up Negro partakes, as regards his intellectual faculties, of the nature of the child, the female, and the senile White....[20]

This misuse of power and these pronouncements continue today: physicians dismiss females as too much "at the mercy of their hormones" to be trusted with serious responsibility, and cite blacks' "low-degree expectations" as a hurdle to parity in medical schools.†

Partly through the sanctity of the private physician/patient relationship, medicine (primarily obstetrics/gynecology and psychiatry) also achieves social control by encouraging us to see personal problems as individual isolated experiences rather than as problems we have in common with other women.

The Doctor-Patient Relationship

The relationship between a woman and her doctor is usually one of profound inequality on every level, an

---

*For example, many poor women are sterilized without their knowledge or consent because they are unmarried or a physician thinks they have "too many babies" (see "Sterilization" p. 256). Physicians have forced some women to accept Cesarean sections, declaring them "unfit mothers" in court when they refuse a recommended section (despite the risk to the mother's own life); some women have had their children taken from them by the courts because a physician judged them "potential child abusers" for refusing medical treatments during pregnancy.[18]
†The kinds of biological (rather than societal) explanations for behavior and social position popular in the nineteenth century are becoming influential once again. Reinforced by such notions as "sociobiology," these myths have dangerous consequences for women, people of color and the poor.[21]

exaggeration of the power imbalance inherent in almost all male-female relationships in our society. The scales are even more unbalanced if the doctor is an ob/gyn with special knowledge about and power over our most intimate bodily selves, or a psychiatrist with the authority to label us crazy or sane, to decide whether we can keep our children or not. *Doctors also frequently doubt our word simply because we are women.*

As in any relationship in which we are less powerful, we tend to evaluate what happens in a medical encounter in terms of *our* behavior rather than the doctor's. If we were embarrassed, we think we shouldn't have been; if we were impatient waiting, we feel ungrateful; if we didn't get all our questions answered, we think we were being too demanding. Often we believe that a doctor's superior education, training, experience, sex and (sometimes) age automatically produce infallible judgment. "Well, he must know," many women say.

We even ask trustingly for advice about how to conduct our lives. Many of us want to believe that we are in the hands of superior physicians—even though this may well not be true.

I knew that my doctor had a reputation for being one of the best in the city, and it made me feel good when I said his name and other people would say, "Oh, right, I've heard of him." I expected that he was going to do the best job he could possibly do. When he criticized me, I shrank inside. Sometimes I'd be annoyed that I had to travel so far for him to look at my stomach. But the mysteries still held. He was going to give me the baby. Once he confused me with someone else, and I was very depressed.

There may always be something about the "laying on of hands" that calls up the child in us and makes us feel dependent, especially when pain and fear are present. Many physicians deliberately work to increase this natural phenomenon into a special kind of dependency (psychiatrists call it "transference") in which the patient turns to the physician for guidance in all kinds of personal problems. Many medical schools and residency training programs teach techniques for eliciting this dependency—with a few vague cautions thrown in—as a useful way of "managing" patients, using the parent-child relationship as a model.* When a woman raises real, matter-of-fact questions, a doctor is apt to say, "What's the matter, don't you trust me?" For most doctors, the fact that the transference develops is justification for it—that is, a woman becomes overly dependent because she "needs" or wants to be.

Dr. G. sighed when he saw me. After examining me he sat down and said, "Let me be direct with you, hon." (I flinched at the "hon.") "You have called me or been here no less than four times this fall. You are complaining about a pain that has no apparent organic basis. Quite frankly, my guess is that there are areas of your life you are having trouble facing, and the result is a funny pain in your chest and shoulder that flits around and is sometimes here and sometimes there and sometimes not anywhere at all."
"But I can feel exactly where it is," I broke in.
"Why don't you just leave the worrying to me?" he admonished. "I am the doctor. I have everything under control."*

We can resist this dependency by pressing for real answers to our questions, using other sources of information besides our doctors (books, magazines, friends, nurses), seeking second opinions (not from a doctor who is our doctor's close colleague, on the same hospital staff or in the same specialty) and by bringing a friend to medical visits. Immersed in the propaganda about women's "need" for dependency, and comfortable with the fatherly, authoritarian role, many physicians react with surprise and even hostility at our "aggressiveness" when we insist on being partners in our health and medical-care decisions. We must not let their reactions prevent us from persisting.

Occasionally, over time, you can build a satisfactory relationship with a doctor.

Friends now marvel at my close relationship with my current doctor and my ability to talk back, question and disagree with him and his colleagues. He respects me and trusts me to tell him what is going on, and I in turn trust him to listen, make suggestions and consult with me before any action is taken. When I don't want a procedure done or feel the psychological burden of making yet another trip to the lab or to his office is just too much for me on an occasion, I will tell him and he understands me most of the time. I have finally after many many years found someone willing to take into account my whole medical history and apply it to my current situation.

Sexual Abuse

Not only have women reported increasing numbers of cases of rape by their doctors, but between 5 and 10 percent of doctors have admitted in surveys and interviews to having sexual relations with their patients,[23] sometimes saying that they believed such relations were either harmless or actually beneficial

---

*As Diana Scully describes in her 1980 landmark study of obstetrician/gynecologists,[22] the training process prepares the surgeon to gain the patient's trust and confidence primarily for the purpose of controlling or "managing" her, and then to *manipulate* her into doing something *the physician wants her to do*—undergoing surgery, for example, or some other procedure. Usually, this is done either to gain experience or to generate income and is frequently not in her interests. (See the sections on hysterectomy and other relevant procedures.)

*From a woman who was later operated on for a rare form of cancer which had spread to her lungs. Stephani Cook, *Second Life*, New York: Simon and Schuster, 1981.

or "therapeutic"' to the women involved. Because of the unequal power relationships involved, this sexual abuse may produce severe damage, akin to father-daughter incest.[24] When the woman turns to or is referred to a psychiatrist, she may be blamed for having "caused" the abuse.* Worse still, a few psychiatrists seduce the woman once again.[25]

It takes enormous courage for women to come forward and speak out about sexual abuse by doctors. Frequently no one believes them, and in one case, even nurses reporting their eyewitness experiences of patient abuse for three years were ignored by hospital administrators until another physician caught his anesthesiologist colleague in the act.[26]

The few cases which do reach state boards of registration in medicine frequently drag on for months and are then resolved with inadequate controls on future abuse. In spite of the fact that the Hippocratic oath and the ethics codes of all medical societies specifically forbid sexual relations with patients, doctors have made no serious effort to discipline those who breach the code. In fact, the medical profession often appears more concerned with covering up for a colleague who commits what are tactfully called "indiscretions." In the words of a woman psychiatrist:

I reported a psychiatrist who had had sex with two of his patients to the medical society. I called back two months later to find out what had been done. They told me the doctor denied everything, and it was his word against the patients; so they were dropping the matter. When I persisted, the chairman of the ethics committee told me, "You know, my dear, we are not a consumer organization."

Physicians themselves may arrange for a problem physician to go to another community, without telling the unsuspecting new community about his assaultive behavior. In one famous case, medical school faculty members wrote glowing letters of recommendation for a convicted rapist who had moved to a new community.†[27]

It is common for women who are sexually abused by a doctor to be persuaded that he has fallen in love with them. This is not a sign of naiveté or psychopathology on our part. The physicians involved have abused a trust which every woman has learned to place in them. (See also Chapter 8, "Violence Against Women.")

We want to encourage women to notice any peculiar or irresponsible behavior and discuss these experiences with one another; to feel entitled to take action if necessary, protect ourselves and others and get our genuine needs for trust met appropriately. Keep a record of what happens; call a local women's group or rape crisis center; give serious consideration to mentioning your experience to a reliable lawyer.

The Profit Motive in Medical Care

Why doesn't the present U.S. medical system provide affordable services and emphasize prevention and primary care? The profit motive has to be the main reason. From the many individuals who still want to be paid "fee for service" and build up a lucrative practice to the profit-making drug and insurance companies, medical care is now an industry in itself—the second-largest in the country—and a virtual monopoly.

The Medical Monopoly

Our present type of medicine created a monopoly at the turn of the century through its control over state licensing laws which defined what the practice of medicine should be and who could be called a doctor. The laws provided state-sanctioned penalties for those who were not "properly" trained and licensed. At the same time the medical profession also gained absolute control over its education process, thus becoming a "legally enforced monopoly of practice."[28] Today medicine continues to set its own priorities and terms, with physicians controlling about 70 percent of the medical decision-making and resource allocation process. The profession decides what will be taught in medical schools, what medical services will be offered and how and where.* Surgeons generate most of their own income by self-referral ("I recommend this procedure and I will also perform it."), a practice judged unethical in other countries. Patients or third-party payers pay for services rendered. With rare exception, there is no one but another doctor to decide whether or not these services are necessary, and no way of knowing whether or not they are effective. When review of costs occurs (as in the case of insurance), it is usually fellow physicians who undertake that review.

Medicine's monopoly was further consolidated when the government made federal funds available for hospital construction (Hill-Burton law), and the "Blues" (Blue Cross/Blue Shield) were created to reimburse in-hospital care. (Many of the Blue Crosses were created

---

*Another 20 percent believe this. In California alone, one survey reported 36 percent of psychiatrists and 46 percent of psychologists had admitted affairs with clients during therapy.

†See also Fox Butterfield, "Doctors' Praise Assailed for Peer in Rape Case," *The New York Times*, September 24, 1981.

*Because medical care should always involve so much more than the application of technical skills and because it always occurs in a social context, society should be able to influence both the quality and quantity of medical care available. For example, we have too many specialists crowded into affluent communities and entirely more doctors than we need, although many inner city and rural areas in greater need have severe shortages of physicians. Yet 95 percent of physicians now specialize, despite a predicted shortage of 16,000 primary-care physicians by 1990, and medical schools take no leadership in rectifying the problem. (See also the footnote on p. 564.) More than 20 million persons now have inadequate access to quality care.[29]

originally by local medical societies and are still physician-dominated.) Backed up by the private insurance industry, hospitals became the base of medical care in this country. Substantial federal funding for Medicare, Medicaid and medical research increased the volume of federal money flowing into medicine. At the same time, profit-making hospital and nursing-home chains also began to proliferate. Today expenditures for medical care grow faster than anything else. The whole system is completely out of control, despite growing cuts. Medicine has been allowed to expand continuously, and virtually without limits or accountability.*

In addition, there has been a phenomenal rise in the "corporatization" of medical care; that is, profit-making medical care chains which operate laboratories, "emergency rooms," mobile CAT scanners, etc., in addition to hospitals and nursing homes—a proliferation of separate services purely for profit.† Academic centers, medical schools and teaching hospitals have themselves created new and unprecedented arrangements amounting to millions of dollars with profit-making drug firms, all in the name of "scientific research"[30]—the "medical-academic-industrial complex."

Those who profit from our illnesses are well-organized politically, and use their ample resources to keep the medical system free from government intrusion. While they do not always agree among themselves, an informal coalition—physicians' lobbying groups like the AMA and ACOG, the pharmaceutical industry, hospital associations, the big voluntary "health" associations (Heart Association, Cancer Society, etc.), among others—tend to support the profit motive, the fee-for-service reimbursement system and the present crisis-care medical model.‡

*Because so much of our tax money is involved, we expect public utilities and our public education system, for example, to be somewhat accountable to the users. Through a public process we participate in decisions about cost, services and salaries, and sometimes even the budget itself. Though medical education, research and hospital operations are heavily subsidized by our taxes at all levels, we have virtually no say in how this money is spent. A few federally funded attempts were made in the past to make medicine more accountable, such as the formation of Health Systems Agencies (HSAs), but further attempts will now have to depend on local funding and initiative.

In addition, when there are errors or abuses in medical practice, physicians insist on "policing" themselves, leaving our range of options for redress short and unsatisfactory. (See "Medical Education and Training," p. 567, and "Our Rights as Patients," p. 584.)

†For example, recent surveys show that half of U.S. physicians are now on salary, many in profit-making corporations which are often physician-owned. The "fee-for-service" system is changing, but not necessarily for the benefit of consumers, since only a few salaried doctors work in nonprofit settings such as health centers. Many can actually earn more on salary than via "fee for service."

‡The Center for Science in the Public Interest has recently launched a Health Charities Reform Project to challenge how these extremely wealthy national organizations spend the money

Health care is becoming a commodity or economic good, with profit as a blatant and legitimate goal. However inadequate government involvement in

---

Where Does the Money Go?

- Today the average U.S. family spends 12 percent of its income on medical care. Inability to pay medical bills is the leading cause of personal bankruptcy.
- Close to 10 percent of our GNP (gross national product) is spent on medical care, 250 billion dollars in 1981 and still rising.
- Our tax dollars support 43 percent of the medical enterprise. This amounts to fifteen cents out of every federal tax dollar.
- Hospital costs in mid-1982 were increasing three times faster than inflation, and now average 2,119 dollars per stay, up from 670 dollars in 1971.
- Despite insurance coverage for 90 percent of Americans, we still pay over a third of our total medical bill out of pocket directly to physicians.
- Technology accounts for 70 percent of the rise in costs over the past decade, most of it of unproven value.
- The hospital industry and the nursing-home industry together account for one-half of all U.S. expenditures on health. Of this amount (138 billion dollars), half is for "ancillary" services (tests, etc.).*

I am retired on a pension of 5,500 dollars a year—no social security. I pay:

Blue Cross/Blue Shield	$ 863.64	
Medicare	122.20	
Deductible	60.00	
Doctors	102.00	*(after subtracting reimbursement)*
Eyeglass frame	50.00	*(no reimbursement so far)*
Eyedrops for glaucoma (2 different types)	110.00	
	$1,307.84	*(27.77 percent of pension)†*

---

donated to them, and to spur them to play a more effective role in health policy directed toward prevention. We can work locally by getting onto boards of chapters to help influence local projects (see Resources in Chapter 25, "Organizing for Change: U.S.A.").

*The above information is from a variety of sources available on request from the Collective office.

†Letter from a woman in Florida. She pays for "Blues" *and* Medicare because Medicare will be inadequate if she gets seriously ill.

medical care was, it did make it possible for us to partially evaluate the system. It increased access to the system in some regions for a percentage of those who most needed it, and helped us to monitor or check a few of the system's most flagrant abuses. Government agencies were forced to respond *somewhat* to citizen pressure in the name of public interest. But federal regulations are evaporating in the eighties, with the result that profit-making enterprises will increase in number and monitoring their practices will be more difficult. In less than ten years the concept of health as a *right*, which had begun to seem reasonably secure, has been threatened as never before.[31]

Our best hope is to form groups of workers and friends in the community, and to work at the state level, making sure that reasonable options for care remain open to as many as possible at reasonable prices.

Insurance

The insurance principle has become increasingly influential in shaping U.S. medical care. All "third-party" reimbursement systems, whether through private, profit-making insurance systems, "nonprofit" Blue Cross/Blue Shield (the "Blues") or public programs (Medicare, Medicaid), reward doctors and hospitals by reimbursing them for doing the most expensive and complicated procedures "fee for service." Yet they pay nothing or even require us to pay out of pocket for basic well-woman or preventive care. The insurance system thus acts as a kind of "blank check": we pay the premiums, directly or through our taxes (both continually rising); the doctors and hospitals bill the third parties (sometimes doctors also bill us for the "difference" between what insurance covers and what their real charges are), and there is no one looking to see if something cheaper or better (or sooner) might have been done. Medical costs skyrocket as a result. The chief beneficiaries of the insurance system are actually the doctors and stockholders, whose incomes and profits are all guaranteed.[32]

The insurance industry discriminates blatantly against women both as health and medical care workers and as consumers. Programs rarely reimburse directly for the services of nonphysician workers like nurse-midwives, nurse-practitioners, physical therapists and nutritionists, the majority of whom are women (though this varies and is slowly changing). Instead they reimburse the physicians, health departments or hospitals who hire or supervise them, and indeed profit from their labor.

In the case of consumers, the Fair Insurance Practices Act outlaws bias on grounds of race, color, religion or national origin, but *not* sex. Companies often assume that "the husband" is a "primary" wage earner, and gear policies around the notion that wife and children are dependents. When marriage ends through death or divorce, benefits often cease automatically.[33] In some parts of the country, single women cannot get coverage for reproductive health in areas such as contraception, childbirth or abortion. Women are often denied access to policies available to men, and are assigned higher costs, different benefits and lesser coverage. (One exception: maternity benefits as part of workplace compensation has been achieved through the courts.) Many unions also omit women's health needs when negotiating for insurance benefits, partly because women participate less in union organizing and partly because covering women is more expensive. (Ironically, this is to some extent due to unnecessary surgery urged on women by physicians.)

What to Do?

Shopping carefully for policies is a first and basic step, but it is hardly enough, and difficult to do. At the very least, look over your policy and have it explained thoroughly. Many people do not discover until they actually use a policy that maternity care, for example, is often inadequately covered, and that there are many exclusions, co-payments (the company pays something and you also pay something) and deductibles (they will pay, but only after you have paid a certain amount, which they then deduct). Get involved with other women in "economic literacy" programs, where the intricacies of this and other finance industries are exposed and explained (life insurance, too). Change policies if you can.

It is no coincidence that the wealthy private insurance industry has contributed more than any other group to campaigns to defeat the ERA. If passed, the ERA would almost certainly require much more equitable treatment of women, both as premium-payers and as beneficiaries. Companies might then have to choose between cutting profits and raising rates for male customers to equalize their contributions.

For all these and many other reasons, a national health *insurance* system is not the answer* to either inadequate coverage or the inflationary fee-for-service system, both of which would be perpetuated (along with the sex discrimination) under this plan. We cannot hope to improve women's coverage without consistent organizing pressure in the companies—large and small—where we are employed. On a state level, getting involved with women's health groups, governors' commissions on the status of women, or NOW (The National Organization for Women) is absolutely necessary to the creation of effective coalitions working to change laws governing the insurance industry

*Presently close to 9 million people have lost insurance coverage as a result of unemployment. A majority of poor and near-poor blacks and Hispanics have no insurance during all or part of the year due to seasonal unemployment, or earnings so marginal they don't qualify for Medicaid but cannot afford insurance.

and thereby eliminate discriminatory practices. OWL (The Older Women's League) has been working in many states to require laws which will continue a woman's insurance coverage after death or divorce of a spouse, or after retirement.* But the best single mechanism is the passage of ERA legislation at the national as well as state level, and what we need is a *nonprofit* national health *service* for all.

The Drug Industry

Almost nowhere is the inherent conflict between profit-making and public safety more obvious than with the manufacture and sale of prescription drugs. Yet it is difficult to control the drug industry, which lies at the heart of both the medical system and the capitalist system. According to Dr. James L. Goddard, former commissioner of the FDA:†

An American buying prescription drugs buys on faith what his doctor has prescribed. He is like a child who goes to the store with his mother's shopping list, which he cannot even read. He is totally unsophisticated as to the workings of the $5,000,000,000 [1972 figures] industry to which he is contributing and which his tax money is already helping to support. The consumer of drugs pays up and takes his medicine, and the Drug Establishment, about which he knows nothing, scores again.

Prescription drug sales in 1981 were estimated at about 10 billion dollars, averaging ten prescriptions for every adult and child in the U.S.[34] Pharmaceutical companies regularly show a return on investment of close to 18 percent (more than half again as much as the nearest competitive industry), outperforming any other part of the industrial sector.[35]

While some drugs do save lives and enhance the quality of life for many sick people, research reveals increasing numbers of both new and older drugs to be dangerous or useless.‡ The GAO (the government's General Accounting Office) reports that Medicare/Medicaid pays 40 million dollars a year for drugs shown to have no effectiveness. Each year, at least 1.5 million people go into the hospital because they have adverse reactions to drugs.[37] Women receive about two-thirds of all prescription drugs, and the most profitable drugs made by the industry are oral contraceptives, injectable contraceptives (like Depo-Provera) and tranquilizers, all dangerous in some ways and all targeted mainly for women.[38]

Drug companies spend well over a billion and a half dollars a year in advertising for physicians, almost four times the amount spent on research and development, despite industry claims to the contrary.[39] Virtually all this advertising is beamed directly to physicians (some to pharmacists) by drug "detail" men or women through personal contact, costing the drug company 4,000 to 5,000 dollars annually for each practicing physician.* Representatives of the drug companies give out free stethoscopes and other gifts to students in the medical schools; sponsor lectures and symposia in teaching hospitals; and in many prestigious medical centers, one salesman is assigned to *each* physician in specialty training, offering samples and getting feedback. Because medical school training in pharmacology is largely inadequate, doctors become permanently dependent on drug companies for information (or misinformation). As a result, physicians often cannot or do not protect us from ineffective or dangerous drugs. Often they don't know the possibly serious negative effects, or they continue to prescribe the drugs anyway,† based on personal observation or the belief that any negative findings (always challenged by the drug companies) have been inaccurate. Doctors also tend to prescribe the advertised brand-name drugs, which are more profitable to the drug companies, rather than using generic drugs, cheaper for the consumer,[41] and often encourage patients' notions that a visit to a doctor is not complete without a prescription to "solve" the problem.

Regulation

The Food and Drug Administration (FDA) was ostensibly designed to protect the public from the dangers of adulterated food and harmful or useless drugs.‡ Over many years, the efforts of some conscientious FDA staff, prompted and encouraged by the pressure of consumer groups, activists, investigative reporters and members of Congress, have sometimes led to effective, though limited, protection, as well as increased consumer participation in the regulatory process.

● Barbara Seaman, a founder of the National Women's Health Network and an early researcher on the Pill and menopausal estrogens, helped alert the

---

*As we go to press, national legislation is also pending which would eliminate sex discrimination in insurance. (See Chapter 22, "Women Growing Older.") Legislation calling for a national health service which would eliminate profit-making insurance has also been filed.

†Quoted in *Science for the People*, Science and Society Series, No. 1 (November 1973).

‡An industry-sponsored study of all drugs approved between 1938 and 1962 showed only 12 percent effective for their prescribed use and at least 15 percent to have no effectiveness whatsoever. *Yet most of these drugs are still on the market.*[36]

*See Dr. James L. Goddard's comments above. These figures are a decade old, but recent figures indicate that about 3,000 to 4,000 dollars is still spent on U.S. doctors (see Maryann Napoli, cited in note 36 [p. 596]). Figures for detail men overseas are more difficult to obtain, but they probably make up the additional sum (see Milton Silverman, cited in note 35 [p. 596]).

†For instance, physicians continued to prescribe progestin for pregnancy tests despite the discovery of a link to birth defects. The FDA warned against the use of the drug in the early stages of pregnancy, yet 75,000 prescriptions for progestin tests were given in 1978, years after the first FDA warning. (Testimony of Sidney Wolfe before Senator Kennedy's subcommittee.)[40]

‡See Chapter 2, "Food," for more on the FDA.

public to the risk of these drugs in her testimony before Congress.

- Doris Haire, founder of the American Foundation for Maternal and Child Health, has repeatedly challenged the FDA, Congress and physician experts to demonstrate the safety to the infant and mother of drugs administered during pregnancy, labor and delivery.
- Nader's Health Research Group has publicized the dangers and ineffectiveness of many drugs, successfully pressured the FDA to get them off the market, testified in Congress and worked extensively with the FDA staff on behalf of consumers.

However, these achievements are being increasingly threatened by the "antiregulatory" climate of a conservative government, and also by the fact that the FDA's small budget has never been able to compete against the huge financial resources the drug industry musters for lobbying, court cases and the production of new products. The FDA is no match for many of the "best" drug companies, which often have substantial criminal records involving bribing of officials in foreign governments, falsifying of test data and failing to comply with FDA requirements to report adverse reactions to drugs.[42] Since drug companies are themselves required to test new drugs for safety and effectiveness, they also hire most of the researchers; if the research lab or doctor can make data look favorable to the company, it is more likely to continue to obtain funding.

At the very least, the drug industry should be required to submit to certain basic reforms, such as the severing of financial connections to those researching the safety and efficacy of the drugs they want to market, and the payment of much more severe penalties for misconduct. Consumer and public-interest groups have to be better watchdogs than ever before, and also must serve as pressure groups to establish better regulatory systems at the state and local levels.

Medical Education and Training

Physicians have unusually broad powers. They decide which patients will be treated and where, who goes to the hospital, what treatment is given and for how long and which drugs are administered and in what quantities. They also have enormous influence in our most personal decisions. Why do so many physicians misuse their power, consciously or unconsciously? Many of the behaviors we complain about in physicians—their authoritarian manner, their insensitivity and condescension—can be traced back to their education and training as doctors.

Who Gets into Medical School?

Traditionally, upper- and upper-middle-class white men have been the ones to survive the fierce competition for medical school entrance. In the words of one prestigious medical educator, "The years of premedical education, once considered so rewarding, have become a battleground of ruthless competition."* Some students tear out textbook pages so others cannot read them, and distort their fellow-students' experiments. Many also cheat, and it is known that those who do so will continue their deceptive behavior as doctors. Experienced educators have believed for some time that medicine is no longer attracting the best and brightest students, one reason being that they are repelled by the typical premed who would become their colleague. Although 1960s and 1970s activism resulted in a surge of women, poor and minority students, this number peaked around 1977, in part due to cutbacks in federal funding and in part to the fact that most medical schools were accepting these other candidates only under pressure.† Therefore, most physicians train alongside people more or less exactly like themselves, with teachers formed from the same mold. The result is a kind of cloning: the medical profession reproduces itself.[43]

The Training

Medical schools ask students to absorb an enormous quantity of highly technical information in compressed form, largely through one-way lectures. They place little emphasis on thinking and reasoning, and none at all on questioning, criticizing or arguing. Few could learn to think critically in this environment if they did not know how before medical school. Students "are being driven to absorb an enormous amount of science at the sacrifice of just about everything else." Recall is poor after even a short period, however, and many in academic medicine admit that much of this material, irrelevant to competent medical practice, has crowded out crucial skills and subject matter.[44] In the words of a woman physician:

The training program is disease-oriented, with life-threatening or rare conditions receiving the most attention, and the acquisition of skill in doing procedures (biopsies, punctures) and using diagnostic machines (EKG, X-ray, lab tests) being prized. The day-to-day ills of the public are ignored as "minor problems." The promotion of health and the prevention of disease are neglected almost entirely.[45]

The training does not challenge students to become more aware of the social and political realities affecting people's health or to work through their own sexism, homophobia, class bias, ageism and racism. A woman doctor, a chief resident at a Philadelphia hospital, who does have a political awareness, wrote:

When I show a student her own cervix with a mirror, she is fascinated. When she is with me as a student and I offer my white middle-class patient the opportunity, the student thinks it is great. But when I offer a sixty-year-

*Dr. John Z. Bowers, as quoted in *Medical Area Focus* (Harvard Medical School), February 11, 1982.

†Enrollments for women are still increasing, however.

old woman the chance or a twenty-five-year-old working-class black woman, the student is amazed that "that kind" of patient would want to see her cervix. When I say, "This could be done in the clinic and would make women feel more in control," students say to me, "Oh, no, there's no time" (one extra minute?) or, worse, " 'Those people' wouldn't be interested."

Glaringly absent from medical training are most of the values, concerns and skills often thought of as "feminine": nurturance, empathy, caring, sensitive listening, encouraging others to take care of themselves, collaboration rather than competition. The medical hierarchy relegates these values and skills to the domain of nurses, other aides and (female) family members of the patients—physicians have "more important" things to attend to. Patients deprived of these elements of caring may not be as quick to recover, may miss absorbing important information about aftercare or preventive care and may end up feeling depressed about their experience because no one has paid attention to the emotional impact of their health problems. Women often complain bitterly of cold, abstract, impersonal or authoritarian doctors. A major study by the Institute of Medicine found that a majority of families were dissatisfied with their doctors and up to half had changed them as a result.* These qualities may have less to do with the physician's original personality than with the one-sidedness of her or his training. Similarly vital knowledge needed for optimum patient care—how to evaluate studies and risks accurately, what tests and treatments really cost, how to recognize a patient's rights and identify the ethical issues involved in medical decisions, what patients could do for themselves to prevent illness— is either absent altogether or relegated to the status of an elective. Students get the message: this material is not important.†

Many medical educators are now alarmed over the erosion of clinical skills caused by the overemphasis on technology in today's training; that is, by the increasing inability of younger physicians to make judgments based on experience, examination and careful listening to the patient rather than on readings from tests and machines.[46]

The focus narrows further at the residency stage, where students aim to specialize because specialization promises more money, prestige and control over one's work.

Specialization and the rapid rate of advancement of knowledge and technology may tend to pre-empt the attention of both teachers and students from the central purpose of medicine, which is to heal the sick and relieve suffering.‡

*Derek Bok, *Harvard Magazine*, May–June 1984, p. 43.
†Ibid.
‡Curriculum review panel for medical school education initiated by the Association of American Medical Colleges. *The New York Times*, October 21, 1982.

Residency programs are grueling, low-paid, often demanding as much as thirty-six hours at a stretch and a hundred hours a week in consistently understaffed conditions, undesirable for both residents and patients alike. Teaching becomes haphazard and, not surprisingly, all types of residents have shown declining scores and performances in recent years, particularly in basic skills.

In short, specialty training is a dehumanizing process. Few working conditions in the industrial age have survived with so little change. Composed of one part sleep deprivation, one part shutting off of all feelings and one part automatic response to orders in what is probably the most militaristic of all civilian disciplines, this training resembles a kind of brainwashing.* The stress contributes to physicians' high rates of mental breakdown, drug addiction, alcoholism, suicide and family disruption.† Rates of incompetence among physicians in practice have also grown alarmingly.‡ In addition to errors, they both perform many useless procedures and fail to perform needed ones.§

*The term "brainwashing" has been used repeatedly by medical educators, students and physicians in conversations with the authors. See also Allan Chamberlain, "Night Life: Sleep Deprivation in Medical Education," *The New Physician* (May 1981), p. 30, for use of this term.
†See Jack D. McCue, "The Effects of Stress on Physicians and Their Medical Practice," *New England Journal of Medicine*, Vol. 306, No. 8 (February 25, 1982), pp. 458–63.
‡*The New York Times* (Series), Boyce Rensberger, et al., "Unfit Doctors Create Worry in Profession," January 26–31, 1976.
§President's Commission for the Study of Ethical Problems in Medicine and Biomedical Research. *Securing Access to Health Care*, 1983. Also see Marcia Millman, *The Unkindest Cut* (see Resources).

Lady as physician   *The Feminist Press*

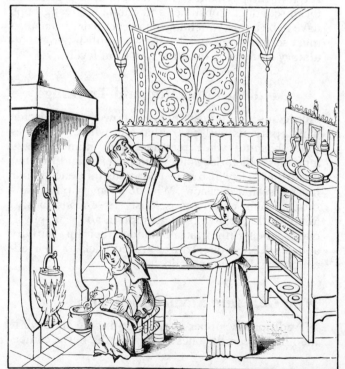

Images of Women in Medical Textbooks

Medical students and physicians in residency training are often referred to ob/gyn and psychoanalysis textbooks as sources of authority on how to determine the character of and how to "manage" women patients. Most practicing physicians today absorbed as students considerable sexist, judgmental and paternalistic dogma from these books.* While there have been some improvements in recent years, the following excerpts are from recent texts currently used in leading medical schools today. The tone of these comments clearly encourages doctors to think of themselves as skilled and powerful counselors who have the right and even the obligation to act as our judges and moral guardians. It is ironic that doctors are looked upon by society as experts on women's psyche and sexuality, yet are typically so ignorant and poorly trained. These passages help perpetuate both the attitudes and errors passed down from one generation of doctors to the next.

1983 The evaluation of the patient's personality need not be a lengthy matter. It begins as she enters the consultation room and sits down. Character traits are expressed in her walk, her dress, her makeup, her responses to questions, and in almost every action, both verbal and non-verbal in nature. The observant physician can quickly make a judgment as to whether she is overcompliant, overdemanding, aggressive, passive, erotic or infantile....

Many physicians hesitate to delve into a patient's emotional state because they fear a negative reaction from the patient or even that their questions might make the patient feel worse. If they question patients gently and watch for signs of resistance, no harm can be done. Certainly the patient who responds with anger or disgust should be allowed to keep her own confidences, but this response in itself indicates that an emotional problem may exist....[48]

1981 With the dawn of female suffrage and equality, the professional prostitute has begun to disappear, but the nonprofessional prostitute has appeared....

In Western culture, education in sexuality had as its proper aim the development of a mature, responsible adult who was, therefore, prepared to enter into a happy, monogamous marriage and become a responsible parent. [Repeated similarly in four places.]...In the Jensen *Handbook*, it is advised to discuss *certain abnormalties of the sex drive, such as homosexuality, exhibitionism and child molesters.* [Emphasis ours.]...The topic of masturbation, however, is one which might be casually introduced as a normal adolescent habit pattern which disappears as the individual reaches adulthood....One should know that intercourse is habit-forming. The nervous system of an adolescent is still plastic, therefore habits are easily established. This is one reason why it is especially unwise for individuals still under the age of 21 to use habit-forming addictive drugs, such as alcohol, pot, glue, etc., likewise with the habit of intercourse....The frequency of intercourse should depend primarily upon the male sex drive, for the male physiology involved requires active physical stress.

The female should be advised to allow her male partner's sex drive to set their pace and she should attempt to gear hers satisfactorily to his. Lack of consideration for the male partner's inherent physical drive is a common cause of impotence and reflects an immature attitude of the female who is using her partner for self-gratification.

The patient should be encouraged to discuss her attitude towards intercouse in order that the phyician may evaluate her maturity and knowledge....*Sexual frigidity*, by which is meant the inability to respond sexually, is not frequent in the female, although there seems to be little doubt that libido, which is well developed among normal males, appears to be somewhat less highly developed among females....[49]

1978 Many women complain bitterly of severe, persistent lower abdominal pelvic pain, which is completely out of proportion to the physical findings. The pain is real to the patient, but she is totally unable to convey to the gynecologist any clear-cut description of its nature, its point of origin or its path of radiation....

It is a difficult matter to pinpoint the trigger mechanism for the production of pelvic pain due to *functional* cause. In general, there seems to be agreement that this kind of pain is related to some form of emotional disorder. The actual cause of the pain is similar to that noted in patients who suffer from hysteria....[Emphasis ours.]

To get a maximum response in the patient with dysmenorrhea it may be necessary to alter her attitude toward femininity and encourage the patient to accept her maturing womanly status with pride. If you can accomplish this the patient may come to feel that the monthly cramps are not so intolerable as she formerly believed. Simple analgesic drugs may then be effective. It is alleged that black women are more likely to take pride in their womanhood and as a consequence have much less dysmenorrhea....

It has been stated and confirmed by competent authority that more successful pregnancies stem from an informative discussion of the problem coupled with a complete physical examination than from any other form of therapy for sterility....The woman who consults her physician because of failure to conceive has an emotional problem, however well adjusted she may appear at first. The measure of success in helping the infertile woman to become pregnant is in direct proportion to the physician's ability to bring about a release from her emotional tension through sympathetic understanding.*

---

*See Diana Scully, *Men Who Control Women's Health: The Mis-Education of Obstetrician-Gynecologists*, for excerpts from texts of the past two decades (see Resources).

*Langdon Parsons and Sheldon C. Sommers, *Gynecology*, Second Edition. Philadelphia: W.B. Saunders Company, 1978, pp. 331, 352 and 378.

Studies have shown that while medical students may begin medical training with idealism and a sincere desire to help people, after years of training in the closed worlds of medical school and residency they become almost invariably more cynical, detached and mechanistic than at entry.[47] Their ability to communicate has actually deteriorated during the process.* Because of the enormous personal sacrifice medical training requires, and because most of the teachers and the doctors they admire are highly paid specialists, young physicians feel entitled to earn very large sums of money and to command interpersonal authoritarian power once the training is completed.† Here is how another distinguished medical educator puts it: "What emerges are physicians without inquiring minds, physicians who bring to the bedside *not* curiosity and a desire to understand but a set of reflexes that allows them to earn a handsome living."‡

These criticisms are not new; indeed, many were voiced as soon as the medical monopoly was created nearly a century ago. When *Our Bodies, Ourselves* came out in 1973, the then President of the American Association of Medical Colleges said every medical student should read it. But interest in community concerns and patient perspectives has declined dramatically since then.

What is new is the pressure on medicine, partly because of soaring costs, to deliver much better quality than present training allows, for the same or less money. Also, the doctor glut may create enough competition so that some can and will offer more comprehensive primary care and develop the skills once delegated to other professionals—counselors, nurses, social workers. But even if all these educational reforms were to be realized, without substantial input from consumers and their communities and without selecting a different type of student and teacher, the experience of health and medical care will continue to be frustrating for women. Meanwhile, we can look to the many alternative and neighborhood facilities created by women and men over the past fifteen years or so for examples of successful efforts to integrate competence, caring and community partnership. (See Chapter 25, "Organizing for Change: U.S.A.")

Women Physicians

Today about 11 percent of all MDs in the United States are women, and this percentage may rise to 25 percent by the year 2000. Women express over and over again the hope and belief that female physicians will be different from their male colleagues, that they will listen, understand, be sensitive and caring. How realistic is this hope?

Within five years of the beginning of the second wave of feminism, women began applying to medical schools in record numbers. From 1960 to 1976 female enrollments increased 700 percent and in 1982 stood at a record high of 27.9 percent.[50] The leadership of medicine, almost entirely male, was at first clearly appalled at this influx, and tried every kind of psychological intimidation to discourage women from applying.* Camouflaging a basic fear of women as economic competitors, arguments against women being doctors focus now (as in the nineteenth century) on women's supposed biological inappropriateness for the role of physician: the menstrual cycle causes emotional instabilities, women in the classroom distract males, women marry and have children and prove their training a waste. In the 1970s, it took a class-action lawsuit charging discrimination against every medical school in the country, plus many individual lawsuits and Affirmative Action legislation, to get medical schools and residency programs to accept women in anything but token numbers.[51]

Once in school, women students "have to work twice as hard as men to be accepted...to be considered equal."[52] Very few women are on the faculty.

Women students must also endure hostility from their male colleagues. In one Ivy League school in 1982 women found obscene and angry graffiti left on their bulletin boards: "Scrotum breaths" and "You are pigs, but we like that in a woman." Plates of excrement appeared outside their doors.[53]

Perhaps worse, women students continuously encounter the demeaning and objectifying way women patients are presented in classrooms, textbooks and actual clinical settings.

I have been told by a surgeon that a twenty-five-year-old female with abdominal pain was *by definition* an "unreliable historian."

A professor who had included a nudie slide in his lecture [said]..."Men need to look down on women, and that's why I show the slide."

Often women are portrayed as hysterical or as nagging mothers or as having trivial complaints. Men are almost never pointed to as having a psychological component to their illnesses.[54]

Such indignities present women students with a painful dilemma. As one said, "Every day we must

*Derek Bok, President of Harvard University, in his annual report to the Board of Overseers, April 1984, as printed in *Harvard Magazine*, May–June 1984, p. 70.

†See Cynthia Carver, note 45. Students are still concerned. The American Medical Student Association (AMSA) has organized "Health Watch," a project to document for Congressional action instances where low-income patients receive inadequate treatment or are denied treatment because of inability to pay. (*AMSA Health Newsletter*, Vol. 13, No. 1 [January 1983], p. 9.)

‡Dr. J. Michael Bishop, in a speech to the American Association of Medical Colleges, November 8, 1983.

*Margaret Campbell (see Resources in Chapter 25, "Organizing for Change: U.S.A.") completely catalogues the many forms of discrimination. In a major study of attitudes toward female applicants, some of the replies from medical schools were "too outrageous to be published." (*Why Would a Girl Go into Medicine?* Old Westbury, NY: The Feminist Press, 1974.)

choose between speaking up in a sexist situation or suffering in silence." The only other alternative is to block off any personal identification with other women students or with women patients.

Many women students keep silent, deciding to concentrate first on performing well: "I felt as a medical student you played by the rules of the game, otherwise you weren't going to keep moving." Later, when fully credentialed, they plan to use their authority to challenge and perhaps change the distressing practices they saw as students. Unfortunately, medical training cuts so deeply into one's prior values that many women may well lose their desire to work for change. Others have no such desire.

A number of women—feminists, minority women and women slightly older than average—have tried to challenge the offensive behavior directed toward women or minority patients, or against themselves. For doing so, some have been dismissed, threatened with dismissal or forced to resign their posts. A few have taken their cases to court. If only one or two women speak out, it is easy for a school or hospital to label them as misfits or troublemakers. Yet overworked women medical students find it difficult to carry out sustained organizing. And the highly individualistic nature of the training also leads them further and further away from the habit of working in groups, which is so central to successful organizing. An equally challenging dilemma for many women is the effort to conform to male styles of emotional detachment. As Jean Baker Miller reports, most women carry with them the socialization to be highly sensitive to others.* However, the very qualities medical reformers claim they are seeking in students—sensitivity, empathy, honesty, humility—are instantly suspect, if displayed by women, as signs of their possible clinical or intellectual incompetence. This tremendous resource women are bringing into medical schools is being smothered by the training. Similarly, more general criticisms of the training process are much less likely to be raised openly by women.

Analysts of the situation insist that once there is a "critical mass" of women, their sheer numbers will put them in a position to make real changes in the system. While it is doubtless true that few changes can be initiated until women no longer feel isolated, unless they resist their training no new consciousness will result. Simply taking over leadership positions as presently constituted, even if that were possible, is not what critics usually mean by change, either. Wisely, few women are choosing the most grueling specialties; their preference is to live like human beings. Unfortunately, most of the influential leadership of medicine is not drawn from specialties women favor. It is only a critical mass in *leadership* positions which may give women power, but only if they all want the same things.

*See Resources in Chapter 6, "Psychotherapy."

Women in medical training need a tremendous amount of support from friends outside the medical world just to be able to survive the training whole, much less resist the injustices. Some women who entered medical school at the height of the women's movement say the support and encouragement they had counted on from feminists have been sadly lacking, especially as women activists have stepped up their criticism of medicine.

Women residents find their work even more arduous. The exhausting routine, originally set up for men who have women at home to take care of them, allows no flexibility for other commitments like family or sick relatives. Many women are unprepared for the deep isolation of the final years of training. They postpone having children or forego motherhood entirely. Those who are mothers find it enormously stressful to combine childbearing and/or marriage with medical training. Part-time residencies are few.

The emotional cost of medical training for most women is tremendous, more so than for most (white) men, because of discrimination, lack of support and intensity of outside demands. With these stresses added to the already dehumanizing training, many women emerge from the process expecting prestige and position just as male MDs do. What's more, many are eager to prove that they can be as good as any male physician according to the male-centered criteria of the profession: clinical competence, emotional detachment and financial success. Since they have not chosen to question the underlying medical ideology, they are virtually indistinguishable from their male counterparts. These women physicians can be a great disappointment if the patients' expectations are high.

At the medical plan I belong to, I chose one of the two women doctors because I believed a woman would be less likely to push drugs and surgery, would look with me first for the less invasive nonmedical alternatives. In the first visit, she suggested not only thyroid medication but also a "routine" breast X-ray; she talked crisply, rapidly, coolly, with many complicated medical terms. I felt like I was sitting across from a medical school curriculum.

It is a mistake, therefore, to assume that women physicians are the answer to the inadequacies of the medical system. The very existence of women physicians may deceive people into believing that medicine has indeed reformed. Unfortunately, the public and even the medical community have quickly elevated women doctors to the status of "experts" on the feelings, experiences and health needs of all women. In health books, talk shows, conferences and magazines, female physicians are replacing the voices of women speaking their own truths. Women MDs sometimes study and write about us, the "patients," in exactly the objective ways we once criticized male doctors for doing.[55]

Yet there are also women doctors who have survived the training, kept alive their warmth and compassion and remember what it's like to be a woman patient. They can make a great difference.

For the first time I left a doctor's office feeling absolutely wonderful. I felt that she was genuinely concerned for my well-being as a person. I knew that if I had any further complications, I could call and discuss them with her without feeling like I was "eccentric."

Rate a woman physician as you would any doctor—for skill, honesty, quality of communication, flexibility, intellectual curiosity, ability to really listen and respect for you as a person.

Women as Workers in the Medical Care System

The medical system in this country is a pyramid, with highly paid male doctors and administrators at the top and women—underpaid and undervalued—forming the vast base. While about 88 percent of doctors are men, *more than 80 percent of all medical-care workers are women*: nurses, physical therapists, medical technicians, secretaries and other clerical workers, service and maintenance staff and more. When we go for care, particularly to a hospital, we encounter mainly women—women whose freedom to offer care and healing is often limited by lack of power.

Physical and occupational therapists, social workers, nutritionists and other allied health workers have such a low position in the medical-care hierarchy in terms of pay and control that the public usually sees them as less skilled or valuable than doctors. Yet each is a profession separate from medicine, setting its own standards and training its own workers in distinct and vital skills. These workers can help us make the daily changes often necessary for a real cure or for preventing illness. Their techniques speed healing, help us live with physical limitations and ease the helplessness, loneliness and fear that often come with sickness. Yet they can rarely fully use their knowledge and skills. The system is set up so that patients do not have easy access to them, and often don't know their services exist unless their doctor tells them. *You will have to learn more about what they do. Remember to ask to see one of these workers if you think they might be at all helpful to you.*

Women health workers are part of a medical system we strongly criticize; like most physicians, some are overly "medicalized," focused on technology, too busy or seemingly uncaring. Yet at the same time women health workers, like most other women workers, work within a structure over which they have little or no control, which means tremendous frustration and overwork. We want to support these women as they fight within the system to be able to deliver more humane, person-oriented care, for better working conditions and for more control over their work.

Nursing

Since the male-physician takeover of health and medical care at the turn of the century, nursing has been one of the few options open to women who want constructive and useful health-related work. Today, of 1.4 million nurses—registered nurses (RNs) and licensed practical nurses (LPNs)—97 percent are women. Nursing has historically been a low-status occupation, like other women's jobs. In 1981, approximately 482 million dollars of federal funds for training health workers went to train physicians and dentists and 64 million dollars to train nurses.[56] Nurses have been seen as doctors' servants or handmaidens, and doctor-nurse relationships have embodied all the worst in male-female inequalities: the female must be obedient and dependent, while the male is (or pretends to be) knowledgeable and has the prestige and power. Class differences exaggerate this imbalance: most nurses come from the middle and lower classes, most physicians from the upper-middle or upper classes.

Hospitals, which employ 80 percent of nurses, use them primarily as sources of inexpensive labor in the "business" of providing medical care. Hospital administrators set nursing rules and regulations in the interests of convenience, profit and prestige for doctors, and for the hospital itself as an expanding enterprise. Working conditions for nurses are often poor, with severe and growing understaffing, occupational hazards, insufficient job mobility and low pay. Within hospitals, nurses are the chief coordinators, administrators and monitors of the patients' experience. Despite this huge responsibility, they lack overall administrative power, as do workers in most other hospital departments.

Nurses themselves see nursing as distinct from medicine. In the "caring versus curing" dichotomy which fragments medical care today, nurses traditionally do the caring—the day-to-day, hands-on work with patients and their families, the listening, soothing, teaching, with a special emphasis on prevention. Partly because hospitals undervalue this work, nurses who want job promotions and higher pay have to move into supervisory or administrative roles. Nurses active in working for change stress that they *want* to be able to care directly for patients, and to be valued and paid well for this work. They believe *medical* care will improve dramatically with this shift, since caring plays

572

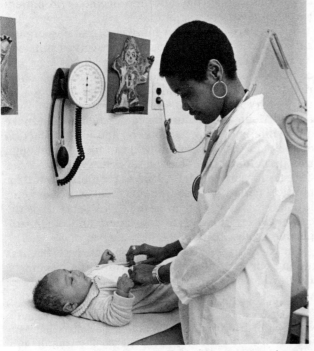

Ellis Herwig/Stock Boston

much more of a role in actual "curing" than medicine has so far been willing to admit.*

Nurses have also increasingly been delegated *medical* functions—doing physical examinations, conducting tests, drawing blood, starting IVs, doing EKGs, etc. Yet they do this medical work without much acknowledgment or control. For instance, many nurses have become skilled in using diagnostic and treatment machines; many see this as a form of expertise which will help them professionally. But physicians retain full control over who uses the technology, when it is used and what diagnoses are made. It is still dangerous to go beyond "doctor's orders."

My friend Jeanie works in a nursing home. One of her patients had a terrible case of bedsores. Both of us have used aloe vera† to cure ourselves of similar kinds of skin irritations. I suggested she use the remedy. "No way," she said. "I could get fired for using something not prescribed by the doctor."

Nurses, who see patients far more than physicians do, have been "making diagnostic decisions for years but protect themselves with elaborate games, which cast physicians in a decision-making role even when

*As Mary Howell, Michelle Harrison and other feminist physicians have pointed out, medicine undervalues caring because of sexism (women's work is less valuable), because of medicine's continual fascination with ever more complex technology and because hospitals are increasingly becoming big businesses. Caring work doesn't use medical supplies, drugs or expensive machines, or generate profits.

†A simple house plant whose juice has healing properties.

the decision has been made by the nurses."[57] To make things worse, a nurse can be sued if she does something which harms a patient, even if she is only obeying doctor's orders.*

Many nurses are now looking for work, and some nursing schools are closing down. The nursing shortage is over, creating an employers' market and more difficult working conditions. Economic hard times have reduced hospital staff and kept down turnover.[59]

Nurses' frustration with the nursing role is on the rise, partly because the women's movement has affirmed women's capabilities and worth and inspired women to express their entitlement to better conditions. Their frustration has led to a number of developments.

1. Within nursing there has been a move toward professionalism. The American Nurses Association (ANA), the most influential of nursing's professional associations, has made a recommendation that all nurses obtain a baccalaureate degree (B.S.), which would put an end to the "diploma" nurse trained at a local hospital.† Certified nurse-midwives, nurse-anesthetists and nurse-practitioners (CNMs, NAs and NPs) have been developing extra skills and a strong professional identity.

Hospitals themselves have tried to attract nurses by promoting various degrees of professionalization; most recently they have developed the idea of the "primary-care nurse," who has full responsibility for providing twenty-four-hour nursing care to a certain number of patients, a situation which may be more satisfying but also more stressful.

Many aspects of professionalization are controversial among nurses themselves, because professionalism emphasizes more education and credentials as well as a doctorlike relationship to patients. Nurses also express the concern that extra responsibilities and functions do not always bring additional recognition or compensation.

Professionalism teaches us to see ourselves as unique and better than other health care workers. The more we talked about professionalism, the more we saw that it was used by administrators to make us work in certain ways which are not beneficial to us or our patients. In other words, professionalism can be used to exploit nurses.[60]

*Mary Daly has called nurses "token torturers" because they have to carry out so many painful procedures ordered by doctors, whereas doctors more often carry out their far more invasive procedures behind the shield of anesthesia.[58] See also Chapter 7 in Daly's *GYN-ECOLOGY: The Meta-Ethics of Radical Feminism*, "American Gynecology: Gynocide and the Holy Ghosts of Medicine and Therapy," Beacon Press, 1978. For decisions establishing liability of hospital personnel, see: Darling vs. Charleston Community Hospital, 33 Illinois, 2d 326, 211 N.E. 2d 253, 1965.

†The NLN (National League for Nursing), whose larger membership includes more "diploma nurses," strongly disagrees with this trend.

Still other critics believe that dividing up nurses as health care workers into increasingly specialized or professionalized subgroups continues to rob nurses of their collective unity and power to work for significant change.

Professionalism doesn't guarantee control over working conditions, job security or access to clients. When specially trained nurses threaten to compete with physicians—when nurse-midwives or nurse-practitioners, for instance, start to attract the same affluent clients who used to fill doctors' private offices

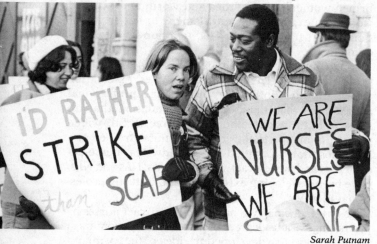

Sarah Putnam

(instead of sticking to poor communities where most doctors don't want to practice)—their existence becomes precarious. Their freedom to work is still in the hands of physicians, administrators and legislators. Nurse-practitioners (about 1 percent of nurses) became popular a decade ago because they saved private physicians' and health maintenance organizations' (HMOs') time, often bringing in more money than they were paid. Today many are being replaced by physicians' assistants (PAs), who charge less and are less of a threat to doctors.*

2. Increasing numbers of nurses are joining "temporary" nursing agencies.[61] Modeled after "Kelly Girl" secretarial agencies, they offer a chance to travel if desired, more money in most cases and freedom from the daily hassles and responsibilities of a staff position in hospitals. The effect of these agencies on the aspirations for nursing as a whole, however, can be disastrous as, for instance, when agency personnel are "imported" to break nursing strikes.

3. Collective action: nurses are seeking change and taking more risks, speaking out against injustices to themselves and to patients. Nurses and other hospital workers are beginning to organize and go out on strike more frequently, asserting their demands for better

*Trained by doctors somewhat like military "medics" or corpsmen, PAs often perform more complex procedures than other primary health-care workers. Many doctors prefer PAs to specially trained RNs, because PAs are never trained to take on the whole care of any patient but only to carry out specific tasks.

conditions, higher pay and improvements in patient care. Some are joining unions.*

4. Legislative action: a number of nursing organizations are lobbying increasingly actively at state and national levels, and groups like Nurses-NOW (a part of the National Organization for Women) seek effective political and legislative strategies. One goal is third-party reimbursement by insurance companies and by Medicaid for nursing care, which would make a big difference in the autonomy and job satisfaction of many nurses with specialized training, even though this perpetuates the "fee for service" system. Nurses have far fewer financial resources for lobbying and for political action than does the medical establishment; legislative change will, at best, be slow, and needs the combined efforts of both consumers and other supportive professionals.

The growing mix of frustration and assertiveness among nurses comes through vividly in a November 1981 article by Rachael Lynch in *New Women's Times*:

The nursing shortage means more than overwork. It means ignoring loneliness, suffering and pain in the people the nurse works with, their friends and families. The dollars and cents demand that you maintain a semblance of giving the necessary physical, technical and miracle care while ignoring the human beings. Nurses watch people live and die alone because they don't have the time to really *be* with the people they work for.

We have put up with so much. Our contributions are barely mentioned, the labor of our backs is never recognized. We have come to the point where we actively discourage others from becoming nurses. We are beginning to question whether we want to continue to be the mainstay of the "health industry" and all its concomitant pollutants.

We nurses must begin to believe in ourselves. We must look at our numbers and consider the sum total of our shared experiences. We must rejoice that our hands can soothe, that our arms can lift those that cannot move, that our eyes can show what is in our hearts....They have made us handmaidens—we will not be machines! The dictatorship of the dollar must end. It is time that we nurses start to define the structure of our work. We can be creative. We know we are strong. And we know we are right.

SURVIVING THE SYSTEM: CHOOSING AND USING MEDICAL CARE

Where to Find (and Not to Find) the Information We Need

To have some control over our lives and to be informed participants in our health and medical care, we need

*Unionization poses another set of problems, since traditional unions tend to be controlled by men, have a "blue-collar" image and are not very responsive to women's problems in the workplace. The public, which often has mixed feelings about unions, may become less sympathetic.

information about our bodies and about the caregiving system. Knowledge gives us the ability to make choices, and some of the control we desire.

Often when we visit doctors what we really come for is solid, factual information, not medical attention. When we have appropriate factual information and even a little skill or a few tools, or can get access to them quickly, we are in a much better position to cope with minor emergencies and to decide whether or not we really need to spend the time and money on a medical visit. Illnesses like toxic shock, pelvic inflammatory disease, strep throat and some ear infections can have serious complications, so we should be aware of the symptoms and get them treated early. Many simple infections and even more complex ones like sexually transmitted diseases are to some extent preventable.

Today there is much more health and medical information available than there was ten years ago, some of it trustworthy, some of it not; this section offers guidance in selecting the most reliable sources. It is crucial for our health that we get information from sources which are both *accurate* and *independent*—that is, sources able to evaluate the material from technical, user *and* feminist perspectives.

Ourselves

We know a lot about our bodies; we must listen to and trust what our bodies are telling us. Our awareness of change in ourselves or our children is the first and most important indicator of sickness. Most of what doctors learn about us we tell them. We learn much from the women in our lives: our mothers, sisters, aunts, grandmothers and friends.

Reading

Reading is important, but we must make sure that our sources are as accurate as possible. Magazines and newspapers, a common resource, have their problems (see below). Consumers can also buy the *Physicians' Desk Reference (PDR)* or ask for it in local libraries to find out what the drug industry says about the drugs it manufactures. *Be sure to see consumer guides to drugs as well* (see Resources in Chapter 25, "Organizing for Change: U.S.A."). Beware of booklets and brochures in your doctor's office.*

Self-Help Groups

These are one of the most important sources of both courage and information. Different from medically run "self-care" groups, these small informal groups of women are meeting throughout this country to help

---

*Usually prepared by drug companies, medical foundations or guilds and the large national health charities, these items tend to downgrade nonmedical or nonpharmacological approaches, and are slow to present innovative alternatives or prevention orientations.

each other learn about birth control, fertility awareness, menopause, breast cancer, DES, cervical self-exam and many other topics as well.

Such groups are organized in ways which reflect values important to us. They are nonhierarchical; every member plays an equal part. Information is free. Implicit in these groups is the belief that we *can* understand medical information, that it "belongs" rightfully to us. Group members' experiences are an important source of information about health, illness and treatment. By comparing notes and trading stories with other women, we learn best how to use the information we get from both medical and nonmedical sources. Independent of medical-care institutions and professionals, these groups are not hampered in exploring nonmedical therapies and practitioners, or in questioning, challenging and evaluating accepted ones.

When groups focus on one specific issue, they are often better able than many physicians to keep abreast of the most current research. Some groups already exist (see Resources in Chapter 25). We have to initiate others as the need arises. When you find one or two other women who want to get together, that is a good beginning.

The Media

These days the media carry more women's health and medical information than ever before. A few women's magazine articles and TV shows are excellent, well researched and responsible in their outlook. Most often, however, a "medical expert" (usually a physician) presents only the medical point of view, with no consumer representation. Reporters, awed by medical "expertise," may spread inaccuracies by quoting as fact what are actually the doctor's opinions, or assuming the doctor is always up to date in her or his information. Sometimes public relations firms hired by drug companies or medical specialty groups pay for such TV shows and articles. And the media cater to the human fascination with drama, highlighting the spectacular "cures" and treatments, the most daring surgery, the most expensive and highly technical procedures. Media coverage usually perpetuates the mistaken assumption that medicine and spectacular medical technology create good health. Look for presentations that focus on what *you* can do. Remember that experts often disagree.

Health Information Centers

There are a few good (and fairly stable) independent health information centers women can turn to. Examples are our Collective office in Watertown, Massachusetts, devoted to all aspects of women and health; the Consumer Health Information Center in Salt Lake City; the Center for Medical Consumers and Health Care Information in New York City; and Plane Tree Health Resource Center in San Francisco. In these centers, a cross between a library and a hotline, anyone can come to read, learn and sometimes talk about health and medical care—what the controversies are, what home remedies women have tried, the risks and possibilities of various medical and nonmedical treatments. They may also try to help you select a practitioner and put you in touch with women who have gone through experiences similar to yours. Many women's health centers and community groups offer similar services on a more limited basis.

Health Information Centers of the Future: Our Vision

As community funds dry up and hospitals take on a larger corporate existence, it is likely that the health information centers of the future will not be community run but hospital run, with all the limits outlined below. We strongly believe that health information centers should be part of each neighborhood and/or region, located in public libraries or other community settings. They should be community controlled, with a definite consumer perspective and plentiful information on where to go for additional resources. We will have to fight for them and convince others they are worthwhile and worth paying for.

Sources within the Medical Establishment

Doctors

While most of us learned while growing up to turn mainly to doctors for health and medical information, our experience reveals that they have limits to what they can or will tell us. Some doctors are happy to give over-the-phone common-sense information which can be extremely helpful. Others send complete reports in writing after a checkup. But the information we get from doctors can be limited by:

- the sexism, racism and homophobia of their training;
- how little time they budget to teach patients;
- their mistrust of our ability to understand or make good use of complex information;
- their tendency not to keep up with the latest research or their inability to evaluate it;*
- pressures from drug company representatives to push certain medications;
- the desire to control information as "belonging" rightfully to MDs;
- the desire to appear "sure" and "dependable," which creates an unwillingness to admit to uncertainty or controversy;
- their unfamiliarity with and distrust of nonmedical alternatives;

*Doctors are not taught skills to keep up with new information; close to half of one group of practicing specialists admitted they could not do so.

- overspecialization: training to focus on an organ or system and not to take into account the whole person.

It can be frustrating, even humiliating, to try to get information over the phone or in person from doctors who don't want to give it, who think of most women as dumb and women who ask a lot of questions as "pushy." We may try to get test results and find that the doctors will not give them to us. We may leave an office or clinic with many questions.

We must remember in these situations not to blame ourselves. We have a right to be treated with respect and to get the information we need.* See "What Can One Woman Do?" (p. 579) for suggestions.

Nurses

Nurses, especially nurse-practitioners, learn in their training to consider teaching patients as one of their roles. If your doctor's office has hired a nurse-practitioner, or if one has set up an independent practice in your community, s/he may be more informative and sensitive than a physician. S/he may, however, be unfamiliar with nonmedical alternatives and too busy to keep up to date on innovative or controversial treatments.

Health Educators

These medical workers, usually hired by hospitals or large medical centers, can help those of us with chronic conditions when we need to change daily habits and adjust to physical limitations. Often, however, the health educator simply makes sure that patients understand and accept medical routines and treatments. As employees, they are frequently restricted in what they are able to say about controversial matters. Also, they are often available only after a person is sick and not always for preventive care.

Classes or Groups Sponsored by Hospitals, Physicians or HMOs (often called "self-care" groups)

Some of the more practical physicians and medical centers have recognized, mainly because of pressure from women's and consumer health activists, that patients want and can use more information than they are getting. One popular solution is groups or classes in everything from childbirth to smoking cessation to weight management or posthysterectomy adjustments. These groups help up to a point, mainly because they give you a chance to talk with other people in your situation, trade ideas, feel less alone and perhaps learn a few skills. Such groups often emphasize "self-care," that is, those activities *doctors* and *nurses* have decided you can carry out for yourself. Be aware that these classes and groups have a major limitation: their main goal is a smoothly functioning medical system with compliant patients who are, in one self-care

*Lab or X-ray results may be available as part of your hospital record, depending on your state's laws.

expert's words, "members of the health care team."[62] They rarely offer nonmedical alternatives or a chance to criticize accepted practices.

Living with Uncertainty

In giving up our unquestioning trust of the information we get from doctors and other medical personnel, we also give up the (often false) comfort that comes from their frequent reassurances that we are getting "the best treatment possible." Often we and our health practitioners have to make decisions without complete information, because no one, not even the "experts," knows enough yet about certain problems to suggest that one approach is necessarily better than another. Yet physicians often believe that they have to act *sure* even when they are not. Especially when we are scared, it can be deeply reassuring to believe them. Learning about the controversies and alternatives rather than blindly trusting what our doctors tell us, therefore, may mean living without the particular kind of certainty or hope that they offer.* Often what we need most is courage in the face of uncertainty.

Choice

When we need medical care, we want as much choice as possible. As in most aspects of our lives, economic status, sex and race limit our choices. There is a severe maldistribution of doctors. Prepaid medical programs, while sometimes convenient, limit our choices. Profit-making incentives limit choice even more for people who need medical care most. For example, more and more hospitals are turning away women in labor if they cannot prove they can pay. In many settings, the elderly are forced to pay for many of their drugs and increasing amounts of their care. Women who are poor, women of color, working-class women, lesbians, older women and disabled women seeking medical care have often faced particular language or culture barriers, physical-access barriers, prejudice and abuse. As our choices evaporate, it becomes more necessary to improve our skill at evaluating care, and to create fair and equitable complaint and grievance systems wherever medical care is given.

Practitioners

Primary-Care Practitioners†

Primary care refers to a basic, general form of caregiving which emphasizes prevention. Ideally we would seek care first from primary-care practitioners who would then refer us to specialists as necessary. A good primary-care practitioner is trained to give well-person care and checkups. S/he monitors mild, uncomplicated conditions and recommends appropriate treatments, recognizes more serious complications which require more expert evaluation and treatment, coordinates specialists' care and institutional treatments, helps act as an advocate in decisions about medical treatment, provides continuity and helps to evaluate our experience afterwards.

Nurse-Practitioners or Certified Nurse-Midwives

You may want to rethink the whole question of seeking a physician as your first choice of practitioner for normal childbirth or well-woman gynecological care. A skilled nurse-practitioner (NP) or nurse-midwife (CNM) may well be more satisfying and appropriate, and less expensive. Both handle routine exams and problems. While both NPs and CNMs always work in consultation with MDs, some have agreements which permit relatively autonomous practices, referring to their backup doctors only rarely; others work within doctors' offices, hospitals or clinics and are in daily consultation with them. Depending on the situation, a specially trained nurse may be able to make referrals and give out health and medical care information relatively independent of doctors. Some have better performance records than doctors.[63]

Many physicians fear that these specially trained nurses threaten both their accustomed roles in medical care and their incomes. However, some doctors accept them when they discover how skilled the nurses are at routine, time-consuming care and answering patients' questions; and that a solo office practice can generate much more income when even one such worker is included. To improve your access to NPs and CNMs, get involved in state legislation and regulation.

Checking Up on Your Doctor

Is s/he licensed to practice in your state? Check the medical society or the state board of regulations.

Does s/he have hospital privileges? Ask her/him or the hospital.

If s/he calls her/himself a specialist, is this self-defined or certified? See the *Directory of Medical Specialists* in your local library, or at your local medical society, for the doctor's training history and qualifications.

Family-Practice Physicians

These practitioners are specialists, different from old-time general practitioners in that they have gone

---

*A very few doctors are learning to admit their uncertainties and share the decision-making with patients. For a sample of how this kind of thinking works in practice, see H. Burstajn, et al., *Medical Choices, Medical Chances*, New York: Delacorte Press/ Seymour Lawrence, 1981.

†Primary-care practitioners are often looked down upon by specialists.

through a residency in family medicine and perhaps taken a specialty board examination as well. Family practitioners treat both families and individuals of all ages, and many specialize in delivering babies, frequently with fewer interventions than their ob/gyn counterparts. Some family-practice physicians set up an office and have admissions privileges at a hospital. Others are prevented by specialists from getting hospital admitting privileges.

Primary-Care Internists

Another reasonable choice for primary care might be an internist, a specialist with residency training in internal medicine. However, most internists actually subspecialize (circulatory, heart, digestive problems, etc.) and only a few have had special training in primary care. Inquire about the kind of diseases and patients s/he is interested in. Traditionally some internists have had an unspoken "gentleman's agreement" to refer most women to ob/gyns for routine care, while they themselves prefer to care for male patients. However, women have serious nonreproductive medical problems which the internist, not the ob/gyn, is specifically trained to treat—work-related or environmental illnesses, for instance; difficulties with basic body functions, such as metabolism, elimination, breathing, etc.; as well as problems created by contraceptive or tranquilizer use.

Physician Specialists

Today about 90 percent of practicing physicians are specialists (graduate training after the MD degree) in fields like surgery, radiology, psychiatry, cardiology, neurology.* Most doctors regard specialty medicine as more important and more dramatic than primary care; it is more lucrative and prestigious. Specialists are less likely to see you as a whole person or oversee your total care than a primary-care practitioner would. However, since there is a shortage of primary-care practitioners and an excess of specialists, most of us rely on nonprimary-care specialists. Three have particular relevance for women: obstetrician/gynecologists, psychiatrists and surgeons. (See "Surgery," p. 482, and Chapter 6, "Psychotherapy.")

Obstetrician/Gynecologists

Today the majority of ob/gyns are seeing healthy women who turn to them for routine well-woman care, and they attend 95 percent of births. *Yet their training is neither necessary nor appropriate for this service.* Ob/gyns are surgical specialists, trained especially to diagnose and treat diseases of the reproductive organs,

manage childbirth complications (about 5 to 15 percent of births) and perform gynecological surgery. With this kind of training and a tendency to suspect a psychological origin for the physical pain women report, ob/gyns may miss important nonreproductive illnesses. They may overprescribe tranquilizers and refer to psychiatrists inappropriately. They are also likely to offer treatment solutions more drastic, invasive and permanent than is always necessary—hysterectomy, for example—and may offer few alternatives, medical or nonmedical. But we often need their surgical talents. Many know little about women past menopause and may not appreciate the nonhormonal aspects of the midlife transition or of aging; they are often insensitive to women's emotional needs while giving birth and to the health concerns of lesbians. Yet, though they have neither the training nor the competence for the role, they are socially sanctioned life advisers and sexual counselors for women. The fact that obstetrician/gynecologists see only women as patients—are "specialists in women"—has caused the public to confuse their surgical skills and knowledge of female reproductive disease with expertise on female sexuality, character and proper place in society. (See "The Doctor-Patient Relationship on p. 561.")

Largely because we return to them so often for expensive, routine office visits, for delivering babies and for surgery, ob/gyns have among the highest incomes of any physicians in office-based practice.[64] As a result, ACOG is one of the most effective medical specialty societies, with the financial resources to maintain lobbyists in an office within walking distance of the Capitol in Washington, DC.

Reporting Problems

Tongue depressors, Band-Aids, tampons, diaphragms, IUDs and cervical caps, as well as the more obvious things like kidney dialysis machines, are classified by the FDA as medical devices. If you have any problems, even minor ones, with a medical device, report them to the FDA, which records complaints in their publicly available Device Experience Network (DEN).* (Your name will not appear in the public report.) Complaints about prescription and over-the-counter drugs are kept in a separate file. These reports are the only way to make public the problems women are having and to assess their frequency, since company complaint files generally are not available to the government or the public. The FDA acts only in response to complaints. It will not initiate investigations. Write to the FDA, 5600 Fishers Lane, Rockville, MD 20857. Keep a copy of your complaint for future reference.

---

*This results in serious, dangerous shortages of primary-care doctors. See D. Steinwachs, et al., "Changing Patterns of Graduate Medical Education," *New England Journal of Medicine*, Vol. 306, No. 1 (January 7, 1982) pp. 10–14.

*Reporting a problem to your physician alone does not guarantee that the FDA will learn about it.

What Can One Woman Do?*
Three Steps to Begin to Get Better Medical Care

1. *Before Your Visit*

Talk to many other women about individual doctors and clinics. Contact women's groups or consumer groups to get more information about costs, attitudes and medical competence of a number of practitioners or clinics. (See "Practitioners," p. 577, and "Evaluating Health/Medical-Care Settings," p. 580.)

2. *At Your Visit*

Know your own and your family's medical history. If possible, bring a written record of your own. If you have a problem, write down when it began, symptoms, etc. When you are in the waiting room, or before that, write down any questions that you want to ask about it.

Bring a friend with you.

Firmly ask the practitioner to explain your problem, treatments, tests and drugs in a clear and understandable fashion.

Take notes, or ask your friend to do so. (A tape recorder, if you have or can borrow one, will help in the case of long, complicated explanations.) Such record-keeping can be invaluable, so try to be assertive even if your doctor reacts defensively.

Ask the doctor to prescribe drugs by their generic names rather than brand names (for example, aspirin, *not* Bayer's). This will save you money.

Talk to nurses and assistants. They are often sources of valuable information and support and may explain things better than the doctor.

Ask for a written summary of the results of your visit and any lab tests.†

Remember, you have a *right* to a second opinion. If a series of expensive tests or surgery is recommended, you can tell the doctor to wait until you consult another doctor. This may prevent unnecessary treatment.

Don't forget—it's your life and your body. You have a right to make decisions about drugs, treatments, methods of birth control, etc.

3. *Afterward*

After the visit, write down an accurate account of what happened. Be sure you know the name of the doctor and/or the other people involved, the date, the place, etc. Discuss your options with someone close to you.

"Shop" drugstores, too. Studies have shown that many drugstores in poorer neighborhoods charge more than those in richer neighborhoods.*

Ask to see the pharmacist's package inserts listing medical indications and contraindications. Request detailed information about interactions with certain foods, beverages, alcohol, aspirin, and other drugs, and get warnings taped onto the medication container.

Have clear instructions written on the label, because of the risk to others who may take it in error, and also because when traveling abroad you may be challenged for possession of pills.

If you get poor treatment, if you are given the wrong drugs, if you are not listened to, it is important for your own care and that of other women that you *protest*. (See "Our Rights as Patients," p. 584.) Then write a letter describing the incident to one or several of the following:

- the doctor involved;
- the doctor who referred you;
- the administrator or director of the clinic or hospital;
- the director of community relations of the clinic or hospital;
- the local medical society;
- the organization that will pay for your visit or treatment (for example, your union, your insurance plan or Medicare);
- organizations that may be paying this doctor for treating other patients (such as Medicaid or Medicare);
- the local health department;
- the neighborhood health council or community boards;
- community agencies;
- local women's groups, women's centers, magazines, newspapers. (See also "The Doctor-Patient Relationship," p. 561.)

And about a hospital:

- Joint Commission on Accreditation of Hospitals, 875 N. Michigan Avenue, Chicago, IL 60611;
- American Hospital Association, 840 N. Lake Shore Drive, Chicago, IL 60611.

However, it is hard for one woman to keep working alone. The medical profession and health institutions are very strong and powerful and will always defend themselves against complaints from the outside. Patients must work together to get the treatment and services they need.

So, to get changes made:
WORK WITH A GROUP...
FIND ONE OR START ONE.

---

*Adapted from HealthRight, Inc.

†Since laboratory quality varies considerably, be sure to ask for at least one more test from a different lab to verify results, especially before agreeing to undergo any invasive procedure.

*For a more detailed discussion, see Alex Gerber, *The Gerber Report*, New York: David McKay Co., Inc., 1971, pp. 158–59.

General Surgeons

See Chapter 23, "Some Common and Uncommon Health and Medical Problems."

Health and Medical-Care Treatment Settings Other than the Practitioner's Office

Clinics

These institutions are generally outpatient departments or "ambulatory care centers" attached to non-profit hospitals. Wealthy industrialists and their wives used their philanthropy to found clinics around the turn of the century. They were spurred by doctors who needed teaching material and saw free care for the poor as an ideal solution.

Almost all specialist physicians (residents), interns and even medical students still get at least part of their training in these teaching-hospital settings.* Since university medical centers' interests are primarily research, teaching or profit, they find ways to attract or discourage patients who do or do not fit in with these priorities. Many centers provide two different types of clinic care: one for the public and poor patients and another for the more affluent.[66]

There are a few clinics (some in hospitals, some not) which offer very high-quality care for all who come. They often attract excellent workers, many of them women drawn to primary care. Workers in these clinics tend to be comfortable in a teamwork situation where one's judgments are always on view and subject to checks and balances by others, health workers and physicians alike. Patients can benefit from this type of setup.

Profit-making enterprises are setting up a wide variety of free-standing walk-in clinics offering hypertension monitoring, primary care, emergency rooms and so on as specific limited services. These are often located in shopping malls. Ask other clients and friends in the community about their experiences. (See "Evaluating Health/Medical-Care Settings," this page.)

Women's Health Centers and Clinics

An excellent option in some cities† and often a good model for quality care, women-run health centers specializing in well-woman care, gyn exams, birth control and abortion services are worth hunting for. The atmosphere is usually different from that of conventional clinics, since clients may see a health worker first and may have a chance to talk with other women clients either informally or in an organized group. Physician care, when needed, is available on site or by referral. The quality of information in many centers is very high; staff will usually answer questions or make information available even if you do not choose to use their services.

At the same time, women-run health centers should be scrutinized with the same care as any other health facility. The informality of some settings and personnel may be uncomfortable for some women accustomed to conventional care, while others may find it reassuring. Because they are run on a not-for-profit basis without regular sources of funding, centers are often understaffed by women who may be underpaid. Services may sometimes suffer as a result.

Some centers also run self-help groups, film showings and classes in addition to offering health and medical services. Most are also involved in political work to improve women's health through legislation, demonstrations and mailings.

---

*There are nonteaching-hospital clinics in many smaller cities which are staffed by fully trained doctors who spend part of their week providing care for poor people for less than their customary fee. Some of the most punitive and moralistic charity may be given at these institutions.[65]

†Though many have closed, new centers are opening each year. Be alert for both conventional medical facilities and antiabortion centers which masquerade as women-controlled centers by using similar names but do not subscribe to self-determination in either reproductive health or medical care.

Evaluating Health/Medical-Care Settings

1. Who is in charge? (Owners, administrators, board?) Do users have a strong voice in planning and evaluating the services? Is management provided by an outside corporation hired by the board or by people within the medical facility itself? Who makes decisions about care, services, staffing, etc., and to whom are the decision makers accountable? How does one become a board member? Does the facility put out public reports and make its records public?

2. Is there a mechanism which brings users/consumers together to discuss common concerns and raise issues to bring to the management or staff? Do clients and management meet together?

3. Is there a grievance procedure and, if so, how does it work? Are nonphysicians involved in reviewing physicians' judgments? What is the ultimate recourse of a dissatisfied client?

4. How are staff members selected and evaluated, and what input, if any, do they have? What are staff working conditions?

5. Is there a directory which describes training and background of providers and staff?

6. If this is a free-standing facility, what are its hospital backup arrangements?

7. Do costs and quality care change over time?

These are only some of the questions you might ask.

Emergency Rooms

If they are part of hospitals, emergency rooms are required by law to take all comers. Accidents and emergencies, alcoholism, drug abuse and mental illness bring many people into emergency rooms, sometimes on a regular basis. For this reason many people who cannot afford doctors and have no insurance turn to emergency rooms for routine care, which can be surprisingly expensive.

The ER staff makes judgments about the legitimacy of both your complaint and your claim on the facilities. Their judgments directly affect the speed with which you are seen and whether or not you receive adequate care. To improve ER care, try to bring someone with you who can explain your emergency and advocate for your care. Try to establish your ability to pay as soon as possible. If you have any contact with regular staff inside the hospital (doctor, nurse or social worker), get in touch with that person as soon as possible; s/he may also advocate for you with the ER staff. Ask for bilingual assistance whenever you need it.

Neighborhood Health Centers

These facilities are part of a program begun in the sixties; some still exist in parts of the U.S., though many are closing due to shrinking federal monies. This model of care has demonstrated several important principles: 1. that comprehensive, primary care at the community level is feasible, and improves outcomes as well as reducing hospitalization; 2. that people in an economically or racially mixed neighborhood can receive a single standard of care; 3. that health and medical care services can be managed and made accountable to the community (through a representative board) in a way that is mutually satisfying to both consumers and providers. Many medical care analysts and consumers feel that NHC care is superior to that given in either hospital clinics or doctors' offices. Consumers can use the principles and standards established by such centers as a yardstick for judging other types of services.

Group Practices

You might want to choose a group practice rather than a solo doctor in office practice. Yet in some places group practice may be almost as rushed and crowded as a clinic, and you may never see the same doctor twice. Some group practices charge so much more than clinics that you may not find them as desirable. On the other hand, when doctors in a group practice exchange opinions and judgments with each other, they will probably give you better diagnoses and treatment options than a physician in solo practice.

There are two kinds of group practice, with impor-

tant differences. In one, a group of the same type of specialist has banded together to share the load and better manage their time and profits by seeking more patients. (Most ob/gyns in metropolitan areas are in this type of practice.) In the other, a collection of different specialists sets out to offer families and individuals more comprehensive care. Yet even this type of group practice is not primary care, but specialty medicine dominated by physicians for those who can afford the office fees or prepayment fees supporting it.

Health Maintenance Organizations (HMOs)

One of the most important options for comprehensive health and medical care is the HMO.* Subscribers enroll as members for an annual premium paid in advance and, except for nominal sums for visits or special services, receive all office or outpatient visits and hospitalizations for this same fee. In principle, the advantages are obvious: "one-stop shopping" for all office visits, which are "free" or obtainable at a nominal fee; one price that you can budget in advance; if you do need specialized services, your HMO will arrange and coordinate them for you, as any primary-care practitioner will do. You are protected from unnecessary hospitalization by an incentive program in which physicians lose money when they hospitalize patients too often.[67]

HMOs: How They Work

HMOs do work: rates of hospitalization are 51 percent lower, regardless of the procedure involved and independent of whether clients are more or less sick to begin with. They are cheaper than conventional hospital insurance plus out-of-pocket payments, and apparently the quality is as good as conventional, fee-for-service care in most of the government-qualified plans. HMOs control their costs mainly through these mechanisms:

- outpatient surgery;
- prescreening hospital admissions (to make certain they are necessary);
- performing most tests prior to admission;
- putting physicians on salary;
- bonus payments to physicians as incentives to keep costs down;
- extensive use of home health care and nursing home programs;
- watching the length of hospital stay carefully.[68]

We have talked with people in HMOs in different parts of the country. Most of them agree that it is a far better system with respect to preventive care and

---

*Other prepaid group plans may also call themselves HMOs, but only federally qualified HMOs require that practitioner practices be audited regularly for quality.

care during mild illnesses than what is available through more expensive conventional health insurance. However, many describe unpleasant or frightening incidents when they tried to get treatment during a crisis, couldn't get through an overloaded switchboard or were discouraged by receptionists or doctors by telephone, and later found that serious medical conditions had been ignored. Others who had to get emergency care at other than the designated facilities were later denied coverage by the plan, even when the emergencies did turn out to be "justified." Others deplore their loss of choice, either when they'd prefer to use a different facility but would have to pay or when they tried to get some flexibility in procedure during hospitalization for maternity or pediatric care. Some HMO practitioners leave out important tests because they are too expensive. From too much doctoring for profit, we may be moving toward too little (also for profit).

Another serious flaw in all group and HMO systems is that a group of physicians or practitioners may decide together that a patient is "deviant" or simply an untrustworthy informant—"a crock," in their language. When they reinforce one another's convictions in this way, there is little a woman can do to reinstate her credibility or to win an advocate from among them.[69]

The HMO principle, for all its advantages, perpetuates many of the negative characteristics of the present system. The HMO offers technical medical services to a diverse membership and has no basic commitment to community-oriented or community-controlled care as neighborhood health centers do. It is a business whose customers have no connection with one another and have great difficulty organizing politically to improve care or find out how their money is being spent. Efficiency becomes a major goal of this system, but efficiency continues the depersonalization, the fragmenting of care and the specialization of labor that is a major frustration of the present system. Finally, the physician is still the dominant figure and the major decision-maker.[70]

Since we want HMOs to be sensitive and responsive to women's needs for primary care and better information, we will have to strive within our workplaces and communities, as well as in the state legislatures, for: 1. one-third consumer representation on HMO boards, or on the boards of the corporations which control them at a distance; 2. "open enrollment," which allows individuals to join a plan (enrollees in some states must come in as part of employee groups, which excludes the small-shop or part-time employee, the poor, elderly, chronically ill or disabled); 3. requirements that HMOs be developed in underserved areas;* and 4. some say in how profits are distributed. If we want to keep profit-making HMOs out (and these are

*These were federal requirements, now dropped.

increasing while federally funded HMOs are decreasing), we will have to pass laws that restrict them (only four states presently inhibit their creation).

Hospitals (Tertiary Care, Acute-Care Institutions)

The so-called nonprofit, private voluntary hospital run by a board of trustees with a separate medical staff is still the most common. However, profit-making or "investor-owned" (proprietary) institutions are growing fast. Most nonprofit hospitals were constructed at least in part by federal Hill-Burton funds, which obliged them to provide free care to those who cannot pay. Most serve a wide range of patients through a variety of reimbursement mechanisms, and use the payments of the affluent to help offset the costs of servicing the sicker and poorer clients. In order to maximize income and enable expansion to take place, most private, nonprofit hospitals concentrate on providing well-reimbursed and "elective" (nonemergency) services. *Investor-owned hospitals* take *only* the paying customers and offer an even narrower range of the most profitable services. Neither type of hospital has any internal mechanisms for accountability for its policies and practices to either the public or its users; however, both have been accused of compromising patient-care quality through cost cutting, primarily through reducing nursing staff. (Profit-making hospitals may also be more unhealthy.)[71]

Public hospitals, meanwhile, are caring for the overwhelming majority of the poor and "medically indigent" and most are also teaching hospitals. Funded by tax money, they have been hovering on the edge of collapse for more than a decade, as city, county and now federal governments suffer increasing cutbacks. Under further Medicaid cuts, some may actually go under, to be taken over by profit-making corporations. Some have already made alliances with state governments to contract for exclusive care of the poor (as teaching material in what may well become a twentieth-century version of the "charity wards" and clinics of the last century). There are many such schemes afoot, and we as taxpayers must get involved in shaping and monitoring them. Our tax dollars and the wellbeing of large segments of the population are at stake.[72]

The Hospitalization Experience: Problems and Survival

The major problems of hospitalization for us as women and consumers have to do with costs, risks, isolation and the lack of provider accountability in almost all settings. Since most of us will continue to use hospitals, we have to be aware of how to use them as well as possible.

First of all, make sure you need to be hospitalized. If the procedure is elective (postponable, nonemergency), get a second or even third opinion. About one-third of Blue Cross/Blue Shield and some Medicaid programs will pay for this. Investigative outpatient surgical possibilities, which may be less invasive, use local anesthesia and may be cheaper. Consider medical *and* nonmedical alternatives.

Once hospitalization seems necessary, find out from your doctor, friends and neighbors what hospitals you can use and what their policies are. For example, one mother was upset to discover that the hospital would not allow her to stay with her seriously ill child; another woman learned that her partner could not be with her during her Cesarean section; still another woman discovered that her lesbian lover was excluded from the intensive-care unit because she was neither "family" nor spouse, and therefore had no "legitimate" claim.

If possible, bring someone with you when you are being hospitalized who can act as your advocate and help you make decisions. (See "Our Rights as Patients," p. 584.) Once you are hospitalized, the following information may be helpful:

- *Whenever you are in a hospital, you have a right to know the name of one doctor in charge of your case.*
- Whenever tests or X-rays are proposed, be sure to ask why. The rapid expansion of technology in hospitals vastly increases overall hospital cost and further depersonalizes care; such technology is often applied inappropriately, creating iatrogenic illnesses and problems.
- Try to forge an alliance with the nursing staff. Nurses are the true coordinators of your total care, and keep their own records which are separate from the doctors'. Nurses' judgments can influence the whole course of your care. Remember that they work under constraints which may severely limit their ability to advocate for you. Also, just because a nurse is a woman does not necessarily mean that she will be able to empathize with you.
- There are nearly continuous outbreaks of infection in most hospitals which are increasingly resistant to antibiotic treatments.* Such infections complicate surgeries, delay recoveries and may cause secondary illnesses which necessitate further treatments; sometimes they are fatal (as in the case of some newborns). If you are hospitalized, try to go home as soon as is reasonable.
- In a wide range of operations, local anesthesia can be used instead of general anesthesia. Local anesthesia enables you to recover more quickly, and doesn't carry the same risk of death. (See "Surgery," p. 482.)
- Since rates of error in administering medications remain high, find out as soon as you can what medicines have been prescribed for you, by whom, for what purpose and how often you must take them. Ask nurses which medications they are giving you, try to keep a record of these and cross-check with your doctor(s). Resist *routine* tranquilizers and sleeping pills if at all possible. Try milk at bedtime instead of juice, because it contains L-tryptophan, a natural relaxant (also available in supplements).
- Since hospital food is frequently not nutritious, ask friends to bring you good food daily. Hospital water at the bedside has repeatedly been shown to be contaminated by bacteria, such as salmonella, so bottled spring water is also a good idea. Also consider taking vitamins, especially Vitamin C, unless your doctor(s) has objections on the grounds that they would interfere with medications or other treatment.
- Wearing your own sleepwear, robes, etc., may make you feel more like yourself.
- As you leave the hospital, ask for a copy of your records; they may be useful in the future, and some hospitals destroy records after a short period of time. (They will send them to your home.)

Nursing Homes

Although the majority are profit-making and many are funded through Medicaid and Medicare, there is a substantial though dwindling number of community-based homes. The quality of nursing homes varies enormously. The past decade has been witness to continuing scandals involving abuse and substandard care in many different parts of the country. Presently, slightly less than 10 percent of the elderly are in nursing homes, but the majority are women. If you are considering nursing-home care for a member of your family, or "home care," be sure to investigate carefully. In addition to a tour of the facility, inquire among different caregivers and social-service agencies in the community about what "home care" options are really

*Called *nosocomial* infections, they are not brought in from outside the hospital, as many hospital personnel imply, but are produced within the hospital environment and carried, largely by doctors and nurses, some of whose antiseptic techniques are careless.

James Holland/Stock Boston

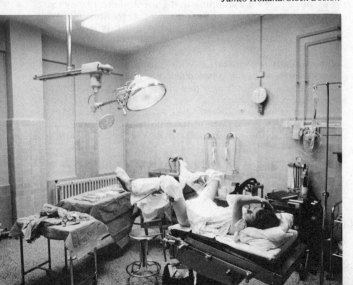

583

available and possible before you decide on a nursing home. If there is an HSA in your region or state, find out what kinds of standards have been established for licensed nursing homes, home care or hospice care in your state. Or call the public health department, since many federal regulations are being dropped. Several books and brochures have been prepared to help you evaluate different settings.* (See Chapter 22, "Women Growing Older.")

Our Rights as Patients

Each of us has specific and inviolate legal rights which protect us in our daily lives, including a number of particular rights as consumers of medical-care services.

In a medical setting, your most important right is the right to control what happens to your body. This includes the right of "informed consent," which means that before you permit anyone in a medical or mental-health setting to do anything to you, they must first inform you fully as to 1. what is being planned, 2. the risks and potential benefits of that treatment plan and 3. the alternative forms of treatment, including the option and outcome of no treatment at all. For consent to be truly informed, you must also understand all that is being explained. It is not enough for a provider to simply catalogue the risks and benefits in a quick or complicated manner, to do it when you are under the effects of medication, or in English if it's not your first language. You should ask as many questions as you have and wait until they are answered to your satisfaction before proceeding. You might ask for a written statement of the treatment plan in order to monitor your care or in case you choose to seek a second opinion later. Where no medical emergency exists, take as much time as you need to think about your decision. You can make a decision and later change your mind, since informed consent includes the right to refuse *during* as well as before any treatment. And you must agree *voluntarily*, without any coercion or pressure applied by physician, family members or others.

Yet despite the fact that it is the *physician's legal duty* to insure informed consent, many doctors and hospitals do not do so. Insist on an unpressured discussion with your provider. It is not uncommon for patients to be told little or nothing about the risks of treatments and medications being proposed for them.

Once you decide to seek medical care or are admitted to any facility, you run the risk of trading away some of your rights. Sometimes hospitals will tell you that unless you sign a "blanket" consent form which authorizes the hospital or physician to do whatever

they consider "necessary," you will not be admitted. Physicians and hospitals frequently take advantage of the few legal exceptions to the informed consent requirements.*

It is essential to read any consent form very carefully and to inquire about any vague or technical terms before signing, since your signature suggests—often incorrectly—that you *were* informed. Some hospitals ask patients to write out their understanding of the proposed procedure in their own words. You may cross out, reword or otherwise amend a prepared form before signing. Insist on getting a second opinion if you have any unanswered questions about proposed treatment or surgery. Remember that signing a general or blanket consent form does not prevent you from refusing a treatment at any time or from bringing a suit afterwards.† Be sure to ask for a copy of any form you sign.

Why do abuses occur? Medical schools teach little about informed consent or respect for patients' rights. Some physicians believe that these rights challenge their superior knowledge, while others resent the loss of total control. Some fear that with full and accurate information the patient will decline treatment or take her/his business elsewhere. Others prefer to discuss treatment choices with the patient's family as well. Many say, "I'm simply too busy to sit down with each person and go into a detailed explanation...."

Some state legislatures or courts have specified what a physician's obligation is with respect to patient consent,‡ but it is usually up to *us*, the patients, to insist on adequate and accurate information. We are the best, and in most situations the only, advocates available. (See "A Model Patients' Bill of Rights," p. 586.)

Experimentation

Under certain conditions medical personnel are obligated, legally and ethically, to give us much more de-

---

*The National Women's Health Network is currently preparing a "Nursing Home Resident's Bill of Rights" (see Resources in Chapter 25, "Organizing for Change: U.S.A.").

*1. In the event of a "medical emergency" (trauma/shock, for example), the physician is supposed to seek the consent of a relative, but if none is available, s/he can proceed without consent. Staff in mental institutions sometimes abuse the informed consent principle by claiming that a medical emergency exists so as to give psychiatric medications or other treatments without patient consent. 2. The so-called "therapeutic privilege" permits a physician—in very limited circumstances—to withhold information when s/he feels that disclosure would have an adverse effect, usually when dealing with critically ill or acutely depressed persons. Many physicians abuse the "therapeutic privilege," assuming that it is in patients' best interest not to know the truth. 3. Each state, and very often each hospital, has its own laws or policies governing at what age and to what procedures minors can consent. (Abortion consent laws in Massachusetts, Michigan, North Dakota, and Rhode Island are examples.)

†This is true even though signed forms are sometimes used as evidence of informed consent.

‡Check with your local branch of the American Civil Liberties Union.

tailed and complete information before we give our consent to treatment, as when:

- the provider uses an unproven (experimental) medical, surgical or psychiatric treatment, and the outcome in this case is therefore unknown (see the discussion of technology evaluation, p. 558.);
- a study is being carried out which may involve giving certain people *no* treatment, or a treatment which may be inferior, in order to compare results with a newer treatment;
- a drug may be used in a research project for a purpose not approved by the FDA. (Check the *PDR—Physicians' Desk Reference*—or package insert for the approved purposes.) *This situation is extremely common among women, since most routinely used obstetric drugs, many hormonal preparations and some psychiatric drugs are given for purposes not specifically approved by the FDA.*

Since so much research goes on in teaching hospitals, it is important to determine whether or not you are being treated with standard or experimental therapies. Also, the line between treatment and experimentation is often unclear, and since researchers are so poorly prepared or unwilling to protect us, we must continually ask questions about recommended treatments in order to make certain we are not unknowingly participating in research. Experimental situations require that researchers keep a record of our statements that we understand and agree to the experiment and realize that the *probability* of a good outcome is uncertain. If the research is taking place in an institution which derives part of its support from public funds, federal regulations require a special committee called an "institutional review board," which includes both medical personnel and nonmedical community representatives, to be created. This board must first grant approval to the project, and then make certain that we are adequately informed and clearly consenting.[73] In this instance the researcher is obligated to give you a copy of any informed consent form you sign. (See *Protecting Human Subjects*, listed in Resources in Chapter 25, "Organizing for Change: U.S.A.")

What Other Rights Do We Have?

The law does not yet recognize all the rights we feel we should have, although women's and consumer health activists are working to expand these rights through lawsuits and legislation. We believe that physicians and institutions should recognize *all* of our rights and not just the ones legally defined.

Certain rights are guaranteed by laws, including the Constitution, federal and state laws and case law, which is developed through lawsuits, and federal or state agency regulations (such as those of the U.S. Department of Health and Human Services [DHHS] and the FDA, Medicare, Medicaid and so forth). A number of decisions made by hospitals or other private groups may also affect our rights as consumers.*

Reproductive Rights

The United States Constitution implicitly guarantees each one of us a right to privacy, and the Supreme Court has ruled that this right protects a woman's ability to make personal decisions concerning abortion, sterilization, contraception and other reproductive matters. Although the Court has delegated to each of the fifty states the right to limit women's reproductive rights where a "compelling state interest" exists, it has confirmed a woman's right to privacy in seeking an abortion.[74] The United States Supreme Court has, however, determined that this right to privacy is not absolute, and that the fifty states have a certain amount of power to limit the exercise of this right. Presently, both federal and state governments are attempting to limit women's access to abortions. Should they succeed, women's already limited choices as consumers of reproductive-related services will be further restricted. (See Chapter 16, "Abortion.")

The Right to Refuse Treatment

Each of us has a legal right to refuse medical treatment at any time, even if we have consented to it previously. In life-or-death matters, however, physicians and hospitals often resist a person's choice to refuse treatment. Several states† have passed laws which, through the use of a "living will," allow terminally ill patients to authorize the withholding or withdrawal of medical treatment, even though such an order may lead to their death. These statutes enable both patients and their families to seek death with dignity and also protect hospitals from any lawsuits which might result.

Courts have generally found that a competent individual has the right to refuse even life-saving treatment, and procedures have been developed to determine whether a person is "competent" to make such a decision. A person is competent if s/he understands the nature of the illness, the risks and benefits of the proposed treatment and the outcome of nontreatment. Simply disagreeing with your physician's recommendation does *not* mean that you are incompetent. The whole area of medical decision-making and competence becomes even more difficult when we are required to make treatment choices for persons

*Many national hospital organizations and local hospitals have issued their own "patients' bill of rights" as public-relations gestures, but these statements can neither give nor take away our constitutional rights, though they may help inform both patients and staff.

†As of mid-1982: Alabama, Arkansas, California, Idaho, Kansas, Nevada, New Mexico, North Carolina, Oregon, Texas, Washington and Washington, DC.

who clearly are incompetent, such as children, or elderly parents who may be senile or comatose. Many courts have refused to permit parents to withhold treatment that would save the life of their child.* This dilemma is most acute in the case of severely handicapped newborns.

Merely seeking medical care in a teaching hospital places you in a subtly coercive environment which sometimes makes it increasingly difficult to refuse the proposed treatment. As a result, it is often difficult to assert your right to refuse, and you must be prepared to explain your position. Remember, too, that accepting one part of the treatment plan does not mean that you must accept it all, and you always have the right to leave the hospital if your wishes are not respected. Enlisting the support of a family member or other advocate may be particularly helpful in such situations.

The Right to Receive Care

The laws in our country do not recognize an affirmative right *to* treatment, except in the case of medical emergencies seen in a hospital emergency room. *If either transfer or discharge will threaten or adversely affect a patient's condition, then treatment must be rendered, regardless of ability to pay.*†

The lack of a legal right to treatment, when combined with the high costs of medical care, means that many people receive either inadequate care or no care at all. There are a few programs for pregnant women and low-income, elderly or physically challenged persons, although many of these are being cut back—for example, Medicare or Medicaid payments (which are constantly being cut, and the eligibility requirements made more stringent) and monthly Social Security payments for those who are temporarily disabled, regardless of age. All hospitals which have received public monies for construction‡ must allocate a certain amount of money each year to the provision of free care. Contact your local legal services office for a full list of the various programs and their eligibility requirements.

We hope that some day everyone's right to receive quality care will be guaranteed, but we realize that such a prospect is not immediately likely. Women's health activists and organizations will continue to advocate for these rights; meanwhile, they may make available lists of nongovernmental resources for those affected by cutbacks.

Rights Regarding Medical Records

In about a third of the states, patients have a legal right to see, obtain or have access to their hospital

*The Chad Green case is the best-chronicled of this type.[75]

†Hospitals refusing such treatment to poor women in labor often assume they will not have the knowledge or resources to bring suit. (See p. 331.)

‡Called Hill-Burton funds.

Following is a *model* patients' bill of rights developed by George Annas for the American Civil Liberties Union. This bill applies to hospitals and clinics, not to doctors in private offices. Its language is precise: where the phrase "legal right" is used, the right is one well recognized by case law or statute. The term "right" refers to one that probably would be recognized if the case were brought to court. "We recognize the right" refers to "what ought to be."

The model bill is set out as it would apply to a patient in his or her chronological relations with the hospital: sections 1–4 for a person not hospitalized but a *potential* patient; 5 for emergency admission; 6–15 for inpatients; 16–22 for discharge and after discharge; and 23 relating back to all 22 rights.

A Model Patients' Bill of Rights

Preamble: *As you enter this health care facility, it is our duty to remind you that your health care is a cooperative effort between you as a patient and the doctors and hospital staff. During your stay a patients' rights advocate will be available to you. The duty of the advocate is to assist you in all the decisions you must make and in all situations in which your health and welfare are at stake. The advocate's first responsibility is to help you understand the role of all who will be working with you, and to help you understand what your rights as a patient are. Your advocate can be reached at any time of the day by dialing———. The following is a list of your rights as a patient. Your advocate's duty is to see to it that you are afforded these rights. You should call your advocate whenever you have any questions or concerns about any of these rights.*

1. *The patient has a legal right to informed participation in all decisions involving his/her health care program.*
2. *We recognize the right of all potential patients to know what research and experimental protocols are being used in our facility and what alternatives are available in the community.*
3. *The patient has a legal right to privacy regarding the source of payment for treatment and care. This right includes access to the highest degree of care without regard to the source of payment for that treatment and care.*
4. *We recognize the right of a potential patient to complete and accurate information concerning medical care and procedures.*

records. But in reality, many patients are never informed of this right, and find it difficult and costly to obtain their records. In addition, many facilities keep medical records only for the limited period of time

5. *The patient has a legal right to prompt attention, especially in an emergency situation.*

6. *The patient has a legal right to a clear, concise explanation in layperson's terms of all proposed procedures, including the possibilities of any risk of mortality or serious side effects, problems related to recuperation, and probability of success, and will not be subjected to any procedure without his/her voluntary, competent and understanding consent. The specifics of such consent shall be set out in a written consent form, signed by the patient.*

7. *The patient has a legal right to a clear, complete, and accurate evaluation of his/her condition and prognosis without treatment before being asked to consent to any test or procedure.*

8. *We recognize the right of the patient to know the identity and professional status of all those providing service. All personnel have been instructed to introduce themselves, state their status, and explain their role in the health care of the patient. Part of this right is the right of the patient to know the identity of the physician responsible for his/her care.*

9. *We recognize the right of any patient who does not speak English to have access to an interpreter.*

10. *The patient has a right to all the information contained in his/her medical record while in the health care facility, and to examine the record on request.*

11. *We recognize the right of a patient to discuss his/her condition with a consultant specialist, at the patient's request and expense.*

12. *The patient has a legal right not to have any test or procedure, designed for educational purposes rather than his/her personal benefit, performed on him/her.*

13. *The patient has a legal right to refuse any particular drug, test, procedure, or treatment.*

14. *The patient has a legal right to privacy of both person and information with respect to: the hospital staff, other doctors, residents, interns and medical students, researchers, nurses, other hospital personnel, and other patients.*

15. *We recognize the patient's right of access to people outside the health care facility by means of visitors and the telephone. Parents may stay with their children and relatives with terminally ill patients 24 hours a day.*

16. *The patient has a legal right to leave the health care facility regardless of his/her physical condition or financial status, although the patient may be requested to sign a release stating that he/she is leaving against the medical judgment of his/her doctor or the hospital.*

17. *The patient has a right not to be transferred to another facility unless he/she has received a complete explanation of the desirability and need for the transfer, the other facility has accepted the patient for transfer, and the patient has agreed to transfer. If the patient does not agree to transfer, the patient has the right to a consultant's opinion on the desirability of transfer.*

18. *A patient has a right to be notified of his/her impending discharge at least one day before it is accomplished, to insist on a consultation by an expert on the desirability of discharge, and to have a person of the patient's choice notified in advance.*

19. *The patient has a right, regardless of the source of payment, to examine and receive an itemized and detailed explanation of the total bill for services rendered in the facility.*

20. *The patient has a right to competent counseling from the hospital staff to help in obtaining financial assistance from public or private sources to meet the expense of services received in the institution.*

21. *The patient has a right to timely prior notice of the termination of his/her eligibility for reimbursement by any third-party payor for the expense of hospital care.*

22. *At the termination of his/her stay at the health care facility we recognize the right of a patient to a complete copy of the information contained in his/her medical record.*

23. *We recognize the right of all patients to have 24-hour-a-day access to a patient's rights advocate who may act on behalf of the patient to assert or protect the rights set out in this document.*

As is apparent from the preamble of this document, it is my view that a statement of rights alone is insufficient. What is needed in addition is someone, whom I term an advocate, to assist patients in asserting their rights. As indicated previously, this advocate is necessary because a sick person's first concern is to regain health, and in pursuit of health patients are willing to give up rights that they otherwise would vigorously assert.

specified by state law. There are also variations from state to state as to medical versus psychiatric records, hospitals' versus doctors' or nurses' records and minors' versus adults' records. It is advisable to have copies of all medical encounters for future reference.

Theoretically, your records are private and only personnel directly involved in your care may see them. However, with the rise of computerization and the large numbers of staff persons with access to records, violations of rights to confidentiality are becoming more common.

Physicians' records, on the other hand, are the doctors' property, though states vary in requiring physicians to make them available to patients. Some physicians will give you copies of your records and test results if you ask, and a few may send you reports voluntarily. Otherwise, your only recourse is to hire a lawyer who will demand the records through either a letter or, in rare circumstances, a lawsuit. When selecting a physician, you might ask how s/he feels about making records available.*

How Can We Enforce Our Rights?†

Our rights as patients mean little if we are unable to enforce them effectively. The method of enforcement will depend on state laws and the right involved. Listed below are some of the most common ways to exercise and enforce our rights.

Patient Advocacy

One way to safeguard your rights is to bring someone as an advocate to all medical encounters. Your advocate may be a friend, relative or women's health worker—anyone you trust enough to share confidential health information with and who will help you assert your rights. Before your medical visit, discuss with your advocate what you expect—and what you *want*—to happen. Make sure you both understand what kinds of diagnostic tests, treatments or surgery are being proposed. Ask your advocate to keep a record of events which occur while you are unable to be aware of them. Try to anticipate those situations which, in the past, made you feel powerless or inadequately informed. Make a list of the questions you want to ask. If there is more than one physician involved in your case, your advocate can help coordinate your care. If the medical staff raises questions about your emotional or psychiatric stability (and thereafter dismisses your concerns and complaints), an advocate can speak up for you.

While some private physicians do not mind the presence of a relative or friend during office visits or examinations, hospitals may be more restrictive. Be as firm as you can about wanting your advocate with you, and if your provider refuses unreasonably, you may want to make a change if you can. Some hospitals have specific policies about advocates.

Large hospitals may employ "patient advocates" or "patient representatives" who can be helpful in cutting through red tape. Yet because they represent the hospital, these advocates are simply not free to represent your interests when they conflict with the interests of the hospital or doctor. While they may help with small or administrative complaints, they are not generally able to provide the kinds of information and control that are essential to pursuing and enforcing your rights.

Complaint Mechanisms

If you are unhappy with the results of a medical encounter, do not be afraid to complain. Make a written record of the events as soon as they occur, and draft a letter which clearly states what happened and when. If friends or family members have firsthand knowledge of the events, ask them to record their thoughts and observations right away. If your complaint is against a licensed health professional, send it to the appropriate licensing board, and send a copy to the relevant county and state professional societies. You can also contact a local women's health group for assistance and encouragement. When complaining about a facility (hospital, nursing home, clinic, etc.) which is licensed by the state, contact the appropriate licensing agency, as well as the consumer protection division of the Attorney General's office. If you have reason to think you have received an experimental drug or experience a strong drug reaction, report this to your local FDA.* The Joint Commission on Accreditation of Hospitals in Chicago should also be sent a copy of any correspondence dealing with the facilities they accredit.†

It is sometimes useful to discuss your intentions with the provider before actually lodging any complaints, since this may provide the incentive necessary to improve the situation. Make certain, though, that all your medical records and supporting materials are in order prior to discussing the matter with your provider, since once they are put on notice as to your discontent, they may become more defensive and limit or manipulate the information included in your record.

Litigation and Malpractice

The number of malpractice suits is increasing rapidly, largely because patients have no other way of expressing their dissatisfaction with medical care. The dollar amounts in damages awarded are also rising, though not as much as insurance companies would like us to believe. These increases give the companies an excuse to raise malpractice insurance premiums, which results in many physicians being unable to afford the hikes. When we analyze the actual lawsuits, however, we find that:

- obstetrician/gynecologists are sued more than any other type of doctor;

*All federally qualified HMOs must make records available.

†Further information and possible assistance can often be obtained by contacting local women's health groups, consumer groups or legal services organizations (see Resources in Chapter 25, "Organizing for Change: U.S.A.").

*See Resources in Chapter 25, "Organizing for Change: U.S.A."
†See Resources in Chapter 25.

- 75 percent of all malpractice claims originate from treatments given in hospitals;
- a *few* doctors are being sued several times, most doctors never;[76]
- the majority of suits are unsuccessful, largely due to doctors' refusal to testify against one another, even when malpractice is obvious.*

Rather than police their colleagues, most doctors prefer to pass the cost of increased premiums on to their patients in the form of higher fees and work with the state legislatures to restrict patients' ability to sue.†

Contrary to the protestations of the medical profession and the insurance companies, patients are not responsible for the skyrocketing cost of malpractice insurance, which in turn drives up the cost of medical care. Doctors who practice bad or careless medicine are responsible, and malpractice suits are one way we as patients can be compensated for the harm those doctors cause. Litigation, though, is an expensive, time-consuming and often frustrating means of recourse. Unless you have suffered serious injury, lost earnings (past *or* future), incurred large medical bills or experienced serious emotional harm, litigation will probably not be worth the effort.

In order to recover in a lawsuit against a provider or drug/device manufacturer, it is necessary to show 1. that the defendant provider had a responsibility to you, the patient (which generally exists as a matter of law); 2. that that responsibility was breached; 3. that you were harmed; and 4. that the harm was a direct result of the breach, or negligent behavior.

If you feel you have been injured, you will probably want to seek a lawyer. Lawyers, like doctors, tend to specialize. Make sure that your lawyer has had extensive experience with malpractice cases. Both NOW and the American Civil Liberties Union usually maintain reliable attorney referral lists. Many attorneys will take malpractice cases on a "contingency fee" basis and will not charge clients for pursuing the matter unless they win (in which case they claim a percentage of the recovery), while others charge the clients for expenses regardless of outcome.

Legislation

Changing a state or federal law is a difficult and time-consuming process, requiring both the skill necessary to negotiate the legislative process and the political clout that comes from forming alliances among diverse groups. Only strong and sustained support can help you resist the attacks of the powerful and well-organized opponents many advocates for women's health have faced across the country. While the legislative route is difficult, it does offer the promise of more permanent and broader solutions than most groups can achieve at the local level.

Women as Healers

The history of women as healers is our history. It tells us where we have come from and casts a revealing light on our present condition. It puts us in touch with a power that has rightfully belonged to women throughout the ages and which we now legitimately reclaim. Without a past, our image is incomplete, and part of our deepest selves is lost.

We are just beginning to discover the true history of women and healing, because history as men have written it ignores women. In particular, midwives and "wise women" (healers) have been primarily poor and working class, and as such have not been recognized as significant matter for history. Women's research is uncovering the missing pieces of our story, and so we learn about ourselves from the way churchmen and medical men viewed women. Many of us have internalized these views.

What has happened in the evolution and suppression of women as healers is critical to our understanding of the relationship between medicine and women today. It helps us to see the vast difference between healing and medicine.

Below are a few selections from early writings by and about women healers, and from recent historical works by women. In the space allotted in this book, all we can do is open a door. *This is our history. These are our historians.*

Foreword

Medicine, like war, is an extension of politics. The story of the old wife is not the story of an inferior practice losing ground with the advances of medical science and technology; rather, it is a story which concerns the politics of medicine— a story of control and access.

—Mary Chamberlain, a
modern historian [78]

The Healers

The practitioners of healing in the pre-classical cultures of the Near and Middle East were also the religious guardians.

About 3000 B.C.
Near East

In nearly all areas of the world, goddesses were extolled as healers, dispensers of curative herbs, roots, plants and other medical aids, casting the priestesses who attended the shrines into the role of physicians of those who worshipped there. [Merlin Stone]

---

*The AMA Principles of Medical Ethics urge doctors to "...strive to expose those physicians deficient in character or competence, or who engage in fraud or deception."

†"Medical whores" is the term doctors use to describe doctors who will testify to another doctor's malpractice or incompetence.[77]

In Sumer, Assyria, Egypt and Greece until about the third millenium the practice of healing was almost exclusively in the hands of priestesses.

—Mary Chamberlain[79]

About 1550 B.C. Egypt

The Ebers Papyrus, which contains guidance on midwifery, indicates that knowledge of gynaecology and obstetrics was quite advanced, including not only childbirth and abortion but a range of other problems from breast cancer to prolapse of the womb.[80]

About 129–201 A.D., Rome

The conversion of the Roman empire to Christianity crystallised attitudes towards women and women healers. The Roman gods were replaced by one all-powerful God whose duties included healing, and who delegated the role of healing to His chosen successors. Thus men were confirmed in their role as official healer and Galenic medicine...was confirmed as Christian medicine.

—Mary Chamberlain[81]

Midwife attending childbearing woman seated on obstetrical stool, 16th century   *The Feminist Press*

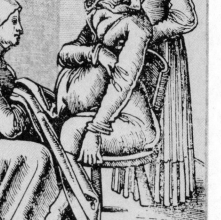

11th–12th century, Europe

In fact, the wise woman, or witch, as the authorities labeled her, did possess a host of remedies which had been tested in years of use. *Liber Simplicis Medicinae*, the compendium of natural healing methods written by St. Hildegarde of Bingen (A.D. 1098–1178), gives some idea of the scope of women healers' knowledge in the early middle ages. Her book lists the healing properties of 213 varieties of plants and 55 trees, in addition to dozens of mineral and animal derivatives.

—Barbara Ehrenreich and Deirdre English, modern historians[82]

14th–16th century, Europe

For all but the very rich healing had traditionally been the prerogative of women. The art of healing was linked to the tasks and spirit of motherhood; it combined wisdom and nurturance, tenderness and skill. All but the most privileged women were expected to be at least literate in the language of herbs and healing techniques; the most learned women traveled widely to share their skills. The women who distinguished themselves as healers were not only midwives caring for other women, but "general practitioners," herbalists, and counselors serving men and women alike.

—Barbara Ehrenreich and Deirdre English[83]

15th century, England

And although women have various maladies and more terrible sicknesses than any man knows, as I said, they are ashamed for fear of reproof in times to come and of exposure by discourteous men who love women only for physical pleasure and for evil gratification. And if women are sick, such men despise them and fail to realize how much sickness women have before they bring them into this world. And so, to assist women, I intend to write of how to help their secret maladies so that one woman may aid another in her illness and not divulge her secrets to such discourteous men.

—Unknown writer[84]

14th–16th century, England

They [Old Wives] were the custodians of communal and community medical knowledge. But this knowledge was free and freely given. With little or no money at stake there was no need to preserve a "closed" profession in terms of entry, training and dissemination of knowledge.

—Mary Chamberlain[85]

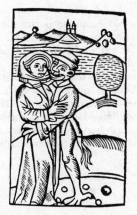

Devil seducing a witch

The Feminist Press

Suppression: *The Witch Trials*

14th century, Europe

An acquaintance of herbs soothing to pain, or healing in their qualities, was then looked upon [by the Church] as having been acquired through diabolical agency. In the fourteenth century the Church decreed that any woman who healed others without having studied, was duly a witch and should suffer death.

—a 19th century feminist historian[86]

14th century, Europe

The exclusion of women from the universities, and therefore from access to learning, was justified on the grounds that their intellects were deficient, largely because they were governed by the senses rather than by reason.

—Mary Chamberlain[87]

All witchcraft comes from carnal lust which is in women insatiable.... Wherefore for the sake of fulfilling their lusts they consort even with devils.... It is sufficiently clear that it is no matter for wonder that there are more women than men found infected with the heresy of witchcraft.... And blessed be the Highest who has so far preserved the male sex from so great a crime.

—Dominican monks Frs. Sprenger and Kramer, authors of the Inquisition's *Malleus Maleficarum*[88]

1484–1700s, Europe and England

And if it is asked how it is possible to distinguish whether an illness is caused by witchcraft or by some natural physical defect, we answer that there are various methods. And the first is by means of the judgement of doctors.

—Frs. Sprenger and Kramer[89]

Moreover...it was shown...that the greatest injuries to the Faith as regards the heresy of witches are done by midwives: and this is made clearer than daylight itself by the confessions of some who were afterwards burned.

—Frs. Sprenger and Kramer[90]

1608, England

For this must always be remembered, as a conclusion, that by Witches we understand not only those which kill and torment, but all diviners, charmers, jugglers, all Wizards, commonly called wise men and wise women...and in the same number we reckon all good Witches, which do no hurt but good, which do not spoil and destroy, but save and deliver.... It were a thousand times better for the land if all Witches, but especially the blessing Witch, might suffer death.

—William Perkins, the leading English Witch Hunter[91]

15th–16th century, Europe

The extent of the witch craze is startling: in the late fifteenth and early sixteenth centuries there were thousands upon thousands of executions—usually live burnings at the stake—in Germany, Italy, and other countries. In the mid-sixteenth century the terror spread to France, and finally to England. One writer has estimated the number of executions at an average of six hundred a year for certain German cities—one or two a day, leaving out Sundays. In the Bishopric of Trier, in 1585, two villages were left with only one female inhabitant each. Many writers have estimated the total number killed to have been in the millions. Women made up 85 per cent of those executed—old women, young women, and children.

The targets of the witch hunts were, almost exclusively, peasant women, and among them female lay healers were singled out for prosecution.

—Barbara Ehrenreich and Deirdre English[92]

15th–16th century, Europe and England

Because the Medieval Church, with the support of kings, princes and secular authorities, controlled medical education and practice, the Inquisition constitutes, among other things, an early instance of the "professional" repudiating the skills and interfering with the rights of the "nonprofessional" to minister to the poor.

—Thomas Szaz, a modern psychiatrist and historian[93]

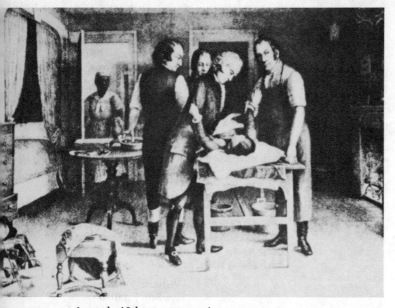

An early 19th century ovariotomy   *The Feminist Press*

Doctor delivering under a sheet, for modesty's sake

The Feminist Press

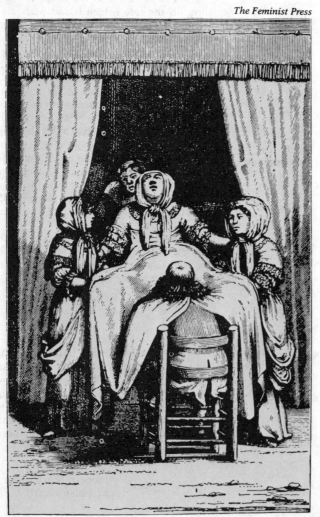

The witch trials established the male physician on a moral and intellectual plane vastly above the female healer. It placed him on the side of God and the Law, a professional on a par with lawyers and theologians, while it placed her on the side of darkness, evil, and magic. The witch hunts prefigured—with dramatic intensity—the clash between male doctors and female healers in nineteenth-century America.

—Barbara Ehreneich
and Deirdre English[94]

Suppression: The Intellectual Arguments

17th century, Europe and England

Between the twelfth and seventeenth centuries the theological arguments which held that the spiritual deficiency of women laid them open to temptation by the Devil were translated into lay terms. By the seventeenth century spiritual deficiency had become intellectual deficiency: women were not merely open to the temptations of sensuality but were motivated by illogicality and irrationality. In both arguments, women's bodies were seen to be the cause of their fundamental weakness.

—Mary Chamberlain[95]

The Hippocratic (medical) tradition held that women were governed by the womb and were therefore "naturally" incapable of logic and reason. Moreover...women took advantage of the sick!

—Mary Chamberlain[96]

1612, England

Such persons are the curse of God and the sinne of man [for they that] persuade the sicke that they have no needs of the Physition, call God a lyar, who expressly saith otherwise! And make themselves wiser than their creator, who hath ordained the Physition for the good of man.

—John Cotta, an early
17th century physician[97]

18th century, England and Europe

The intellectual mood of the eighteenth century meant a move away from the "arts" of the Middle Ages and towards the cognitive sciences and ideas of progress and enlightenment. With this came the desire to protect those areas of knowledge from those unable to comprehend its complexities. Knowledge itself began to be institutionalized, and became expertise. Knowledge without expertise became skillful deceit. "Cunning" changed its meaning from "knowledge" to "craftiness," and the cunning woman, once an expert, was now a charlatan.

—Mary Chamberlain[98]

Suppression: North America

18th–19th century, America

The North American female healer, unlike the European witch-healer, was not eliminated by violence. No Grand Inquisitors pursued her; flames did not destroy her stock of herbs or the knowledge of them. The female healer in North America was defeated in a struggle which was, at bottom, economic. Medicine in the nineteenth century was being drawn into the marketplace, becoming—as were needles, or ribbons, or salt already—a thing to be bought and sold. Healing was female when it was a neighborly service, based in stable communities, where skills could be passed on for generations and where the healer knew her patients and their families. When the attempt to heal is detached from personal relationships to become a commodity and a source of wealth in itself—then

does the business of healing become a male enterprise.

—Barbara Ehrenreich
and Deirdre English[99]

late 19th century, America

But the American medical profession would settle for nothing less than the final solution to the midwife question: they would have to be eliminated—outlawed. The medical journals urged their constituencies to join the campaign: "Surely we have enough influence and friends to procure the needed legislation. Make yourselves heard in the land; and the ignorant meddlesome midwife will soon be a thing of the past."

—Barbara Ehrenreich
and Deirdre English[100]

late 19th–early 20th century, U.S.A.

The obstetricians thought of her as "...The typical, old, gin-fingering, guzzling midwife with her pockets full of forcing drops, her mouth full of snuff, her fingers full of dirt and her *brains* full of arrogance and superstition" (Gerwin, 1906); "filthy and ignorant and not far removed from the jungles of Africa" (Underwood, 1926); "a relic of barbarism" (deLee, 1915); "pestiliferous" (Garrigues, 1898); "vicious" (Titus in Huntington, 1913); "often malicious" (Emmons and Huntington, 1911); "[with] the overconfidence of half-knowledge...unprincipled and callous of the feelings and welfare of her patients and anxious only for her fee" (Emmons and Huntington, 1912); "[earning] $5,888,888...which should be paid to physicians and nurses for doing the work properly" (Ziegler, 1913); and lastly "un-American" (Mabbott, 1907).

—Neal Devitt,
modern physician
and historian[101]

Gynecological exam — *The Feminist Press*

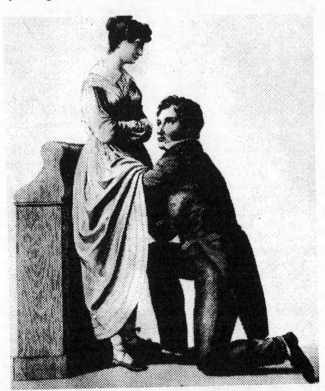

Men doctors teaching about woman patient — *The Feminist Press*

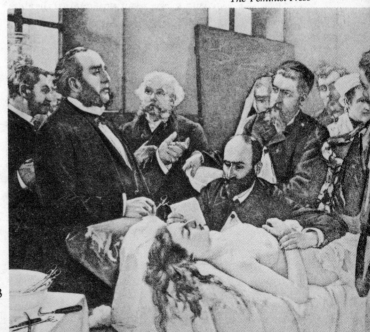

593

The Consequences

With the elimination of midwifery, all women—not just those of the upper class—fell under the biological hegemony of the medical profession. In the same stroke, women lost their last autonomous role as healers. The only roles left for women in the medical system were as employees, customers, or "material."....The male takeover of healing had weakened the communal bonds among women—the networks of skill and information sharing—and had created a model for professional authority in all areas of domestic activity.

20th century, U.S.A. and the western world

—Barbara Ehrenreich and Deirdre English[102]

It is perhaps inevitable that childbirth and areas related to women's sexuality should have become those areas most susceptible to aggressive medical techniques. For not only are these areas ones in which the old wife remained a challenge but they are also areas in which women, as women, remain a challenge to men.

—Mary Chamberlain[103]

The medical system we have inherited today has certain intrinsic features which were accentuated in the struggle for dominance over what came to be termed "illegitimate" practitioners. These practitioners were largely women and the struggle for dominance was, I believe, fundamentally a gender struggle. To that extent, modern medicine is "masculine" medicine, and some of its most dominant features are reactions against healers' practice.

—Mary Chamberlain[104]

An Alternative

This is the vision that is implicit in feminism—a society that is organized around human needs: a society in which healing is not a commodity distributed according to the dictates of profit but is integral to the network of community life...in which wisdom about daily life is not hoarded by "experts" or doled out as a commodity but is drawn from the experience of all people and freely shared among them.

the year 2000 and beyond

—Barbara Ehrenreich and Dierdre English[105]

NOTES

1. See Chapter 3 "Alcohol, Mood-Altering Drugs and Smoking," in this book. See also Karen J. Armitage, Lawrence J. Schneiderman and Robert A. Bass, "Response of Physicians to Medical Complaints in Men and Women," *Journal of the American Medical Association* (Brief Reports), Vol. 241, No. 20 (May 18, 1979), pp. 2186–87; Barbara Bernstein and Robert Kane, "Physicians' Attitudes Toward Female Patients," *Medical Care*, Vol. XIX, No. 6 (June 1981), pp. 600–08. See also "Images of Women in Medical Textbooks" and "Women Physicians," on pp. 568–69 in this book.

2. Gena Corea. *The Hidden Malpractice: How American Medicine Mistreats Women*. New York: Jove/HBJ, 1977, pp. 15–16. See also the discussion of the Pill in this book, pp. 237–47.

3. Arthur Owens. "Who Says Doctors Make Too Much Money?" *Medical Economics* (March 7, 1983), pp. 66–7. See also Peter Conrad and Rochelle Kern, *The Sociology of Health and Illness: Critical Perspectives*, New York: St. Martin's Press, 1981, p. 4; Victor Sidel and Ruth Sidel, *A Healthy State: An International Perspective on the Crisis in United States Medical Care*, New York: Pantheon Books, 1977, p. 42. See figures quoted elsewhere in this chapter for taxpayer expenditures for medical care and training. The estimated annual cost to taxpayers for physician training, for example, is $20,000 a year per student in Massachusetts. About one-third of all U.S. doctors who have been aided by the government in their training are delinquent in repayments or have refused outright to repay. (A. A. Michelson, "Socialized Medicine Nothing New," *The Boston Globe*, December 12, 1981, p. 7.) Also, in 1983, taxpayer costs for kidney dialysis treatments approached $2 billion, most of which was paid out in profits to physician-controlled dialysis centers despite the availability of the cheaper and more desirable option of home dialysis. (Beth Baker and Stuart Kaufer, "Blood Money: A 'Noble Experiment' Turns a Profit on the Pain of Kidney Patients," *The Progressive*, April 1981, pp. 38–41.) Physician incomes are also rising. According to *Medical Economics*, in 1975 only one in eight office-based doctors had a net income of $100,000 or more after expenses. In 1980 that figure was one in three doctors, and one in ten reported earning at least $150,000 after expenses.

4. "Pill No Longer a Menace," *The Evening Post*, Wellington, New Zealand, September 20, 1982, p. 1.

5. The U.S. ranked sixteenth in infant mortality rates (IMRs) internationally in 1978, trailing after Japan and many other industrialized nations at a rate of 13.6; that is, for every 1,000 babies born, 13.6 died within the first year of life (most during the first few days). Low-birth-weight babies are the major cause of such rates. The rate for black babies was 21.7. In 1979 the overall U.S. rate dropped to 13.2, and for the twelve months ending August 1982 it was 11.4 (11.2, provisionally, for the year). Yet in 1981, for the first time in many years, several states (Alabama, Alaska, Kansas, Michigan, Missouri, Nevada, Rhode Island and West Virginia) reported *rises* in their infant death rates; thirty-two urban areas nationwide reported similar upswings. While nationally the 1981 IMR was 11.7, in Washington, D.C., one of the nation's most affluent communities, it was 22.6, 14.1 for whites and 25.5 for blacks. In poorer communities, like the Mississippi Delta and Kankakee County, Illinois, the rates range between from 45.0 for the former and 43.6 for the latter. The meaning is clear: there is what Professor Edward Sparer has called an "infant death gap" between haves and have-nots, which is getting wider. See National Health Law Program, "Infant Mortality and Lack of Prenatal Care," *Hard*

Facts: The Administration's 1984 Health Budget, March 1, 1983, p. 1. See also Geraldine Dallek, "America's Widening Infant Death Gap," *Health and Medicine* (Summer/Fall 1982), pp. 23–27. See Resources in Chapter 25, "Organizing for Change: U.S.A."

6. Kathleen Newland, *Infant Mortality and the Health of Societies* (Worldwatch Paper #47), 1981, pp. 6–11. Washington, DC: Worldwatch Institute, 1776 Massachusetts Avenue NW, Washington, DC 20036. See also U.S. Department of Health, Education and Welfare, *Factors Associated with Low Birth Weight*, HEW, Hyattsville, MD, April 1980, p. 2.

7. John B. McKinlay and Sonja M. McKinlay "Medical Measures and the Decline of Mortality," in Peter Conrad and Rochelle Kern, *The Sociology of Health and Illness: Critical Perspectives*. New York: St. Martin's Press, 1981, pp. 12–30. See also Thomas McKeown, *The Role of Medicine: Dream, Mirage, or Nemesis*, London: Nuffield Provincial Hospitals Trust, 1976; Rene Dubos, *Mirage of Health: Utopias, Progress, and Biological Change*, New York: Harper Colophon, p. 23 ff.

8. "Legal Abortion, Family Planning Services Largest Factors in Reducing Neonatal Mortality Rate," *Family Planning Perspectives*, Vol. 13, No. 2 (March/April 1981).

9. Lack of teaching of scientific method in medical school is documented in David H. Banta, Clyde J. Behney and Jane Sisk Willems, *Toward Rational Technology in Medicine*, New York: Springer Publishing Co., Inc., 1981, p. 30. Additional discussion of the unscientific nature of modern medicine may be found in Rick Carlson, *The End of Medicine*, New York: John Wiley and Sons, Inc. (Wiley Interscience), 1976; Barbara Ehrenreich and Deirdre English, *For Her Own Good: 150 Years of the Experts' Advice to Women*, Garden City, NY: Doubleday/Anchor Books, 1979; Norman Cousins, *Anatomy of an Illness*, New York: W.W. Norton and Co., Inc., 1979. A discussion of how medical decision-making might be brought more into line with modern scientific thinking is presented in Harold Bursztajn, Richard I. Feinbloom, Robert M. Hamm and Archie Brodsky, *Medical Choices, Medical Chances*, New York: Delacorte Press/Seymour Lawrence, 1981. Even the AMA does not call medicine a science. See Maryann Napoli, *Health Facts: A Critical Evaluation of the Major Problems, Treatments, and Alternatives Facing Medical Consumers*, Woodstock, NY: Overlook Press, 1981, p. 14; statement of Terence S. Carden, Jr., of the AMA in *Journal of the American Medical Association*, October 27, 1978; Elliot Mishler, et al., *Social Contexts of Health, Illness and Patient Care*, England: Cambridge University Press, 1981.

10. David H. Banta, et al., *Toward Rational Technology in Medicine*, p. 122.

11. Male prisoners and volunteers are frequently used to test drugs. For nutrition research, see J.S. Garrow, *Energy Balance and Obesity in Man*, New York: Elsevier/North Holland (Biomedical Press), 1978.

12. Leonard S. Syme and Lisa F. Berkman. "Social Class, Susceptibility, and Sickness," in Conrad and Kern, *The Sociology of Health and Illness*, pp. 35–44. See also National Advisory Council on Economic Opportunity, "Women in Poverty," *The Clearinghouse Review*, 500 Michigan Avenue, Chicago, IL, March 1980 (entire issue); "A Growing Crisis: Disadvantaged Women and Their Children," U.S. Commission on Civil Rights, 1121 Vermont Avenue NW, Washington, DC 20425, April 1983.

13. Geraldine Dallek. "America's Widening Infant Death Gap," *Health and Medicine*, Vol. 1, No. 3 (summer–fall 1982), p. 25.

14. National Academy of Sciences, Institute of Medicine, Division of Health Care Services. "Health Care in a Context of Civil Rights: A Report of a Study." Washington, DC: U.S. Government Printing Office, #1804, 1981.

15. Wornie L. Reed. "Suffer the Children: Some Effects of Racism on the Health of Black Infants," in Conrad and Kern, *The Sociology of Health and Illness*, pp. 317–24.

16. Diana Scully. *Men Who Control Women's Health: The Miseducation of Obstetrician-Gynecologists*. Boston: Houghton-Mifflin, 1980. (See the footnote on p. 562.)

17. Irving Zola. "Medicine as an Institution of Social Control," in *Socio-Medical Inquiries—Recollections, Reflections, and Reconsiderations*. Philadelphia: Temple University Press, 1983, p. 262 ff.

18. George J. Annas. "Forced Cesareans: The Most Unkindest Cut of All," *The Hastings Center Report* (June 1982), pp. 16–17. Also personal interviews with the authors of *Our Bodies, Ourselves*.

19. Dorothy Wertz and Richard W. Wertz. "The Decline of Midwives and the Rise of Medical Obstetricians," in Conrad and Kern, *The Sociology of Health and Illness*, pp. 173–74.

20. Barbara Ehrenreich and Deirdre English, *For Her Own Good*, p. 117.

21. Estelle P. Ramey. "Men's Cycles (They Have Them Too, You Know)," in *Beyond Sex-Role Stereotypes*, A. Kaplan and J. Bean, eds. Boston: Little Brown, 1976. See also Ruth Hubbard, Mary Sue Henefin and Barbara Fried, *Biological Woman—The Convenient Myth: A Collection of Feminist Essays and a Comprehensive Bibliography*, Cambridge, MA: Schenkman Publishing Co., 1982 (entire volume). See also Hal Strelnick with Richard Younge, "Double Indemnity: The Poverty and Mythology of Affirmative Action in the Health Professional Schools," A Health/PAC Bulletin (Special Report) (June 1980), p. 35. (See Resources in Chapter 25, "Organizing for Change: U.S.A.")

22. Diana Scully. *Men Who Control Women's Health*. See also Michelle Harrison, *A Woman in Residence*, New York: Random House, Inc., 1982.

23. Kardiner, et al. *American Journal of Psychiatry* (1973). See also Phyllis M. Schaeffer, "Panelists Condemn Psychiatrist-Patient Sexual Activity," *Ob/Gyn News*, Vol. 16, No. 24, p. 13; Robert Sadoff, "Quiz: Physician-Patient Involvement," *Medical Aspects of Human Sexuality*, Vol. 15, No. 12 (December 1981), pp. 9–12; D. Sobel, "Sex with Therapist Said to Harm Client," *The New York Times*, August 29, 1981, p. 9; John Kelly, "Sexually Abusive Doctors: How Women Are Betrayed by the Men They Trust Most," *Ladies' Home Journal*, June 1979, pp. 55–182; Ronald Kotulak, "Doctor-Patient Sex: Professional Suicide?" *Boston Globe*, October 10, 1975.

24. Anita Diamant. "Bedside Manners: Of Doctors, Patient Abuse, and Regulation. Again," *The Boston Phoenix* (Section Two), November 10, 1981, p. 14.

25. Personal communication, women's medical association members investigating physician sexual misconduct. See also "Therapist-Patient Sex Has Negative Effect for Most," *Ob/Gyn News*, Vol. 16, No. 24; D. Sobel, "Sex with Therapist Said to Harm Client"; John Kelly, "Sexually Abusive Doctors"; Ronald Kotulak, "Doctor-Patient Sex."

26. "New Case Alleges Sex Abuse by an M.D. at Rock's Sacramento," *Medical World News* (September 3, 1979), pp. 38–39. See also Anita Diamant, "Bedside Manners," p. 13.

27. "Harvard Medical School Dean's Statement on Letters of Recommendation," *Harvard Medical Area FOCUS* (October 8, 1981), p. 5.

28. E. Freidson, quoted in Conrad and Kern, *The Sociology of Health and Illness*, p. 161.

29. Harvard School of Public Health. "'Retool Medical Education' says Dr. Lythcott," *Health Sciences Report* (summer 1981), pp. 2, 8. See also Sidel and Sidel, *A Healthy State*.

30. Harvard University News Office for the Medical Area.

"$6 Million Du Pont Gift for Genetics Research," September 12, 1981, p. 8; "Johnson & Johnson Gives $500,000 for Basic Research," September 12, 1981, p. 8; "Gift for Unrestricted Cancer Research from Bristol-Meyers," April 8, 1982, p. 5. *Harvard Medical Area FOCUS*, 25 Shattuck Street, Boston, MA 02115. See also Barbara J. Culliton, "The Hoechst Department at Mass General (Hospital)" (News and Comment, second in a series on the Academic-Industrial Complex), *Science*, Vol. 216 (June 11, 1982), pp. 1200–3. All grantees are Harvard-affiliated; similar gifts and awards have been given at other elite schools. For a critique, read Arnold S. Relman, "The New Medical-Industrial Complex" (Special Article), *New England Journal of Medicine*, Vol. 303, No. 17 (October 23, 1980), pp. 963–70. (Relman is the editor of *NEJM*.)

31. John K. Inglehart. "Health Care and American Business" (Health Policy Report), *New England Journal of Medicine*, Vol. 306, No. 2 (January 14, 1982), p. 120. See also "Jeff Goldsmith on: The Shape of Corporate Medicine" (*Health and Medicine* Interviews), *Health and Medicine* (spring 1982), pp. 15–20.

32. William K. Stevens. "High Medical Costs Under Attack as Drain on the Nation's Economy," *The New York Times*, March 28, 1982, pp. 1, 50; Sandra Salmans, "Critics Say Lack of Incentives Hurt Insurers' Efforts to Curb Medical Costs," *The New York Times*, March 31, 1982.

33. "Insurance vs. Equality" (editorial), *National NOW Times*, May 1983, p. 9. See also Christine Madsen, "Insurance for Women: Just a Chip Off the Old Rock?" Boston: *Equal Times*, p. 9.

34. "Prescription Drugs," *Health Facts*, Vol. VI, No. 26 (March/April 1981), p. 1.

35. See remarks of Dr. James L. Goddard, quoted in *Science for the People*, Science and Society Series, No. 1 (November 1973). (Also in Conrad and Kern, *The Sociology of Health and Illness*, p. 248.) See also Milton Silverman, Philip R. Lee and Mia Lydecker, *Prescription for Death: The Drugging of the Third World*, Berkeley: University of California Press, 1982, pp. 99–100; Michael Cooper, "Competition and Controls in International Pharmaceutical Markets" (Foreign Perspectives), *Colloquium*, Vol. 2, No. 2 (May 1982), p. 2.

36. Maryann Napoli, *Health Facts*, p. 15. See also "Ineffective Drugs," *The Public Citizen, 1981 Annual Report* (winter 1982), p. 22; Sidney M. Wolfe, Christopher M. Coley and the Health Research Group, *Pills that Don't Work: A Consumer's and Doctor's Guide to Six Hundred Prescription Drugs that Lack Evidence of Effectiveness*, New York: Warner Books, Inc., 1982.

37. Maryann Napoli, *Health Facts*, p. 17. (These are 1975 figures; today's figure is probably higher.)

38. *Science*, Vol. 216 (June 11, 1982), pp. 1200–3. (See Chapter 13, "Birth Control," in this book.) See also press release, September 7, 1979, The U.S. House of Representatives, Select Committee on Narcotics Abuse and Control, "Narcotics Committee to Hold Hearing on Women's Dependency on Prescription Drugs."

39. See James L. Goddard in Conrad and Kern, *The Sociology of Health and Illness*, pp. 249–50.

40. Maryann Napoli, *Health Facts*, p. 15.

41. *Ibid.*, pp. 225–28.

42. "Informed Consent," *Health Facts*, Vol. IV, No. 22 (July/August 1980), p. 3. See also Chapter 5, "Bribery and Other Strategies," in Lee and Lydecker, *Prescription for Death*, pp. 119–30; Barbara Seaman and Gideon Seaman, *Women and the Crisis in Sex Hormones*, New York: Rawson Associates, 1977, pp. 73–74; Mark Dowie, et al., "The Illusion of Safety," *Mother Jones*, June 1982, pp. 39, 43, 46–48; Ivan Illich, "The Pharmaceutical Invasion," in *Medical Nemesis*, Pantheon

Books, 1976, pp. 63–76; "Eli Lilly Is Accused in FDA Documents of Not Reporting Adverse Drug Reactions," *The Wall Street Journal*, August 4, 1982, p. 6.

43. See Grace Ziem, "Medical Education Since Flexner: A Seventy-Year Tracking Record," *Health/PAC Bulletin* 76 (June 1977), pp. 8–14. See also Hal Strelnick, et al., "Double Indemnity," *Health/PAC Bulletin* (Special Report).

44. William G. Blair. "Scientific Detail Overwhelms Regard for Human Needs at Medical Schools, Panel Says," *The New York Times*, October 21, 1982. See also Dr. John Z. Bowers, Macy Foundation Emeritus, quoted in *Harvard Medical Area FOCUS* (February 4, 1982), p. 6; Prof. William Bossert, quoted in *FOCUS* (February 18, 1982), p. 6.

45. Cynthia Carver. "The Deliverers," in *Childbirth: Alternatives to Medical Control*, Shelly Romalis, ed. Austin, TX: University of Texas Press, 1981, p. 135.

46. Dr. Stephen Muller, President of Johns Hopkins University, as quoted in William G. Blair in *The New York Times*, October 21, 1982.

47. Howard S. Becker, E.C. Geer, Everett C. Hughes and Anselm L. Straus. *Boys in White*. Chicago: University of Chicago Press, 1961. Though over twenty years old, this classic study appears to apply to most of today's male students as well. (See *FOCUS* articles listed in Note 44.) No comparable work has yet been done on women. The work of psychiatrist Harold Lief, M.D., at the University of Pennsylvania over a twenty-year period has provided similar corroboration, with special reference to sexuality. (The SKAT [Sex Knowledge and Attitude Tests] for physicians, was developed by Dr. Lief.) See also Bryce Nelson, "Can Doctors Learn Warmth?" *The New York Times*, September 13, 1983.

48. Robert J. Willson and Elsie Reid Carrington. *Obstetrics and Gynecology*, 6th Ed. St. Louis: C.V. Mosby Co., 1979, p. 51.

49. Edmund R. Novak. *Novak's Textbook of Gynecology*. Baltimore: The Williams and Wilkins Co., 1981, pp. 847, 849, 851.

50. "Female Enrollments Gain, But Fewer Blacks Enter U.S. Med Schools," *The New Physician* (December 1981), p. 12. See also "Women Fill a Record Number of Places in U.S. Medical Schools," *Ob/Gyn News* (May 15–31, 1982).

51. Gena Corea. *The Hidden Malpractice*, p. 40.

52. "Alumni Day Reprise," *Harvard Medical Area FOCUS* (June 7, 1979), p. 12.

53. Personal communication to members of the Boston Women's Health Book Collective in a meeting with women medical students at their school.

54. Mary C. Howell. "What Medical Schools Teach About Women" (Sounding Board), *New England Journal of Medicine*, Vol. 291, No. 6 (August 8, 1974), pp. 304–7.

55. Malkah T. Notman and Carol C. Nadelson, eds. *The Woman Patient: Medical and Psychological Interfaces* (Vol. I: *Sexual and Reproductive Aspects of Women's Health Care*). New York: Plenum Publishing Corp., 1978.

56. "Selected Health Authorities of P.L. 97-35," Congressional Research Service (Library of Congress) Committee on Surgery and Commerce, Subcommittee on Health and Energy, February 28, 1983. (Analysis from staff of the Subcommittee, July 1983.)

57. See Bonnie Bullough's article in *American Journal of Public Health* (March 1976).

58. Quoted in Denise Connors, "Sickness Unto Death: Medicine as Mythic, Necrophilic, and Iatrogenic," *Advances in Nursing Science*, Vol. 2, No. 3 (April 1980), pp. 39–51.

59. Betsy A. Lehman. "Turnabout," *The Boston Globe*, July 23, 1983.

60. Boston Nurses Group. "The False Promise: Profession-

alism in Nursing" (reprint). Somerville, MA: The New England Free Press, Union Square. (Reprinted from *Science for the People*, Vol. 10, No. 3 [May/June 1978], pp. 20–34.)

61. Patricia Moccia. "The Case of the Missing Nurse," *Health/PAC Bulletin*, Vol. 13, No. 5 (1982), pp. 15–23.

62. Quoted in Levin, Lowell, et al., *Self-Care: Lay Initiatives in Health*, New York: Prodist, 1976. For a critical review, see Norma Swenson, "Self-Care" (review), *Social Science and Medicine*, Vol. 12 (May 1978), pp. 183–88.

63. Ellen C. Perrin and Helen C. Goodman. "Telephone Management of Acute Pediatric Illnesses" (special article), *New England Journal of Medicine*, Vol. 298, No. 3 (January 19, 1978), pp. 130–35, as quoted in Reginald Rhein, Jr., "Nurses: Colleagues or Competitors?" *Medical World News* (July 9, 1979), p. 73.

64. Arthur Owens. "Earnings: Where Do You Fit In?" *Medical Economics* (September 13, 1982), pp. 2–13.

65. Personal communication with hospital personnel. See also "A Doctor Practices Justice in the Inner City," *Catholic Agitator*, October 1982, p. 3.

66. John Stoeckle and Jerome Grossman. "Primary Care: Improving Treatment and Learning Outside the Hospital," *American Journal of Public Health*, Vol. 68, No. 9 (September 1978), p. 833–34.

67. Leatrice Hauptman-Berman. "The Political Potential (II in "NorthCare: The Life and Death of a Community-Based HMO"), *Health and Medicine*, Vol. 1, No. 2 (winter 1982) pp. 11–12.

68. "How HMO's Control Cost," *Consumer Health Action Network* (CHAN), Vol. 7, No. 6 (June/July 1982), p. 4. See also Harold Luft, "How Do Health-Maintenance Organizations Achieve Their 'Savings'?" *New England Journal of Medicine* (special article), Vol. 298, No. 24 (June 15, 1978), pp. 1336–43; "HMO's and Cost Containment: The HMO Approach Evaluated," *The California Health Facilities Commission Bulletin* (April 1983), p. 3 (Re: Kaiser-Permanente HMO).

69. Personal communications to members of the Collective.

70. Leatrice Hauptman-Berman. "The Political Potential."

71. CHAN, Vol. 7, No. 6 (June–July 1982), p. 6.

72. Michael Gelder. "Bringing It All Back Home: A Prospectus for the Illinois Health Service Authority," *Health and Medicine* (winter 1982), pp. 9–22. See also "New Reimbursement Plan for New York Hospitals," *CHAN*, Vol. 7, No. 7, p. 3.

73. See "Informed Consent" in Maryann Napoli, *Health Facts*. See also "A Guide for 'Guinea Pigs'" (The Medical Forum), *The Harvard Medical School Health Letter* (February 1983), p. 3.

74. Fred Barbash. "Supreme Court Re-Affirms 1973 Abortion Decision," *The Washington Post*, June 16, 1983.

75. Barry Chowka. "Update!" *New Age Journal* (May–June 1980), p. 16.

76. "Medical Malpractice Insurance," *Health Letter* (Santa Fe, NM), Vol. 4, No. 7 (March 1982); Gerald E. Rubacky, "Let's Not Kid Ourselves About Who Causes Malpractice Suits," *Medical Economics* (December 7, 1981), pp. 84–9; Lloyd Shearer, "On Suing the Doctor" (Intelligence Report), *Parade Magazine*, February 27, 1983, p. 11.

77. Gerald Rubacky, "Let's Not Kid Ourselves About Who Causes Malpractice Suits," p. 89.

78. Mary Chamberlain. *Old Wives' Tales: Their History, Remedies, and Spells*. London: Virago Press, Ltd., 1981, p. 139.

79. *Ibid.*, p. 11. (Contains a quote from Merlin Stone, *The Paradise Papers*, London: Virago/Quartet, 1976, p. 19.)

80. *Ibid.*, p. 13.

81. *Ibid.*, p. 29.

82. Barbara Ehrenreich and Deirdre English, *For Her Own Good*, p. 36.

83. *Ibid.*, p. 34.

84. Richard Smith. "A Fifteenth Century 'Our Bodies Ourselves,'" *British Medical Journal*, Vol. 283, No. 28 (November 1981), pp. 1452–53.

85. Mary Chamberlain, *Old Wives' Tales*, p. 3.

86. Matilda Joslyn Gage. *Woman, Church and State: The Original Exposé of Male Collaboration Against the Female Sex*. Watertown, MA: Persephone Press, 1980 (original ed. 1893), p. 104.

87. Mary Chamberlain, *Old Wives' Tales*, p. 44.

88. Jacob Sprenger and Heinrich Kramer. *Malleus Maleficarum (The Hammer of Witches)*. Germany (1484). Translated by Montague Summers. London: John Rodker, Publisher, 1928, p. 47.

89. *Ibid.*, p. 87.

90. *Ibid.*, p. 140.

91. William Perkins. *A Discourse of the Damned Art of Witchcraft*. England (1608). As quoted in Christina Hole, *Witchcraft in England*, New York: Collier Books, 1966, p. 130.

92. Barbara Ehrenreich and Deirdre English, *For Her Own Good*, p. 35.

93. Thomas Szaz. *The Manufacture of Madness: A Comparative Study of the Inquisition and the Mental Health Movement*. New York: Harper and Row Publishers, Inc., 1970; Harper Torchbooks, 1984 (paper), p. 91.

94. Barbara Ehrenreich and Deirdre English, *For Her Own Good*, pp. 31–2.

95. Mary Chamberlain, *Old Wives' Tales*, pp. 31–2.

96. *Ibid.*, p. 46.

97. John Cotta. *A Short Discoverie of the Unobserved Dangers of Severall Sorts of Ignorant and Unconsiderable Practisers of Physicken in England*. London, 1612, p. 29.

98. Mary Chamberlain, *Old Wives' Tales*, p. 79.

99. Barbara Ehrenreich and Deirdre English, *For Her Own Good*, p. 41.

100. Ann Sablosky. "The Power of the Forceps: A Study of the Development of Midwifery in the United States." Master's Thesis, Graduate School of Social Work and Social Research, Bryn Mawr College, May 1975, p. 17, quoted in Ehrenreich and English, *For Her Own Good*, pp. 96–7.

101. Neal Devitt. "The Transition from Home to Hospital," in *The Elimination of Midwifery, 1900-1935*, p. 8. Unpublished manuscript, Information Center, Boston Women's Health Book Collective; Watertown, MA.

102. Barbara Ehrenreich and Deirdre English, *For Her Own Good*, pp. 98, 191.

103. Mary Chamberlain, *Old Wives' Tales*, pp. 153–54.

104. *Ibid.*, p. 139.

105. Barbara Ehrenreich and Deirdre English, *For Her Own Good*, p. 324.

25

ORGANIZING FOR CHANGE: U.S.A.

By Judy Norsigian, with Jane Pincus

With special thanks to all the groups who sent us descriptions of their history, projects and ways of working together

This chapter in previous editions was called "Coping, Organizing, and Developing Alternatives," and written by Norma Swenson.

GETTING TOGETHER

There is no one recipe for finding others to work with. Sometimes we come together spontaneously, galvanized by a need to learn something about ourselves or to improve a situation which touches all our lives.

In the early seventies, after working in the antiwar movement, I began to talk with other women about the kind of care doctors gave us and also about our bodies, the quality of our sex lives. I'd thought I was the only one to have questions and problems about birth control and childbirth. But it turned out that many other women were concerned with the same things. Our personal discussions began in our living rooms and kitchens. They then blossomed into many kinds of health groups and projects. We all moved easily back and forth between expression of needs and ideas and political action. I felt absolutely elated that what was so important to me personally could also form the basis for political action in

Sarah Putnam

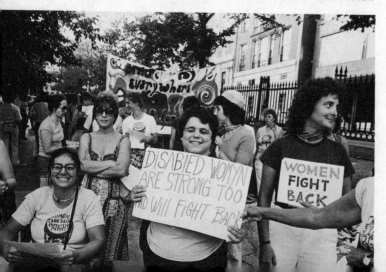

this immediate way. My work created tension in my family: I was away at meetings so often, kept making discoveries which shook up my family as well as myself. Yet my life was so much richer than before, one reason being that woven into every day were friendships which quickly became strong and deep because we touched so many dimensions of our lives through talking, working and playing together.

Why do I keep at it year after year, when progress seems so slow? I keep thinking of how much worse it might be for women in our community if our health information group weren't around. We may not always give out as much information as we would like to, or succeed as we fight for changes in public policy to improve people's health and well-being, but we are always able to raise the issues we believe everyone should be thinking about.

Knowing what I know about the injustices pervading our society, and seeing how racism and sexism ruin the lives of so many, especially women, how could I not contribute at least some of my time and energy to efforts that might change the status quo? It seems immoral not to do so. As long as I don't push myself too much, or forget about my own and my family's day-to-day needs, the work I do enriches my whole life. I love the women in my group, respect the way our collective skills keep creating new solutions to new problems, and value how we change and grow together over the years.

You can meet other women working on health issues through friends and neighbors, at your workplace, at a public meeting, or by placing an ad in a newspaper, a notice on a bulletin board. If you already belong to an organization you may want to become part of a subgroup within it, like the Women's Caucus of the

American Public Health Association, or the reproductive rights committee of a local NOW chapter. You can work from within the system as health workers or from the outside as a "consumer" pressure group seeking institutional change (e.g., a local childbirth group).

Working together with other women to keep *Manushi* alive has been a joyful experience in spite of many, many setbacks and difficulties, because the way *Manushi* is being received (both the love and hostility it provokes) fills me with the hope that, however far away, the future is ours—it belongs to women.

The most encouraging and rewarding aspect of our work is that wherever *Manushi* is reaching, it is acting as a catalyst in the emergence of new women's groups. When the news of struggles in some particular areas reaches areas where women have not yet started organizing, they seem to get the feeling, "If women in that place could do it, why can't we do it here?" And that is often the beginning of a new women's group.

Ever since *Manushi* started, I feel accountable for every minute of my life and feel every day filled with purpose. And through *Manushi*, getting to see and know the strength that is in us as women, and in myself, I feel my struggle has become more joyful.

—Madhu Kishwar of *Manushi*, an Indian women's magazine

For more on what women are doing internationally, see Chapter 26, "Developing an International Awareness."

Once your group starts to meet, your need for information and for taking effective action generates its own energy and fuels your enthusiasm. At first, women may drift in and out, but usually the group settles down to a steady number of people. After you choose a focus (or it chooses you!) and continue to work together, you'll want to ask and answer the many questions which come up about how to proceed. Here's a sampling:*

The Issue(s)

● What will be the scope of our work? What is the background of the issue?
● How many women are affected?
● What research has been done already? By whom?

*Borrowed, reordered and paraphrased from *The Rock Will Wear Away: An Organizing Handbook For Women*. We recommend that you send for this useful handbook (see Resources).

● Who and what is the opposition?
● What approaches to the problem are we considering? What is the possibility of success with these approaches?
● Are there already other organizations or individuals working on the problem?
● Will our work give women a sense of power? Will our work help inform the public and motivate it to work for more improvements in women's health? Will it tangibly improve the quality and accessibility of good health and medical care for women?

The Group

● Should we close it to new members or keep membership open? (The former increases stability and minimizes the need to keep orienting new people, while the latter allows for valuable new resources and energies.)
● How should we make decisions? By consensus? By majority vote?
● When, how often and where should we meet? (It is difficult for mothers of young children to attend dinnertime meetings; inaccessible locations may prevent women with certain physical disabilities from attending.)
● Do we want our group to have diversity in terms of race, class, age and physical ability? How can we go about achieving this?
● How much money do we need? How can we get it? What resources other than money do we need? How much can we achieve without money?
● How will we handle conflict among ourselves? Will we be able to stop discussing business when we have strong, unresolved, maybe even unvoiced feelings or personality clashes?

Some Resources and Tactics

1. *Using the media effectively*—knowing when and how to get publicity when we need it—is essential to all our efforts to bring about change, since most people get almost all their information from TV, newspapers, radio and magazines. To get the best media coverage possible it is essential to develop your *speaking skills*

National Women's Health Network activist testifying before Congress   *Robert Frazier*

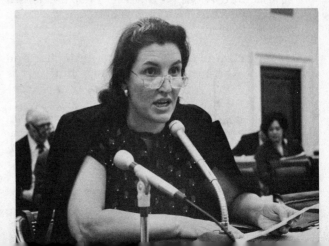

for press conferences and interviews with media people both "on" and "off" stage, *writing skills* for press releases and newspaper articles and *graphic skills* for flyers, posters and brochures.

In our group very few women had experience speaking publicly to or before the media. So we set aside some meetings to role play, to practice speaking before a group and to learn how to say the most important things in the least amount of time. We also practiced saying the things we wanted people to hear even if it was not related to the interviewer's question. Doing all this is a great way to break through shyness and stage fright.

Working with the media can have serious drawbacks. Inevitably, distortions occur, even when you are careful about what you say. You may be quoted out of context, or misquoted so badly that you seem to be saying the opposite of what you intended. When this begins to happen frequently, you may need to pull back for a while. But try again. Over time it becomes clear which reporters are most reliable, sympathetic and trustworthy.*

2. *Allies inside government agencies and health institutions* can be useful sources of information (e.g., about upcoming meetings, proposals for new technologies, studies) and can help to develop strategies for achieving specific goals. Sometimes these contacts can offer invaluable advice about how best to approach a key official. By offering assistance from the "inside," these women and men who support the women's health movement can make significant contributions.

3. *Writing letters* to legislators and key officials about specific legislation, institutional policies and regulatory proposals is an effective way to influence policy makers. Write clearly and concisely, as a group or as private individuals, and point out why your position is in the best interests of women and possibly other constituents of the official addressed.

When I heard that the Massachusetts Medical Society was actively lobbying against the bill which would allow nurse-midwives to practice in free-standing birth centers [birth centers outside of hospitals], I picked up my pen and wrote to my state senator for the first time. I got several friends to send letters and make phone calls, too. I wasn't sure it would help much, but when I saw that the Legislature overrode the Governor's veto and passed the legislation, I knew that enough of us had spoken up to make a difference.

It is important to thank officials for their efforts on your behalf. There will always be a next time!

---

*An excellent media resource is *The Media Book: Making the Media Work for Your Grassroots Group*, available for $8.50 from the Coalition for the Medical Rights of Women (see Resources).

THE WOMEN'S HEALTH MOVEMENT

There are now thousands of women in the women's health movement. Many of us began working on health issues with several other people. Some groups have remained small, while others have expanded into much larger organizations. You will find excellent models to pattern your own group after from the wide range of existing groups and organizations below.

Self-Help Groups

People have always banded together to help one another deal with everyday problems. Self-help means discussing feelings and experiences, supporting each other to learn together; finding out what we *do* know, what we do *not* know, what we *want* to know, and exploring from there; demystifying health professionals' "expertise" and our own bodies; making choices based on our own valid experience and knowledge. Through sharing knowledge, we develop certain skills which enable us to meet medical professionals halfway, and reverse the doctor-as-only-authority versus patient-who-knows-nothing roles. Self-help also stresses that the *ways* in which we learn—from one another in settings where we feel equal, comfortable and respected—are as important as *what* we learn. Finally, self-help is political in that it challenges the medical hierarchy's monopoly of information and care. It gives us more control over what we allow to be done to our bodies.

Self-help groups may be action-oriented; the possibilities are endless, depending only on our needs and creativity.

Carol Downer and Lorraine Rothman, founders of the *Feminist Women's Health Center* in Los Angeles, began one of the first gynecological self-help groups in 1971. Each woman examined her vagina and cervix with a mirror, speculum and flashlight, seeing for the first time those formerly unmentionable, mysterious parts of her own body. They learned to distinguish what was normal for each of them. On the East Coast, *Washington Women's Self-Help* holds community workshops, participates in radio programs, provides cervical caps and generally aims to give women tools for self-education. Another such group, the *Menopause Collective*, began in the late seventies when several women affiliated with a feminist health center in the Boston area started a series of discussion groups about menopause. Members of these groups, in their thirties, forties and fifties, continued working together to offer more self-help groups for community women and to research and write about menopause and other health concerns of older women. In New York City, women in the *Lesbian Illness Support Group* meet to give each other understanding and courage in the face of severe illness. This group has future plans others might like to consider.

...inviting health workers to speak to the group, a Speak-out on Lesbians and Illness, a resource listing of readings and doctors' names we have found useful, the creation of group rituals, joining class action suits against the government and taping some of the meetings to share with other groups.*

Some more suggestions:

- Focus on a specific topic such as infertility, PID, endometriosis, being teenagers, herbal remedies.
- Organize a "Know Your Body" course.
- Start a hotline for birth control and abortion information, postpartum support, help for women who are raped or beaten.
- Publish listings of the better community resources where women can go for basic well-woman care, breast cancer treatment, abortion services, infertility help, midwifery care, etc. Start a childbirth education group to provide information about both hospital and out-of-hospital birthing options.
- Work to change a local health-care facility.
- Get childcare/daycare into clinics and hospitals.
- Mobilize with other parents around issues concerning children's health—immunizations, cost of medications, street safety, violence on TV and in local films, etc.

You can also start a *health information center*. The Health Book Collective's present information center began in one room of a group member's house, and overflowed into the rest of the house as more information and women kept coming in. Books, periodicals, medical journals, newsletters, newspaper clippings piled up. People began phoning for specific health information, or to get support in their dealings with the medical profession. It was only after five years that we rented an office in the basement of a church. We acquired more filing cabinets and hired more staff to help answer phone calls, send out information, file and manage the office.

On a different scale, you can start a *women-controlled health center*. These centers offer a supportive atmosphere for such services as well-woman care and abortions. Some stress learning to do as much as you can for yourself and encourage women to learn about their bodies and health care together in groups. For example, the *New Hampshire Feminist Health Center* began in 1974 as the first free-standing clinic in New Hampshire to offer abortions. Now it provides many services, including gynecological care, women's health courses, a community outreach and education program and an excellent nationally distributed publication called *WomenWise*. These centers can be incredibly exciting places to create and to work in.

*Off Our Backs, May 1981 (see Resources).

ISIS is a *resource and documentation centre* in the international women's movement. It was set up in 1974 to collect materials from women's groups and to make these resources available to other women.

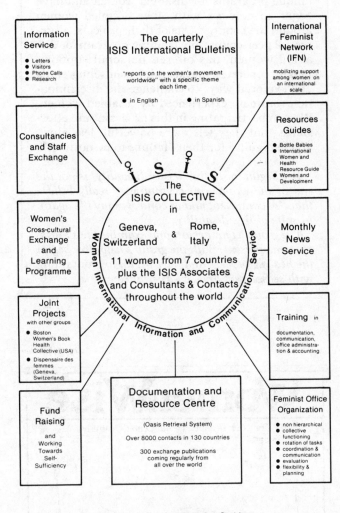

ISIS is the name of an Egyptian Goddess.

ISIS SWITZERLAND

P.O. Box 50 (Cornavin)
1211 Geneva 2 Switzerland
Tel.: 022/33 67 46

ISIS ITALY

Via S. Maria dell'Anima, 30
00186 Roma, Italy
Tel. 06/656 58 42

Still, there are many difficulties and frustrations, including conflicts between the desire to provide skilled, compassionate unhurried services to all women regardless of ability to pay and to earn adequate income to keep workers and centers going. Another conflict arises when workers want to reach and care for lots of women and are also committed to taking time for group process. In the words of the women of the New Hampshire Feminist Health Center:

The *Boston Self-Help Center* incorporated in 1977 as a community-based self-help organization. Women at BSHC have established several unique programs for disabled women and have begun to network with other disabled women around the country. One of their projects, a successful peer-counseling training program for disabled women, has offered personal support, taught concrete "marketable" counseling skills and explored ways to challenge the discrimination routinely experienced by disabled women. Women participating in this program said afterwards that they felt more powerful, less alone and less guilty for their "failure to be normal."

I've begun to see that it [my disability] is not the end of the world. I'm beginning to really believe that I'm competent and in control of my life again, in spite of this disability.

The group let me explore and examine life's hurts, past and present. With the group's help, I've begun the healing process and have begun to grow strong with self-respect and self-assurance.

Loy McWhirter

...For over two years now, we have closed our doors on Thursdays and held day-long staff meetings....Some have called it a waste of time; a more friendly critic calls it idealistic but cost-ineffective. Still, it is the way we...choose to do our work, make our decisions and run our affairs.

The New Hampshire Feminist Health Center, through its abortion rights work, cervical cap research and its leadership role in the National Women's Health Network, has become a resource for many other groups around the country. Many clinics have been picketed, harassed and invaded by antiabortion groups. These pressures also create tension. A number of health-center workers at the *Vermont Women's Health Center* in Burlington fought in the Vermont state legislature to preserve the Apprentice Physician's Assistant system* and to fight the procession of restrictive antiabortion laws which have come up these past few years.

*Being licensed as a PA after apprenticing to a physician, rather than going through a special course of studies at school.

Hope Zanes

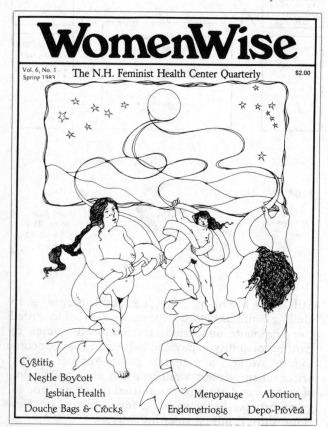

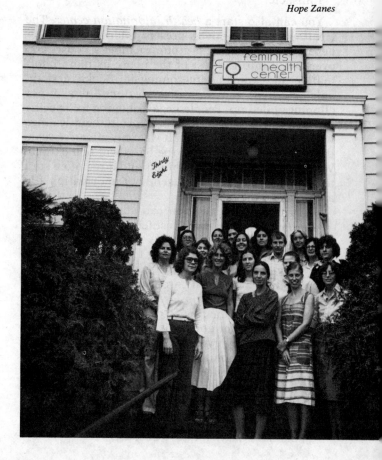

santa cruz women's health center

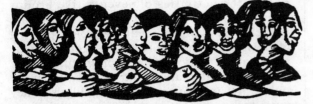

250 locust street
santa cruz, ca 95060
(408) 427-3500

Alliances and Coalitions

Some groups, after working a while on a single issue, take up other issues as well. As you learn more and meet with more women (and men), you may create or become part of *alliances*, larger networks of groups and individuals in which you exchange new infor- mation and ideas, compare different strategies for change and sometimes even organize into a larger or- ganization or movement. In the Northeast, women working in feminist health centers and health-infor- mation groups from Vermont, New Hampshire, Mas- sachusetts, Connecticut, Maine, Rhode Island, New York City and Philadelphia have been meeting to-

The beginning of 1982 marked a turning point in the *Santa Cruz Women's Health Center* (SCWHC) as the Bilingual Outreach Program was launched. Our Mobile Health Unit, a van equipped with medical and educational supplies, provides health information, counseling and referrals directly to three Latino neighborhoods in North Santa Cruz County. The Mobile Health Unit also serves as a link between Latina women and the bilingual health services offered at the SCWHC.

We consist of a multiracial group of women who designed and developed this project for the SCWHC. Our names are Rosamaria Zayas, Lucy Trujillo, Marilyn Marzell, Jody Peugh, Her- malinda Saavedre, Carmela Saavedra, Laura Giges and Martha Ways. We are mentioning our names because it is important for us to empha- size that this project has, from its beginning, been a project for Latina women, designed by Latina women, and initiated by the abovementioned multicultural group of women.

The dream was to create a bilingual outreach program that would serve the desires and needs of Latina women in our community. The goal of the program is to bring basic information about women's health care to the Latino and low-in- come community; to give women the informa- tion they need to have/take more control over their lives and the lives of their children and families.

Our process has been based on the exchange of information, knowledge and experience; we have learned an enormous amount from the women whom we are serving. We started our project by going to the four designated target areas in North Santa Cruz County as a team, literally knocking on every door and talking to women about our dream to bring a mobile health unit to the community. We met with women once a week and our question was always, "Is this service something you feel you can use?" The answer was always overwhelmingly yes; the women always encouraged us.

In addition to the outreach, other work has included translating SCWHC medical and health pamphlets and handouts and designing and pre- paring the van itself. The van is a nine-passenger Dodge van. It contains a minilab and a library, and serves as a resource center with health in- formation and community referrals. The van is staffed by one person working outside the van, talking to women and counseling, and two peo- ple inside the van doing lab work and medical charts. The mobile unit provides health educa- tion classes and counseling in nutrition, high blood pressure, anemia, pregnancy counseling, prenatal care, birth control and abortion coun- seling. It also serves as a link between the com- munity and the bilingual clinic services offered at the SCWHC.

—Rosamaria Zayas and Martha Ways
(excerpts from a letter to the MS Foundation)

gether twice yearly to discuss problems, think up solutions and connect with each other. The *Reproductive Rights National Network* (see p. 612 for its "principles") draws participants from groups nationwide.

In some cities, groups which hold widely different views come together to work on a particular local issue. These *coalitions* may form and dissolve as needed. The *Coalition for Reproductive Freedom* in Boston consisted at one point of more than thirty groups, among them lawyers', teachers', physicians' and community action groups.

In Oakland, California, a community organization called the *Coalition to Fight Infant Mortality* is working to lower the scandalously high infant mortality rates in poor and minority neighborhoods.* From 1978 to 1980, Coalition members conducted a community-based investigation of the problem of infant mortality and, in particular, the quality of care at the county's only public hospital offering obstetrical services to the low-income community. They presented their results to the entire community and finally forced the trustees of the hospital to recognize the problem officially and make certain changes, such as the addition of obstetricians who have a strong commitment to community-based health care. The Coalition also sought a midwifery service and expanded bilingual services. The community clinics also began to offer early prenatal care and the state legislature passed a bill that would help create comprehensive perinatal services. The Coalition and the community continue fighting together to demand quality services that are accessible to all regardless of ability to pay. They are strongly aware that high infant mortality rates reflect racism and discrimination against women and the poor as well as the profit orientation of the health and medical system.

Two Model Organizations

The *Coalition for the Medical Rights of Women* (not a coalition in reality), a remarkably successful project based in San Francisco, California, began as a small group concerned about the absence of state and federal laws regulating the testing and marketing of IUDs. Over the past ten years or so, the Coalition has grown into a large membership organization of both consumers and providers. One of their publications, *The Rock Will Wear Away: Handbook for Women's Health Advocates* (see Resources), offers invaluable advice to those forming new women's health groups. It describes how the Coalition itself was structured, how its main issues have been selected and how several "issue committees" have worked on specific problems. With its phenomenal growth, the Coalition is constantly looking for new ways to develop and build a structure that will allow work to be done as effectively

*There were 26.3 infant deaths per thousand live births in 1976 as compared with 3.5 per thousand in nearby, more affluent Piedmont.

Since 1977, the Northwest Coalition for Alternatives to Pesticides (NCAP) has been coordinating the activities of seventy-five groups throughout the Northwest working to decrease pesticide exposure, especially herbicide spraying of forest lands. Their work involves educating the public about pesticide effects, promoting the use of pesticide alternatives and intervening in the public processes determining pesticide use. They provide the information and strategy advice necessary for citizens to effectively challenge exposure to these toxic chemicals.

The entire staff and 70 percent of the membership are women. Women in NCAP do most of the local community organizing and intervention in government pesticide-use processes.

Women and children are most clearly affected by herbicide exposure and it is therefore women who have provided the impetus and strength for our organization. Women in NCAP are generally either rural residents or forest workers who have united through their communities' NCAP member groups in activities opposing herbicide spraying on the forest lands they live adjacent to or work in. This is a survival issue for us.*

NCAP's first efforts, following investigations of miscarriages which occured after nearby herbicide spraying, helped instigate a national emergency suspension by the EPA of dioxin-containing 2, 4, 5-T and Silvex on forest lands.

as possible without losing the feminist workstyle—hearing all viewpoints, reaching decisions by consensus—that is essential to their work. They have a small, part-time paid staff and many volunteers, do effective fund-raising and hold periodic membership meetings.

The *National Women's Health Network*, this country's only national membership organization devoted exclusively to women's health, influences health policy at the local, national and international level. Founded in 1975, its membership has grown to over 20,000, including several hundred organizations which represent a constituency of half a million people. Today the annual budget is 450,000 dollars, with five staff members at its national headquarters in Washington, D.C., and dozens of interns and volunteers. The members of the Network's board of directors come from different geographical areas, diverse racial and ethnic backgrounds and span forty years in age. Its many committees work on reproductive health; occupational and environmental health; alcohol, smoking and drugs; black women's health; breast cancer; disabled women; health planning; health law and regulations; international issues; lesbian health; midlife and older women's health; women and nutrition; rural women's health; and wholistic health care.

*The complete statement is available from NCAP, P.O. Box 375, Eugene, OR 97440.

Recent Accomplishments of the National Women's Health Network

- Testified at numerous U.S. Senate and House hearings on unsafe birth control pills and devices, drug reform laws, contraceptive research priorities, nurse-midwifery practice, treatment for DES daughters and unsafe hospital childbirth practices.
- Won, with other groups, a precedent-setting lawsuit requiring drug companies to publish patient information on the risks of menopausal estrogen drugs.
- Initiated a national campaign to locate women's health activists to become consumer representatives at FDA hearings.
- Testified at HEW's hearings on sterilization abuse and recommended safeguards to insure informed consent and bilingual patient information.
- Testified before the U.S. Senate against proposed bills that would outlaw abortion services.
- Organized the first major rural women's health conference in Appalachia in June 1981.
- Successfully pressured the federal government to spend 1.5 million dollars to study the effectiveness of the cervical cap and make it available to women nationwide.
- Brought a lawsuit in federal court challenging the Catholic Church's antiabortion political and lobbying activities.
- Filed a worldwide class-action lawsuit against the A.H. Robins company on behalf of all women damaged or potentially damaged by the Dalkon Shield IUD.
- Testified at FDA hearings against approval of Depo-Provera for contraceptive use in the U.S. and also filed a class-action suit against Upjohn Co. on behalf of women damaged by this drug.

Joining the Network is an important way women and men can support the goals of the Women's Health Movement. For more information write to the National Women's Health Network, 224 Seventh Street SE, Washington, DC 20003.

RESOURCES

Books

Annas, George. *The Rights of Doctors, Nurses and Allied Health Professions: A Health Law Primer*. New York: Avon Books, 1981. Another in the ACLU series on civil liberties, this one clarifies why the rights of medical personnel to refuse to administer treatment ultimately limit our rights to medical care. A useful companion to *The Rights of Hospital Patients*, also one of the ACLU series.

———. *The Rights of Hospital Patients: The Basic Guide to a Hospital Patient's Rights*. New York: Avon Books, 1974.

Ashley, Joan. *Hospitals, Paternalism, and the Role of the Nurse*. New York: Teacher's College Press, 1976.

Banta, David H., Clyde J. Behney and Jane Sisk Willems. *Toward Rational Technology in Medicine*. New York: Springer Publishing Co., Inc. (Springer Series on Health Care and Society, Volume 5). The best single source documenting the lack of evaluation of medical care, with precise analyses and recommendations.

Barker-Benfield, G.J. *Horrors of the Half-Known Life: Male Attitudes Toward Women and Sexuality in 19th Century America*. New York: Harper and Row Publishers, Inc., 1976; Harper Colophon (paper), 1978. A fascinating rendering of the mood of the nineteenth century around sexuality, sexism and the rise of gynecology; important to an understanding of today's women's health issues.

Bunker, John P., M.D., Benjamin A. Barnes and Frederick Mosteller, Ph.D. *Costs, Risks and Benefits of Surgery*. New York: Oxford University Press, 1977.

Burack, Richard, M.D., with Fred Fox, M.D. *The New Handbook of Prescription Drugs*, rev. ed. New York: Ballantine Books, Inc., 1976.

Campbell, Margaret. *Why Would a Girl Go into Medicine?* The Feminist Press, Box 334, Old Westbury, NY 11568, 1974. A detailed study by a former Harvard dean of the systematic discrimination against women by U.S. medical educators during the rapid rise of women medical school candidates following the WEAL suit (see p. 569). A classic primer on the mechanisms of prejudice, whatever its object. *Still highly relevant to women medical students in the 1980s.*

Chamberlain, Mary. *Old Wives' Tales: Their History, Remedies, and Spells*. London: Virago Press, Ltd., Ely House, 37 Dover Street, London WIX 4HS, England, 1981. Paper. Available in the U.S. from Merrimack, 458 Boston Street, Topsfield, MA 01983. Part I is an excellent historical and political analysis of the suppression of women healers, from the English perspective, also relevant to the U.S. and the West generally. Part II assembles direct quotes of ancient remedies.

Conrad, Peter, and Rochelle Kern. *The Sociology of Health and Illness: Critical Perspectives*. New York: St. Martin's

Ellen Shub

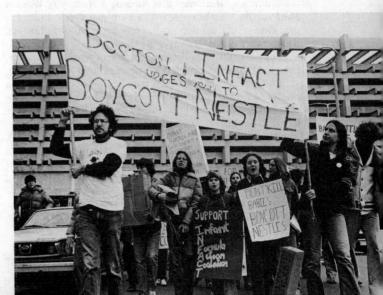

Press, 1981. Paper. An outstanding collection of classic articles by a variety of writers critical of medicine. Provides analysis and documentation of many of the issues which concern the women's health movement today. (New edition forthcoming in 1984.)

————, and Joseph W. Schneider. *Deviance and Medicalization: From Badness to Sickness*. St. Louis: C.V. Mosby Co., 1980. Paper. Traces sickness as sin to sickness as disease, showing medicine's role in defining social values.

Cook, Stephani. *Second Life*. New York: Simon and Schuster, 1981. One woman's personal account of her condescending and dangerous treatment by doctors during diagnosis and treatment of a life-threatening illness.

Corea, Gena. *The Hidden Malpractice: How American Medicine Mistreats Women*. New York: William Morrow and Co., Inc., 1977; Jove/HBJ (paper), 1978. Rev. ed. Harper and Row Publishers, Inc., 1985. Remains the most stunning investigative journalism extant on American medicine's shameful history toward women.

Dreifus, Claudia, ed. *Seizing Our Bodies*. New York: Vintage Books, 1978. A useful selection of classic articles on women's health issues from the early days of the women's health movement.

Dubos, René. *Mirage of Health: Utopias, Progress, and Biological Change*. New York: Harper and Row Publishers, Inc., 1979. Paper. A readable classic, basic for demystification of health, disease, science and medicine.

Ehrenreich, Barbara, and John Ehrenreich. *The American Health Empire: Power, Profits, and Politics*. A Health/PAC book. New York: Random House/Vintage, 1971. Paper. A classic radical account of medicine's transition from a cottage industry dominated by independent entrepreneurs and their guild to a sophisticated empire dominated by specialty medicine and its academic centers—at the expense of patient care and good health.

————, and Deirdre English. *Complaints and Disorders: The Sexual Politics of Sickness*. Old Westbury, NY: The Feminist Press, 1974. Paper. A vivid portrait of nineteenth century class struggle, and the role of medicine and women in it.

————. *For Her Own Good: 150 Years of the Experts' Advice to Women*. New York: Doubleday/Anchor Books, 1978. Paper. No other book makes modern women's manipulation by succeeding generations of male experts appear so credible, or so devastating. Exposes the unscientific basis of "scientific" expertise used to control women; indispensible for an understanding of how women's role has become defined in modern industrial society.

————. *Witches, Midwives, and Nurses: A History of Women Healers*. Old Westbury, NY: The Feminist Press, 1972. Paper. One of the classics of the second wave of feminism, this powerful booklet explains the medieval witch-burnings of the Church as the suppression of female sexuality, female organizing and female healing, in a move to consolidate patriarchal power. A parallel history of American medicine's outlawing of women healers following the popular health movement concludes the work.

Ehrenreich, John, ed. *The Cultural Crisis of Modern Medicine*. Monthly Review Press, 62 W. 14th Street, New York, NY 10011, 1978. The general framework questions medicine's role as exclusively derivative of economic and political structures, and argues that it also has a strong shaping influence on a broad range of fundamental values and human experiences, at least in the West.

Gage, Matilda Joslyn. *Woman, Church and State*. Watertown, MA: Persephone Press, 1980 (original printing 1893). A remarkable account of systematic oppression of women by Christian church teachings (including Judaic influences) through the centuries. By one of the major feminists of the nineteenth century.

Gordon, Linda. *Woman's Body, Woman's Right—A Social History of Birth Control in America*. New York: Penguin Books; Middlesex, England: Penguin Books, 1977. Traces the history and development of the birth control movement in the U.S., covering political, social and economic aspects. An excellent feminist analysis.

Graedon, J. *The People's Pharmacy*. New York: St. Martin's Press, Inc., 1976. Still one of the best practical guides.

Harrison, Michelle. *A Woman in Residence*. New York: Random House, Inc., 1982. A gripping account by a seasoned woman physician of her specialty training in ob/gyn at a major Ivy League teaching hospital; shows clearly how the quality of patient care is undermined by training priorities.

Holmes, Helen B., Betty B. Hoskins and Michael Gross, eds. *Birth Control and Controlling Birth: Women-Centered Perspectives* (Vol. I); *The Custom-Made Child: Women-Centered Perspectives* (Vol. II). Based on the proceedings of Ethical Issues in Human Reproductive Technology: Analysis by Women, June 1980. Clifton, NJ: Humana Press, Inc., 1980. A series of reflections and discussions by women about the use and abuse of technology by powerful forces in our society which intend to control and manipulate human reproduction. Much important detail not available elsewhere.

Hornstein, Francie, and Judith Waxman, eds. *Birthrights: An Advocate's Guide to Ending Infant Mortality*. Los Angeles: National Health Law Program, 1983.

Hubbard, Ruth, Mary Sue Henefin and Barbara Fried, eds. *Women Looking at Biology Looking at Women*. Cambridge, MA: Schenkman Publishing Co., 1979. Valuable reflections on the contributions of biology and social sciences to the denigration of women, and refutations of the "scientific" basis for it. An extremely important work. Also, by the same authors, *Biological Woman: The Convenient Myth*, Cambridge, MA: Schenkman Publishing Co., 1983.

Huff, Barbara B., ed. *Physicians' Desk Reference*. Oradell, NJ: Medical Economics. The industry-sponsored guide to drugs, on which most doctors depend for information. Published annually.

Illich, Ivan. *Medical Nemesis: The Expropriation of Health*. New York: Pantheon Books, 1976; Bantam Books (paper), 1977. A rich and provocative analysis of iatrogenesis (medically-induced illness) on many levels.

Kaufman, Joel, et al. *Over the Counter Pills that Don't Work*. New York: Pantheon Books, 1983.

Kotelchuk, David. *Prognosis Negative: Crisis in the Health Care System*. A Health/PAC book. New York: Random House/Vintage, 1976. Paper. A useful selection of articles from *Health/PAC Bulletin* and other sources which give a radical critique of many aspects of the medical care system.

Law, Sylvia. *Blue Cross: What Went Wrong?* New Haven: Yale University Press, 1974. Comprehensive documentation of the domination of Blue Cross by physician and hospital interests.

Lear, Martha Weinman. *Heartsounds*. New York: Simon and Schuster, 1980; Pocket Books (paper). A powerful and readable book about a doctor's heart disease and death under sophisticated medical care, written by his journalist wife. Extremely valuable criticisms and insights for anyone using the system, especially in preparation for major crises in our lives or the lives of those close to us.

Long, James W. *The Essential Guide to Prescription Drugs*, 2nd rev. ed. New York: Harper and Row Publishers, Inc., 1980. Over 200 of the most commonly prescribed drugs are profiled. Contains such information as year introduced, drug action, symptoms that should be reported to the doctor, side effects, adverse effects, storage instructions, and foods or other drugs to avoid while on medication.

Millman, Marcia. *The Unkindest Cut: Life in the Backrooms of Medicine*. New York: William Morrow and Co., Inc., 1977. Paper. An eyewitness study of doctors' handling of errors, and each other, when "peer review" is instituted.

Moore, Emily C. *Woman and Health: United States 1980*. Washington, DC: U.S. Government Printing Office, 1980. Paper. (A supplement to the September–October 1980 issue of *Public Health Reports*, a publication of the U.S. Public Health Service, Office of the Assistant Secretary for Health and Surgeon General.) A report of women's major health issues, with mortality and morbidity, reproductive health and other concerns presented via data and discussion through 1980. Prepared for the U.S. delegation at the Women's Conference, Copenhagen, 1980. Good bibliography.

Napoli, Maryann. *Health Facts: A Critical Evaluation of the Major Problems, Treatments and Alternatives Facing Medical Consumers*. Woodstock, NY: Overlook Press, 1982. A compilation from materials assembled under the direction of the Center for Medical Consumers and Health Care Information in New York; this is an excellent critical survey.

Newland, Kathleen. *Infant Mortality and the Health of Societies* (Worldwatch Paper #47). Washington, DC: Worldwatch Institute, 1981. Paper. Analysis of the factors affecting infant mortality in different countries, showing unmistakably that outcome is not necessarily the result of expenditures on conventional medical care, and that the education of the mother is the single most important variable which predicts that outcome.

The President's Commission for the Study of Ethical Problems in Medicine and Biomedical and Behavioral Research. *Protecting Human Subjects: The Adequacy and Uniformity of Federal Rules and Their Implementation*. GPO #040-000-00452-1, December 1981. Write to Superintendent of Documents, U.S. Government Printing Office, Washington, DC 20402.

Ruzek, Sheryl. *The Women's Health Movement: Feminist Alternatives to Medical Control*. New York: Praeger Publishers, 1978. A fine feminist study of self-help and its role in changing fundamental attitudes toward medical care. Detailed history, case examples. A useful text.

Sarath, Maria, Melissa Auerbach and Ted Bogue. *Medical Records: Getting Yours, a Consumer's Guide to Obtaining Your Medical Records*, 2nd ed. Published by and available from the Health Research Group (see "Groups"). $2.50 plus 50¢ postage.

Scully, Diana. Men Who Control Women's Health: *The Miseducation of Obstetrician-Gynecologists*. Boston: Houghton Mifflin, 1980. This three-year study of ob/gyn training at two leading U.S. hospitals is outstanding; it shows how all aspects of training ultimately prepare surgeons to manipulate women to accept surgery, and control by doctors during childbirth. A good section on policy change proposals.

Seaman, Barbara. *The Doctors' Case Against the Pill*, rev. ed. New York: Doubleday and Co., Inc., 1980. Paper. Classic background to the Pill cover-up.

———, and Gideon Seaman. *Women and the Crisis in Sex Hormones*. New York: Rawson Associates Publishers, 1977; Bantam Books (paper), 1978. A detailed account of the development of major birth control methods and their hazards and side effects, including information about recovery. Important information about the industry/FDA relations. A basic tool.

Sidel, Victor W., and Ruth Sidel. *A Healthy State: An International Perspective on the Crisis in United States Medical Care*. New York: Pantheon Books, 1977. Systematic comparisons between the U.S. and Sweden, Great Britain, the U.S.S.R. and the People's Republic of China, with suggestions for U.S. changes based on a national health service model emphasizing primary care, as advocated by many feminists.

Walsh, Mary Roth. *Doctors Wanted—No Women Need Apply: Sexual Barriers in the Medical Profession 1835–1975*. New Haven: Yale University Press, 1977. An excellent history of U.S. women doctors and why feminism is essential to their survival, now as then.

Wertz, Dorothy, and Richard Wertz. *Lying-In: A History of Childbirth in America*. New York: Free Press, 1977. The most comprehensive history of the takeover of childbirth by male-dominated technology and medicine from women and midwives, ranging from European roots to modern times.

Wolfe, Sidney M., Christopher M. Coley and the Health Research Group. *Pills that Don't Work: A Consumer's and Doctor's Guide to Six Hundred Prescription Drugs that Lack Evidence of Effectiveness*. New York: Warner Books, Inc., 1982.

Articles

Bell, Susan. "Political Gynecology: Gynecological Imperialism and the Politics of Self-Help," *Science for the People* (September/October 1979). 897 Main Street, Cambridge, MA 02139. Single issue $1.00. The article focuses on the experiences of a group of feminists involved in a program to teach pelvic examinations to medical students. Raises important questions about instituting change in the medical system, working for short-range reforms versus long-term radical change, and the problem of cooptation.

Concerned Rush Students. "A Critical Look at the Drug Industry: How Profit Distorts Medicine." *Science for the People*, 897 Main Street, Cambridge, MA 02139, 1977. $2.50. This excellent paper by U.S. medical students documents the powerful influence of the most profitable industry in the U.S. on the institution and the practice of Western medicine. Described in detail are the mechanisms which consolidate that power—gifts and "help" to students, direct professional affiliation with organized medicine, aggressive advertising and marketing practices beamed at all physicians and the increasing development of pharmaceutical "answers" to all of life's problems. The report shows how the drive for profits ultimately leads to the undermining of responsible research and the evasion of safeguards in the laws of some countries through multinational expansion and production.

Hamilton, Sharon. "More Notes on Restructuring," Emma Goldman Clinic for Women *Newsletter*, No. 2, 1978. 715

N. Dodge Street, Iowa City, IA 52240. $1.00. "There have always been problems with collective structures... inefficiency, lack of direction for many, lack of productivity, little accountability, burnouts, and sometimes chaos." This brief article describes one group's efforts to solve some of these problems (through more job specialization, fewer committee meetings, etc.), creating a more workable collective structure and process.

Lipnack, Jessica. "The Women's Health Movement," *New Age Journal* (March 1980). 32 Station Street, Brookline, MA 02146. Single issue $1.50. An excellent and thorough review of major aspects of the U.S. women's health movement, including historical background, relationship to the wholistic health movement (nonconventional approaches to healing originating *outside* the mainstream of the women's health movement) and a good reading list.

Smith, Beverly. "Black Women's Health: Notes for a Course" in *But Some of Us Are Brave*, Hull, Scott and Smith, eds. New York: The Feminist Press, 1982.

Weaver, Jerry, and Sharon D. Garrett. "Sexism and Racism in the American Health Care Industry: A Comparative Analysis," *International Journal of Health Services*, Vol. 8, No. 4 (1978), pp. 589–617. A clear, detailed analysis of how and where discrimination is applied, including 127 references. Also in Elizabeth Fee, *Women and Health: The Politics of Sex in Medicine*, Farmingdale, NY: Baywood Publishing Co., 1983, pp. 79–104.

Periodicals

The APRS Federal Monitor, Box 6358, Alexandria, VA 22306. $10.00 yearly (minimum of 8 issues). A newsalert providing updates on legislative and regulatory activities relating to the health of women and children.

Coal Mining Women's Support Team News, Coal Employment Project, Box 3403, Oak Ridge, TN 37830. Monthly; often covers health and safety issues of special concern to women.

The Harvard Medical School Letter, Boston, MA 02115. An establishment review and update of current issues in medical practice, sometimes progressive.

Health Facts. (See New York City under "Health Information Centers for Consumers," below.) Regular, clear, in-depth, referenced discussion of key issues for consumers. Excellent.

Health and Medicine, 220 S. State Street, Suite 300, Chicago, IL 60604. A new, outstanding presentation of the important policy questions and practical strategies of current developments in health.

Health Newsletter, 1127 University Avenue, Madison, WI 53715. A helpful collection of short articles and items with both local and national focus, many on women.

Healthsharing, Women Healthsharing, Box 230, Station M, Toronto, Ontario M6S 4T3, Canada. A quarterly newsletter covering a wide range of women's health concerns.

The Medical Letter on Drugs and Therapeutics, Medical Library Association, 56 Harrison Street, New Rochelle, NY 10801. The single best independent source of professional drug evaluation.

Medical Self-Care, P.O. Box 717, Inverness, CA 94937. Each issue on a special theme, with many articles and resources. See No. 12, "Women's Health," for a lively introduction. Ask for the catalogue of medical items.

Off Our Backs, 1841 Columbia Road NW, Room 212, Washington, DC 20009. Probably the best feminist newspaper, with excellent regular coverage of women's health issues.

Science for the People, 897 Main Street, Cambridge, MA 02139. An excellent bimonthly offering analyses of the politics of science. Frequently examines women's health issues.

The Tufts [University School of Nutrition] Diet and Nutrition Letter, P.O. Box 2464, Boulder, CO 80321. This new publication will hopefully carry up-to-date research reports.

Women in Medicine Newsletter, Women in Medicine Task Force, American Medical Student Association, 14650 Lee Road, Box 131, Chantilly, VA 22021.

Womenwise. (See New Hampshire Feminist Health Center under "Organizations for Change," below.) An excellent quarterly.

Special Publications

Children in Hospitals 1982 Consumer Directory, CIH, 31 Wilshire Park, Needham, MA 02192. $2.00. Surveys Massachusetts hospital policies in pediatric, maternity and adult care. A model for similar efforts to monitor and change institutions.

Double Indemnity: The Poverty and Mythology of Affirmative Action in the Health Professional Schools, 2 parts by Hal Strelnick, M.D., and Richard Younge, M.D. From Health/PAC. (See "Groups," below.) A magnificently documented detailed presentation of why and how minorities and women are kept down. Very useful.

How Safe is Safe? by Doris Haire. Available from National Women's Health Network. (See "Groups," below.) A special report on how the FDA determines drug safety, and what consumers need to know to protect themselves. A guide to state laws, regulations. $1.00 postpaid.

Science for the People. (See "Groups.") Special Issue. *Science and the Attack on Women*. 1981.

Self-Help: Resource Guide No. 7, National Women's Health Network. The guide includes philosophy, practical self-examination instructions and critical history and politics. Menstrual extraction is described in detail, and its politics are thoroughly discussed. Companion material on population control is also included. Illustrated, with bibliography and resources.

Audiovisual Materials

Code Gray: Ethical Dilemmas in Nursing, a 28-minute 16-mm. 1983 color film. Available from Fanlight Productions, 47 Halifax Street, Jamaica Plain, MA 02130. Documents situations where nurses confront ethical dilemmas as decision-makers in their daily practice. Good for stimulating discussion.

Healthcaring from Our End of the Speculum, a 35-minute color film available from Women Make Movies, 257 W. 19th Street, New York, NY 10011. A good introductory film covering many different women's health concerns.

Nursing: The Politics of Caring, a 22-minute 16-mm. 1978 color film. Available from Fanlight Productions, 47 Halifax Street, Jamaica Plain, MA 02130. A documentary about the struggles of nurses to increase their voice in the system, especially as advocates of patients. Explores attitudes of nurses toward their work.

La Operación, a 40-minute 16-mm. color film. Order from La Operación, P.O. Box 735, Chelsea Station, New York,

NY 10011, (212) 864-6564. Rental (sliding scale, $35 to $100) or sale. A powerful documentary about sterilization abuse, particularly among Puerto Rican women.

Taking Our Bodies Back: The Women's Health Movement, a 33-minute 1973 color film. Available from Cambridge Documentary Films, Box 385, Cambridge, MA 02139. A classic general film on women's health.

Turning Around: A Humorous Look at Sexism in Medicine, an 18-minute 1983 color film and video. Based on actual experiences of health professionals, students and patients, but the sex roles have been reversed. For rental information contact Maureen Longworth, M.D., P.O. Box 881532, San Francisco, CA 94188-1532.

Health Information Centers for Consumers

Boston (Watertown): Boston Women's Health Book Collective, 465 Mt. Auburn Street, Watertown, MA 02172, (617) 924-0271. Publishes *Nuestros Cuerpos, Nuestras Vidas* and pamphlets on menstruation and STDs. Distributes "Our Jobs, Our Health" (an expansion of Chapter 7, "Environmental and Occupational Health," in this book).

New York City: Center for Medical Consumers and Health Care Information, 237 Thompson Street, New York, NY 10012, (212) 674-7105. Publishes *Health Facts*. (See "Books" and "Periodicals.")

Salt Lake City: Consumer Health Information Center, 680 E. 600 South, Salt Lake City, UT 84102, (801) 364-9318.

San Francisco: The Plane Tree Health Resource Center, 2040 Webster Street, San Francisco, CA 94115, (415) 346-4636.

Groups

Black Women's Health Project
Martin Luther King Community Center, Suite 157
450 Auburn Avenue NE
Atlanta, GA 30312
(404) 659-3854

Boston Self-Help Center
18 Williston Road
Brookline, MA 02146
See p. 602. A counseling, consulting and disability rights organization staffed by and for people with disabilities.

CARASA (Coalition for Abortion Rights and Against Sterilization Abuse)
17 Murray Street, 5th floor
New York, NY 10007
Publishes *CARASA News*.

Cassandra: Radical Feminist Nurses Network
P.O. Box 341
Williamsville, NY 14221-0341
A women's group in which radical feminist nurses share ideas, support and encouragement three times yearly with diverse offerings.

Center for Science in the Public Interest
1757 S Street NW
Washington, DC 20009
(202) 332-9110

Excellent resources, including posters on food and nutrition. Publishes *Nutrition Action*.

Coalition to Fight Infant Mortality
Box 10436
Oakland, CA 94610
(415) 655-2068
See p. 604.

Coalition for the Medical Rights of Women
2845 24th Street
San Francisco, CA 94110
(415) 826-4401
A health advocacy and information resource. Publishes a monthly newsletter, *Second Opinion*, *The Rock Will Wear Away*, *The Media Book* and other publications. Send for their list.

Concern for Dying
250 W. 57th Street
New York, NY 10107
(212) 246-6962
An educational council which provides information and advice for consumers and professionals concerned with dying. Concern has developed a model patient-oriented "living will" act.

DSA Nurses' Caucus, Democratic Socialists of America
P.O. Box 59422
Chicago, IL 60659
(312) 871-7700
Publishes *DSA Caucus Newsletter*. A national group in which activist nurses can link up, discuss nursing issues and provide nursing input into the DSA organization.

Feminist Women's Health Center
6411 Hollywood Boulevard
Los Angeles, CA 90028
(213) 469-4844
A resource for self-help and women-controlled health care.

Gay Nurses' Alliance
44 St. Mark's Place
New York, NY 10003
An active group working for both gay rights and health issues; provides educational resources.

Health/PAC (Health Policy Advisory Center)
17 Murray Street
New York, NY 10007
(212) 267-8890
Analyses and study of health issues from a radical perspective; produces a variety of publications, including the periodical *Health/PAC Bulletin*.

Health Research Group
2000 P Street NW
Washington, DC 20036
(202) 872-0320
Ralph Nader–affiliated research and advocacy group; publishes consumer-oriented books and manuals on drugs, medical devices, occupational and environmental health, health insurance and benefits programs and related topics; testifies in Congress and works with the media to alert the public.

Institute for the Study of Medical Ethics
   P.O. Box 17307
   Los Angeles, CA 90017
   (213) 413-4997
   An active patients' rights group offering advocacy, documentation and research; active in monitoring legislation.

International Childbirth Education Association (ICEA)
   Box 20048
   Minneapolis, MN 55420
   (612) 854-8660
   Offers extensive annotated lists of publications and audiovisual resources; their monthly newsletter covers a wide range of childbirth issues. (See Unit IV, "Childbearing.")

Montreal Health Press
   Box 1000, Station G
   Montreal, Quebec H2W 2N1, Canada
   (514) 272-5441
   Publishes *A Book About Birth Control*, *A Book About Sexually Transmitted Diseases*, *A Book About Sexual Assault* and poster kits on female and male reproduction, birth control methods and abortion. Updated materials, 1979–1980. English and French. Booklets 50¢ each. Send for information on poster kits and bulk orders.

National Black Nurses' Association, Inc.
   P.O. Box 18358
   Boston, MA 02118
   (617) 266-9703
   Membership over 1,000. Influences legislation and policies affecting black people; conducts, analyzes and publishes research about health needs of blacks; maintains a national directory of black nurses; assists the media in the dissemination of information about black nurses; helps black nurses write and publish.

National Health Law Program
   2639 S. La Cienega Boulevard
   Los Angeles, CA 90034
   (213) 204-6010
   Health backup center for the Legal Services Corporation; publishes *Health Advocate* newsletter; covers many issues of concern to women.

National Women's Health Network
   224 7th Street SE
   Washington, DC 20003
   (202) 543-9222
   A national consumer/provider membership organization; monitors and works to influence government and industry policies. Publishes *Network News*.

New Hampshire Feminist Health Center
   38 S. Main Street
   Concord, NH 03301
   (603) 225-2739
   Publishes a periodical, *Womenwise*, which covers a wide variety of topics on women and health.

Northwest Coalition for Alternatives to Pesticides (NCAP)
   P.O. Box 375
   Eugene, OR 97440
   (503) 344-5044
   See p. 604.

Nurses' Network
   c/o Health/PAC
   17 Murray Street
   New York, NY 10007
   (212) 267-8890
   Holds monthly meetings, publishes quarterly newsletter to discuss wages, working conditions, etc.

Reproductive Rights National Network (R₂N₂)
   17 Murray Street
   New York, NY 10007
   (212) 267-8891
   Publishes *Reproductive Rights Newsletter*.

Santa Cruz Women's Health Collective
   250 Locust Street
   Santa Cruz, CA 95060
   See p. 603. Publishes an excellent monthly newsletter and other publications (list available).

Society for the Right to Die
   250 West 57th Street
   New York, NY 10107
   (212) 246-6973
   Works through educational, judicial and legislative action for recognition of the right to die with dignity. Publishes a yearly handbook listing "living will" acts in effect throughout the country.

Taller Salud
   Apdo. 2172
   Hato Rey
   PR 00919
   A self-help and health activist collective in Puerto Rico.

Washington Women's Self-Help
   P.O. Box 1604
   Washington, DC 20013
   (202) 462-3224
   See p. 600. Distributes information packets on the cervical cap and on home remedies.

Women's Dance Health Project
   P.O. Box 8958
   Minneapolis, MN 55408
   By and for Native American women. Offers a range of educational, counseling, advocacy and training programs with self-help and family-centered emphasis. One of the project founders has written a women's health book for native American women which can be ordered directly from her:
   Katsi Cook, P.O. Box 230
   Rooseveltown, NY 13683

Women's Rights Project
   Center for Law and Social Policy
   1751 N Street NW
   Washington, DC 20036
   (202) 872-0670
   General resource on women's rights law.

26

DEVELOPING AN INTERNATIONAL AWARENESS

By Vilunya Diskin

With special thanks to Norma Swenson, Judy Norsigian, Anita Anand, Asoka Bandarage, Elizabeth Coit, Jane Cottingham, Marilee Karl, Una MacLean, and Annie Street

As feminists, we feel a strong bond with all women. We value the solidarity that comes when women in different countries meet, listen and exchange experiences with one another. We believe that feminism as a political perspective must look across national boundaries to address all the issues which affect women's lives.

All of us have been systematically denied access to crucial information about our bodies, bodies which are similar whether we inhabit them in the U.S., Africa, Asia, Australia, Latin America or Europe. We all have fundamental needs for water, food and shelter.

Denial of reproductive rights, domestic violence, rape, sexual harassment in the workplace or on the street, racism, sexism, repression of lesbians, occupational hazards, economic exploitation and the horrors of war—none of these respect national boundaries. From a rural women's health and education group in South India:

When we read about women like us, rural, poor, from other parts of the world, we begin to feel women are similarly placed all over the world. The cultural contexts may differ, but the exploitation of women is the same everywhere.[1]

Women in the U.S. lack information from and about women throughout the world; women in industrialized countries know little about Third World women. There are few communication channels for useful and honest dialogue. An Asian woman observed: "American and European feminists, by being uninformed about their sisters in other countries, contribute unwittingly to their exploitation."[2] Living and voting in the most affluent and industrialized country, we have to take responsibility for the ways this country's policies affect the lives of women elsewhere. For example, if we succeed in removing dangerous contraceptives or other consumer products here, manufacturers may dump them on unsuspecting Third World women, as was the case with the Dalkon Shield and the high-estrogen pills. Our activism must include organizing with women of other countries to prevent such abuses.

Opening our eyes to common issues and being aware and respectful of our different realities, women around the world can better understand and help one another.

SEXISM

Sexism, or discrimination on the basis of sex, is a universal problem. There are differences in the varying forms and degrees, but all patriarchal societies (those dominated by men and organized around their activities and goals) circumscribe girls' and women's basic rights and opportunities. They thereby lose the benefit of our skills, talents and energies.

Women around the world face the imperative to bear

Oxfam, America

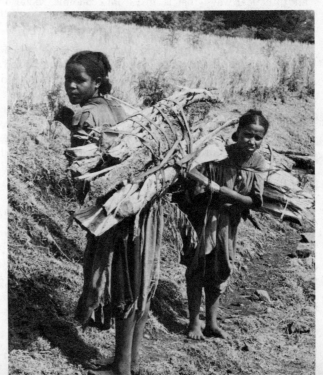

611

and rear children and to take primary responsibility for the home. Cultures value us as reproducers, homemakers and consumers but rarely as workers and producers. This "invisibility" is absurd, considering that women's participation worldwide in the agricultural labor force is between 40 and 50 percent.[3] Women produce 44 percent of the world's food; prepare, process and store food; and are integral to local distribution systems. Wherever water must be carried, young girls and women do it. In many cultures, women also have important roles as traders of foodstuffs.

REPRODUCTION: WOMAN/ COMMUNITY-CONTROLLED REPRODUCTIVE RIGHTS

Control of our bodies is a core feminist issue. Whether it is forced sterilization in Puerto Rico or denial of sterilization in France, "family planning" centers in India or restricted availability of abortion in the U.S., wife-battering, sexual slavery, "crimes of passion"— the result is the same: women are not free to control our own bodies. Patriarchal domination begins here. In the words of an Indian woman:

We are brought up to view our bodies with suspicion and contempt, and this gives us a poor self-image. We are taught to consider our very existence as women as a misfortune; we never understood the way our bodies functioned and always feared or were ashamed of natural happenings like menstruation, pregnancy, childbirth.

A healthy attitude towards our bodies would help us develop our self-respect, and such self-awareness is the first step towards playing an active role in our communities, to change the unjust structures of which we are a part.[4]

When we say women must have reproductive freedom, we mean the possibility of controlling for ourselves, in a real and practical way—that is, free from economic, social or legal coercion—whether and under what conditions we will have children.[5]

Women all over the world increasingly see reproductive-rights issues as central to self-determination. London's International Contraception, Abortion and Sterilization Campaign (ICASC) grew out of women's struggles for the right to control our fertility. Since the forces manipulating women's reproduction are many and powerful—governments, multinational corporations, churches, the medical establishment and antiabortion organizations—we need an international campaign to counteract them effectively.

Many people see overpopulation as the world's priority issue, believing that it causes mass starvation, social disruption, violence and poverty. On the contrary, we believe that it is not overpopulation but the inequitable distribution of the world's resources that has led to a cycle of poverty and misery for many of the world's peoples. The U.S. consumes one-third of the world's resources to support only 6 percent of the world's population. While large populations can put a strain on natural resources, so can high-consumption lifestyles.

Birth control and population control are *not* the same. It is every woman's right to control her fertility through birth control information and services. Population control is a program imposed to lower a country's birth rate with no regard for cultural, social and economic factors which make many families both desire numbers of children and be unwilling or unable to use contraceptives. Those who advocate population control fail to address basic questions about the just distribution of resources. Private and governmental development agencies in the U.S. have already spent millions on population control projects, going so far as to require developing countries receiving economic assistance from the U.S. Agency for International Development (AID) to institute a population policy program.[6] The population control establishment, in its typically Western desire for speedy solutions to complex problems, moves away from human and woman-scale control. It pushes dangerous and invasive drugs and techniques, like Depo-Provera, silastic implants and sterilization rather than safer methods, like the diaphragm, cap, condom or fertility observation, which take more time and money to teach people to use effectively. In one country, family-planning workers go into overcrowded state hospitals and tell women in labor that they can stay there for three days instead of the usual twenty-four hours if they consent to sterilization after the birth. In another country, only the benefits of sterilization are advertised.

In cases where contraceptives are packaged, messages on sterilization can be inserted or printed inside. People who are already spacing or limiting births with a temporary method may be more easily convinced to accept sterilization when constantly exposed to its benefits. The ultimate aim is to print sterilization messages on all mass distribution consumer products and containers.[7]

Population controllers have not considered women's needs. For instance, population funds from the U.S. to programs abroad increased from 10.5 million in 1965 to 140 million in 1977, while funds for maternal and child health decreased.[8] Agencies do not consult users in the disbursement of these funds, and hire too few women to design, implement or evaluate the programs. Women would more likely advise that the monies be spent for health education, especially in reproduction and sexuality, and to train traditional birth attendants (*dais*) who serve 90 percent of the women in developing countries as midwives and health agents in rural communities.

We must ask many questions about birth control programs overseas: Who controls the program being offered? Who funds it, and what strings are attached? Who distributes the contraceptives, and what kind?

What kind of information and instructions are offered? Most important, how much and what kinds of birth control do people really want?

Access to safe abortion is another major problem. We deplore the carnage that results from illegal abortions (still, next to childbirth, the world's major cause of maternal mortality) due to the unavailability of safe, legal procedures. Even where abortions are legal, as in India and Italy, we know from women's groups that the situation can still be dangerous and unfair. In India, few women are aware that abortion is legal, fewer still have access, and those who do get to a facility receive deplorable treatment. In Italy and Greece many doctors refuse to perform abortions in hospitals on grounds of conscience, but manage to overcome their scruples if a woman pays a large sum as a private patient. In the U.S. Medicaid cuts for abortion mean that many minority and poor women must end up being sterilized when that isn't what they really want.

EXPORTING MISGUIDED PRIORITIES

Development

The word "development" usually means modernization. Here we talk about development as the conscious exportation of the process of modernization according to a Western model. Development theory is based on the history of Western industrialization, and assumes that Third World countries could and would choose to follow the same path of economic growth. "Development experts," mostly Western males, study poverty, low productivity and unemployment as "problems of underdevelopment." They conceptualize programs to alleviate these "problems" after talking only with male spokesmen in the countries involved. They then try to get individual governments or international/ multinational agencies like the United Nations or the World Bank (to which they often belong) to fund these programs either with low-interest loans or free assistance. The end products of such aid are often extremely high levels of debt for "developing" nations and dependency on foreign goods and money.

Women worldwide criticize this kind of development policy, which largely ignores both their traditional role as major food producer and the devastating effects of the policy itself on women and children. Since the Western model assumes that only men work in agriculture, these programs usually give land titles only to men, thus denying women access to their traditional family-subsistence plots.

In Africa, for instance, women have the main responsibility to feed their children (i.e., grow, harvest and cook the food), pay school fees and purchase clothes and supplies. How can they accomplish these things when their land is taken away from them? The health of the community also declines, because subsistence crops (women's domain) are the stuff people eat, while cash crops (men's domain) are grown to be sold. Men control the money made from cash crops and are not as likely as women to spend it on food or on the family.

Also, development programs usually offer extension programs and training only to men, thereby denying women opportunities for learning new skills. When women are included, their workload is often increased, as for example in the high-yield grains which require more hours of weeding and harvesting. Planners find it hard to grasp that women need paid work. An Indian woman writes:

> There is a prevailing myth that women live like parasites off the earnings of their husbands, but we found the reverse to be true. The women who came to Saheli [a women's resource center in Delhi, India] were women who had worked before and after marriage—they earned their own living and had often built assets (i.e., dowry) for their new homes—yet when the marriage broke up, they usually lost all these assets.[9]

Western and Third World academic and development experts of the "women and development school" push Western-style development in the name of women's liberation. However, "development theory" will never adequately benefit women if it does not address the question of patriarchy.

> Society's acceptance of male-domination pervades development work. Though much lip-service is paid to the equal participation of women in the male-dominated development circles, there is little thought or real effort toward genuine power sharing with women.[10]

We need a new theory of development which both acknowledges women's central role in production and challenges the economic and political systems which oppress women. More women in every country must be involved in designing and implementing flexible programs to meet women's needs and to reflect their productive roles both inside and outside the home.

Multinational Corporations

The multinational corporations (MNCs) we are discussing here are those which have branches in different countries but retain concentration of capital and authority in the industrialized West. Even though they are often women's only source of paid employment, they have a primarily negative effect on Third World women's lives.

The MNCs force women to compete with one another. For example, women in the U.S. buy products produced by the toil of Third World women under sweatshop conditions. Whenever women (in South Korea, for example) begin to organize for better wages and working conditions, industries pick up and move to another community. U.S. women face unemployment because U.S. industries relocate to the Third World.

Textiles, electronics and agribusiness are three industries which locate in developing countries because of tax incentives and the promise of cheap and docile labor. Women perform 80 to 90 percent of low-skilled assembly jobs. The MNCs pay low wages for long hours in unhealthy working conditions and then claim they are "liberating" women by giving them work.

In the Philippines...starting wages in U.S.-owned electronics plants are between $36-$46 a month, compared to a cost of living of $37 a month; in Indonesia the starting wages are actually about $7 a month less than the cost of living. "Living" is interpreted minimally: a diet of rice, dried fish, and water (a Coke might cost a half-day's wages), lodging in a room occupied by four or more people.[11]

Female workers worldwide earn 40 to 60 percent less than their male counterparts. Single women enlist for these new jobs often at the insistence of their families, who desperately need their earnings. Their move to urban areas means an upheaval—they lose their kin and community networks and in return receive no wage protection, work benefits, priority or seniority. They are the most exploited section of the formal labor force.

Health hazards abound in MNC workplaces. In the electronics industry, one of the safest and cleanest of the exporting industries, toxic chemicals and solvents sit in open containers filling the air with powerful fumes. An AFSC (American Friends Service Committee) worker in Northern Mexico heard about cases where ten or twelve women passed out at once. The newspapers reported this as "mass hysteria." In Malaysia, mass hysteria has become a form of resistance. One young woman sees a *hantu* or *jin* (hideous varieties of ghosts) and falls screaming to the floor in convulsions, and within minutes the hysteria spreads up and down the assembly line. Sometimes the plant has to close for a week or more to exorcise the spirits. Malaysian academics point out that the attacks are likely to be preceded by a speedup or a tightening of plant discipline.[12]

The stress of peering through a microscope at tiny wires for seven to nine hours at a time, straining to meet quotas at a pay rate of two dollars per day, could make anyone hysterical. Electronics workers often lose the twenty/twenty vision required for the job. One study in South Korea found severe eye problems in electronics assembly workers; after only one year of employment, 88 percent had chronic conjunctivitis, 44 percent had become nearsighted and 19 percent had developed astigmatism. In one stage of the electronic assembly process, workers have to dip the circuits into open vats of acid. In Penang, Malaysia, women wear gloves and boots to do dipping, but when these leak, burns are common, and the workers sometimes lose fingers in painful accidents.[13]

Textile and garment industry conditions rival those of any nineteenth or twentieth century Western sweatshop. Workers are packed into poorly lit rooms where summer temperatures rise above a hundred degrees; textile dust, which can cause permanent lung damage, fills the air; rush orders require forced overtime of as much as forty-eight hours at a stretch, with the management supplying pep pills and amphetamine injections as needed. In her diary, published in a magazine now banned by the government, a thirty-year-old South Korean sewing-machine operator describes conditions in the garment factory where she works from seven A.M. to eleven-thirty P.M.

When apprentices shake the waste threads from the clothes, the whole room fills with dust, and it is hard to breathe. Since we've been working in such dusty air, there have been increasing numbers of people getting tuberculosis, bronchitis, and eye diseases....

It seems to me that no one knows our blood dissolves into the threads and seams, with sighs and sorrow.[14]

Stress is probably the most invidious health hazard. Visits to the bathroom are a privilege; in some cases, workers must raise their hands for permission and wait up to half an hour. Working days one week and then nights the next wreaks havoc with sleeping patterns. Stomachaches and nervous problems reflect internalized anxieties and pressures of meeting production quotas. Management actually encourages a high turnover rate in many industries; because wages rise with seniority, it is cheaper to train a new batch of teenagers than to pay for an experienced "older" (i.e., twenty-three- or twenty-four-year-old) woman.

The MNCs say they are contributing to development, but they come into a country for one thing—cheap labor—and when the labor stops being so cheap, they move on. What kind of development is it that depends on people staying poor? Saralee Hamilton, an AFSC staff organizer of a 1978 conference on "Women and Global Corporations,"* says:

The multinational corporations have deliberately targeted women for exploitation. If feminism is going to mean anything to women all over the world, it's going to have to find new ways to resist corporate power internationally.[15]

Infant Formula

After the postwar baby boom (when birth rates declined in the West), infant formula companies looked to the relatively untouched Third World markets. Con-

*Women's Network on Global Corporations, an outgrowth of the 1978 conference, is an independent clearinghouse for technical assistance and information on women's roles as workers, consumers and transmitters of culture in agribusiness, electronics and textile industries. The Network aims to assist grassroots organizing and to alert international development groups about the influence of multinationals on women and development. See also the monthly newsletter of the Pacific Studies Center for the Global Electronics Information Project (865 W. Dana, #204, Mountain View, CA 94101). $5 for subscriptions.

vinced by aggressive and often unethical advertising practices that a bottle-fed baby will be healthier and more likely to survive than a breastfed baby,* millions of Third World mothers stopped breastfeeding, but were unable to maintain the sanitary conditions for mixing and storing the formula, and often couldn't afford to purchase it in sufficient quantities. The result has been ten million cases of severe malnutrition each year and approximately three million infant deaths.[16]

The infant formula industry promotes sexism, convincing women who have borne healthy babies that their bodies cannot keep the babies healthy and that they need an expert, often a male doctor, to tell them what to do.

Citizens around the world have organized a major campaign to stop these unethical practices. The Infant Formula Action Coalition (INFACT) and International Baby Food Action Network (IBFAN) began a boycott against Nestlé, a Swiss company, which is the world's largest multinational food corporation and generates almost half of all infant formula sales in the developing world.[17] This, the largest U.S. nonunion boycott in history, involved over 300 national groups and forty-one countries. The demands: an end to direct consumer advertising; an end to promotion through and to members of the health care professions; an end to company "milk nurses"; and an end to free samples.

The boycott has had an economic impact.† In 1978 the Norwegian Dairy Sales Association canceled its exclusive contract with Nestlé for the distribution of Jarlsberg cheese; when Notre Dame in the U.S. became a "Nestlé-free campus," the food service stopped using 40,000 dollars per week of Nestlé products. The greatest success of the boycott has been the consumer education impact, which has brought the whole issue to the international governmental-agency level for serious debate and action. As a result, the World Health Organization (WHO) developed an "International Infant Formula Code of Marketing Behavior" for the industry. When the World Health Assembly voted on the code in May 1980, every country voted in favor of it except the U.S., whose representatives stated that it infringed upon the free enterprise system.

It's not enough just to get rid of infant formula. Breastfeeding is not always easy or possible, because

*Infant formula manufacturers use a large repertoire of promotion tactics, including billboards and posters showing healthy children next to company products. They send sales personnel dressed in nurses' uniforms to offer mothers advice on infant feeding and give them free samples. Taking advantage of the medicalization of childbirth, they vigorously promote their products to and through health care providers, especially in hospitals.

†The Nestlé boycott ended in early 1984, but the work of investigating other corporations involved in marketing breast-milk substitutes and commercial products for children in developing countries continues. U.S. corporations, in particular, will be under pressure to conform to the terms agreed on by Nestlé, and monitoring of all corporations' compliance will be stepped up.

many women have to work full time outside the home and many have tremendous family responsibilities. Women's fight is not only against a technological culture which says it's better to bottle-feed, but also for alternatives—increased maternity leave with pay, workplaces where breastfeeding is part of the schedule and acceptance of the fact that women have a right to make choices in these matters. As a Senegalese woman puts it:

It's not enough to talk about the natural superiority of breast milk and the advantages to both the mother and infant. We have to create the conditions to make it possible for women to do this. Yes to breastfeeding, but...how?[18]

Drugs—Not Merely a Local Matter: The Impact of the U.S. Drug Industry on Third World Women

Dominated by some of the most powerful and profitable multinational corporations in the world, the pharmaceutical industry is now in a period of rapid international expansion.* By 1980 in the U.S., patents for most of the 200 largest-selling drugs had expired. Having exploited the domestic market thoroughly, U.S. firms are now looking more aggressively to developing countries for new consumers—most especially women.† The U.S. government is eager to encourage export of drugs as a means of improving the balance of international payments. Weak restrictions in under-developed countries mean that these companies can promote their products with impunity. This is not good news for Third World women. Furthermore, efforts to find safe drugs for women in the U.S. often involve testing on poor and Third World women. The birth control pill was first tested on women (usually poor and illiterate) in Puerto Rico and later in El Salvador, sometimes without their knowledge and with severe consequences to their health.

Pharmaceutical companies develop drugs for "rich country" diseases, like heart complaints, depression, insomnia and cancer, but do little research into the tropical diseases affecting approximately a billion people in the Third World.[20] They dump drugs which regulations or consumer complaints make unmarketable in the U.S. Sending a multitude of representatives to the Third World, they sometimes spend more on promotion and advertising than Third World countries spend on health budgets. They promote many drugs which are ineffective and others for the wrong diseases, in which case their use may be hazardous. They provide inadequate information on negative effects and contraindications, even to the professionals who will dispense the drugs.

*From 1.2 billion dollars in 1965 to 4.5 billion dollars in 1976.[19] The U.S. accounts for one-fifth of this trade, Western Europe controlling the rest.

†Third World women are increasingly the targets for psychoactive drugs in particular.

Women health activists and consumer coalition groups are getting together to work against these abuses. Health Action International (HAI) was established in Geneva in May 1981 to coordinate activities and share ideas and resources internationally among consumers and development and public interest groups, as well as to provide the framework for international campaigns. HAI has set up an international clearinghouse for information on the drug industry's structure, ownership and marketing practices, and has established an international consumer product warning network, "The Consumer Interpol." They must be doing something right, because they have the pharmaceuticals worried. The July 17, 1981, *Food and Drug Letter* (Washington Business Information, Inc.) talks about a "group of activists—fresh from their work against infant formula industry marketing practices—[which] has set its sights on [the issue of] selling drugs to consumers in the Third World Nations."[21] The *Letter* is worried that HAI will conduct a media campaign against multinational drug firms along the lines of the Nestlé boycott. But most worrisome for the industry is the possibility that HAI may influence WHO (The World Health Organization) to adopt a regulatory drug code similar to the one on infant formula marketing. The International Federation of Pharmaceutical Manufacturers' Associations (IFPMA) has developed a provisional, voluntary "Code of Pharmaceutical Marketing Practice" in an effort to head off the mounting criticism and avoid regulation. The IFPMA Code is vague, incomplete and difficult to interpret or monitor. It makes no references to gifts or samples, the content of advertising, methods of production or product liability. Also, the requirements are so broad it is safe to assume nothing is likely to change.

Western Medicine Vs. Indigenous Systems

We export Western medicine all over the world, under the guise of sharing "expertise" (the so-called "transfer of technology"). A tragic result is the devaluation and persecution of indigenous health systems. For example, U.S.-assisted health care planning in newly independent India (in 1948) assumed a need for increased

Unknown

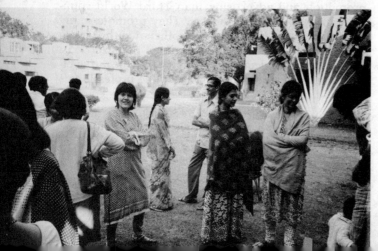

Western medical science and technology, in spite of the historical existence and availability of the traditional Indian system of Ayurveda (use of herbs) and yoga. Ayurvedic medicine, through its wholistic approach, provides effective prevention for a range of health problems untouched by Western medicine. Ayurveda, like many traditional systems, is decentralized, giving individuals more control over their own health, a crucial factor in a country like India where 85 percent of the people live in rural areas.[22] Rural people are most often in need of simple, preventive services. Infectious diseases are still prevalent; public health measures like clean water, sanitation and a proper diet could prevent much more ill health than new machines, drugs and factories ever will.

Women all over the world suffer when governments accept physicians' monopoly over the direction of health policy. Two centuries ago, the medical establishment in the industrialized world began to ostracize and persecute women healers, the midwives and abortionists who had always served poor and rural women. "Development" often means a similar shift in the Third World. Since most women live in rural areas, most countries need to keep health in the hands of community health providers, traditional healers and village health workers and to use doctors as auxiliaries or consultants, the role they should have in any case, based on their narrow, highly technical training.

Tourism

Tourism is an increasingly important source of income in the Third World, in some cases the third or fourth largest source of foreign currency. A strong incentive for tourism is the availability of women in these countries either explicitly as prostitutes or disguised as hospitality girls, massage and bath attendants, performers in sex shows, hostesses and waitresses in clubs. Closely related to the sex-tourism industry is the "rest and relaxation" business which has grown up around many permanent U.S. military bases in Asia. The sex-tourism and R-and-R industries exploit the vast majority of their employees both sexually and economically. Women enter this type of employment out of economic necessity and because there are often no alternatives for them.

In Thailand, the gap in incomes and opportunities between the city and countryside is enormous, setting the way for rural–urban migration. For women from poor rural backgrounds, migration provides an earning power which is simply astounding compared to normal rural budgets. Two or three years' working as a masseuse/prostitute enables a [woman's] family to build a house of size and quality few people in the countryside could hope to achieve with the earnings of a lifetime. Many families, indeed entire villages, have raised their standard of living through the bodies of their daughters.[23]

Most of the money generated by sex tourism goes to tourist agencies, hotels, club owners, tour operators, *(text cont. on p. 618)*

616

Female Circumcision

As part of traditional cultural practices, between 20 and 74 million African females (and an unknown number in Indonesia and Malaysia)—mostly young girls—undergo some form of genital removal every year. The mildest form of reduction is *circumcision*, which involves cutting off the hood (prepuce) of the clitoris. This is often called *sunna*, or traditional circumcision. The next level of removal is *excision*, or *clitoridectomy*, which involves cutting off part or all of the clitoris and part or all of the labia minora. Even more extreme is *infibulation* (Pharaonic circumcision), in which part or all of the middle section of the labia majora is also cut off. The two sides of the vulva are then pinned together with acacia thorns or stitched together with catgut or silk sutures, leaving a small opening for menstrual blood and urine. While not as common, infibulation is still widely practiced in Africa.

The health and medical consequences can be serious: tetanus from unsterilized tools; chronic vaginal and/or urinary infections; very painful menstruation; cysts as large as grapefruits; scar tissue which interferes with sexual arousal and/or response; pain during intercourse; urinary incontinence; and totally obstructed birth, which can result in the death of mother and/or baby. Many now advocate that the procedure be done in a hospital to reduce some of the risks involved; in some places this is already happening.

The infibulated woman is usually reopened before the wedding night by a traditional midwife or in a clinic. In some cases, her husband opens her through repeated attempts at penetration over several days, often with the aid of a sharp instrument to gain access. In communities where women are sewn up again after the birth of every child (to make them "tight" again), women may go through these processes many times.

Circumcision is deeply embedded in a way of life. It is often regarded as a basic part of growing up and is viewed by many adult women with special pride as a unique proof of their womanhood. Usually it is performed because people believe it is proof of virginity and thus will insure marriageability. It is extremely difficult to convince many women and men that this maiming, life-threatening practice ought to stop. People have it done mainly because it was done to them or because they believe their daughters will have no secure future in their community without it.

Those who seek an end to this practice call it "genital mutilation." African protesters now include a small but growing number of women and men, including physicians and public health personnel. Many Western women, including those in our Collective, have also spoken out against this practice, but as the Association of African Women for Research and Development (AAWORD) has cautioned:*

Fighting against genital mutilation without placing it in the context of ignorance, obscurantism, exploitation, poverty, etc....without questioning the structures and social relations which perpetuate this situation, is like "refusing to see the sun in the middle of the day." This, however, is precisely the approach taken by many Westerners, and is highly suspect, especially since Westerners necessarily profit from the exploitation of the peoples and women of Africa, whether directly or indirectly.

Feminists from developed countries must accept that it is a problem for *African women*, and that no change is possible without the conscious participation of African women. They must avoid ill-timed interference, maternalism, ethnocentrism and misuse of power. These are attitudes which can only widen the gap between the Western feminist movement and that of the Third World.

African women must stop being reserved and shake themselves out of their political lethargy. They must make themselves heard on all national and international problems, defining their priorities and their special role in the context of social and national demands.

On the question of traditional practices like genital mutilation, African women must no longer equivocate or react only to Western interference. They must speak out in favour of the total eradiction of all these practices, and they must lead information and education campaigns to this end within their own countries and on a continental level.†

Those working to eradicate genital mutilation deserve international support. All of us can begin by educating ourselves. In the United States, we can write to U.S. AID (Agency for International Development) and ask that any assistance programs concerning family planning or health include, when relevant, specific efforts to disseminate information about the medical consequences of circumcision and infibulation.

---

*AAWORD, whose aim is to carry out research which leads to the liberation of African people, and women in particular, *firmly condemns* genital mutilation and all other practices—traditional or modern—which oppress women and justify exploiting them economically or socially, as a serious violation of the fundamental rights of women.

†AAWORD/AFARD, November 1979.

pimps and other organizers of the business. Tourist agencies and airlines in industrialized countries reap huge profits. Because they see it as an important source of income, some governments condone or encourage sex tourism outright: some officials even exhort their women to prostitution as a form of great patriotism! The most blatant examples are in the Philippines, South Korea and Thailand. Some 700,000 women work in Bangkok's massage parlors, teahouses, nightclubs, brothels and disco-restaurants. From a Dutch travel agency's promotional material:

...Thailand is a world full of extremes and possibilities are unlimited. Anything goes in this exotic country, especially when it comes to girls....However, it may be a problem for visitors to Thailand to find the right places where they can indulge in unknown pleasures. It is frustrating to have to ask the hotel receptionist in broken English where you can pick up pretty girls. Rosie has done something about this. For the first time, you can book a trip to Thailand with erotic pleasures included in the price....[24]

Dutch men board charter flights from Amsterdam to Bangkok where they can buy a woman for twenty-five guilders a night (twelve and a half dollars), a hundred guilders a week. The "girls," on the other hand, earn about eighty guilders a month when they can find work. The fact that 70 percent of the women suffer from sexually transmitted diseases does not serve as a deterrent, and the airplane home has been nicknamed the "gonorrhea express."[25]

Japanese businessmen often fly on one-night *Kisaeng* (i.e., sex) tours to South Korea. The following appeared in a Japanese magazine:

There are only two types of people who don't sleep with South Korean women: those with no money and those with something wrong with a certain part of their body.

A young Japanese male asked this magazine:

"I've heard that you can do absolutely anything you want with South Korean women. Is this true? If I travel, I'd like to taste women to the full, so I'd like to know a little more about South Korean "service."

The magazine answered:

No, it is not an exaggeration to say that South Korea fully deserves its reputation as a "Male Paradise." These special tours cost a little more, but you can still buy a woman for only 75 dollars. In addition, these Korean girls are young, between 18 and 25, and very ripe. If you want our advice, get going to the "Male paradise," South Korea.[26]

Prostitution in the Philippines has always flourished where there is a heavy concentration of foreigners, for example, in the row of "clubs" adjacent to the U.S. military bases in Angeles City (Clark Air Force Base) and Olongapo (Subic Bay Naval Base). About 6,500 American military and civilian personnel come to Olongapo every day for R and R. Average monthly earnings for an Olangapo hostess is between 500 and 600 pesos (seventy to eighty-four dollars). Some girls

(text cont. on p. 620)

Sisterhood Is Powerful; International Sisterhood Is Even More Powerful

The decades of the seventies and eighties can be called the decades of women's organizing. Here are just a *few* examples of what women have been doing to link internationally over the past decade.

1974   ISIS began as a resource and documentation center in the international women's movement. It makes materials from local women's groups available to women all over the world and publishes a quarterly bulletin and several guides.

1975   Designated by the United Nations as International Women's Year. The official conference took place in Mexico; there was an unofficial parallel conference, called the Tribunal, to which NGOs (non-governmental organizations) and women's groups sent delegates.

1976 to 1985   U.N. International Women's Decade. Countries were instructed to look at their national priorities in development and to include women.

1976   International Tribunal of Crimes Against Women, Brussels. Out of this conference the International Feminist Network (IFN) was established. The IFN, coordinated by ISIS, is a communication channel through which women in one country can ask those in others for help—for instance, in the form of telegrams and letters expressing solidarity with an action they are taking.

1977   First International Women and Health Meeting, Rome.

1977   As part of International Women's Decade, there was a National Women's Conference in Houston, Texas, which 20,000 women attended. A delegation from the International Wages for Housework Campaign was represented by the following categories of women: white, Catholic, Protestant, Jewish, Latin-American, Ukranian, Anglo-Saxon, Irish, Italian, Polish, German, Lithuanian, Austrian, Russian, Roumanian, African-American, West Indian and Native American. Together these women—from all races and regions, lesbians, married and single, prostitutes—won passage of the Women, Welfare, and Poverty Resolution, which prompted Sarah Weddington, President Carter's special assistant on Women's Affairs, to state publicly that "the central

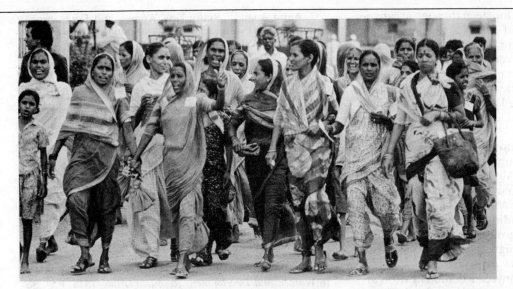

Striking domestic workers of Poona

Navrose Contractor

issue for women is economic, and the nub is paying housewives!" The battle over welfare at Houston represented more money for the *majority* of women vs. token positions for a few professionals. As Wilmette Brown, of Black Women for Wages for Housework (U.S.), stated, "Our fight for money of our own is not so we can join the *man* sitting on top of the world. Our victory is an open invitation to share the wealth."[29]

1979   Feminist Conference, Bangkok. Third World women participants decided to embrace the term "feminism," despite its distorted media image. They recognized an "indigenous feminism" which was comprised in part of Third World women questioning the whole concept of "development" and asking whether women *wanted* integration into this process, no matter how "equally." These women defined feminism in terms of two long-term goals: first, the achievement of women's equality, dignity and freedom of choice through power to control our bodies and lives, inside and outside the home; second, the removal of all forms of inequity and oppression through the creation of a more just social and economic order, nationally and internationally.

1980   International Feminist Workshop to follow up on the Bangkok Conference, Stony Point, New York.

1980   Mid-Decade U.N. Conference on Women, Copenhagen. There was also an NGO Forum, a parallel conference which 8,000 women attended. The theme was "Development, Equality, and Peace."

1980   Second International Health Meeting, Hanover, Germany.

1981   Third International Health Meeting, Geneva, organized by ISIS and Dispensaire des Femmes. Five hundred women, working in self-help in thirty-five countries, convened to exchange knowledge, experiences and ideas. As ISIS explained, "These women represent an international movement responding to the need of women to reappropriate knowledge about health in order to gain direct control over their own lives."

1981   First Latin American/Caribbean Feminist Meeting, Bogota, Colombia.

1982   National New Zealand Women's Health Conference.

One more conference is scheduled to end the International Women's Decade in 1985 in Nairobi, Kenya. Undoubtedly, there will be reports and speeches about the "great strides" governments have made in insuring women a role in national priorities and goals. It will be up to women to monitor and evaluate how real this "progress" is in women's lives and to demand their rightful places in the political processes of their respective countries. The International Women's Decade has served primarily to make all of us more deeply aware of the vast extent of women's *exclusion* from the political process on every continent. A challenge for the next decade is to maintain this new awareness of the need for change and full involvement for women, as well as to push for the implementation of the gains we have so painstakingly won.

start work at age thirteen or fourteen through arrangement with club owners and managers, and women work until their late forties or fifties, or as long as the owners will allow it. Upon retirement, most have no savings or social security benefits, and end up as poor and exploitable as when they began. Analysts have predicted that as long as the U.S. naval base remains, the profitable and powerful existing R and R trade will remain.[27]

Women's and church groups in Asia have begun to protest these activities, many seeking international solidarity. The Third World Movement Against the Exploitation of Women, headquartered in the Philippines with groups in all Southeast Asian countries, has been active on this issue. Responding to appeals by South Korean women, women's groups in Japan have organized information campaigns and actions against the Japanese tourist agencies involved.

South Korean women organized a demonstration at the airport where the Kisaeng airplanes land. They carried placards in Japanese saying: "We will throw you beyond the sea, Japanese sex monsters!"[28]

"TO TALK FEMINISM IS NEVER TO TALK NONSENSE"*

International women's organizations, such as ISIS, IFN, and ICASC, along with the hundreds of local groups in every region on every continent,[30] point to feminist efforts in organizing a strong women's international presence. We must nurture and expand these groups so that women may truly learn about the lives of their sisters by exchanging information, experiences and hopes. The numerous feminist magazines further these goals. *Broadsheet* (New Zealand), *Manushi* (India), *Spare Rib* (England), *Courage* (Germany), *La Revuelta* (Mexico), and *Off Our Backs* (U.S.) are just a few of our important "spokeswomen." This kind of exchange can help diminish some of the barriers of region, race, class and fear that now divide us, and can strengthen the similarities we share. As the Korean garment worker quoted on p. 614 wrote in her diary, "We all have the same hard life. We are bound together by one string."[31] And, from a woman in India:

We will be able to derive strength for all our efforts if all women stand united, convinced of our worth, and angry at our oppression.[32]

*Donna Awatere, a Maori woman, New Zealand.

NOTES

1. T. K. Sundari. "Women's Camp," July 30–August 3, 1981, p. 35. From: Rural Women's Social Education Centre and Rural Development Society, 15/1. Peria Melamaiyur, Chingleput 603 002, Tamilnadu, S. India.

2. ISIS International Bulletin #3, April 1977, p. 3.

3. Anita Anand. "Rethinking Women and Development: The Case for Feminism," In *Women and Development Resource Guide*, ISIS, P.O. Box 50, 1211 Geneva 2, Switzerland, 1983, p. 7.

4. Sundari. "Women's Camp," p. 33.

5. *International Women and Health Resource Guide*. Boston: BWHBC and ISIS, 1980, p. 51. Available for $5 from BWHBC, 465 Mt. Auburn Street, Watertown MA 02172.

6. Bonnie Mass. *Population Target*, Latin American Working Group and The Women's Press, Toronto, 1977, pp. 45–51.

7. Mechai Viravaidya. "My Pigeon Flies High: Some Innovative Approaches to Promoting Voluntary Sterilization," in *Voluntary Sterilization: A Decade of Achievement*, M. Schima and I. Lubell, eds., International Project of the Association for Voluntary Sterilization, 1980.

8. *WIN NEWS*, Vol. 5, No. 1 (Winter 1979).

9. *Saheli*. Indian Women's Resource Center, 10 Mazamudeen East, New Delhi 110013, India.

10. Anita Anand. "Rethinking Women and Development," in *Women and Development Resource Guide*, ISIS, P.O. Box 50, 1211 Geneva 2, Switzerland, p. 6.

11. Barbara Ehrenreich and Annette Fuentes. "Life on the Global Assembly Line," *Ms.* magazine, January 1981, p. 55.

12. *Ibid.*, p. 55.

13. *Ibid.*, p. 56.

14. *Ibid.*, p. 57.

15. *Ibid.*, p. 60.

16. Fred Clarkson. "Growing Nestle Boycott Haunts Infant Formula Makers," *WIN Magazine*, March 1, 1981, p. 12.

17. Sally Austen Tom. "Hazards of Infant Formula," in *Heresies*, Vol. 4, No. 1, Issue 13 (1981), p. 74.

18. Marie-Angelique Savané. "Yes to breast feeding, but…how?" *Assignment Children*, UNICEF 49/50 (Spring 1980), p. 82.

19. Michael Bader. "Hustling Drugs to the Third World," *The Progressive*, December 1979, p. 42.

20. "Women and Health," Part 1, *ISIS International Bulletin* #7, Spring 1978, p. 5.

21. *The Food and Drug Letter*, an independent biweekly from Washington Business Information, Inc., 235 National Press Building, Washington, DC 20045, July 17, 1981, p. 1.

22. J. Bandyopadhyay and V. Shiva. "Alternatives for India, Western or Indigenous Science," in *Science for the People*, Vol. 13, No. 2 (March/April 1981), pp. 22–28.

23. Pasuk Phongpaichit. "Bangkok Masseuses: Holding Up the Family Sky," in "Tourism: Selling Southeast Asia," *Southeast Asia Chronicle*, Issue 78 (April 1981), p. 23.

24. "Tourism and Prostitution," *ISIS International Bulletin* #13, November 1979, p. 9.

25. *Ibid.*, p. 9.

26. *Ibid.*, p. 22.

27. *Ibid.*, p. 20.

28. *Ibid.*, p. 8.

29. Prescod-Roberts and Steele. *Black Women: Bringing It All Back Home*. London: Falling Wall Press, 1980, pp. 43–44.

30. Details on many women's international health groups can be found in the *International Women and Health Resource Guide*, July 1980. Available for $5 from BWHBC, 465 Mt. Auburn Street, Watertown, MA 02172.

31. B. Ehrenreich and A. Fuentes. "Life on the Global Assembly Line," *Ms.* magazine, January 1981, p. 60.

32. Sundari. "Women's Camp." p. 36.

RESOURCES

Books

Arditti, Rita, et al, eds. *Science and Liberation*. Boston, MA: South End Press, 1980.

Atiya, Nayra. *Khul Khaal: Five Egyptian Women Tell Their Stories*. Syracuse, NY: Syracuse University Press, 1982.

Banks, J.A., and Olive Banks. *Feminism and Family Planning in Victorian England*. New York: Schocken Books, 1977.

Barry, Kathleen. *Female Sexual Slavery*. New York: Avon Books, 1981.

Bhagat, Mukarram. *Aspects of the Drug Industry in India*. Centre for Education and Documentation, 3, Suleman Chambers, 4 Battery Street, Bombay 400 039, India, February 1982.

Boserup, Ester. *Woman's Role in Economic Development*. New York: St. Martin's Press, 1970.

Boston Women's Health Book Collective. *Nuestros Cuerpos, Nuestras Vidas* (Spanish-language edition of *Our Bodies, Ourselves*). Published by and available from the Collective (see address below).

——. *Our Bodies, Ourselves*. Over fourteen foreign-language editions. Write to the Collective (see address below).

—— and ISIS. *International Women and Health Resource Guide*. Order from BWHBC, 465 Mt. Auburn Street, Watertown, MA 02172, $5.00.

Boulding, Elise. *Women in the Twentieth Century World*. Halstead Press, 1977. Explores differences between women in the industrialized world and the Third World.

Chen, Martha Alter. *The Quiet Revolution: Women in Transition in Rural Bangladesh*. Lexington, MA: Schenkman Publishing Co., 1983.

Dixon, Ruth B. *Rural Women at Work*. Baltimore: Johns Hopkins University Press, 1978.

El Saadawi, Nawal. *The Hidden Face of Eve*. Boston: Beacon Press, 1980.

Hayter, Teresa. *Aid as Imperialism*. New York: Penguin Books, 1974. An early work exploring aid to developing countries by a World Bank analyst.

Heller, Tom. *Poor Health, Rich Profits: Multinational Drug Companies and the Third World*. Spokesman Books, Bertrand Russell Peace Foundation, Ltd., Bertrand Russell House, Gamble Street, Nottingham, England, 1977.

Hosken, Fran P. *The Hosken Report: Genital and Sexual Mutilation of Females*. WIN News, 187 Grant Street, Lexington, MA 02173, 1979.

——. *Universal Childbirth Picture Book*. WIN News (see address above).

Huston, Perdita. *Third World Women Speak Out*. New York: Praeger Publishers, 1979.

ISIS. *Women in Development: A Resource Guide for Organization and Action*, 1983. Order from ISIS C.P. 50 (Cornavin), 1211 Geneva 2, Switzerland. $12.00. A good feminist source with excellent, detailed resource sections.

Jordan, Brigitte. *Birth in Four Cultures*. Montreal: Eden Press, 1978.

Latin American and Caribbean Women's Collective. *Slaves of Slaves: The Challenge of Latin American Women*. Zed Press, 57 Caledonian Road, London N1 9DN, 1980.

Leghorn, Lisa, and Katherine Parker. *Women's Worth; Sexual Economics and The World of Women*. Boston and London: Routledge and Kegan Paul, 1981.

—— and Mary Roodkowsky. *Who Really Starves? Women and World Hunger*. New York: Friendship Press, 1977.

Mamdani, Mahmood. *The Myth of Population Control: Family, Caste and Class in an Indian Village*. New York and London: Monthly Review Press, 1972.

Mass, Bonnie. *Population Target: The Political Economy of Population Control in Latin America*. Toronto: Women's Press, 1976.

Medawar, Charles. *Insult or Injury: An Inquiry into the Marketing and Advertising of British Food and Drug Products in the Third World*. Social Audit, Ltd., 9 Poland Street, London W1V 3DG 1.5OL, 1979.

Melrose, Dianna. *Bitter Pills: Medicines and the Third World*. Oxfam Press, 274 Banbury Road, Oxford OX2 7DZ, England, 1982.

Mernissi, Fatima. *Beyond the Veil: Women in the Arab World*. New York: John Wiley and Sons, Inc., 1975.

Nash, June, and Helen Icken Safa, eds. *Sex and Class in Latin America*. South Hadley, MA: Bergin and Gorney, 1980.

Newland, Kathleen. *Infant Mortality and the Health of Societies*, Worldwatch Paper #47. Worldwatch Institute, Washington DC, 1981.

——. *The Sisterhood of Man*. New York and London: W.W. Norton and Co., Inc., 1979.

Niethammer, Carolyn. *Daughters of the Earth: Lives and Legends of American Indian Women*. New York: Collier Books, 1977.

O'Kelly, Charlotte G. *Women and Men in Society*. New York, Toronto, London and Melbourne: D. Van Nostrand Co., 1980.

Omvedt, Gail. *We Will Smash This Prison: Indian Women in Struggle*. London: Zed Press (see address above).

Patterns for Change: Rural Women Organizing for Health. Order from National Women's Health Network, 224 Seventh Street SE, Washington, DC 20003. June 1981.

Randall, Margaret. *Sandino's Daughters: Testimonies of Nicaraguan Women in Struggle*. Vancouver, BC: New Star Books, 1981.

——. *Women in Cuba: Twenty Years Later*. New York: Smyrna Press, 1981.

Reiter, Rayna R. *Toward an Anthropology of Women*. New York and London: Monthly Review Press, 1975.

Rogers, Barbara. *The Domestication of Women: Discrimination in Developing Societies*. London and New York: Tavistock, 1980.

Rosaldo, Michelle Zimbalist, and Louise Lamphere, eds. *Woman, Culture, and Society*, Stanford CA: Stanford University Press, 1974.

Sakala, Carol. *Women of South Asia: A Guide to Resources*. Millwood, NY: Kraus International Publications, 1980.

Silverman, Milton, et al. *Prescriptions for Death: Drugging the Third World*. Berkeley, CA: University of California Press, 1982.

SNDT Women's University. *Women in India*. Research Unit on Women's Studies, Sir Vithaldas Vidyavihar, Juhu Road, Santacruz West, Bombay 400 049, India.

Turshen, Meredeth. *Women, Food and Health in Tanzania: The Political Economy of Disease*. Onyx Press, Ltd., 27 Clerkenwell Close, London ECIR OAT, England, 1980. $7.75.

Werner, David. *Donde No Hay Doctor (Where There Is No Doctor)*. The Hesperian Foundation, Box 1692, Palo Alto, CA 94302. Spanish, English, Portuguese, Swahili, Hindi.

Articles

Bruce, Judith and S. Bruce Shearer. "Contraceptives and developing countries: The role of barrier methods." (See p. 261.)

Grant, James M. "The State of the World's Children—1982." Available from the U.S. Committee for UNICEF, 331 E. 38th Street, New York, NY 10016, (212) 686-5522.

Audiovisual Materials

Bottle Babies, a 30-minute, 16-mm., 1975 color film. NCC Audio-Visual, Room 860, 475 Riverside Drive, New York, NY 10115. Sale $225. Illustrates the impact of multinational corporations' infant formula sales techniques on women and children in the Third World. Filmed in Kenya.

Controlling Interest: The World of the Multinational Corporation, a 45-minute color film. Rent $60, sale $550. CA Newsreel, 630 Natoma Street, San Francisco, CA 94103. A look at the multinational corporations (focus on Brazil, Chile and the Dominican Republic), runaway shops, U.S. imperialism and the CIA.

The Double Day (Doble Jornada), a 56-minute 1975 color film. Rent $75, sale $700. Tricontinental Films, 333 Avenue of the Americas, New York, NY 10014, or P.O. Box 4460, Berkeley, CA 94704. The efforts of Latin American working women to achieve equality in the home and workplace—a "double day."

Formula Factor, a 30-minute, 16-mm., 1978 color film, originally a Canadian Broadcasting Co. broadcast. CA Newsreel (see address above). Infant formula abuse in Jamaica.

Global Assembly Line, a 60-minute, 16-mm. color film. Produced by Lorraine Gray, Anne Bohlen and Patricia Fernandez. Transit Media, P.O. Box 315, Franklin Lakes, NJ 07417. A documentary film about the historical, socioeconomic and psychological impact of twin plant production on working women and their families in the U.S. and free trade zones of underdeveloped countries.

Into the Mouths of Babes, a 30-minute, 1978 CBS color documentary by Bill Moyers. Available from NCC Audio-Visual, Room 860, 475 Riverside Drive, New York, NY 10115. On the use and abuse of infant formula. Filmed in the Dominican Republic.

Killing Us Softly: Advertising's Image of Women, a 30-minute 16-mm. color film. Rent $38. Cambridge Documentary Films, Inc., P.O. Box 385, Cambridge, MA 02139. An examination of the advertising industry's manipulation of sex roles to sell products.

La Operación, a 40-minute 16-mm. color film. Order from La Operación, P.O. Box 735, Chelsea Station, New York, NY 10011, (212) 864-6564. Rental (sliding scale, $35 to $100) or sale. A powerful documentary about sterilization abuse, particularly among Puerto Rican women.

Southeast Asian Women Electronics Workers, a slide show from the Southeast Asia Resource Center, P.O. Box 4000 D, Berkeley, CA 94704. Focus on social and economic issues.

Periodicals and Groups

Acción Para la Liberación de la Mujer Peruana (ALIMUPER)
A. A. 2211
Lima, Peru

An autonomous socialist-feminist group which sees women as a socially oppressed sector needing to develop their own line of action. The focus is on health, i.e., the relationship of the couple, whether or not to have children, abortion, mental and physical violence by husbands. Currently working to create an information center for women's health.

Asian Women's Association
Poste Restante
Shibuya Post Office
Tokyo, Japan
One of the major groups involved in campaigns against sex tourism. In their newspaper, *Asian Women's Liberation*, they continually bring the issue up and report on actions taking place.

Boston Women's Health Book Collective
465 Mt. Auburn Street
Watertown, MA 02172
An information center, open to the public, which includes many foreign-language books, periodicals and documents, as well as English-language materials on women's international issues.

Broadsheet
Box 5799
Wellesley Street
Auckland, New Zealand
An excellent in-depth coverage of women's health issues in New Zealand.

Committee on South Asian Women (COSAW)
c/o Dr. T.R. Rao
804 Cherry Lane, Apt. 106
E. Lansing, MI 48824
A recent newsletter (November 1982) identified and reported current events in South Asia (Bangladesh, Bhuton, India, Nepal, Pakistan, Sri Lanka) of special relevance to women's status. They are also interested in problems facing women of South Asian origin living abroad.
Students $5, professionals $10.

Committee on Women in Asian Studies (CWAS)
Association of Asian Studies
c/o Barbara D. Miller
409 Maxwell Hall
Syracuse University
Syracuse, NY 13210
Since 1971, the organization has supported research and dissemination of knowledge concerning gender in Asia and among Asians living outside Asia. Carries news about activities, conferences, profiles of members and their work and book reviews. Membership fee: Students $3, faculty $5.

Comunicación, Intercambio y Desarrollo Humano en America Latina (CIDHAL)
Apartado 579
Cuernavaca, Morelos
Mexico
A documentation center for Latin American women, CIDHAL holds classes, publishes pamphlets on health and education for women and organizes meetings and study groups. The focus is on rural and working-class women.

Creatividad y Cambio
Jr. Callao 573

Apt. 5132
Lima, Peru

Produces practical health guides for women which explain the process of birth and different methods of birth control in simple, clear language.

Health Action International (HAI)
  c/o International Organisation of Consumers' Unions (IOCU)
  P.O. Box 1045
  Penang, Malaysia

An international "antibody" set up in May 1981 to resist ill treatment of consumers by multinational drug companies. It is a broad-based network of consumer and professional groups whose main concern is to look into contraceptive drugs and pharmaceutical companies' activities in this field. Produces *HAI News*, a bimonthly newsletter on current actions, publications and meetings on pharmaceuticals.

Healthsharing
  Women Healthsharing
  Box 230, Station M
  Toronto, Ontario M6S 4T3
  Canada

A quarterly newsletter covering a wide range of women's health concerns.

Interfaith Center on Corporate Responsibility (ICCR)
  475 Riverside Drive
  Room 566
  New York, NY 10115

A sponsored related movement of the National Council of Churches, ICCR tries to make corporations responsible for their policies. They bring stockholder resolutions to try and change policies they don't agree with. Soon they will come out with an information/action packet on the whole issue of pharmaceutical marketing in the Third World. Write to them if you are interested in receiving this packet.

International Baby Food Action Network (IBFAN)
  Current coordinating point (1980): Doug Clement
  1701 University Avenue SE
  Minneapolis, MN 55414

A network of groups active on the baby foods issue. Produces regular information packets on current actions for the use of groups.

International Childbirth Education Association (ICEA)
  Box 20048
  Minneapolis, MN 55420

Offers extensive annotated lists of publications and audiovisual resources; the monthly newsletter covers a wide range of childbirth issues.

International Contraception, Abortion and Sterilization Campaign (ICASC)
  374 Grays Inn Road
  London WC1, England

Set up in 1978, the aims of ICASC are to fight for women's reproductive rights all over the world. Each year they organize an international day of action in support of the struggle for reproductive rights of women, and publish a quarterly newsletter that brings together news of actions of different national groups and campaigns and the status of laws in different countries.

ISIS
  P.O. Box 50 (Cornavin)
  1211 Geneva 2
  Switzerland
  Tel: 022/33 67 46
  or Via S. Maria dell'Anima 30
  00186 Roma, Italy
  Tel: 06/656 58 42

ISIS is an international women's information and communication service with a resource and documentation center. They provide original and in-depth feminist analyses of a wide variety of topics: health, education, food, nutrition, appropriate technology, communication, media, violence against women, employment, migration, tourism, etc. Their publications are excellent with extensive resource and bibliographic sections. This organization is a must for feminists to support. If you only subscribe to one journal, make it ISIS's *Women's International Bulletin* (in both English and Spanish). $15 surface, $20 airmail, for a year's subscription. You may also order *Third International Meeting on Women and Health*, ISIS International Bulletin #20 for $3.50 surface, $5.00 airmail.

Manushi
  C/1202 Lajpat Nagar 1
  New Delhi 110024, India

A feminist magazine (manushi means "woman") which encourages women to write in and tell their stories as well as analyze their situations and move toward a shared understanding. Lively, interesting and sometimes very grim, as it reflects the Indian woman's often harsh reality. Published in English and Hindi, it deserves support and wide circulation. $18 (U.S. bank check).

Medico Friend Circle Bulletin
  c/o National Institute of Nutrition
  P.O. Jamai Osmania
  Hyderabad 500007, India

A monthly newsjournal providing a radical critique of health services and policies in India. Has a membership organization of mostly doctors and health workers with some nurses, social workers and activists. The group meets annually to discuss a previously planned topic in depth. Recently published an excellent book on health in India called *Health Care, Which Way to Go?* which can be ordered for $2.00 from MFC, 50, L.I.C. Quarters, University Road, Pune 411 016, India, or from *VHAI*, address below.

Mujer y Desarrollo
  Mujeres en Desarrollo, Inc.
  Apartado 325
  Santo Domingo, Dominican Republic

A newsletter for women in rural areas. It deals in simple language with basic health issues such as nutrition, growing food, breastfeeding and infant feeding, and explains how to prevent and care for basic illnesses.

Mujeres en La Lucha
  A.A. 52206
  Bogota, Colombia

A group of professional women interested in organizing with all women to reflect on their common problems around health, sexuality and the family. They are working to develop a theory on the situation of women and to make contacts with feminist groups at both the national and international level. They have written a 22-page manuscript giving a

623

glimpse of what Latin America is, which elements compose health policies and the significance of self-help programs within the Latin American context. Title: "Self-Help for Latin American Feminists: A Reformist or a Revolutionary Alternative?" Available in Spanish and English.

National Women's Health Network
224 Seventh Street SE
Washington, DC 20003

The only national membership organization devoted exclusively to women and health, NWHN is the "umbrella" of the U.S. women's health movement. Group and individual members receive *Network News*, "newsalerts" about issues that need immediate attention, and access to the Network's clearinghouse. The Network documents international dimensions of selected women's health issues.

Quest—A Feminist Quarterly
P.O. Box 8843
Washington, DC 20003

Interesting articles on a wide range of topics relevant to women internationally. Active in organizing a two- or three-day workshop on tourism at the upcoming final Conference on the Decade on Women in 1985 in Nairobi.

Radical America
38 Union Square
Somerville, MA 02143

An excellent monthly socialist journal covering a variety of topics not exclusive to women but with a feminist perspective when women are discussed. See especially Volume 15, Numbers 1 and 2, spring 1981.

Reaching Out
Bombay, India

For more information, write to Women's Centre, 5 Bhavana Apartments, S.V. Road, Ville Parlé West, Bombay, 400 056, India. A feminist group which does wonderful graphics. They have put out a calendar for the past two years and do other graphic work also.

Rural Women's Social Education Centre (RWSEC)
15/1, Periya Melamaiyur
Vallam Post
Chingleput 603 002
South India

A group of rural Indian women who meet regularly and plan literacy programs and health education programs for their respective villages. They have been meeting since 1980 and are now a close personal as well as a work group. They give primary health care to village women and their children and also build awareness of how women can obtain basic health services from the government.

Saheli
10 Nizamudeen East
New Delhi, India

A group of feminists working out of a garage to build awareness of women's issues and rights in India. It began as a group organizing against dowry burnings and tortures and now covers a broad range of women's issues. They run workshops and exhibits on health, consciousness raising and family violence and provide counseling to women on legal matters. They are a wonderful group of dedicated women but are too small to solve the gargantuan problems Indian women face.

SNDT
Research Unit on Women's Studies at SNDT Women's University
Sir Vithaldas Vidyavihar
Juhu Road, Santacruz West
Bombay 400 049
India

An excellent newsletter on research being done at the university as well as feminist activities in and around Bombay. The director is a dynamic, outspoken feminist and welcomes exchanges of opinion and information from other groups. The unit publishes a list of the many studies they have done. These are for sale and cover a wide range of concerns for women: education, health, employment, women's organizations, etc. Write to them if you are interested in an exchange of newsletters.

Southeast Asia Resource Center
P.O. Box 4000 D
Berkeley, CA 94704

Publishes *Southeast Asia Chronicle*, an excellent bimonthly journal of timely research and information on current developments in Vietnam, Laos, Kampuchea, Thailand, Malaysia, Indonesia and the Philippines. $10 for a one-year subscription.

Taller Salud
Apartado 2172
Hato Rey
Puerto Rico 00919

A self-help and activist collective devoted to health. They translate, print and reproduce information leaflets on different aspects of health and distribute them to women in various communities. They hope to set up a health center to carry on their work.

Voluntary Health Association of India (VHAI)
C-14 Community Centre
Safdarjung Development Area
New Delhi 110 016
India

VHAI is a nonprofit federation of state and regional voluntary health associations with a goal of making good health a reality for all the people of India, especially its neglected rural population. VHAI publishes an excellent bimonthly journal called *Health For the Millions*, with articles and news of health care in India from a critical perspective. There is a small group of women health professionals within VHAI who have put out a terrific issue, "Women and Health" (Vol. VIII, No. 4 [August 1982]).

WIN News
Women's International Network News
187 Grant Street
Lexington, MA 02173

A quarterly covering a wide range of topics of concern to women, including United Nations actions and conferences, health, violence, development, media, international career opportunities and reports from around the world. Good statistical data and in-depth interviews and book reviews. Includes regular reports on female circumcision.

Women's Centre
5 Bhavana Apartments
Ville Parlé, Bombay 400 056
India

A feminist group concentrating on family violence in Bombay. The Centre is open two days a week, and women come to share problems, work out solutions, get advice and help (including legal and medical help). The group works voluntarily and is now trying to raise funds for a building where women can come and learn together and where battered women can be sheltered. An energetic, dynamic group of women.

INDEX

The letter t denotes a table.

Norway, 615. *See also* Scandinavia
Nose disorders, 80t, 86t, 346, 545
Nosocomial infections (occurring in hospitals), 377, 378, 583. *See also* Iatrogenic disorders
Notre Dame University, 615
"Nova," 320fn
NOW (National Organization for Women), 74, 315, 566, 574, 589
Nuclear power plants, 77–78, 82
Nurse(s), 340, 572–74, 576, 583. *See also* Nurse-anesthetists; Nurse-midwives, certified; Nurse-practioners
Nurse-anesthetists (NAs), 573
Nurse-midwives, certified (CNMs), 334, 336–37, 338, 339t, 340, 352, 395, 576–77; and insurance, 565; physicians and, 328, 337, 557; professionalization of, 573
Nurse-practitioners (NPs), 330, 565, 573, 574, 576–77
Nurses NOW, 574
Nursing homes, 47, 457, 464, 564, 565, 573, 583–84
Nursing of babies, *see* Breastfeeding
Nutrition, 3, 4, 11–32, 73; and aging, 453, 454–56, 460, 461–62; and anemia, 521; and arthritis, 522; for benign breast conditions, 491; for breastfeeding, 17, 18t, 401–2; and cancer, 12t, 16, 23, 24, 490, 491, 524; after childbirth, 398; children's, 11, 15, 16, 20, 24, 27; and diabetes, 12t, 13, 539, 540; and dieting, 20–23; for drug dependence, 35; and heart disease, 12t, 16, 540, 543; and herpes, 276; and hypertension, 12t, 449, 541, 542, 543; and infertility, 421, 422; and intestinal disorders, 23, 455; and menopause, 446, 449, 450, 459; and menstrual problems, 215, 509; and osteoporosis, 12t, 454, 461–62; for PID, 506; and the Pill, 244; and pregnancy, 17, 18t, 329–32, 343–45; and stress, 446; and surgery, 483; and teeth, 12t, 18t, 19t, 23. *See also* Vitamin(s)
Nutritionists, 509, 565, 572

Oakland Feminist Women's Health Center, 152fn
Obesity, *see* Overweight
Obstetrician/gynecologists, 334, 335, 339t, 578; and aging, 456; attitudes toward childbirth, 328, 362–65; and home births, 341fn; and hysterectomies,

512, 578; and infertility, 420, 425; and intervention in childbirth, 342fn, 364, 379–89; and malpractice suits, 588; and menopause, 444; and midwives, 337, 338, 562fn, 590; prenatal visits to, 343, 379; rise of, 337, 362–63; and social control of women, 363, 560–62; training of, 328, 330–31, 364–65, 385–86, 562fn, 578
Occupational health hazards, 3, 4fn, 84–98, 201, 421, 453, 487, 523
Occupational Safety and Health Administration, U.S. (OSHA), 88, 90, 98
Occupational therapists, 572
Odent, Michel, 328
Off Our Backs, 620
Older women, *see* Aging; Menopause; Midlife
Older Women's League (OWL), 436, 438fn, 566
Olympic Marathons, 48fn
Oophorectomy (removal of the ovaries), 188, 511–12, 514–17, 538, 549; and breast cancer, 536; and ectopic pregnancy, 428, 515; prophylactic, 448
Oophoritis, 502
Operating room, 339t
Ophthalmologists, 458
Optometrists, 458
Oral sex, 177, 265, 268
Orgasm, 168, 169, 171–72, 179, 186, 188, 190; and breastfeeding, 400; and chronic diseases, 191–93t; and conception, 255–56; and hysterectomy, 513, 516; and intercourse, 185–86; male, 190, 223; and menstrual problems, 187, 215; and oral sex, 177; and pelvic muscles, 206; and the Pill, 243; problems with, 189
Os, 207
Osteoarthritis, 55–56, 65
Osteomalasia, 461fn
Osteopaths (DOs), 335
Osteoporosis, 12t, 46fn, 448, 543; and aging, 453fn, 454, 455, 461–62; and ovary removal, 515
Ostomy, 193t
Ottawa Marathon, 46
Ovarian cancer, 24, 242, 244, 512, 515, 523, 524, 538
Ovaries, 188, 204, 207–10, 217; abscess of, 503; cancer of, *see* Ovarian cancer; cysts of, 190, 244, 481, 500, 509, 510–511, 515; growths on, 500; infection

of, 502; malfunction of, 421; and menopause, 445, 446; removal of, *see* Oophorectomy
Overmedication, 457, 460
Overpopulation, 201, 220. *See also* Population control
Overweight (obesity), 5, 7–8, 20–23, 31; and cancer, 524, 538, 539; and chronic diseases, 8, 455, 539, 541–43; exercise for, 8, 46, 68
Ovral, 248
Ovulation, 206, 209–10, 211, 217, 223, 239t. *See also* Ovulation method
Ovulation method (of birth control), 236
Ovulation Method Teachers' Association, 235
Ovum, *see* Egg
Oxalic acid, 19t
Oxytocin, 305, 375, 380, 381, 400
Oxytocin challenge tests, 386

Paget's disease, 462
Palpitations, 69
Pancreas, cancer of, 24, 37
Pancreatitis, 33
Pap smear, 244fn, 245, 251, 477–81 *passim*, 485–88, 502, 512; and cervical cancer, 537; and STD, 272, 275, 276, 279
Paracervical block, 388
Paralysis, 79, 358, 545
Paranormal healing, 68–69
Parathyroid gland, 454–55
Parenthood: adjusting to, 396–418; lesbian, 145, 152, 157–63, 396, 413; partnership in, 409–10, 411
Parkinson's disease, 452
Parthenogenesis, 323
Paternity leave, need for, 416
Patients' rights, 568, 583, 584–89
PCBs, 78, 80t, 81t, 82, 83
Pauling, Linus, 528
Peanut butter, 14, 17t, 19t, 20
Peanuts, 12fn, 17t, 18t, 215
Peas, *see* Legumes
Pectins, 19t, 23
Pediatrician, 560
Pediculosis pedis (crabs), 264t, 265, 483
Pelvic bone, 204, 207, 208
Pelvic examination, 285, 423, 476–78, 301
Pelvic-floor muscles, 206; exercises for, 333, 346, 349
Pelvic inflammatory disease (PID), 190, 318fn, 502–6, 509, 575; and DES, 498; and ectopic (tubal) pregnancy, 210, 427, 503; from IUD, 194fn, 249,